health psychology:
biopsychosocial interactions

AN AUSTRALIAN PERSPECTIVE

Marie L. Caltabiano
James Cook University

Don Byrne
Australian National University

Paul R. Martin
University of New England

Edward P. Sarafino
The College of New Jersey

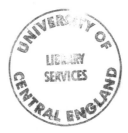

John Wiley & Sons Australia, Ltd

First published 2002 by
John Wiley & Sons Australia, Ltd
33 Park Road, Milton, Qld 4064

Offices also in Sydney and Melbourne

Typeset in 10/12 pt Berkeley

US edition © John Wiley & Sons, Inc. 1998
Australian edition © John Wiley & Sons Australia, Ltd 2002

National Library of Australia
Cataloguing-in-publication data

Caltabiano, Marie, 1959–
   Health psychology: biopsychosocial interactions,
   an Australian perspective.

   Bibliography.
   Includes index.
   For tertiary students.
   ISBN 0 471 34127 4.

   1. Clinical health psychology. I. Title.

610.19

Cover and internal design images:
The Image Bank/Daniel Arsenault

Illustrated by Craig Jackson, Paul Lennon and the
John Wiley Art Department

Printed in Singapore by
Seng Lee Press Pte Ltd

10 9 8 7 6 5 4 3 2 1

Dedication

To my parents Alfio and Rosetta, and my uncle Albert.

In memory and gratitude.

Brief contents

Contents

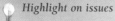

Preface

When I was approached by John Wiley Australia to write an Australian adaptation of Edward Sarafino's *Health Psychology: Biopsychosocial Interactions*, I was extremely excited and felt very privileged to be involved in such a project. I have taught Health Psychology in the Psychology degree program at James Cook University since 1992, and have also taught variations of the subject to Nursing Science and Social Work students. While I have adopted several different texts for these courses, I have often returned to Sarafino's book. This widely respected text is comprehensive, easy to read and well liked by students. Over time, however, I came to recognise the need for a text that was relevant to the experience of students in Australia. Students needed a resource book that was similarly comprehensive, but that cited up-to-date Australian statistics on disease incidence and prevalence, discussed the Australian health care system, examined the findings of national surveys, and reviewed Australian health promotion programs and studies by Australian researchers.

My objective has been to update Sarafino's text with recent research conducted both within and outside Australia. I have incorporated Australian statistics (for example on disease and mortality incidence, and health risk) and documented Australian health programs and health-related research conducted by health psychologists, public health researchers and those working in related fields.

My job was facilitated by the wealth of creative ideas and innovative research in Australia coming out of professions such as public health, psychology and nursing. Although it was not possible to incorporate all these ideas, I believe that the research included represents the high quality of work being done in Australia. I have also incorporated historical material on infectious diseases during the early settlement of Australia, trends over time in eating patterns, smoking and alcohol use in Australia, along with anecdotal data and the recounted experiences of well-known Australians. New sections include those on psychosocial responses to disaster and traumatic events (chapter 3); social support as transactional process (chapter 4); applications of the theories of reasoned action and planned behaviour (chapter 6); and the use of the PRECEDE/PROCEED model as a guiding framework for health promotion in community health psychology (chapter 6). This new material serves to complement Sarafino while maintaining the integrity of the original text.

One additional theme makes this book unique — namely, its sustained focus on lifespan development in health and illness. For example, the book discusses how health and health-related behaviour change with age, and describes health care issues and examples that pertain to pediatric and elderly patients.

The biopsychosocial model remains the basic explanatory theme for understanding the whole person in health and illness. The components of the model interrelate in a dynamic and continuous fashion, consistent with the concept of *systems*. The psychological research cited reflects an eclectic orientation and supports a variety of behavioural, physiological, cognitive and social-personality viewpoints. In addition, gender and sociocultural differences in health and related behaviours are addressed at many points in the book. In these ways, this book presents a balanced view of health psychology, positioning it squarely in the mainstream of current thinking in the field.

Health Psychology: Biopsychosocial Interactions — an Australian Perspective draws on the research and theoretical perspectives of many disciplines to illustrate the interrelationship of psychology and health. This depth makes it a teaching resource suitable for undergraduate and postgraduate courses on health psychology or behavioural medicine taught within Psychology degree programs, Nursing Science or Medicine. The material will be relevant and interesting to students from disciplines other than psychology, such as public health, nursing, medicine, allied health and social work. Undergraduate training in health psychology has developed rapidly and can play an important role in helping students from many disciplines to understand the interplay of biological, psychological and social factors in people's health. The text, and the exhaustive bibliography, will also be a valuable resource for practitioners and researchers in allied health professions.

The field of health psychology is exciting because of its relative infancy in Australia. It can be seen as a focal point for the application of psychological principles and psychological theory emanating from many other fields within psychology. Health psychology is particularly interesting because of its relevance to the lives of students, the researchers who study biopsychosocial aspects of health and illness, and the people students will work with in the future. Researchers from many disciplines, including psychology, are uncovering fascinating relationships between behaviour and health, and learning more about the roles of cognition, emotion and personality in health, adjustment to medical conditions and rehabilitation. Keeping up to date across such a broad field has been a challenge. In addition to some two thousand publications cited by Sarafino, close to another thousand, most published in the past few years, have been cited in this Australian edition.

Writing this book has been both a major undertaking and a very rewarding experience. I have read more deeply in the literature than could possibly be acknowledged here, and I am greatly indebted to all those researchers whose work I have cited. As Sarafino has remarked, without their endeavours there would be no health psychology. I would particularly like to thank Professor Don Byrne, for his work on chapters 13 and 14, and Professor Paul Martin, for chapters 11 and 12.

There are a number of other people whose contribution I would like to acknowledge. At John Wiley & Sons Australia, I am indebted to Judith Fox, who was the publishing editor for much of the duration of this project. Without her enthusiasm, encouragement and support this book would not have been possible. I would also like to extend my appreciation to Janine Burford in her role of publishing editor during the latter part of the project, and for the excitement she brought to the final stages. Special thanks are also extended to project editor Jem Bates, who has been a true gem in the expertise he has brought to the editorial process, his coordinating abilities and most importantly in his generosity with time and his patience. A number of other Wiley people deserve special acknowledgement — namely, developmental editor Rebecca Gollan, senior editor Catherine Spedding, publishing assistant Pam Hollander and the Wiley Production staff.

I have also benefited from the many helpful suggestions made by the following reviewers: Paula Shulz, Australian Catholic University McCauley; Don Byrne, Australian National University; Doug MacLean, University of Newcastle; and John Connors, Charles Sturt University, Wagga Wagga.

Other individuals deserve mention. I would like to thank the Head of the School of Psychology at James Cook University, Professor Colin Ryan, for his support and many kind words of encouragement during the writing of this book. Rebecca Wood, in her role as research assistant in the early phases of this project, contributed many hours in organising inter-library loans and photocopying articles. I would also like to thank the countless academics both within and outside my field who have had a significant influence on my work. Of my family, I would like to thank most especially my best friend, sister and colleague, Dr Nerina Caltabiano, and my niece Amelia for their unwavering support. Finally, thank you to the students, who make all this work worthwhile.

Marie L. Caltabiano
October 2001

To the student

'I wish I could help my father stop smoking,' a student in one of our health psychology courses said. Maybe she did help — he had quit by the end of the semester. This example points out two things that will probably make health psychology interesting to you: (1) the material is *personally relevant* and (2) many of the things you learn can actually be *applied* in your everyday life. Studying health psychology will also help you answer important questions you may have considered about health and psychology in the past. Does the mind affect our health — and if so, how? What effect does stress have on health and recovery from illness? What can be done to help people lead healthier lives than they do? Why don't patients follow their doctors' advice, and what can health care workers do to help? What special needs do children have as patients, and how can parents and health care workers address these needs? How can families, friends, and health care workers help patients adjust to disabling or life-threatening health problems?

As these questions indicate, a knowledge of health psychology can be relevant both now and later when you enter *your future career*. This is so whether you are studying to be a psychologist, medical social worker, nurse or doctor, physical or occupational therapist, public health worker or health educator. You will learn in this book that the relationship between a person's health and psychology involves a 'two-way street' — each affects the other. Psychological factors go hand in hand with medical approaches in preventing and treating illness and in helping patients adjust to the health problems they develop.

THE BOOK

This book was designed for you, the reader. First and foremost, it provides a thorough and up-to-date presentation of the major issues, theories, concepts and research in health psychology undertaken both within and outside Australia. Throughout the book, the major point of view is 'biopsychosocial' — that is, that health and illness influence and result from the interplay of biological, psychological and social aspects of people's lives. Because integrating these aspects involves complex concepts and technical material, we have made special efforts to write in a straightforward, clear and engaging fashion. When a new term is introduced it is defined immediately; important terms are set in bold type, listed as 'key terms' at the end of the chapter and defined in the glossary at the back of the book. Examples and case studies are include to clarify sometimes complex concepts.

Three types of boxed feature are presented throughout the book in order to illustrate or elaborate on surrounding content. These features are identified in the text by the corresponding icons.

Highlight on Issues. Applied, high-interest and new frontier topics are highlighted here. They feature issues such as the effects of second-hand smoke, the burden of caregiving, careers relating to health and psychology, breast and testicular self-examination, and acute pain in burn patients.

Focus on Research. These features spotlight the research methods used in health psychology, reviewing unique or interesting research findings on topics such as heredity and alcohol abuse, the effect on heart disease of changing Type A behaviour, stress and immune response, and inducing pain in laboratory research.

Assess Yourself. Here students are given the opportunity to examine their own health-related characteristics, knowledge and beliefs on issues such as daily hassles, eating self-efficacy, alcohol use, AIDS, responding to pain, emotional support and ethical questions.

To help you absorb the material and remember it longer, the book also includes the following learning aids:

- **Chapter contents and prologue.** Each chapter begins with a contents list that outlines the major topics in the order in which they are covered. The prologue then introduces the chapter with a vignette that is relevant to the material ahead and gives an overview of the ideas you will read about.
- **Illustrations.** The many figures and tables in each chapter are designed to clarify concepts and research findings and help them stick in your mind.

- **Summary and key terms.** Each chapter closes with two features: (1) the summary, which presents the most important ideas covered, and (2) the key terms — a list of the most important terms in the chapter.
- **Glossary.** The glossary at the back of the book gives definitions of important terms and concepts, along with pronunciation keys for the most difficult words. It will be useful when you are studying or reading and are not sure of the exact meaning or pronunciation of a term.

ORGANISATION

The text is organised so that the main focus progresses across chapters from *primary prevention* (parts 1 to 3), through *secondary prevention* (parts 4 and 5), to *tertiary prevention* and care (part 6). The book is divided into seven parts.

Part 1. Chapter 1 presents a history and overview of health psychology, and introduces the main concepts and research methods used. Chapter 2 introduces the body's physical systems to help the student to understand how these systems interrelate. This introduction provides students with a useful resource to refer back to when each system is discussed in later chapters. (You will note in the sections on metabolism and body weight that we have retained the imperial unit of measure the *calorie*, since this term remains more generally recognised than the *kilojoule*. The metric equivalent of one calorie is 4.186 kilojoules.)

Part 2. Chapters 3 and 4 examine stress in relation to illness, and chapter 5 looks at ways of coping with and reducing stress. The position of this discussion early in the book recognises stress's influence on a wide range of health-related problems.

Part 3. The following chapters consider largely non-clinical approaches to enhancing health and preventing illness. Chapter 6 discusses health-related behaviours and public health promotion programs. Chapter 7 focuses on smoking, and on alcohol and drug use and abuse. Chapter 8 considers nutrition, weight control, physical activity and safety issues.

Part 4. Chapter 9 describes the kinds of health services available in Australia, the patient–practitioner relationship, and patients' adherence to medical regimes. Chapter 10 introduces the hospital setting, staff and procedures, how patients cope with the physical and mental stresses they experience there, and the role of health psychologists in this coping process.

Part 5. Pain is the focus of the next two chapters. Chapter 11 explores the nature of clinical pain and its symptoms, while chapter 12 discusses medical and psychosocial approaches to managing and controlling pain.

Part 6. The following two chapters emphasise tertiary prevention through an examination of chronic and life-threatening health problems. Chapter 13 addresses serious chronic illnesses, such as asthma, diabetes and arthritis, along with their medical and psychosocial treatments. Chapter 14 examines four high-mortality illnesses — heart disease, stroke, cancer and AIDS — and people's experiences with terminal illness and death.

Part 7. Finally, chapter 15 looks to the future of health psychology, its goals and controversies and, not least, career opportunities in the field in Australia.

STUDY HINTS

There are many ways you can use the features of this book to learn and study well, and you may want to 'experiment' to find the best way for you. The following is one method that works well for many students.

Survey the chapter first. Read the contents list and browse through the chapter, examining the figures and tables. Some students also find it useful to read the summary first, even though it contains terms they may not yet understand. Then read the prologue. As you begin each new section of the chapter, look at its title and turn it into a *question*. Thus, the heading early in chapter 1, 'An illness/wellness continuum', might become 'What is an illness/wellness continuum?' Doing this helps you focus on your reading. After reading the section, *reflect* on what you have just read. Can you answer the question you asked when you reworded the title?

When you have finished the body of the chapter, *review* what you have read by reading the summary and trying to define the items in the list of key terms. If there is something you do not understand, look it up in the chapter or glossary. Last, *re-read* the chapter at least once, concentrating on the important concepts or ideas. You may find it helpful to underline or highlight selected material now that you have a good idea of what is important. If your exam will consist of 'objective' questions, such as multiple choice, using this approach intensively should be effective. If your exam will have essay items, you will probably find it helpful to develop a list of likely questions and write an outline or a complete answer for each one.

We hope that you enjoy this book, that you learn a great deal from it, and that you will share our enthusiasm and fascination for health psychology by the time you finish the course.

Edward P. Sarafino
Marie L. Caltabiano

About the authors

Dr Marie L. Caltabiano is a senior lecturer in the School of Psychology at James Cook University, Cairns Campus. Her interest in health psychology began with her doctoral research into the stress-moderating benefits of leisure. Her research has been in the areas of the psychosocial aspects of stress, stress management, immunocompetence, burnout, craving and disordered eating, parental coping, adolescent health risk behaviours and women's health. She has published papers in the *Australian and New Zealand Journal of Public Health*, *Climacteric*, *Psychological Reports*, the *Journal of Social Psychology*, the *Australian Journal of Marriage and Family*, *Leisure Studies*, *Society and Leisure* and *Adolescence*. Dr Caltabiano is a member of the Australian Psychological Society, the APS College of Health Psychologists, the American Psychological Society, the Public Health Association of Australia and the International Federation of University Women. She has been on the advisory board of the international journals *Human Relations* and *Perceptual and Motor Skills*.

From 1995 to 1997 Dr Caltabiano was an Associate Dean within the Faculty of Arts at James Cook University. In 1997 and 1998 she was Chair of the Editorial Board of the Centre for Social and Welfare Research. She is co-editor, with Richard Hil and Rosemary Frangos (1996), of the book *Achieving Inclusion: Exploring Issues in Disability*, and co-author of *Menopausal Health and the Family* and *Influences of Healthy Eating Practices in Ethnic Communities* (1997), both published by the Centre for Social and Welfare Research, James Cook University.

Don Byrne is Professor of Clinical and Health Psychology at the Australian National University. He is currently Deputy Dean of the Faculty of Science at the ANU and chairs the University's research grants committee. His research interests include the roles of stress and behaviour in mediating risk of cardiovascular disease; the measurement, causes and management of occupational stress; and the role of coping in response to chemotherapy among women with breast cancer. Research in these and related areas has resulted in the publication of 11 books (as author or editor) and more than 100 papers in refereed journals or as invited book chapters. Professor Byrne is a Fellow of the Academy of the Social Sciences in Australia, the Australian Psychological Society and the International College of

Psychosomatic Medicine, of which he is a past president. He remains on the Executive Council of the College and is also a member of the Australian Academy of Science's National Committee on Psychology.

Paul R. Martin is Professor and Head of the School of Psychology at the University of New England (UNE) and President of the Australian Psychological Society (APS). He completed his doctorate at the University of Oxford. He held a research position at the University of Oxford followed by a lectureship at Monash University, before moving in 1981 to the University of Western Australia (UWA), where he served as Director of Clinical Training and Director of the Adoptions Research and Counselling Service. He introduced professional doctoral programs at both UWA and UNE. He has served as President of the Australian Behaviour Modification Association and Director of Scientific Affairs of APS. He took up his current position in 1996. His research program has been supported by grants from the National Health and Medical Research Council. He is author/editor of the texts *Handbook of Behavior Therapy and Psychological Science* and *Psychological Management of Chronic Headaches*, and co-author/editor of *Behavioural Medicine*, *Clinical Psychology*, *Psychology and Society*, *Treating Postnatal Depression* and *Health and Medical Research: Contribution of the Social and Behavioural Sciences*. In addition to his research and teaching activities, since completing his training in 1977 he has engaged in continuous professional practice as a clinical and health psychologist in a broad range of hospital and community settings.

Edward P. Sarafino received his PhD from the University of Colorado and is Professor and former Chairperson of the Psychology Department at the College of New Jersey. He has published about three dozen professional articles and five books, including *Behavior Modification*, *Behavioral Treatments for Asthma* and *Child and Adolescent Development*. He is a fellow of the American Psychological Association, a member of the APA Divisions of Health Psychology (Division 38) and Experimental Analysis of Behavior (Division 25), and a member of the Society of Behavioral Medicine and the American Psychosomatic Society. He is a former Secretary of Division 38 and has served on and chaired the division's Committee on Education and Training.

Acknowledgements

The author and publisher would like to thank the following copyright holders, organisations and individuals for their permission to reproduce copyright material in this book.

Figures
Page 7 (figure 1.2): from AIHW, *Australia's health, 1998: 6th biennial health report of the AIHW*, AGPS, Canberra; page 46 (figure 2.2): illustrations by Edith Lenneberg, from Eric H. Lenneberg, 1967, *Biological foundations of language*, pp. 160–61, John Wiley & Sons, New York, based on photographs from the postnatal development of the human cerebral cortex by Jesse L. Conel (1939–67); page 160 (figure 4.5): from F. Andrasik, D. D. Blake and M. S. McCarran, *Child health behavior: a behavioral pediatrics perspective*, © 1986, John Wiley & Sons, New York; page 188 (figure 5.1): from E. P. Sarafino, 1986, *The fears of childhood: a guide to recognizing and reducing fearful states in children*, Human Sciences Press, New York. Reproduced by permission of Kluwer/Plenum Publishers; page 198 (figure 5.6): from J. P. Foreyt and D. P. Rathjen (Eds), *Cognitive behavior therapy: research and application*, © 1978. Reproduced by permission of Plenum Publishing; page 223 (figure 6.1): adapted from M. H. Becker and I. M. Rosenstock, 1984, 'Compliance with medical advice', in A Steptoe and A Mathews (Eds), *Health care and human behaviour*, Academic Press, London. Reproduced by permission of the publisher; page 225 (figure 6.2): adapted from I. Ajzen and T. J. Madden, 1986, 'Prediction of goal-directed behavior: attitudes, intentions and perceived behavioral control', *Journal of Experimental Psychology*, 22, 458; page 242 ('Injury Storyboard'): appendix 2 from R. Spark, R. J. Donovan and P. Howat, 1991, 'Promoting health and preventing injury in remote Aboriginal communities', *Health Promotion Journal of Australia*, 1(2), 10–16; page 265 (figure 7.1): from T. Makkai and I. McAllister, *Patterns of drug use in Australia, 1985–95*, 1998, Department of Health and Family Services, © Commonwealth of Australia. Reproduced by permission; page 280 (figure 7.4): reproduced courtesy of CMI, Inc., www.alcohol test.com; page 308 (figure 8.1): reproduced by permission of CSIRO and the Anti-Cancer Foundation of South Australia; page 347 (figure 8.5): derived from NHMRC, 1991, *Health implications of long term climate change*, AGPS, © Commonwealth of Australia. Reproduced by permission; page 364 (figure 9.1): from AIHW, *Australia's health, 2000: the 7th biennial health report of the AIHW*, AGPS, Canberra; page 369 (figure 9.3): from L. Ellington and D. J. Wiebe, 1999, 'Neuroticism, symptom presentation and radical decision making', *Journal of Health Psychology*, 18(6). Reproduced by permission of Sage Publications; page 475 (figure 12.1): from Paul R. Martin, *Psychological management of chronic headaches*, © 1993. Adapted by permission of The Guilford Press.

Text
Page 88 (table 3.1): from T. H. Holmes and R. H. Rahe, 1967, Social Adjustment Rating Scale, *Journal of Psychosomatic Research*, vol. 11, pp. 213–18. Reproduced by permission of Elsevier Science; pages 119–20 (table 3.3): from E. Sarafino, 1997, Hassles Assessment Scale for Students in College (Hass/Col): preliminary version, unpublished manuscript; page 209 (table 6.1): from AIHW, *Australia's Health, 2000: 7th biennial health report of the AIHW*, AGPS, Canberra; page 210 (table 6.2): from AIHW, *Australia's Health, 1996: 5th biennial report of the AIHW*, AGPS, Canberra; page 317 (table 8.1): reproduced from *Allan Borushek's pocket calorie and fat counter*, 28th edition, 2001, Family Health Publications, WA; page 325: from S. M. Glynn and A. J. Ruderman, 1986, 'The development and validation of an eating self-efficacy scale', *Cognitive Therapy and Research Journal*, 10, 403–20. Reproduced by permission of Kluwer Academic Publishers; pages 466–7 (quote): from H. Flor and D. C. Turk, 'Chronic illness in an adult family member: pain as a prototype', in D.C. Turk and R. D. Kerns (Eds), *Health, illness and families: a life-span perspective*, © 1997 John Wiley & Sons Australia; page 481 (quote): from D. C. Turk, D. H. Meichenbaum and M. Genest, *Pain and behavioral medicine: a cognitive-behavioral perspective*, © 1983. Reproduced by permission of Guilford Publications; pages 482–3 (patient–therapist dialogue): from A. D. Holzman and D. C. Turk, *Pain management: a handbook of psychological treatment approaches*, Pergamon, New York, © 1986; page 488 (dialogue between therapist and Mrs Cox): from D. C. Turk, D. H. Meichenbaum and M. Genest, *Pain and behavioral medicine: a cognitive-behavioral perspective*, © 1983. Reproduced by permission of Guilford Publications.

Every effort has been made to trace the ownership of copyright material. Information that will enable the publisher to rectify any error or omission in subsequent editions will be welcome. In such cases, please contact the Permissions Section of John Wiley & Sons Australia, Ltd, who will arrange for the payment of the usual fee.

PART 1

An introduction: basic issues and processes

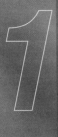

An overview of psychology and health

Prologue

Mandy came from a health-conscious family. Her mother always cooked nutritious meals for the family and encouraged the children to be involved in sporting activities. Breakfast consisted of cereal and juice, with toast. Fruit and vegetables were eaten regularly. Mandy played on the school netball team and loved to go jogging around the neighbourhood. It kept her in shape, and she felt more energetic after her run. Mandy has never had a weight problem. Like her parents she has a slender, athletic frame. Since moving away from home to university, Mandy has found that she does not have time for exercise or team sports. Perhaps she will once assignments settle down. The first few weeks of university were fun. She went out with friends and socialised until late at night. Although she knew she should not drink so much, it didn't seem right to refuse a drink. She was having fun. But the late nights seem to have caught up with her, and now she is struggling to catch up with her studies. Putting in the late hours has its downside as she is so tired the next day in lectures. Mandy has been sleeping in late, so she usually skips breakfast to make class. Fortunately, the campus has a cafeteria that makes good strong coffee to keep her going through the day. Some days Mandy skips lunch, making up for it with a couple of chocolate bars. Although Mandy does not realise it, many of the **health behaviours** she once engaged in back home are slowly being eradicated with her changed circumstances and changed environment.

This story illustrates important issues related to health. For instance, the things that a person does, such as skipping breakfast or not exercising, can affect health. Also, the individual's social relations may encourage unhealthy behaviour, as we saw in Mandy's increased drinking. In this book we will examine the relationships between health and a wide variety of psychological, biological and social factors in people's lives.

This chapter introduces a relatively new and very exciting field of study called *health psychology*. We look at its scope, its history, its research methods, and how it draws on and supports other sciences. As we study these topics, you will begin to see how health psychologists would answer such questions as: Does the mind affect our health? What role does the cultural background of individuals play in their health? Does the age of a person affect how he or she deals with issues of health and illness? But first let's begin with a definition of health.

What is health?

You know what health is, don't you? How would you define it? You would probably mention something about health being a state of feeling well and not being sick. We commonly think about health in terms of an absence of (1) objective *signs* that the body is not functioning properly, such as measured high blood pressure, or (2) subjective *symptoms* of disease or injury, such as pain or nausea (Birren & Zarit 1985; Thoresen 1984). Dictionaries define health in this way, too. But there is a problem with this definition of health. Let's see why.

An illness/wellness continuum

Consider Mandy, the university student in the opening story. You've surely heard people say, 'It's not healthy to skip meals or not to exercise'. Is Mandy healthy? What about someone who feels fine but whose lungs are being damaged from smoking cigarettes, or whose arteries are becoming clogged from eating foods that are high in saturated fats? These are all signs of improper body functioning. Are people with these signs healthy? We probably would say they are not 'sick' — they are simply less healthy than they would be without the unhealthy conditions.

This means health and sickness are not entirely separate concepts — they overlap. There are degrees of wellness and of illness. Medical sociologist Aaron Antonovsky (1979, 1987) has suggested that we consider these concepts as the two ends of a continuum, noting that 'We are all terminal cases. And we all are, so long as there is a breath of life in us, in some measure healthy' (1987, p. 3). He also proposed that we revise our focus, giving more attention to what enables people to stay well than to what causes people to become ill. Figure 1.1 presents a diagram of an **illness/wellness continuum**, with *death* at one end and *optimal wellness* at the other.

We will use the term **health** to mean a positive state of physical, mental and social wellbeing — not simply the absence of injury or disease (WHO 1946) — that varies over time along a continuum. At the wellness end of the continuum, health is the dominant state. At the other end of the continuum, the dominant state is illness or injury, in which destructive processes produce characteristic signs, symptoms or disabilities. Note that this is a 'holistic' definition of health.

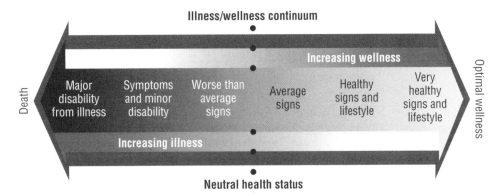

Figure 1.1 An illness/wellness continuum to represent people's differing health statuses. Starting at the centre (neutral level) of the diagram, a person's health status is shown as progressively worse to the left and progressively improved to the right. The segments in the central band describe dominant features that usually characterise different health statuses based on the person's *physical condition* — that is, his or her signs (such as blood pressure), symptoms and disability — and *lifestyle*, such as his or her amount of regular exercise, cholesterol consumption and cigarette smoking. Medical treatment typically begins at a health status to the left of the neutral level and intensifies as the physical condition worsens. Medical treatment can bring the person's health status back to the mid-range of the continuum, but healthy lifestyles can help, too. Increasing wellness beyond the mid-range can be achieved through lifestyle improvements.

Source: Based on information in Antonovsky (1987); Bradley (1993); Ryan & Travis (1981).

Illness today and in the past

People in Australia and other industrialised nations live longer, on average, than they did in the past, and they suffer from a different pattern of illnesses. During the eighteenth and nineteenth centuries, people in Australia suffered chiefly from two types of illness: dietary and infectious illness (Cumpston 1989). **Dietary diseases** result from malnutrition — for example, scurvy was rampant among convicts and the first settlers to Australia because food was inadequate and in short supply, having to be brought by store ships from England. **Infectious diseases** are acute illnesses caused by harmful matter or micro-organisms, such as bacteria or viruses, in the body. In most of the world today, infectious diseases continue to be the main causes of death.

A good example of the way illness patterns have changed in industrialised nations comes from the history of diseases in Australia. In the first years of settlement in Australia, the diseases introduced into the penal colony were associated with insanitary conditions aboard ships transporting convicts to New South Wales. Before the long sea voyage, overcrowded and insanitary conditions in the gaols of England contributed to the spread among convicts of diseases like typhus fever. Outbreaks of cholera, dysentery, typhoid fever and typhus fever were common in the early colonial years (Cumpston 1989). These diseases did not exist among indigenous people of Australia before British settlement. The convicts and settlers brought the infections with them and the death toll among the indigenous people was extremely high. An outbreak of smallpox in 1789 was responsible for many Aboriginal deaths (Cumpston 1989). This high death rate occurred for two reasons. First, the indigenous population had never been exposed to these new micro-organisms, and thus lacked the natural immunity that our bodies develop after lengthy exposure to most diseases (Grob 1983). Second, indigenous people's immune functions were probably limited by a low degree of genetic variation among these people (Black 1992).

In the nineteenth century infectious diseases were still the greatest threat to the health of Australians. The illnesses of the colonial years continued to claim many lives, but new diseases now began to appear. One of these was tuberculosis, or 'consumption' as it was often called. Between 1862 and 1887 the death rate from tuberculosis increased steadily, but after this period and until 1926 the death rate fell rapidly (Cumpston 1989). The other significant disease was influenza, with two pandemics occurring in 1891 and 1919. The pandemic of 1919 was responsible for many deaths in Australia (with 6387 of these deaths occurring in New South Wales alone) despite rigid interstate quarantine measures. Effective maritime quarantine against New Zealand and South African ships prevented the spread of a virulent form of influenza that had claimed many lives in those countries. After 1918 the death rate from influenza declined to a normal level, and though there was another influenza epidemic in 1923, it was not on the same scale as the earlier pandemics (Cumpston 1989).

Did this decrease in tuberculosis and influenza result mostly from advances in medical treatment? Although medical advances helped to some degree, the decrease occurred long before effective vaccines and medications were introduced. This was the case for most of the major diseases we've discussed, including tuberculosis, diphtheria, measles and influenza (Cumpston 1989; McKeown 1979). It appears that the decline resulted mainly from *preventive* measures — such as improved personal hygiene, greater resistance to diseases (owing to better nutrition) and public health innovations, such as quarantine and building water purification and sewage treatment facilities. As a result of sanitary reform, fewer deaths occurred from infectious diseases because fewer people contracted them.

The twentieth century saw great changes in the patterns of illness affecting people in Australia. The death rate from life-threatening infectious diseases continued to decline as a result of advances in preventive measures and in medical care. At the same time, the average life expectancy of people increased dramatically. At the turn of the twentieth century in Australia, the life expectancy of a male at birth was about 55 years, while the life expectancy of a female at birth was about 59 years. In

1998 the life expectancy for a male baby was almost 76 years and for a female baby, 82 years (AIHW 2000). Figure 1.2 shows this change in life expectancy over time, for infants at birth, and for people who have reached the age of 15 or 65. The increased life expectancy of Australians can be attributed mostly to the decrease in infant mortality over time, though reductions in mortality among the elderly in recent times have also contributed to increased life expectancy (AIHW 2000). A male in 1901 who had reached the age of 15 years could expect to live to almost 64 years of age, while a female who had reached the age of 15 could be expected to live to age 67. As the death rate for children is much lower today, only a small difference exists in the expected total life span for newborns and 15-year-olds (AIHW 2000). While life expectancy for mainstream Australians has increased over time, Aboriginal and Torres Strait Islander people do not share the same health status. Life expectancy for indigenous peoples in 1998 was 20 years below that of other Australians (AIHW 2000).

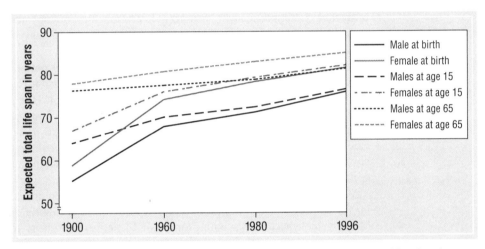

Figure 1.2 Expected total life span at various years since 1900 for Australian males and females who were born in the specified year or had reached 15 years or 65 years of age

Source: AIHW (1998).

Death is still inevitable of course, but people die at later ages now and from different causes. The main health problems and causes of death in Australia are **chronic diseases** — that is, degenerative illnesses that develop or persist over a long period of time. These diseases are also termed lifestyle diseases because the things we do as part of our everyday living, such as smoking, not exercising or not eating a high fibre diet, affect our future health. About two-thirds of all deaths in Australia are caused by three chronic diseases: heart disease, cancer and stroke (AIHW 2000).

Patterns of mortality are different for indigenous Australians compared with other Australians. The leading cause of death for Aboriginal men and women is diseases of the circulatory system (AIHW 2000). The death rate from these diseases was more than double that for the total Australian population. Respiratory diseases, cancer, injury/poisoning and diabetes account for the remainder of indigenous deaths. The mortality rate for injury and poisoning among Aborigines is more than double that for the total Australian population, while for respiratory diseases the death rate is three times higher than the national rate (AIHW 2000). Compared with indigenous groups from other countries, Australian Aborigines have higher mortality rates for heart disease, respiratory diseases and injury (Hogg 1992). Concern with the health of indigenous people in Australia has led to specific priority health targets for Aboriginals, outlined in the *Goals and Targets for Australia's Health in the Year 2000 and Beyond* (Nutbeam et al. 1993).

The health of ethnic minorities in Australia is better than for the rest of the population, though this tends to equalise with length of residence in Australia and with successive generations (AIHW 1996, 1998). Australians aged over 15 years who were born overseas have lower death rates from most of the leading causes of death, and have a higher life expectancy than those born in Australia. Differences exist in disease patterns, however. For example, Asian immigrants have higher death rates from diabetes and infectious diseases than other Australians. Most of the health difference between immigrants and Australian-born persons has been attributed to the **'healthy migrant effect'**, due in part to a number of factors (Taylor & Quine 1992). Immigrants to Australia are selected on the basis of health status. The staple diet of some migrants (in particular those from southern Europe and Asia) has also been found to have a protective function against coronary heart disease, one of the leading causes of mortality in Australia. New immigrants to a country also may be less able to afford luxury foods high in sugar or refined carbohydrate.

Diseases such as cancer, heart disease and stroke are not new, but they were responsible for a much smaller proportion of deaths before the twentieth century. Why? One reason is that people's lives are different today. For example, the growth of industrialisation increased people's stress and exposure to harmful chemicals. In addition, more people today survive to old age, and chronic diseases are more likely to afflict the elderly than younger individuals. Thus, another reason for the current prominence of chronic diseases is that more people are living to the age when they are at high risk for contracting them (AIHW 1998).

What are the main causes of death in Australian children and adolescents today? By far the leading cause is not an illness, but death from accidental injury (AIHW 2000). Motor vehicle accidents account for about 17 per cent of injury-related deaths in children between the ages of one and 15 years, while drowning accounts for about 20 per cent of injury deaths. In childhood, the next two most frequent causes of death are congenital abnormalities and cancer; in late adolescence they are suicide and drug dependence (AIHW 2000). Clearly, the role of disease in death is very different at the two ends of the life span.

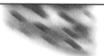

Viewpoints from history: physiology, disease processes and the mind

Is illness a purely physical condition? Does a person's mind play a role in becoming ill and getting well? People have wondered about these questions for thousands of years, and the answers they have arrived at have changed over time.

Early cultures

Although we do not know for certain, it appears that the best educated people thousands of years ago believed physical and mental illnesses were caused by mystical forces, such as evil spirits (Stone 1979). Why do we think this? Researchers found ancient skulls in several areas of the world with coin-size circular holes in them that could not have been battle wounds. These holes were probably made with sharp stone tools in a procedure called *trephination*. This procedure was done presumably for superstitious reasons — for instance to allow illness-causing demons to leave the head. Unfortunately, we can only speculate about the reasons for these holes because there are no written records from those times.

Ancient Greece and Rome

The philosophers of ancient Greece produced the earliest written ideas about physiology, disease processes and the mind, between 500 and 300 B.C. Hippocrates, often called 'the Father of Medicine', proposed a *humoral theory* to explain why people get sick. According to this theory, the body contains four fluids called *humours* (in biology, the term humour refers to any plant or animal fluid). When the mixture of these humours is harmonious or balanced, we are in a state of health. Disease occurs when the mixture is faulty (Stone 1979). Hippocrates recommended eating a good diet and avoiding excesses to help achieve humoral balance.

Greek philosophers, especially Plato, were among the first to propose that the mind and the body are separate entities (Marx & Hillix 1963; Schneider & Tarshis 1975). This view is reflected in the humoral theory: people get sick because of an imbalance in body fluids. The mind was considered to have little or no relationship to the body and its state of health. This remained the dominant view of writers and philosophers for more than a thousand years.

Many people today still speak about the body and the mind as if they were separate. The *body* refers to our physical being, including our skin, muscles, bones, heart and brain. The *mind* refers to an abstract process that includes our thoughts, perceptions, and feelings. Although we can distinguish between the mind and the body conceptually, an important issue is whether they also function independently. The question of their relationship is called the **mind/body problem**.

Galen was a famous and highly respected physician and writer of the second century A.D. who was born in Greece and practised in Rome. Although he believed generally in the humoral theory and the mind/body split, he made many innovations. For example, he 'dissected animals of many species (but probably never a human), and made important discoveries about the brain, circulatory system, and kidneys' (Stone 1979, p. 4). From this work he became aware that illnesses can be localised, with pathology in specific parts of the body, and that different diseases have different effects. Galen's ideas became widely accepted.

The Middle Ages

After the collapse of the Roman Empire in the fifth century, much of the Western world was in disarray. The advance of knowledge and culture slowed sharply and remained at a low level during the Middle Ages, which lasted almost a thousand years. Galen's views dominated ideas about physiology and disease processes for most of this time.

The influence of the Church in slowing the development of medical knowledge during the Middle Ages was enormous. According to historians, in the eyes of the Church the human being

> was regarded as a creature with a soul, possessed of a free will which set him apart from
> ordinary natural laws, subject only to his own willfulness and perhaps the will of God.
> Such a creature, being free-willed, could not be an object of scientific investigation. Even

the body of man was regarded as sacrosanct, and dissection was dangerous for the dissector. These strictures against observation hindered the development of anatomy and medicine for centuries. (Marx & Hillix 1963, p. 24)

The prohibition against dissection extended to animals as well, since they, too, were thought to have souls.

People's ideas about the cause of illness took on pronounced religious overtones, and the belief in demons became strong again (Sarason & Sarason 1984). Sickness was seen as God's punishment for doing evil things. As a result, the Church came to control the practice of medicine, and priests became increasingly involved in treating the ill, often by torturing the body to drive out evil spirits.

It was not until the thirteenth century that new ideas about the mind/body problem began to emerge. The Italian philosopher St. Thomas Aquinas rejected the view that the mind and body are separate. He saw them as an interrelated unit that forms the whole person (Leahey 1987). Although his position did not have as great an impact as others had had, it renewed interest in the issue and influenced later philosophers.

The Renaissance and after

The word *renaissance* means rebirth — a fitting name for the fourteenth and fifteenth centuries. During this period in history Europe saw a rebirth of inquiry, culture and politics. Scholars became more 'human-centred' than 'God-centred' in their search for truth and 'believed that truth can be seen in many ways, from many individual perspectives' (Leahey 1987, p. 80). These ideas set the stage for important changes in philosophy once the scientific revolution began after 1600.

The seventeenth-century French philosopher and mathematician René Descartes probably had the greatest influence on scientific thought of any philosopher in history (Schneider & Tarshis 1975). Like the Greeks, he regarded the mind and body as separate entities, but he introduced three important innovations. First, he conceived of the body as a machine and described the mechanics of how action and sensation occurred. For example, Figure 1.3 shows his concept of how we experience pain. Second, he proposed that the mind and body, although separate, could *communicate* through the pineal gland, an organ in the brain (Leahey 1987). Third, he believed that animals have no soul and that the soul in humans leaves the body at death (Marx & Hillix 1963). This belief meant that dissection could be an acceptable method of study — a point the Church was now ready to concede (Engel 1977).

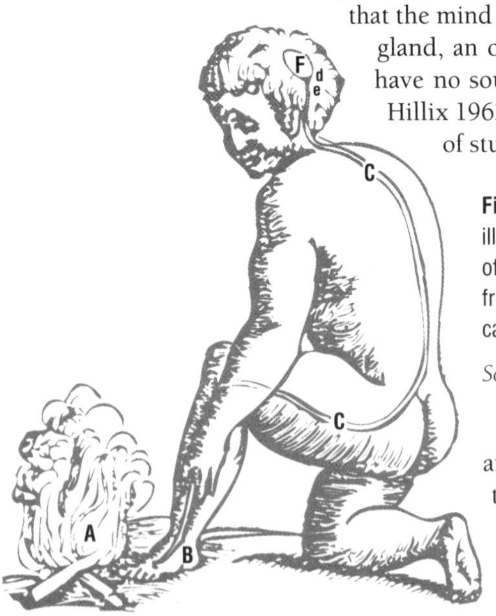

Figure 1.3 Descartes' concept of the pain pathway. Descartes used this drawing to illustrate the mechanisms by which people experience and respond to pain: The heat of the fire (at A) sends tiny particles to the foot (B) that pull on a thread that courses from the foot to the head. This action opens a pore (*de*), releasing spirits from a cavity (F) that travel to the parts of the body that respond (e.g. the leg moves away).

Source: From Descartes (1664, figure 7).

In the eighteenth and nineteenth centuries, knowledge in science and medicine grew quickly, helped greatly by the development of the microscope and the use of dissection in autopsies. Once scientists learned the basics of how the body functioned and discovered that micro-organisms cause certain diseases, they were able to reject the humoral theory of illness and propose new theories.

The field of surgery flourished after antiseptic techniques and anaesthesia were introduced in the mid-nineteenth century (Stone 1979). Before that time hospitals were 'notorious places, more likely to spread diseases than cure them' (Easterbrook 1987, p. 42). Over time, the reputation of physicians and hospitals began to improve, and people's trust in the ability of doctors to heal increased.

These advances, coupled with the continuing belief that the mind and body are separate, laid the foundation for a new approach, or model, for conceptualising health and illness. This approach — called the **biomedical model** — proposes that all diseases or physical disorders can be explained by disturbances in physiological processes, which result from injury, biochemical imbalances, bacterial or viral infection and the like (Engel 1977; Leventhal, Prohaska & Hirschman 1985). The biomedical model assumes that disease is an affliction of the body and is separate from the psychological and social processes of the mind. This viewpoint became widely accepted during the nineteenth and twentieth centuries and still represents the dominant view in medicine today.

Seeing a need: psychology's role in health

The biomedical model has been very useful. Using it as a guide, researchers have made enormous achievements. They conquered many infectious diseases, such as polio and measles, through the development of vaccines. They also developed antibiotics, which made it possible to cure illnesses caused by bacterial infection. Despite these great advances, however, the biomedical model needs improvement.

Overcoming problems with the Australian health care system

In 1997–98 health care expenditure in Australia accounted for 8.3 per cent of the gross domestic product (GDP), having almost doubled over the previous four decades (AIHW 2000). This increase in health expenditure since 1960, which represents an average annual increase of 3.6 per cent per person (AIHW 2000), has been attributed to three factors — population growth, an increase in the number of aged persons and greater use of health services at all ages (AIHW 2000). Total health expenditure in 1997–98 was $47 030 million or approximately $2523 per person (AIHW 2000), with the largest part being directed to hospitals, both public and private, and medical services (AIHW 2000). As medical costs continue to rise, we need to consider new approaches for improving people's health.

One solution to curtailing health costs is to focus effort on health promotion and disease prevention in regard to the major causes of mortality and morbidity. The national health priorities are listed in the report *Goals and Targets for Australia's Health in the Year 2000 and Beyond* (Nutbeam et al. 1993). These targets address preventable morbidity and mortality, healthy lifestyles and risk factors, health literacy and life skills, and healthy environments, thereby acknowledging the importance of biopsychosocial factors in health.

Another solution to reducing health care costs lies in 'best practice'. This can be achieved through correct diagnosis of conditions and appropriate treatment, and through interventions that facilitate speed of recovery. Psychologists can make valuable contributions in the latter area. In a review of the literature on the effects of psychological intervention on surgical recovery and heart attack rehabilitation, Mumford, Schlesinger and Glass (1982) reported that patients in treatment groups spent on average 2.4 days less in hospital than did control groups. The types of treatment used varied from psychological support to relaxation techniques, group therapy, hypnotherapy and systematic desensitisation. Outcome indicators compared across the 34 controlled experimental studies included post-operative pain, use of narcotics, complications, speed of recovery and days spent in hospital. In 85 per cent of the comparisons, the treatment group demonstrated better outcomes. A more recent Australian study by Milgrom, Walter and Green (1994) compared the cost-effectiveness of medical and psychological treatment for cases characterised by frequent outpatient attendances, high medication use, lengthy hospitalisations and conditions with non-organic basis. The cost savings for psychological interventions ranged from $185 to $103 466 with an average saving of $4161. Yet Australian psychologists have not been prominent in acute hospital settings (Groth-Marnat 1988).

Given the importance of psychological factors to patient treatment and recovery, some psychologists (James 1994; Richards 1992; Winefield 1991) see the solution to reducing health care costs as not only providing psychological services for patients, but also the shared training of medical practitioners by psychologists. The latter is seen as a way of ensuring a more holistic mode of medical treatment through the acquisition by medical practitioners of psychological knowledge of importance to understanding the patient's needs and concerns.

These considerations have led to questions within the discipline of psychology that relate to how much responsibility psychologists should assume for the training of non-psychologists (Lee 1994). In a consultant or 'shared care' model of health care, psychologists would support and assist medical practitioners in psychological aspects of medical care, facilitate patient compliance with treatment regimes, teach coping strategies to patients, and be directly involved in the provision of specific psychological procedures currently provided by other professionals (Richards 1992). This differs from a consultancy model in which psychologists wait to be asked to train others in psychological skills and assume no direct responsibility for their application by other health professionals (Richards 1994).

'The person' in health and illness

Have you ever noticed how some people are 'always sick' — they get illnesses more frequently than most people do and get well more slowly? These differences between people can result from biomedical sources, such as variations in physiological processes and exposure to harmful micro-organisms. But psychological and social factors also play a role. Let's look briefly at two of these factors: the lifestyle and personality of the person.

Lifestyle and illness

Earlier we saw that the occurrence of infectious diseases declined sharply in the late nineteenth century mainly because of such preventive measures as improving nutrition and personal hygiene. These measures involved changes in people's *lifestyles* — their everyday patterns of behaviour, such as in preparing and eating better balanced meals. The chief health problems in technological societies today are chronic diseases. These, too, can be reduced by people making changes in their lives. Let's see how.

Characteristics or conditions that are associated with the development of a disease or injury are called **risk factors** for that health problem. Although some risk factors are *biological*, such as inheriting certain genes, others are *behavioural*. For example, it is well known that people who smoke cigarettes face a much higher risk of developing cancer and other illnesses than non-smokers do. Other risk factors for cancer include eating diets high in saturated fat and a family history of the disease. People who 'do more' or 'have more' of these characteristics or conditions are more likely to contract cancer than people who 'do less' or 'have less' of these factors. Keep in mind that a risk factor is *associated* with a health problem — it does not necessarily *cause* the problem. For example, being poor is a risk factor for cancer (Levy 1985), but it does not cause the disease — at least not directly.

Many risk factors result from the way people live or behave, such as smoking cigarettes and eating unhealthy diets. Some behavioural risk factors associated with the five leading causes of death are:

1. *heart disease:* smoking, high dietary cholesterol and lack of exercise
2. *cancer:* smoking, high alcohol use and diet
3. *stroke:* smoking, high dietary cholesterol and lack of exercise
4. *COPD (chronic lung diseases, e.g., emphysema):* smoking
5. *accidents (including motor vehicle):* alcohol/drug use, driving motor vehicles too fast and not using seatbelts (McGinnis 1994).

Many of the people who are the victims of these illnesses and accidents live for at least a short while and either recover or eventually succumb. Part of today's high medical costs result from a failure in personal responsibility by those victims who had lifestyles that contributed to their health problems. The vast majority of Australian health care efforts and funds are directed towards treating illness, not preventing it (Bridges-Webb et al. 1992).

'Why don't people do what's good for them?' There's no simple answer to that question — there are many reasons. One reason is that less healthy behaviours often bring immediate pleasure, as when the person has a 'good-tasting' cigarette or ice-cream. Long-range negative consequences seem remote, both in time and in likelihood. Another reason is that people sometimes feel social pressures to engage in unhealthy behaviour, as when an adolescent begins to use cigarettes, alcohol or drugs. Also, some behaviours can become very strong habits, perhaps involving a physical addiction or psychological dependency, as happens with drugs and cigarettes. Quitting them becomes very difficult. Finally, sometimes people are simply not aware of the dangers involved or how to change their behaviour. As psychologist Carl Thoresen has pointed out, 'People need to be taught how to be more caring and more responsible for their own health and wellbeing, especially when the social environment commonly promotes irresponsible or nonhealthy behaviour' (1984, p. 300).

Personality and illness

Do you believe, as many do, that people who suffer from ulcers tend to be worriers or 'workaholics'? Or that people who have migraine headaches are highly anxious? If you do, then you believe there is a link between personality and illness. The term **personality** refers to a person's cognitive, affective or behavioural tendencies that are fairly stable across time and situations.

Researchers have found evidence linking personality and health. For example, low levels of conscientiousness in childhood and poor mental health in adulthood are associated with dying at earlier ages from diseases such as heart disease and cancer (Friedman, Tucker et al. 1995). In addition, people whose personalities include high levels of *anxiety, depression, anger/hostility* or *pessimism* seem to be at risk for developing a variety of illnesses, particularly heart disease (Everson et al. 1996; Friedman & Booth-Kewley 1987; Scheier & Bridges 1995). These four emotions are reactions that often occur when people experience stress, such as when they have more work to do than they think they can finish or when a tragedy happens.

People differ in the way they deal with stressful situations. Many people approach these situations with relatively positive emotions. Their outlook is more optimistic than pessimistic, more hopeful than desperate. These people are not only less likely to become ill than are people with less positive personalities, but when they do, they tend to recover more quickly (Reker & Wong 1985). A dramatic and well-known anecdotal example of the role of this optimistic and hopeful outlook is the case of Norman Cousins, a former editor of an American newspaper, the *Saturday Review*, who developed an 'incurable', painful and usually fatal illness. His strong knowledge of medicine allowed him to react to his doctors' prognosis by becoming actively involved in decisions regarding his medical treatment. He decided to stop taking massive doses of pain-killers, supplement his treatment with high doses of vitamin C and try to reduce his pain with lots of laughter, which he got by watching comic films like those of the Marx Brothers and Laurel and Hardy. As his condition began to improve, he came to believe he was recovering because his optimism enabled him to mobilise his body's resources to fight the disease (Cousins 1979).

The link between personality and illness is not a one-way process: illness can affect one's personality, too (Cohen & Rodriguez 1995). People who suffer from serious illness and disability often experience feelings of anxiety, depression, anger and hopelessness. But as psychologists Irwin and Barbara Sarason have pointed out:

> A physical illness does not necessarily have to be catastrophic to exert a psychological impact. Anyone who has had the flu, has a sprained ankle, or has had a toothache knows how much psychological damage these relatively minor problems can cause. Of course, the more serious the physical disorder, the greater the likelihood that it will significantly affect a person's thoughts and feelings. These psychological changes compound the detrimental effects of the person's physical condition. (1984, p. 157)

People who are ill and overcome their negative thoughts and feelings can speed their recovery. We will examine this relationship in more detail later in this book.

Our glimpse at the relationships of the person's lifestyle and personality in illness demonstrates why it is important to consider psychological and social factors in health and illness. Next we will see how this recognition came about.

How the role of psychology emerged

The idea that medicine and psychology are somehow connected has a long history, dating back at least to ancient Greece. It became somewhat more formalised early in the twentieth century in the work of Sigmund Freud, who was trained as a physician. He noticed that some patients showed symptoms of physical illness without any organic disorder. Consistent with his psychoanalytic theory, Freud believed that these symptoms were 'converted' from unconscious emotional conflicts (Alexander 1950; Davison & Neale 1994). He called this condition *conversion hysteria*.

What symptoms do patients with conversion hysteria show? The symptoms can include paralysis, deafness, blindness and the loss of sensation in part of the body such as the hand. This last symptom is called *glove anaesthesia* because only the hand has no feeling. When a loss of sensation in the body is inconsistent with the relevant nerve pathways, it probably does not have an organic cause (Davison & Neale 1994). These forms of conversion hysteria occur less frequently in urban than in remote areas, perhaps because urbanites realise that medical tests can generally determine if an organic disorder exists (Rosenhan & Seligman 1984).

Focus on research
Health and lifestyles

In 1965 Nedra Belloc and Lester Breslow began a project to study the importance of personal lifestyles on people's health. The researchers surveyed nearly 7000 adults who ranged in age from about 20 to over 75, and asked them two sets of questions. One set asked about the health of these people over the previous 12 months — for instance whether illness had prevented them from working for a long time, forced them to cut down on other activities, impaired their continued activities or reduced their energy level. The second set of questions asked about seven aspects of their lifestyles: sleeping, eating breakfast, eating between meals, maintaining an appropriate weight, smoking cigarettes, drinking alcohol and undertaking physical activity.

How important were these lifestyle factors? When the researchers compared the data for subjects in different age groups, they found that at each age health was typically better as the number of healthy practices increased. The impact of these lifestyle practices is suggested by the finding that the health of those who 'reported following all seven good health practices was consistently about the same as those 30 years younger who followed few or none of these practices' (Belloc & Breslow 1972, p. 419).

Were these health practices important in the future health of these people? Very much so. Breslow (1983) has described later studies of the same group of subjects. One study determined which people had died in the $9\frac{1}{2}$ years after the original survey. These data were then separated according to the age, sex and number of healthy behaviours the people reported

practising in the original survey. Figure 1.4 presents the results of this analysis for the men. The important finding was that the percentage dying generally decreased with increases in the number of healthy behaviours practised, and this impact was greater for older people than for younger ones. The results for the female subjects were similar, but the impact of these health practices was not as strong.

These findings show that health and survival are strongly influenced by people's lifestyles. Practising healthy behaviours can reduce people's risk of illness and early death substantially. Lifestyle appears to be more critical for the health of men than women, and is particularly important as individuals get older.

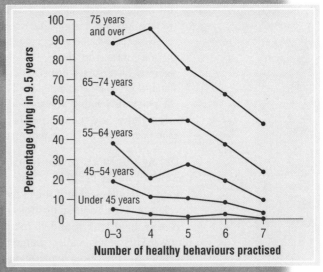

Figure 1.4 Percentage of male adults who died within $9\frac{1}{2}$ years as a function of the number of healthy behaviours they reported practising and of their ages (at the start of the study, in 1965). The findings for women were similar, but the decreases in deaths associated with increasing numbers of healthy behaviours were not as sharp.

Source: Data from Breslow (1983, table 3.6).

The need to understand conditions such as conversion hysteria led some researchers in the 1930s to study the interplay between emotional life and bodily processes (Alexander 1950). The field called **psychosomatic medicine** emerged in association with the US National Research Council, which began publishing the journal *Psychosomatic Medicine* in 1939. Its founders were primarily researchers trained in medicine, and their leaders included the psychoanalyst Franz Alexander and the psychiatrist Flanders Dunbar. Four years later the field was organised as a society, which is now called the American Psychosomatic Society. There was no equivalent professional body in Australia (Oldenburg & Owen 1990).

Nonetheless, Australia has had a long and successful history of research in psychosomatic medicine. Bodies such as the International College of Psychosomatic Medicine have attracted strong membership in Australia, with a recent President of the College being Australian. Australia has also hosted two large World Congresses of that College in recent times — the Ninth World Congress (Sydney, 1987) and the Fourteenth World Congress (Cairns, 1997).

During the society's first 25 years or so research in psychosomatic medicine focused on psychoanalytic interpretations for a specific set of health problems, including ulcers, high blood pressure, asthma, migraine headaches and rheumatoid arthritis. We can see this approach in the case study of a 23-year-old student in therapy who had developed a bleeding ulcer at age 18. His

> most conspicuous personality trait was his extreme casualness, which reflected his marked control over the display of emotion... His casualness and show of imperturbable security were but a defence against insecurity and dependence, which became overwhelming under his mother's exaggerated expectations. This conflict showed itself conspicuously in his relationship to women; he did not allow himself to become emotionally involved, had only casual sexual relationships, and terminated each affair as soon as the woman showed some personal interest in him... He succeeded gradually [in therapy] in renouncing more and more of his excessive dependency and in accepting a more mature attitude. With these internal developments a profound change took place in his relationship to women. He fell in love with a young woman, and for the first time in his life a prolonged happy sexual affair ensued. He later married her. At the same time his stomach complaints diminished and he was able to live on a normal diet. (Alexander 1950, pp. 113–4)

During the 1960s psychosomatic medicine began to focus on new approaches and theories (Totman 1982). It is now a broader field concerned with the interrelationships among psychological and social factors, biological and physiological functions, and the development and course of illness (Lipowski 1986).

A new field was founded in the early 1970s to study the role of psychology in illness. This field, called **behavioural medicine**, grew out of the perspective in psychology called *behaviourism*, which proposed that behaviour results from two types of learning. These are:

- *classical (or respondent) conditioning*, in which a stimulus (the conditioned stimulus) gains the ability to elicit a response through association with a stimulus (the unconditioned stimulus) that already elicits that response
- *operant conditioning*, in which behaviour is changed because of its consequences, such as reward or punishment.

Behaviourism was in its heyday at this time, and conditioning methods had shown a good deal of success as therapeutic approaches in helping people modify problem *behaviours*, such as overeating, and *emotions*, such as anxiety and fear (Sarafino 1996). By this time, physiological psychologists had clearly demonstrated that psychological events — particularly emotions — influence bodily functions, such as blood pressure. And researchers had shown that people can learn to control various physiological systems if they are given *feedback* as to what the systems are doing (Miller 1978).

Why were these findings important? They revealed that the link between the mind and the body is more direct and pervasive than was previously thought. Soon they led to an important therapeutic technique called *biofeedback*, whereby a person's physiological processes, such as blood pressure, are monitored by the person so that he or she can gain voluntary control over them. The feedback serves as a consequence of operant conditioning. As we shall see in later chapters, biofeedback has proven to be useful in treating a variety of health problems, such as headaches.

In the late 1970s the field of behavioural medicine was formally launched in association with the US National Academy of Sciences, the *Journal of Behavioral Medicine* was established, and the Society of Behavioural Medicine was founded. No equivalent professional body existed in Australia. Practitioners and researchers working in the field of behavioural medicine published in the American journal (Oldenburg & Owen 1990). An important characteristic of this field is that its membership is interdisciplinary — they come from a wide variety of fields, including psychology, sociology and various areas of medicine. As a result, the society strives to pool the talents and perspectives of this diverse membership in a 'joint exploration targeted on health issues of mutual concern' (Gentry 1984). These health issues involve all aspects of illness — prevention, diagnosis, treatment and rehabilitation.

A third field also emerged in the late 1970s in the United States, but this one is within the discipline of psychology. It is called **health psychology**. The American Psychological Association has many divisions, or subfields; the Division of Health Psychology was introduced in 1978 (Wallston 1993). The journal *Health Psychology* began publication four years later as the official journal of this division. Joseph Matarazzo, the first president of the division, has proposed the following definition of the field.

> *Health psychology* is the aggregate of the specific educational, scientific, and professional contributions of the discipline of psychology to the promotion and maintenance of health, the prevention and treatment of illness, the identification of etiologic and diagnostic correlates of health, illness, and related dysfunction, and to the analysis and improvement of the health care system and health policy formation. (1982, p. 4)

The last part of this definition describes four goals for health psychology. Let's look at some of the ways psychologists can contribute to these goals.

The first goal is to promote and maintain health. Psychologists study such topics as why people do and do not smoke cigarettes, use safety belts in cars, drink alcohol and follow particular diets. As a result, health psychologists can help in the design of school health education programs and media campaigns to encourage healthy lifestyles and behaviours.

The second goal involves the prevention and treatment of illness. Psychological principles have been applied effectively in preventing illness, such as in reducing high blood pressure and, therefore, the risk of heart disease and stroke. For those people who become seriously ill, psychologists with clinical training can help them adjust to their current condition, rehabilitation program and future prospects, such as reduced work or sexual activity.

The third goal focuses on the causes ('aetiologic correlates') and detection of illness. Psychologists study the causes of disease; the research we saw earlier showing the importance of personality factors in the development of illness is an example of the work towards this goal. Psychologists also study physiological and perceptual processes. This knowledge has been applied to the diagnosis of problems in vision and hearing, for example.

The last goal is to improve the health care system and health policy. Psychologists contribute towards this goal by studying how patients are affected by characteristics or functions of hospitals, nursing homes, medical personnel and medical costs. With the resulting knowledge, they can make recommendations for improvement, suggesting ways to help doctors and nurses become more sensitive and responsive to the needs of patients and to make the system more accessible to individuals who fail to seek treatment.

By now you may be wondering, 'Aren't psychosomatic medicine, behavioural medicine and health psychology basically the same?' In a sense they are. The goals of the three fields are very similar, and the overlap in the knowledge used in these fields is extensive. Perhaps the main distinction among them is the degree to which they are interdisciplinary. Behavioural medicine has the most diverse membership, drawing knowledge directly from a wide variety of disciplines in their research. Psychosomatic medicine continues to be closely allied with medical disciplines, especially psychiatry. And health psychology is a subfield of psychology — almost all of its members are psychologists — and draws directly on the many other subfields within the discipline: clinical, developmental, experimental, physiological and social psychology.

It is important to realise also that these three fields are separate mainly in an organisational sense. Many professionals are members of all three organisations. Although the fields have slightly different perspectives, they share the view that health and illness result from the interplay of biological, psychological and social forces. As this suggests, these fields are interested in knowledge from a wide variety of disciplines and are engaged in a cooperative effort to enhance wellness and reduce illness. Although the main focus of this book is health psychology, we will keep in mind the overlap with and contributions of the fields of psychosomatic medicine and behavioural medicine.

Health psychology in Australia

Although the field of health psychology in the United States has been active for 25 years, with formal recognition as a division of the American Psychological Association in 1978, in Australia the College of Health Psychology came into existence in 1996. This does not mean that the field has had no representation in the past. In the 1980s a series of behavioural medicine conferences were held for the presentation of theoretical and research papers in the field (Sheppard 1982; 1989). This was followed by a Working Party on Health Psychology within the Australian Psychological Society (APS) and later the Interest Group in Health Psychology, which met at annual conferences of the APS. There have also been attempts to survey the expertise and practices of both academics and practitioners in the field (Carlson & Sheppard 1992) along with more recent debate about the contribution health psychologists can make to the health care system (James 1994; Richards 1992; Milgrom, Walter & Green 1994), models of service delivery (Richards 1994), and issues of training and standards (Martin 1988; Richards 1992).

A survey of 3197 Australian psychologists (Carlson & Sheppard 1992) indicated that in 1990 the majority of those who considered themselves to be actively involved in the areas of health psychology/behavioural medicine were in private practice (40.5 per cent) or worked in academic settings (25.2 per cent). The majority of health psychologists in Australia possessed either a master's degree (27 per cent) or a PhD (35.8 per cent). Research and professional interests centred predominantly on stress, pain and their management. Other interests related to rehabilitation, depression, anxiety and therapeutic methods. Of the psychologists who responded to the survey, 19 per cent indicated professional interests in health education, counselling, promotion and health program evaluation.

Currently, health psychologists are employed in a diverse range of settings, with professional involvement in either health promotion or clinical health. Those working in the health promotion area are typically involved in risk factor identification, health promotion, disease prevention and public health advocacy at the family, community or organisational level. Clinical health psychologists apply psychological theory and knowledge to diagnosis, treatment and rehabilitation of illness, in inpatient hospital settings and outpatient medical facilities. Other health psychologists may be actively engaged in formulating new theoretical ideas on the basis of research, which can further advance health interventions or change patterns of health risk behaviours.

With the establishment of the APS College of Health Psychologists, this professional body has been instrumental in defining the core and specialist competencies required for the training of health psychologists, and for membership of the College (see table 1.1). As health psychology is a focal point for many other fields within psychology, health psychologists are expected to have a broad-based knowledge of psychological theory (cognitive, behavioural, social, developmental), psychological processes (motivation, emotion, cognition), and assessment procedures in their application to health promotion/illness prevention, diagnosis, rehabilitation and treatment. A knowledge of the health care system, and relevant Commonwealth/State health regulations and priorities is desirable. Specialisation is encouraged by the APS College in the areas of health promotion/disease prevention, and the application of psychological theory and research to illness diagnosis, treatment and rehabilitation in medical settings (APS 2001). (For more on the College's core and specialist competency requirements, see the appendix to table 1.1, reproduced on page 602.)

Table 1.1 Core and specialist competencies in the training of health psychologists, as specified by the College of Health Psychologists of the Australian Psychological Society

1	Body of knowledge	
	Indicators of competence	Area of competence
1.1	The individual needs to demonstrate a competent understanding of the areas listed, through assessment outcomes of relevant course subjects or professional training programs, documented successful application of these areas in a research project, program evaluation or work environment, or other documented evidence. Examples: • Written articles, books, chapters • Presented seminars, workshops, conference papers, debates • Attendance at professional development activities • Written notes/analyses of tapes, videos or articles • Written position statements on theories, practice and evaluation of the body of knowledge in health psychology.	**Core areas:** • Biological, psychological and social determinants of health and illness • Epidemiology of Australian population groups • Basic physical systems • Models of health behaviours and behaviour change • Psychology of health risk factors • Health beliefs and attitudes • Stress, coping and social support in health and illness. **Specialist competencies — health promotion area:** • Behavioural epidemiology • Health promotion strategies and methods (e.g. applied to exercise, lifestyle and nutrition) • Disease prevention • Systems and organisation for health promotion in Australia • Consumer behaviour. **Specialist competencies — clinical health area:** • Models of health and health care • Processes of acute and chronic illness, and seeking medical care • Developmental issues in acute and chronic illness • Psychosomatic, psychophysiological and behavioural medicine principles • Communication in health settings • The patient–practitioner relationship. *(continued)*

Table 1.1 *Continued*

1.2	The individual will be able to describe the theoretical and practical relevance of these areas. Examples: • Written articles, books, chapters • Presented seminars, workshops, conference papers, debates • Attendance at meetings and professional development activities • Written notes/analyses of tapes, videos or articles • Evidence of having applied knowledge in research, evaluation or service delivery.	**Non-psychological knowledge relevant to the specialist area:** • Australian health care systems, relevant federal and State health regulations and priorities • Interdisciplinary public health • Health service planning • Epidemiological and biostatistical research methods • Media advocacy • Economics and marketing • Basic physiological systems • Other health professions (e.g. medicine, nursing and social work).
1.3	The individual will be able to specify the appropriate application, the validity and reliability qualities, and the theoretical basis of assessment instruments. Examples: • Written reviews on the qualities of test instruments • Written presentation of the use of these tests • Presentation of seminars, workshops, conference papers, debates that include instruments • Attendance at professional development activities • Written notes/analyses on the utility of instruments.	**Major methods and instruments used for assessment:** A range of measures are utilised based on adequate psychometric performance measuring the following domains: • Health status, quality of life • Illness description and symptom assessment • Health behaviours • Health risk assessment • Stress, coping, social support • Social competence • Health care evaluations • Individual differences (e.g. *Type A behaviour, dispositional optimism, neuroticism, self-efficacy*) • Attitudes and beliefs, including cultural differences.
1.4	The individual will be able to demonstrate sound knowledge of the intervention techniques, and critically evaluate application research evidence and the theoretical basis for these interventions. Examples: • Presented a workshop, seminar or discussion group on intervention strategies • Written case analyses • Documentation of community needs analysis, community development or health promotion work undertaken.	**The major psychological approaches and interventions:** • Emotional, social and cognitive skill development • Cognitive-behavioural approaches in health management • System*s* approaches relevant to health and illness • Health behaviour, lifestyle management (e.g. sexual health, nutrition) • Health beliefs and attitudes • *Stress* inoculation and stress management. **Specialist competencies — health promotion area:** • Community needs analysis • Community development, intervention and empowerment strategies • Public health marketing and communication. **Specialist competencies — clinical health area:** • Psychological treatment relevant to health and illness (e.g. pain management, addiction, sleeping, eating problems) • Adjustment (e.g. grief, bereavement, death and dying) • Trauma, disability and rehabilitation.

2	Skills in psychological assessment and interpretation	
	Indicators of competence	Area of competence
2.1	Able to select, administer and interpret assessment instruments. Can provide written or oral critical evaluation of the psychometric qualities of psychological assessment methods and instruments appropriate to the specialist area. Examples: • Evidence of appropriate application, evaluation and interpretation of instruments • Written reports of peer supervision • Written reports from supervisor on work assessments.	• Assessment of health risk factors • Health status assessment • Health behaviour assessment • Assessment of stress and coping resources • Social support and social network assessment. **Specialist competencies — health promotion area:** • Community epidemiological assessment • Community needs assessment • Health care quality assessment. **Specialist competencies — clinical health area:** • Psychological assessment and diagnosis relevant to health and physical illness • Pain assessment • Clinical case assessment and planning • Health service record keeping.
3	Application (intervention skills)	
	Indicators of competence	Area of competence
3.1	Able to select and apply appropriate interventions, and justify the appropriateness of their application to the specialist area. Examples: • Ability to critically review intervention processes and strategies underlying effective prevention, treatment and rehabilitation for an individual, community or organisation. • Evidence of successful achievement of process, impact or outcome targets through the application of intervention techniques and programs.	**Selection and application of interventions for:** • Behaviour change • Stress management • Social skills, social intervention training • Family and workplace health enhancement. **Specialist competencies — health promotion area:** Selection and application of interventions for: • System level (school, peer group, organisational, community) health intervention • Health team development • Public health advocacy. **Specialist competencies — clinical health area:** Selection and application of interventions for: • Psychological and behavioural management in the treatment of illness • Enhancement of rehabilitation • Treatment of health risk behaviours • Enhancement of medical investigation and treatment.
3.2	To undertake the design, development, implementation and evaluation of interventions. Examples: • Sample of case notes, reports and records of intervention designs and implementation strategies • Written reviews of the development and evaluation of programs.	Family and workplace intervention design, development, implementation and evaluation of process, impact and outcome **Specialist competencies — health promotion area:** • System level (school, peer group, organisational, community) health intervention design, development, implementation and evaluation of process, impact and outcome. **Specialist competencies — clinical health area:** • Clinical intervention design, development, implementation and evaluation of process, impact and outcome.

Source: Australian Psychological Society (2001).

Where is health psychology taught in Australia?

Many APS-accredited undergraduate programs offer units in health psychology. No tertiary institution in Australia currently offers a degree specifically in health psychology at undergraduate level. The APS does not accredit an undergraduate degree specifically in health psychology, as no specialist professional qualification in psychology at undergraduate level would meet accreditation guidelines. Several universities offer units in either behavioural medicine or health psychology in their graduate diploma programs, though these units are usually taught within clinical training programs and are generalist rather than specialist in their approach. A number of both master's and doctoral programs in health psychology are offered at universities in Australia (Oldenburg & Owen 1990; Richards 1992; Sanson-Fisher et al. 1990a).

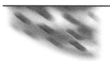

Current perspectives on health and illness

Once we add the person to the biomedical model, we have a different and broader picture of how health and illness come about. This new perspective involves the interplay of biological, psychological and social aspects of the person's life. As a result, this perspective is called the **biopsychosocial model** (Engel 1977, 1980; Schwartz 1982).

The biopsychosocial perspective

We can see elements of the biopsychosocial perspective in the story about Mandy at the beginning of the chapter. Mandy's athletic physique and normal weight can be explained by the biological contribution of inherited genes, but social factors, such as the family's dietary practices and health values, play an important part. Psychological factors, such as learning correct eating behaviour, imitation of such behaviour and maintenance of the behaviour through positive reinforcement, influenced Mandy's healthy behaviour practices early in life. Social factors had an influence on Mandy's drinking behaviour while away from home. Let's look at the elements of the biopsychosocial model in more detail.

The role of biological factors

What is included in the expression *biological factors*? This term embodies the genetic materials and processes by which we inherit characteristics from our parents. It also includes aspects of the person's physiological functioning — for example whether the body (1) contains structural defects, such as a malformed heart valve or some damage in the brain, that impair the operation of these organs; (2) responds effectively in protecting itself, such as by fighting infection; and (3) overreacts sometimes in the protective function, as happens in many allergic reactions to harmless substances, such as pollen or dust.

The body is made up of enormously complex physical systems. For instance, it has organs, bones and nerves, and these are composed of tissues, which in turn consist of cells, molecules and atoms. The efficient, effective and healthy functioning of these systems depends on the way these components operate and interact with each other.

The role of psychological factors

When we discussed the role of lifestyle and personality in health and illness earlier, we were describing behaviour and mental processes — in other words, psychological factors. Behaviour and mental processes are the focus of psychology, and they involve cognition, emotion and motivation.

Cognition is a mental activity that encompasses perceiving, learning, remembering, thinking, interpreting, believing and problem solving. How do these cognitive factors affect health and illness? Suppose, for instance, you strongly believe, 'Life is not worth living without the things I enjoy'. If you enjoy smoking cigarettes, would you quit to reduce your risk of getting cancer or heart disease? Probably not. Or suppose you develop a pain in your abdomen and you remember having had a similar symptom in the past that disappeared in a couple of days. Would you seek treatment? Again, probably not. These examples are just two of the countless ways cognition plays a role in health and illness.

Emotion is a subjective feeling that affects and is affected by our thoughts, behaviour and physiology. Some emotions are positive or pleasant, such as joy and affection, and others are negative, such as anger, fear and sadness. Emotions relate to health and illness in many ways. For instance, people whose emotions are relatively positive are less disease-prone and more likely to take good care of their health and to recover quickly from an illness than are people whose emotions are relatively negative. We considered these relationships when we discussed the role of personality in illness. Emotions can also be important in people's decisions about seeking treatment. People who are frightened of doctors and dentists may avoid getting the health care they need.

Motivation is a term applied to explanations of why people behave the way they do — why they start some activity, choose its direction and persist in it. A person who is motivated to feel and look better might begin an exercise program, choose the goals to be reached and stick with it. Many people are motivated to do what important people in their lives want them to do. Parents who quit smoking because their children plead with them to protect their health are an example.

The role of social factors

People live in a social world. We have relationships with individual people — an acquaintance, a friend or a family member — and with groups. As we interact with people, we affect them and they affect us. But our social world is larger than just the people we know or meet, and it contains levels of social spheres, such as our community and our family, and each level affects the others.

On a fairly broad level, our *society* affects the health of individuals by promoting certain values of our culture. One of these values is that being fit and healthy is good. Often the mass media — television, newspapers and so on — reflect these values by setting good examples and urging us to eat well, not to use drugs, and not to drink and drive. The mass media can do much to promote health. But sometimes these media encourage unhealthy behaviour, such as when we observe celebrities on television smoking cigarettes or drinking excessively. Can individuals affect society's values? Yes. As part of the society, we can affect its values by transmitting our opinions to the mass media, selecting which television shows and movies to watch, and buying healthy products, for example.

Our *community* consists of individuals who live fairly near one another, such as in the same town or suburb. The relationships we have with these people often involve relatively direct and reciprocal influences — we influence and are influenced by each other. This influence can be seen in the research finding that communities differ in the extent to which their members practise certain health-related behaviours, such as smoking cigarettes or consuming fatty diets (Diehr et al. 1993). These differences may develop in many ways. For instance, adolescents often start smoking cigarettes and drinking alcohol as a result of peer pressure (Quine & Stephenson 1990). Sometimes simply observing other teenagers engaged in these behaviours can encourage adolescents to smoke and drink. They want very much to be popular and to look 'cool' or 'tough' to others in their community. These examples involve clear and powerful motivational elements that are social in nature.

The closest and most continuous social relationships for most people occur within the *family*, which can include non-relatives who live together and share a strong emotional bond. As individuals grow and develop in early childhood, the family has an especially strong influence (Sarafino & Armstrong 1986). Children learn many health-related behaviours, attitudes and beliefs from their parents, brothers and sisters. They learn these things when their parents set good examples for healthy behaviour by using seatbelts, serving and eating nutritious meals, exercising, not smoking and so on. They also learn good habits when their families encourage them to perform healthy behaviours and praise them when they do. Moreover, as we have said, the individual can influence the larger social unit. The family may stop eating certain nutritious foods, such as brussels sprouts or fish, because one of the children has a tantrum when these foods are served.

The role of biological, psychological and social factors in health and illness is not hard to see. What is more difficult to understand is how health is affected by the *interplay* of these components, as the biopsychosocial model proposes. The next section deals with this interplay.

The concept of 'systems'

The whole person — as in the sentence, 'We need to understand the whole person' — is a phrase we hear often. It reflects our recognition that people and the reasons for their behaviour are very complex. Many health professionals strive to consider the impact of all aspects of a person's life as a total entity in understanding health and illness. This approach uses the biopsychosocial model and is sometimes called holistic. This term is derived from the Greek word *holos*, which means 'whole' (Lipowski 1986). The holistic approach views health not just as the absence of illness but as a general state of wellbeing. But many people today use the term *holistic* to include a broad range of 'alternative' approaches to promote health, such as treatments that use aromas and herbs to heal.

How can we conceptualise the whole person? George Engel (1980) has proposed that we can do this by applying the concept of 'systems' developed by Ludwig von Bertalanffy (1968). The term **system** refers to a dynamic entity consisting of components that are continuously interrelated. Your body qualifies as a system, and it includes the immune and nervous systems, which consist of tissues and cells. Your family is a system, and so are your community and society. As systems, they are entities that are dynamic — or constantly changing — and they have components that interrelate, such as by exchanging energy, substances and information.

As you can see in figure 1.5, the systems concept places smaller, simpler systems within larger, more complex ones. There are levels of systems. Cells are within the person who is within a society, for instance. In the previous section of this chapter, we saw that a system at one level, such as a person, is affected by and can affect a system at another level, such as the family. Similarly, if we look at levels within the person, illness in one part of the body can have far-reaching effects: If you fell and seriously injured your leg, your internal systems would be automatically mobilised to help protect the body from further damage. In addition, the discomfort and disability you might experience for days or weeks might affect your social relations with your family and community.

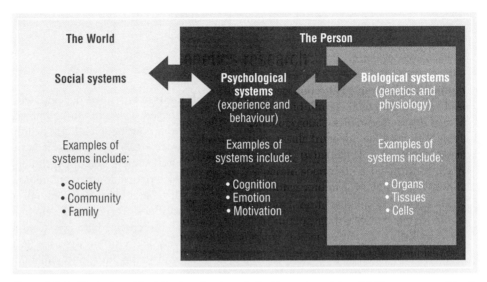

Figure 1.5 An illustration of the interplay of systems in the biopsychosocial model. The person consists of biological and psychological systems, which interrelate; and each of the systems includes component systems. The person interrelates with the social systems of his or her world. Each system can affect and be affected by any of the other systems.

To illustrate how the systems concept can be useful, let's use it to explain how a weight problem in a female adolescent might have come about. Let's assume that the person concerned inherited some factor that affects her weight. The nature of this factor might involve a preference for sweet foods, for instance (Rozin 1989). When she was a toddler, her parents quietened her tantrums by giving her lollies, which almost always calmed her. The parents were not concerned that she was getting heavy because they believed a popular misconception: 'a chubby baby is a healthy baby'. The meals the family ate usually contained lots of high-fat, high-kilojoule foods and a sweet dessert. Being heavy, she was less agile and tired more easily than children who were not overweight. So she usually preferred to engage in sedentary activities, such as playing with dolls or watching television, rather than sports. She and her friends snacked on biscuits while watching television. The commercials on most children's television shows made her weight problem worse, promoting high-fat, sweet breakfast and snack foods, which she got her parents to buy. This hypothetical account shows how different but interacting biopsychosocial systems can contribute to a person's weight problem.

Using the biopsychosocial model as a guide, researchers have discovered new and important ways to promote people's health and recovery from illness. Here is a sample of discoveries that we will discuss in later chapters.

- Using psychological methods to reduce anxiety in patients who are awaiting surgery enables them to recover more quickly and leave the hospital sooner.
- Programs that teach safer sex practices have dramatically reduced risky sexual behaviour and the spread of HIV infection.
- People who have a high degree of social support from family and friends are healthier and live longer than people who do not.
- Stress impairs the functioning of the immune system.

- Applying psychological and educational programs for cancer patients reduces their feelings of depression, improves their immune system functioning and enables them to live longer.
- Biofeedback and other psychological techniques can reduce the pain of people who suffer from chronic, severe headaches.

The life-span perspective

People change over time through the process called development. As people develop, each portion of their life span is affected by events in earlier years, and each affects what happens in years to come. Throughout people's lives, health, illness and the role of different biopsychosocial systems change. This is why it is important to keep the life-span perspective in mind when we examine health psychology.

In the **life-span perspective**, characteristics of a person are considered with respect to their prior development, current level and likely development in the future. How do characteristics relating to health and illness vary with development? One way is that the kinds of illnesses people have tend to change with age. Compared with older individuals, children suffer from relatively few chronic diseases (AIHW 1998). Illnesses that keep children out of school tend to be short-term infectious diseases, such as colds or the flu. In contrast, many people in late adulthood and old age suffer from heart disease, cancer and stroke.

How do the roles of different biopsychosocial systems change as we develop? Biological systems change in many ways. Virtually all systems of the body grow in size, strength and efficiency during childhood and decline in old age. The decline can be seen in the slowing down that older people notice in their physical abilities. They have less stamina because the heart and lungs function less efficiently and the muscles are weaker (Tortora & Grabowski 1993). They also recover from illness and injury more slowly.

Psychological systems change with development, too. As an example, we will look at the role of cognitive processes. Children's knowledge and ability to think are limited during the preschool years but grow rapidly during later childhood. Before children can assume responsibility for their health, they need to understand how their behaviour can affect it. As children get older and their cognitive skills improve, they are more likely to engage in behaviours that promote their health and safety (Maddux et al. 1986). They also become better able to understand the implications of their own illness when they are sick.

People's social relationships and social systems also change with development. How? For one thing, there are some usual progressions: Children usually become parents of their own families in adulthood, and grandparents in old age. They also progress through levels of education and employment, and retire in old age. Some changes in social relationships are related to health and illness. Children's health is largely the responsibility of adult caregivers — parents and teachers. During the teenage years, adolescents take on more and more of these responsibilities. At the same time, social relationships with their peers in the community start to have a very powerful influence on adolescents. The strong need to be accepted by peers sometimes leads teens towards unhealthy or unsafe behaviour. For example, an adolescent who has a chronic illness that can be controlled — as diabetes can — may neglect his or her medical care to avoid looking and feeling different from other adolescents (La Greca & Stone 1985).

The life-span perspective adds an important dimension to the biopsychosocial perspective in our effort to understand how people deal with issues of health and illness.

Relating health psychology to other science fields

Knowledge in health psychology is greatly enriched by information from many other disciplines, including disciplines within *psychology*, such as the clinical and social areas; *medicine*, including psychiatry and paediatrics; and *allied fields*, such as nursing, nutrition, pharmacology, biology and social work. Four other fields are especially important because they provide both information and a context for health psychology. We turn now to a description of these four related fields.

Related fields

To understand health psychology fully, we need to know the context in which health and illness exist. Part of this context is provided by the field of *epidemiology* — the scientific study of the distribution and frequency of disease and injury. Researchers in this field determine the occurrence of illness in a given population and organise these data in terms of when the disease or injury occurred, where, and to which age, gender and ethnic or cultural groups. Then they attempt to discover why specific illnesses are distributed as they are.

Epidemiologists use several terms in describing aspects of their findings (Gerace & Vorp 1985; Runyan 1985). We will define five of these terms.

- **Mortality** means death, generally on a large scale. An epidemiologist might report a decrease in mortality from heart disease among women, for instance.
- **Morbidity** means illness, injury or disability — basically any detectable departure from wellness.
- **Prevalence** refers to the number of cases, such as of a disease or of persons infected or at risk. It includes both continuing (previously reported) and new cases at a given moment in time — for example the number of cases of asthma as of the first day of the current year.
- **Incidence** refers to the number of *new* cases, such as of illness, infection or disability, reported during a period of time. An example is the number of newly diagnosed cases of HIV in Australia in a specific year.
- **Epidemic** usually refers to the situation in which the incidence, generally of an infectious disease, has increased rapidly.

Some of these terms are used with the word *rate*, which adds relativity to the meaning. For instance, the mortality rate refers to the number of deaths per number of people in a given population during a specified period of time. An example might be a mortality rate of 5 babies per 1000 female births dying in their first year of life during 1994 in Australia.

Another discipline of importance to health psychology is *public health*, the field concerned with protecting, maintaining and improving health through organised effort in the community. People who work in public health do research and set up programs dealing with immunisations, sanitation, health education and awareness, and ways to provide community health services (Runyan 1985). This field studies health and illness in the context of the community as a social system. The success of public health programs and the way individual people react to them are of interest to health psychologists.

The third related field is *sociology*, the science of human social life. Sociologists study groups or communities of people and evaluate the impact of various social factors, such as the mass media, population growth, epidemics and institutions. *Medical sociology* is a subfield of sociology. Medical sociologists study a wide range of issues related to health, including the impact of social relationships on the distribution of illness, cultural and social reactions to illness, socioeconomic factors of health care use, and the way hospital services and medical practices are organised (Adler & Stone 1979). Knowledge from sociology gives us a broad social view and describes the social environment in which the individual exists.

The fourth field, *anthropology*, includes the study of human cultures. Its subfield, *medical anthropology*, examines the differences in health and illness across cultures: In what ways do the nature and definition of illness vary across different cultures? How do people in these cultures react to illness, and what methods do they use to treat disease or injury? How do they structure health care systems? If health psychologists did not explore the knowledge of anthropology, our notions of health and illness would be very narrow. Medical anthropology gives us a world view of medical issues and allows us to look at different ways to interpret and treat illness (Adler & Stone 1979).

The combined information that health psychologists receive from the fields of epidemiology, public health, sociology and anthropology paints a broad picture for us. It describes the social systems in which health, illness and the person exist and develop.

Health and psychology across cultures

Health and illness have changed across the history and cultures of the world, as the following excerpt shows.

> Less than a hundred years ago the infant mortality rate in Europe and North America was as high as it is in the developing world now. In New York City in the year 1900, for example, the IMR [infant mortality rate] was approximately 140 per 1000 — about the same as in Bangladesh today. In the city of Birmingham, England, a survey taken in 1906 revealed an IMR of almost 200 per 1000 — higher than almost any country in the world in the 1980s. A look behind these statistics also shows that the main causes of infant death in New York and Birmingham *then* were much the same as in the developing world *now* — diarrheal diseases and malnutrition, respiratory infections, and whooping cough. (UNICEF, cited in Skolnick, 1986, p. 20)

The world view we get from historical–cultural comparisons can be quite dramatic. Each country's present culture is different from one another's and from the culture it had 200 years ago. Lifestyles have changed in each culture, and so has the pattern of illnesses that afflict its citizens.

Sociocultural differences in health

The term **sociocultural** means involving or relating to social and cultural factors, such as ethnic and income variations within and across nations. For instance, it has been found that certain forms of cancer, particularly stomach cancer, have far higher prevalence rates in Japan than in Australia today, but the reverse is true for breast (in females) and prostate (in males) cancers (AIHW 2000). Furthermore, large differences in rates of specific cancers even exist between regions of the same country — for example the incidence of melanoma in Queensland (age standardised rate of 63.2/100 000) compared with Tasmania (34.7) and the Northern Territory (32.8) (AIHW 2000). The differences we see in illness patterns between countries, regions or ethnic groups result from many factors, including heredity, environmental pollution, economic barriers to health care and cultural differences, such as in the diets and health-related beliefs and values of the people (Flack et al. 1995; Johnson et al. 1995). Although people around the world value good health, some people feel that maintaining health is more important than others do. It seems reasonable that the more people value their health, the more likely they are to take care of it.

Sociocultural differences in health beliefs and behaviour

Differences across history and culture can also be seen in the ideas people have about the *causes* of illness. Recall our discussion of the widespread belief in the Middle Ages that evil spirits caused illness. Today, educated people in technological societies generally reject such ideas. But less sophisticated people often do not, as the following excerpt shows.

> I've heard of people with snakes in their body, how they got in there I don't know. And they take 'em someplace to a witch doctor and snakes come out. My sister, she had somethin', a snake that was in her arm. She was a young woman. I can remember her bein' sick, very sick, and someone told her about this healer in another little town. And I do know they taken her there. This thing was just runnin' up her arm, whatever it was, just runnin' up her arm. You could actually *see* it. (Snow 1981, p. 86)

Although this account was given by a disadvantaged person in the United States, it is typical of the level of knowledge generally found in people in underdeveloped regions or countries. This is important to recognise because the large majority of people in the world live in underdeveloped societies.

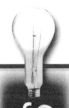

Highlight on issues

Careers relating health and psychology

The process of rehabilitation for a patient who is suffering from a chronic illness, serious injury or disability involves a variety of professionals working together with the physicians as a team. Each professional has specific training for a special role in the rehabilitation process. Most of them have some education in psychology. Let's look at some of these careers and the training they require in Australia.

Health psychologists

Because the field of health psychology is so new, its full potential for careers is developing rapidly. As we noted earlier, most health psychologists work in hospitals, clinics and academic departments of universities. In these positions, they either provide direct help to patients or give indirect help through research, teaching and consulting activities.

The direct help health psychologists provide generally relates to the patient's psychological adjustment to and management of health problems. Health psychologists with clinical training can provide therapy for emotional and social adjustment problems that being ill or disabled can produce — for example in reducing the patient's feelings of depression. They can also help patients manage the health problem by, for instance, teaching them psychological methods, such as biofeedback, to control pain.

Health psychologists provide indirect help, too. Their research provides information about lifestyle and personality factors in illness and injury. They can apply this and other biopsychosocial knowledge to design programs that help people lead more healthful lifestyles, such as by preventing or quitting cigarette smoking. They can also educate doctors and the other health care workers we have discussed towards a fuller understanding of the psychosocial needs of patients.

(continued)

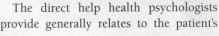

The qualifications for becoming a health psychologist in Australia include an accredited postgraduate (fifth and sixth year) program in health psychology. The APS now requires a full six-year sequence of tertiary study in order to quality for membership. Registration by State Boards is required for the practice of clinical techniques. Only a small number of registration acts allow for specialist registration, none of which are in health psychology.

Nurses

In Australia there are two categories of nurses: registered nurses and enrolled nurses. The completion of the Bachelor of Nursing degree is required to obtain a registered nurse qualification. An enrolled nurse may or may not receive credit for her or his qualification towards a Bachelor of Nursing degree. To become an enrolled nurse requires the completion of 12 months' hospital training or an 18-month TAFE diploma in Queensland.

In hospitals, registered nurses assess and record patients' symptoms and progress, conduct tests, administer medications, assist in rehabilitation, provide education and support for self-treatment, and instruct patients and their families in ways to improve or maintain their health. RNs often deal with mental, spiritual and emotional aspects of the patient as well.

Registered nurses work in a range of employment settings apart from hospitals. They may also work as part of a multidisciplinary health team in the community in child health centres, school health service, domiciliary nursing care, community health centres or public health education. Registered nurses employed in medical practice work alongside general and specialist medical practitioners. In industrial settings they are directly involved in occupational health and safety. Registered nurses may also be employed in the defence services or in overseas service with organisations such as World Health, the Save the Children Fund, Australian Volunteers Abroad and medical missions.

The most significant change in nursing education in the past ten years in Australia has been university education as opposed to hospital-based training, and the encouragement of postgraduate qualifications. Education programs are designed to meet the regulations of the Nurses Board within each State.

Dietitians

Dietitians study and apply knowledge about food and its effect on the body (ADA 1991). They do this in a variety of settings, such as hospitals, clinics, nursing homes, universities and schools. Some dietitians are administrators who hire and supervise food service workers, enforce sanitary and safety codes, and prepare budgets and reports. Other dietitians work directly with patients in assessing nutritional needs, implementing and evaluating dietary plans, and instructing patients and their families on ways to adhere to diets after discharge from the hospital. Some dietitians work for social service agencies in the community, where they counsel people on nutritional practices to help maintain health and speed recovery when they are ill.

Becoming a dietitian requires a bachelor's or master's degree specialising in nutrition sciences. To practise as a dietitian, graduates must be registered with the Dietitians Registration Board of Australia. Professional recognition in the form of membership of the Dietitians Association of Australia is desirable.

Physiotherapists

Many patients need help in restoring functional movement to parts of their body and in relieving pain. If they have suffered a disabling injury or disease, treatment may be needed to prevent or limit permanent disability. Physiotherapists plan and apply treatment for these goals in rehabilitation (APTA 1995).

To plan the treatment, physiotherapists begin by reviewing the patient's records and performing tests or measurements of muscle strength, motor coordination, endurance and range of motion of the injured body part. Treatment is designed to increase the strength and function of the injured part and aid in the patient's adaptation to having reduced physical abilities, which may be quite drastic. People who have suffered severe strokes are sometimes left partially paralysed, for instance. The most universal technique used in physiotherapy involves exercise, generally requiring little effort initially and becoming more and more challenging. Another technique involves electrical stimulation to move paralysed muscles or reduce pain.

Physiotherapists also give instructions on carrying out everyday tasks, such as tying shoelaces or cooking meals. If the patient needs to use adaptive devices, such as crutches or a prosthesis (replacement limb), the therapist provides training.

All physiotherapists must have a degree from an approved training program recognised by the Australian Physiotherapy Association. Practising physiotherapists must be registered with their State Board.

Occupational therapists

Occupational therapists help physically, mentally and emotionally disabled individuals gain skills needed for daily activities in a work setting, at school, in the community and at home (AOTA 1994). Their patients are often people who had these skills at one time, but lost them because of a spinal cord injury or a disease, such as muscular dystrophy. These professionals usually specialise in working with a particular age group, such as the elderly, and a type of disability — physical, for example. Based on the patient's age and the type and degree of disability, a program of educational, vocational and recreational activities is designed and implemented. The program for a child, for instance, might involve academic tasks and crafts; for an adult, it might involve typing, driving a vehicle, or using hand and power tools.

Occupational therapists in Australia must have a degree from an approved training program for registration with the Occupational Therapists Registration Board within each State. Most occupational therapists are members of the Australian Association of Occupational Therapists.

Social workers

The field of *social work* is broad. Probably most social workers are employed in mental health programs, but many others work in hospitals, nursing homes, rehabilitation centres, and public health programs (Boyce & Graff 1983; Watts, Elliott & Mayadas 1995). When working with people who are physically ill or disabled, social workers help patients and their families make psychological and social adjustments to the illness and obtain needed community services, including income maintenance. Thus, social workers may arrange for needed nursing care at home after a patient leaves the hospital or refer a patient for vocational counselling and occupational therapy if the illness or disability requires a career change. These professionals are usually called medical social workers.

Training requires a bachelor's degree in social work accredited by the Australian Association of Social Workers. Undergraduate training usually involves gaining an understanding of related social science fields such as social welfare, psychology and sociology.

Australia has been described as a multicultural nation. Immigrants carry with them health ideas and customs from their former countries. For example, many Chinese immigrants have entered their new country with the belief that illness results from an imbalance of two opposing forces, *yin* and *yang*, within the body (Campbell & Chang 1981). According to this view, too much yin causes colds and gastric disorders, for instance, and too much yang causes fever and dehydration. Practitioners of traditional Chinese medicine treat illnesses by prescribing special herbs and foods or by using *acupuncture*, in which fine needles are inserted under the skin at special locations of the body. These methods are intended to correct the balance of yin and yang. Immigrants and others with these beliefs who are sick will often use these methods instead of or as a supplement to treatment by a doctor. They may pressure their children and grandchildren to do this, too. As an example, a pregnant Chinese woman who was a registered nurse 'routinely followed her obstetrician's orders, but at the same time, under pressure from her mother and mother-in-law, ate special herbs and foods to insure birth of a healthy baby' (Campbell & Chang 1981, p. 164).

Religion is an aspect of culture. Many religions include beliefs that relate to health and illness. For instance, Jehovah's Witnesses reject the use of blood and blood products in medical treatment (Sacks & Koppes 1986). Christian Scientists reject the use of medicine totally, believing that illnesses are cured only by mental processes in the sick person. As a result, the sick person needs prayer and counsel as treatment to help these processes along (Henderson & Primeaux 1981). These beliefs are controversial and have led to legal conflicts between members of these religions and health authorities, particularly when parents reject medical treatments for life-threatening illnesses in their children. In such cases, the doctor and hospital can move quickly to seek an immediate judicial decision (Sacks & Koppes 1986).

Some religions include specific beliefs that promote healthy lifestyles. Seventh-Day Adventists, for example, believe that the body is the 'temple of the Holy Spirit'. They cite this belief as the reason people should take care of their bodies. Adventists abstain from using tobacco, alcohol and non-medically prescribed drugs. In addition, they promote in fellow members a concern for exercise and eating a healthy diet (Henderson & Primeaux 1981). Although it is clear that cultural factors play a role in health, our knowledge about this role is meagre and needs to be expanded through more research.

Research methods

Contemporary mass media constantly bombard us with scientific findings. Diets high in fibre and low in saturated fats are good for your health. Smoking is not. Dozens of toxic, or poisonous, chemicals appear to cause cancer. How do scientists discover these relationships? What methods do they use?

Scientists do research. Often their research is planned and conducted to test a **theory** — a *tentative explanation* of why and under what circumstances certain phenomena occur. For example, a leading theory of the cause of heart disease is that excess *cholesterol*, a fatty substance in the blood, is deposited on artery walls. Because this substance, like other saturated fats, is not water soluble, it builds up on the walls over time. This build-up hardens and narrows the diameter of the artery, thereby reducing the flow of blood and nutrients and causing tissue damage to the heart or arteries. Cholesterol comes from two sources. Most cholesterol in the blood is manufactured by the body; the rest of it comes from the foods we eat — especially red meats, egg yolks, butter and most cheeses.

The cholesterol theory is one of several useful theories of heart disease. By useful we don't necessarily mean that it is correct. We mean that it:

1. is clearly stated
2. brings together or organises known facts
3. relates information that previously seemed unrelated
4. enables us to make predictions, such as what would happen if cholesterol levels were reduced.

Useful theories play an extremely important role in all sciences. Because of the predictions they provide, they guide research programs by suggesting a sort of road map of relationships to study.

As you think about the causes of heart disease, you will realise that both the illness and the theoretical cause — in this case, high levels of cholesterol — can change or vary from one time to another and from one individual to another. That is, the condition of the heart and arteries and the amount of cholesterol in the blood are not constant. Because these things *vary*, they are called *variables*. We will define **variable** as any measurable characteristic of people, objects or events that may change. The variables studied in research are of two types: an *independent variable* is studied for its potential or expected influence, as in the case of cholesterol levels; a *dependent variable* is assessed because its value, such as the condition of the heart, is expected to 'depend' on the independent variable.

Researchers who study heart disease use a variety of *experimental* and *non-experimental* methods to examine variables such as the ones we have discussed.

Experiments

An **experiment** is a controlled study in which researchers manipulate an independent variable to study its effect on a dependent variable. In a well-designed experiment — often called a *trial* in health research — all other variables are controlled or held constant. The term *manipulate* means that the researchers produce or introduce the levels of the independent variable they are studying.

The experimental method: a hypothetical example

To illustrate the experimental method, let's see how researchers might test the cholesterol theory of heart disease. One prediction, or *hypothesis*, from the theory is that the incidence of heart disease should decrease if the levels of cholesterol in people's blood were reduced. We could test this hypothesis by lowering some people's cholesterol levels and seeing if these people develop fewer heart attacks over a suitable period of time than they otherwise would. How can we lower their cholesterol levels? There are two ways to manipulate this independent variable, both of which would require including medical professionals in the research team. One way is to alter the subjects' diets, and the other is to have them take an anti-cholesterol drug regularly. We will use the drug approach for our example.

The first thing we need to do is to select a sample of subjects — preferably middle-aged people, because they have a relatively high risk of having a heart attack in the near future. Then we assign them *randomly* to the conditions, or groups in the experiment. One way to assign them randomly is to put their names on cards in a bowl, mix up the cards, and draw the cards out one at a time. The first name drawn would be assigned to one group, the second name to another group, and so on. By doing this, we distribute other characteristics, such as their personality traits and genetic factors, fairly equally across the groups. As a result, these characteristics will have about the same impact on the dependent variable (heart attacks) for each of the groups.

To test the hypothesis, we will need two groups of subjects. One group receives the experimental treatment, the anti-cholesterol pills, and is called the *experimental group*. The other group does not receive the treatment, and is called the *control group*. By administering the drug to one group and lowering the cholesterol level of that group but not the other, we are manipulating the independent variable. We then observe over time the incidence of heart attacks. If the experimental group has fewer heart attacks than the control group, the hypothesis is supported.

You may be wondering, 'Isn't it possible that a decrease in heart attacks for the experimental group could result *not* from the drug per se, but simply from taking *any* substance a medical person prescribes?' Sometimes people's beliefs or expectations can affect their health (Critelli & Neumann 1984; Sobel 1990). To control for this possibility, we would have a third group of subjects. This group would receive an inert, or inactive, substance — called a **placebo** — in the form of pills that look like medicine. Once again, subjects would be randomly assigned to the anti-cholesterol drug group, the placebo group or the control group to eliminate the potential influence of other variables on our dependent variable. The placebo group would be given the same instructions as the experimental group, and both would have equal expectations about the effectiveness of the pills. Any influence the placebo has on the dependent variable is called a *placebo effect*.

One other control procedure is needed. Just as the subjects should not know which pills contain the active drug, neither should the person who distributes the pills. Why? This person could inadvertently bias the outcome of the experiment, such as by giving instructions offhandedly to the placebo group and emphatically and precisely to the experimental group. Being unaware of which group is getting the experimental treatment is called being *blind* as to the treatment. Since both the subjects and the person who distributes the pills are unaware, the method we are using is called the **double-blind** procedure.

Now that we have included these control procedures, let's look at the outcome of our hypothetical experiment. As figure 1.6 shows, the experimental subjects had far fewer heart attacks than the subjects in the other groups. Thus we can conclude that lowering cholesterol levels in the blood causes a decrease in heart disease, as the theory predicts. Notice also in the graph that the subjects in the placebo group had somewhat fewer heart attacks than the control subjects. This suggests a placebo effect, with expectancy having some effect on heart disease, but not nearly as much as the active ingredient in the anti-cholesterol drug.

You may have noticed that our conclusion used the word *causes*: lowering cholesterol 'causes' a decrease in heart disease. To make a *cause–effect* conclusion, we must be able to see that three criteria have been met: the levels of the independent and dependent variables corresponded or varied together, the cause preceded the effect, and all other plausible causes have been ruled out. Well-designed experiments meet these requirements because the researchers manipulate the independent variable while controlling variables that are not being studied. Other research approaches do not use experimental methods and do not provide the ability to determine what causes what.

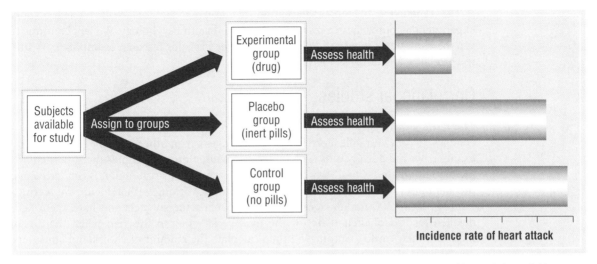

Figure 1.6 The left-hand portion of this diagram shows how the study would be carried out. Subjects are assigned to groups and, after a suitable period of time, the researcher checks whether they have had heart attacks. The right-hand portion illustrates how the results might appear on a graph: subjects who received the anti-cholesterol drug had far fewer heart attacks than subjects in the placebo group, who had somewhat fewer attacks than those in the control group.

Comparing experimental and non-experimental methods

Research always involves the study of variables, but in *non-experimental methods*, the researchers *do not manipulate an independent variable*. In addition, there is frequently less opportunity for precise measurement and for control of variables not being studied. As a result, although non-experimental methods may be used to point out relationships between variables, they do *not* provide direct and unambiguous tests of cause–effect relationships.

Non-experimental methods are nevertheless very valuable and have important advantages. Sometimes it is simply not feasible to assign subjects randomly and manipulate the variable of interest. We cannot manipulate the past lifestyles of people, for instance; the past has already happened. Neither can we have individuals in one group of a study do harmful things they would ordinarily not do simply to test an important theory. For instance, it would be unethical to assign people of a sample, some of whom are not cigarette smokers, to a group in which all subjects must smoke for the next five years. Even if it were ethical, non-smokers might refuse to do it. What if we didn't randomly assign the subjects to groups? If we do not randomly assign subjects, the groups are not likely to be equal at the start of the study with respect to characteristics, such as genetics or past lifestyle, that could affect the outcome of the research. In situations like this in which ethical considerations prevent the use of human subjects, animals are sometimes used.

In many cases, the aim of a research project requires only that an association between variables be demonstrated. We may want to know, for instance, which individuals are at greatest risk for a disease so that we may help them avert it. Studies to determine risk factors are examples. This kind of research has revealed that people who are among the most likely to develop heart disease are male and/or over 50 years old (Susser, Hopper & Richman 1983). Researchers cannot and need not manipulate people's gender or age to arrive at this relationship, and a non-experimental method is, in fact, the most appropriate technique.

The remainder of our examination of research methods will focus on non-experimental approaches in research relating to health psychology. We will continue to use the cholesterol theory of heart disease as the basis for research examples. Let's turn to correlational studies as the first of these methods.

Correlational studies

The term *correlation* refers to the *co* or joint relation that exists between variables — changes in one variable correspond to changes in another variable. Suppose, for example, we did a study of two variables: heart function and people's diets, particularly the amount of cholesterol they consume. A measure of heart function is *cardiac output*, the amount of blood the heart pumps per minute. Working with a doctor, we recruit a sample of, say, 200 middle-aged adults. We contact the subjects and have them keep detailed records of their diets for the two weeks prior to the visit when the doctor measures their cardiac output. We then calculate the amount of cholesterol consumed on the basis of their records.

Once we know the cardiac output and cholesterol intake of each of the subjects, we can assess the degree to which these variables are related. This is expressed statistically as a **correlation coefficient**, which can range from +1.00 through 0.00 to −1.00. The sign (+ or −) of the coefficient indicates the *direction* of the relationship. A plus sign means that the association is 'positive': high scores on one variable — say, cardiac output — tend to be associated with high scores on another variable, such as blood pressure. Conversely, a minus sign means that the association is 'negative': *high* scores on one variable tend to be associated with *low* scores on another variable. For example, high cardiac output is correlated with low concentrations of cells in the blood, because cells thicken the blood (Rhoades & Pflanzer 1996). Thus, there is a negative correlation between cardiac output and concentration of blood cells.

Disregarding the sign of the correlation coefficient, the absolute value of the coefficient indicates the *strength* of association between variables. The higher the absolute value (that is, the closer to either +1.0 or −1.0), the stronger the correlation. As the absolute value decreases, the strength of the relationship declines. A coefficient approximating 0.00 means that the variables are not related. From the information we have just covered, we can now state a definition: **correlational studies** are non-experimental investigations of the degree and direction of statistical association between two variables.

Let's suppose that our study revealed a strong negative correlation — a coefficient of −0.72 — between cardiac output and cholesterol intake. This finding would support the cholesterol theory, because low cholesterol intake should produce less fatty build-up to clog the arteries, thereby allowing the heart to pump more blood per minute. But we cannot say on the basis of our study that these events occurred, and we cannot conclude that low cholesterol intake *causes* high cardiac output. Why? Because we did not manipulate any variable — we simply measured what was there. It may be that some variable we were not studying was responsible for the correlation. For example, the people with low cholesterol intake may also have had low concentrations of blood cells, and it may have been this latter factor that was responsible for their high cardiac output. We don't know. We would know for sure only that the two variables have a strong negative relationship.

Correlational studies, despite their inability to determine cause–effect relations, are useful for examining existing relationships and variables that cannot be manipulated, developing hypotheses that may be tested experimentally and generating predictive information, such as risk factors for health problems.

Quasi-experimental studies

Sometimes researchers conduct non-experimental studies by selecting for or assessing an existing variable and then using it to categorise subjects into one of two or more groups, such as male or female, for example, or high, moderate or low blood cholesterol levels. Investigations of this type are called **quasi-experimental studies** — they *look* like experiments because they have separate groups of subjects, but they are not: the variable — gender or cholesterol level — that defines the groups was *not manipulated*, and the subjects *cannot be randomly assigned* to the groups.

We could do a quasi-experimental study relating to the cholesterol theory of heart disease in the following way. Suppose we wanted to see if people's cholesterol level at the time of a heart attack is associated with the severity of the attack. For this study, we could just consult the medical records of heart disease patients, since it is standard practice to assess both variables. We could categorise the patients as having a high or low cholesterol level at the time they were admitted to the hospital. Then we would determine whether the attacks of one group were more severe than those of the other group.

If we found that the high-cholesterol patients had the more severe heart attacks, could we conclude that higher levels of cholesterol in the blood cause more severe attacks? No — for the same reasons we've discussed before. We cannot tell what caused what. In fact, this particular study could have been turned around. We could have categorised the patients on the basis of the severity of their attacks and then compared these groups for cholesterol levels. We would have found the same relationship: severe heart attacks are associated with a high level of cholesterol in the blood.

In general, the conclusions from quasi-experimental studies are basically correlational. The relationships they reveal do not become causal simply because we categorise subjects. There are many variations to the quasi-experimental method. We will look at a few of the more important ones, beginning with retrospective and prospective approaches.

Retrospective and prospective approaches

The prefix *retro* means 'back' or 'backward', and *spective* comes from the Latin word meaning 'to look'. Thus, the **retrospective approach** uses procedures that look back at the histories of subjects, such as individuals who do or do not have a particular disease. The purpose of this approach is to find commonalities in the people's histories that may suggest why they developed the disease.

How is the retrospective approach used in a quasi-experimental study? We might identify two groups of individuals. One group would consist of people who have already developed a particular illness, such as heart disease. They would be compared against a control group, consisting of similar people without the disease. We would then examine the two groups for characteristics of their histories that are common to one group, but not the other. We might find, for example, that the heart disease victims tended to eat higher-cholesterol diets during the preceding 10 years than the control subjects did. Although the retrospective approach is relatively easy to implement, it has a potential shortcoming: when the procedures rely on people's memories, especially of long-past events, the likelihood of inaccurate reports increases.

The **prospective approach** uses procedures that look *forward* in the lives of people, by studying whether differences in a variable at one point in time are related to differences in another variable at a later time. We could do this to see whether certain characteristics or events in people's lives are associated with their eventual development of one or more diseases. In using the prospective approach, we would start by recruiting a large group of people — say, 2000 — who did not yet have the illness in question, heart disease. Periodically over several years we would interview them, have a doctor examine them, and check their medical records. The interviews would inquire about various events and characteristics, such as cholesterol intake. Then we would categorise the subjects — for instance as having or not having had a heart attack — and determine whether these groups differed in some earlier aspects of their lives.

What might our study show? We might find that, compared with people who did not have heart attacks, those who *did* had eaten diets that were much higher in cholesterol. We might also find that changes in people's diets, becoming higher or lower in cholesterol content over the years, corresponded with their suffering an attack. That is, those who consumed increasing amounts of cholesterol had more heart attacks than those whose cholesterol intake decreased. Because this is a quasi-experimental study, we cannot be certain that high-cholesterol diets caused the heart disease. But the prospective approach gives greater plausibility to a causal link than the retrospective approach would. This is because the diets, and changes in them, clearly preceded the heart attacks.

Retrospective and prospective approaches to studying health were developed by epidemiologists. These approaches have been useful in identifying risk factors for specific illnesses.

Developmental approaches

We saw earlier that the life-span perspective adds an important dimension to the study of health and illness. An essential research approach in studying life-span development is to examine and compare people at different ages. Of course, the age of the subjects cannot be manipulated; we can assign individuals to groups based on their age, but this assignment is not random. This approach is quasi-experimental, and therefore *age* itself cannot be viewed as a cause of health or behaviour.

Two basic approaches are used for studying the age variable. In the **cross-sectional approach**, different individuals of different ages are observed at about the same time. The **longitudinal approach** involves the repeated observation of the *same* individuals over a long period of time. The longitudinal approach is like the prospective method, but it focuses specifically on age as a variable. Let's see how the cross-sectional and longitudinal approaches are used.

Suppose we were interested in examining age-related changes in dietary intake of cholesterol among middle-aged adults. If we use a *cross-sectional* approach, we might evaluate the diets of, say, 50 adults at each of three approximate ages — for example 35, 45 and 55 years — during the current month. On the other hand, if we use a *longitudinal* approach to examine the same age range, we would evaluate the diets of 50 35-year-olds during the current month, and again when they are 45 and 55 years of age. This longitudinal study would take 20 years to complete.

Not all longitudinal studies take so long to do. Often a shorter span of ages — sometimes only a few months — is appropriate, depending on the question or issue the researcher wants to resolve. But the longitudinal approach, and the prospective approach in general, is typically more costly in time and money than the cross-sectional approach. Also the longer a study lasts, the greater the likelihood that subjects in the sample will be lost. Some will move away, others will lose interest in participating, and still others may die. Despite these difficulties, it is a valuable research approach that is unique in its ability to examine *change and stability in the lives of individuals* across time. For example, our longitudinal study could tell us whether individuals who eat a high-cholesterol diet at age 35 will generally continue to do so many years later. In contrast, a cross-sectional approach loses sight of stability and individual changes.

Now, let's suppose we did our cross-sectional study and found that the cholesterol content of adults' diets decreased with age. We would then like to know why this is so. One possible answer is that people change their diets as they get older because they feel more vulnerable to heart disease. So we asked the oldest group, using the retrospective approach, if they feel more vulnerable and eat less high-cholesterol food today than they used to. Sure enough, they said yes. But another reason for the current age differences in diet could be that the older adults never ate diets as high in cholesterol as those of the younger adults. So we asked the oldest group to describe the diets they ate 10 or 20 years ago. The diets they described contained less cholesterol than their current diets (which we already knew) *and* the current diets of the 35- and 45-year-olds in our study! This finding reflects the fact that the older subjects grew up at a different time, when food preferences or availability may have been different.

The influence of having been born and raised at a different time is called a **cohort effect**. The term *cohort* refers to a group of individuals who have a demographic factor, such as age or social class, in common. As a result, they share a set of experiences that are distinct from those of adjacent cohorts. In developmental approaches, the meaning of 'cohort' is similar to 'generation', but the amount of time separating adjacent cohorts can be much shorter than the time separating a generation. For example, suppose researchers at a high school planned to present a drug prevention program to all tenth-graders in a particular year. They might compare attitudes about drug use among the tenth-graders at the end of that year with those of two cohorts: tenth-graders two years before and two years after the program.

How can research methods take cohort effects into account? One way would be to combine the two developmental approaches to produce a *cross-sectional/longitudinal design* (Buss 1973; Schaie 1965). Looking back at our study with middle-aged adults, the combined approach could be carried out by selecting and testing 35-, 45- and 55-year-olds initially. So far the study is cross-sectional, but we would follow most of these same adults longitudinally and add younger subjects along the way. By doing this in a planned and systematic way, we will have information about cross-sectional differences, changes within each cohort and differences between cohorts.

Single-subject approaches

Sometimes studies are done with just one subject. One type of research that uses this approach is the **case study**, in which a trained researcher constructs a systematic biography from records of the person's history, interviews and current observation. This kind of research is useful in describing in depth the development and treatment of an unusual medical or psychological problem. Earlier in this chapter we saw an excerpt from a case study of a university student who had developed an ulcer. Other types of research that use one subject are called **single-subject designs**. This approach is often used for demonstrating the usefulness of a new treatment method for a specific medical or psychological problem. In the simplest of these designs, the statuses of the patient's condition at the beginning and end of therapy are compared. Often, follow-up assessments are made weeks or months later to see if the patient's condition has regressed. Some single-subject designs have additional phases or features that enable them to provide strong evidence for cause–effect relationships.

The principal disadvantage of single-subject approaches is that information gained from only one subject, no matter how detailed it is, may not describe what would be found with other individuals. A major purpose of psychological research is to collect information that can be applied or generalised to other people. Nevertheless, studies using one subject stimulate the development of new treatment procedures and suggest topics for further research.

Genetics research

How do psychologists and other scientists determine whether hereditary factors influence people's health and illness? The methods are based on a distinction between two types of twins. *Monozygotic*, or identical, twins have exactly the same genetic inheritance because they result from the splitting of a single fertilised egg, called a zygote. *Dizygotic*, or fraternal, twins develop from two separate zygotes, each of which was fertilised by a separate sperm. As a result, they are no more genetically similar than any singly born siblings and may, of course, be of different sex.

Most of the research on hereditary factors has focused on the differences in characteristics shown in monozygotic (MZ) twins as compared with dizygotic (DZ) twins. Investigations using this approach are called **twin studies**. The rationale for making these comparisons, although statistically complex, is logically simple. Because the two individuals in an MZ pair are genetically identical, we can assume that differences between them are environmentally determined. Conversely, the greater the similarity between MZ twins, the more likely it is that the characteristic is genetically influenced. Differences between DZ twins, on the other hand, are due to both genetic and environmental factors, even when they are the same sex. If we could assume that both members of each MZ and same-sex DZ pair that we study have had equal environmental experiences, then we could measure genetic influence simply by subtracting the differences for MZs from the differences for DZs.

The assumption that both members of each MZ and DZ pair have had equal environmental experiences presents a problem for researchers. As you might expect, environments are more likely to differ for fraternal pairs than for identical pairs. For instance, MZ children more often dress alike, play together and share the same friends than do same-sex fraternal twins (McClearn 1968). When this kind of problem exists — and it is hard to avoid totally — it makes the influence of heredity less clear. But some studies have been able to take environmental similarity into account, and when they do, important genetic forces are still found (Scarr & Kidd 1983).

Another way to examine hereditary influences is to study children adopted at very early ages. **Adoption studies** compare traits of adopted children with those of their natural parents and their adoptive parents. Why? Adoptive parents contribute greatly to the rearing environment, but are genetically unrelated to the children; the natural parents are genetically related to the children, but play little or no role in rearing them. So, if adopted children are more similar to their natural parents than to their adoptive parents, we then have evidence for heredity's influence.

What conclusions relevant to health psychology have come from twin and adoption studies? For one thing, MZs are not only more similar than DZs for physical characteristics, such as height and weight, but also for physiological functions, including heart rate and blood pressure (Ditto 1993). Also, genetic disorders are known to produce very high levels of cholesterol in the blood, making their victims susceptible to heart disease at very early ages (AMA 1989). Moreover, some evidence indicates that heredity has its greatest impact on people's health early in life, and by old age the role of habits and lifestyle become increasingly important (Harris et al. 1992).

In this chapter we have discussed a variety of research methods that are useful in health psychology. Which one is best? Some scientists might say that the experiment is best because it can uncover cause–effect relationships. But precise control and manipulation do not always yield results that help us understand real-life behaviour. For example, studying behaviour in experimental settings sometimes involves artificial conditions, such as precisely occurring events and special equipment. To the extent that these conditions are unlike the real world, the subjects' behaviour may be influenced. As a result, when reading about an experiment, it is useful to keep two questions in mind: Does the experimental situation approximate anything the subjects might experience in real life? If the experimental situation is highly artificial, what specific effect might this have on the outcome of the experiment?

In a sense, all the research methods we discussed are 'best', since the investigator must select the most suitable method(s) to answer the specific question(s) under study. This leads us to a final point: it is possible and desirable to use experimental and non-experimental methods *simultaneously* in one study. Suppose, for instance, we wanted to find out whether reading information about the health effects of excessive cholesterol would induce people to modify their diets. Using experimental methods, we would manipulate the independent variable in the following way: the experimental group would read the cholesterol information and a control group might read some unrelated material. But isn't it possible that the success of this experiment might depend on a variable that cannot be manipulated, such as the subjects' age or gender? People who are 50 years of age might be more inclined to follow recommendations to lower their cholesterol levels than people who are 20, for example. We could examine both variables by testing experimental and control groups for each of the two ages. Note, however, that the kinds of conclusions yielded by each variable will differ; only the manipulated variable can yield unambiguous causal statements.

Summary

Health and illness are overlapping concepts that exist along a continuum. One end of the continuum is dominated by health — a holistic state of physical, mental and social wellbeing that varies over time. The other end of the continuum is dominated by illness, which produces signs, symptoms and disabilities. The patterns of illness affecting people have changed across history, especially in the twentieth century. Compared with earlier times, today people die at later ages and from different causes. Infectious diseases are no longer the principal cause of death in technological societies around the world. Chronic illnesses constitute the main health problem in Australia now. The health of indigenous people continues to be of concern, although the health of ethnic minorities is better than of mainstream Australians.

Ideas about physiology, disease processes, and the mind have changed since the early cultures thousands of years ago, when people apparently believed that illness was caused by evil spirits and the like. Between the years 500 and 300 B.C., Greek philosophers produced the earliest written ideas about health and illness. They tried to explain how sickness happens and proposed that the mind and body are separate entities. During the Middle Ages the Church had an enormous influence on ideas about illness, and the belief in mystical causes of disease became strong again. Philosophers and scientists from the seventeenth to the twentieth centuries provided the foundation for the biomedical model as a way to conceptualise health and illness.

The biomedical model has been extremely useful, enabling researchers to make great advances in conquering many infectious diseases through the development of vaccines and treatments. Recent dissatisfaction with the biomedical model has centred on the rising cost of health care in Australia. Many researchers today have come to recognise that aspects of individual patients — their histories, social relationships, life-styles, personalities, mental processes and biological processes — must be included in a full conceptualisation of health and illness. As a result, the biopsychosocial model has emerged as the leading theoretical alternative to the biomedical approach as the fields of psychosomatic medicine, behavioural medicine and health psychology have developed. This new model proposes a constant interplay of biological, psychological and social systems — each interrelated with and producing changes in the others. The life-span perspective adds an important dimension to this model by considering the role of the person's development in health and illness.

Health psychology draws on knowledge from a variety of other subfields in psychology and several non-psychology fields, such as medicine, biology, social work, epidemiology, public health, sociology and anthropology. The last four of these fields are especially important in describing the social systems in which health, illness and the person exist and develop. Health psychologists are well positioned to make improvements to the health care system in Australia through their efforts in health promotion and in offering psychological services to surgical patients and those in rehabilitation.

The study of important variables in health psychology involves the use of experimental and non-experimental research methods. Experimental methods usually involve rigorous control and manipulation of variables and lead to cause–effect conclusions. Non-experimental methods focus on the study of relationships between variables. A correlation describes an association between variables but does not indicate whether it is a causal relation. Quasi-experimental approaches are useful in studying variables that cannot be manipulated, such as the subjects' history, age and gender. To study people at different ages, researchers use cross-sectional and longitudinal approaches. The role of heredity in health and illness can be examined through twin and adoption studies.

Key terms

adoption studies	dietary diseases	infectious diseases	psychosomatic medicine
behavioural medicine	double-blind	life-span perspective	quasi-experimental studies
biomedical model	epidemic	longitudinal approach	retrospective approach
biopsychosocial model	experiment	mind/body problem	risk factors
case study	health	morbidity	single-subject designs
chronic diseases	health behaviour	mortality	sociocultural
cohort effect	health psychology	personality	system
correlation coefficient	healthy migrant effect	placebo	theory
correlational studies	illness/wellness continuum	prevalence	twin studies
cross-sectional approach	incidence	prospective approach	variable

2 The body's physical systems

Prologue

When Tom was born 20 years ago, his parents were thrilled. Here was their first child — a delightful baby with such promise for the future. He seemed to be healthy. His parents were pleased that he began to consume large amounts of milk, often without becoming satiated. They took this as a good sign. But, in this case, it wasn't.

As the weeks went by, Tom's parents noticed that he wasn't gaining as much weight as he should, especially since he was still consuming lots of milk. He started to cough and wheeze often and developed one respiratory infection after another. They became concerned, and so did his pediatrician. After a series of tests, the devastating diagnosis was clear: Tom had *cystic fibrosis*, a chronic, progressive and eventually fatal disease. Cystic fibrosis is an inherited disease of the respiratory system for which there is no cure and no effective treatment.

Tom has had a difficult life, and so has his family. The respiratory infections he had in infancy were just the beginning. His disease causes thick, sticky secretions that constantly block airways, trap air in the lungs, and help bacteria to thrive. Other body systems also become affected, causing additional problems, such as insufficient absorption of food and vitamins. As a result, he was sick often and remained short, underweight and weak compared with other children. His social relationships have always been limited and strained, and the burden of his illness has taken its toll on his parents.

When Tom was younger and people asked him, 'What do you want to be when you grow up?' he would answer, 'I'm going to be an angel when I grow up.' What other plans could he have had, realistically? At 20, he has reached the age by which half of the victims of cystic fibrosis die. Physical complications, such as heart damage, that generally afflict several body systems in the last stages of this disease have begun to appear.

We can see in Tom's story that biological factors, such as heredity, can affect health; illness can alter social relationships; and all interrelated physiological systems of the body can be affected. In this chapter we outline the major physical systems of the body. Our discussion focuses on the normal functions of these systems, but we consider some important problems, too. What determines the degree of paralysis a person suffers after injury to the spine? How does stress affect our body systems? What is a heart attack, and what causes it?

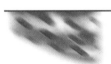

The nervous system

We all know that the nervous system, particularly the brain, in human beings and other animals controls the way we initiate behaviour and respond to events in our world. The nervous system receives information about changes in the environment from sensory organs, including the eyes, ears and nose, and it transmits directions that tell our muscles and other internal organs how to react. The brain also stores information — being a repository for our memory of past events — and provides our capability for thinking, reasoning and creating.

How the nervous system works

The nervous system is constantly integrating the actions of our internal organs — although we are not generally aware of it. Many of these organs, such as the heart and digestive tract, are made of muscle tissues that respond to commands. The nervous system provides these commands through an intricate network of billions of specialised nerve cells called **neurons**.

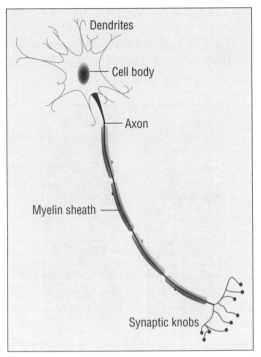

Dendrites

Cell body

Axon

Myelin sheath

Synaptic knobs

Although neurons in different parts of the nervous system have a variety of shapes and sizes, the diagram in figure 2.1 shows their general features. Projecting from the *cell body* are clusters of branches called *dendrites*. Generally, dendrites function as receivers for messages from adjacent neurons. These messages then travel through a long, slender projection called the *axon*, which splits into branches at the far end. The tips of these branches have small swellings called *synaptic knobs* that connect to the dendrites of other neurons, usually through a fluid-filled gap. This junction is called a *synapse*. Messages from the knobs cross the gap to adjacent neurons, and in this way eventually reach their destination.

Figure 2.1 An idealised diagram of a neuron and some of its major parts. Electrochemical messages received by the dendrites are transmitted to the synaptic knobs. The myelin sheath covers the axon of most neurons.

The messages neurons send consist of *electrochemical* activity. Within the neuron, the message begins with chemical changes that occur when a dendrite is stimulated. If these changes produce a sufficient concentration of electrically charged particles, called *ions*, an impulse of electrical potential is triggered. That impulse travels through the axon and stimulates the synaptic knobs to release a chemical called a **neurotransmitter**, which travels to the dendrites of an adjacent neuron. Dozens of different neurotransmitters have been identified. Some of them tend to *excite* the receiving neuron, increasing the likelihood that an electrical impulse will be generated. Others tend to *inhibit* the neuron, making an impulse less likely. Some neurotransmitters can have either effect, depending on certain characteristics of the receiving neuron.

What changes occur in the nervous system as a person develops? By the time the typical baby is born, a basic structure has been formed for almost all the neurons this person will have. But the nervous system is still quite immature — for instance, the brain weighs only about 25 per cent of the weight it will have when the child reaches adulthood (Sarafino & Armstrong 1986). Most of the growth in brain size after birth results from an increase in the number of *glial cells* and the presence of a white fatty substance called *myelin*. The glial cells are thought to service and maintain the neurons. A myelin sheath surrounds the axons of most, but not all, neurons. This sheath is responsible for increasing the speed of nerve impulses and preventing them from being interfered with by adjacent nerve impulses, much the way insulation is used on electrical wiring. The importance of myelin can be seen in the disease called *multiple sclerosis*, which results when the myelin sheath degenerates. People afflicted with this disease have weak muscles that lack coordination and move spastically (AMA 1989).

As the infant grows, the brain forms few, if any, new neurons. But the network of dendrites and synaptic knobs to carry messages to and from other neurons expands dramatically, as figure 2.2 shows. The myelin sheath covering the neurons is better developed initially in the upper regions of the body than in the lower regions. During the first years of life, the progress in myelin growth spreads down the body — from the head to shoulders, to the arms and hands, to the upper chest and abdomen, and then the legs and feet. This sequence is reflected in the individual's motor development: the upper parts of the body are brought under control at earlier ages than the lower parts. Studies with animals have found that chronic poor nutrition early in life impairs brain growth by retarding the development of myelin, glial cells and dendrites. Such impairment can produce long-lasting deficits in a child's motor and intellectual performance (Reinis & Goldman 1980).

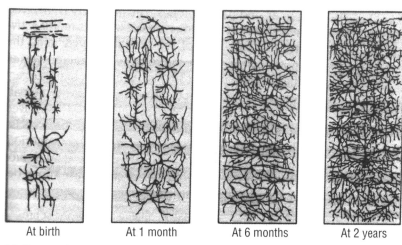

| At birth | At 1 month | At 6 months | At 2 years |

Figure 2.2 The neural structure of a section of the human cortex at four different ages. Notice that the number of cell bodies (dark spots) stays the same, while the network of dendrites expands with age.

Source: Lenneberg (1967, figure 4.6); based on photographs from Conel (1939–67).

Beginning in early adulthood, the brain tends to lose weight with age (Stevens-Long 1984). Decreases occur in the number of brain cells, their water and protein content, and the blood flow to them. At the same time, the chemical composition of the brain changes. For instance, calcium decreases while potassium and phosphorus increase. These alterations in the brain are associated with the declines people often notice in their mental and physical functions after they reach 50 or 60 years of age.

The nervous system is enormously complex and basically has two major divisions — the central nervous system and the peripheral nervous system — that connect to each other. The **central nervous system** consists of the brain and spinal cord. The *peripheral nervous system* is composed of the remaining network of neurons throughout the body. Each of these major divisions consists of interconnected lower-order divisions or structures. We will examine the nervous system, beginning at the top and working our way down.

The central nervous system

The brain and spinal cord race towards maturity early in life. For example, the brain weighs 75 per cent of its adult weight at about two years of age, 90 per cent at five years and 95 per cent at 10 years (Tanner 1970, 1978). The brain may be divided into three parts: the *forebrain*, the *cerebellum* and the *brainstem*. Each of these parts has special functions.

The forebrain

The forebrain is the uppermost part of the brain. As figure 2.3 shows, the forebrain consists of two main subdivisions: the *telencephalon*, which consists of the cerebrum and the limbic system, and the *diencephalon*, which includes the thalamus and hypothalamus. As a general rule, areas towards the top and outer regions of the brain are involved in our perceptual, motor, learning and conceptual activities. Regions towards the centre and bottom of the brain are involved mainly in controlling internal and automatic body functions and in transmitting information to and from the telencephalon.

The **cerebrum** is the upper and largest portion of the human brain and includes the *cerebral cortex*, its outermost layer. The cerebrum controls complex motor and mental activity. It develops rapidly in the first few years of life, becoming larger, thicker and more convoluted. The cerebrum has two halves — the *left hemisphere* and the *right hemisphere* — each of which looks like the left hemispheres drawn in figure 2.4.

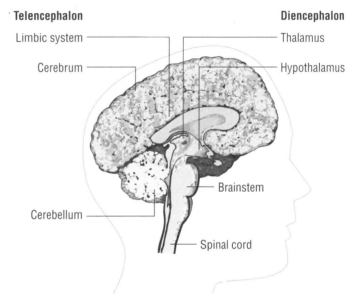

Figure 2.3 A side view of the human brain in cross-section, sliced through the middle from front to back. The forebrain consists of the telencephalon (cerebrum and limbic system) and the diencephalon (thalamus and hypothalamus). The remaining divisions of the central nervous system — the cerebellum, the brainstem and the spinal cord — are also labelled.

Although the left and right hemispheres are physically alike, they control different types of processes. For one thing, the motor cortex (see figure 2.4b) of each hemisphere controls motor movements on the opposite side of the body. This is why damage to the motor cortex on, say, the right side of the brain may leave part of the left side of the body paralysed. The two hemispheres also control different aspects of cognitive and language processes. In most people, the left hemisphere contains the areas that handle language processes, including speech and writing. The right hemisphere usually processes such things as visual imagery, emotions and the perception of patterns, such as melodies (Geschwind 1979).

You will probably notice in figure 2.4 that each hemisphere is divided into a front part, called the frontal lobe, and three back parts: the temporal, occipital and parietal lobes. The *frontal lobe* is involved in a variety of functions, one of which is motor activity. The back part of the frontal lobe contains the motor cortex, which controls the skeletal muscles of the body. If a patient who is undergoing brain surgery receives stimulation to the motor cortex, some part of the body will move. The frontal lobe is also involved in important mental activities, such as the association of ideas, planning, self-awareness and emotion. As a result, injury to areas of this lobe can produce personality and emotional reactions, like those described by the physician of Phineas P. Gage.

> He is fitful, irreverent, indulging in the grossest profanity (which was not previously his custom), manifesting but little deference to his fellows, impatient of restraint or advice when it conflicts with his desires, at times ... obstinate, capricious, and vacillating ... His mind was radically changed, so that his friends said he was no longer Gage. (Cited in McClintic 1985, p. 93.)

Phineas had survived a workplace accident in which a tamping iron was blown through the front of his head.

The *temporal lobe* is involved mainly in hearing, but also in vision and memory. Damage to this region can impair the person's comprehension of speech and ability to determine the direction from which a sound is coming. The *occipital lobe* contains the principal visual area of the brain. Damage to the occipital lobe can produce blindness or the inability to recognise an object by sight. The *parietal lobe* is involved mainly in body sensations, such as of pain, cold, heat, touch and body movement.

The second part of the telencephalon — called the **limbic system** — lies along the innermost edge of the cerebrum and adjacent to the diencephalon (refer back to figure 2.3). The limbic system is not well understood yet. It consists of several structures that seem to be important in the expression of emotions, such as fear, anger and excitement. To the extent that heredity affects a person's emotions, it may do so by determining the structure and function of the limbic system (McClintic 1985).

The diencephalon includes two structures — the thalamus and hypothalamus — that lie below and are partially encircled by the limbic system. The **thalamus** is a truly pivotal structure in the flow of information in the nervous system. It functions as the chief relay station for directing sensory messages, such as of pain or visual images, to appropriate points in the cerebrum, such as the occipital or parietal lobe. The thalamus also relays commands going out to the skeletal muscles from the motor cortex of the cerebrum.

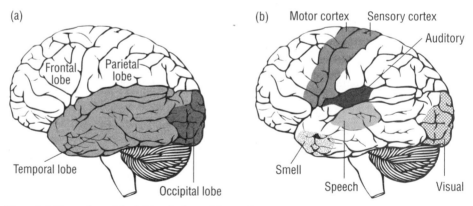

Figure 2.4 The surface of the left hemisphere of the cerebrum. (a) shows the four parts of the hemisphere; (b) points out the areas associated with specific functions. The right hemisphere has the same four parts and functional areas.

The **hypothalamus**, a small structure just below the thalamus, plays an important role in people's emotions and motivation. Its function affects eating, drinking and sexual activity, for instance. Research with animals has shown that if a certain part of the feeding centre is destroyed, the animal will eat incessantly; but if a different centre is destroyed, the animal refuses to eat. Both of these conditions cause the animal to die (Nelson 1989). Occasionally, people become overweight as a result of a disease that affects the feeding centre of this structure.

Another important function of the hypothalamus is to maintain *homeostasis* — a state of balance or normal function among our body systems. Our normal body temperature and heart rate, which are characteristic of healthy individuals, are examples of homeostasis. When our bodies are cold, for instance, we shiver, thus producing heat. When we are very warm, we perspire, thus cooling the body. These adjustments are under the control of the hypothalamus (McClintic 1985). We will see later that the hypothalamus also plays an important role in our reaction to stress.

The cerebellum

The **cerebellum** lies at the back of the brain, below the cerebrum. The main function of the cerebellum is in maintaining body balance and coordinating movement. This structure has nerve connections to the motor cortex and most of the sense organs of the body. Although specific movements may be initiated by areas of the cerebrum, the cerebellum makes our actions precise and well-coordinated.

How does the cerebellum do this? There are at least two ways. First, it continuously compares our intent with our performance, ensuring that a movement goes in the right direction, at the proper rate and with appropriate force. Second, it smooths our movements. Because of the forces involved in movement, there is an underlying tendency for our motions to go quickly back and forth, like a tremor. The cerebellum damps this tendency (McClintic 1985). When injury occurs to the cerebellum, the person's actions become jerky and uncoordinated — a condition called *ataxia*. Simple movements, such as walking or touching an object, become difficult and unsteady.

Figure 2.5 shows the location of the cerebellum relative to the brainstem, which is the next section of the brain we will discuss.

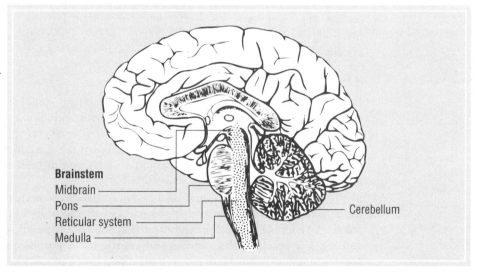

Figure 2.5 A side view of the human brain in cross-section, showing the cerebellum and the brainstem, which includes the midbrain, pons, reticular system and medulla

The brainstem

The lowest portion of the brain — called the **brainstem** — has the form of an oddly shaped knob at the top of the spinal cord. The brainstem consists of four parts: mid-brain, pons, reticular system and medulla.

The **midbrain** lies at the top of the brainstem. It connects directly to the thalamus above it, which relays messages to various parts of the forebrain. The midbrain receives information from the visual and auditory systems and is especially important in muscle movement. The disorder called *Parkinson's disease* results from degeneration of an area of the midbrain (Tortora & Grabowski 1993). People severely afflicted with this disease have noticeable motor tremors, and their neck and trunk postures become rigid, so that they walk in a crouch. Sometimes the tremors are so continuous and vigorous that the victim becomes crippled.

The **reticular system** is a network of neurons that extends from the bottom to the top of the brainstem and into the thalamus. The reticular system plays an important role in controlling our states of sleep, arousal and attention. When people suffer a coma, often it is this system that is injured or disordered (McClintic 1985). *Epilepsy*, a condition in which a victim may become unconscious and begin to convulse, seems to involve an abnormality in the reticular system (Scambler 1997). One type of epileptic seizure called *grand mal* may result from 'reverberating cycles' in the reticular system.

> That is, one portion of the system stimulates another portion, which stimulates a third portion, and this in turn restimulates the first portion, causing a cycle that continues for 2 to 3 minutes, until the neurons of the system fatigue so greatly that the reverberation ceases. (Guyton 1985, p. 356)

Following a grand mal seizure, the person often sleeps at least a few minutes and sometimes for hours.

The **pons** forms a large bulge at the front of the brainstem and is involved in eye movements, facial expressions and chewing. At the bottom of the brainstem is the **medulla**, which contains vital centres that control breathing, heartbeat rate, and the diameter of blood vessels (which affects blood pressure). Because of the many vital functions it controls, damage to the medulla can be life threatening. *Polio*, a crippling disease that was once epidemic, sometimes damaged the centre that controls breathing. Patients suffering such damage needed constant artificial respiration to breathe (McClintic 1985).

The spinal cord

Extending down the spine from the brainstem is the **spinal cord**, a major neural pathway that transmits messages between the brain and various parts of the body. It contains neurons that carry impulses away from (the *efferent* direction) and towards (*afferent*) the brain. Efferent commands travel down the cord on their way to produce muscle action; afferent impulses come to the spinal cord from sense organs in all parts of the body.

The organisation of the spinal cord parallels that of the body — that is, the higher the region of the cord, the higher the parts of the body to which it connects. As a result, the effect of disease or injury to the spinal cord depends on the location of the damage. For example, if an accident severs the lower portion of the cord, the lower regions of the body are paralysed — a condition called *paraplegia*. If the upper portion of the spinal cord is severed, paralysis is more extensive. Paralysis of the legs and arms is called *quadriplegia*.

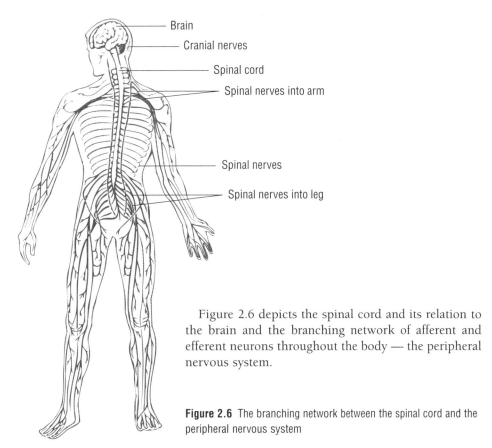

Brain
Cranial nerves
Spinal cord
Spinal nerves into arm
Spinal nerves
Spinal nerves into leg

Figure 2.6 depicts the spinal cord and its relation to the brain and the branching network of afferent and efferent neurons throughout the body — the peripheral nervous system.

Figure 2.6 The branching network between the spinal cord and the peripheral nervous system

The peripheral nervous system

The **peripheral nervous system** has two parts: the somatic nervous system and the autonomic nervous system. The **somatic nervous system** is involved in both sensory and motor functions, serving mainly the skin and skeletal muscles. The **autonomic nervous system** activates internal organs, such as the lungs and intestines, and reports to the brain the current state of activity of these organs.

In the somatic nervous system, afferent neurons carry messages from sense organs to the spinal cord, as figure 2.7 illustrates. Efferent neurons carry messages to, and activate, *striated* (grooved) skeletal muscles, such as those in the face, arms and legs, that we can move voluntarily. A disorder called *myasthenia gravis* can develop at the junction of these muscles and neurons, weakening muscle function of the head and neck. This produces characteristic symptoms — such as drooping eyelids, blurred vision, and difficulty swallowing and breathing — and can lead to paralysis and death. Although medical treatment is effective in restoring muscle function, some symptoms may recur when the person is under stress (AMA 1989).

Figure 2.7 also shows that in the autonomic nervous system, neurons carry messages between the spinal cord and the *smooth* muscles of the internal organs, such as the heart, stomach, lungs, blood vessels and glands. This system itself has two divisions, the sympathetic and parasympathetic, which often act in opposite ways, as figure 2.8 shows. The **sympathetic nervous system** helps us mobilise and expend energy in responding to emergencies, expressing strong emotions and performing strenuous activity. For instance, suppose you are crossing a street, notice a speeding car barrelling towards you and hear its brakes start to squeal. The sympathetic nervous system instantly moves into action, producing several simultaneous changes — for example, it speeds up the heart, dilates certain arteries to increase blood flow to the heart and skeletal muscles, constricts other arteries to decrease blood flow to the skin and digestive organs, decreases salivation and increases perspiration. These changes, in general, enable you to mobilise energy, and you leap to safety out of the car's path. This system is called 'sympathetic' because it acts in agreement with your current emotional state.

What does the parasympathetic division do? The prefix *para* means 'alongside of' — this division acts alongside of, and often in opposition to, the sympathetic division. The **parasympathetic nervous system** regulates 'quiet' or calming processes, helping our individual organ systems to conserve and store energy. One example of parasympathetic activity can be seen in the digestion of food. When you eat a meal, the parasympathetic nervous system carries messages to regulate each step in the digestive process, such as by increasing salivation and stomach contractions. Another example can be seen in the course of emotional or emergency reactions — when an emergency has passed, the parasympathetic division helps restore your normal body state.

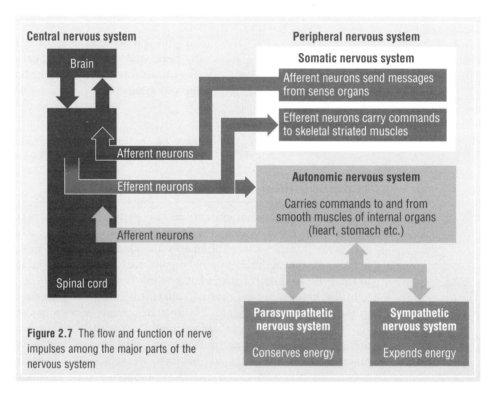

Figure 2.7 The flow and function of nerve impulses among the major parts of the nervous system

Communication within the peripheral nervous system is handled by 12 sets of *cranial nerves*, most of which originate in the brainstem. The *vagus nerve* extends from there to muscles of most major body organs, such as the airways, lungs, heart and intestines, and is directly involved in the regulation of sympathetic and parasympathetic activity (Porges 1992, 1995; Tortora & Grabowski 1993). Efferent messages from the brain can target specific organs to increase or decrease their function.

As you now realise, the nervous system is connected to and regulates all of our other body systems, and the brain is the control centre. The remainder of this chapter examines these other body systems, beginning with the endocrine system.

The endocrine system

The **endocrine system** consists of a set of glands that often work in close association with the autonomic nervous system. These systems share an important function: they communicate with various parts of the body. But they do this in somewhat different ways. Whereas the nervous system uses both electrical and chemical messages, the endocrine system communicates only with chemical substances, which are called **hormones**. Each endocrine gland secretes specific hormones directly into the bloodstream, which carries these chemicals to various parts of the body. Figure 2.9 shows where several of the more important endocrine glands are located. Certain chemicals are produced by both the endocrine and nervous systems and function as both hormones and neurotransmitters.

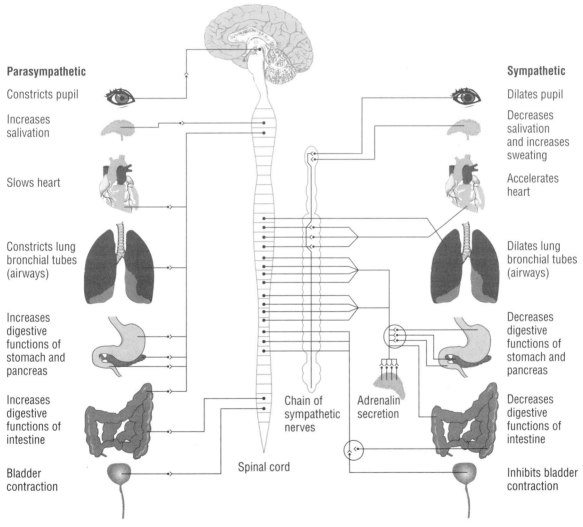

Parasympathetic

Constricts pupil

Increases salivation

Slows heart

Constricts lung bronchial tubes (airways)

Increases digestive functions of stomach and pancreas

Increases digestive functions of intestine

Bladder contraction

Sympathetic

Dilates pupil

Decreases salivation and increases sweating

Accelerates heart

Dilates lung bronchial tubes (airways)

Decreases digestive functions of stomach and pancreas

Decreases digestive functions of intestine

Inhibits bladder contraction

Chain of sympathetic nerves

Adrenalin secretion

Spinal cord

Figure 2.8 The autonomic nervous system and its interconnections between the spinal cord and various organs of the body. The function of the parasympathetic division in conserving energy is shown on the left side of the diagram. The function of the sympathetic division in expending energy is shown on the right side. Notice that each organ connects to both divisions.

The endocrine and nervous systems working together

How are the endocrine and nervous systems associated? The nervous system is linked to the endocrine system by connections between the hypothalamus (in the forebrain) and a gland that lies just below it — the **pituitary gland**. The hypothalamus sends chemical messages directly to the pituitary gland, causing it to release pituitary hormones into the blood. In turn, most of these hormones selectively stimulate the other endocrine glands to secrete. Because the pituitary gland controls the secretion of other endocrine glands, it is called the 'master gland'.

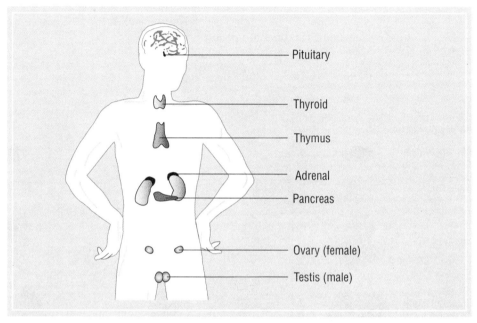

Figure 2.9 Some of the endocrine glands and their locations in the body

Researchers have identified dozens of different hormones that course through our veins and arteries. Each hormone has its own specific effects on cells and organs of the body, thereby directly or indirectly affecting psychological and physical functions. Some hormones, such as oestrogens and testosterone, are produced mainly in females' *ovaries* (where egg cells develop) and males' *testes* (where sperm develop). These hormones are especially important in the development and functioning of female and male reproductive systems. Other hormones affect blood pressure, general body growth, and the balance of various chemicals, such as calcium, in the body. Still other hormones help us react to specific situations we encounter in our lives.

We saw earlier that the autonomic nervous system plays an important role in our reaction to an emergency. So does the endocrine system. Let's see how by returning to the incident in which you leaped out of the path of a speeding car. At the same time that the sympathetic nervous system reacts to your emergency, the hypothalamus immediately sends a hormone called corticotropin-releasing factor to the pituitary gland. This causes the pituitary to release ACTH (adrenocorticotropic hormone) into the blood. The ACTH then travels throughout the body and stimulates the release of a variety of hormones — especially those of the adrenal glands — that affect your reaction to the emergency.

Adrenal glands

The **adrenal glands** are located on top of the kidneys, as figure 2.9 depicts. These glands release several important hormones in response to emergencies and stress (Tortora & Grabowski 1993). One of these hormones, *cortisol*, helps to control swelling when we are injured. If when you leaped to avoid being hit by the car you sprained your ankle, this hormone would help reduce swelling. But continued high levels of cortisol and similar hormones over a long time can be harmful to the body. They can lead to high blood pressure and the formation of ulcers, for example.

Two other important adrenal hormones are *epinephrine* and *norepinephrine* (also called adrenalin and noradrenalin). These hormones work in conjunction with the sympathetic nervous system to produce such bodily reactions as speeding up heart and respiration rates and increasing the liver's sugar output for quick energy. After the emergency has passed and sympathetic activity has subsided, some impact of the hormones may continue for a while because they are still in the bloodstream.

The impact of the nervous and endocrine systems' activities in emergency situations differs in the speed and persistence of their effect. The nervous system responds by sending messages that move instantly to specific locations; once they reach their destination, they become deactivated or dissipated. For example, the nervous system also produces and uses epinephrine and norepinephrine, but these chemicals function as neurotransmitters, relaying their commands from neuron to neuron and having a localised effect. The impact of the message stops quickly and persists only if additional messages are sent. Hormones from the endocrine system move more slowly and broadly through the bloodstream, and their effects can be delayed and long-lasting.

Other glands

Several other endocrine glands are also important. The *thyroid gland*, located in the neck, produces hormones, such as thyroxine, that regulate the body's general activity level and growth. Disorders in thyroid production are of two types: *hypothyroidism*, or insufficient secretion of thyroid hormones, and *hyperthyroidism*, or excessive thyroid secretion (AMA 1989; Butler 1997). Hypothyroidism leads to low activity levels and to weight gain. If the condition is congenital and untreated, dwarfism and mental retardation often result. The condition can be treated medically by having the person take hormone supplements orally. Hyperthyroidism leads to high activity levels, short attention spans, tremors, insomnia and weight loss. Untreated people with a common form of this condition, called *Graves' disease*, act in a highly restless, irritable and confused manner.

The *thymus gland*, which is located in the chest, is quite large in infancy and childhood but diminishes in size and efficiency after puberty (Tortora & Grabowski 1993). The thymus plays an important role early in life in the development of antibodies and immunities against diseases.

Another endocrine gland is the *pancreas*, which is located below the stomach. Its main function is to regulate the level of blood sugar, or glucose. The pancreas does this by producing two hormones, *glucagon* and *insulin*, that act in opposition. Glucagon raises the concentration of glucose in the blood, and insulin lowers it (Tortora & Grabowski 1993). The disorder called *diabetes mellitus* results when the pancreas does not produce sufficient insulin to balance the action of glucagon. This imbalance produces excess blood sugar levels — a condition called *hyperglycemia*. If this condition persists and is untreated, it may cause coma and death. Diabetes can be medically controlled, generally through diet and either medication or daily insulin injections (Kilo & Williamson 1987; Shillitoe 1995).

The digestive system

Whether we eat an apple, drink some milk or swallow a pill, our bodies respond in the same general way. The **digestive system** breaks down what we have ingested, converts much of it to chemicals the body can use, and excretes the rest. The chemicals the body uses are absorbed into the bloodstream, which transports them to all of our body cells. Chemical nutrients in the foods we eat provide energy to fuel our activity, body growth and repair.

Food's journey through digestive organs

Think of the digestive system as a long hose — nearly seven metres long — with stations along the way. The journey of food through this hose begins in the *mouth* and ends at the *rectum*. These digestive organs and the major organs in between are shown in figure 2.10.

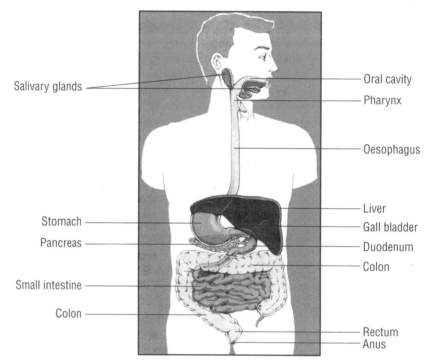

Figure 2.10 Major parts of the digestive system

Digesting food

How does this system break down food? One way is mechanical: for example, we grind food up when we chew it. Another way is chemical: by the action of **enzymes**, substances that act as catalysts in speeding up chemical reactions in cells. How do enzymes work? You can see the effect of an enzyme by doing the following experiment (Holum 1994). Place a bit of liver in some hydrogen peroxide and watch what happens: An enzyme in liver called *catalase* causes the peroxide to decompose, frothing as oxygen is given off as a gas. This is the same reaction you see when you use peroxide to disinfect a wound.

In most cases, the names for enzymes end in the letters -*ase*, and the remainder of each name reflects the substance on which it acts. The following list gives some examples.

• *Carbohydrase* acts on carbohydrates.
• *Lactase* acts on lactose (milk).
• *Phosphatase* acts on phosphate compounds.
• *Sucrase* acts on sucrose (sugar).

As food is broken down into smaller and smaller units in the digestive tract, water molecules become attached to these units (Rhoades & Pflanzer 1996).

When food is in the mouth, there is more digestive action going on than just chewing. Food is moistened with saliva, which contains an enzyme that starts the process of breaking down starches. The salivary glands release saliva in response to commands from the brainstem, which responds primarily to sensory information from tastebuds. Simply seeing, smelling or even thinking about food can produce neural impulses that cause the mouth to water (Rhoades & Pflanzer 1996).

Highlight on issues

issues

Our physiological individuality

Think about some differences between two people you know. Probably the first things that come to mind are their physical and behavioural characteristics. One person is tall and has blond hair, blue eyes and an outgoing personality; the other is short and has dark hair, dark eyes and is shy. But what about their internal physiological structure and functions?

We don't usually think about internal physiological differences between people. This is partly because the pictures of internal organs we see in books are always the same. As a result, we get the impression that if you've seen one heart or stomach, you've seen them all. This impression is wrong. Our individuality exists not only in our external features, but in our internal organs and body chemistry as well. The aorta is a major blood vessel that arches, or curves, over and attaches to the heart. Examples of some of its structural variations are given in figure 2.11 (page 58). The diagram on the left depicts the usual branching that forms at the arch of the aorta, and the other drawings show variations that occur, sometimes quite frequently. Major differences like these occur in virtually all organs (Skolnick 1986).

Our physiological individuality can have major implications for our health and behaviour. For example, people's reactions to medicines differ, sometimes quite substantially. Some people may require many times the normal dose of certain drugs before the desired effect occurs. The age and weight of the person contribute to this variability. Heavy people usually require larger doses of a drug than other people do. Infants and the elderly seem to be particularly sensitive to the effects of drugs, and overdoses are a danger for them (Bennett 1987; USDHHS 1981). Blood pressure medication in the elderly may overshoot and lower the pressure too far, for example.

There are gender differences in many organ systems, too. Males generally have larger hearts and lungs, and higher blood pressure, than females do. Our body systems also react to stress differently. We saw earlier that the adrenal glands respond to stress by secreting hormones — two of which are epinephrine and cortisol. When under stress, males secrete more of these hormones than females do (Collins & Frankenhaeuser 1978; Pollack & Steklis 1986).

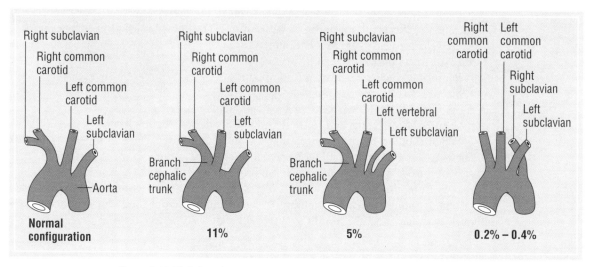

Figure 2.11 Variations in arterial branching of the aortic arch and the approximate percentages of their occurrence

Source: Grant (1972, plate 446.4).

The journey of food advances to the *oesophagus*, a tube that is normally flattened when food is not passing through it. The oesophagus pushes the food down to the stomach by wave-like muscle contractions called *peristalsis*. By the time food enters the oesophagus, the stomach has already begun digestive activities by releasing small amounts of gastric juice even before food reaches it. Tasting, smelling, seeing or thinking about food can initiate this process (Feldman & Richardson 1986). Once food reaches the stomach, this organ amasses large amounts of gastric juices, including *hydrochloric acid* and *pepsin*, an enzyme that breaks down proteins. (This enzyme name is one of the few that does not end in -*ase*.) The stomach also produces a sticky mucous substance to protect its lining from the highly acidic gastric juices. To prepare the food for the next stage in digestion, the muscular stomach walls produce a churning motion — which we are generally not aware of — that mixes the food particles with the gastric juices.

The mixing action in the stomach continues for three or four hours, producing a semiliquid mixture. Peristalsis in the stomach then moves this mixture on, a little at a time, to the beginning section of the small intestine called the *duodenum*. Several important digestive processes occur in the small intestine (Rhoades & Pflanzer 1996; Tortora & Grabowski 1993). First, the highly acidic food mixture becomes chemically alkaline as a result of substances added from the pancreas, the gall bladder and the wall of the small intestine. This is important because the linings of the small intestine and the remainder of the digestive tract are not protected from high acidity, as the stomach is.

Second, the process of breaking down food continues. Enzymes secreted by the pancreas into the duodenum further break down carbohydrates, proteins and fats. The role of the small intestine in the digestion of fats is especially important because fats are not broken down very much before entering the duodenum. The processing of fats in the small intestine is aided by a substance called *bile* that is produced in the liver and stored in the gall bladder. Bile separates fatty materials into tiny particles that enzymes from the pancreas can process efficiently.

The third process that occurs in the small intestine is *absorption*. Most of the ingested substances our bodies use are absorbed into the bloodstream through the lining of the small intestine. Alcohol is one of the few substances that is normally absorbed by the stomach lining, but eating fatty foods before drinking delays absorption of alcohol until it reaches the small intestine (Nelson 1989). By the time food is ready to be absorbed through the intestine wall, the digestive process has broken down nutrients into molecules — carbohydrates are broken down into simple sugars, fats into *glycerol* and *fatty acids*, and proteins into *amino acids*.

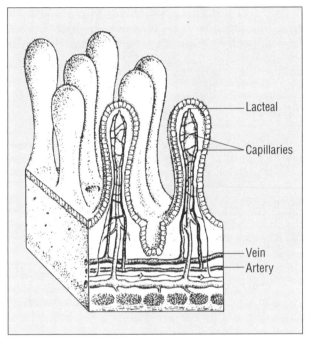

How does absorption occur? The inside of the small intestine is made of a membrane that will allow molecules to pass through. To increase the absorbing surface, the intestine wall has many folds that contain projections, as pictured in figure 2.12. Each of the many thousands of projections contains a network of structures that will accept the molecules and transport them away to other parts of the body. These structures include tiny blood vessels called *capillaries* and a tube called a *lacteal*. Capillaries absorb amino acids, simple sugars and water; they also absorb some fatty acids, vitamins and minerals. Lacteals accept glycerol and the remaining fatty acids and vitamins.

The remaining food material continues its journey to the large intestine, most of which is called the *colon*. Absorption, mainly of water, continues in the first half of the colon, and the remaining material is transported on and converted through bacterial action into faeces. The faeces eventually reach the rectum, where they are stored until defecation occurs.

Figure 2.12 The interior wall of the small intestine. The wall has many tiny projections. The cross-section shows the capillaries and lacteal of each projection.

Disorders of the digestive system

Judging from the television commercials for stomach and 'irregularity' remedies, it seems that many people have a good deal of trouble with their digestive processes. We will consider a few digestive problems.

One disorder of the digestive system is *peptic ulcers*, which are open sores in the lining of the stomach or intestine, usually in the duodenum. These sores appear to result from excess gastric juices chronically eroding the lining when there is little or no food in the stomach, but bacterial infection seems to play a role, too (Rhoades & Pflanzer 1996). Abdominal pain is the chief symptom of the disorder. Although the victims of ulcers are mostly adults, the disorder also occurs in children, particularly boys (Whitehead 1986). People who experience high levels of stress seem to be more susceptible to ulcers than people who do not.

Hepatitis is a class of viral diseases in which the liver becomes inflamed and unable to function well. The first symptoms often are like those of flu. But the symptoms persist, and jaundice, a yellowing of the skin, generally follows. *Infectious hepatitis* (often called 'hepatitis A') appears to be transmitted through contaminated food, water and utensils. *Serum hepatitis* ('hepatitis B') is thought to be transmitted by transfusion of infected blood and by the sharing of contaminated needles by drug addicts, but the mode of transmission may be broader. Occasionally, hepatitis leads to permanent liver damage (AMA 1989).

Another disease of the liver is called *cirrhosis*. In this disease, liver cells die off and are replaced by nonfunctional fibrous scar tissue. The scar tissue is permanent, and when it becomes extensive, the liver's normal functions are greatly impaired. As we will see later, the liver is not only important in the digestive process; it also cleanses and regulates the composition of the blood. Cirrhosis can result from several causes, including hepatitis infection and, particularly, alcohol abuse (AMA 1989).

Cancer may occur in any part of the digestive tract, especially in the colon and rectum (AMA 1989; Levy 1985). People over 40 years of age have a higher prevalence for cancers of the digestive tract than do younger individuals. Early detection for many of these cancers is possible and greatly improves the chances of recovery.

Using nutrients in metabolism

The term **metabolism** refers to all chemical reactions that occur in the body's cells (Holum 1994; Tortora & Grabowski 1993). Three principal outcomes of metabolism are:
- *synthesis* of new cell material from proteins and minerals to build and repair the body
- *regulation* of body processes — by producing enzymes and hormones for example — through the use of proteins, minerals and vitamins
- *energy* to heat the body and fuel its activities.

We now focus on the third outcome, energy production.

Metabolism takes place constantly in the cells of all living organisms. Without the energy it produces, all of our body systems would cease to function. The energy to fuel our internal functions and our physical actions comes mainly from the metabolism of carbohydrates and fats. Although protein can be converted into energy, little of it is used in this way when other sources of energy are available to the body (Tortora & Grabowski 1993).

The amount of energy a food contains is measured in *calories*. One calorie (equivalent to 4.186 kilojoules) is the amount of heat needed to raise one gram of water one degree Celsius. Nutrition researchers measure the calories contained in a given quantity of a food by burning it in a special apparatus. In general, the number of calories per gram of food is more than twice as high for fats as for carbohydrates or proteins, which have about the same calorie content per gram (Tortora & Grabowski 1993).

How much energy do we use to support our basic bodily functions? The number of calories we burn up when our bodies are at rest — an index called the *basal metabolic rate* — depends on the size of the body (Tortora & Grabowski 1993). For this reason, the basal metabolic rate is expressed in terms of calories per area of body surface (in square metres) per hour. A person who is 160 centimetres tall and weighs 59 kilos has a body surface area of about 1.7 square metres, for example. The basal metabolic rate also varies with the person's age and gender: the average rate is higher in males than in females and higher in younger people than in older people, as figure 2.13 indicates.

What other factors affect the basal metabolic rate? People who are under stress, who live in cold climates or whose hormone secretion by the thyroid gland is greater than normal tend to have high basal metabolic rates (McClintic 1985; Tortora & Grabowski 1993). Factors such as these account for the fact that different people of the same size, age and gender may have different metabolic rates.

Activity raises metabolism above the basal rate. Food materials that are not used up by metabolic processes are stored as body fat. This means that people become over-weight generally because they regularly consume more calories than their body uses to fuel their internal functions and physical actions. To maintain normal body weight, people who do not metabolise all the calories they consume need to eat less or exercise more, and preferably both.

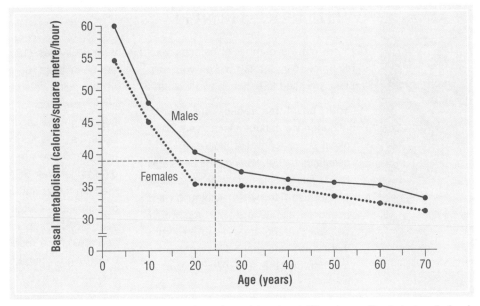

Figure 2.13 Normal basal metabolic rate for males and females at different ages. The dashed vertical and horizontal lines give an illustration: an average 24-year-old male's basic metabolism is 38.7 calories per square metre per hour.

Source: Data from Hafen (1981, table 16.6).

The respiratory system

Breathing supplies the body with oxygen — but why do we need oxygen? The chemical reactions in metabolism require oxygen, some of which joins with carbon atoms from food to form *carbon dioxide* (CO_2) as a waste product. So breathing has another function — it lets us get rid of this waste product. We will begin our examination of the **respiratory system** by looking at its structures.

The respiratory tract

After air enters the body through the nose or mouth, it travels past the *larynx*, down the *trachea* and *bronchial tubes*, and into the *lungs*. These organs are depicted in figure 2.14. The bronchial tubes divide into smaller and smaller branches called *bronchioles* inside the lungs. These branches finally end in millions of tiny air sacs called *alveoli*. Each alveolus looks like a minute bubble made of a membrane that is thin enough to allow oxygen, CO_2 and other gases to pass through. Alveoli are enmeshed in beds of capillaries so that gases can be transferred to and from the bloodstream quickly and efficiently.

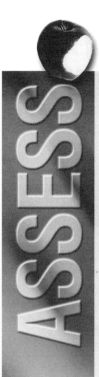

Assess yourself

HOW MANY CALORIES DO YOU BURN WHILE RESTING?

To work out the number of calories your body probably burns while you are resting, we need to estimate two factors.

1. **Your basal metabolic rate (BMR)**. Although we cannot assess your BMR directly, we can use figure 2.13 to estimate it by finding the average BMR for people of your age and gender. Do this by: (a) finding on the horizontal axis where your age would be, (b) drawing a vertical line from that point to the graph for your gender and (c) drawing a horizontal line to the vertical axis. The value at this intersect is our estimate of your BMR, which you should enter in the formula below.

2. **Your body surface area (BSA)**. Estimates of BSA in square metres are usually made by plotting the person's height and weight on complex graphs. We have used one of these graphs (Hafen 1981, figure 16.5) to develop an alternative two-step method. First, start with a BSA score of 1.540 and adjust it based on your height by adding (or subtracting) 0.035 for *each inch* by which you are taller (or shorter)

than 60 inches (152 cm). Thus, if you are 66 inches (168 cm) tall, your score at this point would be 1.750. Second, take your weight into account by adjusting your score in *one* of four ways: (a) if your body has a small frame and you are very slim, subtract 0.08 to get your BSA; (b) if you have a medium frame and an average weight, do nothing — your current score is your BSA; (c) if your frame is large and/or you are moderately heavy, add 0.08 to get your BSA; (d) if you are overweight by 9 kilograms or more, add 0.15 to get your BSA.

Enter your BSA in the formula below and multiply it by your BMR to estimate the number of calories you burn per hour while sleeping or lying down.

_____ BMR × _____ BSA = _____
calories/hour

When engaged in light activities, such as shopping or golfing, you burn two to four times that much, and when doing moderate or heavy activities, such as scrubbing floors or jogging, you burn four to 10 times that much.

When we breathe, what makes the air go in and out? Inhaling and exhaling are caused by diaphragm and rib muscles. When we inhale, the rib muscles draw the ribs up and outward and the diaphragm — a horizontal sheet of muscle below the lungs (see figure 2.14) — contracts, pulling downward on the bottom of the lungs. These actions pull air in and enlarge the lung chambers (Rhoades & Pflanzer 1996). When we exhale, these muscles relax, and the elasticity of the lungs forces the air out, like a balloon.

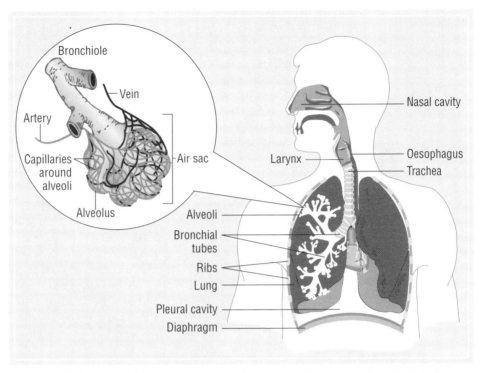

Figure 2.14 Major organs of the respiratory (also called pulmonary) system are shown in the body. The organ shown between the lungs and the pleural cavity is the heart. A close-up of alveoli (air sacs) is presented above.

Respiratory function and disorders

How do the muscles 'know' when it's time to inhale and exhale? Our blood vessels contain sensors that monitor blood gases and send this information to the medulla of the brain, which directs actions of the muscles to cause us to inhale and exhale. When the CO_2 level is high, the medulla increases the breathing rate; when the level is low, breathing rate is decreased (Rhoades & Pflanzer 1996).

Foreign matter, such as airborne particles and micro-organisms, can readily enter the respiratory tract. The respiratory system therefore needs protective mechanisms to prevent foreign matter from reaching the lungs and entering the bloodstream. Two protective mechanisms are *reflexes*: (1) sneezing in response to irritation in nasal passages and (2) coughing in response to irritation in lower portions of the system. Another protective mechanism is the *mucociliary escalator*. How does this mechanism work? Most of the lining of the respiratory system is coated with a sticky mucus that traps foreign matter. Furthermore, the air passages leading from the mouth to the lungs are lined with tiny hairlike structures called *cilia* that move in such a way as to force the mucus coating up towards the mouth — hence the name 'mucociliary escalator'. When the mucus reaches the back of the mouth, it is usually swallowed (McClintic 1985). In this way, the respiratory system cleanses itself and protects the body from harmful matter that we inhale.

The opening story of this chapter is about a young man named Tom who is a victim of cystic fibrosis, a fatal disease of the respiratory system. We will look at several of the many other disorders that attack this system. Some of these disorders mainly affect the alveoli of the lungs, thereby impairing the normal exchange of CO_2 and oxygen. For instance, there are several types of *pneumonia*, which can be caused by either bacterial or viral infection (AMA 1989). Although this disease often affects the bronchial tubes, the most serious types of pneumonia cause the alveoli to become inflamed and filled with fluid. In another respiratory disease called *emphysema* the walls between alveoli are destroyed. This decreases the lungs' surface area for exchanging gases and their elasticity for exhaling CO_2 (Haas & Haas 1990; Tortora & Grabowski 1993). *Pneumoconiosis* is a disease that afflicts people who chronically inhale air containing high concentrations of dust — generally at their workplaces. The black lung disease of coal miners provides an example. Dust that is not removed by protective mechanisms accumulates as thick sheets around the alveoli and bronchioles, damaging these structures and blocking air exchange.

Other disorders of the respiratory system primarily affect the bronchial tubes, usually by narrowing the tubes and reducing air flow. *Asthma* is a disorder in which the bronchial airways narrow because they become inflamed, develop spasms and secrete too much mucus (ALA 1994; Busse 1990). Attacks usually are temporary and occur in response to an irritant, such as an infection or something to which the victim is allergic. Breathing becomes difficult and, in very serious attacks, portions of the lungs may collapse temporarily. In *chronic bronchitis*, inflammation and excess mucus occur in the bronchial tubes for an extended period. This condition may be permanent or occur several times a year, lasting two weeks or more each time it occurs (Burg & Ingall 1985; Haas & Haas 1990).

Lung cancer involves an unrestrained growth of cells that crowd out cells that aid respiration. This process usually begins in the bronchial tubes and spreads to the lungs (Tortora & Grabowski 1993). In its final stages, the diseased cells enter the bloodstream through the capillaries and spread throughout the body. At this point death is almost always near.

Many of the respiratory diseases we have discussed can be caused or worsened by smoking cigarettes. This risk factor is also important in diseases of the cardiovascular system.

The cardiovascular system

The physical design of every complex organism has to deal with a basic problem: How can the body service its cells, supplying the substances they need to function properly and removing the wastes that metabolism produces? In humans and many other animals, this problem is solved by having a **cardiovascular system** to transport these materials. The blood circulates through blood vessels — capillaries, arteries and veins — within a closed system, one in which the blood does not directly contact the cells and tissues it services (Tortora & Grabowski 1993). All transfers of oxygen, nutrients, waste products and other substances occur through membranes that are separated by fluid-filled spaces. The heart is the centre of the cardiovascular system.

The heart and blood vessels

The *heart* is a fist-sized pump made of muscle that circulates the blood throughout the body. It 'beats', or pumps, about 100 000 times a day (AHA 1994). The muscular portion of the heart wall is called the *myocardium*. The interior of the heart has four chambers, as figure 2.15 illustrates. The two upper chambers are called atria, and the two lower ones are called ventricles; the left and right sides are labelled from the body's perspective, not from ours.

Looking at the drawing, we see several blood vessels that connect to the heart. How are arteries and veins different? *Arteries* carry blood *from* the heart, and *veins* carry blood *to* it. You will also notice in figure 2.15 that the shading of some blood vessels is light, and in others it is dark. The vessels with light shading carry blood that is laden with CO_2 towards the lungs; the dark vessels carry blood away from the lungs after it has expelled CO_2 and received oxygen.

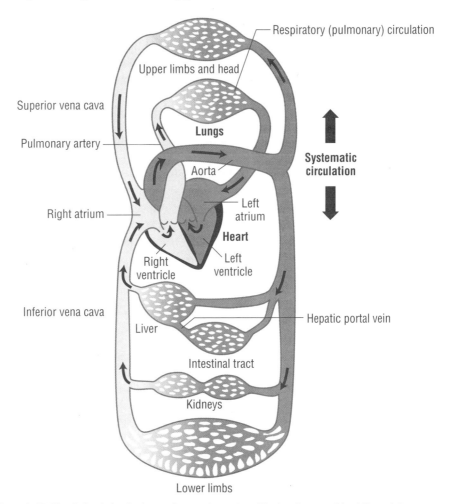

Figure 2.15 Blood circulation in the cardiovascular system. The heart pumps blood through two loops: *respiratory* (pulmonary) circulation and *systemic* (general) circulation. The respiratory loop allows blood to exchange CO_2 for oxygen; the systemic loop transports the blood to and from the rest of the body.

Now, let's follow the route of blood through the body. The blood that enters the *right atrium* of the heart is laden with waste products, such as CO_2, from our cells and is deficient in oxygen, which makes the blood bluish in colour. After the atrium is filled, the blood passes through a valve to the *right ventricle*. The ventricles provide the main pumping force for circulation as the heart muscle contracts, and their valves prevent the blood from going back up to the atria. From the right ventricle, the blood enters pulmonary circulation to the lungs, where it becomes oxygenated and, consequently, red in colour. The oxygenated blood travels to the *left atrium* of the heart and is passed to the *left ventricle*, which pumps it out through the *aorta* into systemic circulation. It then goes to various parts of the body before returning to the heart and beginning the cycle again. The complete cycle takes about one minute in the resting person (Tortora & Grabowski 1993).

Portions of each quantity of blood pumped by the heart travel through the liver and kidneys, where important functions take place (Guyton 1985). The *kidneys* receive blood from the general circulatory system, cleanse it of waste products and pass these wastes on to be eliminated in the urine. The *liver* receives blood from two sources: most of the blood comes from the intestinal tract, and the remainder comes from systemic circulation. What does the liver do to the blood? First, it cleanses the blood of harmful debris, such as bacteria. In fact, it is 'so effective in removing bacteria that probably not one in a thousand escapes through the liver into the general circulation' (Guyton 1985, p. 467). Second, the liver removes nutrients and stores them. The blood that comes from the intestinal tract after we consume a meal is rich in nutrients, such as simple sugars and amino acids. Large portions of these nutrients are retained in the liver until they are needed by the body. In this way, the ebbs and flows of nutrients in the blood are kept relatively even over time.

Blood pressure

Imagine you are holding a long balloon that is filled with air. Its end is tied off. If you squeeze it in the middle, the rest of it expands. This is what happens when pressure is applied to a closed system. The cardiovascular system is also closed, and the myocardium does the squeezing when it pumps blood from the heart. Like the balloon, the cardiovascular system always has some pressure in it. The squeezing increases the pressure.

Our arteries are elastic — they expand when pressure is applied. **Blood pressure** is the force exerted by blood on the artery walls. The heart is at rest between myocardial contractions, while it fills with blood. The resting force in the arteries that occurs at this time is called *diastolic pressure*. When the heart pumps, each contraction produces a maximum force in the arteries, which is called *systolic pressure*. A person's blood pressure is expressed by two numbers: a larger number, representing systolic pressure, followed by a smaller number, representing diastolic pressure. Your doctor might tell you that your blood pressure is '120 over 80', for example. Blood pressure readings are standardised in units of *mm Hg* to reflect the number of millimetres (mm) the pressure can raise a column of mercury (Hg).

Blood pressure varies. It changes from one moment to the next, it is higher in one part of the body than in another, and different people have different blood pressures. What determines blood pressure? We can answer this question in two ways — one involves the laws of fluid dynamics and the other involves factors in people's lives that affect these dynamics. We will start with the first approach and examine five aspects of fluid dynamics that affect blood pressure (McClintic 1985).

1. *Cardiac output* is the volume of fluid being pumped per minute. Blood pressure increases as cardiac output rises.
2. *Blood volume* refers to the total amount of blood circulating in the system. The greater the volume, the higher the blood pressure needed to move it.

3. *Peripheral resistance* refers to the difficulty fluid encounters in passing through narrow tubes or openings. When you put a nozzle on a hose and turn on the water, the pressure is greater at the nozzle than in the hose. Arteries vary in diameter. *Arterioles* are small arteries that connect larger arteries to capillaries. Peripheral resistance is generally greater in arterioles than in larger arteries. Normally arterioles are highly elastic and can expand or contract readily in response to messages from the nervous and endocrine systems. After we eat a meal, extra blood is needed around the small intestine for the absorption of nutrients. Messages to the arterioles in that region cause them to expand and accept more blood.

4. *Elasticity*, as we have seen, describes the ease in expanding and contracting. When blood vessels become less elastic, blood pressure — especially systolic pressure — rises.

5. *Viscosity* refers to the thickness of the fluid. The viscosity of blood depends on its composition, such as whether it contains high levels of red blood cells. Thicker blood flows less easily than thinner blood and requires more blood pressure for it to circulate through the cardiovascular system.

What factors in people's lives affect these dynamics? In our everyday lives we experience a variety of states that affect blood pressure. The *temperature* of our environment defines one of these states. When the temperature is high, the blood vessels in our skin enlarge and our cardiac output and diastolic pressure fall, which makes us feel drowsy. Low temperatures have the opposite effect. Another factor is *activity*. For example, exercise increases blood pressure during the activity and for some time thereafter. Simply changing our posture can also affect blood pressure. When we go from a lying position to standing, blood flow in the veins that feed the heart slows down because of gravity. This causes a drop in cardiac output and blood pressure. As a result, blood flow to the brain drops, sometimes making us feel dizzy (McClintic 1985). A third factor is *emotional experience*. When we experience stress, anger or anxiety, the sympathetic nervous system is activated. This causes a variety of cardiovascular reactions, such as increased cardiac output. Both systolic and diastolic pressures increase when people are emotionally aroused (James et al. 1986).

High blood pressure strains the heart and arteries. Some people have high blood pressure consistently over a period of several weeks or more. This condition is called *hypertension*. How high is 'high' blood pressure? People whose pressures are at or above 160 (systolic) over 95 (diastolic) are classified as hypertensives (Bennett 1995, 1996). When systolic pressure reaches 200, the danger is high that a rupture may occur in a blood vessel, particularly in the brain (McClintic 1985). This is one way by which strokes occur. High diastolic pressure is troubling because the arteries are constantly being strained, even between heartbeats, when they should encounter little pressure.

There are several known risk factors for hypertension. For example, blood pressure shows a positive correlation with body weight, especially in early and middle adulthood (Alexander 1984). Heavy people have more body mass to move when they are active than lighter people do, and they have a larger volume of blood for the heart to pump. Another factor is age — blood pressure generally rises with age. The percentage of individuals who are hypertensive is several times higher among the elderly than among young adults (AIHW 2000). But ageing per se may not be responsible for this relationship. Why? As adults get older, for instance, they tend to get heavier, at least in industrialised countries. In a number of traditional societies where adults do not show an increase in body weight as they get older, blood pressure does not seem to increase with age (Herd & Weiss 1984).

Other risk factors for hypertension among Australians relate to gender, ethnicity and family history (AIHW 1998, 2000). In adulthood, the prevalence rate for hypertension is higher for males than for females, particularly before about 55 years of age.

Thereafter, this gender difference reverses with females having higher prevalence rates (AIHW 1998). Indigenous people have high rates of hypertension (George & Davis 1998). Family history is important, too. People are more likely to become hypertensive if their parents had high blood pressure.

The reasons for these gender, ethnicity and family history differences in hypertension are not fully clear. Evidence from twin studies suggests that genetics plays a role in blood pressure (Rose 1986; Smith et al. 1987). Perhaps hereditary factors are responsible for these differences. Body weight may also be important. After 50 years of age, but not before, females are more likely than males to be overweight. In addition, indigenous people are more likely to be overweight than are other Australians, and this difference is quite pronounced among adult females at all ages (AIHW 1998, 2000). Still other factors, such as stress, may play a role — and so may diet, as we will see in the next section.

Blood composition

Blood is sometimes thought of as a 'liquid tissue' because it consists of cells that are suspended in a liquid. The adult's body contains between four and six litres of blood, and males on average have about 20 per cent more blood than females do (Tortora & Grabowski 1993). Because our bodies can replace blood quickly, we can donate half a litre of blood with no ill effects.

Blood composition can affect blood pressure. As we saw earlier, the thicker the blood, the more pressure is needed to circulate it. What is blood made of, and how does its composition change its thickness? Blood has two components — formed elements and plasma (Holum 1994; Tortora & Grabowski 1993).

Formed elements

Formed elements are the cells and cell-like structures in the blood that constitute about 45 per cent of our blood volume. There are three types of formed elements.

1. *Red blood cells* are the most abundant cells in the blood — there are about 5 million of them per cubic millimetre of blood. They are formed in the bone marrow and have a lifetime of about three months. Red blood cells are important mainly because they contain *haemoglobin*, a protein substance that attaches to oxygen and transports this element to body cells and tissues. *Anaemia* is a condition in which the level of red blood cells or haemoglobin is below normal (AMA 1989).

2. *Leucocytes* are white blood cells. Each of several types of leucocytes serves a special protective function — for example, some engulf or destroy bacteria. White blood cells are produced in the bone marrow and various organs in the body. Although there are normally several thousand leucocytes per cubic millimetre of an adult's blood, they are the least abundant type of formed element. *Leukaemia* is a malignant disease in which abnormal white blood cells are produced in extremely high quantities, crowding out normal leucocytes, which fight infection, and red blood cells, which prevent anaemia (ACS 1996; AMA 1989).

3. *Platelets* are granular fragments, produced by the bone marrow, that enable the body to prevent blood loss. They do this by plugging tiny wounds or helping the blood to clot when the wound is larger. *Haemophilia* is a disease in which the platelets do not function properly, thereby impairing clotting, because the blood lacks a critical protein (AMA 1989; Tortora & Grabowski 1993).

How do formed elements affect the viscosity of blood? The higher the concentration of formed elements suspended in the plasma, the thicker the blood.

Plasma

Plasma is a liquid substance that comprises about 55 per cent of our blood. About 90 per cent of plasma is water, and the remainder consists of *plasma protein* and various other organic and inorganic elements (Holum 1994; Tortora & Grabowski 1993). Plasma protein is a special element, consisting of molecules that are generally too large to be transferred through capillary walls to body tissue. This characteristic is important because this protein is needed within the blood to help other substances pass through capillary walls. Plasma protein increases the thickness of the blood.

Although the remaining elements in plasma constitute only a small percentage of its volume, they are extremely important substances. They include hormones, enzymes and waste products. They also include the nutrients we derive from digestion — vitamins, minerals, simple sugars, amino acids and fatty materials.

Fatty materials make up the broad class of substances in the blood called **lipids**. Two of these fatty materials are triglycerides and cholesterol (Holum 1994; Rhoades & Pflanzer 1996). *Triglycerides* are the material we commonly think of as fat. Made of glycerol and fatty acids, they are the most abundant lipid in the body. Some of the fatty acids in triglycerides are fully hydrogenated — they cannot take up any more hydrogen — and are called *saturated* for that reason. They are usually solid at room temperature and are mostly derived from animal fat. Other fatty acids are *unsaturated* or *polyunsaturated*. They can take up more hydrogen, are usually liquid at room temperature, and are derived from plants.

Cholesterol is a fatty substance that builds up in patches on artery walls over time and narrows the artery (Ross & Glomset 1976a, 1976b). Although most of the cholesterol in the blood is manufactured by the body, the rest comes from the foods we eat. Eating fats that are highly saturated tends to increase blood cholesterol levels. Let's see why this is a problem.

Cardiovascular disorders

The accumulation of fatty patches, or plaques, on artery walls is called **atherosclerosis**. These plaques tend to harden. This is a common process by which the diameter and elasticity of arteries is reduced — a condition called **arteriosclerosis** (Tortora & Grabowski 1993). The narrowing and hardening of arteries increase blood pressure. Although arteriosclerosis becomes an increasing problem as adults get older, plaque begins to form early in life (Clarkson, Manuck & Kaplan 1986). Autopsies on American soldiers killed in Vietnam showed that 45 per cent of these men had some degree of atherosclerosis present in their arteries (McNamara et al. 1971).

Of the many diseases of the heart and blood vessels, we will describe just a few. One of them is *myocardial infarction*, or 'heart attack'. Infarction refers to the death of tissue caused by an obstruction in the supply of blood to it. Thus, a myocardial infarction is the death of heart muscle (myocardium) tissue as a result of arterial blockage, usually resulting from atherosclerosis (Clarkson, Manuck & Kaplan 1986). Another form of heart disease is *angina pectoris*, in which the victim feels strong pain and tightness in the chest because of a brief obstruction in an artery, but little or no damage occurs. This kind of attack is often brought on by overexercise or stress.

One disorder of the blood vessels is an *aneurysm*, a bulge in a weakened section of an artery or vein. If the bulge is in a major blood vessel and it ruptures, the person may die (AMA 1989). Another disorder of the blood vessels — a *stroke* — occurs when the blood supply to a portion of the brain is disrupted. This can be caused by a rupture in a cerebral artery, causing a haemorrhage in the brain, or by a blood clot, called a *thrombosis*, in a cerebral blood vessel. In either case, damage occurs to the brain. The effects of this damage depend on where it occurs and how extensive it is. It may cause paralysis or sensory impairments, for instance, or even death (AHA 1994). Aneurysms and strokes can result from atherosclerosis and hypertension.

The immune system

You may not realise it, but wars are raging inside your body. They happen continuously, every day. Most of the time they are minor skirmishes, and you are unaware of them. When they become major battles, however, you are usually aware something's going on. The 'good guys' are the organs and cells that make up your **immune system**. This system fights to defend the body against 'foreign' invaders, such as bacteria and viruses.

The immune system is quite remarkable. Scientists knew very little about this intricate and enormously important system until recently. But it is now the subject of major research efforts, and new information about how the immune system functions is emerging rapidly. We know, for instance, that this system is highly sensitive to invasions by foreign matter and is able to distinguish between 'self', or normal body constituents, and 'not self' — friend and foe.

Antigens

When the body recognises something as a 'not self' invader, the immune system mobilises body resources and attacks. Any substance that can trigger an immune response is called an **antigen**. Bacteria and viruses are recognised as invaders by telltale aspects of their protein coats and DNA (Krieg et al. 1995).

What triggers an immune response? Some of the first antigens that come to mind are bacteria, fungi, protozoa and viruses. *Bacteria* are micro-organisms that exist in vast numbers throughout the environment — in rivers and oceans, in the air, on and in plants and animals, and in decaying organic matter. Billions of them may populate just one kilogram of rotting garbage. Because they help in breaking down organic matter into simpler units, their activities are essential to the life and growth of all living things. Some bacteria cause illnesses, such as tuberculosis, scarlet fever and food poisoning. They do this by growing rapidly and competing with our cells for nutrients and by excreting *toxic*, or poisonous, substances that destroy our cells or impair their metabolic processes (AMA 1989; Jaret 1986). Although treatment with antibiotics kills bacteria, these drugs are becoming less effective because they have been overused and bacteria are developing drug-resistant strains (Brown 1995).

Fungi are organisms, such as moulds and yeasts, that attach themselves to an organic host and absorb nutrients from the host. Some of them can cause skin diseases through direct contact, as occurs in ringworm and athlete's foot, and internal diseases through inhalation of contaminated air. Other fungi are very beneficial — for example, penicillin is derived from moulds (AMA 1989). *Protozoa* are one-celled animals, such as amoebas, that live primarily in water and insects. Drinking water contaminated with protozoa can cause amoebic dysentery, an intestinal illness, and being bitten by an infected mosquito can cause malaria (AMA 1989; Jaret 1986).

The tiniest antigens are *viruses*, particles of protein and nucleic acid that are smaller than cells and, strictly speaking, may not even be alive. They consist of genetic information that allows them to reproduce. A virus functions by attaching to a cell, slipping inside, and taking over by issuing its own genetic instructions. The invaded cell abandons its own metabolic activities and becomes a 'factory' for making viruses. In short order, enough viruses can be produced to rupture the cell and spread to infect other cells. Viruses can be quite devious, too, developing new strains and lying dormant in the body for periods of time before becoming infectious. They are responsible for a variety of diseases, including flu, herpes, measles and polio (AMA 1989; Jaret 1986, 1994).

The immune system also tends to recognise the tissue of an organ transplant as 'not self' and treat it as an antigen. This is what physicians mean when they say that the body 'rejected' a transplant. There are two basic ways to encourage transplant acceptance. The first is to select the transplant carefully so that the tissues of the donor and the recipient are closely matched. The closer the genetic relationship between the two people, the better the match is likely to be. Identical twins provide the best match, of course. The second approach uses drugs to suppress the immune system so it won't mobilise and reject the organ. A drawback to this approach is that long-term suppression of immune function leaves the patient susceptible to disease.

For many people, the immune system mounts an attack against normally harmless substances, such as pollen, tree moulds, poison ivy, animal dander and particular foods. These people suffer from *allergies*; the specific substances that trigger their allergic reactions, such as sneezing and skin rashes, are called *allergens*. Most allergic people react to some, but not all, of the known allergens. Someone with hay fever is not necessarily allergic to poison ivy, for instance. Some allergies can be reduced by administering regular, small doses of the allergen, usually by injection (Benjamini & Leskowitz 1991).

The organs of the immune system

The organs of the immune system are located throughout the body (Benjamini & Leskowitz 1991; Rhoades & Pflanzer 1996; Tortora & Grabowski 1993). These organs are generally referred to as *lymphatic* or *lymphoid* organs because they have a primary role in the development and deployment of **lymphocytes**, specific white blood cells that are the key functionaries or 'soldiers' in our body's defence against invasion by foreign matter. The main lymphatic organs include the bone marrow, thymus, lymph nodes and vessels, and spleen.

Lymphocytes originate in *bone marrow*, the soft tissue in the core of all bones in the body. Some of these cells migrate to one of two organs where they mature. One of these organs is the *thymus*, which, as we saw earlier in this chapter, is a gland that lies in the chest. The other organ is not known for certain, but it is thought to have the same function in maturing human lymphocytes that a structure called the 'bursa' has in birds (Benjamini & Leskowitz 1991). Most of this processing of lymphocytes occurs before birth and in infancy.

The *lymph nodes* are bean-shaped masses of spongy tissue that are distributed throughout the body. Large clusters of them are found in the neck, armpits, abdomen and groin. What do they do? Each lymph node contains filters that capture antigens and compartments that provide a home base for lymphocytes and other white blood cells. The lymph nodes are connected by a network of *lymph vessels* that contain a clear fluid called *lymph*. These vessels ultimately empty into the bloodstream. Although the lymph nodes and vessels play an important role in cleansing body cells of antigens, they can become a liability in some forms of cancer either by becoming infected with cancer or by distributing cancer cells to other parts of the body through the lymph and blood.

Lymphocytes and antigens that enter the blood are carried to the *spleen*, an organ in the upper left side of the abdomen. The spleen functions like an enormous lymph node except that blood, rather than lymph, travels through it. The spleen filters out antigens and serves as a home base for white blood cells. It also removes ineffective or worn-out red blood cells from the body.

Soldiers of the immune system

White blood cells play a key role in the immune system — they serve as soldiers in our counterattack against invading substances in the body. There are two types of white blood cells. Lymphocytes, as we have seen, are one type; phagocytes are the other.

Phagocytes are scavengers that patrol the body and engulf and ingest antigens. They

> are not choosy. They will eat anything suspicious that they find in the bloodstream, tissues, or lymphatic system. In the lungs, for instance, they consume particles of dust and other pollutants that enter with each breath. They can cleanse lungs that have been blackened with the contaminants of cigarette smoke, provided the smoking stops. Too much cigarette smoking, over too long a time, destroys phagocytes faster than they can be replenished. (Jaret 1986, p. 715)

There are two types of phagocytes: *macrophages* become attached to tissues and remain there, and *monocytes* circulate in the blood (Benjamini & Leskowitz 1991; Rhoades & Pflanzer 1996). The fact that phagocytes 'are not choosy' means that they are involved in *nonspecific immunity* — they respond to any kind of antigen.

Lymphocytes react in a more discriminating way, being tailored for attacks against specific antigens. Figure 2.16 shows that, in addition to the process of nonspecific immunity, there are two types of *specific* immune processes: cell-mediated immunity and antibody-mediated 'humoral' immunity (Bachen, Cohen & Marsland 1997; Benjamini & Leskowitz 1991; Borysenko 1984; Braveman 1987; Jaret 1986; Rhoades & Pflanzer 1996; Tortora & Grabowski 1993). Let's examine these two specific immune processes and how they interrelate.

Cell-mediated immunity operates at the level of the cell. The soldiers in this process are lymphocytes called **T cells** — the name of these white blood cells reflects their having matured in the *thymus*. T cells are divided into several groups, each with its own important function.

- *Killer T cells* (also called CD8 cells) directly attack and destroy three main targets: transplanted tissue that is recognised as foreign, cancerous cells and cells of the body that have already been invaded by antigens, such as viruses.
- *Memory T cells* 'remember' previous invaders. At the time of an initial infection, such as with mumps, some T cells are imprinted with information for recognising that specific kind of invader — the virus that causes mumps — in the future. Memory T cells and their offspring circulate in the blood or lymph for long periods of time — sometimes for decades — and enable the body to defend against subsequent invasions more quickly.
- *Delayed-hypersensitivity T cells* have two functions. They are involved in delayed immune reactions, particularly in allergies such as to poison ivy, in which tissue becomes inflamed. They also produce protein substances called *lymphokines* that stimulate other T cells to grow, reproduce and attack an invader.
- *Helper T cells* (also called CD4 cells) receive reports of invasions from other white blood cells that patrol the body, rush to the spleen and lymph nodes, and stimulate

lymphocytes to reproduce and attack. The lymphocytes they stimulate are from both the cell-mediated and the antibody-mediated immunity (also called 'humoral' immunity) processes.

- *Suppressor T cells* operate in slowing down or stopping cell-mediated and antibody-mediated immunity processes as an infection diminishes or is conquered. Suppressor and helper T cells serve to regulate cell-mediated and antibody-mediated immune processes.

What is antibody-mediated immunity, and how is it different from the cell-mediated process? **Antibody-mediated immunity** attacks bacteria, fungi, protozoa and viruses while they are still in body fluids and before they have invaded body cells. Unlike the cell-mediated process of attacking infected cells of the body, the antibody-mediated approach focuses on the antigens directly. The soldiers in this approach are lymphocytes called **B cells**. Figure 2.16 shows that B cells give rise to *plasma cells* that produce antibodies. This process is often induced by helper T cells or inhibited by suppressor T cells.

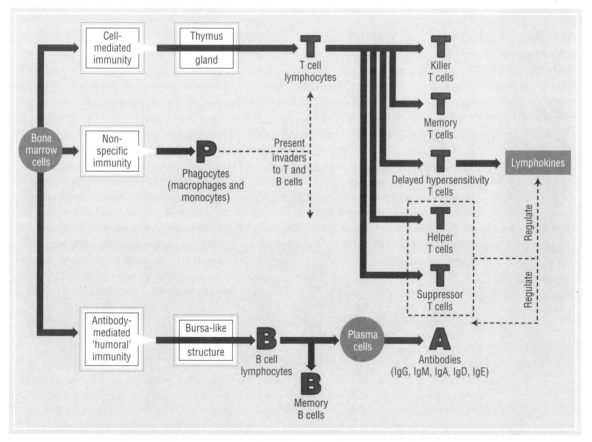

Figure 2.16 Components and interrelationships of the immune system. Bone marrow produces two types of white blood cells (leucocytes): *phagocytes* and *lymphocytes*. There are two kinds of lymphocytes: *T cells*, which are processed by the *thymus* gland; and *B cells*, which are processed by an as yet unknown *bursa*-like structure. (B cells were first discovered in the 'bursa of Facricius' structure of birds.) See text for description.

Sources: Benjamini & Leskowitz (1991); Borysenko (1984); Braveman (1987); Jaret (1986); Rhoades & Pflanzer (1996); Tortora & Grabowski (1993).

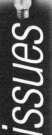

Highlight on issues

When immune functions are absent

I can remember reading for the first time many years ago about a child who had to live in a large plastic 'bubble' because he was born without virtually all major immune defences. The condition he had is very rare and is called *severe combined immunodeficiency disease*. He lived in the bubble because it was germ free — exposure to micro-organisms in the general environment is soon fatal for such children. Transplants of healthy bone marrow tissue early in the child's life can cure this disorder (Benjamini & Leskowitz 1991). More common inborn immune deficiencies involve the absence of only part of the system and can sometimes be treated with injections.

Having little or no immune defence was almost unheard of prior to the 1970s, and people were not very concerned about immune processes. All that changed in the 1980s as people became aware of the disorder called *acquired immune deficiency syndrome* (AIDS). This disorder is not inborn — it is caused by a virus that is transmitted when an infected person's body fluid, such as blood or semen, contacts the body fluid of an uninfected person. This occurs in three major ways: through sexual activity if the body fluids become exposed to each other, in intravenous drug use if syringes are shared, and from an infected mother to her baby (Francis & Chin 1987). Receiving contaminated blood in a transfusion was once a major source of the virus, but in Australia and many other countries close monitoring of hospital blood supplies has sharply reduced this risk.

Although AIDS is a fatal disorder, it does not kill directly. It disables or destroys an extremely important component of the immune system — *helper T cells* — and leaves the victim defenceless against a variety of diseases, including pneumonia and a form of cancer called Kaposi's sarcoma

(Batchelor 1988; Francis & Chin 1987). One of these diseases becomes the actual cause of death. Although researchers have made great progress in finding ways to prevent and treat AIDS, no fully successful methods exist yet.

AIDS is a worldwide epidemic: 21.8 million people have died from AIDS since the beginning of the epidemic, and an estimated 36.1 million are living with HIV. The majority of people infected with HIV (approximately 95 per cent) live in the developing world (National Center for HIV, STD and TB Prevention 2001). In Australia, an estimated 11 800 people were living with HIV at the end of 1998 (AIHW 2000). The number of HIV/AIDS diagnoses has declined since 1994, which is attibuted to the use of effective drug therapies that have delayed the progression from HIV to AIDS (AIHW 2000). So far, most AIDS victims in Australia have been sexually active homosexual males and, to a lesser extent, intravenous drug users. Prevention by changing high-risk behaviour is essential, and studies of these changes have found encouraging results in technologically advanced countries. Gay males have shown substantial changes in their behaviour, such as by avoiding sex with unfamiliar partners and using condoms and other methods to prevent the exchange of body fluids (Kalichman, Carey & Johnson 1996; Stall, Coates & Hoff 1988; Van Griensven et al. 1989). Many intravenous drug users have reduced their risks by decreasing drug use and using sterile or decontaminated (with bleach) needles (Des Jarlais, Friedman & Casriel 1990). But more progress in preventive efforts is needed in these high-risk groups and among people in the larger population, especially since most AIDS victims around the world have been neither gay nor drug users. We will discuss the topic of AIDS again in later chapters.

How are antibodies involved? **Antibodies** are protein molecules called *immunoglob-ulins* ('Ig') that attach to the surface of invaders and accomplish three results. First, they slow down the invader, making it an easier and more attractive target for phagocytes to destroy. Second, they recruit other protein substances that puncture the membrane of an invading micro-organism, causing it to burst. Third, they find new invaders and form *memory B cells* that operate in the future like memory T cells. As you can see, antibodies are like sophisticated weapons in immune system wars. Researchers have identified five classes of antibodies — IgG, IgM, IgA, IgD and IgE — each with its own special function and 'territory' in the body. For example, IgA guards the entrances of the body in fluids, such as saliva, tears and secretions of the respiratory tract.

Defending the body with an immune response

Now that we have seen the soldiers and weaponry of the immune system, let's see how all of this is orchestrated in defending your body. Protection from disease actually involves a series of defences (Benjamini & Leskowitz 1991; Jaret 1986; Rhoades & Pflanzer 1996; Tortora & Grabowski 1993). We will start at the beginning, as the invader tries to enter the body.

Your body's first line of defence is the skin and the mucous membranes that line the respiratory and digestive tracts. The skin serves as a barrier to entry, and mucous membranes are coated with fluids that contain antibodies and other antimicrobial substances. Even though these defences are highly effective, large numbers of antigens get through, either by eluding the antibodies or by entering a wound in the skin or the mucous membrane.

Once an antigen penetrates this barrier, it encounters the second line of defence, which includes nonspecific and specific immune processes. Phagocytes in your blood and tissues attack and consume invading substances of all types. They also have another important function: They present the antigen to B cells and helper T cells, as if to say, 'Here's the enemy. Go get 'em!' The B cells respond to this message and to stimulation from helper T cells by giving rise to plasma cells that produce the needed antibodies. The role of the phagocytes is especially important if the antigen is new and there are no memory B cells yet for this substance. Antibodies in body fluids attach to micro-organisms, thereby aiding the phagocytes and other protein substances that can kill the invaders.

Antigens that manage to get through and invade body cells encounter the third line of defence in which killer T cells destroy the invaded cells. Phagocytes often initiate this process by presenting antigens to T cells, as we have seen. Once again, this is especially important if the antigen is new to the cell-mediated system and there are no memory T cells for the substance. As the invasion subsides, suppressor T cells slow down the cell-mediated and antibody-mediated immune responses. Memory B and T cells are left in the blood and lymph, ready to initiate the immune response if the same antigen invades the body again.

You may be thinking, 'This is a wonderful and complex system that responds when there are antigens in the body, but killer T cells also attack cancer cells. Why? Aren't cancer cells basically normal cells that multiply out of control?' Cancer cells have antigens on their surface to which T cells respond (Benjamini & Leskowitz 1991; Jaret 1986). What scientists don't yet know is why some cancers escape destruction. One reason is that some cancer cells appear to release substances that suppress the immune response (Acevedo, Tong & Hartsock 1995; Mizoguchi et al. 1992). Another possibility is that the antigen is simply not easy for the immune system to recognise. As a result, the immune response may not be strong enough to stop the cells from multiplying wildly. Some researchers are studying approaches for treating cancer that are designed to strengthen the patient's own immune processes. In one of these approaches, for example, researchers manufacture antibodies that are sensitive to and seek out a specific type of cancer cell. These approaches are not yet perfected, but they are very promising.

Less-than-optimal defences

If our immune systems always functioned optimally, we would become sick much less often. Why and in what ways do our defences function less than optimally?

The effectiveness of the immune system changes over the life span, becoming increasingly effective throughout childhood and declining in old age (Rogers, Dubey & Reich 1979). Newborns come into the world with relatively little immune defence. They have only one type of antibody (IgG), for example, which they receive prior to birth from their mothers through the placenta (the filterlike organ that permits the exchange of nutrients and certain other substances between the bloodstreams of the mother and baby). Infants who are nursed receive antibodies, particularly IgA, in their mother's milk (Ashburn 1986).

In early infancy, children in technological societies generally begin a regular schedule of immunisation through the use of vaccines. Most vaccines contain dead or disabled disease micro-organisms that get the body to initiate an immune response and produce memory lymphocytes, but do not produce the full-blown disease (AMA 1989; Benjamini & Leskowitz 1991; Nelson 1989). The efficiency and complexity of the immune system develop very rapidly in childhood. As a result, the incidence of illness serious enough to keep children home from school declines with age (Ashburn 1986).

Throughout adolescence and much of adulthood, the immune system generally functions at a high level. Then, as people approach old age, the effectiveness of the system tends to decline (Braveman 1987). Although the overall numbers of T cells, B cells and antibodies circulating in the blood do not decrease, their potency diminishes in old age. Compared with the T cells and B cells of younger adults, those of elderly people respond weakly to antigens and are less likely to generate the needed supply of lymphocytes and antibodies to fight an invasion.

Unhealthy lifestyles, such as smoking cigarettes and being sedentary, have been associated with impaired immune function (Kusaka, Kondou & Morimoto 1992). Poor nutrition can also lead to less-than-optimal immune function (Braveman 1987; Brody 1987). Diets deficient in vitamins A and E diminish the production of lymphocytes and antibodies; vitamin C is important in the effectiveness of phagocytes. Being overweight and eating diets that are high in fats and cholesterol seem to impair immune function and increase people's susceptibility to infections.

When your immune system functions optimally, it attacks foreign matter and protects the body. Sometimes this process goes awry, and the immune response is directed at parts of the body it was designed to protect. Several disorders result from this condition — they are called *auto-immune diseases*. One of these diseases is *rheumatoid arthritis*, in which the immune response is directed against tissues and bones at the joints. This causes swelling and pain and can leave the bones pitted. In *rheumatic fever*, the muscles of the heart are the target. This disease can damage the heart valves permanently. *Multiple sclerosis*, a disease we considered earlier, results when the immune system attacks the myelin sheath of neurons. Another auto-immune disease is *lupus erythematosus*, which affects various parts of the body, including the skin and kidneys.

What causes auto-immune diseases? Although we are not certain of the causes, it is likely that heredity and immune responses to prior infections play important roles (Benjamini & Leskowitz 1991; Jaret 1986).

The reproductive system and heredity

At one time, many educated people believed that a miniature, completely formed, baby was passed on from a man to a woman during sexual intercourse. In the eighteenth century researchers disproved this and similar ideas and demonstrated that a *sperm* cell from a male had to combine with an egg cell — an *ovum* — from a female before development could begin.

Conception and prenatal development

A human being begins to form at conception, when a sperm cell unites with an ovum. The resulting single fertilised cell, called a *zygote*, starts to divide, forming new cells. It soon attaches to the wall of the mother's uterus, and the *placenta* and umbilical cord develop. These structures allow nourishment, wastes and other substances to be exchanged between the mother's and offspring's separate bloodstreams.

During the next few weeks, the offspring begins to develop all the body systems we have just examined. By the ninth week of prenatal development, for instance, the foetus has a tiny and incompletely formed heart that pumps blood through minute blood vessels, and the basic structures of the brain, liver and kidneys have developed. The body systems undergo continuous improvement in organ structure and functioning during the remainder of gestation (Sarafino & Armstrong 1986).

Pregnancy produces substantial alterations in the mother's anatomy and enormous additional demands on her body systems (Pillitteri 1981). The most obvious changes are to the size and weight of the foetus and the accompanying structures and fluids. But other, less obvious changes also occur. The mother's blood volume increases by 30 per cent, which places heavy demands on her heart. Furthermore, her usual dietary intake of iron is likely to be inadequate for meeting the combined needs of herself and the foetus. This condition can produce *iron deficiency anaemia* — a general physical weakness — in both the mother and baby before and after birth unless she increases her iron intake. Added burdens are also placed on her respiratory and digestive systems.

Genetic processes in development and health

Although researchers in the nineteenth century discovered that each person developed from the union of a sperm and an ovum, no-one knew what forces or substances inside these cells directed the growth processes. Charles Darwin speculated that unseen particles called 'gemmules' were present in the sperm and ovum. Darwin's concept of gemmules formed the basis for the search for genetic materials.

Genetic materials and transmission

What did this search yield? By the early twentieth century, researchers discovered threadlike structures called **chromosomes** and proposed that these structures contained units called *genes*. Soon they determined the basic substance common to all genetic material — *deoxyribonucleic acid*, or DNA for short — and described its structure. Today we know that DNA determines our growth patterns and physical structures. We also know that genes are discrete particles of DNA and that strings of genes are organised into chromosomes.

In what form are these genetic materials passed on to the next generation? Each ovum and sperm contains 23 chromosomes. At conception, the 23 chromosomes of the ovum are paired with those of the sperm, yielding 46 chromosomes in the zygote. As the offspring grows, these 46 chromosomes are duplicated and passed on to each newly formed cell of the body. Sperm and ova, which are produced by the reproductive system, are the only cells in the human body that contain just 23 chromosomes. Thus, half of the genetic information contained in each of your body cells comes from each of your parents, and half of their genetic information comes from each of their parents.

Chromosomes can be identified by certain features. Photographs taken through a microscope can be arranged according to the size and shape of chromosome pairs. One pair is called the *sex chromosomes* because they carry the genes that will determine whether an individual will be female or male. The normal sex chromosomes for males consist of one large chromosome (called an X chromosome) and one small chromosome (called a Y chromosome); females have two X chromosomes. Since the mother can provide only an X sex chromosome to her offspring, the child's gender is determined by the information received from the father. If the sperm that fertilises the ovum carries an X chromosome, the zygote will develop into a female. If the sperm carries a Y chromosome, the child will be a male.

As with chromosomes, genes come in pairs (Tortora & Grabowski 1993). Some of a person's traits are determined by a single pair of genes. Furthermore, some traits occur in the presence of a single gene, with the paired gene making little or no contribution. Such genes are said to be *dominant*. In humans, dominant genes produce such characteristics as freckles and poor visual acuity. On the other hand, when a trait occurs only if two identical genes make up the pair, these genes are called *recessive*. Recessive characteristics include flat feet and albinism (lack of colouration in skin, hair and eyes). When the pair consists of one dominant and one recessive gene — say, one gene for freckles and one for no freckles — the dominant trait appears. This is why it is important to distinguish between the trait we observe, which is called a *phenotype*, and the underlying genetic makeup, which is called the *genotype*.

Not surprisingly, geneticists have discovered that genetic transmission is often far more complicated than the process just described. First of all, paired genes can be *co-dominant* so that the phenotype will show the influence of both genes. This is the case for the ABO blood type. Also, some genes become dominant at different ages in the life span — changes in hair colour and distribution, eruption and loss of teeth, and the production of sex hormones are but a few examples. Second, *mutations* occur that change the chemical or structural composition of a gene. Most mutations are harmful and can be passed on to an offspring as a recessive gene (Gardner, Simmons & Snustad 1991). Such alterations sometimes result from excessive exposure to environmental agents, such as X-rays. In addition, it is likely that many behavioural traits, such as intelligence, are partially determined by the process of *polygenic inheritance*, involving the combined interaction of many gene pairs.

The impact of genetics on development and health

Researchers involved in the Human Genome Project have determined that every human cell contains 50 000 to 80 000 genes and have identified and mapped most of the human system of genes (Foote 1999; Trent 1999). Genes control a vast number of traits, including more than 3000 diseases. For some diseases, researchers have even pinpointed the exact gene locations. We will look at some of these traits and diseases.

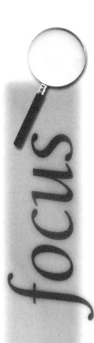

Focus on research
Stress and the immune response

Many people believe stress and illness often are related — and they are right. Research has confirmed this belief, showing, for instance, that the incidence of respiratory illnesses increases when people experience high levels of stress (Jemmott & Locke 1984). Why is this so? One likely answer is that stress suppresses immune functions in some way, leaving the person open to infection. This explanation is consistent with the finding that people who have low levels of the antibody IgA in their saliva — part of the body's first line of defence against respiratory infection — have more respiratory illnesses than people who have high levels of IgA (McClelland et al. 1980).

These findings are provocative, but they do not show a direct relationship between stress and immune function. Psychologist Janice Kiecolt-Glaser and colleagues from a variety of disciplines have done an impressive series of studies to examine this relationship. Let's look at one of their studies in detail (Kiecolt-Glaser et al. 1984). The researchers recruited 75 first-year medical students who were scheduled to take a series of highly stressful final examinations. The study assessed important variables in two sessions: The first session occurred at a time when examination stresses should be relatively low — one month before the finals and one month after their last major exam. The second occurred when stresses should be high, just after the students had taken their first two exams during the final exam week.

In the first session, the researchers took a sample of blood from the students and had them fill out questionnaires that assessed their experience of loneliness and stress during the past year. In the second session, only a blood sample was taken. Both samples of blood were analysed for the degree of killer-T-cell activity and concentrations of antibodies. The results showed that, although antibody concentrations were not consistently related to stress variables, killer-T-cell activity was. Killer-cell activity was considerably lower in the second (high stress) blood sample than in the first. Moreover, in both blood samples, killer-cell activity was lower for students who scored high on the loneliness and stress questionnaires than for those who scored low.

In another study, Kiecolt-Glaser and her co-workers (1987) analysed blood samples of married and separated or divorced women. Among the married women, those who reported less marital satisfaction showed weaker immune function than those who reported greater satisfaction. Among the separated or divorced women, those who refused to accept the fact of the separation or thought excessively about their ex-spouse had weaker immune function than those who did not. In addition, women who had been separated for relatively short amounts of time showed weaker immune function than married women and women separated for a longer time. The findings of these two investigations provide direct evidence of an association between stress and immune suppression.

Studies by other researchers support these results, finding, for example, that immune function is suppressed in individuals several weeks following the deaths of their spouses (Antoni 1987; Jemmott & Locke 1984). How does the suppression occur? One way is through the endocrine system. Earlier in this chapter we saw that stress causes the adrenal glands to produce epinephrine and cortisol. These substances affect immune cells (Antoni 1987; Biondi & Pancheri 1995). Epinephrine appears to increase suppressor T cells and decrease helper T cells in the blood, at least for a short while. Cortisol inhibits the function of phagocytes and lymphocytes — and if stress is chronic, cortisol causes important lymphoid tissues to wither away. The nervous system also can affect immune function: research has shown that chemicals secreted by nerves in the skin can suppress immune function in nearby cells (Hosoi et al. 1993).

Sickle-cell anaemia is a hereditary disease whose victims are usually black people. In the United States, approximately 10 per cent of the black population carry a recessive gene for this disease and do not have the disorder (Holbrook 1985). But when a person has two of these genes, the body manufactures large quantities of sickle-shaped red blood cells. Compared with normal blood cells, these defective cells carry little oxygen and tend to clump together in the bloodstream — often they cannot pass through capillaries. As a result, the oxygen supply to vital organs becomes inadequate, and tissue damage often occurs. The condition, which usually develops in childhood, leads to progressive organ failure and brain damage.

Another recessive disease is *phenylketonuria* (PKU). In this disease, which occurs more frequently among whites than other ethnic groups, the baby's body fails to produce a necessary enzyme for metabolising phenylalanine, a toxic amino acid present in many common foods (Collins & Lipman 1985). If the disease is not treated, the amino acid builds up and causes brain damage. This can be prevented by placing PKU babies on special diets as soon as possible after birth. When the brain is more fully developed after about five years of age, many PKU children can switch to normal diets. PKU provides a good example of an inherited disease that can be controlled by modifying the victim's behaviour.

The X chromosome has a special significance beyond determining a person's gender: it sometimes carries genes for dozens of disorders that are described as *sex-linked* (Gardner, Simmons & Snustad 1991). These disorders include *colour blindness*, *haemophilia* and *mitral stenosis*, a heart valve abnormality. For these disorders, if the child has only one X chromosome — as a boy does — and it carries the sex-linked gene, he will have the phenotype. If the child has two X chromosomes — as a girl does — *both* must carry the gene for the phenotype to show up. It is partly for this reason that females can be carriers of a sex-linked disorder but rarely show the phenotype.

Genetics researchers have made enormous progress in the last few decades in discovering the specific genes that cause certain diseases, such as the muscle-wasting disease called *Duchenne's muscular dystrophy*, and can test for the presence of each gene in a foetus early in pregnancy. This ability recently enabled researchers to discover a surprising finding about the genes for hereditary diseases: they can enlarge across generations. For example, the gene that causes the most common form of muscular dystrophy, *myotonic dystrophy*, grows larger each time it is inherited (Harley et al. 1992). Moreover, the bigger the gene, the more severe the illness. These findings contradict the long-held beliefs that genes are transmitted across generations essentially unchanged and that a gene is either normal or it is not.

Researchers are also closing in on certain *oncogenes*, which are genes that can cause cancer (Williams 1990). Researchers have, for example, found oncogenes for certain types of cancers of the colon (Bodmer et al. 1987), breast (Chen et al. 1995; Wooster et al. 1995), skin (Hussussian et al. 1994), lung (Rodenhuis et al. 1987), and prostate (Lee et al. 1994). Oncogenes can be normal genes or mutations that may result from exposure to harmful environmental agents, such as tobacco smoke. Once the genes are isolated for hereditary disorders, it may be possible to treat the disorders by replacing the defective genes. But tests of this kind of 'gene therapy' have not been successful (Begley 1995).

We know that oncogenes can cause cancer. One of the next steps in research will be to increase our knowledge regarding what causes genes to mutate into oncogenes. Assume for a moment that this mutation can result from engaging in certain behaviours, such as smoking cigarettes and eating diets that are high in fats and low in fibre. If this is true, as many researchers believe, we would have additional evidence that behavioural risk factors for cancer constitute major causal links in its development. The case for believing in biopsychosocial determinants of this disease is already strong; it would be ironclad with this evidence.

A biopsychosocial perspective in our examination of heredity is important in another way. Many researchers believe that we often inherit a predisposition or susceptibility — rather than a certainty — for developing a disease (Syme 1984; Weiner 1977). This might account in part for the observation that not everyone who is exposed to harmful substances and micro-organisms in their environments becomes sick. Someone who inherits a high degree of susceptibility to a form of cancer and has relatively little exposure to relevant antigens may be just as likely to develop the illness as someone who has little genetic susceptibility but high antigen exposure. If doctors could determine whether a patient has a genetic predisposition to a specific disease, they could provide the person with instructions for taking early preventive action.

Summary

To understand health psychology, we need to know how the body systems function. The nervous system provides a communications network for all systems of the body. The central nervous system consists of the brain and spinal cord and is the control centre, sending and receiving electrochemical messages through neurons throughout the body. The brain is divided into the forebrain, the cerebellum and the brainstem. The uppermost regions of the brain are involved in perceptual, motor, learning and conceptual activities. Areas towards the centre and bottom of the brain are important in controlling internal and automatic body functions and the flow of information to and from the brain. The spinal cord is the major neural pathway that connects the brain to the peripheral nervous system.

The peripheral nervous system is a branching network of afferent and efferent neurons throughout the body. It has two divisions, somatic and autonomic. The somatic nervous system is involved in sensory and motor functions. The autonomic nervous system carries messages between the spinal cord and various internal organs, and this system has two parts, sympathetic and parasympathetic. The sympathetic nervous system acts in agreement with our current emotional state and helps us mobilise and expend energy. The parasympathetic nervous system is involved in processes to conserve and store energy and in calming the body following sympathetic arousal.

The endocrine system also communicates with various parts of the body, but does so by sending chemical messages through the bloodstream. This system consists of several glands that secrete hormones. As the 'master gland' in this system, the pituitary gland releases hormones that stimulate other glands to secrete. The adrenal glands secrete hormones such as cortisol and epinephrine (adrenaline), which are important in our response to emergencies and stress. Other glands are important in regulating such factors as general body growth and the level of blood sugar.

The digestive and respiratory systems provide the body with essential nutrients, oxygen and other substances for energy, body growth and repair. These systems are also involved in removing wastes from the body. The outcomes of chemical reactions called metabolism that occur in our body cells include the synthesis of new cells, the regulation of body processes, and the production of energy to heat the body and fuel its activity.

The cardiovascular system uses the heart to pump blood through an intricate network of blood vessels. The blood's circulation takes it to body cells, where it supplies oxygen and nutrients for metabolism and takes away CO_2 and other waste materials. Systolic and diastolic blood pressure are affected by cardiac output, blood volume, peripheral resistance, elasticity and viscosity. Blood consists of plasma and formed elements.

The immune system responds to antigens by attacking and eliminating invading substances and micro-organisms to protect us from infection and disease. It does this by using white blood cells, including phagocytes and two types of lymphocytes: B cells, which produce antibodies, and T cells. The effectiveness of the immune system is impaired by stress and poor nutrition.

The reproductive system and heredity play an important role in development and health by producing a new generation of the species and transmitting genetic information from parents to their offspring. Genetic transmission occurs at conception, when a sperm from the father fertilises an ovum from the mother. The sperm and ovum each contain 23 chromosomes, which are composed of genes. Each of the body systems that we have examined changes across the life span. In general, they are immature at birth, develop during childhood, function relatively effectively during adolescence and early adulthood, and decline in old age.

Key terms

adrenal glands

antibodies

antibody-mediated immunity

antigen

arteriosclerosis

atherosclerosis

autonomic nervous system

B cells

blood pressure

brainstem

cardiovascular system

cell-mediated immunity

central nervous system

cerebellum

cerebrum

chromosomes

digestive system

endocrine system

enzymes

hormones

hypothalamus

immune system

limbic system

lipids

lymphocytes

medulla

metabolism

midbrain

neurons

neurotransmitter

parasympathetic nervous system

peripheral nervous system

phagocytes

pituitary gland

pons

respiratory system

reticular system

somatic nervous system

spinal cord

sympathetic nervous system

T cells

thalamus

PART 2

Stress, illness and coping

3 Stress — its meaning, impact and sources

Prologue

Paul is a 51-year-old executive working for a large Perth advertising firm. Paul has been working for the company for 15 years. He is married to Jan and has three children. Susan has just completed a pharmacy degree and is getting married next month. His son Danny, however, has dropped out of university, cannot seem to hold on to any job and has been caught using marijuana. Kelly, the youngest daughter, has been missing school and is constantly in trouble. Paul feels that he has been a failure as a parent because two of his children are not behaving as he would want them to behave.

Paul's firm recently informed him that he will be transferred to their Sydney office. Jan does not want to move as she has just secured a position as a counsellor. This is the cause of much argument between Jan and Paul. Jan feels that she has always been asked to make career sacrifices for the sake of Paul's career. Putting the family home on the market and making plans for the move has been stressful. Paul feels nervous and has trouble sleeping. However, he believes he must make the move for financial reasons.

Complicating Paul's career problems at this point are some personal problems. Six months ago Paul's best friend died suddenly of cancer; this friend was someone with whom Paul could talk freely and openly. Paul had never really developed any other close friendships, and he belongs to no social organisations. Paul and his wife, although together now, were separated for some months during the past year in an attempt to iron out some of their marital difficulties. Two years ago Paul went through a period of questioning his whole life, its achievements and his fulfilment with family life. This search for meaning resulted in an extramarital affair with a co-worker. The lack of agreement between Paul and Jan about the pending move to Sydney has not helped their relationship.

Paul is overwhelmed with a feeling of loss of control over his life. He feels that many constraints are being placed on him, and he is constantly irritable and anxious. He wonders about the purpose of his life. He is afraid that because of his age he will not be able to find another job if he quits the advertising firm. Being successful is important to Paul's sense of self. To compound these problems, Paul has an intermittent pain in his chest that is accompanied by shortness of breath. Paul is worried about these symptoms as there is a history of heart attack in his family, his father having died in his mid 50s. Paul has always had a hectic work life; he eats take-aways for lunch, drinks five cups of coffee a day, smokes on average two packets of cigarettes per day, and drinks three to four glasses of wine at night to relax.

Like many other people in Australia, Paul is having to cope with the demands of modern living. He is experiencing occupational stress associated with the forthcoming relocation to another city, family opposition to the move, financial stress, problems with his relationship, problems with his children, bereavement stress and health problems. The absence of a support system has increased Paul's vulnerability to emotional breakdown. Additionally, Paul's lifestyle and dietary habits are compounding his risk for a heart attack.

In this chapter we discuss what stress is, where it comes from and the impact it has. As we do, you will find answers to questions you may have about stress. What makes an event stressful? Why does a particular event produce more stress in one person than in another? How does stress affect our bodies and our behaviour? Does the experience of stress change across the life span?

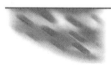

Experiencing stress in our lives

When you hear people say they are 'under a lot of stress', you have some idea of what they mean. Usually the statement means they feel unable to deal with the demands of their environment, and they feel tense and uncomfortable. You understand the meaning because you have had similar experiences, which you labelled 'stress'.

Because of the pervasiveness and commonality of these experiences in our lives, you might expect that defining the concept of stress would be simple. But it isn't. Let's see how psychologists have conceptualised stress and what the prevailing definition is today.

What is stress?

Psychological stress has been conceptualised in three ways (Baum 1990; Coyne & Holroyd 1982; Hobfoll 1989). One approach focuses on the environment, describing stress as a *stimulus*. We see this in people's reference to the source or cause of their tension as being an event or set of circumstances, such as having 'a high-stress job'. Events or circumstances that we perceive as threatening or harmful, thereby producing feelings of tension, are called **stressors**. Researchers who follow this approach study the impact of a wide range of stressors, including (1) catastrophic events, such as tornadoes and earthquakes, (2) major life events, such as the loss of a loved one or a job, and (3) chronic circumstances, such as living with severe pain from arthritis.

The second approach treats stress as a *response*, focusing on people's reaction to stressors. We see an example of this approach when people use the word *stress* to refer to their state of tension, and when someone says, 'I feel a lot of stress when I have to give a speech.' The response has two interrelated components. The psychological component involves behaviour, thought patterns and emotions, as when you 'feel nervous'. The physiological component involves heightened bodily arousal — your heart pounds, your mouth goes dry, your stomach feels tight and you perspire. The person's psychological and physiological response to a stressor is called **strain**.

The third approach describes stress as a *process* that includes stressors and strains, but adds an important dimension: the relationship between the person and the environment (Cox 1978; Lazarus & Folkman 1984a, 1984b; Lazarus & Launier 1978; Sarason & Sarason 1981). This process involves continuous interactions and adjustments — called **transactions** — between the person and the environment, with each affecting and being affected by the other. According to this view, stress is not just a stimulus or a response, but rather a process in which the person is an active agent who can influence the impact of a stressor through behavioural, cognitive and emotional strategies. People differ in the amount of strain they experience from the same stressor, such as being stuck in traffic or losing a job. One person who is stuck in traffic and late for an important appointment keeps looking at his watch, honking his horn and getting angrier by the minute; another person in the same circumstances stays calm, turns on the radio and listens to music.

To define stress, we will borrow ideas from several sources (Cox 1978; Lazarus & Folkman 1984b; Mechanic 1976; Singer & Davidson 1986; Trumbull & Appley 1986). **Stress** is the condition that results when person–environment *transactions* lead the individual to *perceive a discrepancy* — whether real or not — between the *demands* of a situation and the *resources* of the person's biological, psychological or social systems. Let's look at the four components of this definition, starting at the end.

1. Stress taxes the person's biopsychosocial *resources* for coping with difficult events or circumstances. These resources are limited, as we saw when Paul felt unable to cope with his problems and engaged in behaviours that place him at risk of developing heart disease. Sometimes the impact is focused mainly on our biological system — for instance when we tax our physical strength to lift something heavy. More typically, however, the strain has an impact on all three systems; in Paul's stressful experience, his physical, psychological and social resources were strained. He has lost the

social support of his best friend, is experiencing chest pains and feels helpless to change the things happening in his life. Other stressful encounters that strain our biopsychosocial resources include participating in a competitive athletic event, being injured in an accident or becoming nauseated before performing in a play.

2. The phrase 'demands of a situation' refers to the amount of our resources the stressor appears to require. For instance, Paul is overburdened with the job transfer, house sale and family problems.

3. When there is a poor fit, or a mismatch, between the demands of the situation and the resources of the person, a *discrepancy* exists. This generally takes the form of the demands taxing or exceeding the resources, as in Paul's belief that he would be unable to secure another job because of limited skills. But the opposite discrepancy also occurs — that is, our resources may be underutilised — and this can be stressful, too. A worker who is bored by a lack of challenge in a job may find this situation stressful. An important point to keep in mind is that the discrepancy may be either *real* or just *believed* to exist. Suppose you had to take an exam and wanted to do well, but worried greatly that you would not. If you had procrastinated and did not prepare for the test, the discrepancy you see between the demands and your resources might be real. But if you had previously done well on similar exams, prepared thoroughly for this one, and scored well on a pretest in a study guide yet still thought you would not do well, the discrepancy you see would not reflect the true state of affairs. Stress often results from inaccurate perceptions of discrepancies between environmental demands and actual resources. Stress is in the eye of the beholder.

4. In our *transactions* with the environment, we assess demands, resources and discrepancies between them — as Paul has done in evaluating his life at the moment. These transactions are affected by many factors, including our prior experiences and aspects of the current situation. Suppose you are on an athletics team and are running in a race. Relevant transactions for this race actually began long before the race started, such as in your previous wins and losses, your recent training and fitness, and your knowledge of and experience with your competitors. During the race, these prior transactions have an impact on the continuous transactions that occur as you assess your strength and energy reserves, the position you are in relative to the other runners, and the likelihood that another runner will show a surge of speed towards the end of the race.

Appraising events as stressful

Transactions that lead to the condition of stress generally involve an assessment process that Richard Lazarus and his co-workers call **cognitive appraisal** (Cohen & Lazarus 1983; Lazarus & Folkman 1984b; Lazarus & Launier 1978). Cognitive appraisal is a mental process by which people assess two factors: (1) whether a demand threatens their wellbeing, and (2) the resources available for meeting the demand. These two factors form the distinction between two types of appraisal — primary and secondary.

Primary and secondary appraisal

When we encounter a potentially stressful event, such as feeling symptoms of pain or nausea, we first try to assess the meaning of the situation for our wellbeing. This assessment process is called **primary appraisal**. In effect, this appraisal seeks answers to such questions as 'What does this mean to me?' and 'Will I be okay or in trouble?'

Your primary appraisal regarding the pain or nausea could yield one of three judgements.

1. It is *irrelevant* — as you might decide if you had had similar symptoms before that lasted only a short time and were not followed by illness.
2. It is *good* (called 'benign-positive') — which might be your appraisal if you wanted very much to skip work or have a university exam postponed.
3. It is *stressful* — as you might judge if you feared the symptoms were of a serious illness, such as botulism (a life-threatening type of food poisoning).

Events that we appraise as stressful receive further appraisal for three implications: harm-loss, threat and challenge.

Harm-loss refers to the amount of damage that has already occurred, as when someone is incapacitated and in pain following a serious injury. Sometimes people who experience a relatively minor stressor think of it as a 'disaster', thereby exaggerating its personal impact and increasing their feelings of stress (Ellis 1987). *Threat* is the expectation of future harm — for example when hospitalised patients contemplate their medical bills, difficult rehabilitation and loss of income. Stress appraisals seem to depend heavily on harm-loss and threat (Hobfoll 1989). Primary appraisals may be influenced by the personality of the individual. There is some indication that individuals high on the trait of neuroticism perceive situations as more threatening than individuals low on the trait (Shewchuk et al. 1999). Similarly, optimists are less inclined to make stress appraisals than are pessimists (Chang 1998). *Challenge* is the opportunity to achieve growth, mastery or profit by using more than routine resources to meet a demand. For instance, an offer of a higher-level job might be viewed as stressful by a worker, but also as an opportunity to expand her skills, demonstrate her ability and make more money.

Secondary appraisal refers to our ongoing assessment of the resources we have available for coping. Although we generally engage in an assessment of our resources after we appraise an event as stressful, secondary appraisal 'does not necessarily follow primary appraisal in time' (Cohen & Lazarus 1983, p. 609). The two processes are highly interrelated, and sometimes our secondary appraisal of limited resources, or weakness, can lead to primary 'appraisals of threat where they would not otherwise occur' (Coyne & Holroyd 1982, p. 109). Nevertheless, we are probably more aware of secondary appraisal when we judge a situation as potentially stressful and try to determine whether our resources are sufficient to meet the harm, threat or challenge we face. Examples of secondary appraisal judgements include:

• I can't do it — I know I'll fail.
• I'll try, but my chances are slim.
• I can do it if Ginny will help.
• If this method fails, I can try a few others.
• I can do it if I work hard.
• No problem — I can do it.

The condition of stress that we experience often depends on the outcome of the appraisals we make in our transactions with the environment. When we judge the fit between demands and resources to be close, we may experience little or no stress; but when our appraisals indicate a discrepancy, particularly if we appraise greater demands than resources, we may feel a great deal of stress. Like primary appraisals, secondary appraisals may be influenced by personality. Optimists are less likely than pessimists to view personal coping resources as insufficient to meet the demands of situational stressors (Chang 1998).

Can stress occur without cognitive appraisals? According to some researchers, it can, particularly in emergency situations. Suppose you are in your car, stopped at a red light. In a split second you hear the squealing of brakes; your body tenses as you say, 'Oh my God!'; and a car smashes yours in the rear. Your saying, 'Oh my God!' is not really a cognitive appraisal — it's a reflexive response. But a stress reaction has already begun, as the tensing of your body indicates, and this is *'followed* by "feelings" and appraisals' (Trumbull & Appley 1986, p. 34). Often in serious emergencies the stress reaction includes a state of shock in which the person is stunned, dazed or disoriented (Shontz 1975; Leach 1994). This state may last for minutes or hours, or much longer. Because cognitive functioning is impaired during shock, it is unlikely that appraisal processes play an important role in the stress experienced while in that state.

What factors lead to stressful appraisals?

Appraising events as stressful depends on two types of factors — those that relate to the person and those that relate to the situation (Cohen & Lazarus 1983; Lazarus & Folkman 1984b). Let's begin by looking at how personal factors can affect appraisals of stress.

Personal factors include intellectual, motivational and personality characteristics. One example has to do with self-esteem: people who have high self-esteem are likely to believe they have the personal resources to meet demands that require the strengths they possess (Rector & Roger 1997; Whisman & Kwon 1993). This belief pattern relating to confidence in one's ability to solve problems has been termed *self-efficacy* (Bandura 1977). Individuals with a high self-efficacy would most likely interpret a stressful event as a challenge rather than a threat. Another example relates to motivation: the more important a threatened goal, the more stress the person is likely to perceive (Paterson & Neufeld 1987). One other example involves the person's belief system: as the psychologist Albert Ellis has noted, many people have irrational beliefs that increase their stress. For instance:

'Because I strongly desire to have a safe, comfortable, and satisfying life, the conditions under which I live *absolutely must* be easy, convenient and gratifying (and it is *awful* and I *can't bear it* and *can't be happy at all* when they are unsafe and frustrating)!' (1987, p. 373)

A person who has such a belief is likely to appraise almost any sort of inconvenience as harmful or threatening.

What is it about situations that make them stressful? First, events that involve very *strong demands* and are *imminent* tend to be seen as stressful (Cohen & Lazarus 1983; Paterson & Neufeld 1987). Thus, patients who expect to undergo a physically uncomfortable or painful medical procedure, such as surgery, the following day are likely to view their situation as being more stressful than, say, expecting to have a blood pressure test next week.

Ambiguity — a lack of clarity in a situation — can have an effect on stress appraisals. But the effect seems to depend on the type of ambiguity that exists. *Role ambiguity* occurs when the information about a person's function or task is unclear or confusing (Quick & Quick 1984). In the workplace, for instance, this is reflected in unclear guidelines, standards for performance and consequences for job-related activities. Role ambiguity often increases people's stress because they are uncertain about their actions and decisions. *Harm ambiguity* occurs when the likelihood of harm or the availability of resources to meet situational demands is unclear. With this kind of ambiguity, the effect on stress is variable and depends heavily on the person's personality, beliefs and general experience (Lazarus & Folkman 1984a, 1984b; Paterson & Neufeld 1987). One person who is seriously ill and has unclear information about the chances of recovery may draw hope from this ambiguity; another person in the same situation may believe people are deliberately giving ambiguous information because the prognosis is so poor.

Another factor that influences stress appraisals is the *desirability* of the situation (Turner & Wheaton 1995). Some events are typically undesirable to a person in most or all respects — losing your house in a fire is an example. Other events, such as selling a house, are usually viewed as desirable. But either selling a house or losing it in a fire can be stressful because they both produce demands that may tax or exceed the individual's resources. Actually, a wide variety of both desirable and undesirable situations can be stressful. These events include life transitions as well as less momentous circumstances, such as getting a traffic ticket or preparing to throw a party. In general, undesirable events are more likely to be appraised as stressful than are desirable ones (Harris 1997; Sandler & Guenther 1985; Tausig 1982).

One other aspect of the situation that affects the appraisal of stress is its *controllability* — that is, whether the person has the real or perceived ability to modify or terminate the stressor. People tend to appraise an uncontrollable event as being more stressful than a controllable event, even if they don't actually do anything to affect it (Miller 1979; Suls & Mullen 1981; Thompson 1981). There are at least two types of control — behavioural and cognitive. In the case of *behavioural control*, we can affect the impact of the event by performing some action. Suppose, for example, you are experiencing intense pain from a headache. If you have the ability to reduce the pain, you are less likely to be stressed by the headache than if you do not have this ability. In the case of *cognitive control*, we can affect the impact of the event by using some mental strategy, such as by distracting our attention from the stressor or developing a plan to overcome a problem.

Change is also appraised as stressful irrespective of the desirability of an event. Any change demands adaptive effort. The change may be predictable, undesirable, controllable or unpredictable. Change makes demands on physiological systems, psychological processes such as perception and cognition, and social systems. Health psychology is essentially the psychology of change from illness to better health, from limited functioning to enhanced functioning, and from poor coping to adaptive coping with a range of stressors.

Biopsychosocial aspects of stress

In some of the stress experiences we have discussed, we saw that stressors produce strain in the person's biological, psychological and social systems. Let's examine biopsychosocial reactions to stress more closely.

Biological aspects of stress

Anyone who has experienced a very frightening event, such as a near accident or other emergency, knows that there are physiological reactions to stress — for instance, our heartbeat and breathing rates increase immediately and, a little later, our skeletal muscles may tremble, especially in the arms and legs. The body is aroused and motivated to defend itself. As we saw in the previous chapter, the sympathetic nervous system and the endocrine system cause this arousal to happen. After the emergency has passed, the arousal subsides.

Many years ago the distinguished physiologist Walter Cannon (1929) provided a basic description of how the body reacts to emergencies. He was interested in the physiological reaction people and animals make in response to a perceived danger. This reaction has been called the *fight-or-flight* response because it prepares the organism to attack the threat or to flee. In the fight-or-flight response, the perception of danger causes the sympathetic nervous system to stimulate the adrenal glands of the endocrine system to secrete epinephrine, which arouses the body. Cannon proposed that this arousal could have both positive and negative effects: the fight-or-flight response is adaptive because it mobilises the organism to respond quickly to danger, but the state of high arousal can be harmful to health if it is prolonged.

General adaptation syndrome

What happens to the body when high arousal levels are prolonged? Hans Selye studied this issue by subjecting laboratory animals to a variety of stressors — such as very high or low environmental temperatures, X-rays, insulin injections and exercise — over a long period of time. He also observed people who experienced stress from being ill. Through this research, he discovered that the fight-or-flight response is only the first in a series of reactions the body makes when stress is long-lasting (Selye 1956, 1976, 1985). Selye called this series of physiological reactions the **general adaptation syndrome** (GAS). As figure 3.1 shows, the GAS consists of three stages.

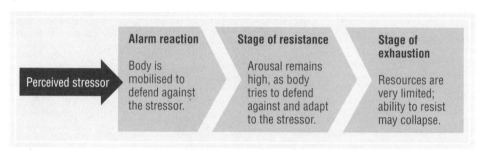

Figure 3.1 General adaptaion syndrome (GAS)

1. **Alarm reaction**. The first stage of the GAS is like the fight-or-flight response to an emergency — its function is to mobilise the body's resources. At the very beginning of the alarm reaction, arousal — as measured by blood pressure for example — drops below normal for a moment, but then rapidly rises to above normal. This fast-increasing arousal results from the release of hormones by the endocrine system: The pituitary gland secretes ACTH, which causes a heightened release of epinephrine, norepinephrine and cortisol by the adrenal glands into the blood-stream. By the end of this stage in the GAS, the body is fully mobilised to resist the stressor strongly. But the body cannot maintain this intense arousal for very long. Some organisms that have experienced a continuous and unrelieved alarm reaction to an extremely intense stressor have died within hours or days.

2. **Stage of resistance**. If a strong stressor continues but is not severe enough to cause death, the physiological reaction enters the stage of resistance. In this stage, the body tries to adapt to the stressor. Physiological arousal declines somewhat but remains higher than normal, and the body replenishes the hormones released by the adrenal glands. Despite this continuous physiological arousal, the organism may show few outward signs of stress. But the ability to resist new stressors may be impaired for long periods of time. According to Selye, one outcome of this impairment is that the

organism becomes increasingly vulnerable to health problems he called *diseases of adaptation*. These health problems include ulcers, high blood pressure, asthma and illnesses that result from impaired immune function.

3. **Stage of exhaustion**. Prolonged physiological arousal produced by severe long-term or repeated stress is costly. It weakens the immune system and depletes the body's energy reserves until resistance is very limited. At this point, the stage of exhaustion begins. If the stress continues, disease and damage to internal organs are likely, and death may occur.

Do all stressors produce the same physical reactions?

Many studies have demonstrated that stressors of various types increase the secretion of hormones by the adrenal glands (Baum, Grunberg & Singer 1982; Ciaranello 1983; Lovallo 1997). These stressors include cold temperatures, noise, pain, athletic competition, failure, taking examinations, flying in an airplane and being in crowded situations.

Selye (1956) believed that the GAS is *nonspecific* with regard to the type of stressor. That is, the series of physiological reactions the GAS describes will occur regardless of whether the stress results from very cold temperature, physical exercise, illness or the death of a loved one. However, although various stressors increase the secretion of adrenal hormones, the notion of nonspecificity does not take important psychosocial processes into account. There are at least two reasons why this is a problem.

One reason is that some stressors elicit a stronger *emotional* response than others do. This is important because the amount of hormone released in reaction to a stressor that involves a strong emotional response, as a *sudden* increase in environmental temperature might produce, appears to be different from the amount released with a less emotional stressor, such as a *gradual* increase in temperature. After conducting extensive studies of various stressors and hormones, John Mason concluded that he and his colleagues 'have not found evidence that any single hormone responds to *all* stimuli in *absolutely* nonspecific fashion' (1975, p. 27). For instance, some stressors led to increases in epinephrine, norepinephrine and cortisol, but other stressors increased only two of these hormones. He also pointed out that research conducted since Selye first described the GAS has shown that stressors are most likely to trigger the release of large amounts of all three of these hormones if the individual's response includes a strong element of emotion. Experimental studies using mental arithmetic and reaction time tasks have demonstrated that increased cortisol levels occur in response to distress, tension and irritability (al'Absi et al. 1994; Lovallo 1997).

The second reason is that cognitive appraisal processes appear to play a role in people's physiological reaction to stressors. This role is suggested by the results of a study by Katherine Tennes and Maria Kreye (1985). The researchers assessed elementary school children's cortisol levels in urine samples taken on regular school days and on days when achievement tests were given. The expected increase in cortisol on test days was found, but not for all children — their intelligence was an important factor. Intelligence test scores were obtained from school records. Cortisol levels increased on test days for children with above average intelligence, but not for children with low to average intelligence. The influence of intelligence suggests that the brighter children were more concerned about academic achievement and, as a result, appraised the tests as more threatening than the other children did.

To summarise, the GAS assumes incorrectly that all stressors produce the same physiological reactions and fails to include the role of psychosocial factors in stress, but its basic structure still appears to be valid.

Psychosocial aspects of stress

At this point, we can begin to see how interwoven our biological, psychological and social systems are in the experience of stress. While stressors produce physiological changes, psychological factors play a crucial role in determining (1) whether or not the stressor is perceived at all — if not perceived, then there is no physiological reaction; (2) the meaning of the stressor, if perceived; and (3) the manner in which the individual responds to the stressor. To give a more complete picture of the interplay among these systems, we will now examine the impact of stress on people's cognitive, emotional and social systems.

Cognition and stress

Many students have had this experience: While taking a particularly stressful exam at university, they may neglect or misinterpret important information in a question or have difficulty remembering an answer they had studied well the night before. It is infuriating to know that an answer is 'on the tip of your tongue', especially since you will probably remember it after the test is over. High levels of stress affect people's memory and attention. Let's see how.

Stress can impair cognitive functioning, often by distracting our attention. For example, noise can be a stressor, and some people live in very noisy environments — next to train tracks or highways for instance. How does chronic noise affect people's cognitive performance? Many people can deal with this kind of stress by changing the focus of their attention from the noise to relevant aspects of a cognitive task — they 'tune out' the noise. Psychologist Sheldon Cohen (1980) has proposed that children who try to tune out chronic noise may develop generalised cognitive deficits because they have difficulty knowing which sounds to attend to and which to tune out. Evidence from several studies supports this position (Cohen et al. 1986; Evans & Lepore 1993). For example, one study tested second- to fifth-grade children who lived in an apartment complex that was built on bridges spanning a busy highway. The children who lived in the noisier apartments had more difficulty discriminating between pairs of words (for example house and mouse) than those who lived in quieter apartments (Cohen, Glass & Singer 1973).

Similar effects of noise on reading and word skills were found for children living near an airport. These children had higher levels of stress hormones, higher blood pressure, impaired motivation and impaired long-term memory compared with children not living near the airport (Evans, Hygge & Bullinger 1995). Improvements in cognitive function occurred in the children when the airport was closed down, although children living in the vicinity of the new airport began to show similar impairments in cognitive functions (Hygge, Evans & Bullinger 1996). Experimental research on the effects of noise on classroom learning (Hygge 1996) has found that short-term memory, but not long-term memory, was impaired from a 15-minute exposure to aircraft and road traffic noise of 66 decibels. No effects on memory occurred from road traffic noise of 55 decibels. Noise that is unpredictable and over which the person has no control has repeatedly been found to have the most impairment on cognitive task performance (Cohen 1980; Jones & Macken 1993; Jones & Morris 1992). So it appears that impaired cognitive function depends on the type of noise experienced, and that the negative effects of noise can be reversed with non-exposure to noise.

But stress can also enhance our attention, particularly towards the stressor. For instance, researchers had people watch a series of pictures while listening to a story about a boy and his mother who go to a hospital (Cahill et al. 1994). For some subjects, the story was emotional: the boy had a terrible accident, his feet were severed and surgeons reattached the feet. For other subjects, the story was neutral: the boy went to the hospital to watch activities there. Before this experience, the subjects with each type of story received an injection of either a placebo or a drug that stops the action of epinephrine and norepinephrine. When tested a week later, the subjects who heard the emotional story remembered more details of it if they had received the placebo rather than the drug. But the drug had no effect on subjects' memory of the neutral story. These findings suggest that epinephrine and norepinephrine enhance the memory of stressors we experience.

Not only can stress affect cognition, but the reverse is true, too. In the story that opened the chapter, Paul believed he had no control over his life, and this was very distressing for him. His thinking was making the stress chronic. Andrew Baum (1990) has studied the thinking patterns of individuals who were living near the Three Mile Island nuclear power plant in Pennsylvania when a major nuclear accident occurred. He found that years later some of these people still experienced stress from the incident, but others did not. One of the main factors differentiating these people was that those who continued to feel this stress had trouble keeping thoughts about the accident and their fears out of their minds. It seems likely that these thoughts perpetuated their stress and made it chronic.

Emotions and stress

Long before infants can talk, they display what they feel by their motor, vocal and facial expressions. You can test this with a little experiment: Place a bit of a bitter food, such as unsweetened chocolate, in a newborn's mouth and watch the baby's face — the eyes squint, the brows drop and draw together, the mouth opens and the tongue juts out. This is the facial expression for the emotion of disgust. Each emotion has a specific facial pattern.

According to Carroll Izard (1979), a prominent researcher of infant emotions, new-born babies do not display all the emotional expressions they will develop, but they do express several emotions, such as disgust, distress and interest. Using procedures like the one with bitter food, he and his colleagues studied two- to 19-month-old infants' emotional reactions to the stress of receiving their regular inoculations at various ages (Izard et al. 1983). The babies' facial expressions following needle penetration were mainly distress and anger. The younger infants' principal emotion was distress, but the older infants' immediate and dominant emotion was anger, probably because infants become more able to act for themselves, such as by pushing at the nurse's hand. Anger spurs this kind of defensive action; distress merely signals the need for help.

Emotions tend to accompany stress, and people often use their emotional states to evaluate their stress. Cognitive appraisal processes can influence both the stress and the emotional experience (Maslach 1979; Schachter & Singer 1962, 1979; Scherer 1986). For example, you might experience stress and fear if you came across a snake while walking in the bush, particularly if you recognised it as poisonous. Your emotion would not be joy or excitement, unless you were studying snakes and were looking for this particular type. Both situations would involve stress, but you might experience fear if your appraisal was one of threat, and excitement if your appraisal was one of challenge.

Fear is a common emotional reaction that includes psychological discomfort and physical arousal when we feel threatened. Of the various types and intensities of fears people experience in everyday life, psychologists classify many into two categories: phobias and anxiety. *Phobias* are intense and irrational fears that are directly associated with specific events and situations. Some people are afraid of being enclosed in small rooms, for instance, and are described as claustrophobic. *Anxiety* is a vague feeling of uneasiness or apprehension — a gloomy anticipation of impending doom — that often involves a relatively uncertain or unspecific threat. That is, the person may not be aware either of the situations that seem to arouse anxiety or of exactly what the 'doom' entails. Patients awaiting surgery or the outcome of diagnostic tests generally experience high levels of anxiety. In other situations, anxiety may result from appraisals of low self-worth and the anticipation of a loss of either self-esteem or the esteem of others.

The things children fear tend to become *less* concrete or tangible and *more* abstract and social as they get older (Harris & Liebert 1991; Peterson, Beck & Rowell 1992; Sarafino 1986). In early childhood, many children develop fears of concrete things, such as animals, doctors and dentists, often because of negative experiences with these things. Cognition can also play a role in these fears. A study of children's fears of dental treatment found that the most fearful children were those who had *not* experienced invasive procedures, such as having a tooth pulled, during the previous few years (Murray, Liddell & Donohue 1989). Not having had these experiences probably allowed the children to imagine that invasive procedures are worse than they are. Later in childhood, concrete fears tend to decline while anxieties relating to school, individual competence and social relations become pronounced. Children who see themselves as less able than their age-mates are likely to appraise their own resources as insufficient to meet the demands of stressors.

Stress can also lead to feelings of sadness or *depression* (Brugha et al. 1997; Dohrenwend 1998; Glass, Kasl & Berkman 1997). We all feel depressed at times, although we may call the feeling something else, like 'sad', or 'blue' or 'unhappy'. These feelings are a normal part of life for children and adults (Quay & La Greca 1986; Rosenhan & Seligman 1984). The difference between normal depression and depression as a serious *disorder* is a matter of degree. Depression becomes a psychological disorder when it is severe, frequent and long-lasting. People with this disorder tend to:
- have a generally unhappy mood
- feel hopeless about the future
- appear listless and passive
- show disrupted eating and sleeping habits
- have low self-esteem, often blaming themselves for the troubles that afflict them (Rosenhan & Seligman 1984).

Having long-term disabling health problems, such as being paralysed by a stroke, often leads to depressive disorders.

Another common emotional reaction to stress is *anger*, particularly when the person perceives the situation as harmful or frustrating. You can see this in the angry response often shown by children whose favourite toy is taken away and by adults who are stuck in a traffic jam. Anger has important social ramifications — it can produce aggressive behaviour, for instance.

Social behaviour and stress

Stress changes people's behaviour towards one another. In some stressful situations, such as train crashes, earthquakes and other disasters, many people may work together to help each other survive. Perhaps they do this because they have a common goal that requires cooperative effort (Leach 1994; Sherif & Sherif 1953). In other stressful situations, people may become less sociable or caring and more hostile and insensitive towards other individuals.

When stress is accompanied by anger, negative social behaviours often increase. Research has shown that stress-produced anger increases aggressive behaviour, and these negative effects continue after the stressful event is over (Donnerstein & Wilson 1976). This increased aggressive behaviour has important implications in real life, outside the laboratory. Child abuse is a major social problem that poses a serious threat to children's health, physical development and psychological adjustment. Studies have found a connection between parental stress and child abuse (Kempe 1976; Kolbe et al. 1986; Rice 1992). Prior to an act of battering, frequently the parent has experienced a stressful crisis, such as the loss of a job. A parent under high levels of stress is at risk of losing control. If, for example, the child runs around the house making a racket, a stressed parent may become very angry, lose control and start beating the child.

Stress also affects helping behaviour. This was shown in an experiment conducted in a shopping centre (Cohen & Spacapan 1978). After each subject completed either a difficult shopping task or an easy one in either a crowded or an uncrowded shopping centre, he or she walked through a deserted hallway to meet the researcher. In the hallway, the subject encountered a woman who feigned dropping a contact lens — a situation in which the subject could provide help. Those subjects who had just experienced the most stress, having completed the difficult shopping task in crowded conditions, helped less often and for less time than those who had completed the easy task in uncrowded conditions.

Gender and sociocultural differences in stress

Does the experience of stress depend on a person's gender and sociocultural group membership? Apparently it does. With respect to gender differences, women generally report having experienced a greater number of major stressors than men (Greenglass & Noguchi 1996). Although this difference may result partly from women's greater willingness to say they have felt distressed, it probably also reflects real variations in experiences. For instance, in today's two-income households, the total daily workload is particularly heavy for mothers because they still do most of the chores at home (Frankenhaeuser 1991; Schwartzberg & Dytell 1996).

Being a member of a minority group or being poor appears to increase the stress people experience (Johnson et al. 1995; Young & Zane 1995). The plight of indigenous Australians with poor health, substandard housing conditions and high unemployment would suggest that stressors are over-represented in their daily existence (McMurray 1999). Differential exposure to stressful situations according to gender, sociocultural background and socioeconomic factors has been linked with more reported physical illness and greater psychological distress (Dohrenwend 1973; Wheaton 1978).

We have seen that the effects of stress are wide-ranging, involving an interplay among our biological, psychological and social systems. Even when the stressor is no longer present, the impact of the stress experience can continue. Some people experience more stress than others, but we all find stress somewhere in our lives. Stress arises from a countless variety of sources.

Sources of stress throughout life

Babies, children and adults all experience stress. The sources of stress may change as people develop, but the condition of stress can occur at any time throughout life. Life has many major events that mark the passing from one condition or phase to another, and they produce substantial changes and new demands in our lives (Moos & Schaefer 1986; Sarason & Sarason 1984). These events are called life transitions, and include:

- starting day care or school
- moving to a new community
- reaching puberty, with accompanying biological and social changes
- starting university, especially away from home
- entering a career

- getting married
- becoming a parent
- losing a spouse through divorce or death
- retiring from a career.

The timing of a life transition can affect the stress it produces. People expect some events, such as marriage or retirement, to occur at certain times in the life span (Neugarten & Neugarten 1987). Deviations from the expected timetable are stressful. Why? For one thing, events that happen too early or too late often leave the person without the support of compatible peers, as a 40-year-old first-time mother might find (Lazarus & Folkman 1984b). Also, the person may interpret being off schedule as a failure, and this is stressful. People who are 'late' graduating from university or advancing on the job may feel as if they have failed.

Where does stress come from, and what are its sources? To answer this question, we will divide up a variety of sources on the basis of the systems from which they arise. That is, we will examine sources that arise within the *person*, in the *family*, and in the *community* and *society*.

Sources within the person

Sometimes the source of stress is within the person. One way stress arises from within the individual is through *illness*. Being ill places demands on the person's biological and psychological systems, and the degree of stress these demands produce depends on the seriousness of the illness and the age of the individual, among other things. Why is the person's age important? For one thing, the ability of the body to fight disease normally improves in childhood and declines in old age (Rogers, Dubey & Reich 1979). Another reason is that the meaning of a serious illness for the individual changes with age. For example, young children have a limited understanding of disease and death. Because of this, their appraisal of stress that arises from their illness is likely to focus on current, rather than future, concerns — such as how well they feel at the moment and whether their activities are impaired (La Greca & Stone 1985). Stress appraisals by ill adults typically include both current difficulties and concerns for the future, such as whether they may be disabled or may die.

Another way stress arises within the person is through the appraisal of opposing motivational forces, when a state of *conflict* exists. Suppose you are registering for next semester and find two courses that you need meet at the same time. You can take only one. Which will you choose? You have a conflict — you are being pushed and pulled in two directions. Many conflicts are more momentous than this one. We may need to choose between two or more job offers, or different medical treatments, or houses we are thinking of buying, for instance. Conflict is a major source of stress.

The pushes and pulls of conflict produce two opposing tendencies: *approach* and *avoidance*. These two tendencies characterise three basic types of conflict (Lewin 1935; Miller 1959).

1. *Approach/approach conflict* arises when we are attracted towards two appealing goals that are incompatible. For example, people who are trying to lose weight to improve either their health or their appearance experience frequent conflicts when delicious, fattening foods are available. Although individuals generally resolve an approach/approach conflict fairly easily, the more important they perceive the decision to be, the greater the stress it is likely to produce.

2. *Avoidance/avoidance conflict* occurs when we are faced with a choice between two undesirable situations. For example, patients with serious illnesses may be faced

with a choice between two treatments that will control or cure the disease, but have very undesirable side effects. People in avoidance/avoidance conflicts usually try to postpone or escape from the decision: a patient might delay or discontinue treatment or change doctors in the hope of getting choices that are more appealing. When delaying or escaping is not possible, people often vacillate between the two alternatives, changing their minds repeatedly. Sometimes they get someone else to make the decision for them. People generally find avoidance/avoidance conflicts difficult to resolve and very stressful.

3. *Approach/avoidance conflict* arises when we see attractive and unattractive features in a single goal or situation. This type of conflict can be stressful and difficult to resolve. Consider, for instance, individuals who smoke cigarettes and want to quit. They may be torn between wanting to improve their health and wanting to avoid the weight gain and cravings they believe will occur.

Conflicts can be more complicated than the examples we have considered. People often have to choose between two or more alternatives, while recognising that each has multiple attractive and unattractive features. Buying a new car is an example because cars differ in many ways, such as cost, 'snazziness', optional equipment, colour, reliability and performance. In general, people are likely to find conflict stressful when the choices involve many features, when opposing motivational forces have fairly equal strength, and when the 'wrong' choice can lead to very negative and permanent consequences. These conditions often apply when people face major decisions about their health.

Sources in the family

The behaviour, needs and personality of each member of a family have an impact on and interact with those of the other members of the family system, sometimes producing stress. Interpersonal conflict can arise from financial problems, from inconsiderate behaviour or from opposing goals. This can be seen when siblings argue over which television program to watch or when a parent confronts an adolescent who plays music at deafeningly loud levels, for example. Living in an overcrowded household increases conflict over privacy and the use of family resources, such as the bathroom. Of the many sources of stress in the family, we will focus on three: adding a new family member, divorce, and illness and death in the family.

An addition to the family

A new child in the family is a joyful event, but it also brings stress — particularly to the mother, of course, during pregnancy and after the birth. But an addition to the family is stressful to other family members, too (Rice 1992). For instance the father may feel the need to earn more money, or worry about his wife's and baby's health, or fear that his relationship with his wife may deteriorate.

After the baby is born, parents experience stress from their new responsibilities in caring for the child. An important factor in parental stress relates to the child's personality. Each baby comes into the world with certain personality dispositions, which are called **temperaments** (Buss & Plomin 1975; Harris & Liebert 1991). Paediatric nurses and physicians, well aware of the unique combinations of temperaments that babies show from birth, describe infants broadly as 'easy' babies and 'difficult' ones. These terms do, in fact, capture the general dispositions of most infants fairly accurately on the basis of differences in the way babies react to feeding, cuddling, bathing, and dressing and undressing.

Temperamentally difficult babies tend to cry a great deal — often very loudly — and efforts to soothe them do not seem to work very well. They resist being introduced to new foods, routines and people, and their patterns of sleep, hunger and bowel movements are hard to predict from day to day. Although only about 10 per cent of babies are classified as 'difficult', displaying most or all of these traits fairly consistently, many others show some of these traits at least occasionally. A child who reacts in a very negative manner to minor irritations is very stressful to parents (Cutrona & Troutman 1986). For these parents, there is bad news and good news: Longitudinal studies have shown that children's temperaments are fairly stable across time — for example, a baby who cried intensely with wet diapers at two months old screamed and kicked when having its temperature taken at one year. But, although aspects of these traits tend to continue for many years, many difficult children show changes towards the development of easy traits (Carey & McDevitt 1978).

The arrival of a new baby can also be stressful to other children in the family (Honig 1987; Rutter 1983). This stress seems to be particularly strong among children who are very young — say, two or three years old — and who may not want to share their parents with the new brother or sister. After the baby arrives, these children tend to show increased clinging to the mother, as well as increased sleeping and toileting problems. If the children are older, they are less likely to view the baby as a rival for their parents' attention, and their stress seems to relate to changes in the pattern of family interaction, such as when the parents introduce new prohibitions.

Divorce

A divorce produces many stressful transitions for all members of the family as they deal with changes in their social, residential and financial circumstances (Grych & Fincham 1990). In the case of the children, they may move to a new neighbourhood, be left with new sitters or have to take on new chores at home. The custodial parent may not be very available to the children because of work or other preoccupations. According to psychologist Judith Wallerstein (1983, 1986), the way children react to the stress of divorce depends in part on their age. Very young children may feel responsible for the divorce, worry that the custodial parent will also leave, and develop sleep disturbances. Older children and adolescents tend to react with anger, often siding with one parent and blaming the other. Adapting to divorce usually takes several years, and some family members may never adjust fully. Parents can do several things to enhance their children's adjustment to a divorce (Sarafino & Armstrong 1986). They can maintain a loving, secure home life and:
- tell the children in advance of the impending separation
- encourage open communication and answer the children's questions truthfully but sensitively
- gear information to the children's levels of understanding, with concrete and accurate explanations of what will happen to all members of the family
- recruit help and advice from others, such as relatives, parent organisations, counsellors and the children's school teachers
- encourage the children to have contact with both parents.

Family illness, disability and death

The following is a familiar story to many parents: In the middle of a frantic day at work, the parent receives a call from the school principal, who says, 'Your child is sick. You'll have to come and pick him up.' Having a sick child adds to the stress in an already stressful day — and chances are the extra stress befalls the mother rather than the father. Even in today's world, if both parents have careers outside the home, the mother usually gets called when their child is sick.

When children have a serious chronic illness, their families must adapt to unique and long-term stresses (Johnson 1985; Kiser, Ostoja & Pruitt 1998; Leventhal, Leventhal & Van Nguyen 1985). Part of the stress stems from the amount of time needed to care for the child and from the reduced freedom family members have in their schedules. For example, children with the respiratory disease called cystic fibrosis generally need physiotherapy two or three times a day to reduce the mucus that collects in their lungs (Burroughs & Dieterle 1985). The family also faces many difficult decisions and must learn about the illness and how to care for the child. The medical needs of chronically ill children are expensive, and this burden adds to the family's stress. Relationships between family members may also suffer. The parents are likely to feel that having a chronically ill child reduces the time they have to devote to each other. In addition, other children in the family may feel isolated and deprived of parental attention.

Adult illness or disability is another source of family stress. The strain on their financial resources is especially severe if the sick adult is a principal breadwinner. Having a physically ill or disabled adult in the family restricts the family's time and personal freedom, lowers quality of life and produces very important changes in interpersonal relationships (Braithwaite 1990; Cairl & Kosberg 1993; Draper et al. 1992; Marsh et al. 1998). For example, when a husband has a heart attack, the wife generally experiences stress from fears that he may have another attack and from his increased irritability and dependency. Although husbands and wives tend to show increased affection for one another during convalescence, their sexual relations are curtailed — often because of fears that sex could induce another attack. And the roles of family members change: the healthy spouse and the children who are old enough take on many of the responsibilities and tasks of the recovering spouse. As the convalescing adult begins to show good physical recovery, the stress generally diminishes in the family.

Does the stress a family experiences when an adult is seriously ill depend on the sick person's age? It can, as the following example illustrates.

> Cancer in an 80-year-old woman has a quite different meaning than the same disease in a 30-year-old woman with two young children. In the former instance, the illness is likely to be seen as striking at an appropriate or expected time in life, after the individual has lived many years, worked, raised children, enjoyed grandchildren... Cancer in the young mother is asynchronous with her roles and functions: It is a threat to the family unit... Chronic illness that is out of step with family and individual life-course processes is likely to generate powerful frustration and intense distress and anger. (Leventhal, Leventhal & Van Nguyen 1985, pp. 132–3)

But if an elderly person who is ill or disabled must live with and be cared for by relatives, the stress for all those in the household can be severe, especially if the person requires constant care and shows mental deterioration (Schulz et al. 1995).

Age is also an important factor in the experience of stress when a family member dies. Some children suffer the loss of a parent during the childhood years — one of the most traumatic events a child can face. Children under about five years of age seem to grieve for the lost parent less strongly and for a shorter time than older children and adolescents do (Garmezy 1983; Rutter 1983). This age difference probably results from their different levels of understanding about the nature of death. Children's concept of death changes between four and eight years of age (Lonetto 1980; Speece & Brent 1984). Young children think death is reversible: the person is simply living somewhere else — such as underground — and can come back. By about eight years of age, most children understand that death is final and involves an absence of bodily functions. Yet children's understanding of death does not depend on cognitive development alone. Eiser (1997) has argued that social and cultural beliefs, as well as experience of death within the family, help children to gain knowledge about illness and death, and so organise that knowledge in a meaningful way.

An adult whose child or spouse dies suffers a tremendous loss (Kastenbaum & Costa 1977; Kosten, Jacobs & Kasl 1985). Losing a child creates other losses — for example, bereaved mothers reported that they had lost important hopes and expectations for the future (Edelstein 1984). A mother who loses her only child loses her identity and role as a mother, too. When a spouse dies, the surviving spouse also loses important hopes, expectations and roles — as well as the one companion who made him or her feel loved, wanted, special and safe. Although the loss of a spouse is difficult at any age, it appears to be especially stressful in early adulthood (Ball 1976–77).

As we have seen, there are many sources of stress within the family. Stressors such as sickness and the addition of a child to the family are intensified when stress occurs in other areas such as at work. The family, however, can be an effective resource system for its members (McCubbin & Patterson 1983; Olson 1997), as we shall see in the next chapter.

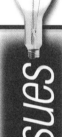

Highlight on issues

issues

The burden of caregiving

Under what conditions does caregiving become a burden? Braithwaite (1990) argues that burden arises when there is a perception by the caregiver that the demands of the care-receiver threaten the fulfilment of the caregiver's basic needs. Braithwaite postulates five crises of decline involving the care-receiver that negatively impact on the wellbeing of the caregiver by threatening basic needs. These are awareness of degeneration, unpredictability of certain illnesses, time constraints, the caregiver–care receiver relationship and choice restrictions.

In a major Australian study into the effects of caregiving in which 144 carers participated, Braithwaite (1990) found that caregiving activities in the form of bathing, household tasks, supervision and decision making were unrelated to burden. Carers in the study, however, reported high levels of anxiety and depression. Burden was experienced by a large proportion of carers in relation to being constantly on call, being unable to get household chores completed and having to change plans at the last minute. Burden was equated with a subjective appraisal of a mismatch between care-receiver demands and caregiver needs. Indicators of burden were sleep deprivation, an inadequate diet, social isolation, financial hardship, lack of freedom and loss of esteem.

All the crises of decline except time constraints were related to burden and poor mental health in caregivers. Caring for someone whose health is deteriorating, being uncertain about the course of the illness, and carer–care recipient relationships characterised by little autonomy in the past and conflict in the present, increased burden. Although many of the carers in the Braithwaite study were involved in multiple roles additional to caring, this did not contribute to burden or psychological distress. Feeling constrained in pursuing outside activities and disruption to family life, however, were related to burden.

Sources of stress in the community and society

The contacts people make outside the family provide many sources of stress. For instance, children experience stress at school and in competitive events, such as in sports and band performances (Passer 1982; Sears & Milburn 1990). Much of the stress adults experience is associated with their occupations, and a variety of environmental situations can be stressful. We will focus on how people's jobs and environments can be sources of stress.

Jobs and stress

Almost all people at some time in their lives experience stress that relates to their occupations. Often these stressful situations are minor and brief and have little impact on the person. But for many people, the stress is intense and continues for long periods of time. What factors make jobs stressful?

The *demands of the task* can produce stress in two ways. First, the workload may be too high, leading to job strain (Karasek & Theorell 1990). Some people work very hard for long hours over long periods of time because they feel required to do so — for example if they need the money or think their bosses would be unhappy if they did not. There is some indication that high job demands and job strain do not have a direct negative impact on health, but rather seem to depend on the type of work (Kristensen 1996; Marshall Barnett & Sayer 1997), personality of the worker (Parker & Sprigg 1999) and skills that impact on job self-efficacy (Schaubroeck & Merritt 1997). Studies have found that excessive workloads are associated with increased rates of accidents and health problems (Mackay & Cox 1978; Quick & Quick 1984). Second, some kinds of activities are more stressful than others. For example, repetitive jobs that underutilise the worker's abilities can produce stress (Melin & Lundberg 1997). As one worker put it:

> I sit by these machines and wait for one to go wrong, then I turn it off, and go and get the supervisor. They don't go wrong very much. Sometimes I think I'd like them to keep going wrong, just to have something to do . . . It's bloody monotonous. (Mackay & Cox 1978, p. 159)

One way to overcome job boredom has been to introduce technological innovations in the workplace. Performance has been found to increase initially under such conditions, although longer-term effects include cognitive and emotional overstrain (Leonova 1996).

Another kind of activity that can produce stress is the evaluation of an employee's job performance — a process that is often difficult for both the supervisor and the employee (Quick & Quick 1984).

Jobs that involve a *responsibility for people's lives* can be very stressful. Medical personnel have heavy workloads and must deal with life-or-death situations frequently. Making a mistake can have dire consequences. In an intensive care unit of a hospital, emergency situations are common; decisions must be made instantly and carried out immediately and accurately. As part of the job,

> the nurse must reassure and comfort the man who is dying of cancer; she must change the dressings of a decomposing, gangrenous limb; she must calm the awakening disturbed 'overdose' patient . . . It is hard to imagine any other situation that involves such intimacy with the frightening, repulsive, and forbidden . . . To all this is added the repetitive contact with death. (Hay & Oken 1985, p. 108)

These and other conditions of jobs in the health professions take their toll, often leading to feelings of emotional exhaustion (Maslach & Jackson 1982). Similar stresses exist in the jobs of police and fire personnel (Grossi et al. 1999).

Several other aspects of jobs can increase workers' stress. For example, stress can result from:

1. *the physical environment* of the job. Stress increases when the job involves extreme levels of noise, temperature, humidity or illumination (Mackay & Cox 1978; Quick & Quick 1984).

2. *perceived insufficient control* over aspects of the job. People experience stress when they have little influence over work procedures or the pace of the work, such as when a machine feeds work to them at a predetermined speed (Steptoe et al. 1993). Low job control has been linked with angina and heart disease in civil servants studied over time (Bosma et al. 1998).

3. *poor interpersonal relationships*. People's stress on the job increases when their boss or a co-worker is socially abrasive, being insensitive to the needs of others or condescending and overly critical of the work other individuals do (Quick & Quick 1984). Stress can also result from an absence of interpersonal support among workers (Warr 1996).

4. *perceived inadequate recognition or advancement*. Workers feel stress when they do not get the recognition or promotions they believe they deserve (Cottington et al. 1986; Quick & Quick 1984). Over-promotion, also known as the **Peter Principle**, can be just as stressful. If a worker lacks the skills to perform at a higher level within the organisation, or cannot keep up with the job, career advancement becomes a source of stress and job security is threatened (Peter 1969).

5. *job loss*. People experience stress when they lose their jobs or think their jobs are threatened. Workers who believe they are likely to be fired or laid off feel a sense of *job insecurity* — and this is stressful, particularly if they have little prospect of finding another job (Cottington et al. 1986; Quick & Quick 1984). Workers' jobs may be threatened with the introduction of new technology. More and more workers have to develop new skills to keep up with their changing jobs. The resulting strain on workers has been described by Craig Brod (1988) as 'techno-stress'. Studies have shown that *unemployment* is associated with psychological and physiological signs of stress, such as loss of self-esteem and heightened blood pressure (Kasl 1997; Lennon 1999; Olafsson & Svensson 1986; Warr & Jackson 1984, 1985).

Apart from the stressful aspects of jobs just discussed, changes in the workplace such as downsizing, relocation (as we saw in Paul's case in the opening anecdote) and outsourcing have been common in recent years in Australia. The nature of the work force has also changed with dual-earner couples, sole parents, workers with dependent children and workers caring for elderly relatives (Fallon 1997). The interplay of these factors needs to be taken into account for a greater understanding of how jobs contribute to stress. Does stress diminish when workers retire?

Many elderly people approach *retirement* with expectations of blissful freedom and leisure. But it does not always turn out that way. Retirees often find that they have lost opportunities for social interaction and an important part of their identity. They may miss the power and influence they once had, the structure and routines of a job, and the feeling of being useful and competent (Bohm & Rodin 1985; Bradford 1986). The stress of these circumstances can affect not only the retirees, but their spouses, too. What's more, many retirees have the added problem that their income is not sufficient for their needs.

Environmental stress

Have you ever been at a big noisy event with thousands of people jammed into an arena and felt physiologically aroused, tense and uncomfortable? Events like these can be stressful partly because noise is a stressor, as we have seen, and also because of the crowded conditions (Jones & Macken 1993). Crowded conditions reduce your control over interpersonal interaction and restrict your ability to move about freely or obtain resources (Pandey 1999), such as seats. Also, you may feel that other people are physically closer than you usually prefer people to be — they are intruding into your *personal space* (Freeman & Stansfeld 1998; Sarafino 1987a). Noise and crowding are two stressors in the environment.

Some environmental conditions are intensely stressful — imagine how you would react to learning that a hazardous substance has seeped into the water supply where you live. How much of it have you and your family already drunk? Has it damaged your bodies already? Will you develop serious illnesses because of it in the future? Can the substance be removed? And after it is, will you believe there is no more danger? Can you sell your house now without suffering a great financial loss? Many people who are exposed to hazardous substances or other continuous threats in their environment worry for years about what will happen to them (Baum 1988; Bland et al. 1996; Specter 1996).

An example of the psychological effects of living in a hazardous environment comes from the nuclear accident at the Three Mile Island power plant in Pennsylvania. More than a year after the accident, researchers compared the stress of nearby residents to that of people who lived near a different nuclear facility that had not had an accident. This comparison revealed greater psychological and physiological evidence of stress among the residents around Three Mile Island than among those near the other facility (Fleming et al. 1982).

So far in this chapter we have seen that stress involves biopsychosocial reactions, and that all sorts of events or circumstances can be stressors. We saw, for instance, that stressors can include extreme temperatures, noise, taking an exam, being stuck in a traffic jam, having a painful medical test, getting married, and losing a job. The possible stimuli and reactions, and the appraisal processes that link them, make for an interesting question: If you were doing research and needed to know whether different people had experienced different amounts of stress, how could you assess this variable? The next section answers this question.

Measuring stress

Researchers have used several different approaches for measuring stress. The three most commonly used approaches involve assessing people's physiological arousal, life events and daily hassles.

Physiological arousal

Stress produces physiological arousal, which is reflected in the functioning of many of our body systems. One way to assess arousal is to use electrical/mechanical equipment to take measurements of blood pressure, heart rate, respiration rate or galvanic skin response (GSR). Each of these indexes of arousal can be measured separately, or they can all be measured and recorded simultaneously by one apparatus called the **polygraph** (see figure 3.2). Miniaturised versions of these devices are available with recording units that can fit in a pocket, thereby allowing assessments during the person's daily life at home, at work or in a stressful situation, such as while flying in an airplane or receiving dental treatment (Carruthers 1983). Using one of these devices, researchers have shown that paramedics' blood pressure is higher during ambulance runs and at the hospital than during other work situations or at home (Goldstein, Jamner & Shapiro 1992).

Focus on research
Stress and measures of physiological arousal

Marianne Frankenhaeuser and her colleagues have conducted many studies of stress, using measures of physiological arousal. In one of their experiments, they studied male and female engineering students' reactions to stress (Collins & Frankenhaeuser 1978). Each subject was tested individually in an experimental (stress) and a control session — each of which lasted 100 minutes and occurred in the morning, a few days apart. The researchers had previously asked the subjects not to smoke or consume any drugs, coffee or alcohol prior to participating.

At the beginning of each session, the subjects gave a urine sample and then ate a light breakfast the researchers provided. In the control condition, the subjects relaxed, read magazines and newspapers, and listened to the radio during the remaining hour or so. In the stress condition, the subjects spent about an hour engaged in a difficult and increasingly stressful cognitive/perceptual task. Heart rate was measured for all subjects continuously during each session, and the subjects gave another urine sample at the end. The urine samples were later analysed for catecholamine (epinephrine and norepinephrine) and corticosteroid (cortisol) concentrations per unit of body weight. The results revealed that heart rate and epinephrine levels increased in both males and females during stress, but other physiological reactions depended on the gender of the subjects.

The outcomes of this and many other studies have led Frankenhaeuser to propose that the pattern of physiological arousal under stress depends on two factors: effort and distress. *Effort* involves the person's interest, striving and determination, and *distress* involves anxiety, uncertainty, boredom and dissatisfaction.

Effort with distress tends to be accompanied by an increase of both catecholamine *and* cortisol excretion. This is the state typical of daily hassles... In working life, it commonly occurs among people engaged in repetitious, machine-paced jobs on the assembly line or in highly routinised work as, for example, at a computer terminal.

Effort without distress is a joyous state, characterised by active and successful coping, high job involvement, and a high degree of personal control. It is accompanied by increased catecholamine secretion, whereas cortisol secretion may be suppressed.

Distress without effort implies feeling helpless, losing control, giving up. It is generally accompanied by increased cortisol secretion, but catecholamines may be elevated, too. This is the endocrine profile typical of depressed patients. (1986, p. 107)

Clearly, psychosocial processes play an important role in physiological reactions to stress.

Research on physiological reactions to stress has shown that it is important to measure more than one index of arousal and to examine psychological and social factors, too.

Another way to measure arousal is to do biochemical analyses of blood, urine or saliva samples to assess the level of hormones that the adrenal glands secrete profusely during stress (van Eck & Nicolson 1994). Using this approach, researchers can test for two classes of hormones: **corticosteroids**, the most important of which is cortisol, and **catecholamines**, which include epinephrine and norepinephrine. The analysis is done by a chemist using special procedures and equipment.

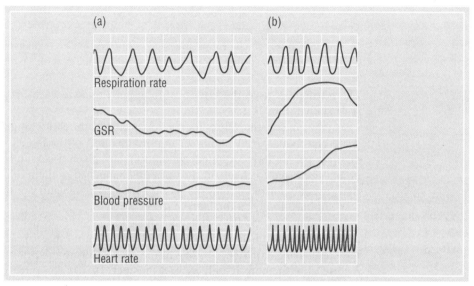

Figure 3.2 A typical polygraph makes a graphical record of several indexes of arousal, including blood pressure, heart rate, respiration rate and galvanic skin response (GSR measures skin conductance, which is affected by sweating). A comparison of the two graphs depicts the difference in arousal between (a) someone who is calm and (b) someone who is under stress.

There are several advantages to using measures of physiological arousal to assess stress (Baum, Grunberg & Singer 1982; Cacioppo, Petty & Marshall-Goodell 1985). Physiological measures are reasonably direct and objective, quite reliable and easily quantified. But there are disadvantages as well. Assessing physiological arousal can be expensive, and the measurement technique may itself be stressful for some people, for example when blood is drawn or when electrical devices are attached to the body. Lastly, measures of physiological arousal are affected by the person's gender, body weight, activity prior to or during measurement, and consumption of various substances, such as caffeine.

Life events

If you wanted to know whether people were feeling stress, you might simply ask them. Using a self-report method is easy to do. But in doing research, you would probably want to get a more precise answer than, 'Yes, I am,' or even, 'Yes, I'm under a lot of stress.' For this reason, a number of different scales have been developed to measure people's stress and assign it a numerical value.

The social readjustment rating scale

One approach many scales have used is to develop a list of **life events** — major happenings that can occur in a person's life that require some degree of psychological adjustment. The scale assigns to each event a value that reflects its stressfulness. One of the most widely used scales of life events has been the *Social Readjustment Rating Scale* (SRRS) developed by Thomas Holmes and Richard Rahe (1967). To develop this scale, these researchers constructed a list of events they derived from clinical experience. Then they had hundreds of men and women of various ages and backgrounds rate the amount of adjustment each event would require, using the following instructions.

> *Use all of your experience* in arriving at your answer. This means personal experience where it applies as well as what you have learned to be the case for others. Some persons accommodate to change more readily than others; some persons adjust with particular ease or difficulty to only certain events. Therefore, strive to give your opinion of the average degree of readjustment necessary for each event rather than the extreme. (p. 213)

The researchers used these ratings to assign values to each event and construct the scale shown in table 3.1.

As you can see, the values for the life events in the SRRS range from 100 points for death of a spouse to 11 points for minor violations of the law. To measure the amount of stress people have experienced, subjects are given a survey form listing these life events and asked to check off the ones that happened to them during a given period of time, usually not more than the past 24 months. The values of the checked items are then summed to give a total stress score.

How commonly do life events like those in the SRRS occur? A study of nearly 2800 adults used a modified version of the SRRS and found that 15 per cent of the subjects reported having experienced none of the events during the prior year, and 18 per cent reported five or more (Goldberg & Comstock 1980). The three most frequent events reported were 'took a vacation' (43 per cent), 'death of a loved one or other important person' (22 per cent), and 'illness or injury' (21 per cent). The number of life events the subjects reported *decreased* with age from early adulthood to old age and *increased* with the number of years of schooling. Single, separated and divorced people reported larger numbers of events than married and widowed individuals did.

Strengths and weaknesses of the SRRS

When you examined the list of life events included in the SRRS, you probably noticed that many of the events were ones we have already discussed as stressors, such as the death of a spouse, divorce, pregnancy and occupational problems. One of the strengths of the SRRS is that the items it includes represent a fairly wide range of events that most people do, in fact, find stressful. Also, the values assigned to the events were carefully determined from the ratings of a broad sample of adults. These values provide an estimate of the relative impact of the events, distinguishing fairly well between such stressors as 'death of a close family member' and 'death of a close friend'. Another strength of the SRRS is that the survey form can be filled out easily and quickly.

One of the main uses of the SRRS has been to relate stress and illness. Many studies have addressed this issue by using retrospective approaches — for example by asking subjects to recall events and illnesses they experienced over the past year. Other studies have combined retrospective and prospective methods — for instance by having subjects report recent life events and then checking their medical records over the next months. Studies using these approaches have generally found that people's illness and accident rates tend to increase following increases in stress (Holmes & Masuda 1974; Johnson 1986; Rahe 1974, 1987; Rahe & Arthur 1978). But the correlation between subjects' scores on the SRRS and illness is only about 0.30 — which means that the relationship is not very strong (Dohrenwend & Dohrenwend 1981).

Table 3.1 Social readjustment rating scale

Rank	Life event	Mean value
1	Death of spouse	100
2	Divorce	73
3	Marital separation	65
4	Gaol term	63
5	Death of close family member	63
6	Personal injury or illness	53
7	Marriage	50
8	Fired at work	47
9	Marital reconciliation	45
10	Retirement	45
11	Change in health of family member	44
12	Pregnancy	40
13	Sex difficulties	39
14	Gain of new family member	39
15	Business readjustment	39
16	Change in financial state	38
17	Death of close friend	37
18	Change to different line of work	36
19	Change in number of arguments with spouse	35
20	Mortgage over $10 000	31
21	Foreclosure of mortgage or loan	30
22	Change in responsibilities at work	29
23	Son or daughter leaving home	29
24	Trouble with in-laws	29
25	Outstanding personal achievement	28
26	Wife begins or stops work	26
27	Begin or end school	26
28	Change in living conditions	25
29	Revision of personal habits	24
30	Trouble with boss	23
31	Change in work hours or conditions	20
32	Change in residence	20
33	Change in schools	20
34	Change in recreation	19
35	Change in church activities	19
36	Change in social activities	18
37	Mortgage or loan less than $10 000	17
38	Change in sleeping habits	16
39	Change in number of family get-togethers	15
40	Change in eating habits	15
41	Vacation	13
42	Christmas	12
43	Minor violations of the law	11

Source: From Holmes & Rahe (1967, table 3).

One reason that the relationship is not stronger is that some individuals may take longer to resolve the same or similar events. One person may still be distressed by marital infidelity of a partner that occurred five years ago, while another may show no distress to a recent divorce. If a 12-month time frame is used to study the relationship between life event stress and illness, the relationship would be reduced because the second person has been able to resolve the event, while the first person would be reporting distress in the absence of an event. Timing of measurement and event resolution can therefore affect the results obtained (Thoits 1994; Turner & Avison 1992). People may also get sick and have accidents for many reasons other than stress. Another reason for the low association between life event stress and illness is that the SRRS has several weaknesses.

Some researchers have criticised items in the SRRS as being vague or ambiguous and thus limiting the validity of the scale (Hough, Fairbank & Garcia 1976). For example, the item 'personal injury or illness' receives a weight of 53 regardless of the severity or nature of the illness or injury. Someone with a life-threatening illness would receive the same score as another person with a headcold or knee sprain. Fifteen of the items ask the individual if a change has occurred in relation to a life task, life domain, relationship or personal habit. The item 'change in responsibilities at work' does not distinguish between a person whose workload has increased and the decreased work demands of another person. Both receive the same weight for the item. Change in the number of arguments with spouse does not indicate whether arguments have increased or decreased. Similarly, 'change in financial state' does not distinguish between the bankrupt person and the million-dollar lotto winner. The SRRS does not assess whether the changes have been positive or negative, welcomed or unwelcomed by the person, expected or unexpected. Vague or ambiguous items reduce the precision of an instrument and the correlation it is likely to have with other variables (Cohen & Swerdlik 1999).

Another criticism is that the scale does not consider the meaning or impact of an event for the individual (Cohen, Kamarck & Mermelstein 1983; Lazarus & Folkman 1984b). For example, two people who each had a mortgage for $50 000 would get the same score for 'mortgage over $10 000' even though one of them made ten times the income of the other. Divorce receives a weight of 73 in the SRRS. Individuals in abusive or unfulfilling relationships may view divorce not as negative or stressful, but rather as a liberating event. Even events like 'death of spouse' would have a very different impact depending on the nature of the death, the age of the spouse and dependence on the spouse. Death may be welcomed for the spouse suffering from terminal cancer. Yet the score people get for this item is the same. These items do not take the person's subjective appraisal into account, and this may also reduce the precision of the instrument.

The SRRS has also been criticised for its inclusion of life events that may be con-founded with measures of illness (Sarason, Sarason & Johnson 1985). Some of the items, such as changes in eating habits, changes in sleeping habits, and personal injury or ill-ness, may strengthen correlations between life event stress and illness. Some researchers (Thoits 1983) have adopted the strategy of removing these life events before correlating total stress and illness. Care must be taken when doing so not to alter the psychometric properties of the scale, or change the life domain being assessed for stress (Cohen, Kessler & Underwood Gordon 1995). Where confounding may be an issue, adjusted correlations should be reported along with correlations for total life stress and illness.

Another criticism of the SRRS concerns its failure to take into account the desir-ability of events for the experience of stress (Sarason et al. 1985). The SRRS assumes that change per se is stressful, but it is the nature of the change that is more important. Research findings indicate that undesirable events are associated with illness, whereas desirable events are not (Harris 1997; Ross & Mirowsky 1979). The SRRS does not distinguish between desirable and undesirable events. Some events, such as death of spouse, gaol term and being fired at work, would be viewed as undesirable by most persons. Similarly, outstanding personal achievement is viewed by most people as a desirable event. Other events may be desirable or undesirable. Whether or not change to a different line of work is perceived as desirable or undesirable depends on expectations of the worker, whether the changed conditions were sought by the person or imposed on the person, and whether or not the work fulfils an individual's personal and financial needs. These aspects of life events important in the experience of stress can only be addressed through more precise wording.

The SRRS has been revised by Hobson et al. (1998) to address the above criticisms. The new instrument contained 51 life events. Confounding of life events with symptoms was eliminated, and items were worded to be less ambiguous. Weighting of life events (unit weighting, community weights or subjective weights) was also considered. The revised inventory was administered to 3122 respondents. The findings indicated strong agreement regarding the perceived stressfulness of life events regardless of gender, age or income level. Differential weights were favoured over unit weights (items weighted 1 for present and 0 for absent) for assessing the impact on health, as they more adequately reflected meaningful differences in the way respondents evaluated the stressfulness of life events. Other research (Turner & Wheaton 1995) has found that the SRRS is just as good a measure when unit weighting is used, and that unit weights predict illness symptoms and psychological distress.

Other life events scales

Several life events scales that have attempted to improve on the method of the SRRS are outlined below.

1. *The Life Experiences Survey* (LES) contains 57 items that are stated relatively precisely, for example 'major change in financial status (a lot better off or a lot worse off)'. Subjects rate each event on a seven-point scale, ranging from extremely negative (-3) to extremely positive ($+3$). The items perceived as positive or as negative can be examined separately or combined for a total change score (Sarason, Johnson & Siegel 1978).

2. *The PERI Life Events Scale* contains 102 items that describe events involving a gain, a loss or an ambiguous outcome. The items are stated clearly and organised into 11 topic areas, including work, finances, family and health. For example, an item dealing with work is, 'took on a greatly increased workload'. Like the SRRS, each item has an assigned value, and the subject simply indicates which events occurred within a given time period (Dohrenwend et al. 1978).

3. In Australia, Tennant and Andrews (1976) extended the work of Holmes and Rahe (1967) and Paykel, Prusoff and Uhlenhuth (1971) by developing a scale for measuring the stress of life events that accounts for life change produced by the event and the amount of distress caused by the event. The scale consists of 67 life events relating to health, bereavement, family and social, friends and relatives, education, work and moving house. Sets of events applicable only to males, females, the single, those who are or were married, and those who have or have had children are incorporated in the scale. The events are worded so as to minimise the likelihood of confounding with stress reactions. The *Life Events Inventory* has good validity and is suitable for an Australian urban sample.

New scales such as these are being used extensively in research today. Through this research, we should be able to determine which scales are likely to be most useful as measures of stress.

The instruments we have discussed so far have been designed to measure stress mainly in adults. Other scales have been developed to measure stress in children and adolescents. The most widely used scale for children is the *Life Events Record*, which is very similar to the SRRS in its format and scoring (Coddington 1972a, 1972b). The items are relevant to children, such as 'divorce of parents' and 'change to a different school', and are assigned separate values for children of different age groups. When children are not old enough to respond to the items themselves, their parents complete the scale for them. Because the Life Events Record has many of the same problems as the SRRS, other instruments for children have been developed (Johnson 1986).

A more recent approach to assessing life event stress is the use of the personal interview method, as in the *Life Events and Difficulties Schedule*, a semi-structured survey instrument (Harris 1991; Wethington, Brown & Kessler 1995). Detailed information is collected about events experienced by the respondent in the previous 12 months. This information is then evaluated along with social and biographical data on the person to give a contextual rating of threat associated with each event. The approach uses trained raters to evaluate contextual threat, rather than individual subjective reactions.

Daily hassles

Some researchers have argued that life events tap a specific type of stress, namely stress due to one-off events. Although the incidence of divorce and remarriage has increased in the past 20 years, many individuals may not experience these events. At worst, they may divorce once and choose to remarry, cohabit or remain alone. Death of spouse may occur only once in a lifetime for most people. Many of the life events assessed in psychological instruments are rare in occurrence and spread out over the life span. Stress may result from minor incidents in a person's everyday life, such as losing one's car keys or being late for an appointment. Other stressors may be a constant part of our lives — for example traffic congestion, urban pollution, unfriendly neighbours, competitive co-workers, or concern about one's weight and physical appearance. These ongoing everyday stressors that are a constant feature of our lives are called **daily hassles** and may be more damaging to our health than the major life events, which occur with less frequency.

Richard Lazarus and his associates have constructed a scale to measure people's experiences with day-to-day unpleasant or potentially harmful events (Kanner et al. 1981). This instrument — called the *Hassles Scale* — lists 117 of these events that range from minor annoyances, such as 'silly practical mistakes', to major problems or difficulties, such as 'not enough money for food'. The subjects indicate which hassles occurred in the past month and rate each event as having been 'somewhat', 'moderately' or 'extremely' severe. These researchers tested 100 middle-aged adults monthly over a nine-month period. The half-dozen most frequent hassles reported were:

- concerns about weight
- rising prices of common goods
- too many things to do
- health of a family member
- home maintenance
- misplacing or losing things.

In the course of developing the Hassles Scale, these researchers proposed that having desirable experiences makes hassles more bearable and reduces their impact on health. So they developed another instrument, the *Uplifts Scale*, which lists 135 events that bring peace, satisfaction or joy. This instrument was administered along with the Hassles Scale to the same adults, who indicated which uplifts they experienced in the past month and whether each event had been 'somewhat', 'moderately' or 'extremely' strong. Some of the most frequently occurring uplifts were 'relating well to your spouse or lover', 'completing a task' and 'feeling healthy'.

The measurement of hassles has continued in the past decade with the work of Kohn and co-researchers, who have developed hassles measures for specific subgroups, such as university students (Kohn, Lafreniere & Gurevich 1990), adolescents (Kohn & Milrose 1993) and adults (Kohn & Macdonald 1992). Recent refinement of existing hassles measures has been conducted by Australian researchers (Maybery 1998; Maybery & Graham 2001) to include daily interpersonal sources of distress and uplifting experiences.

Are hassles and uplifts related to health? Several studies have examined this issue. One study tested middle-aged adults, using four instruments: (1) the Hassles Scale; (2) the Uplifts Scale; (3) a life events scale that includes no desirable items; and (4) the Health Status Questionnaire, which contains questions regarding a wide variety of bodily symptoms and overall health (DeLongis et al. 1982). Both hassles scores and life events scores were associated with health status — both correlations were weak, but hassles were more strongly associated with health than life events were. Uplifts scores had virtually no association with health status. Daily hassles can also impact on health indirectly through reduced physical activity, smoking (Twisk et al. 1999), alcohol consumption (Steptoe, Lipsey & Wardle 1998) and eating behaviour (Conner, Fitter & Fletcher 1999). Other studies generally support these findings regarding the relationship of hassles and uplifts to health (Gortmaker, Eckenrode & Gore 1982; Holahan, Holahan & Belk 1984; Weinberger, Hiner & Tierney 1987; Zarski 1984).

What effect do daily hassles have on psychological wellbeing? An Australian study (Caltabiano & Caltabiano 1992) addressed this question for a group of first-year university students six months after admission. A subset of 91 hassles from Kanner et al.'s (1981) scale were used so as to be more relevant to the life experiences of students. The hassles were categorised into social, family, financial, personal failings, general concerns, personal concerns about future, time management, general health and appearance, and drug related. On average the students reported experiencing 50 of the 91 hassles and that they were moderate in severity. Chronic ongoing stress for students was associated with family problems, time-management problems, personal concerns about the future, personal failings and general appearance. Compared with the general population, students were relatively unconcerned about general hassles relating to traffic, pollution, crime or the weather. The percentage of students who reported experiencing moderate to severe hassles within each category is presented in table 3.2. Females reported more hassles relating to personal failings, time-management problems and concern about family members. Total number of hassles was highly correlated with symptoms of psychological distress ($r = 0.51$), indicating that the more hassles reported by students, the more symptoms experienced. Daily hassles have also been found to be associated with psychological aspects of health such as negative mood (Dennerstein et al. 1999) and diminished life satisfaction (Hart 1999). Recent evidence (Maybery & Graham 2001) indicates that daily interpersonal sources of distress may be more important than other daily hassles in determining mood and global distress.

An overview regarding measures of stress indicates that the instruments available either have shortcomings or have not been sufficiently tested to confirm how accurate they are. Researchers have found that self-report measures of life events are unreliable: A study had subjects fill out a scale regarding life events they experienced during the prior year and then fill out the same scale each month during the next year. The extent to which their later reports agreed with the first measurement declined sharply over time (Raphael, Cloitre & Dohrenwend 1991). Stress is a difficult concept to define, and it is even more difficult to measure. Still, judging from the evidence, stress seems to have a consistent but moderate relationship to health. Stress is one of many factors that contribute to the development of illness.

Table 3.2 Percentage of undergraduate university students reporting experiencing different hassles as severe in intensity

Hassles	% Reporting
Social	18
Family	41
Financial	13
Personal failings	23
General concerns	9
Personal concerns about the future	26
Time management	29
Health and appearance	22
Drugs	12

Source: Caltabiano & Caltabiano (1992–93, table 2).

Disaster and traumatic events

On Christmas Eve, 1974, residents of the city of Darwin were victims to one of the worst cyclones to hit northern Australia. Most of the residents were unprepared for the disaster. Homes were totally destroyed in the cyclone. Survivors had to rebuild their lives, much as Darwin had to be rebuilt physically. Many adults suffered psychological disturbance in the form of nervousness, depression, restlessness and worry about the future. Darwin residents who were evacuated seemed to suffer the most. Young children displayed fearful reactions to wind and rain and reminders of the cyclone. (Milne 1977a, 1977b)

On Ash Wednesday, 1983, fire destroyed an area of 2804 square kilometres of land in the adjoining Australian states of Victoria and South Australia, causing damage to bushland and national parklands, grazing pastures and orchard farms. Seventy-two people lost their lives and more than 2000 homes were destroyed. Damage to livestock incurred a substantial financial loss for graziers and herdsmen, with 335 000 sheep and 10 000 cattle dead. A follow-up of 1515 victims of the fire found 40 per cent to have some psychiatric impairment 12 months later. (Clayer 1984; Leach 1994)

On the morning of 28 December 1989, Newcastle experienced an earthquake measuring 5.6 on the Richter Scale. Thirteen people died and 163 people were treated for injuries. Thousands of businesses and homes sustained damage from the earthquake, whose impact spanned an area of 300 000 square kilometres. Many received counselling for psychological distress. The most common symptoms were recurring thoughts of the disaster, avoidance of recurring thoughts, sleep disturbance, depressed mood, diminished concentration and diminished interest in life. (Carr et al. 1992; Cotton & Anderson 1991)

What do all of these incidents have in common? So far in this chapter the events inducing stress in individuals have been associated with life-span transitions, have been relatively expected and have affected the individual, and at most the immediate family. Traumatic events are broad in their impact, often affecting whole communities; they may last several hours to several days, usually involve devastation to the physical environment, and may affect the very social structure of the community. Major traumatic events include natural disasters such as cyclones, earthquakes, flood and fire as well as human-initiated events like the civil war in the former Yugoslavia, the Tiananmen Square massacre in 1989 and atrocities inflicted on prisoners of war. Often overlooked are events due to accident or mishap involving one individual or a small group of people, but which are traumatic in their effects. These are events such as the Moura underground mine disaster, plane crashes, car accident pile-ups, the collapse of a bridge or dam. Other events involving threats to survival and psychological trauma include being adrift at sea, being lost in dense bushland and being trapped under fallen building debris.

Psychosocial responses to disaster and trauma

What conditions are necessary for an event to be classified as a disaster? Some researchers (Barton 1969; Berren, Beigel & Ghertner 1980; Gleser, Green & Winget 1981) have used a **structural approach** to describe the properties or dimensions of disasters. For example, disasters have been differentiated along the dimensions of degree of impact, duration, preparedness of the community, proportion of the community affected and the nature of suffering. Others (Tyhurst 1951; Leach 1994) have used a **dynamic approach** to understanding reactions to disaster before, during and after the event. Leach (1994) has proposed a five-dimensional model of *pre-impact phase* (threat stage, warning stage), *impact phase*, *recoil phase*, *rescue phase* and *post-trauma phase*. The period of impact refers to the actual experience of disaster, such as when a train is derailed, a tropical cyclone hits a coastal town, a person is trapped under falling rubble in an earthquake, or a fire in an apartment block prevents escape. The period of recoil occurs when the immediate threat has subsided but secondary threats to survival exist. For instance, people who have escaped a sinking ship by resorting to a life raft have to face the ordeal of many hours or even days at sea in a confined space without food and water. The immediate threat of danger during a cyclone may appear to have passed to those with little experience with such natural disasters. Wind speed may intensify with impact, coming from the opposite direction. The period of post-trauma refers to the last phase in the course of a disaster, when the victim has either been rescued or has physically survived the disaster. Psychological and physiological recovery are nevertheless important during this period for full functioning of the individual and integration back into society.

In a review of response patterns across a diverse range of disaster situations, Leach (1994) found that the human reaction to disaster is consistent irrespective of the nature of disaster. In the pre-impact stages, the typical psychological response is denial of the impending threat, while the typical behavioural pattern is one of inactivity. Warnings are ignored and few precautions taken. During impact of the disaster, only a small percentage of the population remains calm and shows appropriate behaviour. In the period of recoil, confusion in survivors gives way to awareness of death and injury of family members, and the extent of damage to property. Survivors give vent to emotions and exhibit a psychological dependency on rescue workers. In the post-trauma phase, survivors attempt to rebuild their lives. Psychological symptoms associated with this stage include anxiety, depression and recurrent dreams of the event.

Although there is individual variability in emotional reactions and behaviour over the course of a disaster, some typical reactions have been identified (Leach 1994). Panic may occur when there is a perceived time and space limit on survival, for instance when a person is trapped beneath rocks and the incoming tide will make drowning inevitable. Anxiety is a common emotion that can paralyse the victim, rendering him or her unable to move or to think. Depression and apathy are typically experienced in association with denial as a coping mechanism. In the recoil phase these emotional reactions can be life threatening as they prevent protective actions, for instance against hypothermia and dehydration. Anger is a universal reaction among disaster victims. This anger is often irrational and is misdirected towards rescue workers. Perceptual distortion is also common during disaster situations. This involves a narrowing of perception and awareness to facilitate concentration on a specific task. However, the behaviour selected may be ineffective for survival. Hyper-activity is typical immediately after impact. Behaviour may appear purposeful although ineffective. Since dependency in victims is high following impact, hyperactivity in individuals may be mistaken for leadership and knowledge, with adverse effects on survival. Guilt is a common emotion in the recoil and post-trauma phases, especially if the individual has survived family and friends.

Are certain coping behaviours and resources associated with survival in arduous circumstances? One of the strongest predictors of survival is the 'will to live', or a sense of purposefulness in the victim. This personality resource is commonly seen in the survivors of Nazi concentration camps and in prisoners of war (Wilner 1976). Sense of purpose is most likely tied in with another characteristic of long-term survivors — attachment to family. Those victims who have a family to return to are more likely to endure torture, fatigue and injury in the hope of being reunited with loved ones. Long-term survival is a process of adaptation to circumstances. Leach (1994) argues that active-passiveness in victims facilitates adaptation in that the person must accept the situation but not give in to it. Other personality resources that facilitate coping and hence survival include self-efficacy and a sense of humour. Those for whom the above coping resources are absent are more likely to experience psychological breakdown and even death. Psychological breakdown is characterised by irritability, sleep disturbance, mild startle reaction, social withdrawal, loss of interest, apprehension, general psychomotor retardation and confusion (Joseph, Williams & Yule 1997; Leach 1994).

Post-traumatic stress disorder (PTSD) is the diagnostic label given to persons who have been affected by a major traumatic event. Also referred to as 'shell shock' or 'battle fatigue', PTSD is well known as a disorder of war veterans. The disorder can, however, result from a range of traumatic events such as sexual assault, serious accident, natural disaster, acts of terrorism or major surgery (Blanchard et al. 1998; Joseph et al. 1997; Pinkowish 1999). Children as well as adults can experience PTSD. An event does not have to be experienced personally for symptoms of PTSD to occur. Persons who witness a horrific event are also susceptible to the symptoms of PTSD. So what are the symptoms necessary for a classification of PTSD?

The Diagnostic Statistical Manual (DSM) IV, revised in 1994, requires that one or more of the following symptoms be present for a diagnosis of PTSD: flashbacks in which the person relives the traumatic event; distressing recurrent dreams about the event; or intense psychological distress when exposed to events associated with the trauma. Two or more avoidance symptoms are required for diagnosis. These can take the form of psychological numbing or diminished interest in former activities, inability to recall the event, not talking about the event, emotional detachment from family and a sense of a foreshortened future. At least two symptoms of increased arousal also need to be present. Increased arousal is demonstrated by startle reactions, sleeping problems, memory problems, difficulty in concentrating, moodiness and violence. Symptoms need to have persisted for more than three months to indicate chronic PTSD. Persons displaying PTSD often have other psychological problems such as an anxiety or personality disorder (Pinkowish 1999), or may show substance abuse (Kofoed, Friedman & Peck 1993). PTSD is debilitating not only for the sufferer but also for the families of those with the disorder (Westerink & Giarratano 1999). Psychologists who work with sufferers of PTSD acknowledge the importance of assessing the psychological aftermath of exposure to trauma and disaster.

Post-traumatic stress disorder does not always occur in response to traumatic events. Some persons are able to maintain normal and productive lives even after experiencing extreme trauma. What theoretical explanations have been offered for the occurrence of

PTSD symptoms? Post-traumatic reactions could be the result of classically conditioned associations between fear and traumatic stimuli, which are maintained through avoidance of memories of the event, and of situations that resemble the event. Some psychologists have argued that PTSD is an analogue of learned helplessness, as the affected individual is subjected to an aversive event over which he or she has no control (van der Kolk 1987; Cotton & Anderson 1991). Information processing theories have also been offered. Horowitz (1975) proposed that traumatic events cause individuals to re-evaluate existing schemas of the world. Active memory of the event leads to emotional distress, which is regulated through an information control system. PTSD intrusion symptoms such as nightmares and flashbacks occur when inhibitory control is weak. When inhibitory control is strong, avoidance symptoms such as inability to recall occur. Foa, Steketee & Rothbaum (1989) postulate a fear network in memory consisting of information about the traumatic event, and information about cognitive, behavioural and physiological reactions to the event. When the fear network is activated, the traumatic event is relived. Avoidance symptoms represent efforts to suppress activation of the fear network. Some theorists, such as Creamer, Burgess and Pattison (1992), argue that activation of the fear network, which they term **network resolution processing**, is important for recovery. High-level intrusions (recurring thoughts, flashbacks) following a traumatic event, and avoidance coping, indicate that the person is reappraising the event and actively working through the trauma. Australian research by McFarlane (1992) has found contradictory evidence for the theorised benefit of network resolution processing. In a study of 290 firefighters, intrusive thoughts at four months were predictive of greater distress at 11 months, and intrusive thoughts at 11 months were predictive of distress at 29 months.

Post-traumatic stress disorder can affect persons present at the scene of tragedy, although they may not have directly experienced the traumatic event. Emergency service workers are just as likely to experience PTSD as are the victims of tragedy. Some occupations are also more likely than others to expose the worker to danger or critical incidents that can have a traumatic effect on the person. For example, police officers are at risk of losing their lives in a shoot-out, or being the victims of criminal aggression. Mitchell (1983) has advocated that some form of crisis intervention occur in the first 72 hours following a critical incident. **Critical incident stress debriefing** (CISD) involves seven phases. These are:

1. *introduction.* Ground rules are established, confidentiality emphasised and participants urged to talk if they so desire.
2. *facts.* Participants provide a description of the incident from their own perspective.
3. *thoughts.* Personal discussion of first thoughts of the event is encouraged.
4. *emotions.* Participants are encouraged to discuss their emotional reactions.
5. *assessment.* Physical and psychological symptoms are recorded.
6. *education.* Stress reactions and coping strategies are discussed.
7. *re-entry.* Question time — a facilitator summarises and concludes debriefing session, providing contact phone numbers.

Leonard and Alison (1999) studied the benefits of CISD in relation to coping and anger management in Australian police officers involved in shooting incidents. They found some support for the effectiveness of CISD, in that police officers who received CISD engaged in more adaptive coping strategies and showed less anger, compared with those officers who did not receive the debriefing.

Can stress be good for you?

Another reason why measures of stress do not correlate very highly with illness may be that not all stress is unhealthy. Is it possible that some types or amounts of stress are neutral or, perhaps, *good* for you? There is reason to believe that this is the case (Seliger 1986).

How much stress may be good for people? Some theories of motivation and arousal propose that people function best, and feel best, at what is *for them* an optimal level of arousal (Fiske & Maddi 1961; Hebb 1955). People differ in the amount of arousal that is optimal, but too much or too little arousal impairs their functioning. Figure 3.3 gives an illustration of how stress, as a form of arousal, relates to the quality of functioning. Let's consider an example of how different levels of stress affect functioning. Imagine that you are in class one day and your instructor passes around a surprise test. If the test would not be collected or count towards your final grade, you might be underaroused and answer the questions carelessly or not at all. But if it were to count as 10 per cent of your grade, you might be under enough stress to perform well. And if it counted a lot, you might be overwhelmed by the stress and do poorly.

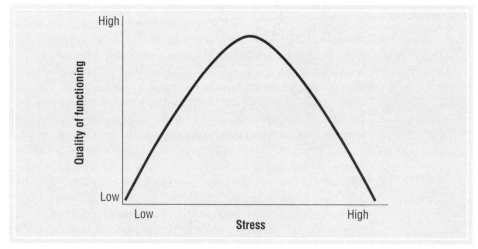

Figure 3.3 Quality of functioning at varying levels of stress. Functioning is poor at very low and very high levels of stress but is best at some moderate, 'optimal' level.

Source: Based on material in Hebb (1955).

Are some types of stress better than others for people? Three prominent researchers on stress have taken very similar positions on this question, claiming that there are at least two kinds of stress that differ in their impact. Selye (1974, 1985), for instance, claimed one kind of stress is harmful and damaging, and is called *distress*; another kind is beneficial or constructive, and is called *eustress* (from the Greek *eu*, which means 'good'). Similarly, as we saw earlier, Frankenhaeuser (1986) has described two components of stress, *distress* and *effort*. Distress with or without effort is probably more damaging than effort without distress. Last, Lazarus has described three types of stress appraisals — *harm–loss*, *threat* and *challenge* — and noted:

> Challenged persons are more likely to have better morale, because to be challenged means feeling positive about demanding encounters, as reflected in the pleasurable emotions accompanying challenge. The quality of functioning is apt to be better in challenge because the person feels more confident, less emotionally overwhelmed, and more capable of drawing on available resources than the person who is inhibited or blocked. Finally, it is possible that the physiological stress response to challenge is different from that of threat, so that diseases of adaptation are less likely to occur. (Lazarus & Folkman 1984b, p. 34)

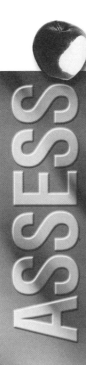

Assess yourself

HASSLES IN YOUR LIFE

Table 3.3 gives a list of circumstances you may sometimes find unpleasant because they make you irritated, frustrated or anxious. Beside each item, estimate its frequency and the usual degree of unpleasantness it produces for you, using the following two scales:

- **FREQ** (*frequency* in last *three months*):
  1 = rarely or not at all,
  2 = occasionally,
  3 = often,
  4 = very often,
  5 = extremely often.

- **UNPL** (*unpleasantness* — usual degree):
  1 = mildly or not unpleasant,
  2 = moderately unpleasant,
  3 = very unpleasant,
  4 = extremely unpleasant.

Multiply the FREQ and UNPL scores for each item, and sum the products for a total score. You can evaluate your relative hassles with the following schedule: Compared with the stress other university students have from hassles, a total score of 300 is about average, 450 indicates much more stress, and 150 indicates much less stress.

Table 3.3 Hassles Assessment Scale for Students in College (HASS/Col)

FREQ	UNPL	
_____	_____	Annoying social behaviour of others (e.g. inconsiderate, rude, sexist/racist)
_____	_____	Annoying behaviour of self (e.g. habits, temper)
_____	_____	Appearance of self (e.g. attractiveness, clothing, grooming)
_____	_____	Accidents/clumsiness/mistakes of self (e.g. spilling beverage, tripping)
_____	_____	Athletic activities of self (e.g. performance, time demands)
_____	_____	Bills/overspending
_____	_____	Boredom (e.g. nothing to do, current activity uninteresting)
_____	_____	Car problems (e.g. breaking down, repairs)
_____	_____	Crowds/large social groups (e.g. at parties, while shopping)
_____	_____	Dating (e.g. lack of, uninteresting partner)
_____	_____	Environment: physical living or working conditions
_____	_____	Extracurricular groups (e.g. responsibilities, activities)
_____	_____	Exams (e.g. preparing for, taking)
_____	_____	Exercising (e.g. unpleasant routines, time to do)
_____	_____	Facilities/resources unavailable (e.g. computers, library materials)
_____	_____	Family: obligations or activities
_____	_____	Family: relationship problems
_____	_____	Fears of physical safety (e.g. walking alone, flying, heights)
_____	_____	Fitness: inadequate physical condition
_____	_____	Flatmate(s)/housemate(s): conflicts with
_____	_____	Food/meals (e.g. unappealing, unhealthful)
_____	_____	Forgetting to do things (e.g. to tape TV show, send cards, do homework)
_____	_____	Friends/peers: relationship problems

(*continued*)

Table 3.3 *Continued*

FREQ	UNPL	
———	———	Future plans (e.g. career, marital)
———	———	Getting up early (e.g. for class or work)
———	———	Girl/boyfriend: relationship problems
———	———	Goals/tasks: not completing enough
———	———	Grades (e.g. not high enough, pressure to do well)
———	———	Health/physical symptoms of self (e.g. flu, PMS, allergies, headaches)
———	———	Homework demands or difficulty (e.g. exams, assignments, reading text)
———	———	Housing: finding/getting or moving
———	———	Injustice: seeing examples of or being a victim of
———	———	Job: searching for or interviews
———	———	Job/work: problems (e.g. demands of, dislike of work or boss)
———	———	Lateness of self (e.g. for appointment or class)
———	———	Lecturers/tutors (e.g. unfairness, unavailability, demands of)
———	———	Losing or misplacing things (e.g. keys, books)
———	———	Loneliness (e.g. lack of friends, missing distant friends or family)
———	———	Medical/dental treatment (e.g. unpleasant, time demands)
———	———	Money: lack of
———	———	New experiences or challenges
———	———	Noise of other people or animals
———	———	Oral presentations/public speaking
———	———	Parking problems (e.g. on campus, at work, at home)
———	———	Peer pressure/social acceptance
———	———	Personal confidence
———	———	Pregnancy: symptoms suggesting (e.g. of self or girlfriend)
———	———	Privacy: lack of
———	———	Registering for or selecting classes to take
———	———	Sex: lack of or problems having
———	———	Sexually transmitted diseases (e.g. concerns about, efforts to reduce risk of AIDS)
———	———	Sleep: lack of
———	———	Sports team/celebrity performance (e.g. favourite professional or recreational team losing)
———	———	Studying: problems with motivation or concentration
———	———	Substance use problems of self or others (e.g. drinking too much, quitting smoking)
———	———	Tedious everyday chores (e.g. shopping, cleaning apartment)
———	———	Time demands/deadlines
———	———	Traffic problems (e.g. traffic jams, inconsiderate or careless drivers)
———	———	Traffic tickets: getting (e.g. for moving or parking violations)
———	———	Waiting (e.g. for appointments, in lines, on the phone)
———	———	Weather problems (e.g. snow, heat/humidity, storms)
———	———	Weight/dietary control problems

Source: Based on Sarafino (1997b).

There is a commonality to these three positions: To state it in its simplest form, there is good stress and bad stress — bad stress generally involves a strong negative emotional component. Cognitive appraisal processes play an important role in determining which kind of stress we experience.

Finally, in discussing whether stress is harmful, one other point should be made: individuals seem to differ in their susceptibility to the effects of stress. John Mason (1975) has proposed that these differences are like those that people show to the effects of viruses and bacteria. That is, not all people who are exposed to a disease-causing antigen, such as a flu virus, develop the illness — some individuals are more susceptible than others. Susceptibility to the effects of antigens and to stress varies from one person to the next and within the same individual across time. These differences result from biological variations within and between individuals, and from psychosocial variations, as we will see in the next chapter.

Summary

Researchers have conceptualised stress in three ways. In one approach, stress is seen as a stimulus, and studies focus on the impact of stressors. Another approach treats stress as a response and examines the strains that stressors produce. The third approach views stress as a process that involves continuous interactions and adjustments — or transactions — between the person and the environment. These viewpoints have led to the definition of stress as the condition that results when person/environment transactions lead the individual to perceive a discrepancy between the demands of a situation and the resources of the person's biological, psychological and social systems.

Transactions that lead to the condition of stress generally involve a process of cognitive appraisal, which takes two forms. One type of appraisal, called primary appraisal, focuses on whether a demand threatens the person's wellbeing. It produces one of three judgements: the demand is irrelevant, it is good or it is stressful. A stressful appraisal receives further assessment for the amount of harm or loss, the threat of future harm and the degree of challenge the demand presents. The other type of appraisal, called secondary appraisal, assesses the resources available for meeting the demand. When primary and secondary appraisals indicate that the fit between demands and resources is close, we may experience little stress. But when we appraise a discrepancy — especially if the demands seem greater than our resources — we may feel a substantial amount of stress.

Whether events are appraised as stressful is influenced by two types of factors — those that relate to the person and those that relate to the situation. Factors of the person include intellectual, motivational and personality characteristics, such as the person's self-esteem, neurotic tendencies and belief system. With regard to situational factors, events tend to be appraised as stressful if they involve strong demands, are imminent, are undesirable and uncontrollable, involve major life transitions, or occur at an unexpected time in the life span.

Stressors produce strain in the person's biological, psychological and social systems. Emergency situations evoke a physiological fight-or-flight reaction, by which the organism prepares to attack the threat or flee. When stress is strong and prolonged, the physiological reaction goes through three stages: the alarm reaction, the stage of resistance and the stage of exhaustion. This series of reactions is called the general adaptation syndrome. According to Selye, continuous high levels of stress can make the person vulnerable to diseases of adaptation, including ulcers and high blood pressure. Psychosocial factors influence the physiological reaction to stress.

Stress can affect psychosocial processes. It can impair cognitive functioning and may lead to generalised cognitive deficits in children. Various emotions can accompany stress — these emotions include fear, anxiety, depression and anger. When stress is accompanied by anger, aggressive behaviour tends to increase and remain at a relatively high level even after the stressful experience is over. Stress also reduces people's helping behaviour.

Although the sources of stress may change as people develop, the condition of stress can occur at any time in the life span. Sometimes stress arises from within the person, such as when the person is ill or experiences conflict. The family can be another source of stress, through the behaviour, needs and personality of each of its members. The whole family can experience stress (1) when one of its members is seriously ill, becomes disabled or dies; (2) if the parents separate or divorce; and (3) if there is an addition to the family, particularly if the addition is a baby who has a difficult temperament. How the family reacts to these stressors depends on the ages of the people involved. The source of stress can also be the community and society — for example from problems related to people's jobs or environmental hazards. Sometimes traumatic events can have a broad impact on entire communities as they cope with disaster. Psychologists using a structural approach try to classify disasters in terms of their impact and duration and the preparedness of the community. Psychologists using a dynamic approach assess social-psychological responses during the pre-impact phase, impact phase, recoil phase, rescue phase and post-trauma phase. Post-traumatic stress disorder can afflict anyone who experiences intense trauma. It is characterised by avoidance behaviours, recurring images of the event as in dreams, and heightened arousal. Some theoretical explanations that have been offered to account for PTSD centre on conditioned fear to traumatic stimuli, learned helplessness, information processing involving fear networks and regulatory control of information in active memory. Emergency service workers and police officers involved in critical incidents are at increased risk of developing PTSD. Critical incident stress debriefing has been advocated as a method of crisis intervention in the first 72 hours following a critical incident.

Researchers measure stress in three ways. One way involves assessing physiological arousal. Blood pressure, heart rate, respiration rate and galvanic skin response can be measured with an apparatus called the polygraph. Biochemical analyses of blood or urine samples can test for corticosteroids (for example cortisol) and catecholamines (for example epinephrine and norepinephrine). Another method of measuring stress uses a survey of people's life events. The most widely used scale of life events has been the Social Readjustment Rating Scale, but newer instruments have been developed to correct some of its weaknesses. A more recent approach to assessing life events stress is the use of the personal interview method. The third method for measuring stress involves assessing the daily hassles people experience. Although stress can contribute to the development of illness, many psychologists believe that not all stress is harmful.

Key terms

alarm reaction	dynamic approach	polygraph	strain
catecholamines	general adaptation syndrome	post-traumatic stress disorder (PTSD)	stress
cognitive appraisal			stressors
corticosteroids	life events	primary appraisal	structural approach
critical incident stress debriefing (CISD)	network resolution processing	secondary appraisal	technostress
		stage of exhaustion	temperaments
daily hassles	Peter Principle	stage of resistance	transactions

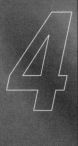

4 Stress, biopsychosocial factors and illness

Prologue

They were best friends, Liz and Sally, on their way to an art museum a year ago when a car accident ended their lives. Their husbands, Steve and Peter, were devastated, not only by their individual losses but for each other's. These men were also friends — both worked as engineers for the same company and shared hobbies and other interests. The four of them used to go out together often, leaving the kids with one babysitter. How did the terrible loss of their wives affect these men?

The initial impact of their loss was similar, but the amounts of stress that followed were different. Steve's stress was not as severe as Peter's. One thing that helped Steve was that he had an extended family that lived nearby. They provided consolation for his grief, a place to go to get out of the house and to socialise, and help in caring for his children. After school, the kids would go to either Steve's or Liz's parents' house, and Steve would pick them up on his way home from work. Sometimes he and the children would stay there for dinner. This helped save him time and money, both of which were in short supply. How was Steve doing a year later? He had made a good adjustment, had a good relationship with his children, was starting to go out with women, and was in good health.

Peter was not so fortunate. For one thing, he had no nearby family to rely on. Compared with Steve, Peter had little emotional support in his grief, and being a single parent made his workload and financial situation very difficult. Peter had little time or money for socialising, and virtually all of his adult contacts were at work. Although he and Steve often had lunch together, their interests were drifting apart. Unlike Steve, Peter had never been very outgoing, and he felt awkward and insecure in meeting women. A year after Sally died, he was isolated and lonely. His relationship with his children was deteriorating, and so was his health. He had developed migraine headaches, neck problems, and high blood pressure. The stress in Peter's life was taking its toll.

This chapter examines the effects of stress on health. We begin by looking at psychosocial factors that can modify the stress people experience. Then we consider how stress affects health and the development of specific illnesses. And in this chapter we address many questions about stress and illness that are of great concern today. Why can some people experience one traumatic event after another without ill effects, but others cannot? Are hard-driving people more likely to have a heart attack than people who are easygoing? Can people actually 'die of a broken heart'? Can stress retard people's recovery from illness?

Psychosocial modifiers of stress

Reactions to stress vary from one person to the next and from time to time for the same person. These variations often result from psychological and social factors that seem to *modify* the impact of stressors on the individual. Let's look at some of these modifiers, beginning with the role of social support.

Social support

We saw in the bereavement experiences of Steve and Peter how important social ties and relationships can be during troubled times. The social support Steve got from his family tempered the impact of his stressful loss and probably helped him adjust. **Social support** refers to the perceived comfort, caring, esteem, or help a person receives from other people or groups (Cobb 1976; Gentry & Kobasa 1984; Wallston et al. 1983; Cohen & Wills 1985). This support can come from many different sources — spouse or lover, family, friends, co-workers, doctor or community organisations. According to researcher Sidney Cobb (1976), people with social support believe they are loved and cared for, esteemed and valued, and part of a social network, such as a family or community organisation, that can provide goods, services and mutual defence in times of need or danger.

Types of social support

What specifically does social support provide to the person? To answer this question, researchers have tried to classify various types of support (Cohen & McKay 1984; Cutrona & Russell 1990; House & Kahn 1985; Schaefer, Coyne & Lazarus 1981). These classifications have emphasised the existence and structure of social networks, or the functions served by social relationships. Other distinctions have been made between available and received support (Barrera 1986; Gottlieb 1985; Dunkel-Schetter & Bennett 1990). The perception that support is available if required may be as health protective as actually receiving support. Although social support has been classified in many ways, there are five basic types of social support.

1. *Emotional support* involves the expression of empathy, caring and concern towards the person. It provides the person with a sense of comfort, reassurance, belonging, and being loved in times of stress. We saw earlier how Steve's family gave him emotional support after the death of his wife.

2. *Esteem support* occurs through people's expression of positive regard for the person, encouragement or agreement with the individual's ideas or feelings, and positive comparison of the person with others, such as people who are less able or worse off. This kind of support serves to build the individual's feeling of self-worth, competence and being valued. Esteem support is especially useful during the appraisal of stress, such as when the person assesses whether the demands exceed his or her personal resources.

3. *Tangible or instrumental support* involves direct assistance, as when people give or lend the person money or help out with chores in times of stress. Steve's family helped with child care, for example, which reduced the demands on his time and finances.

4. *Informational support* includes giving advice, directions, suggestions, or feedback about how the person is doing. For example, a person who is ill might get information from family or a doctor on how to treat the illness. Or someone who is faced with a very difficult decision on the job might receive suggestions or feedback about his or her ideas from co-workers.

5. *Network support* provides a feeling of membership in a group of people who share interests and social activities.

The type of support a person receives and needs depends on the stressful circumstances (Wortman & Dunkel-Schetter 1987). For instance, figure 4.1 shows that cancer patients find emotional and esteem support especially helpful, but patients with less serious chronic illnesses find different types of support equally helpful (Martin et al. 1994).

What type of support do people generally get? Carolyn Cutrona (1986) studied this issue by having university students fill out a questionnaire, rating the degree to which their current relationships provided them with different types of support, and then keep a daily record of their stress and social experiences for two weeks. The daily records revealed that most of the stressors were relatively minor, such as having car trouble or an argument with a flatmate, but one-fifth of the subjects reported a severe event, such as a parent's diagnosis of cancer or the ending of a long-term romantic relationship. As you might expect, the subjects received more social support following stressful events than at less stressful times, and those who initially perceived themselves as having high levels of social support reported receiving more support during the two weeks. Tangible support occurred very infrequently, but emotional, informational and esteem support occurred often. Students who received more frequent esteem support tended to report less depression following stressful experiences, suggesting that esteem may protect people from negative emotional consequences of stress. While Cutrona found perceived support to be related to actual support received, other research has found these concepts to be unrelated (Lakey & Heller 1988) or only moderately related (Bennett, Gottlieb & Cadman 1987; Sarason et al. 1987; Wethington & Kessler 1986).

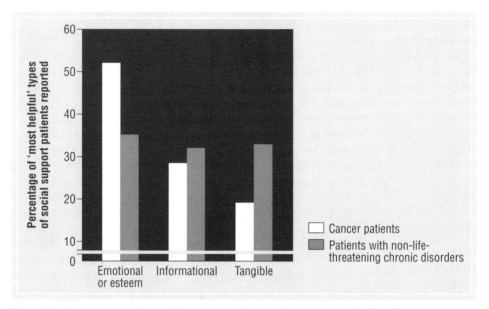

Figure 4.1 Percentage of patients with cancer and with non-life-threatening disorders (chronic headache or irritable bowel syndrome) whose reports of the 'most helpful' social support they received described the emotional/esteem, instrumental or tangible types of support. Notice that the cancer patients found emotional or esteem support especially helpful.

Source: Data from Martin et al. (1994, figure 1).

Who gets social support?

Not everyone gets the social support they need. Many factors determine whether people receive support (Dunkel-Schetter & Bennett 1990; Connell & D'Augelli 1990; Wortman & Dunkel-Schetter 1987). Some factors relate to the potential *recipients* of support. People are unlikely to receive support if they are unsociable, don't help others and don't let others know that they need help. Some people are not assertive enough to ask for help, or feel that they should be independent and not burden others, or feel uncomfortable confiding in others, or don't know whom to ask. Other factors relate to the potential *providers* of support. For instance, they may not have the resources needed, or may be unsure about how best to help, or may be under stress and in need of help themselves, or may simply be insensitive to the needs of others.

Whether people receive social support also depends on the composition and structure of their **social network** — that is, the linkages they have with people in their family and community (Mitchell 1969; Schaefer, Coyne & Lazarus 1981). These linkages can vary in *size* — the number of people with whom you have regular contact; *frequency of contact* — how often you see these people; *composition* — whether these people are family, friends, co-workers and so on; and *intimacy* — the closeness of individual relationships and mutual willingness to confide in each other. Expectations people have of their social support networks may explain why a discrepancy sometimes exists between perceived and available social support (Dunkel-Schetter & Bennett 1991). Some individuals may inaccurately perceive support to be available only to find that it does not materialise, while others may underestimate available support and receive more support than expected. Perceiving more support than is actually available may serve to protect the person's self-esteem and reduce their sense of personal vulnerability. Inaccuracies in perception may also occur because the individual has overestimated the skills and resources of those in his or her social networks. While most supportive networks initially meet the person's expectations, support may decline over time, because support providers may believe that the recipient's needs are being met by others, they may have different beliefs about what constitutes effective support, or they may have their own personal problems and feel overburdened.

People's need for, sources of and ability to provide social support change throughout the life span (Antonucci 1985; Broadhead et al. 1983; Bruhn & Phillips 1987; Sarafino & Armstrong 1986). For example, most young children readily ask for and receive help from older people, but their immature cognitive and social skills hamper their ability to recognise other people's needs easily and provide effective help themselves. As children's social contacts expand outside the family, their peers become an increasingly important source of both stress and social support, particularly during the adolescent years. Although teenagers generally have strong cognitive and social skills, and can provide very effective support, many are reluctant to ask for help or confide in others. Adulthood is a time for taking on increasing levels of responsibility in a family, on the job and in the community. The intimacy and caring that usually characterise adult loving relationships, such as in marriage, give adults the opportunity for a continuous source of support. Old age is a time when social support sometimes declines. Although people's social networks do not get smaller in old age, the elderly exchange less support, perhaps because of the loss of a spouse or because they may feel reluctant to ask for help if they become unable to reciprocate.

How can we assess people's social support, given the different types of support and the complex relationships that are involved? Questionnaires have been developed, but none currently provides a strong measure of all aspects of social support (Heitzmann & Kaplan 1988; Wortman & Dunkel-Schetter 1987). One of the more highly regarded instruments is the *Social Support Questionnaire* developed by Irwin Sarason and his colleagues (1983). It consists of 27 items, such as, 'Who helps you feel that you truly have something positive to contribute to others?' For each item, the respondents list the people they can rely on and then indicate their overall degree of satisfaction with the support available. Using this instrument, these researchers have found that some people report high levels of satisfaction with support from a small number of close friends and relatives, but others seem to need a large social network. Other often-used social support measures include Cutrona and Russell's (1987) Social Provisions Scale and the Interpersonal Support Evaluation List (Cohen & McKay 1984).

Social support as transactional process

Recent approaches to the study of social support have emphasised the dynamic nature of stress-related transactions between support providers and recipients. Such an approach acknowledges that social support is provided within the context of personal relationships (Duck & Silver 1990; Gottlieb & Wagner 1991; Heller 1979; Morgan 1990; Pierce, Sarason & Sarason 1990) and is derived from recurring interaction patterns. The seeking of support and the amount of support provided depend on a number of interpersonal factors such as the stage within the relationship, the anticipated effect of the stressor on the support provider, the ability to communicate needs, and how both parties respond to stress (Gottlieb & Wagner 1991). Barbee (1990) has proposed a model of interactive coping that incorporates affective, cognitive, relationship and personal factors in predicting whether or not transactions will be supportive. Affective variables include the helper's mood, and feelings of empathy or annoyance towards the person in need of support. Cognitive factors relate to the nature of the problem, the attributions made by the helper regarding the cause of the problem, and controllability of the problem, as well as the ability to offer effective support. Supportiveness also depends on the nature of the relationship, the closeness of the relationship and the length of time in the relationship. Among personality factors that affect provision of support are extraversion and neuroticism. For example, one would expect extraverted persons to be more likely to ask for help in times of need. Neuroticism may affect help seeking in that persons high on the trait may be more guarded in revealing their need for help. It could also be the case that neurotic persons may be ineffective in their support seeking, and could make potential support providers feel uncomfortable in assisting them. Evidence for the model suggests that whether the potential support provider helps to solve the problem, dismisses it, is supportive or escapes from helping depends on the interplay of these factors (Barbee & Cunningham 1988). Let's consider an example. Sarah, a second-year Psychology student, is more likely to help her friend Rachael with a late assignment if there were uncontrollable circumstances that caused Rachael to have problems submitting the assignment. Rachael may have been ill, or family responsibilities may have prevented her working on the assignment. However, if Rachael is always late with assignments because she goes out most nights with her boyfriend, Sarah might be less inclined to offer help. Sarah is also more likely to assist Rachael if she feels competent to help with the assignment.

Research suggests that women receive less support from their spouses than men do, and seem to rely heavily on women friends for social support (Greenglass & Noguchi 1996). These gender differences may result from the greater intimacy that seems to exist in the friendships of females than those of males, and may reflect mainly differences in the emotional and esteem support males and females seek out and give (Heller, Price & Hogg 1990).

The transactional nature of social support serves to modify appraisals of events and affects the nature of coping by participants. Supportiveness is negotiated through actions and the verbal exchange of both participants. Wagner and associates (1986; Gottlieb & Wagner 1991) studied the interspousal coping of parents of children diagnosed with cystic fibrosis or juvenile diabetes. They were interested in what each partner said or did to modify appraisals, emotions or coping behaviour of the other partner. Verbal statements were found to range from forceful directives to become more emotionally involved, or to participate more with care, to leading questions such as 'Why are you bothering with this [regimen]? She's not going to live anyway', to suggesting options for communicating with doctors or managing the illness. Not all interactions were supportive. Where verbal exchanges were supportive, they served to affirm coping ability, and confirm shared emotions. Husbands communicated esteem for their partner's ability to cope with their child's illness, and for their dedication to caregiving. Wives' supportive influences were emotionally protective of their husbands, shielding them from adverse changes in the child's health, or allowing the husband to engage in anticipatory coping by preparing them for bad news. Supportive exchanges involved reciprocal influences whereby partners engaged in coping approved by the other, that was supportive to the other partner and that posed no threat to the coping of either partner. The interactional nature of supportive behaviour is also seen in situations where support is not sought because the person anticipates disapproval for a certain action. Pearlin and McCall (1990) found this to be the case with marital support for occupational problems where the spouse did not approve of the other taking the job.

Social support, stress and health

It has been said, 'Friendship is to people what sunshine is to flowers.' What benefits do we get from the social support of friends, relatives and other people? To answer this question, we will look at how social support relates to stress and health.

Research findings suggest that social support may reduce the stress people experience. A study by James LaRocco, James House and John French (1980) examined data from questionnaires assessing the job stress and social support of more than 2000 men in a variety of white- and blue-collar occupations. The measure of social support included its availability from three sources: the employee's supervisor; co-workers; and wife, family and friends. Correlational analyses revealed that the greater the social support available to the employees, the lower the psychological strain they reported. Although lower job stress was linked to social support from home, it was more strongly related to the support the employees received from their supervisors and co-workers. Similar associations between social support and reduced job stress have been found in several other studies (Constable & Russell 1986; Cottington & House 1987). Social support also appears to reduce stress from a variety of other sources. Experiments in which university students engaged in a stressful activity, such as giving a speech, either alone or in the presence of a supportive person found that the increase in blood pressure while speaking was much smaller for subjects with the supportive person than alone (Kors & Linden 1995; Lepore, Allen & Evans 1993).

Having social support also seems to benefit people's health (Berkman 1995; Uchino, Uno & Holt-Lunstad 1999). This has been shown in the death rates for people who have different amounts of social support (Avlund, Damsgaard & Holstein 1998; Tucker et al. 1999). Lisa Berkman and S. Leonard Syme (1979) conducted a prospective study of more than 4700 men and women between 30 and 69 years of age. The subjects were asked about four aspects of social support: marital status, contacts with family and friends, church membership, and formal and informal group associations. Mortality data collected over the next nine years revealed that the greater the degree of social support the subjects had, the lower the likelihood of their dying during the period of the study. Figure 4.2 on the next page shows an example of these findings. In each age category, subjects with few contacts with friends and relatives had higher mortality rates than those with many contacts. In addition, social support was not only associated with deaths from all causes, but also with mortality from several specific diseases, including cancer and heart disease.

The relationship between social support and mortality in these studies is correlational. How do we know whether social support leads to better health and lower mortality or whether the influence is the other way around? That is, could the people who had less social support be less active socially because they were already sick at the start of the study? Berkman and Syme provided some evidence that this was not the case. For instance, the subjects had been asked about past illnesses at the initial interview, and those with high levels of social support did not differ from those with low levels of support. But better evidence comes from a similar study of more than 2700 adults (House, Robbins & Metzner 1982). The subjects in this study were medically examined at the start of the research. These researchers found essentially the same relationship between social support and mortality as Berkman and Syme did, and the initial health of the subjects with low social support was the same as that of those with high support.

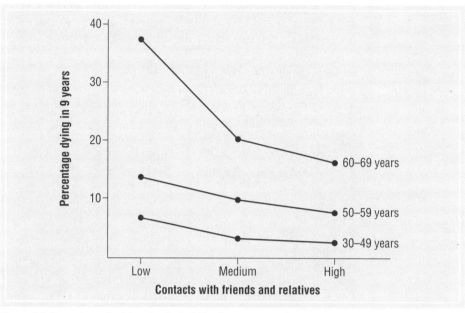

Figure 4.2 Percentage of adults who died within nine years as a function of the number of contacts with friends and relatives and the subjects' ages at the start of the study, in 1965

Source: Data from Berkman & Syme (1979, table 2).

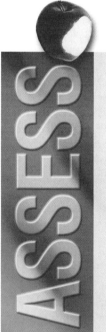

Assess yourself
HOW MUCH EMOTIONAL SUPPORT DO YOU GET?

Think of the ten people to whom you feel closest. For some of them, you may not feel a strong bond — but they are still among the closest ten people in your life. Write their initials in the following spaces.

— — — — — — — — — —

In the *corresponding* spaces below each of the following four questions, rate each person on a 5-point scale, where **1** = 'not at all' and **5** = 'extremely'.

• How reliable is this person? Is this person there when you need him or her?

— — — — — — — — — —

• How much does this person boost your spirits when you feel low?

— — — — — — — — — —

• How much does this person make you feel he or she cares about you?

— — — — — — — — — —

• How much do you feel you can confide in this person?

— — — — — — — — — —

Add together all of the ratings you gave across all of the people and questions. A total score between 120 and 150 is fairly typical and suggests that you can get a reasonably good level of emotional support when you need it.

Source: Based on material in Schaefer, Coyne & Lazarus (1981).

Researchers have also studied the association between social support and the likelihood that people will develop illnesses and recover quickly when they do. Some early studies found an association between support and illness or recovery, but others did not (Wallston et al. 1983). These results were mixed probably because of weaknesses and variations in research methodology, such as in the way support was defined and measured (Friis & Taff 1986; Wortman & Dunkel-Schetter 1987). More recent research has produced more consistently positive results — showing, for example, that heart disease and surgery patients with high levels of social support recover more quickly than comparable patients with less support (Berkman 1995; Fontana et al. 1989; Kulik & Mahler 1989; Reifman 1995). Supportive social relationships also appear to protect against the progression of cancer or relapse (Spiegel, Sephton & Stites 1998). These findings indicate that social support may reduce the likelihood of illness and speed recovery. But the connection between social support and health is not always very strong, probably because support is only one of many factors involved (Kobasa et al. 1985; Smith et al. 1994). Social support appears to have a strong impact on the health of some individuals and a weak influence on the health of others. For instance, some evidence indicates that the recovery of many patients who believe they can cope with the emotional demands of their illness does not benefit from social support (Wilcox, Kasl & Berkman 1994).

Separate from the beneficial effects social support exerts on physical health are its effects on psychological wellbeing. Anxiety and depression have been found to be more elevated in individuals who do not belong to large networks or who have poor-quality support (van der Voort 1999). Depression has also been linked to negative social exchanges and low perceived support satisfaction (Finch et al. 1999).

How may social support affect health?

To explain how social support may influence health and wellbeing, researchers have proposed two theories: the 'buffering' and the 'direct effects' hypotheses. Studies have found evidence consistent with both theories (Cohen & Wills 1985; Pearlin 1999; Payne & Jones 1987; Thoits 1982; Wortman & Dunkel-Schetter 1987). We will begin with the buffering hypothesis.

We saw in chapter 3 that prolonged exposure to high levels of stress can lead to illness. According to the **buffering hypothesis**, social support affects health by *protecting* the person against these negative effects of high stress. A graphical illustration of the buffering hypothesis appears in figure 4.3a. As the graph shows, this protective function is effective only or mainly when the person encounters a strong stressor. Under low-stress conditions, little or no buffering occurs.

How does buffering work? There are at least two ways (Cohen & Wills 1985). One way involves the process of cognitive appraisal. When people encounter a strong stressor, such as a major financial crisis, those individuals with high levels of social support may be less likely to appraise the situation as stressful than those with low levels of support. Individuals with high social support may expect that someone they know can and will help, such as by lending the needed money or giving advice on how to get it. As a result, they judge that they can meet the demands and decide that the situation is not very stressful (Peirce et al. 1996). The second way social support can buffer the effects of stress is by modifying people's response to a stressor after they have appraised the situation as stressful. For instance, people with high social support might have someone provide a solution to the problem, convince them that the problem is not very important, or cheer them on to 'look on the bright side' or 'count their blessings'. People with little social support are much less likely to have any of these advantages — so the negative impact of the stress is greater for them than for those with high levels of support. Buffering effects of social support have been found even at the cellular level, with supported students having greater natural killer immune activity during examination stress (Kang et al. 1998).

The **direct effects hypothesis** maintains that social support is beneficial to health and wellbeing regardless of the amount of stress people experience. According to this hypothesis, the beneficial effects of social support are similar under high and low stressor intensities, as depicted in figure 4.3b. Evidence exists for the direct effects hypothesis (Dolbier & Steinhardt 2000). There are several ways by which direct effects may work (Cohen & Wills 1985; Wortman & Dunkel-Schetter 1987). For example, people with high levels of social support may have a greater sense of belongingness and self-esteem than those with little support. The positive outlook this produces could be beneficial to health independently of stress experiences, such as by making individuals more resistant to infection. Some evidence suggests that high levels of support may also encourage people to lead more healthful lifestyles than low social support does (Broman 1993). People with social support may feel, for example, that because others care about them and need them, they should exercise, eat well and seek medical attention before a problem becomes serious.

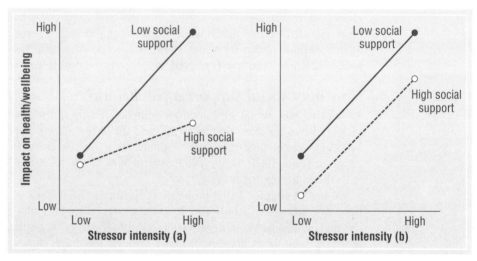

Figure 4.3 Two ways social support may benefit health and wellbeing. Graph (a) illustrates the *buffering hypothesis*, which proposes that social support modifies the negative health effects of high levels of stress. Graph (b) depicts the *direct effects hypothesis*, which proposes that the health benefits of social support occur irrespective of stress.

Does social support always help?

Social support does not always reduce stress and benefit health. Why? For one thing, although support may be offered or available to us, we may not *perceive* it as supportive (Dunkel-Schetter & Bennett 1990; Wilcox, Kasl & Berkman 1994). This may happen because the help is insufficient or we may not want help or are too emotionally distraught to notice it, for instance. Also, the nature of some stressors may make difficult the supportive efforts of others. Bereavement, for instance, may be equally traumatic for the support provider if that person is a relative or close friend, as they too have to come to terms with the loss. In such situations, interpersonal coping may disrupt the provision of adequate support, as alluded to by Gottlieb and Wagner (1991).

> Although they are one step removed from the loss, they, too, are bereaved by the death of a loved one and therefore are also attempting to maintain their own emotional equilibrium. To accomplish this goal of safeguarding their own emotional well-being, they may offer forms of support that either minimise or attempt to improve the bereaved's emotions. But in doing so, they may inadvertently invalidate the bereaved's feelings of loss that arise from their unique privileged relationship to the deceased. Accordingly, the support the bereaved receive from their close associates is unhelpful because it invalidates both their unique feelings of mourning and their unique identities as mourners. It meets the providers' coping needs, not the bereaved's supportive needs. (p. 167)

When we do not perceive help as supportive, it is less likely to reduce our stress.

Another reason why social support does not always help is that the type of support we receive may not *match* the needs that the stressor has produced. For example, if your car broke down, your passenger's emotional consolation probably would not reduce your stress very much. Cutrona and Russell (1990) have outlined a pattern for matching support with need. Instrumental support is particularly valuable for stressful events that are *controllable* — that is, we can do something to achieve a goal or prevent the situation from becoming worse, such as when we feel ill. Emotional support is especially important for *uncontrollable* stressful events, such as when a loved one dies. But other types of support may also be needed — for instance, if the uncontrollable event involved losing your job, esteem and tangible support might help, too. As we have seen, not all support-seeking transactions result in positive consequences. Seeking assistance for personal problems involves costs. When a person asks for help, others learn about that person's weaknesses and private information becomes public. Goldsmith and Parks (1990) have argued that the support process is characterised by opposing motivations to disclose and withhold information, as well as conflicting interactive goals of autonomy and dependence. Risks associated with seeking help include creating a bad impression on the potential supporter, confidentiality being violated, being viewed as having made an inappropriate disclosure or being perceived as a burden. In communicative transactions with others, the person seeking help engages in a number of strategies to manage these risks. In seeking support for a relationship problem, Goldsmith and Parks found that people concerned with negative outcomes tend to adopt the role of either Cautious Discloser or Strategist (using many strategies, moderating the amount of information disclosed, preceding it with qualifying statements), in favour of Expressive Discloser, or a Gatekeeper (alternating between being open and closed) strategy. The receiving of social support also carries with it an obligation to reciprocate support, which may sometimes detract from any benefits to the individual (La Gaipa 1990) as recipients may feel that they lack the resources to reciprocate.

Marriage is often thought to convey a protective health benefit to people by providing social support. Consistent with this idea, studies have found that married people live longer than divorced and never married individuals (Berkman & Syme 1979; House, Robbins & Metzner 1982). James Lynch (1990) has argued that being lonely or having a 'broken heart' is a risk factor for heart disease because widowed, divorced and never married individuals have higher death rates from heart disease than married people do. But more recent research has found that individuals who had not married by midlife were not at greater risk of dying before 80 years of age and that differences in death rates for married and divorced people result in part from differences in their personality characteristics (Tucker et al. 1996). Longitudinal data from the Terman Life-Cycle Study found males to be at greater risk for mortality prior to age 70 if they were separated, divorced or remarried. Marital dissolution seemed to have a long-term detrimental effect on the health of these men (Tucker et al. 1999). Marriage by itself probably does not protect people's health.

Last, there are many circumstances in which social ties with people can harm an individual's health (Burg & Seeman 1994; Kaplan & Toshima 1990; La Gaipa 1990). One circumstance is when people set a bad example for the person. We see this when smoking and drinking behaviour by friends and family lead an adolescent to engage in these behaviours. Friends and family can also set bad examples by not engaging in healthy behaviours, such as using seatbelts, eating a balanced diet or exercising. Other circumstances in which social support can be harmful arise when the person has developed a health problem. For instance, someone who is overweight and has high blood pressure may be encouraged by family to eat prohibited foods. They may say, 'Doctors don't know everything', or, 'A little more cheesecake can't hurt', or, 'You can make up for it by dieting next week.' Also, when someone suffers a long and serious illness, such as heart disease, families may be overprotective and discourage the patient's desire to become more active or to go back to work. This can interfere with a program of rehabilitation and make the patient increasingly dependent and disabled (Kaplan & Toshima 1990).

In summary, people receive various types of support from friends, family and others in their lives. Social support usually tends to reduce people's stress and benefit their health. We turn now to another psychosocial factor that modifies the stress people experience — namely, the degree of control people feel they have in their lives.

A sense of personal control

People generally like the feeling of having some measure of control over the things that happen in their lives, and they take individual action when they want to influence events directly. In doing these things, people strive for a sense of **personal control** — the feeling that they can make decisions and take effective action to produce desirable outcomes and avoid undesirable ones (Folkman 1984; Rodin 1986). Several studies have found that people who have a strong sense of personal control report experiencing less psychological distress and less strain from stressors (Elliott, Trief & Stein 1986; Malik & Sabharwal 1999; Moyle & Parkes 1999; Sapolsky 1999).

Types of control

How can feelings of personal control reduce the stress people experience? Let's see by considering the process of giving birth — a stressful event. Women who attend natural childbirth classes learn many techniques that enhance their personal control in the birth process. They, like other people in stressful situations, can influence events in their lives and reduce the stress they experience in many ways. These ways include four types of control (Averill 1973; Cohen et al. 1986; Miller 1979; Thompson 1981).

1. **Behavioural control** involves the ability to take concrete action to reduce the impact of a stressor. This action might reduce the intensity of the event or shorten its duration. During childbirth, for example, the mother can use special breathing techniques that reduce the pain of labour.

2. **Cognitive control** is the ability to use thought processes or strategies to modify the impact of a stressor. These strategies can include thinking about the event differently

or focusing on a pleasant or neutral thought or sensation. While giving birth, for instance, the mother might think about the event differently by going over in her mind the positive meanings the baby will give to her life. Or she could focus her attention on the sensation of the baby's movements or on an image, such as a pleasant day at the beach.

3. **Decisional control** is the opportunity to choose between alternative procedures or courses of action. The mother and father have many choices to make about the birth process before it occurs. For many of these decisions, the mother usually has the final word — such as in the choice of the obstetrician, whether to use conventional or natural childbirth methods, and whether the birth will occur in a hospital, at home or at an alternative birth centre. In other medical situations, the patient may be given a choice regarding which treatment procedure to use, when the treatment will occur and so on.

4. **Informational control** involves the opportunity to get knowledge about a stressful event — what will happen, why and what the consequences are likely to be. For example, a pregnant woman may get information about the sensations she will experience during labour and delivery, the procedures she can expect to happen and the range of time the process generally takes. Informational control can help reduce stress by increasing the person's ability to predict and be prepared for what will happen and by decreasing the fear people often have of the unknown.

Each of these types of control can reduce stress, but one of them — cognitive control — seems to have the most consistently beneficial effect (Arbuckle et al. 1999; Cohen et al. 1986).

Beliefs about oneself and control

People differ in the degree to which they believe they have control over their lives. Some people believe they have a great deal of control, and others think they have almost none. The latter is shown in the case study of a chronically unemployed man named Karl, who was referred to therapy by the US Veterans Administration with

> an almost total lack of social and interpersonal skills . . . After much coaching and discussion, Karl applied for a job and got it. But this did not raise his expectancies of being able to get another job should he have to do so. Indeed, he attributed his success entirely to good fortune. He believed that the employer probably was partial to veterans or just happened to be in a good mood that day . . . After several comparable episodes, it began to dawn upon the therapist that here was a person who believed that the occurrence of reinforcement was outside his own personal control. (Phares, 1984, pp. 505–6)

People who believe they have control over their successes and failures are described as possessing an *internal* **locus of control**. That is, the control for these events lies within themselves — they are responsible. Other people, like Karl, who believe that their lives are controlled by forces outside themselves — for example by luck — have an *external* locus of control (Phares 1987; Rotter 1966). Positive health states have been found to be associated with the possession of an internal locus of control (Horner 1998).

Certainly it is unrealistic for people to assume everything in their lives is under their control. But the degree to which they attribute responsibility to themselves, versus other forces, determines their locus of control. Julian Rotter (1966) has developed the *I-E Scale*, a test that is used for measuring the degree of internality or externality of a person's beliefs about personal control. This scale presents a series of paired items, such as 'The average citizen can have an influence in government decisions,' and, 'This world is run by a few people in power, and there is not much the little guy can do about it.' For each pair of internal/external items, the respondent selects the one with which he or she most agrees. Most people have moderate beliefs about the influence they have on events in their lives. Their locus of control falls in the midrange between being highly internal and being highly external.

There is another aspect of personal control besides internality/externality that is important, too. This aspect is our sense of **self-efficacy** — the belief that we can succeed at something we want to do (Bandura 1977, 1986). People estimate their chances of success and failure on the basis of their prior observations of the effects that a given activity had for themselves and others. They decide whether to attempt the activity according to their expectations that (1) the behaviour, if properly carried out, would lead to a favourable outcome, and (2) they can perform the behaviour properly. For example, you may know that by taking and doing well in a series of honours courses at university you can graduate with some recognition of that accomplishment, such as a special certificate. But if you estimate the likelihood of achieving that feat as zero, you are not likely to try. People with a strong sense of self-efficacy show less psychological and physiological strain in response to stressors than do those with a weak sense of efficacy (Bandura, Reese & Adams 1982; Bandura et al. 1985; Horner 1998).

Determinants and development of personal control

On what basis do people judge that they have control over things that happen in their lives? We make these assessments by using a wide variety of information and knowledge that we gain from our experiences throughout life (Bandura 1986; Phares 1987; Rodin 1987; Schunk & Carbonari 1984). One of the most important sources is our own performance — the successes and failures we perceive in the activities we attempt. Infants begin to learn about personal control from their own performance as they coordinate their sensory experiences with their motor activity. An example of this is when babies learn that they can make a noise with a rattle by shaking it.

Throughout the life span, we assess our personal control through the process of *social learning*, in which we learn by observing the behaviour of others (Bandura 1969, 1986). During early childhood, the family is particularly important in this process, with members serving as models of behaviour, as agents of reinforcement and as standards for comparison. Parents who are caring, encouraging and consistent in their standards for behaviour tend to have children who develop an internal locus of control and a strong sense of efficacy (Harter 1983). After children enter day care or school, their peers become increasingly important, and they compare themselves for academic ability, naughtiness, talents, popularity and so on. In adolescence, the sense of personal control is strongly affected by, and will in turn affect, social and sexual relationships and decisions about higher education and careers. People who reach adulthood with poor intellectual and social skills and many self-doubts often find these events and many other aspects of adult life stressful. From adulthood to old age, locus of control tends to become more external — that is, people's beliefs that chance and powerful others affect their lives increase (Lachman 1986). As a result, when elderly individuals develop serious illnesses, many of them are more inclined than younger people to prefer having professionals make health-related decisions for them (Woodward & Wallston 1987). Yet this relinquishing of internal control has been found to be linked to increased distress and anxiety in the elderly (Frazier & Waid 1999).

You may have noticed that the information people use in determining their personal control is usually retrospective, can be very complex, and is not always clear-cut. As a result, the judgements we make about our control are not always very objective or based on fact. We sometimes develop what Ellen Langer (1975) calls an *illusion of control* — a belief in our control over an event that is really determined by chance. An experiment demonstrated this illusion by finding that individuals often claim they have control in winning a game of chance if they are given the opportunity to perform part of the activity in the game, even though their actions obviously do not influence the outcome (Wortman 1975).

Gender and sociocultural differences in personal control

Gender and sociocultural differences in personal control often develop, depending on the social experiences individuals have (Taylor & Seeman 1999). Sometimes parents and teachers inadvertently lead girls more than boys towards beliefs in external control and low self-efficacy (Dweck & Elliott 1983). Because various identity groups and poor people generally have limited access to power and economic advancement, they tend to have external locus of control beliefs (Lundin 1987).

When people lack personal control

What happens to people who experience high levels of stress over a long period of time and feel that nothing they do matters? They feel helpless. They feel trapped and unable to avoid negative outcomes. A worker who cannot seem to please her boss no matter what she does, a student who cannot perform well on exams, or a patient who is unable to relieve his severe low back pain — each of these examples describes a situation that can produce apathy. As a result, these people may stop striving for these goals, come to believe they have no control over these and other events in their lives, and fail to exert control in situations in which success is possible. This is the condition Martin Seligman (1975) has called **learned helplessness**, which he describes as a principal characteristic of depression.

An experiment by Donald Hiroto and Martin Seligman (1975) demonstrated that people learn to be helpless by being in uncontrollable situations that lead to repeated failure. The researchers assigned university students to one of three training groups that experienced an unpleasant loud noise. In one group, the *controllable-noise* condition, the subjects were told that a noise would come on from time to time and 'there is something you can do to stop it'. They were given an opportunity to discover that pressing a button on an apparatus would stop it, which they did. The *uncontrollable-noise* group had the same instructions and apparatus, but nothing they did affected the presence of the noise. In a *comparison* group, the subjects were simply told 'From time to time a loud tone will come on for a while. Please sit and listen to it.' All the subjects were tested later for helplessness in a uniform way: they were told that a noise would come on and off and that 'there is something you can do to stop it'. The apparatus was new — it had a sliding knob that, when manipulated correctly, would stop the noise. In this test, students in the uncontrollable-noise group performed much more poorly than those in the controllable-noise and comparison groups. Learning that the noise is uncontrollable with the push-button apparatus impaired the subjects' discovering how to control the noise with the knob apparatus.

Seligman and his colleagues have extended the theory of learned helplessness to explain two important observations (Abramson, Seligman & Teasdale 1978). First, being exposed to uncontrollable negative events does not always lead to learned helplessness. Second, depressed people often report feeling a loss in self-esteem. The theory needed to answer the question of why people would blame themselves for negative events that are beyond their control. The revised theory attempts to deal with these observations by proposing that when people experience uncontrollable negative events, they ask themselves, 'Why am I unable to affect these events, and how long will they continue?' They answer this question through the cognitive process called **attribution**, in which people try to arrive at causes or judgements regarding events, such as their own or others' actions, motives, feelings or intentions.

How does attribution work? When uncontrollable negative events happen, people consider possible judgements and causes by assessing three dimensions of the situation.

1. *Internal–external.* People who feel trapped and unable to control negative events assess whether this situation results from their own personal inability to control outcomes or whether it is due to external causes that are beyond anyone's control. For example, suppose a boy receives physical therapy for a serious injury but cannot seem to meet the goals each week. He might attribute this failure either to his own lack of fortitude or to the rehabilitation program the physical therapist designed. Both judgements may make him stop trying. He is likely to suffer a loss of self-esteem if he attributes the difficulty to a lack of personal strength, but not if he attributes the difficulty to external causes.

2. *Stable–unstable.* Individuals who experience uncontrollable negative events assess whether the situation results from a cause that is long-lasting (stable) or temporary (unstable). If they determine that it is long-lasting, as when people develop a chronic and disabling disease, they are more likely to feel helpless and depressed than if they think their condition is temporary.

3. *Global–specific.* People in unpleasant situations that they cannot control try to assess whether these events result from factors that have global and wide-ranging effects or specific and narrow effects. Someone who is unable to stop smoking cigarettes and arrives at a global judgement — for example, 'I'm totally no good and weak-willed' — is more likely to feel helpless and depressed than a similar individual who makes a specific judgement such as, 'I'm not good at controlling this part of my life.'

Thus, people who tend to attribute negative events in their lives to *stable* and *global* causes are at high risk of feeling helpless and depressed. If their judgements are also *internal*, their depressive thinking is likely to include a loss of self-esteem as well. People who believe bad events result from internal, stable and global factors while good events result from external, unstable and specific factors have a very *pessimistic* view of life (Kamen & Seligman 1989).

How does the lack of personal control affect people in real-life stressful conditions? Some studies have examined this question by testing students in university colleges (Baum, Aiello & Calesnick 1978; Baum & Gatchel 1981; Rodin & Baum 1978). Stress and control were defined on the basis of differences in crowding that result from two types of college floor plans: (1) *short-corridor* designs cluster residents in small numbers around shared areas, and (2) *long-corridor* designs have large numbers of residents along a long hallway. Surveys of college residents have shown that those who live in long-corridor designs report more stress and less ability to control unwanted social interaction than those in short corridors. Furthermore, these differences are associated with helplessness. When tested in social situations, students who live in long corridors show more evidence of helplessness than those who live in short corridors — for example, long-corridor residents initiate fewer conversations with strangers and show less cooperation and a greater tendency to give up in competitive games. Another real-life stressful situation is the crowding that occurs in high-density city areas. Research has shown that perceived cognitive control declines in high-density areas, as does health status, whereas in less crowded areas perceived control and health are higher (Pandey 1999).

Carol Dweck and her associates have examined attributions and learned helplessness in schoolchildren. In one study, fifth-graders were given multicoloured blocks and asked to arrange the blocks to match a pictured design (Dweck & Repucci 1973). The task was actually impossible — the design could not be made with the blocks given. Children who attributed their failure to stable, uncontrollable factors, such as their own lack of ability, showed poorer performance on subsequent problems than those who attributed failure to unstable, modifiable factors, such as a lack of effort. Thus, the children's attributions were linked to their feelings of helplessness. Another study found evidence that some teachers provide feedback that leads girls to feel more helpless than boys (Dweck et al. 1978). Children's experiences often lead them to acquire feelings of helplessness.

Personal control and health

There are two ways in which personal control and health may be related. First, people who have a strong sense of personal control may be more likely or able to maintain their health and prevent illness than those who have a weak sense of control. Second, once people become seriously ill, those who have a strong sense of control may adjust to the illness and promote their own rehabilitation better than those who have a weak sense of control. Both types of relationship have been examined.

To study these relationships, researchers have used several approaches to measure people's personal control. For instance, some researchers have constructed questionnaires or interviews to assess the degree to which people use specific types of control — such as cognitive, behavioural or informational control. Others have examined people's locus of control, either by applying the I-E Scale or by using scales developed to assess specifically health-related control. One of the best-developed health-related measures today is called the *Multidimensional Health Locus of Control Scales* (Wallston, Wallston & DeVellis 1978). This instrument contains 18 statements; the person responds to each item with ratings ranging from 'strongly agree' to 'strongly disagree'. These statements are divided into three scales.

1. *Internal health locus of control.* This scale measures the degree of internality of the person's beliefs with items such as, 'The main thing that affects my health is what I myself do.'
2. *Powerful-others' health locus of control.* This scale assesses the belief that health is controlled by other people, such as doctors. One item for measuring this is, 'Whenever I don't feel well, I should consult a medically trained professional.'
3. *Chance locus of control.* This scale measures the belief that health is controlled by luck or fate, using items such as, 'Luck plays a big part in determining how soon I will recover from an illness.'

As you can see, the powerful-others' and chance scales are directed towards assessing the degree to which people believe important external sources have control over their health.

Does a sense of personal control influence people's health? Studies have shown that pessimistic people — those who believe they have little control — have poorer health habits, have more illnesses and are less likely to take active steps to treat their illness than are people with a greater sense of control (Kamen & Seligman 1989; Lin & Peterson 1990; Scheier, Botuin & Miller 1999). A strong sense of control may also help people adjust to becoming seriously ill and promote their recovery, particularly if the patients perceive their conditions as very severe. Patients with illnesses such as kidney failure or cancer who score high on either internal or powerful-others' health locus of control suffer less depression than those with strong beliefs in the role of chance (Devins et al. 1981; Marks et al. 1986). The belief that either they or someone else can influence the course of their illness allows patients to be hopeful about their future. Moreover, patients with strong internal locus of control beliefs probably realise they have effective ways of controlling their stress.

Some types of control may be more effective than others in helping people adjust to serious illness. One study investigated the relationship between adjustment to breast cancer and the patients' use of different types of control, three of which were cognitive, behavioural and informational (Taylor, Lichtman & Wood 1984). This study found that adjustment was most strongly associated with patients' use of cognitive control, such as by thinking about their lives differently and taking life more easily. Also, patients who used behavioural control — for example by exercising more than before — showed better adjustment than those who did not. But adjustment was not related to their use of informational control, such as by reading books on cancer. It may be that seeking information about the illness either leads the patients to materials that increase their fears or simply has little influence if the patients have no cognitive or behavioural possibilities for control. Other research has indicated that locus of control and social support from relatives interact to affect immunological natural killer cell activity in response to the acute stress of receiving the results of a breast biopsy (Gerits & Ce-Brabander 1999).

Personal control also affects the efforts patients will make towards their own rehabilitation — in particular, feelings of self-efficacy enhance their efforts. A study demonstrated this with older adult patients who had serious respiratory diseases, such as chronic bronchitis and emphysema (Kaplan, Atkins & Reinsch 1984). The patients were examined at a clinic and given individualised prescriptions for exercise, based on their performance on a treadmill exercise test. They also rated on a questionnaire their exercise self-efficacy — that is, their belief in their ability to perform specific physical activities, such as walking different distances, lifting objects of various weights, and climbing stairs. Correlational analyses revealed that the greater the patients' self-efficacy for doing physical activity, the more likely they were to adhere to the exercise prescription.

Health and personal control in old age

Here are two things we know about elderly people who live in nursing homes: First, they often show declines in their activity and health after they begin living in nursing homes. Second, residents of nursing homes frequently have few responsibilities or opportunities to influence their everyday lives. Could it be that the declines in activity and health among nursing-home residents result in part from their dependency and loss of personal control that the nursing home procedures seem to encourage?

Ellen Langer and Judith Rodin (1976) studied this issue by manipulating the amount of responsibility allowed residents of two floors of a modern, high-quality nursing home. The residents on the two floors were similar in physical and psychological health and prior socioeconomic status. On one floor, the residents were given opportunities to have responsibilities — for example, they were given small plants to care for and encouraged to make decisions about participating in activities and rearranging furniture. In comparison, the residents of the other floor continued to have little personal control. For example, they were assigned to various activities without choice, and when they were given plants, they were told that the staff would take care of them. Measures of the activity and happiness of the residents revealed that the residents who were given more responsibility became happier and more active and alert than the residents who had little control. A year and a half later the residents who were given responsibility were still happier and more active than those who had little control (Rodin & Langer 1977). Moreover, comparisons of health data for the residents of the two floors during these 18 months showed that the residents with responsibility were healthier and had half the rate of mortality.

Other research with residents of a retirement home also demonstrated the importance of personal control on physical and psychological wellbeing and showed that withdrawing opportunities for personal control may impair people's health (Schulz 1976; Schulz & Hanusa 1978). The results of these studies suggest two important conclusions. First, personal control — even over relatively simple or minor events — can have a powerful effect on people's health and psychological condition. Second, health care workers and researchers need to consider the nature of the personal control they introduce and what the impact will be if it is removed.

To summarise the material on personal control, people differ in the degree to which they believe they have control over the things that happen in their lives. People who experience prolonged, high levels of stress and lack a sense of personal control tend to feel helpless. Having a strong sense of control seems to benefit people's health and helps them adjust to becoming seriously ill. A sense of personal control contributes to people's hardiness, which is the next psychosocial modifier of stress we will examine.

A hardy personality

According to researchers Suzanne Kobasa and Salvatore Maddi, individual differences in personal control provide only part of the reason why some people who are under stress get sick whereas others do not. They have proposed that a broader array of personality characteristics — called **hardiness** — differentiates people who do and do not get sick under stress (Kobasa 1979, 1986; Kobasa & Maddi 1977). Hardiness includes three characteristics: (1) *Control* refers to people's belief that they can influence events in their lives — that is, a sense of personal control. (2) *Commitment* is people's sense of purpose or involvement in the events, activities and people in their lives. For instance, people with a strong sense of commitment tend to look forward to starting each day's projects and enjoy getting close to people. (3) *Challenge* refers to the tendency to view changes as incentives or opportunities for growth rather than threats to security.

Pollock and Duffy (1990) extended Kobasa's hardiness construct for a health-specific context. Health-related hardiness (HRH) comprises similar components to the hardiness construct as originally formulated by Kobasa, but differs in that commitment and challenge define one dimension of HRH, while control defines the other dimension. The term 'control' is used to refer to a sense of mastery or self-confidence needed to appraise and interpret health stressors appropriately. Adjustment to health problems by committed persons involves appraising ill-health as a challenge rather than as a threat. Health-related hardiness has been found to be associated with positive appraisals of illness and problem-focused coping (Pollock 1989). Even in healthy populations, hardiness has been reported to be associated with higher levels of perceived health, involvement in health promotion activities and supportive social relations (Pollock, Christian & Sands 1990).

Hardiness, coherence and resilience

Other researchers have described similar personality traits that, like hardiness, might protect people from the effects of stress. Aaron Antonovsky (1979, 1987) has described the *sense of coherence*, which involves the tendency of people to see their worlds as comprehensible, manageable and meaningful. A sense of coherence has been found to be positively related to possession of internal resources such as dispositional optimism and self-efficacy (Korotkov 1998). Sense of coherence can act as a personal coping resource in times of stress. Those with a high sense of coherence tend to have lower levels of anxiety and depression, better physical health, appraise situations positively and rely more on problem-focused coping (McSherry & Holm 1994; McSherry, Holm & Popinga 1991). Enhanced health outcomes are reported for diverse groups. For example, fewer symptoms of menopause are reported by midlife women with the dispositional SOC resource (Caltabiano & Holzheimer 1999). Another concept — that of *resilience* — has been applied to children who develop into competent and well-adjusted individuals despite growing up under extremely difficult conditions (Garmezy 1983; Werner & Smith 1982). Resilient children bounce back from life's adversities and recover their strength and spirit.

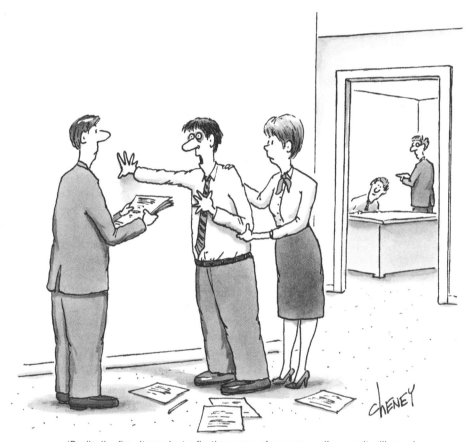

'Really, I'm fine. It was just a fleeting sense of purpose — I'm sure it will pass.'

Source: © 2001 *The New Yorker*, Tom Cheney. Collection from cartoonbank.com. All rights reserved.

Cases have been described of children who flourished or were well-adjusted despite being abused by their parents, or growing up in concentration camps, or living in societies with civil strife and wars (Garmezy 1983; Hartup 1983; Werner 1987).

Studies of resilient children have found that they share important characteristics (Garmezy 1983; Pines 1979; Werner 1987; Rouse, Ingersoll & Orr 1998; Werner & Smith 1982). These children have good social skills, being friendly and at ease with their peers and adults. Their temperaments tend to be easy, rather than difficult, and this promotes positive relationships with family and community members. They have strong feelings of self-esteem and personal control, and they are high achievers, generally doing well in the things they undertake.

Why are some children resilient and others not? Part of the answer may lie in their genetic endowments. Resilient children may have inherited traits, such as their relatively easy temperaments, that enable them to cope better with stress and turmoil. Another part lies in their experiences. Resilient children who have a history of stressful events often have compensating experiences and circumstances in their lives, such as special talents or interests that absorb them and give them confidence, and close relationships with friends or teachers. For instance,

> often they make school a home away from home, a refuge from a disordered household. A favourite teacher can become an important model of identification for a resilient child whose own home is beset by family conflict. (Werner, 1987, p. 95)

Sometimes these compensating relationships occur within the family, such as with older siblings or grandparents. Hardiness, resilience and coherence have a great deal in common and may be basically the same thing.

Hardiness and health

Kobasa (1979) has proposed that hardy people will remain healthier when under stress than those whose personalities are less hardy because they are better able to deal with stressors and are less likely to become anxious and aroused by these events. As a result, the spiralling process that can lead from stress to illness never takes hold.

The results of some studies support this prediction. For instance, retrospective and prospective research has found that hardy individuals report having developed fewer illnesses during extended stressful periods than less hardy people, and utilise health services less (Kobasa 1979; Kobasa, Maddi & Puccetti 1982; Kobasa et al. 1985; Manning & Fusilier 1999; Mathis & Lecci 1999). Other studies have found that people who are high in hardiness tend to deal more effectively with stressful situations than low-hardiness people do — for example by working through problems or transforming negative situations into positive ones (Holahan & Moos 1985; Williams, Wiebe & Smith 1992). In addition, hardy people show less physiological strain when under stress than less hardy individuals (Contrada 1989) and have lower blood pressure (Maddi 1999). Research conducted on staff from Monash University (Sharpley et al. 1995) has found that those staff with high levels of hardiness experienced less job stress, fewer daily hassles, lower anxiety, fewer injuries, fewer accidents and better overall physical health compared to staff with lower hardiness. Hardiness has also been found to have a protective function on psychiatric health — in diminishing, for instance, the negative effects of combat-related stress (Bartone 1999) and preventing the development of post-traumatic stress disorder (Taft et al. 1999). But other studies have found conflicting results, and some evidence indicates that tests used in assessing hardiness may simply be measuring negative affect, such as the tendency to be anxious, depressed or hostile (Funk 1992; Hull, Van Treuren & Virnelli 1987). We saw in chapter 1 that people with these personality characteristics are at risk for developing heart disease and other illnesses.

Although the status of the concept and measurement of hardiness is uncertain at this time, related aspects of personality are clearly involved in maintaining health. Researchers in the future will need to clarify what these personality variables are and how they operate.

Hardiness in old age

As individuals develop, they learn to deal with change by trying and succeeding, failing or compromising. Old age is a time when some very difficult life events occur, particularly those that involve reduced income, failing health and disability, and the loss of one's spouse and close friends. What are hardy people like in old age, and how did they get that way?

Elizabeth Colerick (1985) studied 70- to 80-year-old men and women for the quality she called *stamina*, which is similar to hardiness. This research was undertaken to determine how people who do and do not have stamina in later life deal with setbacks, such as the loss of a loved one. By using questionnaires and interviews, she was able to identify two groups: one with high stamina and one with low stamina. She found that stamina in old age is characterised by 'a triumphant, positive outlook during periods of adversity', as illustrated by the following interview excerpts from two different high-stamina people.

> The key to dealing with loss is not obvious. One must take the problem, the void, the loneliness, the sorrow and put it on the *back* of your neck and use it as a driving force. Don't let such problems sit out there in front of you, blocking your vision . . . Use hardships in a positive way. (p. 999)
>
> I realise that setbacks are a part of the game. I've had 'em, I have them now, and I've got plenty more ahead of me. Seeing this — the big picture — puts it all into perspective, no matter how bad things get. (p. 999)

In contrast, low-stamina people described a negative outlook and feelings of helplessness and hopelessness in the face of changes they experienced in old age. One woman who had undergone surgery for colon cancer said:

> I was certain that I would die on the table . . . never wake up . . . I felt sure it was the end. Then I woke up with a colostomy and figured I have to stay inside the house the rest of my life. Now I'm afraid to go back to the doctor's and keep putting off my checkups. (p. 999)

Elderly persons who are resilient are more satisfied with their ageing experience irrespective of economic hardship or diminished physical health (Staudinger et al. 1999).

Little available research bears directly on the question of how people become hardy, but the study by Colerick found some interesting relationships. Compared with low-stamina individuals, those with high stamina reported healthier pasts, more years of schooling, and more activities in their current lives involving social service and personal growth — for example visiting museums and travelling. More research is needed on a variety of biopsychosocial factors that are likely to shape hardy personalities.

In summary, people with a high degree of hardiness, coherence or resilience — or some related personality traits — may have some protection against the harmful effects of stress on health. The last psychosocial modifier of stress we will consider is people's tendency towards the Type A or Type B behavioural and emotional style.

Type A and Type B behaviour patterns

The history of science has many stories about researchers accidently coming upon an idea that changed their focus and led to their making major discoveries. Such was the case for bacteriologist Alexander Fleming, for instance. When the bacteria cultures he was studying developed unwanted moulds, he happened to notice some properties of the moulds that led to his discovery of penicillin. Serendipity also led to the discovery of the 'Type A' behaviour pattern by cardiologists Meyer Friedman and Ray Rosenman. They were studying dietary differences in cholesterol intake between male heart disease victims and their wives when one of the wives exclaimed, 'If you really want to know what is giving our husbands heart attacks, I'll tell you. It's stress, the stress they receive in their work, that's what's doing it' (Friedman & Rosenman 1974, p. 56). These researchers began to study this possibility by looking at differences between heart disease patients and similar people who were healthy, focusing on the subjects' stress and related behavioural characteristics. This comparison revealed differences in behavioural and emotional style: the patients were more likely than the non-patients to display a pattern of behaviour we now refer to as Type A.

What is the Type A behavioural and emotional style? The **Type A behaviour pattern** consists of three characteristics (Chesney, Frautschi & Rosenman 1985; Friedman & Rosenman 1974):

1. *Competitive achievement orientation.* Type A individuals tend to be very self-critical and to strive towards goals without feeling a sense of joy in their efforts or accomplishments.
2. *Time urgency.* Type A people seem to be in a constant struggle against the clock. Often, they quickly become impatient with delays and unproductive time, schedule commitments too tightly, and try to do more than one thing at a time, such as reading while eating or watching TV.
3. *Anger/hostility.* Type A individuals tend to be easily aroused to anger or hostility, which they may or may not express overtly.

In contrast, the **Type B behaviour pattern** is characterised by low levels of competitiveness, time urgency and hostility. People with the Type B pattern tend to be more easygoing and 'philosophical' about life — they are more likely to 'stop and smell the roses'.

Measuring Type A and Type B behaviour patterns

Researchers measure people's Type A and Type B behaviour either by using a standard interview procedure or by having the people fill out questionnaires. The most widely used interview procedure is called the *Structured Interview*, a standard procedure in which a trained interviewer asks individual subjects a series of questions about their behavioural and emotional styles, particularly regarding their competitiveness, impatience and hostility (Chesney, Eagleston & Rosenman 1980; Rosenman 1978; Rosenman, Swan & Carmelli 1988; Tallmer et al. 1990). For instance, subjects are asked, 'When you play games with people your own age, do you play for the fun of it, or are you really in there to win?' Although the specific answers people give to these questions contribute to the assessment of their behaviour pattern, their style of interaction with the interviewer also contributes. Some features of the interview are designed to encourage Type A behaviours, such as interrupting and talking fast and loudly. For example, the interviewer asks slowly and with hesitations, 'Most people who work have to get up fairly early in the morning. In your particular case, uh, what time, uh, do you, uh, ordinarily, uh-uh-uh, get up?' (You can imagine the Type A person saying, 'Six o'clock!' at the second 'uh'.) The interviewer also does things to annoy or challenge the subjects, thereby encouraging Type A behaviour. This is done by interrupting the subjects often and asking for clarifications in a harsh manner — asking, for instance, 'What do you mean by that?' rather than, 'Could you tell me a bit more about that?'

Structured Interview sessions are audiotaped or videotaped and scored by a trained rater who knows nothing about the subjects beyond what the tapes present. In the scoring process, the rater considers specific answers given to questions, speech characteristics and a variety of behaviours that suggest annoyance — for example sighing frequently or attempting to hurry the interviewer. Videotapes allow the rater to consider other behavioural features also, such as facial expressions, sitting on the edge of the chair and fidgeting. The rater's overall scores for subjects determine their classification as Type A or B.

The questions used in the Structured Interview have been adapted to construct a 52-item self-report questionnaire called the *Jenkins Activity Survey* (JAS) (Jenkins, Zyzanski & Rosenman 1979). Factor analysis of the JAS has revealed three components of Type A behaviour: *hard driving and competitiveness*; *job involvement*; and *speed and impatience*. Some items inquire about the person's usual way of responding to situations that can produce stress as a result of, for example, competition, time pressure or frustration. A sample question is: 'Would people who know you well agree that you tend to do most things in a hurry?' Other questions ask about the person's speed of eating, tendency to hurry someone who talks slowly, and work habits. This questionnaire was designed to test adults, but versions have also been developed for university students (Yarnold, Bryant & Grimm 1987). Another questionnaire for measuring the Type A and B behaviour patterns is the *Framingham Type ·A Scale* (Haynes et al. 1978). It contains only 10 items and has slightly different versions for testing students, homemakers and people who are employed (Powell 1987). Researchers have also developed instruments by which adults can rate Type A and B behaviour patterns in children. Probably the most widely used of these methods is the *Matthews Youth Test for Health* (Matthews & Angulo 1980).

Is one approach for measuring Type A and B behaviour better than the others? Each approach has its own strengths and weaknesses (Carver, Diamond & Humphries 1985; Matthews 1982; O'Rourke et al. 1988; Powell 1984, 1987). The Structured Interview has two important strengths. Its assessment of behaviour patterns seems to involve all three Type A characteristics: competitiveness, time urgency and anger/hostility. In addition, the Type A classification using this method has been associated fairly consistently with health outcomes, particularly heart disease (Booth-Kewley & Friedman 1987; Matthews 1988). But the Structured Interview is time-consuming and expensive to use, and details of the interviewer's and rater's methods can affect the outcome (Tallmer et al. 1990). The strengths of self-report methods rest mainly in their time- and cost-efficiency. But they have three important weaknesses. First, the relationship between health outcomes and Type A classification with existing self-report methods appears to be weak and inconsistent. Second, because characteristics such as impatience and hostility are socially undesirable, people may under-report these behavioural or emotional tendencies. Third, Type A measurements with the Jenkins Activity Survey and Framingham Type A Scale rely very little on and provide poor measures of the anger/hostility dimension of the behaviour pattern. Because of these problems, researchers generally favour the Structured Interview approach when studying connections between Type A behaviour and illness.

Behaviour patterns and stress

Individuals who exhibit the Type A behaviour pattern react differently to stressors than do those with the Type B pattern. That is, Type A individuals respond more quickly and strongly to stress, often interpreting stressors as threats to their personal control (Carver, Diamond & Humphries 1985; Glass 1977). But the Type A behaviour pattern may have another kind of impact on stress: it may actually increase the person's likelihood of encountering stressful events (Byrne & Rosenman 1986; Smith & Anderson 1986). For example, Type A individuals tend to seek out demanding situations in their lives. What's more, people who are often in a hurry and impatient with delays — as is the case for Type A individuals — tend to have more accidents than people who are more easygoing (Suls & Sanders 1988). In these ways the Type A and B patterns can affect the transactions of people in their environments and modify the stress they experience in their lives.

People's response to a stressor — or strain — includes both psychological and physiological components. The physiological portion of the response to stress, such as in blood pressure or cortisol levels, is called **reactivity**, which is measured against a baseline, or 'resting', level of arousal (Matthews 1986). Do Type A individuals show greater reactivity to stressors than Type Bs? In general, yes. One study examined the reactivity of men who each competed in a video game against an individual who was a confederate of the researchers (Glass et al. 1980). Although the instructions indicated that the winner would receive a prize, the game was rigged so that a subject could never win. The subjects were assigned to two groups, Type A or Type B, on the basis of their performance in the Structured Interview. Half of the men in each group played the game while being harassed and insulted by the confederate; for the remaining subjects, the confederate was silent. Several physiological measures were used, including blood pressure, heart rate, and plasma catecholamine levels. In the absence of harassment, both Type A and Type B subjects showed substantial and equal increases in physiological arousal over their baseline levels. But in the harassment condition, the Type A subjects showed greater reactivity than did the Type Bs.

Some research suggests the intriguing possibility that people's Type A behaviour may be caused, in part, by their physiological responses to stress (Contrada, Krantz & Hill 1988; Krantz & Durel 1983; Krantz, Lundberg & Frankenhaeuser 1987). For example, researchers conducted a study with Type A patients who were either taking or not taking a type of medication called *beta-blockers*, which dampen sympathetic nervous system transmission. This research demonstrated that Type A patients who were taking a beta-blocker exhibited less Type A behaviour in the Structured Interview than those who were not taking the drug (Krantz et al. 1982). This suggests that physiological reactions to stressors may influence Type A behaviour.

Gender and sociocultural differences in reactivity

Studies have examined gender differences in reactivity and found that males show more reactivity than females when psychologically stressed (Collins & Frankenhauser 1978; Kirschbaum, Wüst & Hellhammer 1992; Pollack & Steklis 1986; Ratliff-Crain & Baum 1990). Other studies have compared the reactivity of Type A and Type B people, using male and female subjects and a variety of tasks, ways to induce stress, and measures of Type A and B behaviour. Although there are some inconsistencies in their outcomes, most of these studies have found greater reactivity among Type A individuals, especially males (Carver, Diamond & Humphries 1985; Contrada & Krantz 1988; Houston 1986). Other researchers have examined reactivity in Type A and Type B boys and girls and found results similar to those found in adults (Lawler et al. 1981; Lundberg 1986; Matthews & Jennings 1984; Thoresen & Pattillo 1988). This suggests that males are more reactive to stress than females are, and the tendency of Type A individuals to be highly reactive may begin in childhood.

There appear to be sociocultural differences in reactivity, too. Research in the United States has revealed that blacks show greater reactivity than whites when under stress

(Calhoun et al. 1993; McAdoo et al. 1990; Miller et al. 1995). And a study found greater similarity in the degree of reactivity in siblings from black families than from white families, suggesting that part of this difference is inherited (Wilson et al. 1995). These sociocultural and gender differences are important because of the relationships researchers have found between reactivity and health, such as in the development of heart disease.

Type A behaviour and health

How are people's health and behaviour patterns related? To answer this question, researchers have used two approaches. First, studies have examined whether Type A individuals are at greater risk than Type Bs for becoming sick with any of a wide variety of illnesses. One study, for instance, found that Type A people reported having experienced more respiratory symptoms, such as asthma attacks and coughing spells, and more gastrointestinal symptoms, such as ulcers, indigestion and nausea (Woods & Burns 1984). Although several other studies have found similar results, the overall evidence for a link between Type A and B behaviour and general illnesses is weak and inconsistent (Orfutt & Lacroix 1988; Suls & Sanders 1988). The second approach has focused on the Type A pattern as a risk factor for **coronary heart disease (CHD)** — illnesses that result from the narrowing or blocking of the coronary arteries, which supply blood to the heart muscle. These illnesses include *angina*, *arteriosclerosis* and *myocardial infarction* (commonly called 'heart attack').

Dozens of studies have been done to assess the link between Type A behaviour and CHD, and most studies have confirmed the link when behaviour patterns were evaluated with the Structured Interview (Booth-Kewley & Friedman 1987; Haynes & Matthews 1988; Matthews 1988). Type A women and men, particularly white-collar workers, have a much greater chance of developing CHD than Type B adults do. An example of the convincing evidence of this link comes from a large-scale prospective study of healthy men. The Western Collaborative Group Study determined the health status and behaviour patterns (using the Structured Interview) of more than 3000 39- to 59-year-old employed men, most of whom had white-collar jobs (Rosenman et al. 1975; Rosenman et al. 1976). A follow-up on these men $8\frac{1}{2}$ years later showed that the Type A subjects were twice as likely as Type Bs to have developed CHD and to have died of CHD. Because of these and similar results, Type A behaviour has been called 'coronary prone behaviour'.

But some studies assessed behaviour patterns with the Structured Interview and did *not* confirm the link to CHD. Why? These studies have generally used subjects who either were at *high risk* for developing heart disease or were *already coronary patients* (Matthews 1988). An example study comes from a large-scale project called the Multiple Risk Factor Intervention Trial (MRFIT). This research began by identifying more than 12 000 middle-aged men who showed no evidence of CHD but still had a moderately strong risk for heart disease on the basis of their cigarette smoking, high blood pressure and so on (Shekelle et al. 1985). The Type A and Type B subjects did not differ in the incidence of heart disease over the next seven years. Other studies have found that coronary patients with the Type A behaviour pattern either were no more likely than Type Bs to suffer a heart attack following acute myocardial infarction (Palmer et al. 1992) or had a lower mortality rate from CHD over a 12-year period than the Type Bs (Ragland & Brand 1988). To explain why these studies didn't find the expected association between behaviour patterns and CHD, Karen Matthews (1988) has suggested several convincing reasons, and we'll consider two. (1) Type A high-risk and CHD subjects may have been misclassified as Type Bs in those studies if they were taking certain medications, such as beta-blockers, or trying to change their stress-related behaviour. (2) For subjects who were coronary patients, the main cause of the CHD may have been different for Type A and Type B subjects. If the Type Bs' CHD resulted mainly from atherosclerosis, their risk of a recurrent heart attack or death might be fairly high. As we saw in chapter 2, this condition involves the build-up of fatty patches on artery walls. And if the Type A subjects' CHD resulted from an acute precipitating factor, such as coronary spasms, their risk of recurrent attacks might be fairly low. This would be the case if Type A behaviour is linked more closely to developing acute precipitating factors than to atherosclerosis.

Why is the Type A behaviour pattern linked to CHD? We don't have a complete answer yet, but part of it seems to involve the relatively high physiological reactivity of Type A people (Carver, Diamond & Humphries 1985; Krantz, Lundberg & Frankenhaeuser 1987; Wright 1988). Frequent episodes of high arousal produce a lot of wear and tear on the cardiovascular system. One way this may occur is through the hormones that are released during arousal. Research has shown that chronically high levels of certain hormones, such as epinephrine and norepinephrine, can injure the heart and blood vessels. Another way wear and tear may lead to CHD in Type A people is through blood pressure. Studies have recorded higher blood pressure reactivity among Type A individuals — particularly those who score high on measures of anger and hostility — than among Type Bs during stressful situations (Diamond 1982; Diamond et al. 1984; Spiga 1986). High blood pressure strains the heart and arteries.

Behavioural factors may also contribute to the link between Type A behaviour and CHD. For instance, Type A individuals drink considerably more alcohol than Type Bs do, and excessive alcohol use is associated with CHD (Carmargo et al. 1986; Dielman et al. 1991). Another important risk factor for CHD is cigarette smoking. Of adults who smoke, Type A people not only smoke more (Twisk et al. 1999) but also inhale the smoke for a much longer time than Type Bs do, which provides more time for the lungs to absorb the harmful elements of smoke (Lombardo & Carreno 1987). And Type A individuals have more difficulty quitting smoking than Type Bs do (Caplan, Cobb & French 1975). Last, compared with Type Bs, Type A individuals are more likely to suppress or ignore their symptoms of fatigue and exert themselves to their limits despite having been injured (Carver, Coleman & Glass 1976; Carver, DeGregorio & Gillis 1981; Weidner & Matthews 1978). It may be that Type A individuals often drive themselves far beyond the point at which they should slow down, and that their frequent physical exhaustion leads to illness, such as CHD (Carver, Diamond & Humphries 1985).

Type A's 'deadly emotion'

As we have seen, the Type A behaviour pattern consists of three components. Is one component more damaging than the others? Redford Williams (1989; Williams & Barefoot 1988) has argued that the anger/hostility component is the most important factor. One of several studies that support this idea examined the records of 255 men (Barefoot, Dahlstrom & Williams 1983). These men were doctors who had taken a psychological test that included a scale for hostility while they were in medical school 25 years earlier. For the doctors with high scores on the hostility scale, the rates of both CHD and overall mortality during the intervening years were several times higher than for those with low hostility scores. Several other studies have examined the hostility–CHD connection and, although a few studies have not confirmed the link, most have (Byrne 1992; Smith, 1992; Weeks & Waterhouse 1991). Hostility seems to be a deadly emotion that may be especially damaging to health when it is expressed outwardly and when it involves a cynical or suspicious mistrust of others (Siegman 1993; Williams 1989; Williams et al. 1980).

A person's tendency towards hostility can be assessed in several ways, including the Structured Interview and various self-report questionnaires, like the *Cook–Medley Hostility Scale*, which has 50 true/false items, such as 'It is safer to trust nobody' and 'Some of my family have habits that bother and annoy me very much' (Cook & Medley 1954). This scale measures anger, as well as cynicism, suspiciousness and other negative traits (Friedman, Tucker & Reise 1995). By using such measures to identify hostile and non-hostile people, researchers have discovered physiological differences that help account for the CHD link with hostility. For instance, hostile individuals have higher resting blood pressure, and when harrassed or stressed they show poorer heart pumping efficiency and higher heart rate, blood pressure and blood platelet activity (Everson, McKey & Lovallo 1995; Ironson et al. 1992; Markovitz et al. 1996; Powch & Houston 1996; Suls, Wan & Costa 1995; Vitaliano et al. 1993). But these factors may form only part of the picture of why hostility and CHD are related. As psychologist Timothy Smith (1992) has pointed out, a person with cynical and suspicious beliefs about and behaviours towards other people is likely to provoke and worsen social conflicts and undermine his or her social support. A vicious circle emerges: as the social environment becomes less supportive and more stressful, the person's hostility and reactivity are maintained or increased. Research on college students confirmed this scenario, finding that hostile individuals tend to experience excessive anger in many situations and not to seek or accept social support (Houston & Vavak 1991).

Behaviour patterns and development

Research has addressed some important questions relating to the development of Type A behaviour and hostility. For example, do people's behaviour patterns change over the life span? Longitudinal studies have found that although people's behaviour patterns often change over time, many individuals exhibit the same pattern across many years. This has been shown for both children and adults (Bergman & Magnusson 1986; Carmelli et al. 1991; Carmelli, Rosenman & Chesney 1987; Visintainer & Matthews 1987). In addition, cross-sectional studies have found that the Type A behaviour pattern becomes more prevalent with age from childhood through middle age or so and then declines (Amos et al. 1987; Moss et al. 1986; Powell 1987). But it is currently uncertain whether the decline in the prevalence in old age is the result of Type A individuals dying at earlier ages than Type Bs.

Other studies have been conducted to determine the origins of the Type A pattern and factors that influence its development. One promising approach for determining the origins of Type A behaviour is to study how its development relates to the early temperaments of children. This is because behaviour patterns and temperaments involve some similar characteristics, such as the impulsiveness and intensity with which the person reacts and his or her ease in adjusting to changes in the environment. One longitudinal study found that temperament ratings taken in early childhood were related to measures of Type A behaviour taken 20 years later (Steinberg 1985). Another longitudinal study examined this relationship in adults and found an association between measures of temperament and Type A behaviour both at the beginning of the study and 10 years later (Carmelli, Rosenman & Chesney 1987). These results suggest that adult Type A behaviour has roots in the person's early temperament, which remains influential over time in at least some individuals.

Biopsychosocial factors in Type A behaviour

Do both biological and psychosocial factors affect the development of Type A and B behaviour patterns? It appears that they do. Research with identical (monozygotic) and fraternal (dizygotic) twins has demonstrated a genetic contribution in the development of temperament (Buss & Plomin 1975, 1986) and of Type A behaviour (Carmelli, Rosenman & Chesney 1987; Matthews et al. 1984; Pederson et al. 1989). That is, identical twins are more similar to each other in temperament and behaviour patterns than are fraternal twins. And they are much more similar than fraternal twins in their reactivity to stressors, too (Ditto 1993; Turner & Hewitt 1992).

Research has also examined the influence of various psychosocial factors on Type A behaviour. One finding from this research is that children's behaviour patterns are related to the parenting styles they experience. For example, compared with Type Bs, Type A boys who are working on a task receive less praise from their mothers and more statements to strive for improvement, such as, 'That was fine, but next time try harder' (Krantz, Lundberg & Frankenhaeuser 1987; Matthews & Woodall 1988). Another study found that hostile subjects reported that their parents had been less accepting, more punitive and more interfering with the subjects' desires during childhood (Houston & Vavak 1991). Psychological factors may interact with medical risk factors early in life to predispose individuals to coronary disease. Type A behaviour, especially impatience-aggression is much higher in adolescents who are overweight or obese, and who have elevated cholesterol levels (Oginska-Bulik 1998). Some evidence suggests that social support may reduce people's reactivity, but not if they are cynically hostile (Kamarck, Manuck & Jennings 1990; Lepore 1995).

Research with employed adults has shown that stressful work experiences affect people's behaviour patterns. Type A individuals work longer hours and have less supportive relationships with co-workers than Type Bs do (Sorensen et al. 1987). Also, a longitudinal study found that workers exhibit less Type A behaviour a year after retirement than they did shortly before retiring (Howard et al. 1986). Type A persons may experience psychological and physical distress when work environments do not allow them to exert sufficient control (Byrne & Reinhart 1990). Finally, there seem to be cultural differences in the prevalence of the Type A behaviour pattern. For instance, one study found that only a small percentage of Japanese-American men living in Hawaii exhibited the Type A pattern (Cohen et al. 1975). Research on psychosocial factors has revealed a wide variety of environmental influences on the development of Type A behaviour.

The relationships between psychosocial factors and Type A behaviour are very complex and seem to involve multiple levels of human experience. To describe these relationships, we can use a systems or 'ecological' approach with four levels (Margolis et al. 1983). The first level is *intrapersonal*: within the person, Type A behaviour is linked to many psychological factors, such as personal control. Type A behaviour seems to represent an effort by individuals to control stressful experiences in their lives (Glass 1977; Matthews 1982).

At the *interpersonal* level, social processes and Type A behaviour affect each other. This can be tested by having pairs of Type A subjects or Type B subjects engage in tasks together. Studies using this approach with children or university students who could either cooperate or compete in a game found that Type A pairs showed more competitive behaviour and less cooperation than the Type B pairs (Spiga 1986; Van Egeren, Sniderman & Roggelin 1982). Similarly, a study of married couples found that Type A pairs showed more hostile and dominant behaviour than Type Bs when discussing a marital conflict (Sanders, Smith & Alexander 1991). In general, people who display Type A behaviour tend to elicit reactions from others that create more demands and stimulate more Type A behaviour (Smith & Anderson 1986).

The third level is *institutional* and includes the experiences of people in educational and occupational settings. There are several ways these experiences can foster Type A behaviour. One way involves reward structures that promote aggressive competition, as can happen when many individuals are vying for a small number of rewards, such as job promotions or high grades. Another way involves time or work demands by a boss or teacher that encourage the feeling of time urgency. Research has found that employees with high scores on the Jenkins Activity Survey for Type A behaviour have longer work hours and less supportive relationships with co-workers than Type B workers do (Sorensen et al. 1987). More recent evidence indicates that the time pressure and hard-driving/competitiveness components of Type A behaviour in particular are associated with employee burnout, job dissatisfaction and turnover intention (Jamal 1999).

The fourth level of relationships between psychosocial factors and Type A behaviour is *cultural*. Some cultures place greater emphasis than others on the work ethic, getting ahead, status and accumulating goods that reflect status. People in cultures that emphasise these values are likely to display more Type A behaviour than those who live in cultures that do not.

As a summary of the role of psychosocial modifiers of stress, we have seen that social support, personal control, hardiness, and the Type A and B behaviour patterns are factors that can modify the impact of stress on health. High levels of social support, personal control and hardiness are generally associated with reduced stress and resulting illnesses; Type A behaviour is associated with increased stress and illness. The remainder of this chapter focuses on health problems that are affected by people's experience of stress. We begin by considering how stress leads to illness.

How stress affects health

Researchers conducted an interesting experiment: they gave subjects nasal drops that contained a 'common cold' virus or a placebo solution and then quarantined them to check for infection and cold symptoms (Cohen, Tyrrell & Smith 1991). Before the nasal drops were administered, the subjects had filled out questionnaires to assess their stress. Of these subjects, 47 per cent of those with high stress and 27 per cent of those with low stress developed colds. Other evidence indicates that people who show high reactivity to stress are at greater risk of respiratory infections when stressed than less reactive people (Bulcourf, Unrod & Adams 1996). What is it about stress that leads to illness? The causal sequence between stress and illness can involve either of two routes: (1) a direct route, resulting from the changes stress produces in the body's *physiology* or (2) an indirect route, affecting health through the person's *behaviour*. Let's look first at the behavioural route.

Stress, behaviour and illness

Stress can affect behaviour, which, in turn, can lead to illness or worsen an existing condition (Baum 1994). We can see the behavioural links between stress and illness in many stressful situations, such as when a family undergoes a divorce. In many cases, during the first year following the separation the parent who has the children is less available and responsive to them than she or he was before — a situation described as 'diminished parenting' (Wallerstein 1983). Behavioural changes during stressful times often make conditions for all family members less healthy, with haphazard meals, less regular bedtimes, delays in getting medical attention and failures to follow doctors' recommendations for example.

Research has shown that people who experience high levels of stress tend to perform behaviours that increase their chances of becoming ill or injured (Wiebe & McCallum 1986). For instance, they consume more alcohol, cigarettes and coffee than people who experience less stress (Baer et al. 1987; Conway et al. 1981). Consumption of these substances has been associated with the development of various illnesses. In addition, behavioural factors, such as alcohol use and carelessness, probably play a role in the relatively high accident rates of people under stress. Studies have found that children and adults who experience high levels of stress are more likely to suffer accidental injuries at home, in sports activities, on the job and while driving a car than individuals under less stress (Johnson 1986; Quick & Quick 1984).

Stress, physiology and illness

Stress produces many changes in the body's physical systems that can affect health. Clear connections have been found between illness and the degree of reactivity people show in their cardiovascular, endocrine and immune systems when stressed.

Cardiovascular system reactivity and illness

Cardiovascular reactivity includes any physiological change that occurs in the heart, blood vessels and blood in response to stress. Although researchers have not yet demonstrated a clear causal link between chronically high cardiovascular reactivity and the development of either CHD or hypertension, a strong association exists (Manuck 1994; Sherwood & Turner 1995). For example, research has shown that high levels of job stress are associated with high blood pressure and abnormally enlarged hearts (Schnall et al. 1990), and people's laboratory reactivity to stress in early adulthood is associated with their later development of high blood pressure (Menkes et al. 1989). The heightened blood pressure reactivity that people display in laboratory tests appears to reflect their reactivity in daily life (Turner et al. 1994).

Studies have also revealed that stress produces other cardiovascular changes that are related to the development of CHD. For instance, the blood of people who are under stress contains high concentrations of activated platelets (Malkoff et al. 1993; Patterson et al. 1994) and unfavourable levels of lipids, such as cholesterol (Patterson et al. 1995; Vitaliano, Russo & Niaura 1995). These changes in blood composition tend to promote atherosclerosis — the growth of plaques (fatty patches) on artery walls. As these plaques build up, they narrow and harden the arteries, thereby increasing blood pressure and the likelihood of a heart attack or stroke.

Endocrine system reactivity and illness

Part of reactivity involves the release of hormones — particularly catecholamines and corticosteroids — by the endocrine system during stress (Evans et al. 1994; McCann et al. 1993). The increased endocrine reactivity that people display in these tests appears to reflect their reactivity in daily life (Williams et al. 1991). One way in which high levels of these hormones can lead to illness involves their effects on the cardiovascular system. For example, an intense episode of stress with extremely high levels of these hormones can cause the heart to beat erratically and may lead to sudden death.

In addition, chronically high levels of catecholamines and corticosteroids appear to increase atherosclerosis.

Stephen Manuck and his colleagues (1988, 1995) have demonstrated this link between stress and atherosclerosis in research with monkeys. In one study, some of the subjects were relocated periodically to different living groups, thereby requiring stressful social and psychological adjustments to retain their dominant social status; the remaining subjects stayed in stable groups. Regardless of whether the monkeys' diets had high or low levels of cholesterol, the stressed subjects who had to retain their dominant status developed greater atherosclerosis than the subjects in the low stress condition. This effect of stress is probably very similar in humans, and studies have shown that people who have chronically high stress are more likely to develop atherosclerosis than those who do not (McKinney et al. 1984). Studies have also found that people with high levels of social support tend to exhibit lower endocrine reactivity than people with less support (Seeman & McEwen 1996).

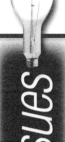

Highlight on issues

issues

Sudden 'voodoo' death

Can a person die from extreme psychological distress? Aborigines believe that 'poison sticks' can be used to sing *yarda* sorcery into people, by which solid objects are projected into their bodies. Such sorcery is usually the result of jealousy. Fear of *yarda* sorcery can lead to high levels of anxiety, and **sudden death** — the abrupt death from cardiac dysfunction of a seemingly healthy person (AHA 1994; Strathern & Stewart 1999). Sudden death was originally called 'voodoo death' (Cannon 1942), perhaps because many of the cases described were associated with voodoo practices in the Caribbean and southern United States.

Sudden death usually results from cardiac failure of some sort and frequently involves two factors: a pre-existing cardiovascular disorder and a severe physical or psychological stressor, such as extreme anger or fear (Allan & Scheidt 1990; Kawachi et al. 1994; Mittleman et al. 1995). Type A individuals seem to be at high risk for sudden death (Perini et al. 1993). The underlying cardiovascular disorder may take two forms (McKinney et al. 1984; Schneiderman & Hammer 1985; Verrier, DeSilva & Lown 1983). First, the disorder may involve damage to the myocardium caused by high levels of catecholamines in the blood. Second, the disorder typically involves the occurrence of *cardiac arrhythmia* — an abnormal rhythm of the heart's functioning. Arrhythmias can take the form of an extremely high heart rate, called *flutter*, or of uncoordinated heartbeats, called *fibrillation* (Tortora & Grabowski 1993).

Immune system reactivity and illness

The release of catecholamines and corticosteroids during arousal affects health in another way: Some of these hormones impair the functioning of the immune system (Jemmott & Locke 1984; Schleifer et al. 1986). For example, increases in cortisol and epinephrine are associated with decreased activity of T cells and B cells against antigens. This decrease in lymphocyte activity appears to be important in the development and progression of a variety of infectious diseases and cancer (Kiecolt-Glaser & Glaser 1995). Sandra Levy and her co-workers (1985) tested women diagnosed with breast cancer and found that patients with high levels of killer-T-cell activity exhibited less spread of the cancer to surrounding tissue than those with low levels of lymphocyte activity.

Immune processes also protect the body against cancers that result from excessive exposure to harmful chemical or physical agents called **carcinogens**, which include radiation (nuclear, X and ultraviolet types), tobacco tars and asbestos (AMA 1989). Carcinogens can damage the DNA in body cells, which may then develop into mutant cells and spread. Fortunately, people's exposure to carcinogens is generally at low levels and for short periods of time, and most DNA changes probably do not lead to cancer (Glaser et al. 1985). When mutant cells develop, the immune system attacks them with killer T cells. Actually, the body begins to defend itself against cancer even before a cell mutates by using enzymes to destroy chemical carcinogens or to repair damaged DNA. Research has shown that high levels of stress, however, reduce the production of these enzymes and the repair of damaged DNA (Glaser et al. 1985; Kiecolt-Glaser & Glaser 1986; Kiecolt-Glaser et al. 1985).

Psychoneuroimmunology

We have seen in this and earlier chapters that psychological and biological systems are interrelated — as one system changes, the others are often affected. The recognition of this interdependence and its connection to health and illness led researchers to form a new field of study called **psychoneuroimmunology**. This field focuses on the relationships between psychosocial processes and the activities of the nervous, endocrine and immune systems (Ader & Cohen 1985; Bachen, Cohen & Marsland 1997; Dunn 1995; Maier, Watkins & Fleshner 1994). These systems form a *feedback loop*: the nervous and endocrine systems send chemical messages in the form of neurotransmitters and hormones that increase or decrease immune function, and cells of the immune system produce chemicals, such as ACTH, that feed information back to the brain. The brain appears to serve as a control centre to maintain a balance in immune function, since too little immune activity leaves the individual open to infection and too much activity may produce auto-immune diseases.

Emotions and immune function

People's emotions — both positive and negative — play a critical role in the balance of immune functions. Research has shown that pessimism, depression and stress from major and minor events are related to impaired immune function (Biondi & Pancheri 1995; Dunn 1995; Leonard 1995; Levy & Heiden 1991; Zautra et al. 1989). For example, a study comparing caregiver spouses of Alzheimer's disease patients with matched control subjects found that the caregivers had lower immune function and reported more days of illness over the course of about a year (Kiecolt-Glaser et al. 1991). But positive emotions can also affect immune function, giving it a boost (Futterman et al. 1994; Stone et al. 1994). In the study by Arthur Stone and his co-workers, adult men kept daily logs of positive and negative events and gave saliva samples for analyses of antibody content. Negative events were associated with reduced antibodies only for the day the events occurred, but positive events enhanced antibody content for the day of occurrence and the next two.

Some stressful situations start with a crisis, and the ensuing emotional states tend to continue and suppress immune processes over an extended period of time. This was demonstrated with healthy elderly individuals who were taking part in a longitudinal study of the ageing process (Willis et al. 1987). The subjects were asked to contact the researchers as soon as they were able if they experienced any major crises, such as the diagnosis of a serious illness in or the death of a spouse or child. Fifteen subjects did so. A month after the crises, and again several months later, the researchers assessed the subjects' cortisol and lymphocyte blood concentrations, recent diets, weights and psychological distress. Because the subjects were already participating in the longitudinal study, comparable data were available from a time prior to the crisis. Analysis of these data revealed that lymphocyte concentrations, caloric intake and body weight decreased, and cortisol concentrations and psychological distress increased, soon after the crises. By the time of the last assessment several months later, however, all of these measures had returned almost to the pre-crisis levels.

When people are reacting to short-term, minor events, such as doing difficult math problems under time pressure, changes in the number and activity of immune cells occur for fairly short periods of time — minutes or hours (Delahanty et al. 1996). The degree of change seems to vary with the event's intensity, duration and type — for example whether the event is interpersonal or nonsocial (Herbert & Cohen 1993). Long-lasting, intense, interpersonal events seem to produce especially large immune changes. Of course, immune system reactivity varies from one person to the next, but an individual's degree of response to a type of event seems to be much the same when tested weeks apart (Marsland et al. 1995). This suggests that a person's reaction to specific stressors is fairly stable over time.

Psychosocial modifiers of immune system reactivity

We saw earlier that psychosocial factors in people's lives may modify the stress they experience. Such factors seem to affect immune system responses, too. For instance, research has shown that people under long-term, intense stress who have strong social support systems have stronger immune systems and smaller immune impairments in response to the stress than others with less support (Esterling, Kiecolt-Glaser & Glaser 1996; Kennedy, Kiecolt-Glaser & Glaser 1990; Kiecolt-Glaser et al. 1991; Levy et al. 1990). Research has also demonstrated that aerobic exercise training and therapy to reduce stress can enhance immune function in people infected with the AIDS virus (Antoni et al. 1990).

A related psychosocial modifier involves describing one's feelings about stressful events, which may help by altering stress appraisals. An experiment using this approach examined the effect of expressing such feelings on blood concentrations of antibodies against the Epstein-Barr virus, a widespread virus that causes mononucleosis in many of those who are infected (Esterling et al. 1994). The university student subjects were randomly assigned to three conditions that met in three weekly 20-minute sessions in which they either described *verbally* a highly stressful event they had experienced, or described *in writing* a highly stressful event they had experienced, or wrote about a trivial (nonstress-related) topic, such as the contents of their bedrooms. The subjects in each condition had the same level of immune control against the virus before the start of the study. But analysis of blood samples taken a week after the last session revealed that immune control improved substantially in the verbal condition, moderately in the written condition, and declined slightly in the control (trivial topic) condition, as figure 4.4 depicts. Other research has found that describing feelings about stressful events is more effective in enhancing immune function in cynically hostile than in non-hostile individuals (Christensen et al. 1996).

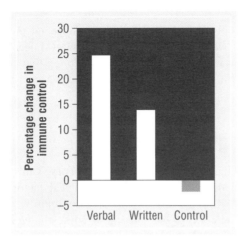

Figure 4.4 Percentage change in immune control against the Epstein-Barr virus, as reflected in blood concentrations of specific antibodies, for subjects having sessions for verbal expression of stress feelings, written expression of stress feelings or a control condition

Source: Based on data from Esterling et al. (1994, figure 3).

Lifestyles and immune function

Do people's lifestyles affect the functioning of their immune systems? Some evidence suggests that they do. People with generally healthy lifestyles — including exercising, getting enough sleep, eating balanced meals and not smoking — show stronger immune functioning than those with less healthy lifestyles (Kusaka, Kondou & Morimito 1992). Other studies have found that sleeping poorly impairs immune function the next day (Irwin et al. 1994) and people who smoke are more susceptible to catching colds (Cohen et al. 1993).

Conditioning immune function

Research on psychoneuroimmunology with animals has revealed that the influence of psychological processes on immune function is not limited to the effects of stress. The impact may be far more broad and pervasive. Robert Ader and Nicholas Cohen (1975, 1985) have described research showing that *immunosuppression can be conditioned*. In their original research, they were actually studying how animals learn to dislike certain tastes. The procedure used a single conditioning trial: the subjects (rats) received saccharin-flavoured water to drink (which they seemed to like) and then got an injection of a drug that induces nausea. To see if the rats' subsequent dislike of the taste depended on its strength, some subjects received more saccharin flavouring than others in this conditioning trial. Over the next several weeks, the drug was not used, but the animals continued to receive saccharin-flavoured water. During this time, the researchers noticed a curious thing: a number of rats had fallen ill and died — and these animals tended to be the ones that had consumed the greatest amount of saccharin in the conditioning trial.

How did these deaths relate to immunosuppression? Since the nausea-inducing drug used in the conditioning trial was also known to suppress immune function temporarily, Ader and Cohen hypothesised that the continued intake of saccharin water served as a conditioned stimulus, suppressing the ability of the rats to fight infection. Subsequent experiments by these researchers and others confirmed this hypothesis and demonstrated that conditioning can influence both antibody-mediated and cell-mediated immune processes (Ader & Cohen 1985). Although the extent to which this kind of conditioning impairs immune function is fairly moderate, the effect is clear. Moreover, similar conditioning effects have been demonstrated in cancer patients who receive chemotherapy substances that impair immune function (Lekander et al. 1995).

Psychoneuroimmunology is a very exciting field, and researchers are discovering fascinating connections between biological and psychosocial processes very quickly. And they are developing ways to apply this knowledge (Maier, Watkins & Fleshner 1994). For instance, Ader and Cohen (1982) demonstrated that conditioned immuno-suppression may be useful in treating auto-immune diseases, in which the immune system attacks parts of the person's own body.

Psychophysiological disorders

The word *psychosomatic* has a long history, and was coined to refer to symptoms or illnesses that are caused or aggravated by psychological factors, mainly emotional stress (Lipowski 1986). Although this term is still commonly used by professionals and the general public, the concept has undergone some changes and now has a new name. The term **psychophysiological disorders** refers to physical symptoms or ill-nesses that result from the interplay of psychosocial and physiological processes. This definition clearly uses a biopsychosocial perspective. We will briefly discuss several ill-nesses that have been traditionally classified as psychosomatic. Some of these illnesses will be examined in greater detail in later chapters.

Digestive system diseases

Ulcers and **inflammatory bowel disease** are two illnesses that involve wounds in the digestive tract that may cause pain and bleeding (P. Bennett 1995). Ulcers are found in the stomach and the duodenum, or the upper section of the small intestine. Inflamma-tory bowel disease, which includes disorders such as *colitis*, can occur in the colon (large intestine) and the small intestine. Although ulcers and inflammatory bowel disease afflict mostly adults, these illnesses also occur in childhood and adolescence (Schwartz & Blanchard 1990; Whitehead 1986). Another digestive system illness, **irritable bowel syndrome**, produces abdominal pain, diarrhoea and constipation without organic evidence of disease (P. Bennett 1995).

Researchers generally believe most ulcers are produced by a combination of excess gastric juices chronically eroding the lining of the stomach and duodenum that has been weakened by bacterial infection (Rhoades & Pflanzer 1996). But stress seems to play a role, too. In a classic study, a patient (called Tom) agreed to cooperate in a lengthy and detailed examination of gastric function (Wolf & Wolff 1947). Tom was unique in that many years earlier, at the age of nine, he had had a stomach operation that left an opening to the outside of the body. This opening, which provided the only way he could feed himself, was literally a window through which the inside of his stomach could be observed. When Tom was subjected to stressful situations, causing feelings of hostility and anxiety, his stomach-acid production greatly increased. When he was under emotional tension for several weeks, there was a pronounced reddening of the stomach lining. Another study reported similar effects with a 15-month-old girl, Monica, who had a temporary opening to her stomach. Her highest levels of acid secretion occurred when she experienced rage (Engel, Reichsman & Segal 1956).

The physical causes of inflammatory bowel disease and irritable bowel syndrome are not yet known. Some studies have found that flare-ups of these illnesses are related to stress, but other studies have not (Drossman 1994; Schwartz & Blanchard 1990; Suls, Wan & Blanchard 1994). The role of stress in these digestive system diseases is currently unclear.

Asthma

Asthma is a respiratory disorder in which inflammation, spasms and mucus obstruct the bronchial tubes and lead to difficulty breathing, with wheezing or coughing. This ailment is more common in children than in adults, and in boys than in girls. About 20 per cent of children and 8 per cent of adults in Australia suffer from asthma (Bauman et al. 1995; AIHW 1998). Asthma attacks appear to result from some combination of three factors: allergies, respiratory infections and biopsychosocial arousal, such as from stress (Busse 1990). In most cases, the cause of an attack is largely physical, but sometimes it may be largely psychosocial.

Professionals working with hospitalised children have noted an interesting phenomenon that suggests a role for psychosocial factors, and in particular dysfunctional family relations, in asthma (Liebman, Minuchin & Baker 1974). About one-third of asthmatic children show reduced symptoms shortly after admission to the hospital even though their medication is not changed. When they return home, the symptoms reappear (Bakwin & Bakwin 1972; Purcell, Weiss & Hahn 1972). Does this happen because the children are allergic to something in their own houses, such as dust, or because of other factors? This question was tested in an ingenious study with asthmatic children who were allergic to house dust (Long et al., 1958). Without the children knowing, the researchers vacuumed the children's homes and then sprayed the collected dust from each house into their individual hospital rooms. None of the children had respiratory difficulty when exposed to their home dust, which suggests that psychosocial factors may be involved. The results of other research indicate that stress can trigger asthma attacks (Brantley & Jones 1993; Miller & Wood 1994; Sarafino & Goldfedder 1995).

Chronic headache

Many people suffer chronically from intense headaches. Although there are many types of chronic headache, two of the most common are called tension-type and migraine headache (Andrasik, Blake & McCarran 1986; Lipton, Silberstein & Stewart 1994;. Pothmann et al. 1994). **Tension-type** (or *muscle-contraction*) **headaches** seem to be caused by persistent contraction of the head and neck muscles, which is a typical feature of people's reaction to stressors (Martin 1993). The pain it produces is a dull and steady ache that often feels like a tight band of pressure around the head. Chronic tension-type headaches occur twice a week or more, and may last for hours, days or weeks (Dalessio 1994).

Migraine headaches seem to involve the dilation of blood vessels surrounding the brain (Martin 1993). The pain often begins on one side of the head near the temple, is sharp and throbbing, and lasts for hours or, sometimes, days (Dalessio 1994). One form of migraine either begins with or is preceded by an *aura*, a set of symptoms that signal an impending headache episode. These symptoms usually include sensory phenomena, such as seeing lines or shimmerings in the visual field. This may be accompanied by dizziness, nausea and vomiting. Chronic migraine is marked by periodic debilitating symptoms, which occur about once a month, with headache-free periods in between (Dalessio 1994; Stewart, Shechter & Lipton 1994).

The great majority of adults and children have headaches at least occasionally, and frequent tension-type headaches are common (Andrasik, Blake & McCarran 1986; Lipton, Silberstein & Stewart 1994; Pothmann et al. 1994). The prevalence of migraine varies widely across cultures, but is about 10 per cent overall, is far greater in females than males, and increases with age from childhood to middle age, and then declines (Stewart, Shechter & Rasmussen 1994). Many children experience their first headaches in the preschool years, and chronic headaches have been reported in boys and girls as young as six years of age (Andrasik, Blake & McCarran 1986). Figure 4.5 presents a drawing by an 11-year-old girl named Meghan to describe her experience of migraine headache pain.

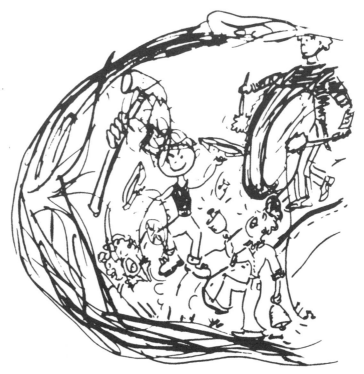

Figure 4.5 Drawing by 11-year-old Meghan of her experience of migraine headache pain. The lower left-hand corner has a self-portrait with a dramatic facial expression. When a headache begins, Meghan typically retreats to her bedroom 'to ride out the storm', lying down in a darkened room.

Source: From Andrasik, Blake & McCarran (1986, figure 18.1).

What triggers headaches? They often are brought on by weather changes, missing a meal, sunlight, sleeping poorly and consuming certain substances, such as alcohol or chocolate. Research has also shown that stressors — particularly the hassles of everyday living — are among the most common triggers of migraine and tension-type headaches (Gannon et al. 1987; Köhler & Haimerl 1990; Robbins 1994). Yet some chronic-headache patients have attacks when they are not under great stress, and others fail to have headaches when they are under stress. Stress appears to be one of many factors that produce headaches, but the full nature of these causes is not yet known.

Other disorders

There are several other psychophysiological disorders for which stress appears to be involved in triggering or aggravating episodes. One of these illnesses is *rheumatoid arthritis* — a chronic and very painful disease that produces inflammation and stiffness of the small joints, such as in the hands. It afflicts about 2.9 per cent of Australians, and its victims are primarily women (AIHW 1996, 1998). Another disorder, called *dysmenorrhoea*, affects millions of women. It is characterised by painful menstruation, which may be accompanied by nausea, headache and dizziness (Calhoun & Burnette 1983; Schuster 1986). A third stress-related problem involves skin disorders, such as *hives*, *eczema* and *psoriasis*, in which the skin develops rashes or becomes dry and flakes or cracks (Grossbart 1982). In many cases, specific allergies are identified as contributing to episodes of these skin problems (Burg & Ingall 1985).

Although current evidence implicates both biological and psychosocial causes for each of the psychophysiological disorders we have considered, the evidence is sketchy and the nature of the interplay of these factors is unclear. For the remainder of this chapter we will focus on the role of stress in the development of cardiovascular disorders and cancer.

Stress and cardiovascular disorders

Earlier in this chapter, we saw that psychosocial modifiers of stress can affect health — for instance, the risk of developing CHD is greater for people with the Type A than the Type B behaviour pattern. Such findings indirectly implicate stress as a factor in the development of cardiovascular disorders, the leading cause of death in Australia. Is there more direct evidence for this link? A large body of evidence indicates that stress plays a role in the development of two types of cardiovascular disorders, hypertension and CHD.

Hypertension

Hypertension — the condition of having high blood pressure consistently over several weeks or more — is a major risk factor for CHD, stroke and kidney disease (AIHW 1998; Knox 1992; Schneiderman & Hammer 1985). In Australia, about one-quarter of the adult population is classified as hypertensive, having blood pressures that consistently exceed 160 (systolic) over 95 (diastolic). The prevalence rates for hypertension increase in adulthood, particularly after about 40 years of age. Fortunately, the percentage of Australian adults with high blood pressure has declined markedly since the late 1960s (P. Bennett 1995). Some cases of hypertension are caused by, or are *secondary* to, disorders of other body systems or organs, such as the kidneys or endocrine system. Secondary hypertension can usually be cured by medical procedures. But the vast majority — over 90 per cent — of hypertensive cases are classified as *primary* or **essential hypertension**, in which the mechanisms causing the high blood pressure are unknown.

To say that the causes for essential hypertension are unknown is somewhat misleading. In cases of essential hypertension, doctors are unable to identify any biomedical causes, such as infectious agents or organ damage. But many risk factors are associated with the development of hypertension — and there is evidence now implicating several of these risk factors as determinants of hypertension (AIHW 1998; Knox 1992; Shapiro & Goldstein 1982). These determinants include:

• obesity
• dietary elements, such as salt, fats and cholesterol
• excessive alcohol use
• physical inactivity
• family history of hypertension
• psychosocial factors.

The psychosocial factors that have received the most research attention involve stress and emotional behaviours such as anger and hostility. One interesting finding is that just the anxiety involved in having blood pressure tested can increase the reading in some individuals, leading to a false diagnosis of hypertension (McGrady & Higgins 1990).

Stress, emotions and hypertension

People's occupations provide sources of stress that can have an impact on their blood pressure. Traffic controllers at airports have an occupation that is often described as stressful. Sidney Cobb and Robert Rose (1973) compared the medical records of thousands of men employed as air traffic controllers or as second-class airmen. Both occupations require yearly physical examinations for renewal of their licences. The medical records were separated so that comparisons could be made for different age groups, since blood pressure increases with age. These comparisons for each age group revealed prevalence rates of hypertension among the traffic controllers that were several times higher than those among airmen. The researchers also compared the records of traffic controllers who experienced high and low levels of stress, as measured by the traffic density at the air stations where they worked. Figure 4.6 depicts the results of this analysis: For each age group, the prevalence rates of hypertension were higher for traffic controllers working at high-stress locations than for those at low-stress sites.

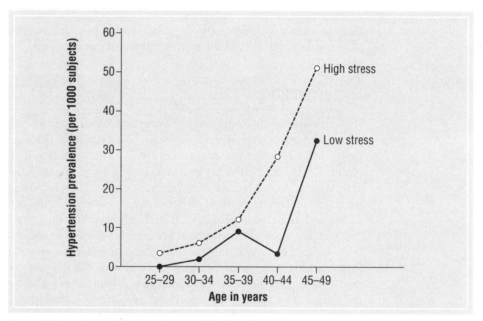

Figure 4.6 Prevalence of hypertension per 1000 air traffic controllers as a function of stress and age. Hypertension rates increase with age and stress.

Source: Data from Cobb & Rose (1973, table 3).

Stress is also related to individuals' social environments, such as crowding and aggression. Experiments with animals have shown that living in crowded, aggressive conditions induces chronic hypertension (Henry et al. 1993). Research with humans compared cardiovascular reactivity among people who live in crowded and uncrowded neighbourhoods to see if living in these conditions influences blood pressure (Fleming et al. 1987). The subjects from the two types of neighbourhoods were similar in important characteristics, such as age, gender and family income. While working on a stressful cognitive task, residents from crowded neighbourhoods showed greater increases in heart rate and systolic and diastolic pressure than those from uncrowded neighbourhoods. Findings of other research indicate that high cardiovascular reactivity may be a risk factor for, or even a cause of, hypertension (Fredrikson & Matthews

1990; Manuck 1994; Menkes et al. 1989). Taken together, the evidence suggests that chronic stress plays an important role in the development of hypertension.

Other research on emotional factors in the development of essential hypertension has focused on the role of anger and hostility. Some studies have found that hypertensives are more likely to be chronically hostile and resentful than are *normotensives* — that is, people who have normal blood pressure (Diamond 1982). Further evidence for the role of emotion in hypertension comes from the Normative Aging Study (Spiro et al. 1995), a longitudinal study that monitored 2280 men over 17 years. Hypertension was found to be linked to emotional instability, even when controlling for baseline hypertension, alcohol consumption and education. Other studies have shown that systolic and diastolic blood pressure increase more when people experience anger and hostility in their everyday lives than when they experience positive emotions, such as happiness (James et al. 1986; Southard et al. 1986). In some families, interpersonal conflicts among parents and children can be major sources of chronic anger, which may lead to hypertension (Ewart 1991a). These findings indicate that chronically high levels of anger and hostility may contribute to the high blood pressure of many hypertensives.

Moderating factors in hypertension

There is some evidence that appraisal support is beneficial in reducing age-related hypertension. Appraisal support refers to the perceived availability of others with whom one can discuss problems. In a study by Uchino et al. (1995), age was found to be related to elevated blood pressure for women low in appraisal support. Uchino et al. (1995) offered the following explanation for their findings.

> ...one mechanism by which appraisal support may be associated with beneficial outcomes is through self-disclosure...one reason self-disclosure may be beneficial is that it allows individuals to understand and assimilate traumatic and stressful events. Talking with others may also provide social comparison information and reduce intrusive or ruminative thinking. Appraisal support, therefore, may be important because it provides an individual with the opportunity to discuss, disclose, and compare one's personal problems during the life span. (p. 560)

Other variables such as personality appear to be associated with hypertension. In a large-scale Australian study of 4870 female and 2746 male twins, hypertension was found to be related to interactive influences between personality, stress and lifestyle variables such as lack of exercise and smoking (Mellors, Boyle & Roberts 1994). Male hypertensive twins were high on neuroticism, low on psychoticism and either introverted or extraverted. Female hypertensives tended to be neurotic introverts, low on psychoticism.

Stress and sociocultural differences in hypertension

The impact of occupational and environmental stressors on hypertension may be particularly relevant for indigenous Australians who have a much higher prevalence rate of high blood pressure than Caucasians do (AIHW 1998; Hogg 1992). Compared with mainstream Australians, indigenous people have to cope with unemployment, limited job prospects, low job security, crowding and inadequate housing conditions. But Aboriginals are not alone in their cardiovascular disease risk. Other Australians of low socioeconomic status share an increased risk of mortality from heart disease and stroke (S. Bennett 1995). The role of racial discrimination in hypertension is suggested by the US finding that blood pressure and darkness of skin colour are correlated for black men and women of low socioeconomic status, but not for blacks with higher income or education. For lower-class black people, those with darker skin probably have fewer economic and social resources available, thereby worsening their stress (Klag et al. 1991).

Few, if any, cases of essential hypertension are likely to be caused by emotional factors alone (Schneiderman & Hammer 1985). Most cases of high blood pressure probably involve several of the determinants listed earlier in this section.

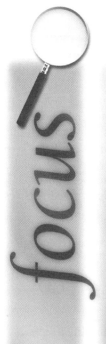

Focus on research
Reactivity and hypertension: a meta-analysis

Meta-analysis is a statistical research method that pools the results of prior studies to create an integrated overview of their findings. Although the purpose of meta-analysis is fairly easy to understand, doing one can be very complex because decisions that can alter the outcome need to be made (Suls & Swain 1993). For example, if you were doing a meta-analysis, would you use only studies that have been published? Will you want to restrict the included studies to only those that had control groups or tested people of certain ages or genders? How broadly will you define your variables — for instance, for the variable of fear, will you include anxieties and phobias?

Mats Fredrikson and Karen Matthews (1990) did a meta-analysis to clarify the connection between reactivity and hypertension. They knew that some studies had found greater reactivity to stressors in hypertensive people than in normotensives, but other studies had not. They decided to focus their meta-analysis on *cardiovascular reactivity* — blood pressure and heart rate — and to include only studies that, for instance, tested hypertensive patients who were not currently taking antihypertensive drugs; had a normotensive control group; and measured reactivity in a laboratory with a psychological stressor, such as performing mental arithmetic or watching a stressful film, rather than a physical one, such as exercising. Then they searched the medical and psychological literature using the restrictions they had decided on, found dozens of studies that qualified, and analysed relevant data with a computer program.

Fredrikson and Matthews organised the meta-analysis to examine several important issues. This analysis revealed two previously unknown patterns: (1) Patients with relatively mild hypertension exhibit heart rate and blood pressure reactivity mainly to psychological stressors that require them to be *active*, such as doing arithmetic, rather than *passive*, as in watching a stressful film. (2) Patients with more severe hypertension show reactivity to *all* types of psychological stressors. Many earlier studies had found no link between cardiovascular reactivity and hypertension because they tested mild hypertensives with passive stressors.

Coronary heart disease

Epidemiologists have studied the distribution and frequency of CHD over many decades in many different cultures. The data they have collected suggest that CHD is, to some extent, a disease of modernised societies — that is, the incidence rate of heart disease is higher in technologically advanced countries than in other nations (Susser, Hopper & Richman 1983). In Australia, mortality from coronary heart disease reached its peak prior to 1960 but has declined since the late 1960s (S. Bennett 1995, 1996). While older Australians appear to have changed risk factors — especially smoking, dietary behaviours and to a lesser extent exercise — the increase in mortality for young men does not demonstrate comparable changes (Wilson & Siskind 1995).

There are many reasons why modernised societies have higher rates of CHD. For one thing, people in technologically advanced societies live longer than those in less-developed countries, being less likely to die of infectious diseases such as malaria for instance. As a result, people in advanced societies live long enough to become victims of CHD, which afflicts mainly older individuals. Also, people in modernised societies are more likely than those in less-developed countries to have certain risk factors for CHD, such as obesity and low levels of physical activity. Last, the psychosocial stressors of modernised societies are different from those in other societies and may be more conducive to the development of heart disease.

The link between stress and CHD has considerable support. For example, studies of occupational stress have shown that high work loads, job responsibility, and job dissatisfaction are associated with a high incidence of CHD (Cottington & House 1987; Quick & Quick 1984). Other research has examined the relationship between heart disease and major life stressors, as measured by life events scales. Retrospective studies have found that victims of myocardial infarction tended to have high levels of life events in the months preceding the attack (Garrity & Marx 1979). Prospective research has also supported the link between stress and CHD. For instance, researchers carried out periodic follow-up assessments over an eight-year period with patients who had recovered from their first myocardial infarctions (Theorell & Rahe 1975). These patients were separated into two groups — those who did and those who did not have subsequent attacks. The group who suffered subsequent infarctions — some of whom died — had experienced a substantial build-up in life events over the year or so preceding the attacks. But the group who had no recurrence of heart attack reported no increase in life events during the study.

We have seen that stress increases catecholamine and corticosteroid release by the endocrine glands and that chronically high levels of these hormones can damage the arteries and heart, promote atherosclerosis, and lead to the development of hypertension and arteriosclerosis (hardening of the arteries). Stress can also produce cardiac arrhythmia, which can cause a cardiac episode and sudden death. These are some of the physiological connections between stress and CHD. There are behavioural connections, too. Stress is associated with cigarette smoking and high levels of alcohol use, for example, which are behavioural risk factors for CHD (Epstein & Jennings 1986; Levenson 1986). In later chapters we will examine in greater detail various risk factors and issues relating to CHD and the next stress-related illness, cancer.

Stress and cancer

The idea that stress and other psychosocial factors contribute to the development of cancer has a long history. The physician Galen, who practised in Rome during the second century A.D., believed that individuals who were sad and depressed, or 'melancholy', were more likely to develop cancer than those who were happy, confident and vigorous (Sklar & Anisman 1981). Similar ideas have appeared in the writings of doctors in later eras.

Cancer is a term that refers to a broad class of disease in which cells multiply and grow in an unrestrained manner. As such, cancer does not refer to a single illness, but to dozens of disease forms that share this characteristic (ACS 1996; Levy 1985; Williams 1990). It includes, for instance, *leukaemias*, in which the bone marrow produces excessive numbers of white blood cells, and *carcinomas*, in which tumours form in the tissue of the skin and internal organ linings. Some cancers take longer to develop or follow more irregular courses in their development than others. Because cancer appears in so many different forms, each with its own characteristics, it is very difficult to study its causes (Fox 1978). Nevertheless, some evidence suggests that stress may play a role in the beginnings and progression of cancer.

Early evidence linking stress and cancer came from research using retrospective methods (P. H. Blaney 1985; Sklar & Anisman 1981). This research generally had cancer patients fill out life events questionnaires to assess the stress they experienced during the year or so preceding the diagnosis. A number of studies found that the appearance of several forms of cancer in children and adults was associated with their reports of high levels of prior stress. But there are problems with retrospective methods that cloud the interpretation of the results of these studies (Fox 1978; Sklar & Anisman 1981). For one thing, the diagnosis of cancer is typically made years after — sometimes many years after — the disease process starts. As a result, the patients' cancers were probably present prior to and during the year for which they reported high levels of stress. Also, the patients' perceptions or recollections of prior stress may have been distorted by their knowledge that they have cancer.

A better approach for implicating the role of stress in the development of cancer would be to use prospective methods: measure or introduce psychosocial factors and follow up on the subjects' health over time. Some studies have used this approach, either by monitoring the incidence of cancer in individuals who were healthy at the start of the research or by following the progress of the disease in people who were already diagnosed with cancer. An overview of the findings from this research suggests four conclusions: First, although some studies with initially healthy subjects have found that people who experienced high levels of stress during the intervening years were more likely to develop cancer than those with less stress, other studies have not, making the role of stress unclear (Sklar & Anisman 1981; Temoshok 1990b; Watson & Ramirez 1991). Moreover, experimental research with animals has produced inconsistent outcomes, too (P. H. Blaney 1985; Sklar & Anisman 1981). Second, studies of people already diagnosed with cancer have found that patients who suffered relapses within a subsequent time period, such as a year, tended to have experienced more stressful life events or received less social support than those who did not have relapses (Rogentine et al. 1979; Sabbioni 1991; Watson & Ramirez 1991). Third, people who generally respond to stressors with appeasing, compliant and unexpressive behaviours (sometimes called the Type C behaviour pattern) seem more likely than others to develop cancer (Temoshok 1990b; Temoshok & Dreher 1992). Fourth, some evidence indicates that cancer patients who receive therapy to reduce their stress live longer than those who do not (Kiecolt-Glaser & Glaser 1995).

The effects of stress on cancer seem to be influenced by many factors, such as the stressor's source or type, whether it is chronic, the way the person reacts to it, and whether it is experienced before or after initiation of the carcinogen or tumour. If stress plays a causal role in the development of cancer, it probably does so by impairing the immune system's ability to combat the disease and by increasing behavioural risk factors, such as smoking cigarettes.

Summary

Researchers have identified several psychosocial factors that modify the impact of stress on the individual. One of these factors is social support — the perceived comfort, caring, esteem or help a person receives from other people or groups. There are five basic types of support: emotional, esteem, tangible or instrumental, informational and network. Whether people receive social support depends on characteristics of the recipients and providers of support, on stress-related transactions in personal relationships, and on the composition and structure of the social network.

Social support appears to reduce the stress people experience and generally enhance their health. The greater the degree of support people have, the lower their mortality rates and likelihood of becoming ill. These benefits seem to accrue in two ways. First, social support may buffer the person against the negative effects of high levels of stress. Second, social support may enhance health regardless of the level of stress by simply providing encouragement for leading healthy lifestyles, for instance.

Another psychosocial modifier of stress is the sense of personal control people have over the events in their lives. Personal control includes beliefs about one's locus of control — that is, whether control is internal or external to the person — and self-efficacy. People acquire a sense of personal control from their successes and failures and through the process of social learning. Individuals who experience prolonged high levels of stress and have a weak sense of personal control tend to feel helpless. The cognitive process of attribution seems to be important in the development of learned helplessness. A strong sense of personal control tends to benefit people's health and help them adjust to a serious illness if it occurs. Hardiness is another psychosocial modifier of stress that may help people remain healthy when under stress.

One other psychosocial modifier of stress is people's tendency towards either the Type A or the Type B behaviour pattern. The Type A behaviour pattern consists of three characteristics: competitive achievement orientation, time urgency, and anger or hostility. Compared with Type Bs, Type A individuals respond more quickly and strongly to stressors both in their overt behaviours and in their physiological reactivity. The Type A pattern — particularly the anger/hostility component — is associated with the development of coronary heart disease (CHD) and hypertension. Both biological and psychosocial factors affect the development of the Type A and B behaviour patterns.

Stress affects health in two ways. First, stress can affect health-related behaviours, such as alcohol and cigarette use. Second, it produces changes in the body's physical systems, as when the endocrine system releases catecholamines and corticosteroids, which can cause damage to the heart and blood vessels and impair immune system functioning. The physiological effects of intense stress can even lead to sudden death. Psychoneuroimmunology is a field of study that focuses on how psychosocial processes and the nervous, endocrine and immune systems are interrelated. Stress also plays a role in many psychophysiological disorders, such as ulcers, asthma, chronic headache, rheumatoid arthritis and several skin disorders. In addition, stress is implicated in the development of hypertension, CHD and cancer.

Key terms

asthma	direct effects hypothesis	meta-analysis	social support
attribution	essential hypertension	migraine headaches	sudden death
behavioural control	hardiness	personal control	tension-type headaches
buffering hypothesis	hypertension	psychoneuroimmunology	Type A behaviour pattern
carcinogens	inflammatory bowel disease	psychophysiological disorders	Type B behaviour pattern
cognitive control	informational control	reactivity	ulcers
coronary heart disease (CHD)	irritable bowel syndrome	self-efficacy	
decisional control	learned helplessness	social network	
	locus of control		

5 Coping with and reducing stress

Prologue

One morning while taking a shower, Karen felt a small lump in her breast. She was sure it had not been there before. It didn't hurt, but she was momentarily alarmed — her mother had had breast cancer a few years before. 'It could be a pimple or some other benign growth,' she thought. Still, it was very worrying. She decided not to tell her husband or her doctor about it yet because, as she thought, 'it may not be anything.' Over the next several days, she examined the lump daily. This was a very stressful time for her, and she slept poorly and seemed preoccupied. After a week without the lump changing, she decided to take action. She told her husband and made an appointment to see her doctor.

Another woman, Liz, had a similar experience. She was also alarmed by finding a lump on her breast, but she didn't deal with the stress as rationally as Karen had. Liz's initial fright led her to re-examine her breast just once, and in a cursory way. She told herself, 'There isn't really a *lump* on my breast, it's just a rough spot.' And she convinced herself that she should not touch it because, she thought, 'That will only make it worse.' During the next few months, Liz was quite worried about the 'rough spot'. She studiously avoided touching it, even while washing. She became increasingly moody, slept poorly and developed many more headaches than usual. She also told her husband that she didn't like him to fondle her breasts in lovemaking. When he asked why she was acting so differently in recent weeks, she denied that anything was wrong. Liz finally mentioned the 'rough spot' to a friend who convinced her to have her doctor examine it.

People vary in the ways they deal with stress. Sometimes people confront a problem directly and rationally, as Karen did, and sometimes they do not. For these two women, the way they dealt with their stress had the potential for affecting their health. Because Liz did not face up to the reality of the lump, she delayed seeking medical attention and experienced high levels of stress for a long time. If the lump were malignant, delaying treatment would allow the cancer to progress and spread. As we have seen, prolonged stress can have adverse health effects even in healthy people.

In this chapter we discuss the ways people can and do deal with stress. Through this discussion, you will find answers to questions you may have about the methods people use in handling stress. Are some methods for coping with stress more effective than others? How can people reduce the potential for stress in their lives? When people encounter a stressor, how can they reduce the strain it produces?

Coping with stress

Individuals of all ages experience stress and try to deal with it. During childhood years, people learn ways to manage feelings of stress that arise from the many fearful situations they experience (Sarafino 1986). One of the more common fears of childhood is of thunderstorms. Psychologist Lois Murphy (1974, p. 76) has described the progress a little girl named Molly made in dealing with the terror she felt during thunderstorms. At three years of age, Molly's efforts to gain control of her fear during a storm were reflected in her trying to reassure herself and her baby brother by saying, 'It's just noise and it really won't hurt you a bit.' But a month later,

> Molly was again terrified as a jet plane flew unusually low overhead; she cried and clung to her sister for comfort. A few hours later she repeated several times to herself, 'Thunder really doesn't hurt you; it just sounds noisy. I'm not scared of planes, only thunder.'

At the age of four, her behaviour during two storms, four months apart, showed that she was gaining substantial control over her fear. In the first instance,

> she was awakened from a nap during a thunderstorm, but remained quietly in bed. Afterward she said to her sister, 'There was lots of thunder, but I just snuggled in my bed and didn't cry a bit.'

On the second occasion,

> Molly showed no open fear herself during a storm, and comforted her frightened brother, saying, 'I remember when I was a little baby and I was scared of thunder and I used to cry and cry every time it thundered.'

Although Molly's progress had some setbacks, such as when the plane flew very low, she became better able to cope effectively with this stressor as she grew older. What's more, in the last steps of her progress she showed pride in having mastered her fear.

What is coping?

Because the emotional and physical strain that accompanies stress is uncomfortable, people are motivated to do things to reduce their stress. These 'things' are what is involved in coping.

What is coping? Several definitions of coping exist (Lazarus 1987; Lazarus & Folkman 1984b). We will use a definition that is consistent with the way we defined stress earlier. In chapter 3 we saw that stress involves a *perceived discrepancy* between the demands of the situation and the resources of the person. Since people engage in coping in an effort to neutralise or reduce stress, coping activities are geared towards decreasing the person's appraisal of, or concern for this discrepancy. Thus, **coping** is the process by which people try to *manage the perceived discrepancy* between the demands and resources they appraise in a stressful situation.

The word *manage* in this definition is important. It indicates that coping efforts can be quite varied and do not necessarily lead to a solution of the problem. Although coping efforts can — and, some would argue, should — be aimed at correcting or mastering the problem, they may also simply help the person alter his or her perception of a discrepancy, tolerate or accept the harm or threat, or escape or avoid the situation (Lazarus & Folkman 1984b; Moos & Schaefer 1986). For example, a child who faces a stressful exam in school might cope by feeling nauseated and staying home.

We cope with stress through our cognitive and behavioural transactions with the environment. Suppose you are overweight and smoke cigarettes, and your doctor has asked you to lose weight and stop smoking because several factors place you at very high risk for developing heart disease. The threat is that you may become disabled or die. This is stressful, but you don't think you can change your behaviour. How might you cope with this? Some people would cope by seeking information about ways to improve their ability to change. Other people would simply find another doctor who is not so directive. Others would attribute their health to fate or 'the will of God', and leave the problem 'in His hands'. Still others would try to deaden this and other worries with alcohol, which would add to the risk. People use many different methods to try to manage the appraised discrepancy between the demands of the situation and their resources.

The coping process is not a single event. Because coping involves ongoing trans-actions with the environment, the process is best viewed as a dynamic series

> of continuous appraisals and reappraisals of the shifting person–environment relationships.
> Shifts may be the result of coping efforts directed at changing the environment, or coping
> directed inward that changes the meaning of the event or increases understanding. They
> may also be the result of changes in the environment that are independent of the person
> and his or her coping activity. Regardless of its source, any shift in the person–environment
> relationship will lead to a reevaluation of what is happening, its significance, and what can
> be done. The reevaluation process, or reappraisal, in turn influences subsequent coping
> efforts. (Lazarus & Folkman, 1984b, pp. 142–3)

And so, in coping with the threat of serious illness, people who make efforts to change their lifestyles may receive encouragement and gain better relationships with their doctor and family. But individuals who ignore the problem are likely to experi-ence worse and worse health and relations with these people. Each shift in one direc-tion or the other is affected by the transactions that preceded it and affects subsequent transactions.

Functions and methods of coping

You have probably realised by now that people have an enormous number of ways of coping with stress. Because of this, researchers have attempted to organise coping approaches on the basis of their functions and the methods they employ.

Functions of coping

According to Richard Lazarus and his colleagues, coping can serve two main functions (Cohen & Lazarus 1979; Lazarus & Folkman 1984b; Lazarus & Launier 1978). It can alter the *problem* causing the stress or it can regulate the *emotional* response to the problem.

Emotion-focused coping is aimed at controlling the emotional response to the stressful situation. People can regulate their emotional responses through behavioural and cognitive approaches. Some examples of behavioural approaches are using alcohol or drugs, seeking emotional social support from friends or relatives, and engaging in activities, such as sports or watching TV, that distract one's attention from the problem. Cognitive approaches involve how people think about the stressful situation. In one cognitive approach, people change the meaning of the situation — for example by deciding, 'There are worse things in life than having to change jobs because of my heart condition,' or, 'Now that my girlfriend has left me, I realise that I really didn't need her.' Another cognitive approach involves denying unpleasant facts, as Liz did with the lump in her breast.

People tend to use emotion-focused approaches when they believe they can do nothing to change the stressful conditions (Lazarus & Folkman 1984b). A clear example of this is when a loved one dies — in this situation, people often seek emo-tional support and distract themselves with funeral arrangements and chores at home or at work. Similarly, pain-coping strategies of arthritis patients tend to be emotion-focused (Affleck et al. 1999). To cope with the intense joint pain, rheumatoid arthritis patients may vent their emotions, or seek emotional understanding and comfort from others. Patients may use emotion-focused strategies in coping with surgery. Terry (1992), however, found that emotion-focused coping did not facilitate adaptation in heart attack patients. Other examples can be seen in situations in which individuals believe their resources are not and cannot be adequate to meet the demands of the stressor. A child who tries very hard to be the 'straight A' student his or her parents seem to want, but never succeeds, may reappraise the situation and decide, 'I don't need their love.'

Assess yourself
YOUR FOCUSES IN COPING

Think about a very stressful personal crisis or life event you experienced in the last year — the more recent and stressful the event, the better for this exercise. How did you handle this situation and your stress? Some of the ways people handle stressful experiences are listed below. Mark an 'X' in the space preceding each one you used.

____ Tried to see a positive side to it

____ Tried to step back from the situation and be more objective

____ Prayed for guidance or strength

____ Sometimes took it out on other people when I felt angry or depressed

____ Got busy with other things to keep my mind off the problem

____ Decided not to worry about it because I figured everything would work out fine

____ Took things one step at a time

____ Read relevant material for solutions and considered several alternatives

____ Drew on my knowledge because I had a similar experience before

____ Talked to a friend or relative to get advice on handling the problem

____ Talked with a professional person (e.g. doctor, clergy, lawyer, teacher, counsellor) about ways to improve the situation

____ Took some action to improve the situation

Count how many of the first six ways you marked — these are examples of 'emotion-focused' ways. How many of the second six — 'problem-focused' — ways did you mark? When you read the text material entitled 'Functions of coping', answer these questions: Did you use mostly emotion- or problem-focused methods? Why, and what functions did your methods serve?

Source: Based on material in Billings and Moos (1981).

Problem-focused coping is aimed at reducing the demands of the stressful situation or expanding the resources to deal with it. Everyday life provides many examples of problem-focused coping, including quitting a stressful job, negotiating an extension for paying some bills, devising a new schedule for studying (and sticking to it), choosing a different career to pursue, seeking medical or psychological treatment, and learning new skills. People tend to use problem-focused approaches when they believe their resources or the demands of the situation are changeable (Lazarus & Folkman

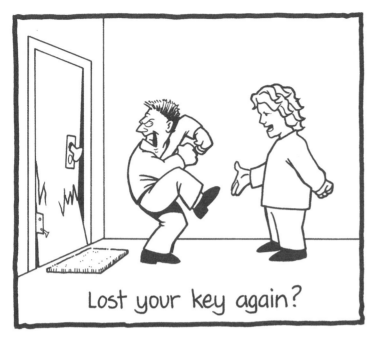

Lost your key again?

1984b). For example, caregivers of terminally ill patients use problem-focused coping more in the months prior to the death than during bereavement (Moskowitz et al. 1996).

To what extent do people use problem-focused and emotion-focused approaches in coping with stress in their lives? Andrew Billings and Rudolf Moos (1981) studied this issue by having nearly 200 married couples fill out a survey. The subjects described a recent personal crisis or negative life event that happened to them and then answered questions that were very similar to the ones you answered in the self-assessment exercise. The outcomes of this research revealed some interesting relationships. Both the husbands and the wives used more problem-focused than emotion-focused methods to cope with the stressful event. But the wives reported using more emotion-focused approaches than the husbands did. Subjects with higher incomes and educational levels reported greater use of problem-focused coping than those with less income and education. Last, the subjects used much less problem-focused coping when the stress involved a death in the family than when it involved other kinds of problems, such as illness or economic difficulties.

Some occupations may foster one type of coping over the other. Research by Evans et al. (1993) on Australian police officers found that problem-focused, direct action strategies were used frequently to cope with occupational stress. These strategies included 'Making action plans and following them', 'Working through situations one step at a time' and 'Standing one's ground and fighting for what one wants'. While officers reported having asked someone they respected for advice on a job-related matter, emotional experiences were usually not shared with families, the item 'Keeping one's feelings to oneself' being reported by a large number of officers. The coping strategies used by these officers were consistent with the image of strong, self-reliant, responsible upholders of the law.

Can problem-focused and emotion-focused coping be used together? Yes, and they often are. Let's look at an example that involves a case in which an employee experienced stress when he was accused by a co-worker of not sending out the appropriate letters for a job. In describing how he reacted to this accusation, he said:

> 'Well, it burned me up . . . My immediate first reaction was to confirm . . . that what he was saying was not true, that everything [letters] had gone out. There's always a chance you might be wrong so I checked first. Then I told him. No, everything had gone out. My immediate reaction was to call him on the carpet first. He doesn't have any right to call me on something like this. Then I gave it a second thought and decided that that wouldn't help the situation.' (Kahn et al., cited in Lazarus & Folkman 1984b, p. 155)

This example shows problem-focused coping in confirming that the letters had gone out, and emotion-focused coping in controlling his angry impulse 'to call him on the carpet'.

Methods of coping: skills and strategies

What types of skills and strategies do people use in altering the problem or regulating their emotional response when they experience stress? Table 5.1 describes several commonly used ways of coping that Susan Folkman, Richard Lazarus and their colleagues (1986) identified from their research. The table labels the strategies as serving problem- or emotion-focused coping functions and gives examples of cognitive or behavioural efforts a hospital patient might make when using each strategy. Coping methods that focus on emotions are important because they sometimes interfere with getting medical treatment or involve unhealthy behaviours, such as using cigarettes, alcohol or drugs to reduce tension. People often use these substances in their efforts towards emotion-focused coping (Wills 1986).

Each of these strategies is quite broad and can be applied in many ways and situations. To clarify how people use emotion-focused methods, we can describe some variations on the strategies in the table. For instance, people may engage in a coping method called *emotional discharge*, which involves expressing or releasing their feelings about a stressful situation. This approach usually occurs in conjunction with seeking social support, such as with friends or family or in support groups, and can also involve using jokes or gallows humour (Moos & Schaefer 1986). For instance, a man jokingly nicknamed himself 'Semicolon' after part of his cancerous colon was removed. Humour can effectively reduce people's stress (Newman & Stone 1996). Although using emotional discharge can help people cope, many people who suffer from chronic stress fail to express their feelings. Instead, they have *intrusive thoughts* and images that perpetuate their stress (Baum 1990). For example, they may think repeatedly about how they or others are to blame for their problems, or have 'flashbacks' of painful or traumatic events. People who often have intrusive thoughts report having poorer health habits and health than individuals who seldom have such thoughts (Nowack 1989). James Pennebaker (1990) has found that people's talking or writing about the problems and negative feelings they have may reduce their stress and benefit their health. Other studies have confirmed that these beneficial effects of expressing one's feelings can occur (Christensen et al. 1996; Esterling et al. 1994). But other researchers have found that expressing emotions to reduce tension, anxiety or frustration can worsen one's mood (Stone, Kennedy-Moore & Neale 1995). It may be that the intentions of the person for expressing feelings influences the outcome.

Cognitive redefinition is a strategy whereby people try to put a good face on a bad situation, such as by noting that things could be worse, making comparisons with individuals who are less well off, or seeing something good growing out of the problem (Pearlin 1991). We can see this approach in the following statements by women with breast cancer (Taylor 1983):

> What you do is put things into perspective. You find out that things like relationships are really the most important things you have — the people you know and your family — everything else is just way down the line. It's very strange that it takes something so serious to make you realize that. (p. 1163)
>
> The people I really feel sorry for are these young gals. To lose a breast when you're so young must be awful. I'm 73; what do I need a breast for? (p. 1166)

People who want to redefine a stressful situation can generally find a way to do it, since there is almost always *some* dimension or aspect of one's life that can be viewed positively (Taylor 1983). Cognitive reappraisal may explain why traumatic events can result in positive growth experiences for some people. Stress-related growth may involve the interplay of appraisal, personal characteristics and coping (Park 1998).

Table 5.1 Ways of coping with stressful situations

Strategy	Coping function	Description	Example
Planned problem-solving	Problem focused	Analysing the situation to arrive at solutions and then taking direct action to correct the problem	Steve, a hospital patient who needs to choose a specialist for a serious illness, might seek and study information about different specialists before choosing.
Confrontative coping	Problem focused	Taking assertive action, often involving anger or risk-taking, to change the situation	If Steve's medical insurance company declines the rebate on a medical treatment, he might stand his ground and fight for payment.
Seeking social support	Problem or emotion focused	Trying to acquire informational or emotional support	Steve might ask friends and nurses about different specialists (informational support with a problem-focused function) and describe his worries to get comfort and encouragement from people he loves (emotion-focused function).
Distancing	Emotion focused	Making cognitive efforts to detach oneself from the situation or create a positive outlook	Steve might try not to think about the health-related problems he is facing, or try to make light of them.
Escape–avoidance	Emotion focused	Thinking wishfully about the situation or taking action to escape or avoid it	Steve might engage in fantasies of miracles or other external events that would make his problems go away, or he might try to avoid dealing with the problems by sleeping or using alcohol a lot.
Self-control	Emotion focused	Attempting to modulate one's own feelings or actions in relation to the problem	Steve might hide his feelings to avoid emotional interactions with others or slow down the pace of decision making to prevent impulsive choices.
Accepting responsibility	Emotion focused	Acknowledging one's own role in the problem while also trying to put things right	Steve might lecture himself for not having sought medical attention sooner, and promise to respond to symptoms more promptly in the future.
Positive reappraisal	Emotion focused	Trying to create a positive meaning from the situation in terms of personal growth, sometimes with a religious tone	Steve might become a better or stronger person from the experience, or feel that he has developed a stronger faith.

Source: Based on Folkman & Lazarus (1988); Folkman et al. (1986).

Other coping processes include the cognitive strategies Freud called 'defence mechanisms', which involve distorting memory or reality in some way. For instance, when something is too painful to face, the person may deny that it exists. This defence mechanism is called *denial*. In medical situations, individuals who are diagnosed with terminal diseases often use this strategy and refuse to believe they are really ill. Another defence mechanism, called *intellectualisation*, consists of dealing with or confronting a stressor on an abstract, intellectual level. Nurses and physicians who have to deal with enormous amounts of human suffering need some way to detach their emotions from these situations. They may intellectualise, for example, by referring to a patient dying of liver cancer as 'the liver in 203'. These approaches are similar to those of distancing and escape–avoidance described in table 5.1.

You may have noticed that some of the methods people use in coping with stress tend to increase the *attention* they give to the stressful situation. Problem-focused methods generally do this. Other methods, particularly some emotion-focused methods, tend to promote *avoidance* of the problem. Both attention to and avoidance of a stressor can be beneficial under some circumstances. Avoidance-promoting approaches, such as distancing, are beneficial when there is little the person can do about the problem (Cohen & Lazarus 1979; Lazarus 1983). For instance, a study examined the coping strategies of women after they had undergone mastectomies for breast cancer. Patients who avoided thinking about cancer and minimised the impact of their illness showed less evidence of distress than those who did not use avoidance-promoting strategies (Meyerowitz 1983). But if the person *can* do something about the problem, failing to give it attention can be more harmful than helpful, as we saw in Liz's denial of the lump in her breast at the beginning of the chapter.

The time frame for using strategies that promote attention to or avoidance of the problem is also important. Jerry Suls and Barbara Fletcher (1985) pooled the results of a large number of studies in a meta-analysis to clarify the effects of attention-promoting and avoidance-promoting strategies. Their analysis led to two conclusions. First, avoidance-promoting strategies can benefit coping mainly in the short run, such as during an early stage of a prolonged stress experience. This is the case for individuals who are diagnosed with a serious illness, for instance. Second, as time goes by, attention-promoting strategies become more effective than avoidance in the coping process. As a rule of thumb, the effectiveness of avoidance-promoting methods seems to be limited to the first couple of weeks of a prolonged stress experience. Thereafter, coping is better served by attention-promoting strategies.

Our discussion indicates that there is no one best method of coping. No single method is uniformly applied or effective with all stressful situations (Ilfeld 1980; Menaghan 1982; Pearlin & Schooler 1978). Research has revealed two important patterns in the way people cope. First, individuals tend to be consistent in the way they cope with a particular type of stressor — that is, when faced with the same problem, people tend to use the same methods they used in the past (Costa, Somerfield & McCrae 1996; Hewitt & Flett 1996). Much of the consistency in coping has been demonstrated by Terry (1994) to be dependent on cross-situational consistency in the type of event experienced, and how such events are appraised. Second, people seldom use just one method to cope with a stressor. Their efforts typically involve a combination of strategies, such as planned problem-solving and denial (Holahan & Moos 1985). The degree to which individuals rely on strategies that promote avoidance of the problem may have important health implications. A one-year prospective study compared people who differed in their reported use of avoidance-promoting approaches. Of the subjects who experienced a high degree of stress during the intervening year, those who had reported a greater tendency to use avoidance-promoting methods had, at the end of the study, more psychosomatic symptoms — for example headaches and acid stomach (Holahan & Moos 1986).

Developing methods of coping

Psychologists have long assumed that coping changes across the life span. But the nature of these changes is unclear because there is little systematic research, especially longitudinal studies, charting the changes (Lazarus & DeLongis 1983; Lazarus & Folkman 1984b).

Some aspects of the changes in coping that occur in the early years are known. Infants and toddlers do not cope very effectively with stress. For example, when being examined by their pediatricians, infants and toddlers often react by trying to stop the examination, and preschoolers tend to protest after it's over (Hyson 1983). We saw earlier in the case of Molly that young children develop coping skills that enable them to overcome many of their fears. The skills she acquired often made use of her expanding cognitive abilities, such as in thinking logically and stating her ideas. Over the next several years, children come to rely increasingly on cognitive strategies for coping (Brown et al. 1986; Miller & Green 1984). So, for example, they learn to think about something else to distract themselves from stress. More and more, they regulate their feelings using emotion-focused methods, such as cognitive redefinition — for instance saying to themselves, 'I can do it', while preparing to give a speech. In coping with their parents having a serious illness, such as cancer, children and adolescents rarely use problem-focused methods — but as they develop they rely more on emotion-focused methods, such as playing with toys or watching TV, to cope (Compas et al. 1996).

Australian research on adolescent coping has indicated that coping strategies are directed towards dealing with the problem while maintaining physical fitness and social connections (Frydenberg & Lewis 1999). Older adolescents tend to use more tension-reduction techniques such as smoking and drinking, seek social support and engage in self-blame, rather than using more productive strategies such as problem solving and focusing on the positive. Female adolescents tend to seek social support (Frydenberg & Lewis 1993; 1999) in favour of professional advice for their problems, and engage in more self-blame and tension-reduction strategies. Boys are more likely to ignore the problem or use distraction in the form of physical recreation or relaxing activities. Research by Gomez (1998) and Frydenberg and Lewis (1996) has found that among adolescents, use of non-productive, avoidance coping strategies, such as self-criticism, giving up or ignoring the problem, is associated with higher levels of anxiety and depression.

Few studies have examined changes in methods of coping from adolescence to old age. One study used interviews and questionnaires to compare the daily hassles and coping methods of middle-aged and elderly men and women (Folkman et al. 1987). The middle-aged men and women used more problem-focused forms of coping, whereas the elderly subjects used more emotion-focused approaches. For example, the middle-aged people were more likely to report coping with stress in a confrontative and planned manner — claiming such actions as, 'I stood my ground and fought for what I wanted,' and, 'I made a plan of action and followed it.' The elderly individuals were more likely to report passive, emotion-focused methods — claiming such approaches as, 'Went on as if nothing had happened,' and, 'Wished that the situation would go away or somehow be over with.'

Why do adults tend to shift from problem-focused to emotion-focused coping as they get older? These changes probably result at least in part from differences in what people must cope with as they age. The elderly subjects in this study were retired from full-time work and reported more stress relating to health and home maintenance than the middle-aged people did; the middle-aged individuals reported more stress relating to work, finances, family and friends. Planned and confrontative action are probably more effective strategies for coping with the kinds of stressors encountered by middle-aged than by elderly people. But there was also a difference in the outlook of the two age groups: regardless of the source of stress, the elderly people appraised their problems as *less* changeable than the middle-aged subjects did. As we saw earlier, people tend to use problem-focused approaches when they believe the situation is changeable and rely on emotion-focused coping when they do not.

Gender and sociocultural differences in coping

Studies of gender differences in coping have generally found that men are more likely to report using problem-focused strategies and women are more likely to report using emotion-focused strategies in dealing with stressful events (Caltabiano & Caltabiano 1992; Ptacek, Smith & Zanas 1992). Men are also more likely to use alcohol and drugs as escape coping, while women vent and express emotions, seek social support or avoid stressful situations (Ptacek, Smith & Dodge 1994). These gender differences appear to be consistent from adolescence (Frydenberg & Lewis 1993) through to young adulthood (Caltabiano & Caltabiano 1992). But when the men and women are similar in occupation and education, no gender differences are found (Greenglass & Noguchi 1996). In research on coping strategies used by men and women specifically in regard to their work, females have reported more coping aimed at control of the stressor (brainstorming solutions, gathering information, taking action) compared with men. The only notable difference appears to be that men are more likely to cope with stress at work by exercising (Christie & Shultz 1998). These results suggest that societal sex roles play an important role in the coping patterns of men and women.

The findings of Billings and Moos (1981) that individuals with higher incomes and educational levels report greater use of problem-focused coping than those with less income and education suggests that the social experiences of disadvantaged people lead many of them to believe they have little control over events in their lives. Consistent with this finding is research by Frydenberg and Lewis (1999), which reported that adolescents from lower socioeconomic backgrounds were more likely to rely on wishful thinking and prayer as a way of coping with problems rather than taking direct action. In general, disadvantaged individuals — a category that typically includes disproportionately more identity group members and indigenous persons — are more likely to experience stressful events and less likely to cope with them effectively than other people are (Gottlieb & Green 1987).

We have examined many ways people cope with stress. Each method can be effective and adaptive for the individual if it neutralises the current stressor and does not increase the likelihood of future stressful situations. Some ways of coping can reduce the potential impact of stressors. For instance, many people who receive a bill that has an error would appraise this situation as a hassle. But a person who often uses humour to cope may appraise this situation differently, perhaps finding it almost amusing (Folkman et al. 1987). In the next section, we consider how people can reduce the potential for stress for themselves and for others.

Reducing the potential for stress

Can people become 'immune' to the impact of stress to some extent? Some aspects of people's lives can reduce the potential for stressors to develop and help individuals cope with problems when they occur. Prevention is the first line of defense against the impact of stress. We will look at several ways people can help themselves and others prevent and cope with stress. The first approach makes use of the beneficial effects of social support.

Enhancing social support

We have all turned to others for help and comfort when under stress at some time in our lives. If you have ever had to endure troubled times on your own, you know how important social support can be. But social support is not only helpful after stressors appear, it also can help avert problems in the first place. Consider, for example, the tangible support newlyweds receive when they get married. The gifts they receive include many of the items they will need to set up a household, without which the couple would be saddled either with the financial burden of buying the items or with the hassles of not having them.

Although there are people in all walks of life who lack the social support they need, some segments of the population have less than others (Antonucci 1985; Broadhead et al. 1983; Heller, Price & Hogg 1990; Ratliff-Crain & Baum 1990; Rook & Schuster 1996).

- Although men tend to have larger social networks than women, women seem to use theirs more effectively for support.
- Many elderly individuals live in isolated conditions and have few people on whom to rely.
- Network size is related to social prestige, income and education: the lower the prestige, income and education level of individuals, the smaller their social networks tend to be.

Furthermore, the networks of people from lower socioeconomic classes are usually less diverse than those of people from higher classes — that is, lower-class networks contain fewer non-kin members. In contemporary Australian society, the traditional sources of support have shifted to include greater reliance on individuals in social and helping organisations. As psychologist Marc Pilisuk has noted, 'The geographic proximity and the functions of the modern extended family have changed substantially, and do not typically provide the same protective buffer associated with large families in the preindustrial era' (1982, p. 26).

Social support, as we saw in chapter 4, is a dynamic process. People's needs for, giving of and receipt of support change over time. Some factors within the individual determine whether he or she will receive or provide social support when it is needed (Broadhead et al. 1983; Coble, Gantt & Mallinckrodt 1996; Cutrona 1996; Wortman & Dunkel-Schetter 1987). One factor is the person's temperament. People differ in their need for and interest in social contact and affiliation. Those individuals who tend to seek interaction with others are more likely to give and receive support than those who do not. To some extent, these tendencies are determined by the experiences people have. Children who grow up in caring families and have good relations with peers learn the social skills needed to seek help and give it when needed. But research has found that people who report that they are coping well with stressful events in their lives 'are more likely to be regarded as attractive by others and less likely to be avoided than those who indicate that they are having some difficulties coping. The implications of these results are depressing, because they suggest that those in greatest need for social support may be least likely to get it' (Wortman & Dunkel-Schetter 1987, p. 98).

It is not necessarily the case that persons with low perceived social support lack basic social skills. Coble, Gantt & Mallinckrodt (1996) have argued that higher order social competencies such as the ability to form emotionally intimate relationships, a willingness to trust others and social efficacy beliefs (beliefs that efforts to obtain support will be successful) are required for supportive interactions. These social competencies are believed to be linked to secure attachment experiences in both childhood and adulthood (Sarason, Pierce & Sarason 1990).

Efforts to enhance people's ability to give and receive social support can begin in early childhood, particularly at school (Broadhead et al. 1983). One approach teachers can use is to have boys and girls engage in cooperative games that promote prolonged interactions with one another. Mara Sapon-Shevin (1980) has identified four types of specific behaviours teachers can help children learn: (1) talking nicely to and complimenting classmates, (2) sharing and taking turns, (3) including children who have been left out in games and activities, and (4) helping classmates who are injured or having difficulty. Teachers can encourage these and other positive social behaviours by reading appropriate storybooks to the class and by having the children play suitable games, such as having them sit in a circle and construct a story, with each child contributing a little piece to it in sequence.

In adulthood, people can enhance their ability to give and receive social support by joining community organisations, such as social, religious, special interest and self-help groups. These organisations have the advantage of bringing together individuals with similar problems and interests, which can become the basis for sharing, helping and friendship. In Australia, there are many widely known self-help groups, including Alcoholics Anonymous and Parents without Partners, special interest groups and support groups for people with specific illnesses, such as arthritis or AIDS. Isolated people of all ages — especially the elderly — can be encouraged to join suitable organisations.

Communities can play a valuable role in enhancing people's resources for social support by creating programs to help individuals develop social networks (Lakey & Lutz 1996). A number of different intervention programs have been developed by psychologists to increase social support. These include having trained volunteers or program staff provide social support, establishing support groups based on a shared characteristic (e.g. support group for families with a disabled child), social skills training to help develop social networks, and restructuring social environments by training persons to offer more effective support. While project-provided support (Kennell et al. 1991) and support group interventions (Toseland, Rossiter & Labrecque 1989) have been successful in producing changes to social networks, they have not been effective in producing changes in naturally occurring social support, or in altering perceived support. Social skills training has been found to improve social support somewhat (Brand, Lakey & Berman 1995; Wolchick et al. 1993), though more interventions of this type are required before firm conclusions can be made about the effectiveness of this social support intervention. Many of the interventions have not produced changes in psychological symptoms largely because perceived social support remained unaltered (Lakey & Lutz 1996). Research has consistently found perceived social support rather than enacted or actual support to be associated with health outcomes (Barerra 1986; Cohen & Wills 1985). It has been suggested by Lakey and Lutz (1996) that social support interventions should target the determinants of perceived support, namely characteristics of the social environment, personality characteristics of the perceiver and their interaction. Such an intervention could include, for example, cognitive approaches to correct biased interpretations of social information or distorted views of social relations; skills training in initiating social interaction; self-disclosure expressing positive emotion; and matching persons for support (Lakey & Lutz 1996).

Social support can also be encouraged in occupational settings (Quick & Quick 1984). Employers can do this in many ways, such as by organising workers in teams or work groups, providing facilities for recreation and fitness training during lunch time or other non-work hours, arranging social events for workers and their families on weekends, and providing counselling services to help employees through troubled times. Some bosses get so caught up in the role of manager that they fail to give the personal support their subordinates need. A supportive boss discusses decisions and problems with employees, compliments subordinates and gives them credit for good work, and stands behind reasonable decisions they make (Kobasa 1986). Less supportive bosses can make a conscious effort to improve these behaviours.

Although social support is generally helpful and appreciated, it isn't always. As we saw in chapter 4, well-meaning efforts by friends and relatives can undermine good health habits and impair the recovery of people who are ill. Social support can also be ineffective if the recipient interprets it as a sign of inadequacy, feels uncomfortable about not being able to reciprocate, or believes his or her personal control is limited by it (Goldsmith & Parks 1990; La Gaipa 1990). Providing effective social support requires sensitivity and good judgement.

Improving one's personal control

When life becomes stressful, people who lack a strong sense of personal control may stop trying, thinking, 'Oh, what's the use.' Instead of feeling they have power and control, they feel helpless and afraid that their efforts will lead to failure and embarrassment. Many patients with chronic painful or disabling illnesses stop trying to improve their conditions, for instance. The main psychological help they need is to bolster their self-efficacy and reduce their passivity and helplessness (Smith & Wallston 1992). A pessimistic outlook increases a person's potential for stress and can have a negative effect on his or her health.

How can people's sense of control be enhanced? The process can begin very early. Parents, teachers and other caregivers can show a child their love and respect, provide a stimulating environment, encourage and praise the child's accomplishments, and set reasonable standards of conduct and performance that he or she can regard as challenges, rather than threats. Doing these things is likely also to enhance the child's resilience or hardiness, and hardy individuals tend to use coping strategies that manage their stress effectively (Holahan & Moos 1985; Williams, Wiebe & Smith 1992).

Adults' personal control can be enhanced, too. Employers can help by giving workers some degree of control over aspects of their jobs (Quick & Quick 1984). One approach involves having employees work in groups to make certain managerial decisions or solve problems, such as how to improve the quality of the product they manufacture. Other approaches include allowing workers to have some control over their work hours, which tasks to work on and the order in which they do them. Similarly, nursing homes and families can allow elderly individuals to do things for themselves and have responsibilities, such as in cleaning, cooking and arranging social activities. One woman described the prospect of living with her children in the following way: 'I couldn't stand to live with my children, as much as I love them, because they always want to take over my life' (Shupe 1985). Because personal control is a central component of hardiness, enhancing it is likely to make people more hardy or resilient and promote their health (Kobasa 1986).

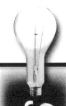

Highlight on issues

The Amish way of social support in bereavement

The Amish people in North America form a conservative religious sect that settled originally in Pennsylvania in the eighteenth century. Amish families generally live in colonies that now exist in about 20 states and Canada. These families have a strongly religious orientation and a serious work ethic that revolves around farming. Their way of life is quite distinctive: they wear uniquely simple and uniform clothing; speak mainly a Pennsylvania-German dialect; and reject modern devices, using horse-driven buggies instead of automobiles for example. Their social lives require their adherence to strict rules of conduct and obedience to patriarchal authority.

One feature of Amish life is that community members give assistance to one another in all times of need. Their way of dealing with death provides a good example, as Kathleen Bryer (1986) has studied and described. Before death, a person who is seriously ill receives care from his or her family. This almost always occurs at home, rather than in a hospital. The Amish not only expect to give this care, but see it as a positive opportunity. A married woman who was asked about caring for a dying relative replied, 'Oh yes,

we had the chance to take care of all four of our old parents before they died. We are both so thankful for this' (p. 251). The experience of death typically occurs at home, in the presence of the family.

Upon someone's death, the Amish community swings into action. Close neighbours notify other members of the colony, and the community makes most of the funeral arrangements. The family receives visits of sympathy and support from other Amish families, some of whom come from other colonies far away and may not even know the bereaved family. In contrast to the social support most Americans receive in bereavement, Amish supportive efforts do not end shortly after the funeral — they continue at a high level for at least a year. Supportive activities include evening and Sunday visiting, making items and scrapbooks for the family, and organised quilting projects that create fellowship around a common task. Moreover, Amish individuals often give extraordinary help to bereaved family members. For instance, the sister of one widower came to live with him and care for his four children until he remarried. The community encourages widowed individuals to remarry in time, and they often do so.

Organising one's world better

'Where did I put my keys?' you have surely heard someone ask frantically while running late for an appointment. People often feel stress because they are late or believe they don't have enough time to do the tasks of the day. They need to organise their world to make things happen efficiently. This can take the form of keeping an appointment diary, designating certain places for certain items, or putting materials in alphabetised file folders, for instance. Organising one's world reduces frustration, wasted time and the potential for stress.

An important approach for organising one's time is called **time management**. It consists of three elements (Lakein 1973). The first element is to *set goals*. These goals should be reasonable or obtainable ones, and they should include long-term goals, such as getting a job promotion next year, and short-term ones, such as meeting a weekly sales quota. The second element involves making daily *To Do* lists with priorities indicated, keeping the goals in mind. These lists should be composed early each morning or late in the preceding day. Each list must be written — trying to keep the list in your head is unreliable and makes setting priorities difficult. The third element is to set up a *schedule* for the day, allocating estimated time periods to each item in the list. If an urgent new task arises during the day, the list should be adjusted to include it.

Exercising: links to stress and health

You have probably heard from TV, radio, magazine and newspaper reports that exercise and physical fitness can protect people from stress and its harmful effects on health. These reports cite a wide range of benefits of exercising, from increased intellectual functioning and personal control to decreased anxiety, depression, hostility and tension. Do exercise and fitness reduce the potential for stress and its effects on health?

Most studies of this question have used correlational or retrospective methods, and show that people who exercise or are physically fit often report less anxiety, depression and tension in their lives than do people who do not exercise or are less fit (Abele & Brehm 1993; Blumenthal & McCubbin 1987; Hays 1999; Holmes 1993). In a review of 80 studies that examined the effects of both aerobic and anaerobic exercise on depression (North, McCullagh & Tran 1990), beneficial effects were found for both types of exercise for all age groups, and for males and females. Exercise had both immediate and longer-term effects in reducing depression, with the most benefit occurring for persons who had the highest initial psychophysiological ill health. Although these results are consistent with the view that exercise and fitness reduce the potential for stress, there are two problems in interpreting them. First, some evidence indicates that part of the reduction in self-reported stress and emotion may have resulted from a placebo effect — that is, the subjects' expectations that psychological improvements would occur (Desharnais et al. 1993). Second, the results of correlational research do not tell us what causes what. Do exercise and fitness cause people to feel less stress? Or are people more likely to exercise and keep fit if they feel less stress and time pressures in their lives? Or are other factors involved? These questions cannot be answered using correlational or retrospective methods. Fortunately, there is stronger evidence for the beneficial effects of exercise and fitness on stress and health.

An experiment by Bram Goldwater and Martin Collis (1985) examined the effects of exercise on cardiovascular fitness and feelings of anxiety in healthy males between 19 and 30 years of age. The subjects were randomly assigned to one of two groups. In one group, the subjects worked out 5 days a week in a vigorous fitness program, including swimming and active sports, such as soccer. Subjects in the second group had a more moderate fitness program. They met twice a week and engaged in less demanding exercise activities, such as badminton. Both groups participated in their programs for six weeks and were tested for cardiovascular fitness and anxiety before and after participating. Compared with the subjects in the moderate program, those in the vigorous program showed greater gains in fitness and reductions in anxiety. Other researchers have found similar beneficial effects of exercise on anxiety among middle-aged adults (Blumenthal et al. 1982). More recent research has demonstrated significant anxiety reduction following vigorous aerobic exercise (Petrozello et al. 1991).

Research has also assessed the effects of exercise on blood pressure and heart rate. Once again, most of the evidence is correlational, revealing that people who exercise or are physically fit show less cardiovascular reactivity to stressors and are less likely to be hypertensive than individuals who do not exercise or are less fit (Dimsdale, Alpert & Schneiderman 1986; Martin & Dubbert 1985). But some studies have used experimental methods. Garry Jennings and his colleagues (1986) conducted an experiment with healthy 19- to 27-year-old individuals who had sedentary occupations and had not regularly engaged in vigorous physical activity in the previous year. Over the next four months, the subjects spent one month at each of four levels of activity: (1) their sedentary normal activity; (2) below-normal activity, which included two weeks of rest in a hospital setting; (3) above-normal activity, which involved their normal activity plus three sessions of vigorous exercise weekly; and (4) much-above-normal activity, consisting of their normal activity plus daily vigorous exercise. Each exercise period lasted 40 minutes. Measurements of heart rate and blood pressure were taken after each month, when the subjects came into the laboratory and rested before beginning the next activity level. Compared with data for the sedentary activity level, the two exercise conditions reduced heart rate by 12 per cent and systolic and diastolic blood pressure by 8 per cent and 10 per cent. Below-normal activity levels did not alter heart rate or blood pressure. Race has been linked with increased risk of hypertension, obesity and low physical activity. Experimental research with at risk American blacks found that an acute aerobic exercise of 40 minutes' duration was an effective buffer of psychosocial stressors (Rejeski et al. 1992). Other researchers have found similar beneficial effects of exercise on blood pressure with normotensive elderly people (Braith et al. 1994).

We need to consider one more link in reviewing the protective effects of exercise and fitness against the impact of stress on health. That is, do exercise and fitness prevent people from developing stress-related illnesses? The results of two studies suggest they do. One of these studies used retrospective methods with men who reported having experienced either high or low levels of stress in the previous three years (Kobasa, Maddi & Puccetti 1982). Those men who scored higher on a survey of their exercise practices reported less illness during the three-year period than those who had lower scores on exercise, and these protective effects were greater for subjects with high levels of stress than for those with less stress. The other study used prospective methods by first assessing the subjects' recent life events and fitness, and then having them keep records concerning their health over the following nine weeks (Roth & Holmes 1985). The results revealed that individuals who reported high levels of stress had poorer subsequent health if they were not fit; stress had little impact on the health of fit subjects.

The evidence that engaging in regular exercise can promote health by reducing stress is fairly strong. Does participating in sports games, such as tennis or soccer, have similar effects? Some evidence exists on this issue. Australian correlational research found evidence for direct health benefits of sport participation, rather than stress-moderating effects (Caltabiano 1995). Fewer physical and psychological illness symptoms were reported by respondents who engaged in more outdoor active sports, irrespective of the amount of coexisting stressful life circumstances. Other research findings indicate that sports activities arouse emotions, especially before participation, and arouse anger and sadness for losers (Abele & Brehm 1993). The health effects of these emotional experiences are not yet clear.

Preparing for stressful events

In this and previous chapters we have discussed a wide variety of stressful events, ranging from being stuck in traffic, to starting day care or school, being overloaded with work, going through a divorce and experiencing a disaster. The potential for stress often can be reduced by preparing for these events. For instance, parents can help prepare a child for starting day care by taking the child there in advance to see the place, meet the teacher and play for a while (Sarafino 1986).

Irving Janis (1958) pioneered the psychological study of the need to prepare people for stressful events, such as surgery. In one study, he found that patients with moderate levels of anxiety before the surgery showed better adjustment after the operation than did those with either very high or very low anxiety. From this finding, Janis proposed that some degree of anticipatory worry about a stressful event is adaptive because it motivates coping via the process he called the *work of worrying*. He described three steps in this process: The person first receives information about the event, which generates anxiety; then develops expectations by rehearsing the event mentally; and then mobilises coping techniques in an effort to become reassured of a successful outcome. Patients with too little anxiety are not motivated enough to complete the process, and those with too much anxiety are distracted or immobilised by their fear.

Subsequent research has confirmed some, but not all, of Janis's findings and theory. In particular, these studies have shown that low levels of anxiety do not impair patients' success in coping with or recovery from surgery. The overall picture from this research indicates that the higher the patients' *pre-operative* fear, the worse their *post-operative* adjustment and recovery tend to be (Anderson & Masur 1983; Johnson 1983). These post-operative outcomes have been shown for a variety of measures, including:

- the patient's self-reported pain
- the amount of medication taken to relieve pain
- self-reported anxiety or depression
- the length of the hospital stay after surgery
- ratings by hospital staff of the patient's recovery or adjustment.

The poorer post-operative outcomes of patients with high levels of anxiety suggest that helping patients cope with their pre-operative concerns could enhance later adjustment and recovery.

Many studies have been done to determine what methods are effective in preparing people psychologically for surgery. Some methods have involved brief *psychotherapy*, in which patients express their worries and receive emotional support and reassurance. But the effectiveness of these approaches is not clear (Anderson & Masur 1983). Other methods have involved *hypnosis*, such as by giving the patient the suggestion under hypnosis that the post-operative pain will not be very severe. These methods seem promising for patients who are hypnotically suggestible, but more research is needed to determine when and how best to apply them (Anderson & Masur 1983; Barber 1986).

The most clearly effective methods of preparing people for the stress of surgery are those designed to enhance the patients' feelings of *control* (Anderson & Masur 1983; Mathews & Ridgeway 1984). One approach attempts to improve patients' *behavioural control* by teaching them how to reduce discomfort or promote rehabilitation through specific actions they can take, such as by doing leg exercises to improve strength or deep breathing exercises to reduce pain. Another method is designed to enhance patients' *cognitive control*, for instance by instructing them on ways to concentrate on the pleasant or beneficial aspects of the surgery, rather than the unpleasant aspects. One other method involves *informational control*, in which patients receive information about the procedures and/or sensations they will experience. Cognitive control can also be effective following surgery by facilitating recovery and reducing the recurrence of a condition. For example, in a study by Helgeson and Fritz (1999) the risk of restenosis (a new cardiac event within six months) following coronary angioplasty was reduced in patients who perceived themselves as having control over their future health, who held positive expectations about their future and who had a positive view of themselves. Each of these and other control-enhancing methods is effective in promoting post-operative adjustment and recovery. (We will examine these methods in greater detail in chapter 10, when we discuss hospital treatment.)

Although enhanced control can be helpful in reducing the potential for stress, these methods need to be applied carefully to prevent some possible negative effects. One consideration is that sometimes information that is meant to reassure people and reduce stress can have the opposite effect. Another consideration is whether a person can have *too much* control. There is some evidence that having too much information, for example, can be confusing and actually arouse fear. Young children who receive a great deal of information about the medical procedures they will undergo often become more anxious (Miller & Green 1984). With children in dental or medical settings, it is generally best not to give a lot of detail, particularly distressing detail. Describing some sensory experiences to expect is especially helpful, such as the sounds of equipment or the tingly feeling from the dental anaesthetic.

In summary, we have discussed several methods that are helpful in reducing the potential for stress and, thereby, benefiting health. These methods take advantage of the stress-moderating effects of social support, personal control, exercise, being well organised, and being prepared for an impending stressor. In the next section, we consider ways to reduce the reaction to stress once it has begun.

Reducing stress reactions: stress management

People acquire coping skills through their experiences, which may involve strategies they have tried in the past or methods they have seen others use. But sometimes the skills they have learned are not adequate for a current stressor because it is so strong, novel or unrelenting. In some cases, the approaches they have acquired reduce stress in the short run — as alcohol or drug use can do — but are not adaptive and increase stress in the long run. These problems in coping often arise in individuals whose potential for stress is high because of a lack of social support, personal control and so on; but coping problems also occur among people whose potential for stress is relatively low. When people cannot cope effectively, they need help in learning new and adaptive ways of managing stress.

Many techniques are available to help individuals manage stress. These *stress management* techniques are mainly psychological, but sometimes *pharmacological* approaches are used under medical supervision.

One such psychological program is that developed by Australian psychologists Barlow and Rapee (1997), which uses a lifestyle approach to help people identify the sources of stress in their lives, and apply relevant techniques to help manage their stress. The program describes a systematic approach for monitoring daily stress, recording thoughts, reality testing and thought substitution, how to manage one's time, learning to become more assertive, effective problem solving and learning how to relax. Before discussing specific behavioural and cognitive methods in managing stress, we will consider the role of medication in reducing arousal.

Medication

Of the many types of drugs doctors prescribe to help patients manage stress, we will consider two: benzodiazepines and beta-blockers. Both of these drugs reduce physiological arousal and feelings of anxiety (Priest 1986; Shapiro, Krantz & Grim 1986). *Benzodiazepines*, which include drugs with the trade names Valium and Librium, appear to work by activating a neurotransmitter that decreases neural transmission in the central nervous system. *Beta-blockers*, such as Inderal, appear to block the activity of sympathetic neurons in the peripheral nervous system that are stimulated by epinephrine and norepinephrine. Beta-blockers cause less drowsiness than benzodiazepines, probably because they act on the peripheral rather than central nervous system. Using drugs to manage stress should be only a temporary measure, either to help during an acute crisis, such as in the week or two following the death of a loved one, or while the patient learns new psychological methods for coping. But more and more people are relying on drugs for long-term control of their stress and emotions (Begley 1994).

Behavioural and cognitive methods

Psychologists have developed methods they can train people to use in coping with stress. Some of these techniques focus mainly on the person's behaviour, and some give greater attention to the person's thinking processes. People who use these methods usually find them helpful.

Relaxation and systematic desensitisation

The opposite of arousal is relaxation — so relaxing should be a good way to reduce stress. 'Perhaps so,' you say, 'but when stress appears, relaxing is easier said than done.' Actually, relaxing when under stress is not so hard to do when you know how. One technique people can learn to control their feelings of tension is called **progressive muscle relaxation** (or just *progressive relaxation*), in which they focus their attention on specific muscle groups while alternately tightening and relaxing these muscles (Sarafino 1996).

The idea of teaching people to relax their skeletal muscles in order to reduce psychological stress was proposed many years ago by Edmund Jacobson (1938). He developed a device to measure electrical activity in muscle fibres. Using this device, he found that subjects would reduce the tension in their muscles when simply asked to 'sit and relax'. He later found that muscle tension could be reduced much more if the subjects were taught to pay attention to the sensations as they tense and relax individual groups of muscles. Research findings indicate that one reason muscle relaxation reduces psychological stress is that the technique tends to arouse pleasant thoughts in the person (Peveler & Johnston 1986).

Although there are various versions of the progressive muscle relaxation technique, they each outline a particular sequence of muscle groups for the person to follow. For example, the sequence might begin with the person relaxing the hands, then the forehead, followed by the lower face, the neck, the stomach and, finally, the legs. For each muscle group, the person first tenses the muscles for 7–10 seconds, and then relaxes them for about 15 seconds, paying attention to how the muscles feel. This is usually repeated for the same muscle group two or three times in a relaxation session, which generally lasts 20 or 30 minutes. The relaxation technique works best in a quiet, non-distracting setting with the person lying down or sitting in a comfortable position.

Stress management has been applied mainly with adults, but children also experience stress without being able to cope effectively. Fortunately, many behavioural and cognitive methods are easy to learn and can be adapted so that an adult can teach a young child to use them (Siegel & Peterson 1980). The relaxation procedure provides a good example. An adult could start by showing the child what relaxing is like by lifting and then releasing the arms and legs of a rag doll, allowing them to fall down. Then, the adult would follow a *protocol*, or script, giving instructions like those in figure 5.1. When children and adults first learn progressive muscle relaxation, they sometimes don't actually relax their muscles when told to do so. Instead of letting their arms and legs *fall* down, they *move* them down. They also sometimes tense more muscles than they are asked to — for example tightening facial muscles when they are supposed to tense only hand muscles. These errors should be pointed out and corrected. Relaxation and stress management training has been demonstrated to be effective in the treatment of migraine in children when compared with drug treatment (Sartory et al. 1998).

Often, after individuals have thoroughly mastered the relaxation procedure, they can gradually shorten the procedure so they can apply a very quick version in times of stress, such as when they are about to give a speech (Sarafino 1996). This quick version might have the following steps: (1) taking a deep breath, and letting it out; (2) saying to oneself, 'Relax, feel nice and calm'; and (3) thinking about a pleasant thought for a few seconds. In this way, relaxation methods can be directly applied to help people cope with everyday stressful events.

Figure 5.1 Progressive muscle relaxation protocol for children

1. 'OK. Let's raise our arms and put them out in front. Now make a fist with both your hands, really hard. Hold the fist tight and you will see how the muscles in your hands and arms feel when they are tight.' (hold for 7–10 seconds)

    'That's very good. Now when I say relax I want the muscles in your hands and arms to become floppy, like the rag doll, and your arms will drop to your sides. OK, relax.' (about 15 seconds)

2. 'Let's raise our legs out in front of us. Now tighten the muscles in your feet and legs, really hard. Make the muscles really tight, and hold it.' (7–10 seconds)

    'Very good. Now relax the muscles in your feet and legs, and let them drop to the floor. They feel so good. So calm and relaxed.' (15 seconds)

3. 'Now let's do our tummy muscles. Tighten your tummy, really hard — and hold it.' (7–10 seconds)

    'OK. Relax your tummy, and feel how good it feels. So comfortable.' (15 seconds)

4. 'Leave your arms at your sides, but tighten the muscles in your shoulders and neck. You can do this by moving your shoulders up towards your head. Hold the muscles very tightly in your shoulders and neck.' (7–10 seconds)

    'Now relax those muscles so they are floppy, and see how good that feels.' (15 seconds)

5. 'Let's tighten the muscles in our faces. Scrunch up your whole face so that all of the muscles are tight — the muscles in your cheeks, and your mouth, and your nose, and your forehead. Really scrunch up your face, and hold it.' (7–10 seconds)

    'Now relax all the muscles in your face — your cheeks, mouth, nose and forehead. Feel how nice that is.' (15 seconds)

6. 'Now I want us to take a very, very deep breath — so deep that there's no room left inside for more air. Hold the air in. (use a shorter time: 6–8 seconds)

    'That's good. Now slowly let the air out. Very slowly, until it's all out ... And now breathe as you usually do.' (15 seconds)

Source: Sarafino (1986, pp. 112–3).

Research has demonstrated that progressive muscle relaxation is highly effective in reducing stress (Carlson & Hoyle 1993; Lichstein 1988). Although relaxation is often successful by itself in helping people cope, it is frequently used in conjunction with **systematic desensitisation**, a useful method for reducing fear and anxiety (Sarafino 1996). This method is based on the view that fears are learned by *classical conditioning* — that is, by associating a situation or object with an unpleasant event. This can happen, for example, if a person associates visits to the dentist with pain, thereby becoming 'sensitised' to dentists. Desensitisation is a classical conditioning procedure that *reverses* this learning by pairing the feared object or situation with either pleasant or neutral events, as figure 5.2 outlines. According to Joseph Wolpe (1958, 1973), an originator of the desensitisation method, the reversal comes about through the process of *counterconditioning*, whereby the 'calm' response gradually replaces the 'fear' response. Desensitisation has been used successfully in reducing a variety of children's and adults' fears, such as fear of dentists, animals, high places, public speaking and taking tests (Lichstein 1988; Morris & Kratochwill 1983; Sarafino 1996).

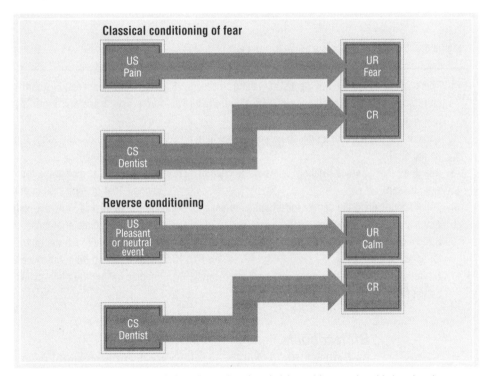

Figure 5.2 Classical conditioning in learning to fear dental visits and in reversing this learning. In conditioning the fear, the unconditioned stimulus (US) of pain elicits the unconditioned response (UR) of fear automatically. Learning occurs by pairing the dentist, the conditioned stimulus (CS), with the US so that the dentist begins to elicit fear. The reverse conditioning pairs the feared dentist with a US that elicits calm.

One of the most important features of the systematic desensitisation method is that it uses a *stimulus hierarchy* — a graded sequence of approximations to the conditioned stimulus, the feared situation. The purpose of these approximations is to bring the person gradually into contact with the source of fear in about 10 or 15 steps. To see how a stimulus hierarchy might be constructed, we will look at the one in figure 5.3, which deals with the fear of dentists. The person would follow the instructions in each of the 14 steps. As you can see, some of the steps involve real-life, or *in vivo*, contacts with the feared situation, and some do not. Two types of non-real-life contacts, of varying degrees, can be included. One type uses *imaginal* situations, such as having the person think about calling the dentist. The other involves *symbolic* contacts, such as by showing pictures, films or models of the feared situation.

In the systematic desensitisation procedure, the steps in a hierarchy are presented individually, while the person is calm, relaxed and comfortable (Sarafino 1996). The steps follow a sequence from the least to the most fearful for the individual. Each step may elicit some wariness or fear behaviour, but the person is encouraged to relax. Once the wariness at one step has passed and the person is calm, the next step in the hierarchy can be introduced. Completing an entire stimulus hierarchy and reducing a fairly strong fear can be achieved fairly quickly — it is likely to take several hours, divided into several separate sessions. In one study with dental-phobic adults who simply imagined each step in a hierarchy, the procedure successfully reduced their fear in six $1\frac{1}{2}$-hour sessions (Gatchel 1980). Individual sessions for reducing fears in children are usually much shorter than those used with adults, especially for a child who is very young and has a short attention span.

Figure 5.3 Example of a stimulus hierarchy for a fear of dentists

1. Think about being in the dentist's waiting room, simply accompanying someone else who is there for an examination.
2. Look at a photograph of a smiling person seated in a dental chair.
3. Imagine this person calmly having a dental examination.
4. Think about calling the dentist for an appointment.
5. Actually call for the appointment.
6. Sit in a car outside the dentist's office without having an appointment.
7. Sit in the dentist's waiting room and hear the receptionist say, 'The dental nurse is ready for you.'
8. Sit in the examination room and hear the dental nurse say, 'I see one tooth the dentist will need to look at.'
9. Hear and watch the drill run, without its being brought near the face.
10. Have the dentist pick at the tooth with an instrument, saying, 'That doesn't look good.'
11. See the dentist lay out the instruments, including a syringe to administer an anaesthetic.
12. Feel the needle touch the gums.
13. Imagine having the tooth drilled.
14. Imagine having the tooth pulled.

Biofeedback

Biofeedback is a technique in which an electromechanical device monitors the status of a person's physiological processes, such as heart rate or muscle tension, and immediately reports that information back to the individual. This information enables the person to gain voluntary control over these processes through operant conditioning. If, for instance, the person is trying to reduce neck-muscle tension and the device reports that the tension has just decreased, this information reinforces whatever efforts the individual made to accomplish this decrease.

Biofeedback has been used successfully in treating stress-related health problems. For example, an experiment was conducted with patients suffering from chronic muscle-contraction headaches (Budzynski et al. 1973). Those who were given biofeedback regarding muscle tension in their foreheads later showed less tension in those muscles and reported having fewer headaches than subjects in control groups. What's more, these benefits continued at a follow-up after three months. Biofeedback seems to be about as effective as progressive muscle relaxation methods for treating headache (Blanchard & Andrasik 1985; Holroyd & Penzien 1985; Sartory et al. 1998). But research on approaches for reducing stress itself has found that biofeedback is no more effective than progressive muscle relaxation techniques, which are less expensive to use (Hatch, Gatchel & Harrington 1982; Masters et al. 1987). Still, some research findings are encouraging and suggest that some individuals may benefit from biofeedback methods more than others.

According to Virginia Attanasio, Frank Andrasik and their colleagues (1985), children may be better candidates for biofeedback treatment than adults. In using biofeedback with children and adults who suffer from muscle-contraction headaches, these researchers have found that 'children exhibit greater self-regulatory abilities than adults, quicker acquisition of the response, and better overall improvement' (p. 135). Why? These researchers have offered some reasons. First, children are generally more enthusiastic about the equipment and procedures than adults, often regarding biofeedback as a game. In fact, some children become so interested and motivated in the game that their arousal interferes with relaxation if the therapist does not help them remain calm. But in about 10 per cent of the cases, the children — especially younger ones — may be frightened by the equipment initially. The therapist can usually eliminate these fears by sensitively explaining and demonstrating that the procedure does not hurt and presents no danger. Second, children are usually less sceptical about their ability to succeed in biofeedback training and to benefit from doing so. Adults often say, 'Nothing else I've ever tried has worked, so why should biofeedback?' This difference in scepticism probably reflects their differences in experience: adults are likely to have had more failure experiences with other treatments than children. Third, children are more likely than adults to practise their training at home, as they are instructed to do.

Although children have many characteristics that make them well suited to biofeedback methods, they also have some special difficulties (Attanasio et al. 1985). For one thing, children — particularly those below the age of eight — have shorter attention spans than adults. If biofeedback sessions last more than 20 minutes or so, it may be necessary to divide each session into smaller units with brief breaks in between. A related problem is that children sometimes perform disruptive behaviours during a session, disturbing the electrodes and wires or interrupting to talk about tangential topics, for instance. The therapist can reduce the likelihood of these unwanted behaviours, such as by providing rewards for being cooperative. Clearly, the difficulties some children have in biofeedback training can usually be overcome. But research is needed to determine whether children benefit more from biofeedback methods than from other approaches for reducing stress-related illnesses.

Modelling

People learn not just by doing, but also by observing. They see what others do and the consequences of the behaviour these models perform. As a result, this kind of learning is called **modelling**, and sometimes 'observational' or 'social' learning.

People can learn fears and other stress-related behaviour by observing fearful behaviour in other individuals. In one study, children (with their parents' permission) watched a short film showing a five-year-old boy's reaction to plastic figures of the cartoon characters Mickey Mouse and Donald Duck (Venn & Short 1973). In the film, when the boy's mother showed him the Mickey Mouse figure, he screamed and withdrew; but when she showed him the Donald Duck figure, he remained calm and displayed no distress. While the subjects watched the film, physiological measures of stress were taken, confirming that the children were more aroused while watching the episode with Mickey Mouse (fearful) than while watching the one with Donald Duck. After the children watched these scenes, they each participated in a task that involved the two figures from the film. At this time, they tended to avoid the Mickey Mouse figure (the stressful one) in favour of Donald Duck. This avoidance reaction was pronounced initially, but a day or two later the children showed no avoidance of or preference for either figure.

Since people can learn stressful reactions by observing these behaviours in others, modelling should be effective in reversing this learning and helping people cope with stressors, too. A large body of research has confirmed that it is (Masters et al. 1987; Thelen et al. 1979). The therapeutic use of modelling is similar to the method of desensitisation: The person relaxes while watching a model calmly perform a series of activities arranged as a stimulus hierarchy — that is, from least to most stressful. The modelling procedure can be presented *symbolically*, using films or videotapes, or *in vivo*, with real-life models and events. Using symbolic presentations, for example, Barbara Melamed and her co-workers have shown that modelling procedures can reduce the stress experienced by hospitalised four- to 17-year-old children and improve their recovery from surgery (Melamed, Dearborn & Hermecz 1983; Melamed & Siegel 1975). But the child's age and previous experience with surgery were also important factors in the results. Children under the age of eight who had had previous surgery experienced increased anxiety rather than less. These children may benefit from other methods to reduce stress, such as activities that simply distract their attention.

Approaches focusing on cognitive processes

Because stress results from cognitive appraisals that are frequently based on a lack of information, misperceptions, or irrational beliefs, some approaches to modifying people's behaviour and thought patterns have been developed to help them cope better with the stress they experience. To achieve this goal, these methods guide people towards what Arnold Lazarus (1971) has called a 'restructuring' of their thought patterns. **Cognitive restructuring** is a process by which stress-provoking thoughts or beliefs are replaced with more constructive or realistic ones that reduce the person's appraisal of threat or harm.

A widely known approach that focuses on cognitive restructuring is **rational-emotive therapy** (RET), which was developed by Albert Ellis (1962, 1977, 1987). RET is based on the view that stress often arises from faulty or irrational ways of thinking. These ways of thinking affect stress appraisal processes, increasing the appraisal of threat or harm. According to Ellis, commonly used irrational ways of thinking include:

• *awfulising* — for example, 'It is *awful* if I get turned down when I ask someone out.'
• *can't-stand-itis* — as in, 'I *can't stand* not doing well on a test.'
• *musterbating* — for instance, 'People *must* like me, or I'm worthless.'

These thoughts exaggerate the person's negative view of a situation and are upsetting. The purpose of RET is to change these thoughts and beliefs.

The procedures used in RET focus on several aspects or stages of the person's thought processes, using Ellis's (1977) A-B-C-D-E paradigm. Figure 5.4 describes the basic outline of this paradigm by using the case of a woman we will call Sue, who is in therapy and is upset at having been fired from a job. An important feature of RET is that it uses homework assignments — the person might be asked to read some materials about irrational beliefs or do desensitisation exercises, for instance. Research into the effectiveness of RET has found it successful in treating anxiety and depression (Engels, Garnefski & Diekstra 1993; Haaga & Davison 1993). But the evidence is far from conclusive, and many questions remain as to why it works and whether improvements persist.

Figure 5.4 Ellis's A-B-C-D-E paradigm for rational emotive therapy

- **A** stands for the *activating* experience, the event Sue describes as having precipitated her upset: Her boss said, 'I've warned you time and again about your lateness and sloppy work. I don't want you to work here any more. You're fired.'
- **B** refers to the *beliefs* and thoughts that go through the person's mind in response to A. These thoughts may be rational, as in, 'I guess I deserved to be fired. I need to be more responsible and careful about my work.' But Sue focused on irrational beliefs, thinking, 'I can't do anything right. I wish I had behaved better; that was a good job. I'm totally worthless and useless. I can't stand myself, and I can't bear facing people and telling them I was fired.'
- **C** symbolises the emotional and behavioural *consequences* of feelings of disappointment and a determination to improve in her next job. But Sue's consequences were inappropriate — she felt depressed, ashamed and helpless, and has not tried to find a new job in the several months since she was fired.
- **D** refers to the *disputing* of irrational beliefs that goes on in therapy. It includes discriminating between true ideas, such as 'I wish I had behaved better,' and irrational ones, such as 'I'm totally worthless.' Irrational beliefs are critically and logically examined in RET so that they can be disproven.
- **E** stands for the therapy's *effect*, which consists of a restructured belief system and philosophy. With this effect, Sue should be able to cope with her world more sensibly in the future.

Another cognitive restructuring approach — called **cognitive therapy** — has been proposed by Aaron Beck (1976; Beck et al. 1990; Beck & Shaw 1977). Its approach is similar to RET's in attempting to change maladaptive thought patterns. Although it was developed originally to treat psychological depression, it is also being applied in treating anxiety. Cognitive therapy attempts to help clients see that they are not responsible for all of the problems they encounter, the negative events they experience are usually not catastrophes, and their maladaptive beliefs are not logically valid. For instance, the following dialogue shows how a therapist tried to counter the negative beliefs of a woman named Sharon.

> THERAPIST: . . . what evidence do you have that all this is true? That you are ugly, awkward? Or that it is not true? What data do you have?
>
> SHARON: Comparing myself to people that I consider to be extremely attractive and finding myself lacking.
>
> THERAPIST: So if you look at that beautiful person, you're less?
>
> SHARON: Yeah.
>
> THERAPIST: Or if I look at that *perfect* person, I'm less. Is that what you're saying? . . .
>
> SHARON: Yeah. I always pick out, of course, the most attractive person and probably a person who spends 3 hours a day on grooming and appearance . . . I don't compare myself to the run-of-the-mill . . . (Freeman 1990, p. 83)

One technique cognitive therapy uses, called *hypothesis testing*, has the person treat an erroneous belief as a hypothesis and test it by looking for evidence for and against it in his or her everyday life. Research has shown that cognitive therapy is clearly effective in treating depression (Hollon, Shelton & Davis 1993; Robins & Hayes 1993) and appears to be a very promising approach for treating anxieties (Chambless & Gillis 1993).

Not all cognitive-based approaches for helping people cope with stress have restructuring irrational thought patterns as the principal focus. Donald Meichenbaum and his colleagues have developed a procedure called **stress-inoculation training** that is designed to teach people skills for alleviating stress and achieving personal goals (Meichenbaum & Cameron 1983; Meichenbaum & Turk 1982). The training program involves three phases.

1. *Conceptualisation.* In this phase, the person learns about the nature of stress and how people react to it. This learning occurs through discussions of the person's past stressful experiences. These discussions can be done on an individual basis or in groups, with each member contributing. They consider such questions as: Under what specific circumstances do you experience stress? What did you do to reduce stress, and what do you believe could be done instead? What seems to make a problem worse or better? What would you have to do to change the way you deal with stress?

2. *Skills acquisition and rehearsal.* In the second phase, the person learns behavioural and cognitive skills to use in emotion-focused and problem-focused coping. Some of these skills are general ones that all individuals in the program would learn, such as skills in relaxation, desensitisation, emotional discharge, seeking social support and cognitive redefinition. Other skills may depend on the individual's personal circumstances and problems. Thus, some people might learn communication skills, or parenting techniques, or study skills, and so on. The person practises the skills he or she has learned under the therapist's supervision.

3. *Application and follow-through.* The last phase involves making the transition to using the learned coping skills in the real world. To achieve this transition, the person responds to stressors that are introduced in the therapy setting in a graded sequence, as in a stimulus hierarchy. A variety of stressors are used to promote effective coping in diverse real-world situations. Follow-up sessions are held periodically during the subsequent year.

The methods used in stress-inoculation training are well thought out and include a number of well-established techniques, such as relaxation, desensitisation and modelling. Although research on the effectiveness of stress-inoculation training in alleviating stress has produced encouraging results, much more evidence is needed to demonstrate its value relative to other approaches (Meichenbaum & Deffenbacher 1988).

Multidimensional approaches

The coping difficulties individuals have are often multidimensional and multifaceted. As a result, one particular technique is not sufficient in helping that person, and the most effective approach usually draws upon many techniques. The method of stress-inoculation training provides an example of an approach that teaches people to use a variety of techniques. When designing a multidimensional approach, the program for helping an individual cope better with stress would be tailored to the person's specific problems (Sarafino 1996). The program may make use of any of the methods we have considered, many methods that would take this discussion too far afield, and the methods we are about to examine.

Meditation and hypnosis

A person's mental activity changes constantly. Some of these changes are obvious, such as the shifts in consciousness when we go from wakefulness to sleep or if we drink alcohol. When our mental functioning changes from its usual pattern of wakefulness, we are said to be in an *altered state of consciousness*. Variations from our usual pattern of wakefulness can occur in several ways other than by going to sleep or drinking alcohol. Two of these ways are meditation and becoming hypnotised. Because people generally report that altered states of consciousness affect their arousal, psychologists have examined the usefulness of meditation and hypnosis in stress management.

Meditation

Transcendental meditation is a method in the practice of yoga that was promoted by Maharishi Mahesh Yogi as a means of improving physical and mental health and reducing stress (Benson 1984, 1991; Nystul 1987). Individuals using this procedure are instructed to practise it twice a day, sitting upright but comfortably relaxed with eyes closed, and mentally repeating a word or sound (such as 'om'), called a *mantra*, to prevent thoughts from occurring.

Similar meditation methods have been advocated by psychologists and psychiatrists for reducing stress. For example, Herbert Benson has recommended that the subject:

> Sit quietly in a comfortable position and close your eyes... Deeply relax all your muscles... Become aware of your breathing. As you breathe out, say the word *one* silently to yourself... Maintain a passive attitude and permit relaxation to occur at its own pace. Expect other thoughts. When these distracting thoughts occur, ignore them by thinking, 'Oh well,' and continue repeating, 'One.' (1984, p. 332)

The purpose of this procedure is to increase the person's ability in the face of a stressor to make a 'relaxation response', which includes reduced physiological activity, as an alternative to a stress response. According to Benson, the relaxation response enhances health, such as by reducing blood pressure, and may be achieved in many different ways. For example, a religious person might find that a meditative prayer is the most effective method for bringing forth the relaxation response.

Although meditation helps people relax, it has a broader purpose: to develop a clear and *mindful awareness*, or 'insight' regarding the essence of one's experiences, unencumbered by cognitive or emotional distortions (Hart 1987; Solé-Leris 1986). Jon Kabat-Zinn (1982; Kabat-Zinn, Lipworth & Burney 1985) has stressed the mindful awareness component of meditation to help individuals who suffer from chronic pain to detach themselves from the cognitive and emotional distortions they have with their pain. The patients were trained to pay close attention to their pain and other sensations without reacting to them in any way, thereby enabling the people to be aware of the pain itself, unembellished by thoughts or feelings about it. Using this technique led to a reduction in the patients' reports of physical and psychological discomfort.

Many people believe that meditation enables the person to reach a state of profound rest, as is claimed by popular self-help books. Many quasi-experimental studies have examined this issue by measuring the physiological arousal of experienced meditators while they practised meditation and of non-meditators while they simply rested. Reviews of these studies do not support the view that meditation produces an uncommonly profound level of rest — that is, research has revealed no consistent differences in blood pressure, heart rate or respiration rate between the meditating and the resting subjects (Holmes 1984; Lichstein 1988). But the quasi-experimental nature of these studies leaves open the possibility that the failure to find consistent differences in arousal may be due to other differences between individuals who do and do not meditate. Research has shown, for instance, that Buddhist monks in South-East Asia can dramatically alter their body metabolism and their brain electrical activity through meditation (Benson et al. 1990).

Still, the main question of concern for stress management is whether meditation — especially Benson's 'relaxation response' approach — is a useful procedure for alleviating stress. Research has generally found that Benson's approach effectively reduces stress for many individuals (Lichstein 1988).

Hypnosis

The modern history of hypnosis began with its being called 'animal magnetism' and 'Mesmerism' in the eighteenth and nineteenth centuries. The Austrian physician Franz Anton Mesmer popularised its use in treating patients who had symptoms of physical illness, such as paralysis, without having a detectable underlying organic disorder. Today, *hypnosis* is considered to be an altered state of consciousness that is induced by special techniques of suggestion and leads to varying degrees of responsiveness to directions for changes in perception, memory and behaviour (Orne 1989).

Not everyone can be hypnotised. People differ in their *suggestibility*, or the degree to which they can be hypnotised. Perhaps 15 to 30 per cent of the general population is easily and deeply hypnotisable (Evans 1987; Hilgard 1967). Suggestibility appears to change with age, being particularly strong among children between the ages of about 7 and 14, and then declining in adolescence to a level that remains stable throughout adulthood (Hilgard 1967; Place 1984). People who are reasonably suggestible can often learn to induce a hypnotic state in themselves — a process called *self-hypnosis*. Usually they learn to do this after they have experienced hypnosis under the supervision of a skilled hypnotist.

Because subjects who have been hypnotised usually claim that it is a relaxing experience, some researchers have examined whether it can help in reducing stress. But there are two interwoven problems with doing therapy and research with hypnosis: most people are not highly suggestible, and the success of the treatment depends heavily on how suggestible the subjects are. Despite these problems, studies have found that hypnosis can be helpful in stress management, but it is not necessarily a more effective method than other relaxation techniques (Tapp 1985; Wadden & Anderton 1982).

In summary, we have seen that many different behavioural and cognitive methods, meditation and hypnosis offer useful therapeutic approaches for helping people cope with stress. Research is also revealing more and more clearly the important benefits of stress management in preventing illness. For instance, one study showed that immune and endocrine system reactions to a stressor depend on ways people cope with it (Olff et al. 1995). And a study by Angele McGrady and her colleagues (1992) found that subjects who received relaxation training showed stronger immune function than control subjects a month later.

Using stress management to reduce coronary risk

Of the many risk factors that have been identified for CHD, a few of them — such as age and family history — are beyond the control of the individual. But many risk factors for CHD are directly linked to the person's experiences and behaviour, which should be modifiable. One of these risk factors is stress. In the remainder of this chapter, we will consider how stress management techniques can be applied to reduce coronary risk.

Modifying Type A behaviour

When the Type A behaviour pattern was first established as a risk factor for CHD, researchers began to study ways to modify the behaviour in an effort to reduce coronary risk (Roskies 1983; Suinn 1982). The task is a difficult one because we don't yet know for certain exactly what makes Type A individuals vulnerable to heart disease (Byrne 1992; Johnston 1992).

Ethel Roskies and her colleagues (1978, 1979, 1986) began a research and therapy program in the 1970s to modify Type A behaviour in healthy professional or managerial men. In the initial research (Roskies et al. 1978, 1979), Type A men were identified with the Structured Interview and randomly assigned to two types of therapy: (1) progressive muscle relaxation and (2) brief psychotherapy, in which a therapist discussed with the men how their childhood experiences may have led to their competitive, hard-driving behaviour. Each group had weekly therapy sessions over 14 weeks, during which time the subjects were asked to try to maintain their usual dietary, exercise, smoking and work habits. The results showed that the groups improved during treatment with respect to their feelings of time pressure, blood cholesterol levels and blood pressure. During a six-month follow-up period, the men who received relaxation therapy maintained their improvements better than the psychotherapy group did.

Although these results were encouraging, Roskies and her co-workers decided they could increase the impact of the intervention on Type A behaviour by using a multidimensional approach (Roskies 1983). They added a variety of cognitive and behavioural components, so that the revised program included progressive muscle relaxation and most aspects of RET and stress-inoculation training. Their rationale was to combat Type A individuals' *physical tension* through relaxation, *emotional outbursts* through RET, and *interpersonal friction* through stress-inoculation training in problem-solving and communication skills. They then tested the revised program with Type A men who were employed in managerial jobs (Roskies et al. 1986). The men were randomly assigned either to the revised program or to one of two physical exercise groups. One exercise group focused on aerobic training (mostly jogging) and the other followed a weight-training program. After 10 weeks, the men were retested for Type A behaviour (Structured Interview) and their cardiovascular reactivity (blood pressure and heart rate) to stressors, such as doing mental arithmetic, for comparison with measures taken earlier. Although none of the three treatments reduced the men's physiological reactivity, the multidimensional program was substantially more successful than either of the exercise programs in reducing the three components of Type A behaviour. Its beneficial effect on the subjects' hostility, for example, can be seen in figure 5.5.

Research by Raymond Novaco (1975, 1978) has also demonstrated the usefulness of stress-inoculation training and relaxation in helping people control their anger. He trained individuals who were both self-identified and clinically assessed as having serious problems controlling anger. In this treatment program, the subjects first learned about the role of arousal and cognitive processes in feelings of anger. Then they learned muscle relaxation along with statements — like those in figure 5.6 — they could say to themselves at different times in the course of angry episodes, such as at the point of 'impact and confrontation'. Finally, they practised the techniques while imagining and role-playing realistic anger situations arranged in a hierarchy from least to most provoking. The results showed that this treatment improved the subjects' ability to control anger, as measured by their self-reports and their blood pressure when provoked in the laboratory.

Some researchers have investigated the possibility of using pharmacological approaches to modify Type A behaviour, particularly by prescribing beta-blockers. In one experiment, male hypertensive patients were randomly assigned to either a group treated with beta-blockers or a control group (Schmeider et al. 1983). The groups were equivalent in Type A behaviour before treatment, but after treatment the subjects treated with beta-blockers showed less Type A behaviour and lower cardiovascular reactivity than the controls. Although the use of beta-blockers may not be the treatment of choice for most Type A individuals, it may be an appropriate alternative for people who are at coronary risk who do not respond to behavioural and cognitive interventions (Chesney, Frautschi & Rosenman 1985).

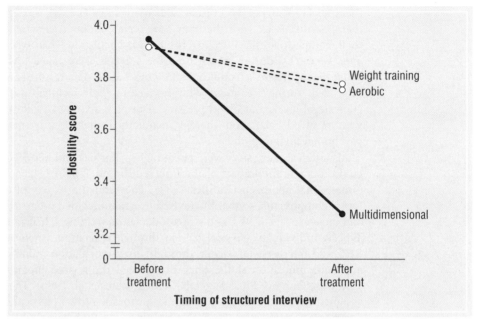

Figure 5.5 Hostility of Type A men measured by the Structured Interview method before and after a 10-week multidimensional, aerobic exercise or weight-training treatment program

Source: Data from Roskies et al. (1986, table 4).

Figure 5.6 Examples of anger management self-statements rehearsed in stress-inoculation training

Preparing for a provocation
This could be a rough situation; but I know how to deal with it. I can work out a plan to handle this. Easy does it. Remember, stick to the issues and don't take it personally. There won't be any need for an argument.
I know what to do.

Impact and confrontation
As long as I keep my cool, *I'm* in control of the situation. You don't need to prove yourself. Don't make more out of this than you have to. There is no point in getting mad. Think of what you have to do. Look for the positives and don't jump to conclusions.

Coping with arousal
Muscles are getting tight. Relax and slow things down. Time to take a deep breath. Let's take the issue point by

point. My anger is a signal of what I need to do. Time for problem solving. He probably wants me to get angry, but I'm going to deal with it constructively.

Subsequent reflection
a. Conflict unresolved
Forget about the aggravation. Thinking about it only makes you upset. Try to shake it off. Don't let it interfere with your job. Remember relaxation. It's a lot better than anger. Don't take it personally. It's probably not so serious.

b. Conflict resolved
I handled that one pretty well. That's doing a good job. I could have got more upset than it was worth. My pride can get me into trouble, but I'm doing better at this all the time. I actually got through that without getting angry.

Source: Novaco (1978, p. 150).

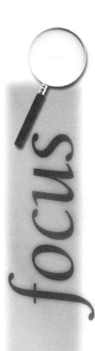

Focus on research
Effect of changing Type A behaviour on CHD

Does decreasing Type A behaviour with stress management techniques decrease the incidence of CHD? Meyer Friedman, Lynda Powell and Carl Thoresen worked together and with other colleagues in an ambitious intervention program called the Recurrent Coronary Prevention Project to examine this question (Friedman et al. 1986; Powell 1984; Powell & Friedman 1986; Powell et al. 1984; Thoresen et al. 1985). The researchers recruited more than 1000 patients who had suffered a myocardial infarction and who agreed to participate in the study for five years. The subjects were primarily married, middle-aged males, and about half were university educated. They were *not* selected on the basis of their exhibiting Type A behaviour, and they continued to be treated by their own doctors throughout the study. More than 860 of the subjects were randomly assigned to two intervention groups; the remaining subjects served as a control group, receiving no special intervention. The purpose of this study was to determine whether Type A behaviour can be modified in a general sample of cardiac patients and whether this modification will lower their subsequent cardiac morbidity and mortality rates.

Subjects in one of the two intervention groups received a program of frequent *cardiac counselling,*which provided information about the causes of myocardial infarction; the importance of altering standard coronary risk factors, such as cigarette smoking (Type A behaviour was not discussed); surgical and drug treatment of CHD; and the importance of avoiding activities, such as excessive physical exertion, that may precipitate another attack. The second group — called the *Type A/cardiac group* — had the same cardiac counselling, but also participated in a multidimensional program to modify Type A behaviour. Type A modification sessions met very frequently at first, and then monthly for the remainder of the study. The multidimensional program included progressive muscle relaxation and cognitive restructuring techniques, as well as several other methods.

The outcome of the study demonstrated the importance of modifying Type A behaviour, which was measured with Structured Interview and questionnaire methods. The Type A/cardiac subjects showed a much larger decrease in Type A behaviour than those in the other groups and had substantially lower rates of cardiac morbidity and mortality (Friedman et al. 1986). For example, subsequent infarctions occurred in about 13 per cent of the Type A/cardiac subjects, 21 per cent of the cardiac counselling subjects, and 28 per cent of the control subjects during the $4\frac{1}{2}$-year follow-up.

Byrne (1992) suggested that interventions to modify Type A behaviour need to be tailored to individual components of the behaviour pattern, since the construct comprises distinct elements that are not evident to the same degree among those exhibiting Type A behaviour, and the different components have different associations to coronary risk. Interventions for modifying Type A behaviour have been outlined extensively by Byrne (1987, 1992). Some of the psychological strategies recommended for modifying Type A behaviour include:

(a) the use of *cognitive restructuring* to alter cognitions that initiate and maintain Type A behaviour — for example the belief that one has to achieve more and more in less time to be successful

(b) *environmental management* to change aspects of work environments that reinforce Type A behaviour, such as training the patient to be more selective in the number of tasks undertaken

(c) *direct behaviour change* — for example monitoring Type A behaviour, learning alternative ways of responding, role playing and rehearsal of response substitution

(d) *time management*, such as learning how to structure time effectively to reduce time urgency

(e) *hostility management* involving monitoring of hostile cognitions and incorporating more passive responses

(f) *stimulus control* or the dissociation of Type A behaviours from situational determinants

(g) *stress management* for emotional distress.

Treating hypertension

As we discussed in chapter 4, essential hypertension is an important risk factor for CHD. Patients with diagnosed hypertension above the borderline level usually receive medical treatment that includes the use of prescription drugs, such as *diuretics*, which lower blood pressure by decreasing blood volume. In addition, doctors generally try to get all hypertensive patients to reduce their body weight, exercise regularly, and reduce their intake of sodium, cholesterol, caffeine and alcohol (AHA 1994; Herd & Weiss 1984). Sometimes doctors and others urge hypertensive patients to 'try to relax' when hassles and pressure occur. But there is a danger in this advice: untrained people who make an effort to relax often end up increasing their blood pressure rather than decreasing it (Suls, Sanders & Labrecque 1986).

Because the development of essential hypertension has been linked to the amount of stress people experience, researchers have examined the utility of stress management techniques in treating high blood pressure. Garcia-Vera, Labrador and Sanz (1997) assessed the effectiveness of stress management training on systolic and diastolic blood pressure for a group of hypertensive patients randomly allocated to either a treatment group or a waiting-list control group. Treatment consisted of a modified version of Jacobson's progressive muscle relaxation, problem-solving training and information on hypertension provided through a self-help booklet. Following treatment, blood pressure was clinically reduced for the treatment group compared with the control patients, and the percentage of patients who achieved a normotensive level of blood pressure was higher in the treatment group. In general, studies have found that blood pressure can be reduced to some degree with certain stress management techniques, such as progressive muscle relaxation, biofeedback and meditation (Johnston 1992; McCaffrey & Blanchard 1985). Some findings suggest that using only relaxation to lower blood pressure is unlikely to help individuals with certain characteristics, such as high levels of anger (Larkin, Knowlton & D'Alessandri 1990). But more recent evidence suggests that the effectiveness of stress management approaches can be strengthened by using multi-dimensional programs: a study using several behavioural and cognitive methods found substantial blood pressure reductions in mildly hypertensive Type A men (Bennett et al. 1991). A meta-analysis by Wolfgang Linden and Laura Chambers (1994) of dozens of studies found that multidimensional programs consisting of behavioural and cognitive methods for stress management are highly effective — as effective as diuretic drugs — in reducing blood pressure. It is now clear that psychological approaches have considerable value in treating hypertension, making effective treatment possible without drugs or with lower doses for most patients.

Other researchers have examined the usefulness of stress management methods in modifying cardiovascular reactivity. Recall from chapter 4 that reactivity refers to the physiological response to a stressor, as when blood pressure rises during a confrontation, and that frequent and prolonged high reactivity may lead to CHD. Some studies have shown that biofeedback, progressive muscle relaxation and cognitive restructuring methods can reduce reactivity, but other studies have produced inconsistent or negative findings (Blanchard et al. 1988; Jacob & Chesney 1986; Seraganian et al. 1987). Why are the outcomes of these studies so inconsistent? The reason may involve differences in the studies' methodological details, such as the duration of the intervention training or therapy, the specific stressors used, and whether the participants liked or believed in the particular intervention they received (Seraganian et al. 1987). Even without intervention, people appear to adapt to repeated exposure to the same stressor, showing decreased reactivity over time (Frankish & Linden 1991).

In an effort to improve the health of employees, many large organisations have introduced voluntary stress management programs for their workers. Most studies of these programs have found that they produce improvements in measures of workers' psychological and physiological stress (Alderman 1984; Gomel et al. 1993; Sallis et al. 1987). Despite the success of stress management programs in reducing coronary risk by modifying Type A behaviour and lowering blood pressure, they are not yet applied widely — partly because the evidence supporting the use of these programs is relatively new, and partly because they cost money to run. Other reasons relate to the participants: although people typically recognise the seriousness of heart disease, Type A individuals probably don't see any connection between CHD and their hard-driving lifestyles (Roskies 1983). Also, people with high blood pressure either don't know they have it or say they 'feel good anyway'. For these and similar reasons, many people who could benefit from stress management programs don't join one when it is available. And many of those who do join drop out before completing the programs or don't adhere closely to their recommendations, such as to practise relaxation techniques at home (Alderman 1984; Hoelscher, Lichstein & Rosenthal 1986).

Minimising risk of cardiac recurrence

So far we have considered the different interventions that have been used to modify coronary risk factors such as Type A behaviour, stress and hypertension. Psychological interventions have also been adopted for the rehabilitation of the cardiac patient to prevent another heart attack. These interventions have taken many forms including counselling for emotional distress, graded exercise programs to increase cardiac efficiency, education on coronary heart disease and the role of Type A behaviour, biofeedback, stress management and relaxation training. Most of these interventions are offered on an outpatient basis, though some interventions in the acute phase of recovery have had some success. Oldenburg and Perkins (1984), for example, provided a brief hospital-based intervention to heart disease patients within the first days of admission to coronary care. One group of patients received counselling, education on heart disease and associated risks, and relaxation training. A second group received education and relaxation but no counselling, while the third group acted as a control receiving only routine medical and nursing care. Although no differences were observed between the three groups in terms of length of hospital stay, patients who received both counselling and education had fewer cardiac complications while in hospital, and both intervention groups had less chest pain compared with the control patients.

There is some indication that emotional distress is evident both in the acute and post-phases of myocardial infarction (Byrne 1987) and can affect recovery. Anxiety has been found to be the predominant emotional response in the acute phase and is higher in patients with a neurotic predisposition, in females and in some patients for whom a definite diagnosis of myocardial infarction (MI) has not been made (Byrne 1987). Depression following MI has also been documented to be higher in females (Frasure-Smith, Lesperance & Talajic 1995). In a study by Byrne, Whyte and Lance (1979), which explored the illness behaviours of MI patients using cluster analysis, an affective component was identified in at least two of the four clusters. These groups of patients exhibited depression and anxiety with disruption to interpersonal relationships. This would seem to substantiate inclusion of a stress management component in interventions for coronary heart disease patients.

A meta-analysis of psychoeducational programs for coronary disease patients (Dusseldorp et al. 1999) reported a 34 per cent reduction in mortality and a 29 per cent reduction in recurrence of heart disease to be associated with stress management and health education programs. Other benefits of these programs included reductions in blood pressure, cholesterol and body weight, as well as changes in smoking and eating habits and physical exercise.

Summary

Coping is the process by which people try to manage the real or perceived discrepancy between the demands and resources they appraise in stressful situations. We cope with stress through transactions with the environment that do not necessarily lead to solutions to the problems causing the stress.

Coping serves two types of functions. The function of emotion-focused coping is to regulate the person's emotional response to stress. This regulation occurs through the person's behaviour, such as using alcohol or seeking social support, and through cognitive strategies, such as denying unpleasant facts. People tend to rely on emotion-focused coping when they believe they cannot change the stressful conditions. The function of problem-focused coping is to reduce the demands of the stressor or expand the resources to deal with it, such as by learning new skills. People tend to use problem-focused coping when they believe they can change the situation. Adults report using more problem-focused than emotion-focused coping approaches when they experience stress. People use a wide variety of strategies to cope with stress. Some of these methods tend to increase the attention the person gives to the problem, and other methods promote avoidance of the problem. There is no one best method of coping, and no method is uniformly applied or effective with all stressors. People tend to use a combination of methods in coping with a stressful situation.

Although coping changes across the life span, the exact nature of these changes is unclear. Young children's coping is limited by their cognitive abilities, which improve throughout childhood. Australian adolescents tend to cope with problems by dealing with the situation while maintaining physical fitness and being socially connected. Female adolescents tend to seek social support more than males, and older adolescents resort more to tension-reduction strategies such as smoking and drinking. During adulthood, a shift in coping function occurs as people approach old age — they rely less on problem-focused and more on emotion-focused coping. Elderly people seem to regard stressors as less changeable than middle-aged individuals do.

People can reduce the potential for stress in their lives and others' lives in several ways. First, they can increase the social support they give and receive by joining social, religious and special interest groups. Second, they can improve their own and others' sense of personal control and hardiness by giving and taking responsibility. Also, they can reduce frustration and waste less time by organising their world better, such as through time management. And by exercising and keeping fit, they can reduce the experience of stress and the impact it has on their health. Last, they can prepare for stressful events, such as a medical procedure, by improving their behavioural, cognitive and informational control.

Sometimes the coping skills individuals have learned are not adequate for dealing with a stressor that is very strong, novel or unrelenting. A variety of stress management techniques is available to help people who are having trouble coping effectively. One technique is pharmacological — that is, using prescribed drugs such as beta-blockers. Stress management methods include progressive muscle relaxation, systematic desensitisation, biofeedback, modelling and several cognitive approaches. Rational-emotive therapy (RET) and cognitive therapy attempt to modify stress-producing, irrational thought patterns through the process of cognitive restructuring. Stress-inoculation training is designed to teach people skills to alleviate stress and achieve personal goals. Stress-inoculation training is an example of a multidimensional approach in that it uses a variety of techniques that are designed to reduce specific components of the person's problems. Beneficial effects on people's stress have been found for all of the behavioural and cognitive stress management methods, particularly relaxation. Meditation and hypnosis have shown promise for reducing stress, too. Stress management techniques can reduce coronary risk by modifying Type A behaviour and by treating hypertension. Psychoeducational programs with a stress management component have also been found to facilitate recovery in heart attack patients, and reduce the recurrence of heart disease in those who have suffered a first heart attack.

Key terms

biofeedback	emotion-focused coping	progressive muscle relaxation	systematic desensitisation
cognitive restructuring	modelling	rational-emotive therapy	time management
cognitive therapy	problem-focused coping	stress-inoculation training	
coping			

PART 3

Lifestyles to enhance health and prevent illness

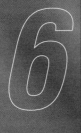

6 Health-related behaviour and health promotion

Health and behaviour

Lifestyles, risk factors and health

Interdisciplinary perspectives on preventing illness

Problems in promoting wellness

What determines people's health-related behaviour?

General factors in health-related behaviour

The role of beliefs and intentions

The role of non-rational processes

Developmental, gender and sociocultural factors in health

Development and health-related behaviour

Gender and health-related behaviour

Sociocultural factors and health-related behaviour

Programs for health promotion

Methods for promoting health

Promoting health in the schools

Work-site wellness programs

Community-wide wellness programs

Prevention with specific targets: focusing on AIDS

Prologue

'It's getting worse — those health freaks are all over the place these days, trying to sell us nuts and seeds to live on,' said Tom as he passed by the health food store of the shopping complex. 'Give me a fat juicy steak and lots of beer to go with it. I don't think you can do better than that!' Things are not necessarily worse, but they have changed. Unlike Tom, many Australians are health-conscious, as can be seen by the increased numbers of people preoccupied with their weight, jogging and walking in the suburbs.

Although the nature of health concerns may have changed over time, interest in health is not new. In the late nineteenth century most developed countries believed that the physical health of their citizens was vital for national power and stability. Notions of preventive health, though, have had a different historical evolution in Australia given its relatively recent settlement. Some of the earliest efforts at public health intervention centred on the survival of a British-administered penal colony in the early 1800s. During this colonial period, quarantine procedures were used to prevent the spread of disease. Outbreaks of infectious disease did occur often, however, with devastating effects on the indigenous people. Environmental sanitation and the control of infectious disease became the responsibility of local government and State-appointed public health commissioners. During the Federation of Australia, preventive efforts and the control of disease were directed towards the productive and reproductive sectors of the community — that is, mothers and their infants, and industrial workers. The post–World War 1 period to 1930 saw the establishment of the Federal Department of Health. Later developments in health focused on the creation of a national health service, health education and the provision of preventive health services. The new public health movement in the 1990s has emphasised the enhancement of life skills through supportive environments, and government policy to promote the health of all Australians (Gordon 1976; Cumpston 1989; O'Connor & Parker 1995).

This chapter begins our examination of health enhancement and illness prevention. We first consider what health habits people practise and how their lifestyles affect their health. Then we turn our attention to factors that influence the health-related behaviours individuals adopt. In the final section of this chapter, we discuss programs to help people lead healthier lives. As we study these topics, you will find answers to questions you may have about health-related behaviour and health promotion. Are people leading healthier lives today than they did in the past? Why is it that some people take better care of themselves than others do? How effective are health-promotion programs that try to motivate healthy behaviour through fear?

Health and behaviour

The role of behaviour in health has received increasing attention in Australia since the turn of the century, as the causes of death have shifted from infectious and dietary diseases to chronic diseases. Mortality from most of today's leading causes of death could be substantially reduced if people would adopt lifestyles that promote wellness, such as by eating healthy diets and not smoking.

The percentage of deaths resulting from any specific cause changes over time. Table 6.1 depicts the pattern of changes in Australia that have occurred since the late 1960s. These changes resulted partly from the modifications people made in their behavioural risk factors for major chronic diseases, especially cardiovascular disease. Of course, making all of the lifestyle changes health experts recommend won't enable us to live forever. Even if researchers found cures for most of the leading fatal diseases, the average life expectancy of people in technologically advanced countries would increase by perhaps a decade or so to its likely upper limit of about 85 years (Olshansky, Carnes & Cassel 1990).

Table 6.1 Death rate per 100 000 Australian males and females for selected causes of death, 1961 and 1998

	1961		1998	
Causes of death	Males	Females	Males	Females
Cancer	197	139	220	133
Circulatory diseases (heart disease, stroke)	759	514	284	187
Respiratory diseases	108	45	77	43
Digestive disease	39	23	22	15
Injuries	104	42	61	22
Infectious diseases	17	9	8	5

Source: AIHW (2000).

Lifestyles, risk factors and health

The typical person's lifestyle includes many behaviours that are risk factors for illness and injury. For instance, millions of people in Australia smoke cigarettes, drink excessively, use drugs, eat high-fat and high-cholesterol diets, eat too much and become overweight, undertake too little physical activity and behave in unsafe ways, such as by speeding in cars. Many people realise the danger these and other risk factors present and adjust their behaviour to protect their health.

Health-protective behaviour

Health-protective behaviour refers to any activity people perform to maintain or promote their health, regardless of their perceived health status or whether the behaviour actually achieves that goal. What health-protective behaviours do Australians actually do? Information on health behaviours practised comes mostly from national health surveys. Table 6.2 presents the percentage of Australians reporting health protective and risk behaviours. Dietary intake as assessed by the 1995 National Nutrition Survey indicated that 90 per cent of Australians had consumed cereal products during the day before the interview (AIHW 1996). More than half the males, and about one-third of children under 12 years of age, had not consumed any fruit. Of concern was the finding that 20 per cent of young children had not eaten any vegetables on the day assessed by the survey. Australians are, however, adopting healthier food alternatives. Nutrition surveys conducted on a random sample of adults in Victoria (CSIRO 1993) indicated that consumption of low-fat dairy products increased between 1985 and 1990, as did the consumption of meat, fruit and vegetables over this period. In regard to weight, about half of adult Australian males are overweight by 20 per cent, while one-third of females are overweight (ABS 1999b). In regard to physical activity, only one-third of Australians do no exercise (AIHW 1996). Walking is the preferred form of physical activity for both males and females, and increased by 10 per cent between 1989 and 1995. The proportion of persons doing aerobics and vigorous exercise remained the same. More males than females drink alcohol and smoke cigarettes (AIHW 2000).

Who practises health-protective behaviour and why? We are far from a complete answer to these questions, but evidence has revealed gender, sociocultural and age differences in practising healthy behaviours (Schoenborn 1993; USBC 1995). For instance, an international survey of adults in European countries found that women perform more healthy behaviours than men (Steptoe et al. 1994). One reason for such differences is that people seem to perform behaviours that are salient to them. For instance, comparisons were made of licensed practical nurses (LPNs), high school teachers and university students for the practice of 30 behaviours. The LPNs gave the highest ratings for keeping emergency numbers near the phone; the teachers gave the highest ratings for watching their weight; and the students gave the highest ratings for getting enough exercise. Another study compared the lifestyles of medical and non-medical students and found that the medical students exercised more and were much less likely to smoke cigarettes, drink alcohol excessively and use drugs (Golding & Cornish 1987).

Table 6.2   Percentages reporting selected health-related behaviours or health-risk characteristics

Behaviour	Men %	Women %
Exercise	66.4	65.6
Smoke regularly	27.3	20.3
Drink alcohol in excess	17.6	10.8
Overweight by at least 20%	46.1	30.3

Sources: AIHW (1996); ABS (1999b).

You probably know some individuals who are highly health-conscious and others who seem to have little concern about their health. Because of these contrasts, some people expect that individuals who practise certain behaviours that benefit their health (1) also practise other healthy behaviours and (2) continue to perform these behaviours over time. To some extent these expectations are true (Schoenborn 1993). Many individuals lead very healthy lifestyles, and the number of health-protective behaviours people practise remains fairly constant over many years. But many other people show little consistency in their health habits (Harris & Guten 1979; Langlie 1977; Mechanic 1979). These research results suggest three conclusions. First, although people's health habits are fairly stable, they often change over time. Second, particular health-protective behaviours are not strongly tied to one another — that is, if we know a person practises one specific health habit, such as keeping to the speed limit in the car, we cannot accurately predict that he or she practises another specific habit, such as exercising. Third, health-protective behaviours do not seem to be governed in each person by a single set of attitudes or response tendencies. Thus, a female who keeps to a safe speed limit to protect herself from injury may watch her weight to be attractive and not smoke because she is allergic to it.

Why are health-protective behaviours not more stable and strongly linked to one another? There are at least four reasons. First, different habits may serve different purposes. For example, people practise some habits, such as getting enough sleep and eating breakfast, to *promote health* but engage in other health-protective behaviours, such as limiting their use of alcohol and cigarettes, to *avoid health risks* (Leventhal, Prohaska & Hirschman 1985). Second, various factors at any given time in people's lives may differentially affect different behaviours. For instance, a person may have lots of social encouragement to eat heartily ('Have some more, you need the energy!') and fatteningly and, at the same time, to limit drinking and smoking. Third, people change as a result of experience and the acquisition of skills to enable change. For example, many people did not avoid smoking until they learned that it was harmful or were able to receive help through a quit smoking program. Fourth, people's life circumstances change; thus, factors such as peer pressure that may have been important in initiating and maintaining exercising or smoking at one time may no longer be present, thereby increasing the likelihood that the habit will change (Leventhal, Prohaska & Hirschman 1985). Some behaviours may be resistant to change even in the absence of peer pressure. Behaviour once patterned is difficult to change, and the mere absence of reinforcers that were useful in the establishment of a habit may not be sufficient, as these reinforcers are not necessarily the ones that will maintain the habit once the pattern is established.

Health status and behaviour

An important perspective in studying health-related behaviour is to consider how it changes with the health status of the individual. Public health researchers Stanislav Kasl and Sidney Cobb have defined the types of behaviour that characterise three stages in the progress of disease:

1. **Health behaviour** refers to 'any activity undertaken by a person believing himself to be healthy, for the purpose of preventing disease or detecting it in an asymptomatic stage' (1966a, p. 246). These activities might include healthy people's exercising, eating healthy diets, having regular dental checkups and getting vaccinations against diseases.

2. **Illness behaviour** involves 'any activity, undertaken by a person who feels ill, to define the state of his health and to discover a suitable remedy' (1966a, p. 246). These activities generally include complaining about symptoms and seeking help or advice from relatives, friends and medical practitioners. A person who feels stomach pains and complains to friends or makes an appointment with a doctor is displaying illness behaviour.

3. **Sick-role behaviour** refers to 'activity undertaken, for the purpose of getting well, by those who consider themselves ill. It includes receiving treatment from appropriate therapists, generally involves a whole range of dependent behaviours, and leads to some degree of neglect of one's usual duties' (1966b, p. 531). A patient who gets a prescription filled, uses it as the doctor directed and stays home from work to recover is exhibiting sick-role behaviour.

Health behaviour has a preventive function — engaging in it helps to maintain or improve current good health and avoid illness. But when people are well, they may not feel inclined to devote the effort and sacrifice that health behaviour entails. They may take the view, 'If it ain't broke, don't fix it.' Thus, whether a person engages in health behaviour depends heavily on motivational factors, particularly with regard to the individual's perception of a threat of disease, the value in the behaviour in reducing this threat, and the attractiveness of the opposite behaviour. Unhealthy behaviours, such as drinking or smoking, are often seen as pleasurable or the 'in' thing to do. As a result, many individuals do not resist beginning unhealthy behaviours and may reject efforts or advice to get them to quit. Some people think health and pleasure are incompatible, feeling that a life that stresses health behaviour is doomed to dullness and fear of illness.

People acquire healthy and unhealthy behaviours through learning processes, which occur by way of direct experience and through observing the behaviour of others. If the behaviour becomes well established, it tends to become *habitual* — that is, the person often performs it automatically and without awareness. For example,

> a confirmed smoker working at his desk may, despite a severe head cold, respond to the sight of an open pack of cigarettes by automatically reaching out, taking one, and starting to smoke without at all being aware of what he has done. Only when the irritation produced in his nose and throat . . . by the smoke 'captures his attention' is he likely to disengage in smoking behavior. (Hunt et al. 1979, p. 115)

Even though the behaviour may have been learned because it was reinforced by positive consequences, it is now less dependent on its consequences and more dependent on cues, called antecedents, with which it has been associated in the past (Sarafino 1996). *Antecedents* are internal or external stimuli that precede and set the occasion for a behaviour. A smoker who says, 'I have to have a cigarette with my coffee after breakfast,' is pointing out an antecedent. Behaviours that become habitual can be very difficult to change.

Because habitual behaviours are hard to change, people need to develop health behaviours as early as possible and eliminate unhealthy activities as soon as they appear. The family system plays a major role in children's learning of health-related behaviours (Baranowski & Nader 1985). Children observe, for example, the dietary, exercise and smoking habits of other family members and often receive encouragement to behave in similar ways. Children who observe and receive encouragement for healthy behaviour at home are more likely to develop good health habits than children who do not.

Illness behaviour has a problem-solving function. The person is concerned about symptoms he or she is experiencing and seeks information and help. People do not always engage in illness behaviour when symptoms appear, and some people are more likely to complain and seek help than others (Kasl & Cobb 1966a; Rosenstock & Kirscht 1979). There are many reasons for these differences. For example, some individuals may be more afraid than others of doctors, hospitals or the serious illness a diagnosis may reveal. Also, some people are more stoic or less concerned than others about the aches and pains they experience. In addition, some people simply have less money than others to pay for medical care and, therefore, do not seek help when they need it. Chapter 9 will examine in more detail these and other reasons why people do and do not use health care services.

Sick-role behaviour is what people do when they believe they are ill. The concept of a sick role was first described by sociologist Talcott Parsons (1951, 1964). By adopting the sick role, people are exempt from their normal obligations and life tasks, such as going to work or school. But a special obligation ordinarily accompanies this status — that of trying to get well. Patients perform most sick-role behaviours in order to get well, as in taking medication as directed. Unfortunately, many patients drop out of treatment, particularly if it is inconvenient to continue or is impersonally administered (Rosenstock & Kirscht 1979). Other sick-role behaviours seem to serve emotional functions, as when patients moan or sigh and receive sympathy as a result.

How people behave when they are sick depends in large measure on what they have learned. As an example, a study of female college students assessed whether they had been encouraged during adolescence to adopt the sick role for menstruation or had observed their mothers exhibit menstrual distress. Compared with students who did not have these experiences, those who *did* reported more menstrual symptoms, disability and clinic visits for these symptoms as adults (Whitehead et al. 1986). Other research has found that there are cultural differences in the way people respond to their symptoms and go about trying to get well (Chrisman & Kleinman 1983; Zola 1973). For example, studies in the United States have found differences among groups of immigrants in their willingness to tolerate pain, but these differences diminish in succeeding generations (Chapman & Brena 1985). It has been noted that Aboriginal people tend to become apprehensive about a part of the body only when it fails to function, often ignoring any symptoms of pain. According to Spark, Donovan and Howat (1991):

> Aboriginal people are more likely to think as collectives rather than as individuals, and family and community and one's place within them may have a higher value than individual health. This could derive from a different conceptualisation of health among Aboriginal people. 'Health' to Aboriginal people traditionally meant 'life'. Traditional Aboriginal life was an integrated system directed towards survival, whose main elements were land, law, culture and family. (p. 11)

Interdisciplinary perspectives on preventing illness

According to public health expert Lester Breslow, although medical science and technology have made great progress in treating disease, 'the principal advances in health have come about through health promotion and disease prevention rather than through diagnosis and therapy' (1983, p. 50). Using tooth decay as an example, we can illustrate three preventive approaches. These are:

• *behavioural influence*, such as encouraging and demonstrating good brushing and flossing techniques

• *environmental measures*, which can involve fluoridating water supplies

• *preventive medical efforts*, such as removing tartar from teeth and repairing cavities.

Comprehensive and effective efforts for health promotion and disease prevention consist of some combination of these three approaches. In the world's industrialised nations, the greatest opportunity for health promotion probably lies in influencing behaviour, such as by reducing cigarette smoking, excessive alcohol use and unhealthy dietary practices (Breslow 1983).

We usually think of prevention as occurring before an illness takes hold. Actually, there are three levels of prevention, only one of which applies before a disease or injury occurs (Leventhal, Prohaska & Hirschman 1985; Runyan 1985; Sanson-Fisher 1993). These levels are called *primary*, *secondary* and *tertiary* prevention. Each level of prevention can include the efforts of oneself, one's social network and professionals who are working to promote health. One's own preventive efforts can include health, illness and sick-role behaviours.

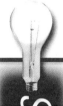

Highlight on issues

Two health behaviours: breast and testicular examinations

Breast cancer is a leading cause of women's deaths around the world. For women in Australia it is predicted that approximately one in 16 will develop breast cancer during their lifetime, especially after the age of 50, and one in 24 will die of it (Agars & McMurray 1993). Breast cancer is the leading cause of cancer death among Australian women, accounting for 17 per cent of all female cancer deaths (ABS 1999a). Compared with breast cancer, testicular cancer is somewhat less prevalent, representing 13 per cent of all male cancer deaths for men in midlife (ABS 1999a). Breast and testicular cancers are treated with some combination of radiation therapy, chemotherapy and surgery, and both cancers have very high cure rates if treated early.

Individuals can detect cancer of the breast or testicles in its early stages by self-examination. Breast and testicular self-examinations are done with the fingers, searching mainly for abnormal lumps. For breast self-examination (BSE), the woman lies on her back and, before examining a breast, places the arm of the same side of the body as that breast behind her head. With her other hand, she presses the ends of the middle three fingers flatly against the breast tissue and moves them in ten cent-sized circular forms.

(continued)

Although women can choose from different search patterns to examine the region, a pattern that has the hand follow a series of vertical strips to cover a square area that includes the breast seems to produce the most thorough search (Atkins et al. 1991; Saunders, Pilgrim & Pennypacker 1986). The standard method for testicular self-examination (TSE) is relatively simple. The man first locates the tubelike structures that extend behind the testicle. Then he rotates the entire surface of each testicle between the fingers and thumbs of both hands, looking for lumps.

Do people practise BSEs and TSEs? Most of what we know about the practice of these health behaviours comes from research on BSEs. For example, almost all American women know of the BSE, and the great majority have tried it at least once. Yet less than half of them practise it at the recommended monthly frequency (Newcomb et al. 1991; Shepperd et al. 1990; USBC 1995). Research shows that a similar situation exists in Australia (we discuss this later in the chapter). This is disheartening because the procedure appears to be effective, and more than 90 per cent of breast cancers are detected by the women themselves. Although past evidence indicated that women who do practise BSE on a regular basis tend to come from higher socioeconomic groups, have more education and feel more vulnerable to cancer than those who do not (Kegeles 1983; Strauss et al. 1987), more recent data suggest that sociocultural factors no longer impair BSE practice (USBC 1995). Research has revealed several reasons why most women do not practise BSE regularly: some women lack the knowledge or confidence to do it correctly, do not know how important early detection can be, are afraid they will find a malignant lump, feel embarrassed by the method, or simply forget and have no reminders to do it (Alagna & Reddy 1984; Champion 1990; Craun & Deffenbacher 1987; Kegeles 1983; Shepperd et al. 1990). Similar factors seem to be involved in men's practice and non-practice of TSE (Brubaker & Wickersham 1990; Friman et al. 1986; Rosella 1994).

How can we encourage the practice of BSE and TSE? One way is through mass communication. BreastScreen Australia has used a well-known rural identity, Sara Henderson, to convey information about the benefits of breast screening and to motivate women to have a mammogram. Reports concerning breast and testicular cancer should compare the very high cure rates (about 90 per cent) when detected in early stages with the much lower rates when detected later. People also need to know that treatment for cancer is often less extensive, traumatic and disfiguring in earlier than later stages. For example, breast cancer in its early stages can often be treated without removing the entire breast.

Another way to encourage these health behaviours is for health practitioners, such as doctors or nurses, to provide information and training through individual and group contacts, such as at universities, work sites and medical offices. TSE is easy to learn by following simple written instructions (Friman et al. 1986). BSE is harder to learn, and many women receive little or no training to do it correctly. An Australian program known as Mammacheck consists of a 60- to 90-minute session for a small group of women led by a female facilitator. Educational information is provided on the physiology of the breast, breast cancer and the rationale underlying BSE. Women are trained in correct BSE technique through the presentation of a video. The facilitator then checks for correctness of the technique as the women practise BSE on themselves, and on artificial breast models. Discussion of barriers to BSE practice and the development of action plans are also incorporated in the session (Clarke et al. 1991). Having reminders to do examinations increases the frequency with which they are done. It is especially important that men and women with family histories or other risk factors for cancer devise effective BSE or TSE reminders, such as by writing them in a calendar.

Primary prevention

Primary prevention consists of actions taken to avoid disease or injury. In avoiding motor vehicle injuries, for example, primary prevention activities include our personal action of keeping to the speed limit, a friend reminding us to stick to the speed limit and public health reminders on TV to avoid speeding. Similarly, primary prevention includes actions taken that help people brush and floss their teeth proficiently, resist beginning to smoke or gain immunity against a contagious disease.

Primary prevention for an individual can begin before he or she is born, or even conceived. Today it is possible to estimate the risk of a child's inheriting a genetic disorder and, in some cases, to diagnose genetic abnormalities in the unborn foetus. Through **genetic counselling**, prospective and expectant parents may obtain information to help them make important family planning decisions (Emery & Pullen 1986; Harper 1981). If the child has not yet been conceived, the counsellor can use several types of information to estimate genetic risks. For some inherited diseases or defects, the incidence increases with the parents' ages; for others, there are biological tests for carriers of the gene (Kopp 1983). If conception has already occurred, these same techniques may be used for determining whether biological tests on the foetus are warranted. These tests, *amniocentesis* and *chorion biopsy*, are expensive and may present some degree of risk of injury to the foetus. If the likelihood of the child inheriting a serious health problem greatly exceeds the risk of injury during the test, the procedure is usually recommended. Genetic counselling and biological tests can be applied to determine the risk of many serious and potentially fatal problems, such as the metabolic disorder *Tay-Sachs disease*, the red blood cell disorder *sickle-cell anaemia*, and *Duchenne muscular dystrophy*. Clearly, the use of genetic counselling and biological tests on the foetus can play an important role in primary prevention, allowing prospective and expectant parents to make informed decisions regarding future pregnancies and abortion. Doctors can help in selecting genetic counsellors.

Another way parents can exercise primary prevention for children is by following the recommended immunisation schedule of the National Health and Medical Research Council (NHMRC). Although many prevalent illnesses, such as pneumonia and the common cold, cannot yet be controlled through immunisation, several diseases can. These diseases include diphtheria, tetanus, whooping cough, measles, rubella, mumps and polio. The proportion of Australian preschool children who lack full immunisation from currently controllable diseases has declined in recent years to 25 per cent (AIHW 1996), but children of non-English speaking backgrounds and Aboriginal children have lower immunisation rates. Australia experienced a measles outbreak over the 1992–93 period, which peaked at 23.9 cases per 100 000. This incident was responsible for a full-scale national immunisation program in 1998 to eliminate the disease (ABS 1996a).

Several promising approaches to primary prevention exist. One involves having medical professionals give health-promotion advice to patients, but doctors have difficulty incorporating this approach in their practices (Levine et al. 1992; Radecki & Brunton 1992). Perhaps other medical staff would be better able to do it. The second approach helps people recognise the need for improvements in their health behaviours by using questionnaires to assess their risk factors (Weiss 1984). You may have seen magazines with versions of questionnaires to assess the reader's life expectancy or risk of heart disease. These are simple self-completed and self-scored tests. Other tests are more elaborate, are scored and analysed by computer, and may need interpretation by a health professional. The questionnaires typically ask about the person's past and current health; family history of illness; personal characteristics, such as age, height and weight, sex and race; and lifestyle, such as personal hygiene, eating habits, use of tobacco and alcohol, physical activity and so on. Using these data in conjunction with mortality and epidemiologic information, these tests estimate the person's risk and, sometimes, how much risk could be eliminated if he or she made certain lifestyle changes. Another approach involves structural changes to promote health, as in the rescheduling of sporting events away from the middle of the day to reduce the incidence of melanoma resulting from overexposure to ultraviolet radiation from the sun. Last, social change might be used to progressively encourage negative attitudes to smoking through a concerted campaign to associate smoking with undesirable attributes such as lack of cleanliness.

Secondary prevention

In **secondary prevention**, actions are taken to identify and treat an illness or injury early with the aim of stopping or reversing the problem. In the case of someone who has developed an ulcer, for example, secondary prevention activities include the person's illness behaviour of seeking medical care for abdominal pain, the doctor's pre-scribing medication and dietary changes, and the patient's sick-role behaviour of following the doctor's prescriptions. Instances of secondary prevention for other health problems can be found in many different settings — examination of the mouth and jaw regions for early cancer detection during dental visits, free blood pressure measurements at shopping centres, and assessments of children's vision and hearing at school, to cite a few.

Many doctors and adult patients practise secondary prevention through complete physical examinations each year. These checkups are costly in time and money — they consist of a medical history, examination of the body, assessment of vital signs (blood pressure, heart rate etc.), and a variety of X-ray and laboratory tests. Because evidence now suggests that several components of the traditional annual physical are not very useful in preventing illness, most medical and public health groups today no longer recommend a complete physical every year (CSA 1983; Shuchman & Wilkes 1986). Instead, they recommend six to ten specific tests, each with recommended schedules ranging from one to five years, depending on the person's age. For instance, the Aus-tralian Cancer Society recommends that women should have *mammograms* (breast X-rays) annually after the age of 50, but less frequently at younger ages. For sexually active women, Pap smear tests every two years are recommended for the detection of cervical cancer (AHMAC 1991). All adults over the age of 50 should have a *sigmoidos-copy* (colon inspection) every three to five years or so. Individuals who are not healthy or are considered to be at high risk, for example because of past illnesses, family history or hazardous work conditions, should be examined more often.

These medical examinations are recommended because they detect the disease earlier and save lives. In the case of mammograms, their accuracy in detecting breast cancer increased dramatically in the 1970s (Smart 1994), and women who follow the recommended schedules for examinations after age 50 reduce their mortality rates by 26 per cent in follow-ups of 10 years or so after diagnosis (Kerlikowske et al. 1995). In regard to cervical cancer, it is estimated that Pap smear testing results in the preven-tion of this cancer for 700 to 750 Australian women each year (Medley 1995). Yet, as is the case in the United States, few Australian women over the age of 40 engage in the recommended screening. Australian national surveys have found that less than 70 per cent of women have had a Pap smear in the last three years, and less than 12 per cent have had a mammogram (Medley 1995; Nutbeam et al. 1993). Women with limited education, older women and those from non-English speaking backgrounds have the lowest rates of screening (Straton 1992). High-risk women with a family history of breast cancer do not have more mammograms than other women, unless their risk is explicitly described to them (Curry et al. 1993).

Reported reasons for not undergoing medical examinations depend on the type of examination and the patient group. Among elderly middle- and upper-middle-class women, the main reasons for not having mammograms are fears of pain and radiation (Fullerton et al. 1996). Different reasons are given for not having a Pap smear. These include embarrassment and inconvenience (Hennig & Knowles 1990; Ruge & Lee 1995); discomfort during the procedure (Bowman 1991), and forgetting or under-estimating the time that has elapsed since the last Pap test (Dickinson, Leeder & Sanson-Fisher 1988). Attendance rates, however, have been found to increase through reminder letters from a general practitioner (Pritchard, Straton & Hyndman 1995), with increases of as much as 40 per cent through direct-mail intervention strategies (Byles & Sanson-Fisher 1996; Mitchell et al. 1991), although beneficial effects appear to lessen with repeated direct mailing strategies (Byles & Sanson-Fisher 1996).

Tertiary prevention

When a serious injury occurs or a disease progresses beyond the early stages, the condition often leads to lasting or irreversible damage. **Tertiary prevention** involves actions to contain or retard this damage, prevent disability and rehabilitate the patient. For patients with severe arthritis, for instance, tertiary prevention includes doing exercises for physical therapy and taking medication to control inflammation and pain. In the treatment of incurable forms of cancer, the goal may be simply to keep the patient reasonably comfortable and the disease in remission as long as possible. And people who suffer disabling injuries may undergo intensive long-term physical therapy to regain the use of their limbs or develop other means for independent functioning.

Problems in promoting wellness

The process of preventing illness and injury can be thought of as operating as a *system* in which the individual, his or her family, health professionals and the community each plays a role. According to health psychologist Craig Ewart (1991b), the effectiveness of each component can be impaired by a wide variety of factors and problems that interrelate and affect each other. Let's look at some of these factors, beginning with those within the individual.

Factors within the individual

People who consider ways to promote their own health often face an uphill battle with themselves. One problem is that many healthy behaviours are less pleasurable than their unhealthy alternatives, which may produce a state of conflict. Many people deal with this conflict by maintaining a balance in their lives, setting reasonable limits on the unhealthy behaviours they perform. But most people probably do not — they opt too frequently in favour of pleasure, sometimes vowing to change in the future: 'I'll go on a diet next week,' for example. On the other hand, some people become obsessed with illness prevention, sometimes doing more harm than good (Brownell 1991).

Another problem is that adopting wellness lifestyles may require individuals to change long-standing behaviours that have become habitual and may involve addictions, as in cigarette smoking. Habitual and addictive behaviours are very difficult to modify. A third problem is that people who are currently healthy often have little immediate incentive to practise health behaviour, particularly if the behaviour is unappealing or inconvenient. The desirable consequences of health behaviour, such as being healthier and fitter, are not immediate, and the undesirable consequence of not practising health behaviour — that is, developing a serious illness — may never materialise. Even when individuals know they have health problems, all too frequently they drop out of treatment or fail to follow some of the recommendations of their doctor (DiMatteo & DiNicola 1982; Rosenstock & Kirscht 1979).

Several other factors within the individual are also important. For one thing, people need to have certain cognitive resources, such as the knowledge and skills, to know what health-protective behaviours to adopt, to make plans for changing existing behaviour, and to overcome obstacles to change, such as dealing with having little time or nowhere to exercise. In addition, individuals need sufficient self-efficacy regarding their ability to carry out the change. Without self-efficacy, their motivation to change will be impaired. Also, being sick or taking certain drugs can affect people's moods and energy levels, which in turn may affect their cognitive resources and motivation.

Interpersonal factors

Many social factors influence people's likelihood of adopting health-protective behaviours. These factors include whether they have friends or family who model the behaviours and receive social support and encouragement for trying to change their lifestyles.

People living in a family system may encounter problems in their efforts to promote wellness. These problems often come about because the family is composed of individuals, each with his or her own motivations and habits. Suppose, for instance, that a member of a family wants to consume less cholesterol, but no-one else in the family is willing to stop eating high-cholesterol foods, such as butter, eggs and red meats. Or suppose the person has begun exercising three times a week, but this disrupts the daily routine of another family member. The interpersonal conflicts that circumstances like these can create in the family may undermine preventive efforts that the majority of family members support. Similar interpersonal conflicts can undermine prevention efforts among friends, classmates at school or university, and fellow employees at work.

Factors in the community

People are more likely to adopt health-protective behaviours if these behaviours are promoted or encouraged by community organisations, such as government agencies and the health care system.

Health professionals face unique problems in trying to promote wellness. One problem is that their knowledge regarding their patients' health-related behaviour comes mainly from the patients, whose reports may be distorted (Beach & Mayer 1990). Second, the knowledge professionals need to help people lead healthier lives is incomplete — they need more information to know when and how to intervene to change unhealthy behaviours effectively. Last, medical practitioners have traditionally focused their attention on treating, rather than preventing, illness and injury. But this focus has begun to change, and doctors are becoming increasingly interested in prevention (Radecki & Brunton 1992).

Finally, the larger community's role in preventing illness and injury is challenged by an enormous array of problems, such as having insufficient funds for public health projects and research, needing to adjust to and communicate with individuals of very different ages and sociocultural backgrounds, and providing health care for those who need it most. Also, Australian health insurance usually does not cover preventive medical services. Among the most difficult problems communities face is trying to balance public health and economic priorities. For example, in some industries, workers are subjected to potentially unhealthy conditions, such as toxic substances, which may also pose a threat to the community as a whole. Such was the case in the asbestos mining industry in Australia in the early 1950s. Thousands of workers were exposed to harmful doses of asbestos dust, later linked to lung cancer. At that time asbestos was also commonly found in most Australian homes, cars and workplaces, putting the community at risk. Asbestos is no longer used because of its link with lung cancer (Giles, Gill & Silver 1991).

What determines people's health-related behaviour?

If people were all like Mr Spock of the TV show *Star Trek*, the answer to the question of what determines people's health-related behaviour would be simple: facts and logic, for the most part. These people would have no conflicting motivations in adopting wellness lifestyles to become as healthy as they can be. In this section we examine the complex factors that affect health-related behaviour.

General factors in health-related behaviour

The 'average' person can describe healthy behaviours and generate a fairly complete list: 'Don't smoke,' 'Don't drink too much, and don't drive if you do,' 'Eat balanced meals, and don't overeat,' 'Get regular exercise,' and so on. But practising these acts is another matter. Several processes affect people's practice of health-related behaviour, and one factor is *heredity*. Genetic factors influence some health-related behaviours, and excessive alcohol use provides a good example. Twin studies and adoption studies have confirmed that heredity plays a role in the development of alcoholism (Ciraulo & Renner 1991; Schuckit 1985). But the exact nature of this role and the relative degree to which genetic and psychosocial factors are involved are unknown.

Learning

People also learn health-related behaviour, particularly by way of *operant conditioning*, whereby behaviour changes because of its consequences (Sarafino 1996). Three types of consequences are important.

- **Reinforcement.** When we do something that brings a pleasant, wanted or satisfying consequence, the tendency to repeat that behaviour is increased or *reinforced*. A child who receives something she wants, such as ten cents, for brushing her teeth at bedtime, is more likely to brush again the following night. The ten-cent coin in this example is a positive reinforcer partly because it was wanted and partly because it was *added* to the situation. But reinforcement can also occur in a different way. Suppose you have a headache, you take aspirin and the headache goes away. In this case, your headache was unpleasant and your behaviour of taking aspirin *removed* it from the situation. The headache is called a 'negative' reinforcer because it was *unwanted* or *unpleasant* and it was *taken away* from the situation. In both cases of reinforcement, the end result is a desirable state of affairs from the person's point of view.

- **Extinction**. When the consequences that maintain a behaviour are eliminated, the response tendency gradually weakens. The process or procedure of extinction exists only if no alternative maintaining stimuli (reinforcers) for the behaviour have supplemented or taken the place of the original consequences. In the above example of toothbrushing behaviour, if the money is no longer given, the child may continue brushing if another reinforcer exists, such as praise from her parents or her own satisfaction with the appearance of her teeth.
- **Punishment**. When we do something that brings an unpleasant consequence, the behaviour tends to be suppressed. A child who gets a scolding from his parents for playing with matches is less likely to repeat that behaviour, especially if his parents might see him. The influence of punishment on future behaviour depends on whether the person expects the behaviour will lead to punishment again. Take, for example, people who injure themselves (punishment) jogging — those who think they could be injured again are less likely to resume jogging than those who do not.

We have seen before that people can learn by observing the behaviour of others — a process called *modelling*. In this kind of learning, the consequences for the model affect the behaviour of the observer (Bandura 1965a, 1965b). If a teenager sees people receiving and enjoying social attention for smoking cigarettes, these people serve as powerful models and increase the likelihood that the teenager will begin smoking, too (Quine & Stephenson 1990). But if models receive punishment for smoking, such as being avoided by classmates at school, the teenager may be less likely to smoke. These social learning principles have formed the basis of peer-led interventions of the Australian National Campaign Against Drug Abuse (NCADA). During a videotaped discussion on smoking, students act as role models for their peer group by making a commitment to remain non-smokers (Miller, Hamilton & Flaherty 1992). In general, people are more likely to perform the behaviour they observe if the model is *similar to themselves* — that is, of the same sex, age or race — and is a *high-status person*, such as a physically attractive individual, movie star or well-known athlete (Bandura 1969, 1986). Advertisers of products such as alcoholic beverages know these facts and use them in their commercials.

Social, personality and emotional factors

Many health-related behaviours are affected by *social* factors (Baranowski & Nader 1985; Kirscht 1983). One of these factors is the degree of support or encouragement individuals receive from other people for health-related behaviours such as smoking and exercising. Friends and family promote or discourage a health-protective behaviour by providing consequences, such as praise or complaints, for it, modelling it and conveying a value for good health (Burg & Seeman 1994; Weiss, Larsen & Baker 1996). These processes probably also lead to gender differences, such as the greater physical activity of Australian boys than girls (Jobling & Cotterell 1990). Although this difference may be determined partly by biology, right from birth, many parents' perceptions of their newborn son or daughter seem to be biased (Rubin, Provenzano & Luria 1974). Even when male and female babies are matched for size, weight and general health, fathers and mothers rate sons as firmer, stronger, better coordinated and more alert. These perceptions tend to continue, and seem to affect how parents treat boys and girls, such as by playing more roughly and vigorously with their sons than with their daughters (Block 1983; Huston 1983). Very different patterns of encouragement may lead boys more than girls towards healthy physical activity.

Two other factors that are linked to health-related behaviour are the person's *personality* and *emotional state*, particularly stress. One personality characteristic associated with practising health-protective behaviour is conscientiousness. People who score high on a test of conscientiousness are more likely to take prescribed medications and follow the recommended schedule for getting mammograms than those who score low on this trait (Christensen & Smith 1995; Siegler, Feaganes & Rimer 1995). The role of emotions can be seen in the findings that people who experience high levels of stress consume more alcohol, cigarettes and coffee than those who experience less stress (Baer et al. 1987; Conway et al. 1981). If you ask people why they smoke, many will say, 'To relieve tension.' People cite coping with stress as their most important reason for continuing to smoke (Gottlieb 1983).

Perception and cognition

People's *perceived symptoms* of illness also influence their health-related behaviours. The way people react varies from ignoring the problem to seeking immediate professional care for it. Certainly when the symptoms are severe — as with excruciating pain, obvious bone fractures, profuse bleeding or very high fever — almost everyone who has access to a health care system will decide to use it (Rosenstock & Kirscht 1979). But how do symptoms affect behaviour when they are not so severe? People who are ill report performing more health-protective behaviour, such as limiting certain foods and not drinking, than people who are healthy (Harris & Guten 1979). Many people react to illness in reasonable ways, adjusting their health-related behaviours to meet the needs of their health problems.

Cognitive factors play an important role in the health-related behaviours people perform. As we saw earlier, people must have correct knowledge about the health issue and the ability to solve problems that arise when trying to implement healthy behaviour, such as how to fit an exercise routine into their busy schedules. People also make many judgements that have an impact on their health. They assess the general condition of their health: Is it good or bad? They also make decisions about other questions, such as: Should I cut back on the salt in my diet? Should I begin an exercise program? And, will I stick with these health behaviours if I start them?

But the answers are sometimes based on misconceptions, as when hypertensive patients overestimate their ability to know intuitively when their blood pressure is high (Baumann & Leventhal 1985; Meyer, Leventhal & Gutmann 1985; Pennebaker & Watson 1988). Hypertensive patients generally report that they can tell when their blood pressure is up, citing symptoms such as headache, warmth or flushing face, dizziness and nervousness. But research has shown that these symptoms are poor estimators of blood pressure. When hypertensive and normotensive individuals are asked to assess their blood pressure, their assessments correlate strongly with their symptoms and moods, but very modestly with their actual blood pressure. The potential harm in their erroneous beliefs is that patients often alter their medication-taking behaviour, and sometimes drop out of treatment, on the basis of their subjective assessments of their blood pressure. Clearly, beliefs are important determinants of health-related behaviour. The next section examines the role of beliefs in people's health.

The role of beliefs and intentions

Suppose your friend believed in *reflexology*, a 'healing' method that involves massaging specific areas of the feet to treat illnesses. The belief that underlies this method is that each area of the foot connects to a specific area of the body — the toes connect to the head, for instance, and the middle of the arch is linked to certain endocrine glands (Livermore 1991). For a patient with a head tumour, a reflexologist's treatment might include massaging the toes. Your friend would probably try ways to prevent and treat illness that are different from those most other people would try.

People's thinking may affect how they feel. Barbara Fradkin and Philip Firestone (1986) conducted an experiment with 25- to 40-year-old women to determine how women's beliefs about premenstrual symptoms affect how they feel during the premenstrual period. The subjects were assigned to three informational groups: a *control* group, which received no information, and two experimental groups. Both experimental groups received information on premenstrual tension by reading an article on the topic, seeing a videotape of a gynaecologist discussing it, and taking part in a discussion group. Each experimental group received information with a different orientation — either biological or psychological. For women in the *biological* group,

> the information strongly endorsed a physiological etiology for universal, unavoidable fluctuations in mood and concentration. Detailed information on hormonal and chemical changes was given, with the intent of enhancing symptom expectations. (p. 249)

In contrast, the women in the *psychological* group received information arguing that

> premenstrual tension was due not to biology but to negative societal myths. The information indicated that self-fulfilling expectations, cognitive bias, misattribution, and the negative labelling of ambiguous physiological arousal combine to create an illusion of premenstrual tension without biological basis. This information was designed to lower symptom expectancy. (p. 249)

The symptoms subjects reported in a questionnaire were equivalent for the three groups initially, and remained the same for the control and biological groups after receiving the information. But the women in the psychological group reported a dramatic decline in their symptoms during the month after getting the information. The information may have changed their beliefs and reduced the symptoms they experienced.

Researchers have also been interested in the role of health beliefs in people's practice and non-practice of health, illness and sick-role behaviours. The most widely researched and accepted theory of why people do and do not practise these behaviours is called the health belief model (Becker 1979; Becker et al. 1977; Becker & Rosenstock 1984; Rosenstock 1966). Let's see what this theory proposes.

The health belief model

According to the **health belief model**, the likelihood that individuals will take *preventive action* — that is, perform some health, illness or sick-role behaviour — depends directly on the outcome of two assessments they make. One of these evaluations pertains to the *threat* of a health problem, and the other weighs the *pros and cons* of taking the action. What factors go into these assessments?

Figure 6.1 shows that several factors influence a person's *perceived threat* of illness or injury. These factors include:

• *perceived seriousness* of the health problem. People consider how severe the organic and social consequences are likely to be if they develop the problem or leave it untreated. The more serious they believe its effects will be, the more likely they are to perceive it as a threat and take preventive action.

- *perceived susceptibility* to the health problem. People evaluate the likelihood of their developing the problem. The more vulnerable they perceive themselves to be, the more likely they are to perceive it as a threat and take action. For example, those persons with a family history of osteoporosis are more likely to make dietary changes to dairy products high in calcium because they perceive themselves as vulnerable to the disorder.
- *cues to action*. Being reminded or alerted about a potential health problem increases the likelihood of perceiving a threat and taking action. Cues to action can take many forms, from a public service announcement of an approaching category 5 cyclone to a reminder phone call for an upcoming dental appointment.

In addition, three other factors are implicated in people's perceived threat of illness or injury. These factors are: *demographic variables*, which include age, sex, race and ethnic background; *sociopsychological variables*, including personality traits, social class and social pressure; and *structural variables*, such as knowledge about or prior contact with the health problem. Thus, for example, elderly individuals whose close friends have developed severe cases of cancer or heart disease are more likely to perceive a personal threat of illness than young adults whose friends are in good health.

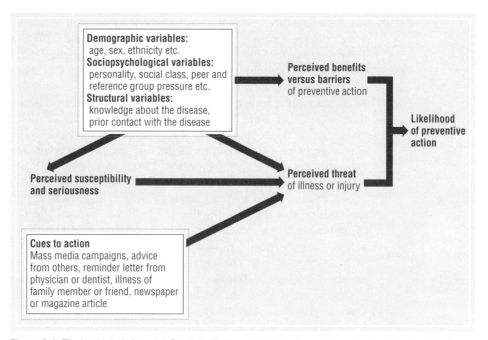

Figure 6.1 The health belief model. People's likelihood of taking preventive action is determined by two assessments they make: their perceived threat of the health problem and the sum of pros and cons they perceive in taking action. Many factors contribute to these assessments.

Source: Adapted from Becker & Rosenstock (1984, figure 2).

In weighing the pros and cons of taking preventive action, people arrive at a decision as to whether the *perceived benefits* — such as being healthier or reducing health risks — of the action exceed its *perceived barriers* or costs. The barriers involved in the health behaviour of getting a periodic physical checkup, for instance, might include financial considerations ('Can I afford the bills?'), psychosocial consequences ('People will think I'm getting old if I start having checkups', 'the doctor may find something serious.') and physical considerations ('My doctor's office is across town, and I don't have a car'). As these costs suggest, people's assessments are related to demographic, sociopsychological and structural variables. Thus, for example, individuals from lower economic classes are more likely than people from higher classes to feel that affording the bills or getting to the doctor's office is very difficult. The connection between these factors and the assessment process can be seen in figure 6.1. The outcome of weighing the benefits against the barriers is an assessed *sum*: the extent to which taking the action is more beneficial for them than not taking the action.

The perceived threat of illness or injury combines with the assessed sum of benefits and barriers to determine the likelihood of preventive action. For the health behaviour we have been considering, people who feel threatened by an illness and believe the benefits of having a periodic checkup outweigh the barriers are likely to go ahead with it, taking action for primary prevention. But people who do not feel threatened or assess that the barriers are too strong are unlikely to have the checkup. According to the health belief model, the processes we described for health behaviour also determine people's illness behaviour in secondary prevention, such as going to the doctor when sick or taking curative medication, and sick-role behaviour in tertiary prevention, such as sticking with a rehabilitation program following a stroke.

Has research generally supported the health belief model's explanation of health-related behaviour? The model has generated a great deal of research, most of which has upheld its predictions (Agars & McMurray 1993; Becker 1979; Becker & Rosenstock 1984; Cody & Lee 1990; Curry & Emmons 1994; Kirscht 1983; O'Brien & Lee 1990; Rosenstock & Kirscht 1979). Let's consider the case of primary prevention. Studies have found that compared with people who do *not* get vaccinations, have regular dental visits, get regular breast and cervical cancer tests, and take part in exercise programs, those who *do* are more likely to believe that they are susceptible to the related health problem, that developing the problem would have very serious effects and that the benefits of preventive action outweigh the barriers. Similar relationships have been found for secondary and tertiary prevention. That is, compared with people who do not take medication as directed and do not stick with prescribed dietary and weight loss programs, those who do are more likely to believe they are susceptible to a worsening of their health, that the resulting illness would have serious effects, and that the benefits of protective action exceed the costs. Furthermore, studies have shown that cues to action, such as reminders to perform breast self-examinations (Agars & McMurray 1993; Craun & Deffenbacher 1987), and demographic and sociopsychological variables (Becker 1979) influence people's practice of preventive measures.

Despite the success that the health belief model has had, it has some shortcomings. One shortcoming is that it does not account for health-related behaviours people perform habitually, such as toothbrushing — behaviours that probably originated and have continued without the person's considering health threats, benefits and costs. Sometimes people may recognise the benefits of a health behaviour but simply forget to perform it, or may not feel competent to perform the behaviour, as was found for breast self-examination (Clarke et al. 1991). Some behaviours, such as unsafe sexual practices, do not appear to be rationally governed but instead are highly dependent on domain-specific factors such as the meaning of love and relationships, or ability to communicate about sexual matters. Even when adolescents hold beliefs consistent with safe behaviour and are knowledgeable, these do not predict safe sexual practices (Moore & Rosenthal 1991; Rosenthal, Hall & Moore 1992). Another problem is that there is no standard way of measuring components of the health belief model, such as perceived susceptibility and seriousness. Different studies have used different questionnaires to measure the same factors, thereby making it difficult to compare the results across studies. These problems do not mean the theory is wrong, but that it is incomplete. We now turn to another theory that focuses on the role of people's beliefs on their practice of health-related behaviour.

The theory of reasoned action

Suppose you are having dinner at a restaurant with Dan, a friend who is overweight, and you wonder whether he will order dessert. How could you predict his behaviour? That's simple — you could ask what he *intends* to do. According to the **theory of reasoned action** (see figure 6.2), people decide their intention in advance of most voluntary behaviours, and intentions are the best predictors of what people will do (Ajzen & Fishbein 1980; Fishbein 1980, 1982).

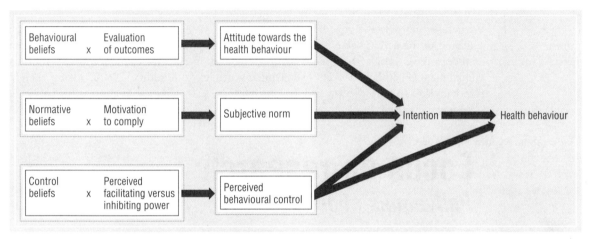

Figure 6.2 Theories of reasoned action and planned behaviour

Sources: Based on Ajzen & Madden (1986); Azjen & Fishbein (1980).

What determines people's intentions to perform a behaviour? The theory indicates that a person's intention is determined by two attitudes, which we'll illustrate with a girl named Ellie who has decided to start exercising.
- *Attitude regarding the behaviour.* This is simply a judgement of whether or not the behaviour is a good thing to do. Ellie's judgement that exercising 'would be a good thing for me to do' is based on her beliefs about (1) the likely *outcome* of the behaviour, such as, 'If I exercise, I will be healthier and more attractive,' and (2) whether the outcome would be *rewarding*, such as, 'Being healthy and good looking will be satisfying and pleasant.'
- *Attitude about a subjective norm.* This opinion reflects the impact of social pressure or influence regarding the behaviour's acceptability or appropriateness. Ellie's attitude is that exercising 'is a socially appropriate thing for me to do'. And this judgement is based on her beliefs regarding (1) *others' opinions* about the behaviour, such as, 'My family and friends think I should exercise,' and (2) her *motivation to comply* with those opinions, as in, 'I want to do what they want.'

The theory of reasoned action proposes that these two attitudes combine to produce an intention, which leads to performance of the behaviour. Suppose Ellie's attitudes were different because she had the following beliefs:
- 'Exercising is inconvenient and uncomfortable, and can cause injury.'
- 'I suffer enough inconvenience and discomfort in my life without having to exercise.'

- 'Nobody I know seems to want me to exercise, and they don't exercise either.'
- 'I value the opinion of my friends and family and want to be like them.'

With these beliefs, Ellie almost certainly would not generate an intention to exercise, and thus would not do so.

The theory of reasoned action was originally formulated to explain a wide variety of behaviours, particularly those of interest to social psychologists. Applying the theory to health psychology has been successful, and research has found support for aspects of the theory in explaining several health-related behaviours. A study by Richard Bagozzi (1981), for example, examined the attitudes, intentions and behaviour of adults regarding donating blood during an annual Red Cross blood drive. In the week prior to the drive, the subjects filled out a questionnaire that asked them to rate the strength of their intentions and their attitudes, such as the degree of pleasantness or unpleasantness, towards giving blood. The Red Cross provided information on whether they actually gave blood. As the theory predicts, attitudes about giving blood related to the actual behaviour through their impact on the subjects' intentions. Other studies have found that people's attitudes and intentions influence their smoking cigarettes (Fishbein, 1982), exercising (Wurtele & Maddux 1987), losing weight (Schifter & Ajzen 1985), and practising testicular self-examinations (Brubaker & Wickersham 1990).

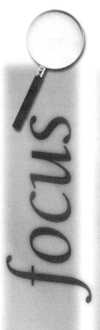

Focus on research
Pollyannas about health

'Compared with other people your age and sex, are your chances of getting lung cancer greater than, less than or about the same as theirs?' This is the kind of question Neil Weinstein has used in his research to examine how optimistically people view their future health. Through this research, he has shown that people tend to be Pollyannas — or *unrealistically optimistic* — about their health.

In one of these studies, Weinstein (1982) had students fill out a questionnaire with a long list of health problems. The subjects were asked to indicate their own risk for developing each problem, relative to other students of the same sex at the university, using a seven-point scale ranging from 'much below average' to 'much above average'. The results revealed that the students believed they were less likely than others to develop three-quarters of the health problems listed, including:

- alcoholism
- arteriosclerosis
- diabetes
- drug addiction
- heart attack
- lung cancer
- overweight by 18 kilos
- skin cancer
- venereal disease.

They believed they were more susceptible than other students to only one of the health problems, that of ulcers.

In a later study, Weinstein (1987) used very similar questions in a mailed survey with 18- to 65-year-old adults in the general population. These subjects also believed they were less likely to develop over three-quarters of the listed health problems, as compared with other adults of their own age and sex. Furthermore, they did not believe they were more susceptible than others for developing any of the problems. What is it about people's thinking that makes them so optimistic? This study found four cognitive factors that affect people's optimism.

(1) the belief that if the problem has not yet appeared, one is exempt from future risk; (2) the perception that the problem is preventable by individual action; (3) the perception that the hazard is infrequent; and (4) lack of experience with the hazard. If a hazard had such characteristics, people had a strong tendency to conclude that their own risk was less than the risk faced by their peers. (Weinstein 1987, p. 496)

Note that the thinking described by these factors is not very logical. For instance, the frequency with which a health problem occurs does not affect one's risk relative to that of others.

Do people remain optimistic about their health when they are sick or when a threat of illness is clear? Evidently not. Using a procedure similar to Weinstein's, a study found that university students who were waiting for treatment at the student health centre were less optimistic about their future health than were healthy students in a psychology course (Kulik & Mahler 1987b). Another study was conducted with students in Poland, just after the radioactive cloud reached their community from the explosion of the atomic power plant at Chernobyl in the Soviet Union (Dolinski, Gromski & Zawisza 1987). Although these subjects believed they were less likely than others to have a heart attack or be injured in an accident, they believed they were equally likely to develop cancer and *more* likely than others to suffer illness effects of the radiation over the next several years. Thus, in the face of a real threat, they showed 'unrealistic pessimism' regarding their health.

Other studies have revealed similar biases in children and teenagers, indicating that feelings of invulnerability are not a unique feature of adolescence (Cohn et al. 1995; Whalen et al. 1994). Clearly, people's beliefs play a powerful role in their perceptions of health risks, and their beliefs are not always logical. Studies of optimistic and pessimistic beliefs are important because research has shown that people who practise health-protective behaviours tend to feel susceptible to associated health problems (Becker & Rosenstock 1984).

What shortcomings does the theory of reasoned action have? One problem is that intentions and behaviour are only moderately related — people do not always do what they plan (or *claim* they plan) to do. When intentions are measured closer to the behaviour in question, the relationship between the two is increased (Boldero, Moore & Rosenthal 1992). Individuals may not always act on their intentions because some behaviours, such as using condoms, are not under their control, but dependent on the partner's attitudes and commitment to safer sex. People's attitudes predict some health-related behaviours, such as alcohol use, but not others, such as smoking, drink driving or safe sexual behaviour (Ross & McLaws 1992; Stacy, Bentler & Flay 1994). Furthermore, the extent to which attitudes and norms influence intentions appears to depend on specific groups and contexts (Gallois et al. 1994). Kippax and Crawford (1993) have criticised the theory of reasoned action for its failure to predict safe sexual behaviour. They argue that the theory needs to take into account the effect of culturally shared meanings and discourses regarding sexual behaviour, and the collective practice of different groups. Another problem is that the theory is incomplete; it does not take into account, for example, the important role of people's prior experience with the behaviour. Studies have found that people's history of performing a health-related behaviour, such as exercising, using a condom or using alcohol or drugs, is a strong predictor of their future practice of that behaviour (Bentler & Speckart 1979;

Gallois et al. 1994; Godin et al. 1987; Kashima, Gallois & McCamish 1992). Thus, for example, compared with adults who have engaged in little exercise in the past, those who have exercised regularly are much more likely to carry out their promises to exercise in the future.

The health belief model and the theory of reasoned action each provide valid explanations for parts of the process that determines people's practice of health-related behaviour. At their core, both theories assume people weigh perceived benefits and costs and behave according to the outcome of their analysis. But neither approach is sufficient and both have limitations (Janis 1984; Kirscht 1983; Weinstein 1988). One weakness in these theories is that they assume people think about risks in a detailed fashion, knowing what diseases are associated with different behaviours and estimating the likelihood of becoming seriously ill. In reality, people may modify their lifestyles, such as reducing coffee consumption, for very vague reasons, such as, 'My doctor says coffee is bad for you.'

Beliefs in personal control

In chapter 4 we examined how a sense of personal control can modify the stress people experience. In this section, we will consider how people's health-related behaviour relates to their beliefs in two aspects of personal control: *locus of control* and *self-efficacy*.

You might expect that people whose health locus of control is strongly *internal* — as measured by a locus of control scale — would tend to practise behaviours that prevent illness and promote their health. Because these individuals believe they can influence their health, they should practise healthier behaviour than those who score high on external control. This seems to be so. Compared with people who score high on external control beliefs, those who score high on internal control tend to perform more health-protective behaviours, such as getting physical examinations and dieting for health reasons (Seeman & Seeman 1983). They also tend to be more successful in reducing cigarette smoking and seek out more information on some health issues, such as high blood pressure (Strickland 1978; Wallston & Wallston 1982). A meta-analysis has revealed that these relationships are fairly strong, particularly for individuals from the middle and upper social classes (Reisch, Wiehl & Tinsley 1994). Why is locus of control not more strongly associated with health-protective behaviour? One reason is that locus of control is just one of many factors that influence the practice of healthy behaviour. Another reason is that the belief in internal control appears to have a greater impact on the behaviour of people who place a high value on their health than on that of those who do not (Lau, Hartman & Ware 1986).

In some cases, performing a healthy behaviour is hard to do — for instance, it may be strenuous or complicated. Therefore, people's belief that they can succeed at something they want to do — or self-efficacy — may be an important determinant of whether they choose to practise specific behaviours (Bandura 1986). Individuals acquire a sense of efficacy through their own successes and failures, observations of others' experiences and assessments of their abilities that other people communicate. When deciding to practise a health-protective behaviour, people appraise their efficacy on the basis of the effort required, complexity of the task and other aspects of the situation, such as whether they are likely to receive help from other people (Schunk & Carbonari 1984).

Research has found that self-efficacy does influence people's health, illness and sick-role behaviour. Cigarette smokers who believe they are incapable of kicking the habit typically don't try, but smokers who believe they can succeed in quitting often break the habit (DiClemente, Prochaska & Gilbertini 1985; Stuart, Borland & McMurray 1994). Similarly, individuals who believe they can succeed in losing weight are more likely to try and to succeed than those who do not (Schifter & Ajzen 1985). Moreover, patients with chronic respiratory illnesses who believe they can perform a prescribed program of physical exercise, such as walking various distances, are more likely to adhere to the program than those who have less self-efficacy (Kaplan, Atkins & Reinsch 1984).

The theory of planned behaviour

The theory of reasoned action was revised by Ajzen and Madden in 1986 to include the notion of perceived behavioural control. The revised theory was called the **theory of planned behaviour**, and is presented in figure 6.2. The theory of planned behaviour is similar to the theory of reasoned action in all respects except for the addition of the measure of perceived control, which is directly related to intentions and actual behaviour. The concept of behavioural control was introduced to account for behavioural intentions, not always predicting actual behaviour. It was argued that intentions would predict behaviour when the behaviour is under the control of the individual. However, not all behaviour is directly under the control of the person. This is most often the case in social contexts that involve communication and cooperation between partners. Although the person may intend to act in a way that is consistent with their behavioural intentions, the actual behaviour may be very different.

Let's apply the theory of planned behaviour to an example. If a person intends to lose weight, the likelihood that he or she will make the desired changes to eating behaviour depends not only on their attitude to dieting, and having the belief that losing weight would be desirable (i.e. having a positive attitude), but also on the motivation to comply with pressure from others to lose weight. However, intentions to lose weight and making the necessary dietary changes depend on the person's perception that dieting is under their personal control, and a belief that he or she can succeed in losing weight.

Applications of the theory of reasoned action and planned behaviour

Australian researchers at the University of Queensland (Deborah Terry and associates) have been instrumental in suggesting extensions to both the theory of reasoned action and the theory of planned behaviour, in relation to predicting safer sexual behaviour (Terry, Gallois & McCamish 1993). Their suggestions for proposed changes are based on extensive studies. One of the proposed changes to the theory relates to the normative component (White, Terry & Hogg 1994). In the current theories, the **subjective norm** refers to an individual's motivation to comply with perceived pressure from significant others to perform a behaviour, and is thought to influence behavioural intentions. The normative influence of membership in a group may exert more subtle effects on behavioural intentions than perceived pressure to perform a behaviour. Because self-concept and social identity derive from group membership, perceptions that significant others consider the behaviour desirable (group attitude), and perform the behaviour themselves (behavioural norm), may have a substantial impact on behavioural intentions. The behavioural norm and group attitude can be thought of as the **group norm**, or the extent to which behaviour is judged to be normatively appropriate. White, Terry and Hogg (1994) found support for the group norm to predict intentions to practise safer sex behaviours, such as using a condom and discussing using a condom with a new partner. These findings have implications for intervention programs as they emphasise the need to assess beliefs about condom use and facilitate a normative climate that is supportive of safer sex.

The other proposed change to the two theories has been in regard to the control component. The notion of perceived behavioural control was incorporated into the theory of planned behaviour (Ajzen & Madden 1986) to account for situations where behaviour is not completely under the person's control, and was proposed to exert an effect on both intentions and behaviour (see figure 6.2). Perceived behavioural control referred to both the person's perception of having control over performing the behaviour, and their appraisal of ability to perform the behaviour (Ajzen 1991), otherwise known as *self-efficacy*.

White, Terry and Hogg (1994) have found that perceived behavioural control is conceptually different from self-efficacy. Their research has also demonstrated different effects of perceived behavioural control and self-efficacy on both behavioural intentions and actual behaviour. Intentions were predicted more by self-efficacy than by perceived behavioural control, although the latter predicted the specific behaviour of discussing use of condoms. Further support for the conceptual difference between perceived behavioural control and self-efficacy has been reported by Terry and O'Leary (1995) for other health behaviours such as exercise.

Research on the effects of self-efficacy and control has implications for educational programs on safer sexual behaviour and AIDS prevention. Such programs should foster in participants beliefs in their ability to perform a behaviour. Such beliefs can be formed through role modelling and skill training. For example, developing assertiveness skills to negotiate safer sex with a partner serves to increase levels of self-efficacy necessary to act on behavioural intentions. Educational strategies for increasing perceived behavioural control (e.g. purchasing and carrying condoms) in sexual relationships can also be incorporated in intervention programs.

A further refinement to the theory of planned behaviour concerns the distinction between generalised control beliefs (internality/externality) and situation-specific measures of perceived behavioural control. Terry, Galligan and Conway (1993) found that generalised control beliefs moderated the effects of intentions on behaviour, rather than having a direct impact on intentions or behaviour. That is, subjects with internal control beliefs were more likely than those with external control beliefs to adhere to specific behavioural intentions such as engaging in an exclusive sexual relationship, or asking partners about their sexual and drug use history.

The research conducted by Terry and associates has helped to extend further the predictive ability of the theories of reasoned action (TRA) and planned behaviour, in regard to safer sexual behaviour. As a result of this research and refinements to the theories, interventions have been designed to promote safer practices and help stop the spread of AIDS in Australia. A comprehensive description of the TRA-based intervention can be found in McCamish et al. (1993).

The stages of change model

Why do some people persist with unhealthy behaviours? Even heart attack patients have been known not to follow doctors' recommendations to lose weight and exercise (Byrne 1987). Although there may be many reasons for why individuals do not change their risk behaviour, one reason may be that they are simply not 'ready'. Readiness to change is the main focus of a theory called the **stages of change model** (also called the *transtheoretical model* because it includes factors described in other theories) (DiClemente et al. 1991; Prochaska & DiClemente 1984; Prochaska, DiClemente & Norcross 1992). This descriptive model outlines five *stages* of intentional behaviour change:

1. *Precontemplation.* People in this stage are not considering changing, at least during the next several months or so. These people may have never thought about changing or decided against it.
2. *Contemplation.* During this stage, people are aware a problem exists and are seriously considering changing to a healthier behaviour within the next several months. But they are not yet ready to make a commitment to take action.
3. *Preparation.* At this stage, individuals are ready to try to change and plan to pursue a behavioural goal, such as stopping smoking, in the next month. They may have tried to reach that goal in the past year without being fully successful. For instance, these people might have reduced their smoking by half, but did not yet quit completely.
4. *Action.* This stage spans a period of time, usually six months, from the start of people's successful and active efforts to change a behaviour.
5. *Maintenance.* People in this stage work to maintain the successful behavioural changes they achieved. Although this stage can last indefinitely, researchers often define its length as, say, six months, for follow-up assessment.

The stages of change model provides a useful framework for classifying individuals' current actions and their future intentions. For example, an Australian survey of physical activity conducted by the National Heart Foundation indicated that 13 per cent of the public could be classified as belonging to the precontemplation stage of change, 10 per cent to the contemplation stage, 16 per cent were in preparation for change, 23 per cent were in the action stage, and 38 per cent were in the maintenance stage (Booth et al. 1993). Stage of exercise adoption has been found to be related to the practice of other health behaviours. Costakis, Dunnagan & Haynes (1999) found that smokers are more likely to be in the precontemplation stage for exercise. Those in contemplation, preparation, action and maintenance are more likely to use seatbelts, while those in the maintenance stage of exercise are more likely to use stress reduction techniques.

According to the stages of change model, people who are currently in one stage show different psychosocial characteristics from people in other stages. For instance, progress along the stages of change for physical activity in the Booth et al. (1993) study increased with higher levels of education and decreased with age. People in the precontemplation stage regarding an unhealthy behaviour, such as eating a high-cholesterol diet, are likely to have less self-efficacy and see more barriers than benefits for changing that behaviour than people in the more advanced stages. Efforts of their own or of others to change the behaviour are not likely to succeed until these individuals advance through the stages. Is it possible to help them advance? One of the values of the stages of change model is that it enables an intervention to *match* useful strategies with important characteristics of people at each stage to help them advance to the next stage (Oldenburg 1994; Patrick et al. 1994; Perz, DiClemente & Carbonari 1996; Prochaska, DiClemente & Norcross 1992; Prochaska, Johnson & Lee 1998). Suppose you are a nurse providing care to an elderly woman with heart disease who doesn't exercise, even though her doctor advised her to do so. If she is at the precontemplation stage, you might talk with her about why exercise would help her physically, for instance, and have her generate ways this would improve her general functioning. The goal at this point is just to get the person to consider changing the behaviour. If she is at the contemplation stage, the goal might be to help her decide to change soon. Discussing the benefits and barriers she perceives in exercising, finding ways to overcome barriers, and showing her that she can do appropriate physical activities would help. The stages of change model is a relatively new theory, but studies have already confirmed its predictions regarding quitting smoking (DiClemente et al. 1991), getting breast cancer testing (Rakowski et al. 1992), and using safer sex practices (Bowen & Trotter 1995).

In the preceding sections, we have examined many aspects of people's beliefs and intentions that appear to influence their health-related behaviour. These aspects include people's perceived susceptibility to illness, perceived barriers and benefits to changing unhealthy behaviour, ideas about what behaviours are socially acceptable and encouraged by family and friends, self-efficacy beliefs and readiness to change. But these factors do not adequately account for *irrational* decisions people often make about their health, so that

> many important aspects of patients' decisions fall between the cracks. For example, the model does not provide an adequate explanation for the widespread tendency of patients who have painful heart attacks to delay obtaining medical aid... Typically, when the afflicted person thinks of the possibility that it might be a heart attack, he or she assumes that 'it couldn't be happening to me.' The patients' delay of treatment is not attributable to unavailability of medical aid or transportation delays; approximately 75% of the delay time elapses before a patient decides to contact a physician... The important point is that the health belief model, like other models of rational choice, fails to specify under what conditions people will give priority to avoiding subjective discomfort at the cost of endangering their lives, and under what conditions they will make a more rational decision. (Janis 1984, pp. 331–2)

In the next section we examine how non-rational processes, such as illogical thinking and stress, affect people's likelihood of taking preventive action.

The role of non-rational processes

Although body builders generally know that using anabolic steroids can harm their health, some may try to justify using these substances to build muscles with statements like, 'Experts have told us almost everything is bad for us and later found out lots of things aren't.' Why are the decisions people make regarding health-related behaviour not more rational? Non-rational motivational and emotional factors can influence cognitive processes.

Motivational factors in beliefs

Research findings indicate that people's desires and preferences influence the judgements they make of the validity and utility of new information, through a process called **motivated reasoning** (Kunda 1990). In one form of motivated reasoning, individuals who prefer to reach a particular conclusion, such as to continue to eat fatty foods or smoke cigarettes, tend to search for reasons to accept supportive information and discount disconfirming information. What's more, the reasons they choose seem 'reasonable' to them, even if the logic is actually faulty. And so, a study found that people who use defence mechanisms a lot to cope with stressful information are more likely than other individuals to deny that they are at risk for AIDS, especially if their risk of infection is high (Gladis et al. 1992). It may be that the high threat motivates their use of denial. Similarly, people who smoke cigarettes give lower ratings of risk than non-smokers do when asked to rate their own risk of developing smoking-related diseases, such as lung cancer (Lee 1989; McCoy et al. 1992). Other research has found that beliefs like these are very resistant to change (Kreuter & Strecher 1995; Weinstein & Klein 1995).

Emotional factors in beliefs

Stress also affects the cognitive processes people use in making decisions. **Conflict theory** presents a model to account for both rational and irrational decision making, and stress is an important factor in this model (Janis 1984; Janis & Mann 1977). The model describes the cognitive sequence by which people make important decisions, including health-related decisions. According to conflict theory, the cognitive sequence a person uses in arriving at a stable decision starts when an event challenges the individual's current course of action or lifestyle. The challenge can be either a *threat*, such as a symptom of illness or a news story about the dangers of smoking, or an *opportunity*, such as the chance to join a free program at work to quit smoking. The first step in the cognitive sequence involves *appraising the challenge*, basically answering the question, 'Are the risks serious if I don't change?' If the judgement is 'no', the behaviour stays the same and the decision-making process ends; but if the answer is 'yes', the process continues — for instance with a survey of alternatives for dealing with the challenge.

Conflict theory proposes that people experience stress with all major decisions, particularly those relating to health, because of conflicts about what to do. According to Irving Janis, these individuals may 'realise that whichever course of action or inaction they choose could lead to serious material or social losses, such as becoming physically incapacitated or losing the esteem of loved ones' (Janis 1984, p. 335). Since people decide whether or not to perform many health-related behaviours, the way they cope with stress may play an important role in health, illness and sick-role behaviour.

What determines how effectively individuals deal with health-related decisions? Conflict theory indicates that people's coping with decisional conflict depends on their perceptions of the presence or absence of three factors: *risks*, *hope* and *adequate time*. Different combinations of these three factors produce different coping patterns, two of which are:

- *hypervigilance*. People sometimes see serious risks in their current behaviour *and* those alternatives they have considered. If they believe they may still find a better solution *but* think they are fast running out of time, they experience high stress. Under these circumstances, people tend to search frantically for a solution — and may choose an alternative hastily, especially if it promises immediate relief.
- *vigilance*. People who perceive serious risks in all possibilities they have considered *but* believe they may find a better alternative and have the time to search experience only moderate levels of stress. Under these conditions, people tend to search thoroughly and make rational choices.

According to the theory, vigilant coping is the only consistently adaptive pattern for decision making. When the challenge consists of a doctor's warning or obvious symptoms of illness, other coping patterns can be highly maladaptive. For example, hypervigilance involves a harried decision-making process in which the person may overlook the full range of consequences and choose impulsively. In other coping patterns, people may try to deny the threat or decide on a course of action without carefully examining the situation. Although the conflict theory model was developed on the basis of an existing and extensive body of research, studies have not yet directly tested its predictions to the point that its strengths and weaknesses are clear. Still, there is little question that the impact of stress is an important determinant of preventive action, particularly in people's illness and sick-role behaviour.

We have examined how each of many different psychological and social factors can affect people's health-protective behaviour. But these factors constitute only part of the picture. A full understanding of this issue requires a detailed description of all relevant biopsychosocial factors and the way they interact with one another, using a *systems* approach, which we discussed in chapter 1. We next examine the relationships that exist between individuals' lifestyles and three factors — age, sex and sociocultural background.

Developmental, gender and sociocultural factors in health

It comes as no surprise that people's health changes across the life span, that women and men have some differences in health risks and needs, and that variations in preventive behaviour occur between individuals of different social classes and ethnic backgrounds. What are some of these changes and differences, and why do they exist? Let's examine these health issues, starting with the role of development.

Development and health-related behaviour

The biological, psychological and social factors that affect people's health change throughout the life span, causing individuals to face different health risks and problems as they develop. For instance, adolescents and young adults are at relatively high risk for injury from motor vehicle accidents, but older adults are at relatively high risk for hypertension and heart disease. As a result, people's preventive needs and goals change with age. Figure 6.3 presents main preventive goals for each period in the life span. During the beginning of the life span, and sometimes towards the end, the individual may lack the ability to take preventive action, and other people assume that responsibility.

During gestation and infancy

In 1996 about 22.8 per 10 000 Australian babies were born with birth defects resulting from chromosomal abnormalities (AIHW 2000). Chromosomal abnormalities accounted for 13 per cent of all congenital malformations, the remainder (e.g. spina bifida, congenital heart disease) being attributed to genetic factors. Harmful factors in the foetal environment may also contribute to birth abnormalities. Birth defects range from relatively minimal physical and mental abnormalities to gross deformities; some are not apparent until months or years later, and some are fatal. The Human Genome Project, an international project concerned with identifying human genes and their functions, may help to reduce the numbers of babies born with defects in the future, through improved diagnostic testing for genetic disorders, and new treatments for such disorders (AIHW 2000; Trent 1999).

For the most part, the mother can control the foetal environment through her behaviour. Early in gestation, a *placenta* and *umbilical cord* develop and begin to transmit substances to the foetus from the mother's bloodstream. These substances typically consist mostly of nourishment, but they can also include hazardous micro-organisms and chemicals that happen to be in her blood. We will consider three main hazards. First, the mother may be malnourished, because of inadequate food supplies or knowledge of nutritional needs. Babies born to malnourished mothers tend to have low birth weights, poorly developed immune and central nervous systems, and a high risk of mortality in the first weeks after birth (Chandra 1991; Huffman & del Carmen 1990; Pilliteri 1981; Smart 1991).

Figure 6.3 Health goals over the life span

Health goals of gestation and infancy
- to provide the mother with a healthy, full-term pregnancy and rapid recovery after a normal delivery
- to facilitate the live birth of a normal baby, free of congenital or developmental damage
- to help both mother and father achieve the knowledge and capacity to provide for the physical, emotional, and social needs of the baby
- to establish immunity against specified infectious diseases
- to detect and prevent certain other diseases and problems before irreparable damage occurs.

Health goals of childhood and adolescence
- to facilitate the child's optimal physical, emotional and social growth and development
- to establish healthy behavioural patterns (in children) for nutrition, exercise, study, recreation and family life, as a foundation for a healthy lifetime lifestyle
- to reinforce healthy behaviour patterns (in adolescents), and discourage negative ones, in physical fitness, nutrition, exercise, study, work, recreation, sex, individual relations, driving, smoking, alcohol and drugs.

Health goals of adulthood
- to prolong the period of maximum physical energy and to develop full mental, emotional and social potential
- to anticipate and guard against the onset of chronic disease through good health habits and early detection and treatment where effective
- to detect as early as possible any of the major chronic diseases, including hypertension, heart disease, diabetes and cancer, as well as vision, hearing, and dental impairments

Health goals in old age
- to minimise handicapping and discomfort from the onset of chronic conditions
- to prepare in advance for retirement
- to prolong the period of effective activity and ability to live independently, and avoid institutionalisation so far as possible
- when illness is terminal, to assure as little physical and mental stress as possible and to provide emotional support to patient and family.

Source: Based on Breslow & Somers (1977).

Second, certain infections the mother may contract during pregnancy can also attack her gestating baby, sometimes causing permanent injury or death (LaBarba 1984; Moore 1983). For example, infection with *rubella* (German measles) in the first several weeks of pregnancy may cause the baby to die or be severely malformed, and infection with *toxoplasmosis* can cause brain damage or death. Pregnant women can protect the foetus from rubella through vaccination and from toxoplasmosis by avoiding contact with major sources of infection (cats, cat litter and undercooked meats).

Third, various substances the mother uses may enter her bloodstream and harm the baby (Cook, Petersen & Moore 1990; LaBarba 1984). Babies exposed prenatally to addictive drugs, such as cocaine and heroin, are far more likely than others to die in infancy or be born with very low weights or malformations, such as of the heart (Lindenberg et al. 1991; MDBDF 1993). Also, cigarette smoke exposure from the mother's smoking or from her environment — for instance if the father smokes — is associated with low birth weight and other health problems in babies (DiFranza & Lew 1995; Eliopoulos et al. 1994; Martinez, Wright & Taussig 1994). And drinking alcohol excessively has been linked to the birth of babies with *foetal alcohol syndrome*, which has several symptoms: (1) low birth weight and retarded subsequent growth, (2) subnormal intelligence and (3) certain facial characteristics, such as small eye openings (Burns & Arnold 1990; NIAAA 1993). Ideally, expectant mothers should use *none* of these substances. Health education for pregnant women can help, such as by getting those who smoke to quit (Windsor et al. 1993).

Birth catapults the newborn into a new world, where risks continue. The rate of infant mortality in Australia is lower than in the United States or the United Kingdom, having declined since 1960 from 19.5 to 3 per 1000 live births for the first year of life (AIHW 1996; AIHW 2000). Out of these, more than half die within the first week of life. The infant mortality rate for indigenous babies is about three times higher than for other babies (Cunningham & Paradies 2000). This high mortality rate among indigenous infants is more likely to be a function of socioeconomic status than of race.

In early infancy, the baby's immunity to disease depends largely on the white blood cells and antibodies passed on by the mother prenatally and in her milk if she breast-feeds (Moore 1983). Because of the immunity it gives to the baby, breast milk is sometimes called 'nature's vaccine'. Parents should arrange for the baby to begin a vaccination program early in infancy for such diseases as diphtheria, whooping cough and polio.

Childhood and adolescence

In the second year of life, toddlers are walking and beginning to 'get into everything'. Although children's advances in motor development are important, they place children at increasing health risk for accidents around the house, such as with sharp objects and chemicals, and outdoors, such as with swimming pools, cars and skateboards. Today accidental injury is the leading cause of death during childhood and adolescence (AIHW 1996). Parents, teachers and other caregivers can reduce the likelihood of injury by teaching children safety behaviours, supervising them when possible, and decreasing their access to dangerous situations, such as by keeping chemicals and sharp kitchen utensils or garden tools out of reach.

The role of cognitive processes in the practice of health-related behaviour has important implications here, since cognitive abilities are immature in early childhood and become increasingly sophisticated as children get older. With these advances, children are more able to engage in health-protective behaviour and to assume responsibility for promoting their own health and safety (Burbach & Peterson 1986; Maddux et al. 1986). As part of this ability, children need to understand the relationship between behaviour and health. This understanding develops gradually, often progressing through the six stages outlined in figure 6.4. As individuals enter adolescence, they become more aware of the complex interaction of internal and external factors in health, illness and recovery (La Greca & Stone 1985). But the amount of knowledge children have about one illness, such as cancer, is not related to the amount they know about other illnesses, such as colds or AIDS (Sigelman et al. 1993). Caregivers and health professionals need to adjust their explanations and expectations for preventive action in light of young children's cognitive limitations and the progress they make as they get older (Burbach & Peterson 1986).

Adolescence is a particularly critical time in the development of preventive behaviour. Although teenagers have the cognitive ability to make the logical decisions leading to healthy behaviour, they face many temptations and forces — especially peer pressure — that lead them in other directions (Brunswick & Merzel 1986; Jessor 1984; La Greca & Stone 1985). This is the time when they stand the greatest chance of starting to smoke, drink, use drugs and have sexual relations. Teenagers also learn to drive, and too often combine this new skill with drinking and using drugs. The large majority of deaths in adolescence result from accidents and violence. Death rates for motor vehicle accidents are highest for males aged 15 to 24 years. In 1998 the accident death rate for male adolescents was 27 per 100 000 compared with 9.4 for the total population. Although death rates for accidents are declining among adolescents, suicide has increased by 40 per cent over the last 20 years, and is four times higher among males than among females (AIHW 2000).

Behaviours acquired during adolescence, such as smoking, drinking and driving, involve substantial health risks, which teenagers are highly susceptible to taking. In performing these behaviours, the immediate experience and impressing peers seem to be more important to adolescents than the possible long-term consequences.

Figure 6.4 Six stages in children's understanding of the relationship between health and behaviour

1. *Phenomenism.* In children's earliest understanding of the relationship between health and behaviour, they tend to define an illness in terms of a single symptom they associate with it. The cause they cite for the illness is likely to be remote; for example, a three-year-old might say the sun causes heart attacks.

2. *Contagion.* At this stage, children continue to describe an illness in terms of a single symptom, but they know a little more about its cause. They attribute a person's sickness to the proximity of a person or object that is its source — without understanding how nearness is important. If a child at this stage says that 'you get measles from people', and you ask how, he or she might simply answer, 'When you walk near them.'

3. *Contamination.* Children at this stage define an illness with multiple symptoms and understand still more about its cause. Most children progress this far by seven years of age. They state that contact with dirt or germs causes illness, and they recognise that behaviour can play a role, saying that people catch colds from 'taking your jacket off outside'. But they also say that just doing something 'bad' can cause illness.

4. *Internalisation.* At this stage, children conceptualise illness in terms of a problem inside the body. They also know that the problem can result from contaminants getting inside when the person swallows or inhales. And they realise the direct effect that behaviour can have, such as that people get heart attacks 'from lifting heavy stuff and working too hard'. Children now view themselves as being able to prevent illness through proper care.

5. *Physiological.* By about 11 years of age, most children can define illness in terms of specific body organs, giving details of how internal functions break down and citing multiple physical causes. They might say, for example, 'Cancer is when cells grow too fast. It happens because of air pollution or chemicals.'

6. *Psychophysiological.* In the last stage, children realise that illness can result from both physiological and psychological sources. They may say, for instance, that people get headaches 'from problems and aggravation'.

Source: Based on Bibace & Walsh (1979).

Adulthood and ageing

When people reach adulthood, they become less likely than they were in adolescence to adopt new behavioural risks to their health. In general, older adults are more likely than younger ones to engage in various health behaviours, such as eating healthy diets and getting medical checkups (Belloc & Breslow 1972; Leventhal, Prohaska & Hirschman 1985).

Do these age-related improvements in health behaviour indicate that adults become more concerned about health habits as they get older? Probably, but this is not clear for two reasons. First, developmental research on the practice of health behaviour has generally used cross-sectional methods. Age-related increases in the percentages of individuals who practise healthy behaviours may simply reflect an increased rate of survival among people who engage in these habits. Second, older and younger adults have very similar beliefs regarding the effectiveness of these behaviours in preventing such chronic illnesses as high blood pressure, heart attacks and cancer (Leventhal, Prohaska & Hirschman 1985). Older adults are likely to perceive themselves as more vulnerable to these illnesses than younger adults, and may engage in preventive acts for that reason.

Old age is not what it used to be. Older people, as a group, are living longer and are in better financial and physical condition than in the past (Horn & Meer 1987; Kolata 1996). One health behaviour that generally declines as adults get older is regular substantial exercise (Booth et al. 1993; Leventhal, Prohaska & Hirschman 1985). Many elderly people avoid physical exercise because they tend to exaggerate the danger that exertion poses to their health, underestimate their physical capabilities and feel embarrassed by their performance of these activities (Woods & Birren 1984).

Gender and health-related behaviour

Life expectancy for an Australian male born in 1998 is 75.9 years, while a female infant would be expected to live to 81.5 years. The expected life span for a female is 5.6 years longer than for a male. For those who survive to 65 years of age, a woman's remaining life expectancy is 3.7 years longer than a man's (AIHW 2000). Why is this so? The answer involves both biological and behavioural factors (Cataldo et al. 1986; Greenglass & Noguchi 1996; Reddy, Fleming & Adesso 1992; Verbrugge 1985). Some of these factors are outlined below.

- Physiological reactivity, such as blood pressure and catecholamine release, when under stress is greater in men than women, which may make men more likely to develop cardiovascular disease.
- Males have shorter life expectancies in most developed countries of the world, and boys have higher death rates than girls even in infancy. These relationships suggest that biological factors play a role in gender differences in mortality.
- Behavioural factors are implicated in the fact that boys have far higher rates of injury than girls — such as from drowning or bicycling and pedestrian traffic accidents.
- In adolescence and adulthood, males have far higher rates of injury and death from motor vehicle accidents than females do.
- Men smoke more and drink more than women do, thereby making men more susceptible to cardiovascular and respiratory diseases, some forms of cancer and cirrhosis of the liver.
- It may be that men's jobs and leisure activities pose greater health hazards than women's, but little or no research has been done on these issues.

One of the few behavioural advantages men have is that they get more strenuous exercise than women do. The practice of most other health-related behaviours is similar for men and women.

Women's longer lives do not mean that they have fewer health problems than men. Actually, the opposite is true (Reddy, Fleming & Adesso 1992; Verbrugge 1985). Women have much higher rates of acute illnesses, such as respiratory and digestive ailments, and non-fatal chronic diseases, such as varicose veins, arthritis, anaemia and headache. They also use medical drugs and services much more than men do, even when pregnancy and other reproductive conditions are not counted.

Sociocultural factors and health-related behaviour

People seem to be increasingly health conscious today, at least in some cultures. Have people's health behaviours been improving in Australia and other countries? A survey on improvements in health behaviours in the United States and Europe across two years found that the percentage of people who reported having increased exercising and decreased alcohol and red meat intake was much greater among Americans than Britons, whose percentage was greater than that of the French (Retchin et al. 1992). People's health behaviours are improving in industrialised nations, but the rates vary across cultures.

Cultural differences also exist within nations. Most Australians feel they are in pretty good health — for instance, a recent national health survey of males and females of all ages and backgrounds found that 85 per cent claimed to be in 'good' to 'excellent' health (ABS 1997a). But this was not true for all segments of the population. Compared with the population as a whole, people were much more likely to rate their health as 'fair' or 'poor' if they were over 45 years of age, from lower income households, unemployed or had migrated to Australia more than five years ago. As it turns out, these lower assessments reflect real health problems among the individuals of these groups. In this section, we examine how health and health-related behaviour are linked to sociocultural factors.

Social class and minority group background

The concept of *social class*, or *socioeconomic status*, describes differences in people's resources, prestige and power within a society (Filsinger 1987; Fitzpatrick & Scambler 1984). These differences are reflected in three main characteristics: income, occupational prestige and education. The lowest social classes in industrialised societies contain people who live in poverty or are homeless. By almost any gauge of wellness, health correlates with social class (Adler et al. 1994; Anderson & Armstead 1995; Marmot, Kogevinas & Elston 1987). Individuals from lower classes are more likely than those from higher classes to:
- be born with very low birth weight
- die in infancy or in childhood
- die in adulthood before age 65
- develop a longstanding illness in adulthood
- experience days of restricted activity because of illness.

Not coincidentally, individuals from the lower classes have poorer health habits and attitudes than those from higher classes — for instance, they smoke more, participate less in vigorous exercise, and are less likely to feel that people can actively promote their own health (Adler et al. 1994; Fitzpatrick & Scambler 1984; Marmot, Kogevinas & Elston 1987). Research has also shown that people from the lower classes have less knowledge about risk factors for disease. They are less likely than individuals from upper classes to know, for example, that people can reduce their cardiovascular risk by controlling their blood pressure, stopping smoking and eating a low-cholesterol diet (Hossack & Leff 1987). As you probably know, members of minority groups usually are disproportionately represented in the lower social classes.

Minority group background is an important risk factor for poor health, largely because such groups are disadvantaged socioeconomically. A baby born in Malaysia stands a better chance of reaching the age of 12 months than the average newborn Aboriginal or Torres Strait Islander (AIHW 1996). Birth weight for babies born to Aboriginal and Torres Strait Islander mothers is about 200 grams lower than that of other Australian babies (AIHW 1996). The rate of infant mortality for indigenous groups in Australia is three to five times higher than for other Australian babies. Among babies who survive the first year, the life expectancy for Aboriginal and Torres Strait Islander babies is 15 to 20 years shorter than for non-indigenous babies (AIHW 1996). Moreover, regardless of the gender of these indigenous babies, they are far more likely to develop a major chronic disease in their lifetime and to die of that disease. Death rates from heart disease, respiratory illness and diabetes are disproportionably higher for Aboriginal and Torres Strait Islanders than for other Australians (AIHW 1996). Smoking, alcoholism, injury and violence resulting from alcohol abuse are highest in Aboriginal communities. Many indigenous people live in environments that do not support healthy behaviour changes or encourage the practice of health-protective behaviour. Aboriginals living in remote communities have restricted food choices in regard to the availability of fresh fruit and vegetables, or dairy products. Unsatisfactory living conditions, and lack of facilities for food storage and preparation, compound the problem for remote dwellers (Spark, Donovan & Howat 1991). These problems are disturbing, and correcting them will take a great deal of time, effort and social change.

Promoting health with diverse populations

How can societies help their diverse populations live healthy lives? Part of the solution would involve broad programs to reduce poverty. And because communities contain people of different ages, genders and sociocultural backgrounds, professionals who are trying to prevent and treat illness need to take a biopsychosocial perspective (Flack et al. 1995; Johnson et al. 1995; Young & Zane 1995). Let's see what this means by focusing on sociocultural differences to illustrate factors of three types that professionals need to consider.

- *Biological factors.* Sociocultural groups can differ in their physiological processes, as reflected in African Americans' high risk of developing the genetic blood disease of sickle-cell anaemia. Some evidence also indicates that black people metabolise a carcinogen in tobacco smoke less efficiently than whites, which may partly explain why they are more likely to develop cardiovascular disease and cancer (Blakeslee 1994). This metabolic difference may result from hereditary or environmental factors, such as diet.
- *Cognitive and linguistic factors.* People of different sociocultural groups seem to have different ideas about the causes of illness, give different degrees of attention to their body sensations, such as pain, and interpret symptoms differently. Chinese people believe that life energy is the source of physical and mental wellbeing, aids health improvement and is what enables the healing process. Professionals who try to refute these beliefs may drive their patients away (Belluck 1996). Language differences between professionals and the people they serve impair their ability to

communicate with each other. In traditional Aboriginal society there was no word for health. The Western notion of health as referring to only one aspect of life does not reflect the importance in Aboriginal society of interrelationships between people, land and creator beings. The closest translation of health in Aboriginal languages is 'life is health is life' (O'Connor & Parker 1995). Health care and health promotion for Aboriginal people need to take this holistic aspect of health into account if effective outcomes are to occur.

• *Social and emotional factors.* Sociocultural groups differ in the amount of stress they experience, their physiological reactivity to it, and the ways they cope with it. They also differ in their amount and use of social support.

These examples describe some of the issues that need to be considered in providing culturally sensitive health-promotion services. The feature below looks at one Aboriginal health promotion program that took a culturally appropriate approach. The remainder of this chapter focuses on techniques and program designs for enhancing health and preventing illness.

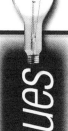

Highlight on issues

issues

Kimberley Aboriginal health promotion project

According to Spark, Donovan and Howat (1991) a culturally appropriate health promotion program for Aboriginals must:

1. acknowledge Aboriginal cultural influences on attitudes to health and health issues
2. use educational and environmental strategies that have cultural relevance
3. involve the Aboriginal community in the health promotion process.

The Kimberley Aboriginal Health Promotion Project sought to 'enable people to gain control over the determinants of their own health' (p. 11). This was done by empowering Aboriginal communities to identify health issues of concern to themselves and developing health promotion messages relevant to those issues. Aboriginal health promotion workers then assisted motivated individuals and groups within the community to develop action plans to address the environmental and behavioural changes required. Health promotion programs were generated by Aboriginal community groups with only consultancy support from Aboriginal health workers.

One important health issue identified by Aboriginal women in the Kimberley region was the potential for injury when young men from the community drink and drive. The men would drive into the nearest town to drink at the pub. Injuries from motor vehicle accidents on the return trip were common, as was fighting between the men and abuse of women on returning home in a drunken state. The storyboard on the following page was created by one of the Aboriginal women and later made into a 60-second television advertisement filmed by a local Aboriginal production company. It depicts the problems associated with drink driving, and how the safety of those who drink can be ensured by having a non-drinker drive the group back home and break up any fighting. This approach to health promotion is more likely to achieve desired outcomes because it addresses a health issue of concern to the community, involves members of the community and uses culturally appropriate resources.

(continued)

Injury Storyboard

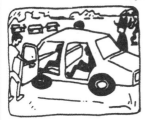

1. Five young men leaving community sober.

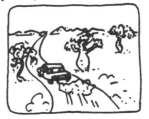

2. Heading to town.

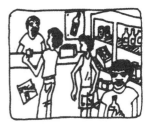

3. At the pub getting takeaway grog.

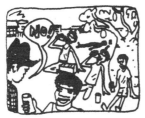

4. One person in the group is a non-drinker.

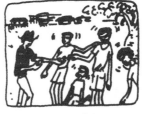

5. Non-drinker getting money from drinkers as they stagger around. He leads them away.

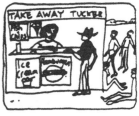

6. Non-drinker buying food for the drinkers.

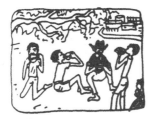

7. Group all eating hamburgers.

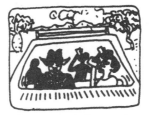

8. Driving back to the community (non-drinker at wheel)

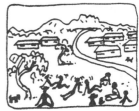

9. Back in community all drinkers sitting around with other people.

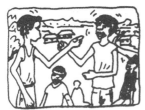

10. Two fellas start to argue.

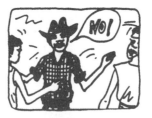

11. Man stands between them and breaks up fight.

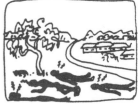

12. Drinkers go off to sleep.

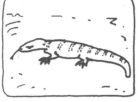

13. Lizard (symbolic).

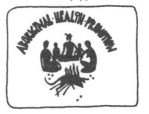

14. Caring and Sharing logo.

Source: Spark, Donovan & Howat (1991).

Programs for health promotion

In 1993 the National Health and Medical Research Council (NHMRC) released a national immunisation strategy to help increase the number of Australian children immunised against preventable diseases. Later initiatives of the Immunise Australia program have linked the maternity allowance, the Childcare Assistance Rebate and the Childcare Cash Rebate to age-appropriate immunisation of the child. While such strategies, in effect since 1997, have the wellbeing of children in mind, some would argue that they are an infringement of civil liberties. In other countries creative approaches by public health agencies have been used for the same purpose. We will begin our discussion of programs for health promotion by looking at some of the methods they use.

Methods for promoting health

Programs for health promotion try to encourage the practice of healthy behaviour by teaching individuals what these behaviours are and how to perform them, and by persuading people to change their current unhealthy habits. An important step in this effort is motivating individuals to *want* to change, and this often requires modifying their health beliefs and attitudes. What methods do these programs use to encourage health-protective behaviour?

Fear-arousing warnings

According to the health belief model, people are likely to practise healthy behaviour if they believe that by not doing so they are susceptible to serious health problems. In other words, they are motivated by fear to protect their health. Many studies have found that fear-arousing warnings can be effective in motivating people to adopt a variety of healthier attitudes and behaviour, for example regarding dental health, safe driving and smoking cigarettes (Sutton 1982; Sutton & Hallett 1988).

How threatening should the warning be? There is some controversy about this. Irving Janis (1967, 1984) has argued that each person and circumstance has an optimal level of fear arousal to motivate a change in attitude or behaviour. Too much fear may stimulate the person to use avoidance coping processes — by ignoring, minimising or denying the threat. This seems most likely to happen when warnings become personally and directly threatening (Lee 1989). Although some studies of warnings support this view, others do not, sometimes finding that very upsetting appeals are more likely to induce people to change their attitudes than weaker appeals (Janis 1984; Sutton 1982). More research is needed to identify the conditions under which fear appeals work.

What can be done to make fear appeals more effective? A study by Carol Self and Ronald Rogers (1990) found that self-efficacy is a crucial factor. Highly threatening appeals were associated with strong intentions to change an unhealthy behaviour only if the subjects received information indicating that they could perform the healthy behaviour, such as exercising, and succeed in protecting their health. People who received highly threatening appeals with information that minimised their ability to protect their health tended to use avoidance processes to cope with the threat. Other research has shown that fear appeals are more effective with adolescents and adults than children (Sturges & Rogers 1996) and if appeals emphasise the organic and social consequences — that is, the perceived seriousness — of developing the health problem (Banks et al. 1995; Kalichman & Coley 1995; Klohn & Rogers 1991).

An important problem with using fear-arousing warnings is that the attitudinal changes they produce often do not lead to behavioural changes. Programs to change unhealthy behaviour are more likely to be successful if they provide specific instructions for performing the behaviour and if they help bolster people's self-confidence before urging them to begin the plan (O'Connor & Parker 1995; Sutton 1982). We look at the fear-arousing campaign run in 1987 in Australia to raise awareness of AIDS later in this chapter.

Providing information

People who want to lead healthy lives need information — they need to know what to do and when, where and how to do it. Consider, for example, the issue of dietary cholesterol. People need to know what cholesterol is and that it can clog blood vessels, which can produce heart disease. They also need to know where they can have their blood tested for cholesterol level, what levels are high, how much cholesterol is in the foods they currently eat, which foods might be good substitutes for ones they should eliminate from their diets, and how to prepare these foods.

Television, radio, newspapers and magazines can play a useful role in promoting health by presenting warnings and providing information, such as to help people avoid or stop smoking (Flay 1987). One approach the mass media have used simply provides information to the general population about the *negative consequences* of an activity — smoking for instance — and tries to persuade people not to smoke, as public service announcements often do. This approach seems to have very limited success in affecting behaviour (Flay 1987; Lau et al. 1980). One reason information may not work is that people often misunderstand the health reports they read (Yeaton, Smith & Rogers 1990). Another reason may be that they just don't want to change the behaviour at issue. Mass communication strategies are more likely to be effective for people in the contemplation stage of DiClemente et al.'s (1991) model of behaviour change. An American newspaper columnist who did not want to change his diet railed against warnings, writing:

> Cholesterol, shmolesterol! . . . Almost everything [experts] say is good for you will turn out bad for you if you hang around long enough, and almost everything they say is bad for you will turn out not to matter. (Baker 1989, p. A31)

This quote is a good example of motivated reasoning.

Other approaches the mass media have used focus on people who already want to stop an unhealthy habit. For example, programs conducted on TV have been effective in getting smokers to take the first steps in quitting by offering free printed materials or kits with hints on how to stop and contact persons at a community agency (Flay 1987). One program on TV in the United States, called CableQuit, was successful in helping people stop smoking by showing them how to prepare to quit, helping them through the day they quit, describing ways to maintain their success, and giving them opportunities to call for advice (Valois, Adams & Kammermann 1996). Of those who started the program, 17 per cent continued to abstain from smoking a year later. In Australia a similar smoking cessation program called Quit has been successful in assisting smokers to give up their habit. We will discuss this program more fully later in the chapter.

Medical settings, particularly doctors' offices, can and should be a major source for information and warnings to promote preventive behaviour. There are advantages and disadvantages in using medical settings as sources of information for health promotion. One advantage is that four out of every five Australians visit their general practitioner at least once a year (AIHW 1996; Ward 1994). Moreover, health care workers are respected as experts. But two disadvantages are that these efforts take up time in already busy practices and that medical personnel may not know how to help people overcome problems they have in following recommendations for prevention (Radecki & Brunton 1992). Figure 6.5 presents responses that doctors and health care workers can use to combat rationalisations smokers commonly give for not quitting. Studies have shown that counselling delivered by doctors or by nurses with video materials can help many smokers to quit (Hollis et al. 1993; Ockene et al. 1994). Unfortunately, less than half of patients who smoke report in surveys that their doctor advised them to quit, and some of the doctors were unaware of the problem behaviour in their patients (Anda et al. 1987; Dickinson 1989; Frank et al. 1991).

Figure 6.5 Common rationalisations of patients who smoke and responses medical staff can give

PATIENT: *I am under a lot of stress, and smoking relaxes me.*

STAFF: Your body has become accustomed to nicotine, so you naturally feel more relaxed when you get the nicotine you have come to depend on. But nicotine is actualy a stimulant that temporarily raises heart rate, blood pressure and adrenaline level. After a few weeks of not smoking, most ex-smokers feel less nervous.

PATIENT: *Smoking stimulates me and helps me to be more effective in my work.*

STAFF: Difficulty in concentrating can be a symptom of nicotine withdrawal, but it is a short-term effect. Over time, the body and brain function more efficiently when you don't smoke, because carbon monoxide from cigarettes is displaced by oxygen in the bloodstream.

PATIENT: *I have already cut down to a safe level.*

STAFF: Cutting down is a good step toward quitting. But smoking at any level increases the risk of illness. And some smokers who cut back inhale more often and more deeply, thus maintaining nicotine dependence. It is best to quit smoking completely.

PATIENT: *I only smoke safe, low-tar/low-nicotine cigarettes.*

STAFF: Low-tar cigarettes still contain harmful substances. Many smokers inhale more often or more deeply and thus maintain their nicotine levels. Carbon monoxide intake often increases with a switch to low-tar cigarettes.

PATIENT: *I don't have the willpower to give up smoking.*

STAFF: It can be hard for some people to give up smoking, but for others it is much easier than they expect. Many smokers quit every year. It may take more than one attempt for you to succeed, and you may need to try different methods of quitting. I will give you all the support I can.

Source: Adapted from USDHHS (1986a).

Medical professionals now have another avenue for providing health promotion information: They can give individuals who are at risk for inherited illnesses, such as some forms of breast cancer, estimates of their chances of getting the disease and advise them to undergo tests, such as periodic breast examinations and genetic testing. Are there psychological risks for people who receive this information and undergo the tests? Although most women who receive this information and testing for breast cancer do not show adverse psychological effects, those who were already very anxious about health threats before receiving the information often become more distressed (Lerman, Audrain & Croyle 1994; Lerman et al. 1996). Research is needed to determine how to prevent these adverse effects.

Behavioural methods

Behavioural methods focus directly on enhancing people's performance of the preventive act itself. These methods include providing specific instructions or training for performing the behaviour, calendars to indicate when to perform infrequent preventive actions, and reminders of appointments. Research has shown that these techniques enhance the effectiveness of programs for health promotion (Kegeles 1983; Sarafino 1996).

Behavioural methods in health promotion also include manipulating the consequences of people's health-related behaviour, particularly by providing reinforcers for practising preventive action. Although reinforcers can be useful for increasing health behaviour, such as practising good dental hygiene, the effectiveness of this method depends on many factors, including the types of reward used, the age and sociocultural background of the individual, and the person's interest in performing the activity (Lund & Kegeles 1984; Sarafino 1987b, 1996; Suls 1984). For instance, people differ in their reward preferences — tickets for a rock concert might be very enjoyable for you, but your friend might prefer hearing a recital by the Australian Chamber Orchestra; and attending either of these events might be very unpleasant for someone else. The consequences need to be matched to the person. There is also some evidence that reward preferences change with age: kindergarten children tend to prefer material rewards (a charm, money, lollies) over social rewards such as praise, but this preference seems to reverse by third grade (Witryol 1971). Other findings indicate that material rewards generally enhance performance of a behaviour when the person's interest in practising it is low, but they sometimes *reduce* motivation when interest is very high (Sarafino & DiMattia 1978). Programs for health promotion need to consider the point of view of the individual with regard to the preventive action and any consequences that the program introduces to enhance performance of that behaviour.

Community approaches

All of the methods discussed assist health promotion planners in developing behaviour change procedures. Psychological theories like the health belief model and the theory of reasoned action are useful to program developers because they help identify factors such as attitudes and beliefs that predict the behaviour. And the stages of change model indicates how elements of a program can best be targeted to specific groups of individuals. But how do we go about implementing these procedures at the community level, and how do we evaluate our program?

The PRECEDE/PROCEED model

Developed by Green and Kreuter (1991), the **PRECEDE/PROCEED model** provides guidelines for health promoters in designing, implementing and evaluating programs conducted on a large number of people. Figure 6.6 outlines the different phases involved in program planning.

Phase 1 of the model directs the health planner to focus on outcomes or 'quality of life' issues before moving on to consider specific details of the program or resources. In order to understand the quality of life issues of importance to a community, some form of social diagnosis is required. Information can be obtained through focus group meetings or community surveys of needs and concerns. The advantage of focusing the health program on issues of concern to community members is that they will be more motivated to change behaviour.

Phase 2 identifies the health problems that appear to contribute to quality of life for individuals. Epidemiological data on mortality and morbidity can be useful in identifying important health problems so that resources can be assigned more efficiently. The first two phases of the model help to clarify the program goal. This may be, for instance, to reduce the incidence of infectious disease in children.

Phase 3 identifies the behaviours and environmental factors that appear to be related to the health problems identified. For example, if an assessment of environmental factors reveals that there are few immunisation service providers within an area, then the program may need to address service provision in order to increase child immunisation rates. This stage in program planning helps to identify program objectives and sub-objectives.

In Phase 4, three sets of factors are identified as having an effect on behavioural change. The first of these are *predisposing factors* or knowledge, attitudes and beliefs that can affect motivation to change. *Enabling factors* are those that increase the likelihood of the behaviour occurring. Sometimes environmental conditions such as limited facilities, or high health insurance premiums, act as barriers to change. The third set of factors are *reinforcing factors* like social feedback that either encourage or hinder the behaviour change. Steps 1 to 4 deal with the design of the health program.

Phase 5 considers the feasibility of implementing the program within the constraints of limited time, financial resources and skills of program staff. Phase 6 deals with implementation of the program, while phases 7 to 9 are concerned with evaluation of the program. Notice that the type of evaluation used should measure different elements of the health program. **Process evaluation** is concerned with the activities of the program — that is, it measures how well the program was delivered. **Impact evaluation** assesses the program objectives — whether behavioural and environmental factors were altered successfully. **Outcome evaluation** determines whether the program achieved its goal — was the intervention successful in improving the health and life quality of participants? Health psychologists often conduct health promotion on an individual basis, but more and more they are becoming involved in multidisciplinary team approaches to health promotion.

Traditionally, psychologists have used a clinical approach to facilitate lifestyle changes in the at-risk individual in settings such as hospitals, psychiatric units and community centres. A range of behavioural approaches have been used, such as monitoring behaviour, devising a behaviour change plan with appropriate reinforcers and teaching skills such as assertiveness in high-risk situations. While this intensive approach has been effective at the individual level, it does not reach large sections of the community that could benefit from the interventions (Sanson-Fisher, Schofield & Perkins 1993). Also, the clinical approach has been criticised for not taking into account the social context within which risk behaviours occur, or the social factors (social support, social networks and socioeconomic class) that have an impact on the behaviour change process (Oldenburg 1994). A more integrative approach to health promotion by health psychologists has been advocated (Oldenburg 1994; Winett 1995) in which psychological theories and models are incorporated into a broader public health approach of program development, implementation and evaluation. The PRECEDE/PROCEED model is a useful guide for psychologists conducting health promotion as part of a multidisciplinary team in settings as diverse as the school, the workplace and the wider community.

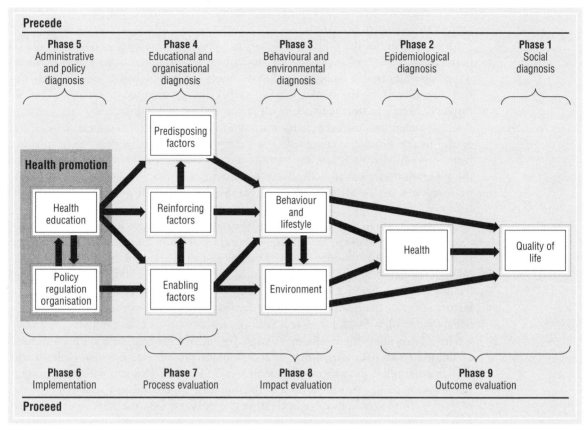

Figure 6.6 The PRECEDE/PROCEED planning model

Source: Green and Kreuter (1991). Reproduced with permission of the publishers.

Many types of programs have been carried out to promote health in different settings and with a variety of goals, methods and populations. We will examine different types of programs, beginning with health education efforts that are designed to reach children and adolescents in schools and establish healthful habits at early ages.

Promoting health in the schools

Public and private schools have a unique opportunity to promote health. In developed nations, schools have access to virtually all individuals during the years that are probably most critical in the development of health-related behaviour. Effective school-based health education teaches children what healthy and unhealthy behaviours are and the consequences of practising them. This can produce two benefits. First, children may avoid developing unhealthy habits at the time when they are most vulnerable to these behaviours taking hold. Second, children may acquire health-protective behaviours that become established or habitual aspects of their beliefs and lifestyles that may stay with them throughout their lives.

So how is health promotion conducted in a school setting? Health education can be incorporated into the school curriculum. Students are taught about good nutrition, the effects of alcohol and drugs on the body, the importance of exercise and the need to protect skin from the damaging effects of the sun. Health education alone is not sufficient to change behaviour. Classroom health education needs to be reinforced through healthy school policy such as making the school a smoke-free environment, providing shade areas for play and making healthy food available at low cost in the school canteen. Providing school health services further allows both students and teachers to act on information acquired. Whether or not health behaviour change occurs as a result of health education depends on a number of other factors such as the attitudes, beliefs and knowledge of parents, cultural differences, and collaboration of community organisations and retailers (Reynolds, Dommers & Spillman 1994; Shilton 1993).

School heart health

Let's take a look at one successful school health promotion endeavour. The National Heart Foundation of Western Australia (NHFWA) used a comprehensive model of health promotion to guide health education programs and to develop resource materials and health services aimed at cardiovascular primary prevention in children and adolescents (Shilton 1993). Most primary and secondary schools, both government and non-government, in the State participated in the NHFWA initiative. Heart health education has centred on the heart, nutrition, smoking and physical activity. Health education was incorporated in home economics courses, teaching food purchasing, nutrition and heart healthy cooking methods. Jump Rope for Heart, an exercise program that began in Western Australia in 1982, has since been implemented in schools across Australia. NHFWA has also been active in changing school policy and in lobbying governments to introduce a smoke-free policy to schools. Impact evaluation studies have indicated up to 90 per cent usage of the resource manuals by schools. Environmental changes were made by 56 per cent of primary schools, and 39 per cent of secondary schools in Western Australia adopted a healthy canteen policy. In 1991 a smoke-free school policy was issued by the Western Australian ministry.

Are school programs effective? Some, like the NHFWA program, are. Attitude and behavioural change to minimise risk factors can still occur even when less comprehensive programs are used, or when changes are made to one area, for example in regard to a healthy food canteen. In a study by McBride and Browne (1993) that used a quasi-experimental design, dietary behaviour and attitudes to nutrition were found to differ depending on the type of food available in the school canteen. Compared with students in schools that did not have a healthy canteen policy, students in schools with a healthy canteen had more positive attitudes to healthy food and consumed more fibre, less sodium and less fat. Other research has indicated the benefits of health education in the practice of safety behaviour (Parcel, Bruhn & Cerreto 1986). But some schools provide little health education, or their programs are underfunded, poorly designed, and taught by teachers whose interests and training are in other areas.

Work-site wellness programs

There is a new 'epidemic' in the health field — wellness programs are spreading rapidly in workplaces in industrialised countries. A survey of more than 1300 American work sites with 50 or more employees found that nearly two-thirds offered some form of health promotion activity, such as for fitness and weight control (Fielding & Piserchia 1989). Workplace health promotion in Australia is a more recent development. Findings from a 1992 survey indicated that 34 per cent of all Australian workplaces and 96 per cent of those with at least 500 employees provide some health promotion activities (National Coordinating Committee for Health Promotion in the Workplace 1992). Some programs use incentives, such as prizes or bonuses for losing weight, stopping smoking or staying well. By doing this, employers are helping their workers and saving a great deal of money. Workers in Australia with poor health habits cost employers substantially more in reduced productivity and absenteeism than those with good habits. These savings offset and often exceed the expense of running a wellness program (Winett, King & Altman 1989).

Work-site wellness programs vary in their aims, but they usually address some or all of the following risk factors: hypertension, cigarette smoking, unhealthy diets and obesity, poor physical fitness, alcohol abuse and high levels of stress. Information is provided about healthy lifestyles, changes are made to the workplace environment to facilitate healthy choices, and skills are taught to participants to bring about changes. Housing these programs in workplaces has several advantages.

> (a) Most employees go to the workplace on a regular schedule, facilitating *regular* partici-
> pation in the programs; (b) contact with co-workers can provide reinforcing social support,
> which is believed by many to be a primary force in sustaining a lifestyle change; (c) the
> workplace offers many opportunities for environmental supports, such as healthy food in
> the cafeteria and office policies regarding smoking; (d) opportunities abound for positive
> reinforcement for individuals participating in the programs; (e) programs in the workplace
> are generally less expensive for the employee than comparable programs in the community;
> and (f) programs in the workplace are convenient. (Cohen 1985, p. 215)

These advantages suggest that work-site programs can attract high levels of partici-
pation and that employees who choose to participate are likely to succeed in improving their health behaviour. Unfortunately, the employees who do not participate are often the ones who need it most — those who report having poor health and fitness (Alexy 1991). We will look at two Australian workplace wellness programs and how effective they are.

Ericsson Australia

A workplace with a comprehensive approach to health promotion is Ericsson Aus-
tralia, a large manufacturer, developer and exporter of telecommunications products (O'Conner & Parker 1995; VicHealth 1993). This company has a work force of 2000 with six locations in Melbourne. Ericsson Australia has had an Occupational Health and Safety (OHS) policy in place since 1975. Part of the health management strategy consists of providing a range of services to employees and their families, and establishing a health centre, a gymnasium, exercise and rehabilitation programs. Other environmental changes have been made in relation to health food items being made available at reduced costs in the company canteen. Ericsson Australia has a drug and alcohol policy, and a policy on being a smoke-free environment.

Cardiovascular risk reduction trial in the NSW Ambulance Service

Some work-site health promotion programs have been designed to target risk reduc-
tion in a specific health area. This was the case with the cardiovascular risk reduction trial conducted by Gomel et al. in 1993 for the Ambulance Service of New South Wales, Australia. A total of 431 employees from 28 stations participated. Four

interventions were trialled to examine their effectiveness in reducing cardiovascular risk among employees. One intervention condition involved assessing major risk factors and providing feedback to each participant. In the second intervention participants received the same health risk assessment and feedback as those in the first condition but were given advice on lifestyle changes required to reduce risk factors. Participants in the third behavioural counselling intervention received risk factor education and participated in up to six lifestyle counselling sessions over a 10-week period following baseline assessment. They also received a self-instructional manual to help with making lifestyle changes in regard to diet, smoking and exercise. Behavioural counselling and the lifestyle change manual were based on Prochaska and DiClemente's (1984) stages of change model. A fourth condition involved behavioural counselling plus incentives. Participants in this condition received monetary incentives for making lifestyle changes or if they succeeded in meeting their projected three-month risk reduction goals. All participants were assessed for cardiovascular risk before intervention and at three, six and 12 months.

The experimental nature of the cardiovascular risk reduction trial allowed two types of evaluation to be performed. First, the program was able to be evaluated in terms of its overall effectiveness in changing risk factors of employees. Second, information could be obtained about the best intervention strategy (risk assessment and feedback, education, behavioural counselling) for changing cardiovascular risk. Of the interventions, the two behavioural counselling conditions resulted in the greatest changes for some risk factors, when compared with education and screening alone. More participants in the two behavioural counselling conditions had quit smoking by three months and had reduced body fat. Long-term reductions in blood pressure were better for the behavioural counselling group without incentives. The cardiovascular risk factor reduction trial demonstrated that health promotion programs in the workplace need not be intensive or large-scale for desired changes to occur.

Community-wide wellness programs

Community-wide programs for health promotion are designed to reach large numbers of people and improve their knowledge and performance of preventive behaviour. These programs may use any or all of the methods we have considered. They may, for instance, use a media blitz to warn people of the dangers of drinking and driving, or provide information regarding free blood pressure testing, or offer people a chance to win a prize for stopping smoking or getting vaccinations.

One of the first disease prevention programs to demonstrate that community approaches to health promotion could be useful was the Three Community Study (Farquhar et al. 1977). Intervention in two of the communities involved media-based and individual programs for those at high risk for heart disease, while the third community acted as a control and received no intervention. Findings from the Three Community Study indicated that people's overall risk for heart disease increased in the control community and decreased in the two campaign towns. The success of the Three Community Study led other researchers in the United States to undertake larger-scale and longer-term projects with more advanced methods for reducing cardiovascular risk factors. Projects that have shown favourable outcomes so far include the Minnesota Heart Health Program (Blackburn et al. 1984), the Pawtucket Heart Health Project (Lasater et al. 1984), the Pennsylvania County Health Improvement Program (Stunkard, Felix & Cohen 1985) and the Stanford Five City Project (Farquhar et al. 1984; Farquhar, Maccoby & Solomon 1984). In Australia, the North Coast Healthy

Lifestyle Program (Egger et al. 1983) compared interventions consisting of media and media plus community programs in altering smoking, dietary fat intake and exercise for the three communities of Lismore, Coffs Harbour and Tamworth, the latter acting as the control community. Lifestyle behaviour change was higher in the intervention communities compared with the control community, the greatest impact being evidenced by the media plus community programs intervention.

Environmental manipulations have also been incorporated in community approaches to heart disease prevention. The North Karelia Project in Finland (Salonen 1987) used this approach. Researchers worked with local food manufacturers and distributors to produce and promote low-fat meat and dairy products. Healthy restaurants and 'no smoking' areas were also established in the Karelia community. Risk factor assessment at five and 10 years into the project has indicated significant reductions for most of the risk factors. Let us now look at Australian health programs that have targeted specific priority areas and evaluate the effectiveness of the methods used.

The SunSmart program

Australia has the highest incidence of skin cancer in the world. In 1996 there were 4313 new cases of melanoma diagnosed in males, and 3448 new cases in females (AIHW 2000). As melanoma skin cancer is linked to ultraviolet radiation, the risk of such cancer can be reduced by adopting sun-protective behaviours. These behaviours consist of avoiding the sun during the middle of the day, wearing a hat and protective clothing, and using a sunscreen with a sun protective factor (SPF) of 15+. In 1980 the Anti-Cancer Council of Victoria (ACCV) launched the Slip! Slop! Slap! campaign, which used an animated seagull called Sid to encourage the public to reduce their ultraviolet exposure through three actions — slipping on a shirt, slopping on some sunscreen and slapping on a hat. The educational campaign took the form of short TV and radio advertisements to convey its message. Throughout the eighties the slogan and message was adopted by each State cancer council. For instance, in New South Wales skin cancer awareness campaigns have targeted specific groups such as outdoor workers and carers of children under the age of five years. Other strategies have included free skin checks at beaches to facilitate secondary prevention of skin cancer (ACCV 1989).

The success of the Slip! Slop! Slap! campaign led to the implementation of a SunSmart public education campaign in 1988 (ACCV 1989). The objective of this campaign was to effect individual change through structural and policy changes within the community. The campaign included four strategies — the use of media and public education, a community program, a schools program and a sponsorship program. The media launches served to increase awareness and knowledge of Australians about skin cancer and prevention behaviours. The community programs relied for their effectiveness on collaboration between local health centres, local government and workplaces. The community strategy was initially concerned with the provision of information, but later assisted workplaces in adopting sun protection practices. SunSmart programs were also incorporated into the Victorian school curriculum. These school programs taught SunSmart behaviour, developed policies such as 'No hat, play in the shade' and were instrumental in providing shade areas in school playgrounds. Sponsorship of sporting groups and role models further helped to convey SunSmart messages (Sinclair et al. 1994). Today the SunSmart program is a comprehensive skin cancer control program involved in information dissemination, education about sun protection, the early detection of skin cancer, scientific research, and policy and program development and evaluation that affects a broad spectrum of the Australian community (ACCV 1995).

Have these public educational programs been effective in increasing knowledge and in changing attitudes and behaviour? Evaluation studies have indicated that the Slip! Slop! Slap! campaign had almost universal awareness up to 14 years after the program was implemented. Following the SunSmart program, more than 95 per cent of individuals surveyed could recall advertisements about sun protection, and were knowledgeable about strategies for protecting oneself from the sun. Preventive behaviours such as wearing a hat and sunscreen have increased over time, while sunburn rates have decreased (Borland, Hill & Noy 1990). Attitudes towards suntans have become more negative (Hill et al. 1993), while sales of sunscreens with an SPF of 15+ have increased markedly since the initial skin cancer educational campaign (White 1990). Sun safety messages appear to have had an impact on much of the Australian community, the only exceptions being adolescent beach-goers (Pratt & Borland 1994) and young males (Marks 1995). These findings point to the substantial impact that a public health campaign can have on knowledge, attitudes and behaviour.

The National Tobacco Campaign

Another extensive health initiative has targeted smoking as a risk factor for heart disease and lung cancer. Smoking is arguably the largest single preventable cause of death in Australia, and is responsible for an estimated 18 000 deaths each year (AIHW 1996). The National Tobacco Campaign combines a public education approach to increase the community's awareness of the dangers of smoking with a nationally coordinated Quitline service for smokers (http://www.quitnow.info.au, accessed August 1999). A resource video and booklet are available to help smokers to quit. Strong graphic images in TV advertising are used to convey the message that 'every cigarette you smoke is doing you damage'. The *Artery* advertisement focuses on the build-up of fat deposits on artery walls, to convey the damage caused to arteries by smoking. Another advertisement, *Lung*, uses an inside the body filming technique to demonstrate the damage caused to lungs, the viewer being taken along the airways into the lung surrounded by tobacco smoke. *Tumor* shows the damage caused to a tumour-suppressing gene in the lung tissue, while *Brain* describes smoking-related stroke.

While early campaigns focused on informing the public about the dangers of smoking, more recent efforts have aimed to change behaviour of smokers by personalising the risk of smoking to health. Public awareness of the tobacco campaign messages has been consistently high with around 85 per cent of people having seen the advertisements, though awareness of the Quitline service was low (34 per cent) in the 1993 campaign (Mullins & Borland 1993). Success rates for campaign awareness of quit services have improved substantially, with nearly 100 000 smokers calling Quitline in the 10-month period up to April 1998 (http://www.quitnow.info.au).

Prevention with specific targets: focusing on AIDS

Sometimes prevention programs focus on reducing people's risk of developing a specific health problem and centre these efforts on specific segments of the population. One example of this approach is the Multiple Risk Factor Intervention Trial (MRFIT), a project that recruited and provided health promotion programs for thousands of men across the United States who were at substantial risk for heart disease (Caggiula et al. 1981; Shekelle et al. 1985). Another example involves efforts to reduce the spread of *acquired immune deficiency syndrome* (AIDS), an incurable and fatal disease. We will focus this section on efforts to prevent infection with the *human immunodeficiency virus* (HIV), which causes AIDS.

HIV infection

The magnitude of the AIDS threat is astounding — it has been estimated that 21.8 million people around the world have died from AIDS since the epidemic began, and about 36.1 million are living with HIV (National Center for HIV, STD and TB Prevention 2001). More than 160 countries have reported cases of AIDS, but the infection is unevenly distributed worldwide. The largest concentration of infections is currently in Africa, where the outlook is cataclysmic, and the incidence is soaring in developing countries in Asia and South America. But the rate of infection appears to have slowed down in industrialised countries. About 17 600 Australians have been infected (AIHW 2000). The number of new diagnoses has declined in recent years with the use of effective drug therapies.

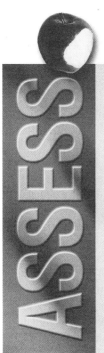

Assess yourself
YOUR KNOWLEDGE ABOUT AIDS

Answer the following true/false items by circling the T or F for each one.

T F 1. People who develop AIDS usually die within a couple of years.

T F 2. Blood tests can usually tell within a week after infection whether someone has received the AIDS virus.

T F 3. People do not get AIDS from using swimming pools or rest rooms after someone with AIDS has.

T F 4. Some people have contracted AIDS from insects, such as mosquitoes, that have previously bitten someone with AIDS.

T F 5. AIDS can now be prevented with a vaccine and cured if treated early.

T F 6. People who have the AIDS virus can look and feel well.

T F 7. Gay women (lesbians) get AIDS much more often than heterosexual women, but not as often as gay men.

T F 8. Health workers have a high risk of getting AIDS from or spreading the virus to their patients.

T F 9. Kissing or touching someone who has AIDS can give you the disease.

T F 10. AIDS is less contagious than measles.

Check your answers against the key below that is printed upside down — a score of 8 items correct is good, 9 is very good, and 10 is excellent.

(*Sources:* Items based on material in DiClemente, Zorn & Temoshok 1987; Grieger & Ponterotto 1988; Vener & Krupka 1990).

Answers:
1.T 2. F 3. T 4. F 5. F 6. T 7. F 8. F 9. F 10.T

There is no vaccine against the HIV virus, and there is not likely to be one in the near future. The virus spreads to an uninfected person only through contact of his or her body fluids with those of an infected person, generally either through sexual practices or when intravenous drug users share needles. The likelihood of infection increases if the person has wounds or inflammation from other sexually transmitted diseases, such as syphilis, herpes or chlamydia (Peterman 1990). Infected mothers sometimes transmit the virus to their babies during gestation, delivery or later during breast-feeding (European Collaborative Study 1991; Fathalla 1990). Changing people's behaviour is virtually the only means of reducing the risk of infection, and worldwide public health efforts for prevention have concentrated on using fear-arousing warnings and providing information. These efforts also try to correct misconceptions about HIV transmission — for instance, that AIDS can only happen to homosexuals and drug users, that all gay men are infected, that mosquitoes can spread the virus, that health care personnel are usually at high risk of becoming infected when working with AIDS patients, or that the virus can be transmitted through casual contact, such as by touching or hugging infected individuals or by sharing office equipment they have used (Batchelor 1988; DiClemente, Zorn & Temoshok 1987). Research on health care workers has found that their becoming infected is rare even when they are accidently stuck with a needle that had been used on an AIDS patient (Clever & LeGuyader 1995; Henderson et al. 1990).

It is true that a large proportion of AIDS victims in Australia are gay men (AIHW 1996). This is probably because many gay men have tended to be very promiscuous and have engaged regularly in certain sexual practices, especially anal intercourse, that involve a high risk of transmission (Darrow et al. 1987; Francis & Chin 1987). But many gay men do not lead high-risk lifestyles, lesbians have a very low prevalence of AIDS and the vast majority of victims in Africa are heterosexuals. A person's sexual orientation is not a guarantee of high or low risk. People are much more likely to have very unsafe sex if they are promiscuous or have sex while under the influence of alcohol or drugs (Cooper, Peirce & Huselid 1994; Leigh 1990; Lowry et al. 1994). In men, intoxication seems to increase negative attitudes and decrease self-efficacy about using condoms (Gordon & Carey 1996).

Efforts to prevent HIV infection

Major efforts have been introduced in most countries around the world to prevent HIV infection. A national campaign was launched in Australia in 1987 to raise awareness and concern about AIDS in the general public. This campaign differed from AIDS prevention strategies in other countries in its use of shock tactics to arouse fear in the general public. The message underlying the campaign was that all members of the Australian community were at risk of AIDS through sexual and drug-using behaviour, not just homosexual males. The campaign relied on a one-week televised commercial that featured the 'Grim Reaper', a skeleton-like figure carrying a scythe, bowling with deadly intent 'pins' in the form of men, women and children. The text that accompanied the 'Grim Reaper' commercial ran as follows:

> 'At first only gays and i.v. drug users were being killed by AIDS, but we now know every one of us could be devastated by it. The fact is, over 50 000 men, women and children in Australia now carry the AIDS virus, that in three years nearly 2000 of us will be dead, and that if not stopped it could kill more Australians than World War 11. But AIDS can be stopped, and you can help stop it. If you have sex, have just one safe partner, or always use condoms — always.' (Rosser 1991; p. 130)

How successful was the use of a fear-arousing message in changing the Australian public's awareness and knowledge of AIDS? Did the community engage in safer sexual practices as a result of exposure to the campaign? While the 'Grim Reaper' campaign appeared to have some desired effects in relation to increasing awareness in the public about HIV and AIDS (with 93.5 per cent recall at five months' follow-up) and changing attitudes towards HIV-infected persons (Ross et al. 1990), post-evaluation findings indicated that the campaign was counterproductive in increasing knowledge (Rigby et al. 1989) or changing behaviour of at-risk groups (Winn 1991). New Zealand male homosexuals not exposed to the 'Grim Reaper' AIDS campaign reported safer sexual practices than Australian homosexuals exposed to the television campaign (Rosser 1991). The use of fear-arousing information, moreover, increased the number of low-risk people compared with active male homosexuals undergoing HIV antibody testing, which placed extreme demands on these specialised health services.

Despite some of the unintended effects of the Australian national AIDS campaign, the lessons learned can guide the development of future AIDS education programs. Efforts to inform the public are continuing, with wide media coverage of new information about AIDS. Public health agencies are involved in the preparation of educational material for schools, and local health organisations have made available speakers for various community groups and work organisations. Three basic messages have been conveyed in most AIDS prevention campaigns around the world:

1. Use 'safer sex' practices by selecting sexual partners carefully, avoiding practices that may injure body tissues, and using condoms in all forms of sexual intercourse with individuals outside of very long-term monogamous relationships. Not all people who have the virus know they do, and not all of those who know they do tell their sexual partners (Marks, Richardson & Maldonado 1991; Simoni et al. 1995).
2. Do not share needles or syringes. If you do, make sure they are sterile.
3. Women who could have been exposed to the virus through sexual practices or drug use should have their blood tested for the HIV antibody before becoming pregnant and, if the test is positive, avoid pregnancy.

Much of this information has been designed to arouse fear, and it has in many people.

Have AIDS educational efforts had lasting effects on knowledge and behaviour? As many public health campaigns have been directed towards the general population, intravenous drug users and their sexual partners, and gays and bisexuals, let us examine the research on each of these groups. Of people in the general population, adolescents and young adults are most vulnerable to infection because of their relatively high levels of sexual promiscuity and drug use. Evidence suggests that their knowledge about AIDS has improved over the years (Dorman & Rienzo 1988; Holtzman et al. 1994). But most sexually experienced adolescents do not seem to take the precautions they should (Hernandez & Smith 1990; Ku, Sonenstein & Pleck 1993; Leigh et al. 1994). Some fail to take precautions because they have incorrect beliefs about the transmission of the virus and their likelihood of infection.

Australian research has indicated that even when adolescents have a good knowledge of AIDS and AIDS precautions, and hold favourable attitudes to condoms, this does not predict safe sexual behaviour (Rosenthal, Hall & Moore 1992). Perceived susceptibility alone, as a health belief, was found to predict reduced risk behaviour for females with casual partners. Most heterosexual adolescents and adults believe themselves to be invulnerable to AIDS if in a steady relationship, ignoring the short duration of these relationships, and placing a great deal of trust in their partner to have engaged in safe sex or safe drug-injecting behaviours in the past (Boldero, Moore

& Rosenthal 1992; Moore & Rosenthal 1991). Adolescents appear to hold one of two beliefs — perceived invulnerability to AIDS, or 'risk and be damned'. These belief patterns are associated with risky sexual practices (Moore & Rosenthal 1991). Risk behaviours in adolescents have also been linked to contextual factors such as alcohol (Ross & Rosser 1989), sexual arousal, condom availability and lack of communication about commitment to safe sex (Boldero, Moore & Rosenthal 1992).

Research findings on intravenous drug users suggest that over 90 per cent of these people know that sharing needles can transmit AIDS and that most of them are now using sterile needles, reducing their drug use, or using drugs in other ways, such as by inhaling (Des Jarlais & Friedman 1988; Des Jarlais, Friedman & Casriel 1990). Australia's low incidence of HIV infection in injecting drug users has been credited to the early introduction by the federal government of needle and syringe exchanges (Nutbeam, Blakey & Pates 1991; Wodak & Des Jarlais 1993), and the later expansion of methadone facilities through the efforts of the NCADA (Wodak 1992). Such exchange schemes have facilitated low-risk behaviour in intravenous drug users (Groseclose et al. 1995; Leary 1995). However, risky sexual behaviour in drug users has been more resistant to change. This is an area where health psychologists can contribute their expertise in helping drug users change their risk behaviours. Few drug users and their sexual partners use condoms (Krajick 1988). Most drug users are heterosexual men, and their sexual partners often are women who know about the risks but feel powerless and are willing to go along with having unprotected sex (Fullilove et al. 1990).

Perhaps the best-organised efforts to change sexual practices have been directed towards gay men, particularly in gay communities in large cities. This is partly because many gay social, political and religious organisations existed before the AIDS epidemic began, and these groups have become actively involved in public health campaigns to prevent the spread of the disease. Studies have found that these efforts have had a substantial impact on gay sexual behaviour across the United States (Joseph et al. 1987; Martin 1990; Catania et al. 1991; Coates 1990). Today, only about a third of new infections in the United States are in gay men (CDC 1995). Similar changes in gay men's behaviour and rates of infection have also been found in Amsterdam, Holland (Van Griensven et al. 1989). Australian research also noted a change to safer sexual behaviour in male homosexuals compared with the heterosexual community (Connell et al. 1989). AIDS education and prevention campaigns with gay and bisexual men have produced 'the most profound modifications of personal health-related behaviours ever recorded' (Stall, Coates & Hoff 1988, p. 878). But a new and ominous trend has appeared: young gays are engaging more in unsafe sex, and their infection rate is increasing (Gold 1995; Rogers 1994; Visser & Antoni 1994).

Making HIV prevention more effective

Studies have shown that interventions to prevent HIV infection have been moderately effective in decreasing people's risky behaviour (Kalichman, Carey & Johnson 1996). But many individuals who should reduce their risky sexual behaviour do not, and the reasons they don't seem to be similar for homosexual and heterosexual individuals. We need to keep in mind that over 40 per cent of today's new infections are in individuals who are neither gay nor intravenous drug users (CDC 1995).

Why do many people engage in risky sexual behaviour? The reasons include people's maladaptive beliefs about their own low self-efficacy and risk of infection, other people's sexual behaviour, and the effect that using a condom would have on sexual pleasure and spontaneity (Gold, Skinner & Ross 1994; Kegeles, Adler & Irwin

1989; Kelly et al. 1991; Kelly et al. 1995; White, Terry & Hogg 1994; Wulfert, Wan & Backus 1996). These beliefs are often clear when people recognise that their behaviour contradicts what they know experts say, so they add qualifiers, such as, 'I know that's what they say but...' or, 'but in my case...' (Maticka-Tyndale 1991). In minority groups, there can be added problems of lesser knowledge about risky behaviour and suspicions concerning information from health care systems they believe have treated them badly (Dula 1994; Lollis et al. 1996; Nyamathi et al. 1993).

Although programs to reduce the spread of HIV infection have helped, they can be made more effective by making sure to provide information about HIV transmission and prevention, use techniques to enhance people's motivation to avoid unsafe sex, and teach the skills needed to perform preventive acts (Fisher et al. 1996). Some ways to incorporate these features include:

- tailoring the program to meet the needs of the sociocultural group being addressed (Kalichman et al. 1993)
- giving strong emphasis to training the actual skills individuals will need to resist having unsafe sex (Kalichman, Rompa & Coley 1996; St. Lawrence, Brasfield et al. 1995; St. Lawrence, Jefferson et al. 1995).
- making sure the training is geared towards bolstering self-efficacy and advancing the individuals through the stages of change (Galavotti et al. 1995)
- making use of popular individuals as leaders to endorse the program's information and training and promote its acceptance by the group being addressed (Kelly et al. 1992).

Although more needs to be done in gay urban communities in Australia, efforts must be sharply intensified in the general population — especially among adolescents and minority groups (Coates 1990; Mays & Cochran 1988; Peterson & Marín 1988).

Summary

People's behaviour has an important impact on their health. Mortality from today's leading causes of death could be markedly reduced if people would adopt a few health-protective behaviours, such as not smoking, not drinking excessively, eating healthy diets and exercising regularly. Although some individuals are fairly consistent in their practice of health-related behaviours, these behaviours can be quite changeable over time, and practising one habit is not strongly related to practising other habits. A person's practice of health-protective behaviours does not seem to be governed by a single set of attitudes or response tendencies. Health-related behaviours that become well established tend to become habitual or automatically performed.

Health problems can be averted through three levels of prevention, one of which applies before a disease or injury occurs. Each level can involve efforts by the individual and by his or her social network, doctor, and other health professionals. Primary prevention consists of actions taken to avoid illness or injury. It can include public service announcements, genetic counselling and a wide variety of health behaviours, such as using seatbelts and performing breast or testicular self-examinations. Secondary prevention involves actions taken to identify and stop or reverse a health problem. It includes tests and treatments health professionals may conduct, as well as illness and sick-role behaviours, such as visiting a doctor when ill and taking medication as prescribed. Tertiary prevention consists of actions taken to contain or retard damage from a serious injury or advanced disease, prevent disability and rehabilitate the patient.

People acquire health-related behaviours through modelling and through operant conditioning, whereby behaviour changes because of its consequences: reinforcement, extinction and punishment. Other determinants of these behaviours include genetic, social, emotional and cognitive factors. Errors in people's perceived symptoms and ideas they have about illnesses can lead to health problems. People's thinking about health and illness is not always logical — it often includes motivated reasoning and unrealistic optimism about their health.

Some theories focus on the role of health beliefs to account for people's performance of health-related behaviour. The health belief model proposes that people take preventive action on the basis of their assessments of the threat of a health problem and the pros and cons of taking the action. The perception of threat is based mainly on the perceived seriousness of and susceptibility to the health problem. Assessing the pros and cons of the action involves weighing its perceived benefits and barriers. These assessments combine to determine the likelihood of preventive action. The theory of reasoned action proposes that people's health-related behaviours are determined by their intentions, which are a function of their attitudes regarding the behaviours (for example, 'Is it a good thing to do?') and their subjective norms. Modifications have been made to the theory of reasoned action to include the influence of perceived behavioural control, the new theory being labelled the theory of planned behaviour. Extensions to both theories in relation to predicting safer sexual behaviour have been made by Australian researchers. The stages of change model emphasises people's readiness to modify their behaviour, and other approaches include an emphasis on the role of stress (conflict theory) and on the role of personal control.

People's age, sex and sociocultural background also affect health-related behaviour and need to be considered in programs for health promotion. Methods for promoting health include fear-arousing warnings, providing information and behavioural approaches. The PRECEDE/PROCEED model offers useful guidelines for planning, implementing and evaluating health promotion programs. Programs for health promotion can be effective in the schools and in work sites. Community-wide wellness programs are designed to reach large numbers of people and improve their knowledge and practice of preventive behaviour. The SunSmart program demonstrated that media campaigns can promote health, and subsequent research has also integrated extensive efforts by community organisations towards improving people's preventive actions, for example in the control of smoking and in stemming the spread of AIDS.

Key terms

conflict theory	health-protective behaviour	primary prevention	stages of change model
extinction	illness behaviour	process evaluation	subjective norm
genetic counselling	impact evaluation	punishment	tertiary prevention
group norm	motivated reasoning	reinforcement	theory of planned behaviour
health behaviour	outcome evaluation	secondary prevention	theory of reasoned action
health belief model	PRECEDE/PROCEED model	sick-role behaviour	

7 Reducing substance use and abuse

Prologue

The stakes were high when Graham signed an agreement to quit smoking for a year beginning on January 2. The contract was with a community health program. For each cigarette Graham smoked, he agreed to give $25 to charity, with a maximum of $100 dollars for any day. Graham knew stopping smoking would not be easy for him — he had smoked more than a pack a day for the last 20 years, and he had tried to quit a couple of times before. The contract could have required that he submit to medical tests to verify that he did in fact abstain, but the health psychologist was willing to trust his word and that of his family, friends and co-workers. These people were committed to helping him quit, and they agreed to be contacted by someone from the program weekly and give honest reports. Did he succeed? Yes, but he had a few lapses — that cost him $325. By the end of the year, Graham had not smoked for 8 months continuously.

People voluntarily use many different substances that can harm their health. This chapter focuses on people's use of three of the most common of these substances: tobacco, alcohol and drugs. For each substance, we examine who uses it and why, how the substance can affect health, and what can be done to help prevent people from using it and abusing it once they start. And we address questions of concern to people who want to enhance their own and others' health. Do people smoke tobacco, drink alcohol and use drugs more than in the past? Why do people start to smoke, drink excessively or use drugs? Why is it so difficult to quit these behaviours? If individuals succeed in stopping smoking, will they gain weight?

Substance abuse

'I just can't get started in the morning without a cup of coffee and a cigarette — I must be addicted,' you may have heard someone say. The term *addicted* used to have a very limited meaning, referring mainly to the excessive use of alcohol and drugs. It was common knowledge that these chemical substances have *psychoactive effects*: they alter the person's mood, cognition or behaviour. But we now know that other substances, such as nicotine and caffeine, have psychoactive effects, too — and people are commonly said to be 'addicted' also to eating, gambling, buying and many other things. How shall we define addiction?

Addiction is a condition, produced by repeated consumption of a natural or synthetic substance, in which the person has become physically and psychologically dependent on the substance. **Physical dependence** is a state in which the body has adjusted to a substance and incorporated it into the 'normal' functioning of the body's tissues. This state has two characteristics.

- **Tolerance** is the process by which the body increasingly adapts to a substance and requires larger and larger doses of it to achieve the same effect. At some point these increases reach a plateau.
- **Withdrawal** refers to unpleasant physical and psychological symptoms people experience when they discontinue using a substance on which the body has become physically dependent. The symptoms experienced depend on the particular substance used, and can include anxiety, irritability, intense cravings for the substance, hallucinations, nausea, headache and tremors.

Different substances appear to have different degrees of *potential* for producing physical dependence: the potential is very high for heroin but appears to be lower for other substances, such as LSD (Schuster & Kilbey 1992; Winger, Hofmann & Woods 1992).

Psychological dependence is a state in which individuals feel a compulsion to use a substance for the pleasant effect it produces, without necessarily being physically dependent on it. They rely heavily on it — often to help them adjust to life and feel good — and they centre many activities on obtaining and using it. People learn to depend on substances through repeated use. Individuals who become addicted to alcohol first become psychologically dependent on it; later they become physically dependent as their bodies develop a tolerance for it. The potential for producing psychological dependence differs from one substance to another — it seems to be high for heroin and cocaine and low for LSD (Schuster & Kilbey 1992).

Whether a person is *abusing*, or overusing, such substances as tobacco, alcohol and drugs depends on the extent and impact of the use. Psychiatrists and clinical psychologists are concerned primarily with the psychosocial functioning of the person. They diagnose **substance abuse** on the basis of two criteria (Davison & Neale 1994). First, the person shows a *clear and persistent pattern of pathological use*, such as heavy daily use and an inability to stop or decrease using the substance. Second, the *abuse has produced at least one of the following* problems:

- failing to fulfil important obligations, such as in repeatedly neglecting a child or being absent from work
- putting oneself or others at risk for physical injury, for instance by driving while intoxicated
- having legal difficulties, such as being arrested for disorderly conduct
- having serious social or interpersonal problems, for instance repeated arguments with family or co-workers.

These four problems clearly apply to alcohol and drug use, and not to tobacco use.

Psychologists in general share a concern about people's psychosocial functioning, but health psychologists give special emphasis to the impact of substance use on illness and injury. As a result, we might want to add the issue of increased risk factors for illness to the second problem, which would then read: 'putting oneself or others at risk for physical injury *or for illness* ...'. Individuals who meet the criteria, as revised, would be considered 'substance abusers' from a health psychology point of view. Smoking cigarettes on a regular basis would qualify as abuse.

Smoking tobacco

When Columbus explored the Western Hemisphere, he recorded in his journal that the inhabitants would set fire to leaves — rolled up or in pipes — and draw in the smoke through their mouths (Aston & Stepney 1982). The leaves these people used were tobacco of course. Other early explorers tried smoking and in the early 1500s, probably because they liked it, took tobacco leaves back to Europe, where tobacco was used mainly for 'medicinal purposes'. Smoking for pleasure spread among American colonists and in Europe later in that century. In the 1600s, pipe smoking became popular, and the French introduced *snuff*, powdered tobacco that people consumed chiefly by inserting it in the nose and sniffing strongly. Upper-class males and females used snuff. In the late eighteenth century, cigar smoking, and later cigarette smoking, were introduced to England from officers who had acquired a taste for these during their war experiences in Spain and Turkey. By this stage pipe smoking was considered ungentlemanly, although the practice of smoking pipes was common among working men.

The values and habits of the upper classes in England served as a model for the early colonists in Australia. Women tended not to smoke unless they were convicts.

Much of the tobacco in the early colonial days was brought in as cargo on convict ships calling in at Rio de Janeiro on the voyage to Botany Bay. With the introduction of import duty and excise tax, in the early 1800s, preference changed to smoking a cheaper colonial leaf. Tobacco was cultivated in penal settlements, until this was banned in 1829, leaving cultivation and manufacture of tobacco to individual land-owners. Before British settlement, Aboriginal peoples in certain areas of Australia sucked or chewed the leaves of native plants containing nicotine. Leaves were dried, roasted and packed in string bags for easy trading. In Arnhem Land the practice of smoking (usually a dry porous root) had been introduced by Macassan visitors before European settlement. Aborigines, however, developed a liking for the white man's tobacco. Missionaries, pastoralists and landowners often used tobacco as an induce-ment or gift for Aborigines attending mass, acting as guides or working on their prop-erties. In the early 1900s inventors made a machine for mass-producing cigarettes, and growers developed mellower tobacco for easier inhaling. As a result, the popu-larity of smoking grew rapidly in Australia over the next 50 years. By the mid-1950s, American and British tobacco companies had established factories in Australia for the manufacture of cigarettes (Walker 1984).

Cigarette smoking reached its greatest popularity in Australia in the mid-1960s, when about 58 per cent of adult males and 28 per cent of adult females smoked regu-larly (Walker 1984). Before that time, people generally didn't know about the serious health effects of smoking. The Australian National Health and Medical Research Council had made recommendations to the government in 1962 for a prohibition of tobacco advertising, and for an official statement that cigarette smoking contributed to lung cancer. These recommendations were reinforced in 1964 by a report from the Surgeon General of the United States linking cigarette smoking with lung cancer, chronic bronchitis and cardiovascular disease. However, it was not until 1972 that health warnings appeared on cigarette packages, and cigarette advertising was phased out within the next four years (Winstanley & Woodward 1992). Since that time the prevalence of adult smokers has dropped steadily, and today about 27 per cent of men and 20 per cent of women in Australia smoke (AIHW 2000).

Do these trends mean cigarette manufacturers are on the verge of bankruptcy? Not at all — their profits are still quite high! In Australia, there are still about 3.2 million smokers, the retail price of cigarettes has increased and manufacturers have sharply increased sales to foreign countries. At the same time that smoking has declined in many industrialised countries, it has been increasing in developing nations, such as in Asia and Africa (Fiore, Newcomb & McBride 1993; Jones 1991).

Who smokes?

Although many Australians smoke, a substantial number do not. Forty per cent of men and 57 per cent of women report having never smoked (AIHW 1999c). Are some people more likely to smoke than others?

Age and gender differences in smoking

Smoking habits vary with age. Very few individuals in Australia begin to smoke regularly before 15 years of age, though children as young as nine years of age experiment with cigarettes (Glicksman et al. 1989). The habit generally develops gradually, and several years may pass before an individual's rate of smoking reaches its eventual adult level (Pechacek et al. 1984). Since 1984 the Centre for Behavioural Research in Cancer has conducted a series of triennial surveys on the use of tobacco by Australian youth. For

12- to 15-year-olds, there has been little change in involvement with tobacco from 1993 to 1996, although smoking has increased since 1987 (Hill, White & Letcher 1999). The proportion of current smokers (those who have smoked in the last week) among 16- and 17-year-olds was greater in 1996 than in 1987 or 1990 (Hill, White & Letcher 1999). The percentage of adults in the population who smoke reaches its highest level among individuals between 25 and 34 years of age, with 34 per cent of men and 28 per cent of women in this age group being smokers, and declines among older individuals (AIHW 2000). Many people stop smoking in adulthood. About 32 per cent of the men and 23 per cent of the women in Australia today are former smokers (AIHW 2000).

We have mentioned gender differences in smoking, and these differences are significant. Before the 1970s the prevalence of smoking among Australian males had always been far greater than that among females, but this gender gap has narrowed considerably for two reasons (McGinnis, Shopland & Brown 1987). First, much larger numbers of men than women stopped smoking after starting. Second, although the number of individuals who started smoking has declined, the percentage of male smokers decreased by more than half between 1950 and 1986, while the percentage of female smokers remained relatively constant at around 30 per cent, dropping to 25 per cent in 1989, with only small decreases up to the present time (AIHW 1998, 2000; Mattick & Baillie 1992; Walker 1984). Gender differences in the smoking behaviour of Australian youth over time indicates that a decade ago more boys than girls aged 9–10 years had smoked at least one cigarette in the previous week (Glicksman et al. 1989), although these gender differences appear to have equalised by age 12, in 1996 (Hill, White & Letcher 1999). However, the gender trend is reversed in later adolescence, with more females than males reporting smoking (Byrne, Byrne & Reinhart 1993; Hill et al. 1987; Hill, White & Letcher 1999). There is a similar trend in the United States, where the percentage of high-school senior girls who smoke daily has exceeded that of boys (Johnston, O'Malley & Bachman 1995). Cigarette advertising targeted at one gender or the other, such as by creating clever brand names and slogans, played a major part in these gender-related shifts in smoking (Pierce & Gilpin 1995). Here is a slogan designed to induce young females to smoke.

> 'You've come a long way, baby,' with its strong but still subtle appeal to the women's liberation movement. The 'Virginia Slims' brand name artfully takes advantage of the increasingly well-documented research finding that, for many female (and male) smokers, quitting the habit is associated with gaining weight. (Matarazzo 1982, p. 6)

Trends in smoking are projected to change in the future. While the prevalence of smoking in 1992 was higher for Australian males than females, it is estimated that from the year 2001 there will be more female smokers than male smokers (Hill & White 1995). There is an important and hopeful point to keep in mind about the changes we have described in smoking behaviour: they demonstrate that people can be persuaded to avoid or quit smoking.

Sociocultural differences in smoking

Sociocultural factors are also associated with smoking (McGinnis, Shopland & Brown 1987; AIHW 1998). In Australia smoking prevalence is twice as high in indigenous people (47 per cent) than in other Australians (23 per cent) (AIHW 1998). Differences in smoking rates are also related to social class. The percentage of people who smoke tends to decline with increases in education, income and job prestige. Thus, the highest rates of smoking are likely to be found among adults who did not complete high school, have low incomes and have blue-collar occupations, such as carpentry, maintenance work and truck driving. In general, racial and social class differences in smoking are more pronounced among males than among females.

How much smokers smoke

Australians spend millions of dollars each year on cigarettes. You may be wondering why the cost of tobacco use is so high, if the number of Australians who smoke has decreased over time. Part of the answer lies in the increased cost of a packet of cigarettes to the smoker. But we also need to examine trends in the percentage of smokers who smoke infrequently, those who smoke between one and 20 cigarettes per day and those who smoke more than 20 cigarettes per day. Between 1985 and 1995 the percentage of infrequent smokers (those who do not smoke daily) has remained constant at around 2 per cent. For those who smoke between one and 20 cigarettes, the most notable change has been for smokers who smoke between 16 and 20 cigarettes daily. In the 10 years to 1995 the proportion of these smokers declined from 8 to 5 per cent. For the group of smokers who smoke more than 20 cigarettes per day, there has been a decrease from 11 per cent in 1985 to 8 per cent in 1995. When these figures are taken into account, the overall reduction in the average number of cigarettes smoked daily over the 10-year period has been minimal, from 18 to 17 cigarettes (Makkai & McAllister 1998). The decline in smoking has been greater in males than females in the heaviest smoking categories. While reductions in smoking for heavy smokers have occurred for those aged between 20 and 29 years, middle-aged smokers (40- to 59-year-olds) have not changed tobacco usage. What this means, of course, is that the people who continue to smoke today are the ones who most need to quit.

Why people smoke

Cigarette smoking is a strange phenomenon in some respects. If you ever tried to smoke, chances are you coughed the first time or two, found the taste unpleasant and, perhaps, even experienced nausea. This is not the kind of outcome that usually makes people want to try something again. But many teenagers do, even though they know that smoking is harmful to people's health (Johnston, O'Malley & Bachman 1995). Given these circumstances, we might wonder why people start to smoke and why they continue.

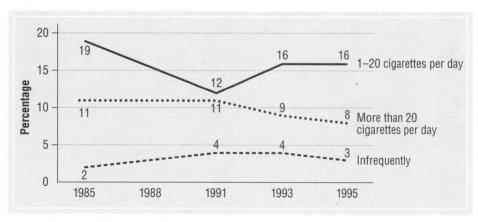

Figure 7.1 Levels of tobacco use, 1985–95

Sources: Makkai & McAllister (1998, figure 1.4); data from 1985–95 NDS surveys.

Starting to smoke

Smoking usually starts during the teenage years, and psychosocial factors provide the primary forces that lead adolescents to begin. Several aspects of the social environment are influential in shaping teenagers' attitudes, beliefs and intentions about smoking. For instance, studies have found that adolescents are more likely to begin smoking if their parents, siblings and friends smoke (Byrne, Byrne & Reinhart 1993; McInman & Grove 1991; Quine & Stephenson 1990). In a longitudinal study of the influence of parents and peers on the initiation of smoking in children, Stanton and Silva (1992) found that smoking status at age 15 was more likely to be correctly classified using a statistical technique called discriminant analysis, if a parent started or resumed smoking when the child was 13. At earlier ages, namely 7–9 years, correct classification was more likely if parents did not smoke. The influence of peers began around age 11 and was most evident at age 13. When teens try their first cigarette, they typically smoke it in the company of peers, and with the peers' encouragement (Leventhal, Prohaska & Hirschman 1985). These findings suggest that modelling and peer pressure are important determinants of smoking.

Personal motivations for smoking help explain why adolescents begin smoking and why they may not heed health warnings. Research on Australian adolescents (Ho 1994) has found that the reasons for smoking can be classified on the basis of *social acceptance* ('Smoking allows me to be part of a crowd'), *pleasure* ('I find smoking enjoyable') and *addiction/habitual needs* ('I smoke because I am addicted to cigarettes'). Female adolescents who smoked for pleasure tended to perceive health warnings as not effective in deterring people from smoking, did not believe that the warnings would influence them personally to give up smoking, or that smoking would lead to increased risk of health problems. For male adolescents, the addiction motive influenced the perceived deterrent effectiveness of cigarette health warnings. The more addicted adolescent males perceived themselves to be, the less effective they believed the health warnings to be in deterring people in general, or themselves, to quit and the less likely they were to believe that smoking caused health problems. Other research by Stanton et al. (1993) has found adolescent smokers to give relaxation/pleasure, friends and image as reasons for smoking.

Adolescents at different stages of the acquisition of smoking behaviour also have different perceptions of risk associated with smoking (Virgili, Owen & Severson 1991). Current smokers perceived less personal risk associated with cigarette smoking than did experimenters, ex-smokers and never-smokers. Experimenters perceived themselves to be at less personal risk of illness, compared with the never-smokers and ex-smokers. This led Virgili, Owen & Severson (1991) to suggest that

> those who have never smoked, but who hold 'smokerlike' beliefs about personal risk and avoidability may be the individuals who are most likely to go on to become smokers, whereas current smokers who hold 'nonsmokerlike beliefs' may be those most likely to be nonsmokers in the future. (p. 321)

Personal characteristics, such as being rebellious and a risk-taker, seem to influence whether adolescents begin to smoke (Conrad, Flay & Hill 1992; Lipkus et al. 1994). As Leventhal and Cleary have suggested, teenagers

> who are less successful in school ... more rebellious, and doing less well in meeting expectations of parents and traditional authorities ... are more likely to be attracted to smoking at an early age and begin using cigarettes as a means of defining themselves as tough, cool, and independent of authority. (1980, p. 384)

Other personal characteristics distinguish Australian adolescents who begin to smoke from those who do not. Longitudinal research by Winefield et al. (1989) found feelings of hopelessness to precede smoking initiation in 19-year-olds. Smokers were also characterised by an external locus of control. Heaven (1989) reported regular adolescent smokers to be more tough-minded and male smokers to possess the characteristic more so than female smokers. Findings from a large representative sample of Australian adolescents (Byrne, Byrne & Reinhart 1993) linked neuroticism and low self-esteem with smoking. Adolescent non-smokers generally have a more positive self-concept than smokers (McInman & Grove 1991).

Social factors influence smoking in adolescents. In the study by Byrne, Byrne and Reinhart (1993) boys were more likely to smoke if the father's occupation was of low status. Also, their decisions to smoke in the future were influenced by teacher role models who smoked. For girls, smoking was more likely if the mother smoked, school performance was poor or there was a concern with self-presentation — for example, perceived body weight was high.

The 'smoker's image' also seems to be important. Studies have found that boys and girls between the ages of 11 and 15 often associate smoking with being attractive to and interested in the opposite sex, looking mature, and being 'glamorous' and 'exciting' (Barton et al. 1982; Dinh et al. 1995). This is reinforced by research which has found that adolescent smokers tend to have a more positive opposite sex self-concept (McInman & Grove 1991). Smoking appears to provide them with feelings of sexual competence. Social images, models and peer pressure are not easily overlooked by teenagers, who are very concerned with how they are viewed by others.

Becoming a regular smoker

There is a rule of thumb about beginning to smoke that seems to have some validity: individuals who smoke their *fourth* cigarette are very likely to become regular smokers (Leventhal & Cleary 1980). Although the vast majority of youngsters try at least one cigarette, most of them never get to the fourth one and don't go on to smoke regularly. Becoming a habitual smoker often develops slowly, sometimes taking a year or more (Ary & Biglan 1988).

Why is it that some people continue smoking after the first tries, and others don't? Part of the answer lies in the psychosocial influences that got them to start in the first place. Two longitudinal studies examined the role of psychosocial factors in the development of smoking by having thousands of adolescents fill out questionnaires in at least two different years (Chassin et al. 1991; Murray et al. 1983). The responses for the different years were then examined to determine whether the subjects' social environments and beliefs about smoking were related to changes in their smoking behaviour. Smoking tended to continue or increase if the subjects:

- had at least one parent who smoked
- perceived their parents as unconcerned or even encouraging about their smoking
- had siblings or friends who smoked
- socialised with friends very often
- felt peer pressure to smoke — for example reporting, 'Others make fun of you if you don't smoke,' and, 'You have to smoke when you're with friends who smoke.'
- held positive attitudes about smoking, such as, 'Smoking is very enjoyable,' and, 'Smoking can help people when they feel nervous or embarrassed.'
- did not believe smoking would harm their health — for instance feeling, 'Smoking is dangerous only to older people,' and, 'Smoking is only bad for you if you have been smoking for many years.'

Other research has shown that teenagers usually smoke in the presence of other people, especially peers, and that smokers consume more cigarettes when in the company of someone who smokes at a high rate rather than a low rate (Antonuccio & Lichtenstein 1980; Biglan et al. 1984). Adolescents who smoke also receive many more offers of cigarettes from friends than non-smokers do (Ary & Biglan 1988).

Psychologist Silvan Tomkins (1966, 1968) has outlined four psychological reasons why people who begin to smoke on a regular basis continue to smoke. One reason focuses on achieving a *positive affect* — smoking for stimulation, relaxation or pleasure. Another reason centres on reducing *negative affect*, such as to relieve anxiety or tension. The third explanation is that smoking may become a *habitual* or automatic behaviour that the person performs without awareness. Fourth, a person may develop a *psychological dependence* (which he called 'addiction') on smoking to regulate positive and negative emotional states. According to Tomkins, one or another of these reasons is the chief controlling factor in a particular person's smoking behaviour. As a result, the person can be categorised as a 'positive affect smoker' or a 'habitual smoker', and so on.

Australian research by Ho (1989) has identified four motives for smoking in the adult population. One motive was *social acceptance* (e.g. 'I smoke because most of my friends smoke'). Another reason for smoking was *addiction/habitual needs* ('I smoke because I find it difficult to quit', 'Lighting up a cigarette is a habit to me'). The third motive identified was *pleasure* ('I enjoy the taste of cigarettes'), while the fourth motive was *boredom* ('Smoking gives me something to do with my hands', 'Smoking gives me a lift'). Males and females smoked for similar reasons. The motives for smoking predicted current smokers' perceptions of difficulty in quitting. The more smokers perceived themselves as addicted, the more difficult they thought it would be to quit the habit. Males who smoked for pleasure believed that it would be difficult to stop smoking.

Findings of other research also indicate that people use smoking as a means of coping with stress. One study found that smoking among young adolescents is related to the amount of stress in their lives — the greater the stress, the more likely they are to smoke (Wills 1986). Another study found that adult smokers reported less anxiety and greater effectiveness in expressing their opinions if they smoked during stressful social interactions than if they did not smoke (Gilbert & Spielberger 1987). But this does not mean that smoking is a 'good' way to relax and reduce tension. Although smokers often perform better and feel more relaxed in stressful situations when they are allowed to smoke than when they are not, some evidence indicates that they do not perform better or feel more relaxed than non-smokers do (Schachter 1980).

In addition to personal motivations for smoking, the belief that an individual will not be negatively affected by smoking, despite knowing that smoking carries negative effects, serves to maintain the habit. Such beliefs are called self-exempting beliefs. Chapman, Leng Wong and Smith (1993) found that five beliefs distinguish smokers from non-smokers.

1. Most lung cancer is caused by air pollution and petrol fumes.
2. Cigarette smoking is not an important enough health hazard for the government to do something about it.
3. The medical evidence that smoking causes cancer is not convincing.
4. Most people smoke.
5. It's safe to smoke low-tar cigarettes.

These self-exempting beliefs were the same for smokers at each stage of behaviour change. As we saw in chapter 6, these stages are precontemplation, contemplation, preparation, action and maintenance. Self-exempting beliefs were only discarded when the smoker quit smoking.

Smokers may distort the health risk to themselves of continued smoking as evidenced by perceptions of personal invulnerability to the harmful effects of their smoking. Lee (1989) found that while smokers accepted their own risk to be higher than that of non-smokers for lung cancer, heart disease and chronic lung diseases such as emphysema or bronchitis, they tended to minimise the risk of disease for the average smoker, and for themselves compared with the average Australian smoker. In a large-scale study of 3000 patients who had seen a doctor at one of 12 participating medical practices, individual perceptions of risk for lung cancer, heart attack and stroke were compared for smokers and non-smokers against actual risk (Strecher, Kreuter & Kobrin 1995). Smokers were found to have optimistically distorted perceptions of risk for all diseases, and in particular in relation to cancer.

Biological factors are also involved in sustaining smoking behaviour. The fact that adolescent smoking is strongly associated with parental and sibling smoking shows that smoking runs in families. Certainly, part of this relationship results from social learning processes. And some evidence suggests that nicotine passed on by a smoking mother to her baby in pregnancy may make the child more susceptible to the addictive effects of nicotine (Kandel, Wu & Davies 1994). Does heredity also play a role? Twin and adoption studies have demonstrated that genetic factors influence people's acquisition and maintenance of smoking (Hughes 1986). Although researchers do not yet have a clear picture of the specific ways heredity influences smoking, tentative evidence suggests three possible pathways. First, genetic factors may underlie certain personality traits, such as rebelliousness, that are associated with smoking. Second, heredity may influence the degree to which a person finds tobacco pleasant or unpleasant. Third, genetic factors may affect how easily and strongly a person becomes physically dependent on tobacco (Pomerleau et al. 1993). As people become regular smokers, they generally show the phenomenon of tolerance, using increasing amounts of tobacco; and if smokers try to quit, they often suffer withdrawal symptoms, such as irritability and difficulty concentrating (Jarvik & Henningfield 1993; Jones 1991).

The role of nicotine

People become physically dependent on tobacco because of the chemical substances their bodies take in when they use it. A person who smokes a pack a day takes more than 50 000 puffs a year, with each puff delivering a wide assortment of chemicals into the lungs and bloodstream (Pechacek et al. 1984). These chemicals include carbon monoxide, tars and nicotine. Cigarette smoke has high concentrations of **carbon monoxide**, a gas that is readily absorbed by the bloodstream and rapidly affects the person's physiological functioning, such as by reducing the oxygen-carrying capacity of the blood. It is possible that these physiological changes influence whether people like or dislike smoking. **Tars** exist as minute particles of residue, suspended in smoke. Although tars have important health effects, there is no evidence that they affect people's desire to smoke. **Nicotine** appears to be the addictive chemical in cigarette smoke and clearly produces rapid and powerful physiological effects.

Nicotine is a substance that occurs only in tobacco. When a person smokes, nicotine penetrates cell membranes of the mouth and nose on the way to the lungs, where alveoli quickly absorb it and transmit it to the blood (Henningfield, Cohen & Pickworth 1993; Jones 1991; Pechacek et al. 1984). In a matter of seconds the blood carries the nicotine to the brain, where it triggers the release of various chemicals that activate both the central and sympathetic nervous systems. One effect of these changes is to arouse the body, increasing the person's alertness, heart rate and blood pressure. While the person is smoking a cigarette, nicotine accumulates very rapidly in the blood. But it soon decreases through metabolism — in about two hours, half of the nicotine inhaled from a cigarette has decayed.

Biological explanations of people's continued cigarette smoking have focused chiefly on the role of nicotine. One prominent explanation, called the **nicotine regulation model**, is based on the addictive quality of nicotine. According to this model, established smokers continue to smoke to maintain a certain level of nicotine in their bodies and to avoid withdrawal symptoms. Stanley Schachter and his associates (1977) conducted an ingenious series of studies with adult smokers that provides evidence for this model. In one study, the researchers had subjects smoke low-nicotine cigarettes during one week and high-nicotine cigarettes during another week. As the model predicts, the subjects smoked more low- than high-nicotine cigarettes. This effect was especially strong for heavy smokers, who smoked 25 per cent more of the low- than high-nicotine cigarettes. Consistent with these results, other researchers have found that people who regularly smoke ultra-low-nicotine cigarettes do not consume less nicotine than those who smoke other cigarettes — ultra-low smokers simply smoke more cigarettes (Maron & Fortmann 1987).

Although the nicotine regulation model has received research support, there are reasons to think it provides only part of the explanation for people's smoking behaviour (Leventhal & Cleary 1980). One reason is that people who quit smoking typically continue to crave it, and often return to smoking, long after all the nicotine is gone from their bodies. Another reason is that some people who smoke regularly for years don't become addicted. These people smoke a few cigarettes a day, don't show the tolerance and withdrawal characteristics of addiction, and absorb as much nicotine from a cigarette as heavier smokers do (Shiffman et al. 1990; Shiffman et al. 1995). Why do people who smoke regularly but who don't become addicted continue to smoke? One explanation may be that nicotine has direct reinforcing effects.

The **biobehavioural model** of Ovide and Cynthia Pomerleau (1989) proposes that people continue to smoke and often have a hard time quitting because they use and come to depend on the effects of nicotine to regulate their cognitive and emotional states. As we saw earlier, nicotine quickly reaches the brain and triggers the release of chemicals that activate body systems. These chemicals include *acetylcholine* and *norepinephrine*, which, independent of smoking, do two things: they (1) *increase* alertness, concentration, memory and feelings of pleasure and (2) *decrease* symptoms of nicotine withdrawal and feelings of anxiety, tension and pain. These very desirable, reinforcing effects begin very soon after the first puff of a cigarette and are temporary (McGehee et al. 1995). According to the biobehavioural model, smokers learn to use nicotine to supplement or fine-tune the other coping processes they use to regulate these states. Habitual smokers have trouble quitting partly because they have come to rely on nicotine to help them cope.

Researchers today generally recognise that a complete explanation of the development and maintenance of smoking behaviour involves the interplay of biological, psychological and social factors (Fisher, Lichtenstein & Haire-Joshu 1993; Galizio & Maisto 1985).

Smoking and health

Australian cigarette packs are required to carry health warnings such as 'Smoking causes lung cancer', 'Smoking damages your lungs', 'Smoking causes heart disease' and 'Smoking reduces your fitness'. Smoking-related illness results in about 18 000 deaths (AIHW 1998) and costs millions of dollars in health care costs each year in Australia (ACIL 1994). Smoking reduces people's life expectancy by several years and increases their risk of many illnesses, particularly cancer and cardiovascular diseases (Thun et al. 1995). No other single behaviour takes such a toll. To what extent do your odds of dying of lung cancer or heart disease increase if you smoke? Figure 7.2 shows that the odds increase greatly, especially for lung cancer (Mattson, Pollack & Cullen 1987). The more you smoke, the worse your odds become — and if you quit, your odds improve steadily, in 15 or 20 years becoming similar to those of people who never smoked (LaCroix et al. 1991; Ockene et al. 1990).

Cancer

In the late 1930s two important studies were done that clearly linked smoking and cancer for the first time (Ashton & Stepney 1982). One study presented statistics showing that non-smokers live longer than smokers. In the other study, researchers produced cancer in laboratory animals by administering cigarette tar. By producing cancer with experimental methods, these researchers demonstrated a causal link between cancer and a chemical in tobacco smoke and identified tar as a likely *carcinogen*. Today the evidence is overwhelming that tobacco tars and probably other by-products of tobacco smoke cause cancer (Denissenko et al. 1996).

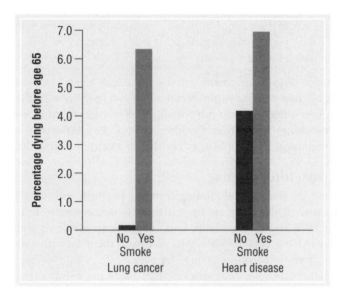

Figure 7.2 Probability of a 35-year-old man dying of lung cancer or heart disease before the age of 65 as a function of smoking heavily or not smoking. Data for women were less complete but probably would reveal similar risk increases.

Source: Data from Mattson, Pollack & Cullen (1987, p. 427).

Hundreds of retrospective and prospective studies have consistently demonstrated the link between tobacco use and cancer in humans. Prospective research provides strong evidence for a causal relationship because the subjects are identified as smokers or non-smokers and then followed over a long period of time to see if they develop cancer. Many large-scale prospective studies have linked smoking with cancers of various body sites, including the lung, mouth, oesophagus, bladder and kidney (Levy 1985; Shopland & Burns 1993). The latter two may result because carcinogenic chemicals in tobacco smoke are absorbed into the blood and conveyed to the urine. Cancers of the mouth and oesophagus can also result from using smokeless tobacco — chewing tobacco or snuff (Severson 1993). Thus, carcinogenic substances exist not only in smoke, but in tobacco products themselves.

Smoking accounts for 30 per cent of all cancer deaths in Australia (AIHW 2000, 1996). As recently as the 1950s, lung cancer in Australia was less prevalent than many other forms of cancer, such as cancer of the breast, stomach and colon (Giles,

Thursfield & Staples 1994). Over the years, the mortality rates for most forms of cancer have either declined or remained fairly constant, but not for lung cancer. For males, the annual death rate for lung cancer increased steadily over time, until 1982 when the death rate began to decline from around 69 per 100 000 to 55 per 100 000 in 1998 (AIHW 2000). For females, the death rate from lung cancer has increased gradually over time, reaching 19 per 100 000 in 1998 (AIHW 2000). Lung cancer is almost three times higher in males than females. The gender difference in mortality from lung cancer over time can be explained by the greater number of male than female smokers, and by the decline in the number of males smoking since the 1970s compared with the relatively stable smoking rates for women, with the exception of increased smoking by younger women. Lung cancer claimed close to 7000 Australians in 1998, with about 80 per cent of these deaths being attributed to smoking (AIHW 2000).

How does smoking harm the lungs? When smoke recurrently passes through the bronchial tubes, the lining of the tubes begins to react to the irritation by increasing the number of cells just below the surface. Then,

> the fine, hairlike growths, or cilia, along the surface of the lining, whose function is to clear the lungs of foreign particles, begin to slow or stop their movement. In time, the cilia may disappear altogether, and as a consequence carcinogenic substances remain in contact with sensitive cells in the lining of the bronchi instead of being removed in the mucus ... At this stage, a *smoker's cough* may develop. It is a feeble attempt by the body to clear the lungs of foreign particles in the absence of functioning cilia. (La Place 1984, p. 326)

Lung cancer usually originates in the bronchial tubes. In most cases, it probably develops because of the continual contact of carcinogens with the bronchial lining.

Smoking is a major risk factor for all forms of cancer, but its role is more direct and powerful in lung cancer than in other cancers. People's environments contain many other carcinogens, and smoking is not the only cause of these diseases.

Cardiovascular disease

Cardiovascular disease — including coronary heart disease (CHD) and stroke — is the leading cause of death by far in Australia. It was responsible for 40 per cent of all deaths in 1998 and claimed more lives than cancer, accidents and several other causes combined (AIHW 2000). When you point out these facts to some smokers, they say, 'Well you have to die of *something*.' Of course, that's true — but *when* you will die is the real issue. Cardiovascular disease takes many male lives early.

Many Australians suffer from CHD and stroke. The risk of having a heart attack is about twice as high for smokers as for non-smokers (AIHW 1998). A prospective study examined the impact of smoking on the incidence of CHD across $8\frac{1}{2}$ years (Rosenman et al. 1976). More than 3000 men participated in the research, beginning when they were 39 to 59 years of age. Compared with non-smokers, the incidence of CHD was more than 50 per cent higher for men who smoked about a pack a day and more than twice as high for those who smoked more than a pack a day. These higher risks for smokers also depend on, or interact with, several other factors (Epstein & Jennings 1986; Khaw & Barrett-Connor 1986; Perkins 1985). In general, the risks that smoking presents for developing CHD are especially strong for people who:
- are males
- are 45 to 55 years of age, rather than older
- have a family history of heart disease
- have high levels of cholesterol in their blood
- have high blood pressure.

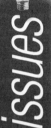

Highlight on issues

Does someone else's smoking affect your health?

Wayne had been a smoker for 25 years, when smoking regulations came into effect. He couldn't smoke in government buildings or while commuting to work. Even now it annoyed him that he had to go outside at work to have a cigarette. It seemed that he craved a cigarette more when being prevented from smoking, especially with all those 'No Smoking' signs everywhere. Why were these regulations introduced?

Not all tobacco smoke goes into the smoker's body, and much of what does comes back out. All this excess smoke gets into the environment for others to consume and is called *second-hand smoke* or *environmental tobacco smoke*. Breathing second-hand smoke is called **passive smoking** or involuntary smoking. In the mid-1980s the United States Surgeon General issued a report on the effects of passive smoking, based on a careful examination of available evidence by dozens of physicians and scientists. This examination led to three conclusions:

1. Involuntary smoking is a cause of disease, including lung cancer, in healthy non-smokers.
2. Compared with the children of non-smoking parents, children of parents who smoke have a higher frequency of respiratory infections, increased respiratory symptoms, and slightly lower rates of increase in lung function as the lungs mature.
3. The simple separation of smokers and non-smokers within the same air space may reduce, but does not eliminate, the exposure of non-smokers to environmental tobacco smoke. (USDHHS 1986b, p. 7)

The smoke that comes from the burning tip of a cigarette — or *sidestream smoke* — makes up most of environmental tobacco smoke and contains high concentrations of known carcinogens (Eriksen, LeMaistre & Newell 1988). High levels of sidestream smoke are found in some workplaces where smoking is permitted (Hammond et al. 1995).

The available evidence of the harmful effects of second-hand smoke is quite substantial. Some of the strongest evidence relates passive smoking to lung cancer (Eriksen, LeMaistre & Newell 1988; USDHHS 1986b). Many studies of this relationship in a variety of countries around the world have examined the development of cancer in non-smokers who had spouses who smoked. These studies have typically found that passive smokers' risk of lung cancer increases, and the amount of increase can range from 10 per cent to 300 per cent. Given that the dose of smoke inhaled from the environment is less concentrated than that inhaled by smoking a cigarette, these results are very compelling. Studies attempting to relate passive smoking to other cancers have produced mixed or inconclusive results so far. But research has found a higher risk of cardiovascular disease in non-smoking spouses of smokers than non-smokers (Humble et al. 1990).

Passive smoking also has other health effects. For instance, an experiment with animals showed that being exposed to sidestream smoke accelerates the development of atherosclerosis (Penn & Snyder 1993). What's more, for people with existing cardiovascular conditions, such as angina, and respiratory problems, such as asthma and hay fever, environmental tobacco smoke can bring on attacks or aggravate acute symptoms (Eriksen, LeMaistre & Newell 1988). In Australia, smoking has been banned for some time now from government buildings, enclosed public places, supermarkets, restaurants and on public transport (Walsh, Paul & Tzelepis 2000). There has been wide support both among non-smokers and smokers for these bans to reduce second-hand smoke (Trotter & Mullins 1998; Wakefield, Roberts & Miller 1999; Walsh, Paul & Tzelepis 2000).

Two other points are important in the link between smoking and CHD. First, the greater risks for CHD among smokers than among non-smokers may be aggravated by stress, since smoking increases when people are under stress. Second, smokers tend to have lifestyles that include other risk factors for CHD, such as being physically inactive (Castro et al. 1989).

How does smoking cause cardiovascular disease? Researchers generally believe the disease process involves several effects that the nicotine and carbon monoxide in cigarette smoke have on cardiovascular functioning (USDHHS 1986a). Nicotine constricts blood vessels and increases heart rate, cardiac output, and both systolic and diastolic blood pressure. Carbon monoxide reduces the availability of oxygen to the heart, which may cause damage and lead to atherosclerosis. Studies have found that the more cigarettes people smoke per day the greater their level of serum cholesterol and the size of plaques on artery walls (Haapanen et al. 1989; Muscat et al. 1991; Tell et al. 1994). The risk of heart attack or stroke declines greatly in the first few years after stopping smoking (Kawachi et al. 1993; Negri et al. 1994).

Other illnesses

Smoking can lead to a wide variety of other illnesses — particularly emphysema and chronic bronchitis — which are classified together as *chronic obstructive pulmonary disease* (COPD) (AMA 1989; Haas & Haas 1990). People with COPD experience permanently reduced airflow, which is especially evident when they try to exhale with force. Death rates for COPD have declined for males but have increased for females since 1960. For males the death rate in 1998 was 38 per 100 000 while for females it was 17 per 100 000 (AIHW 2000). The decline in male deaths has resulted mostly from a reduction in the number of males who smoke. As we saw earlier, recurrent smoking irritates and damages respiratory organs. Research has shown that more damage occurs from smoking high-tar than low-tar cigarettes and that regularly smoking non-tobacco (marijuana) cigarettes also damages the respiratory system (Bloom et al. 1987; Paoletti et al. 1985). COPD can incapacitate its victims, often forcing relatively young individuals to retire from work. It also causes hundreds of deaths each year, particularly among its victims who smoke (AIHW 1998).

Smoking may also increase acute respiratory infections. This has been shown in two ways. First, studies have found that children of smokers are more likely to develop pneumonia than are children of non-smokers (Doyle et al. 1996). Second, when exposed to common cold viruses, smokers are much more likely to catch cold than non-smokers, probably because their immune functions are impaired (Cohen et al. 1993).

Preventing smoking

How can we prevent people from smoking? Effective public health and legislative approaches include increasing the price of cigarettes through taxation, restricting the advertisement and purchase of cigarettes such as by underage adolescents, banning smoking in government buildings, and using taxation revenue from cigarette sales for health promotion (Owen & Halford 1988). Other approaches try to help people avoid beginning to smoke. To do this effectively, prevention programs need to consider two important factors: *when* and *why* individuals start to smoke. The first factor is straightforward and easily addressed by prevention programs. Because people's likelihood of starting to smoke rises during the junior high school years, increases sharply in the high school years and is very low in adulthood, prevention programs should begin early (Oei & Burton 1990). Programs to prevent smoking are often conducted in schools before children reach the age of 12 or so.

School programs to prevent smoking focused originally on giving fear-arousing warnings of the health consequences of smoking (Evans 1984). These programs did not take into account the past social experiences and current psychosocial forces that exert very strong influences on teenage behaviour. Although knowing the health consequences can change children's beliefs and attitudes about smoking, it is usually not sufficient to stop them from starting to smoke (Bruvold 1993; Flay 1985). This failure points up the need of smoking-prevention programs to consider more fully *why* children and adolescents begin to smoke.

As we saw earlier, researchers have identified several psychosocial reasons why young people start to smoke. Social influences and associated social skills appear to have stronger effects on teenage smoking than long-range health consequences that seem remote, both in time and in likelihood. Recognising this, Richard Evans and his colleagues designed and tested a school-based program to deter teenage smoking by addressing psychosocial factors (Evans 1976, 1984; Evans et al. 1978). The program focused on the immediate consequences of smoking, such as how much it costs and its physiological effects. Films with same-age peers as narrators gave information to help students understand how modelling, peer pressure and cigarette advertising influence their willingness to smoke and to teach them how to resist these forces. The purpose of the program was to provide the knowledge and skills to 'immunise' teenagers against forces that lead to smoking. This psychosocial approach produced very encouraging results and has since served as the basis for developing increasingly effective methods for deterring smoking (Best et al. 1988; Flay 1985; Severson & Lichtenstein 1986).

The psychosocial perspective became the foundation for two types of smoking prevention efforts.

- *Social influence approaches* focus on training skills to help individuals resist social pressures to smoke. They include (1) discussions and films regarding how peers, family members and the media influence smoking by teenagers, (2) modelling and role-playing of specific refusal skills, such as saying, 'No thank you, I don't smoke,' and (3) requiring that each student decide his or her intention regarding whether or not to smoke and announce that decision publicly to classmates (Flay et al. 1985).
- *Life skills training approaches* address general social, cognitive and coping skills. Because many individuals who begin smoking seem to lack these general skills, this approach focuses on improving (1) personal skills, including critical thinking for making decisions, techniques for coping with anxiety and basic principles for changing their own behaviour, and (2) general social skills, including methods for being assertive and making conversation (Botvin, Renick & Baker 1983; Botvin & Wills 1985).

Longitudinal studies have tested these approaches for smoking prevention for one to six years. Although the exact procedures varied somewhat from one study to the next, they were fairly similar. Most of the programs began when the children were in sixth or seventh grade (about age 12). They used a large number of schools, which were assigned to *program* or *control* groups in ways to assure comparability of the schools' size and social class across conditions. The programs gave information about the short- and long-term health and social consequences of smoking. The subjects' self-reports of their smoking were verified, using biochemical analyses of saliva or breath samples.

Were these approaches successful? Compared with the control subjects, children who received each type of program were less likely to begin to smoke during the next couple of years or so (Bruvold 1993). In the case of social influence programs, these benefits were found at assessments after one to three years (Best et al. 1988; Flay et al. 1985; Johnson et al. 1986; Murray et al. 1988; Murray et al. 1987; Severson & Lichtenstein 1986). The life skills approaches showed these benefits in several junior high schools over a two-year period (Botvin, Renick & Baker 1983; Botvin & Wills 1985).

Despite the encouraging early results of these psychosocial approaches to the prevention of smoking, there are three reasons to be cautious about their effectiveness at this time. First, some psychosocial programs have not been successful and have had high subject attrition rates, particularly among smokers and those at high risk of becoming smokers (Ary et al. 1990; Biglan et al. 1987). Second, long-term follow-ups have been conducted with adolescents in studies of social influence programs and found that the programs' beneficial effects do not last beyond four years or so (Flay et al. 1989; Murray et al. 1989). In the junior or senior high school year, a surge in smoking occurred among program subjects, wiping out their earlier advantages over the controls. Third, a study has found that by the time children enter fifth grade many already have positive attitudes about smokers, and having these attitudes at that time was associated with beginning to smoke by the ninth grade (Dinh et al. 1995). This finding suggests that smoking prevention programs may have started too late for many children.

These findings suggest four conclusions. First, programs to prevent smoking probably need to include 'booster' sessions in high school. Second, students who already smoke occasionally at the start of the program require special efforts because they are especially likely to become regular smokers. Third, programs need to start before the fifth grade and focus on attitudes about smokers. Fourth, programs should assess and provide special components for the psychosocial characteristics that put each child at risk for smoking. Getting parents involved may also be useful. The successes these programs have had suggest that psychosocial approaches should be applied in schools more widely to prevent smoking.

Quitting smoking

People are finding that cigarette smoking is not only harmful to their health, but it has negative social effects, too. Smoking in Australia has become something like a deviant behaviour — many non-smokers resent people smoking in their presence, and many smokers feel guilty when they smoke because they know it offends others and believe it is unhealthy, irrational behaviour. Smokers today probably want to quit more than smokers ever did before. In Australia, more than 120 000 smokers quit smoking in the last 12 months (National Tobacco Campaign 2001). What methods do they use to quit, and which ones work?

Stopping on one's own

You probably know people who were smokers — perhaps heavy smokers — and who have quit. Chances are they stopped without any sort of professional help. In a meta-analysis of 14 samples of smokers, Baillie, Mattick and Hall (1995) estimated that the quit rate for stopping smoking without intervention was 7.3 per cent over a 10-month period. Are people really effective at stopping on their own, and does it take enormous effort?

Stanley Schachter (1982) interviewed 161 16- to 79-year-old men and women about their experiences in stopping smoking if they had ever smoked cigarettes regularly. Of these people, 94 had been or were currently smokers — 73 were classified as heavy smokers (smoking at least three-quarters of a pack a day), and the remainder were classified as light smokers. These interviews revealed that over 60 per cent of the smokers who tried to quit eventually succeeded — virtually all had not smoked in the last three months, and the average length of abstinence was more than seven years. Was it harder for the heavy smokers to quit than the light smokers? Yes, much harder. Nearly half of the heavy smokers who quit reported severe withdrawal symptoms, such as intense cravings, irritability, sleeplessness and cold sweats; less than 30 per cent reported having no difficulties. In contrast, almost all of the light smokers said quitting had been easy, even if they had failed! A similar study conducted by researchers at another university found very similar results (Rzewnicki & Forgays 1987).

The results of these studies suggest that most people can stop smoking on their own, even if they smoke heavily. Other studies have clarified the process of quitting on one's own: most people do not succeed in one attempt, but eventually succeed after several tries, and certain factors differentiate those people who do and don't succeed (Carey et al. 1993; Cohen et al. 1989; Curry, Wagner & Grothaus 1990; DiClemente et al. 1991; Gritz, Carr & Marcus 1991; Pallonen et al. 1990; Rose et al. 1996). Compared with smokers who do not succeed in quitting, those who do are likely to:

- have decided that they want and are ready to quit
- feel confident that they can succeed
- have smoked less than a pack a day
- experience less stress
- feel less nicotine dependence and experience less craving for tobacco and fewer and less severe withdrawal symptoms, such as restlessness and tension
- be highly motivated to quit. Although being motivated by *extrinsic* factors, such as financial incentives, can help, people are more likely to succeed if they are motivated by *intrinsic* factors, such as a feeling of self-control or a concern about their health
- be willing to try again if they don't succeed. Many people fail the first few times they try, but learn from their mistakes.

Many people decided to quit when legislation and workplace regulations restricted smoking in public places and at work, especially if there were public health and community quit smoking programs to help them (Borland et al. 1994).

What methods do smokers use when trying to quit? To answer this question, researchers interviewed participants in a month-long, community-wide stop-smoking contest that had a grand prize of a trip to Disney World (Glasgow et al. 1985). These interviews revealed the following data.

- The vast majority of the men and women attempted to quit cold turkey rather than trying to reduce their smoking gradually before the contest began.
- Most participants used oral substitutes, such as lollies or mints, in place of cigarettes.
- Most tried to go it alone, without involving other people, but many others used a buddy system or made bets with others.
- Most used cognitive strategies, such as telling themselves, 'I don't need a cigarette,' or reminding themselves of the health risks in smoking, the commitment they made to quit or the possibility of winning a prize.
- A minority of individuals provided themselves with material rewards for sticking with quitting or punishment for backsliding.

Fifty-five participants — about 40 per cent — remained abstinent throughout the month (which was verified through biochemical saliva or breath analyses). Some methods were more strongly related to successful quitting than others. Although some of the strategies were probably effective in helping particular individuals to quit, only a few methods stood out as being effective for many participants. Compared with individuals who failed, those who succeeded tended to quit cold turkey rather than gradually, provided themselves with rewards for abstaining and used positive cognitive statements to themselves (for example, 'Think of the example I'll set by stopping smoking') rather than negative ones (for example, 'Think how weak I'll be if I give in and smoke').

What about smokers who cannot seem to succeed in stopping on their own even after many attempts? Many of them stop trying to quit and continue to smoke, of course. Many others seek professional help in trying to stop.

Treatment for stopping smoking

Of the smokers who are willing to try to stop smoking, the ones who seek help are likely to be psychologically and physically very dependent on smoking, decreasing the chances that they will succeed. Interventions for smokers range from those in primary health care settings, to brief interventions in the form of advice to quit, or a self-help manual, to nicotine substitution and pharmacotherapies, or behavioural methods. Smokescreen is an intervention delivered by medical practitioners that consists of advice to quit, in the presence of evidence of current health problems linked to smoking, information about quitting strategies, and follow-up appointments (Richmond & Webster 1985). Compared with no-treatment controls, between 24 and 36 per cent of smokers recruited into the Smokescreen program had stopped smoking (Copeman et al. 1989; Richmond & Webster 1985). Community-based approaches to smoking cessation also exist. The Fresh Start program was developed by the Anti-Cancer Council of Victoria (1983) to provide support to participants making a 'fresh start' without tobacco, provide information about the benefits of not smoking and offer strategies to assist smokers to quit. The program's success has been found to depend on participants' commitment to quitting and their perceived likelihood of quitting, or self-efficacy. Meta-analytic data (Mattick & Baillie 1992) have found that two or more brief interventions are more effective in helping smokers to quit than no treatment. Therapists in clinics can design programs that use a variety of methods to help smokers.

One approach therapists have tried involves the use of *drugs* that might combat the conditions that maintain or increase smoking behaviour (Jarvik & Henningfield 1993; Kozlowski 1984). People report many reasons for smoking, including wanting to become aroused or to reduce tension. As a result, therapists have tried using tranquillisers and stimulants to reduce people's smoking, but these drugs have not been effective. The most promising drug approach involves having the smoker take nicotine directly, such as by chewing *nicotine-containing gum* or wearing a *nicotine patch* on the skin. The addition of a nicotine patch to a behavioural intervention can increase abstinence by about 20 per cent (Buchkremer et al. 1989). The nicotine dose is gradually tapered off over a few months. Using nicotine in this way decreases withdrawal symptoms, such as sleeplessness, and helps in achieving short-term and long-term quitting success (Cepeda-Benito 1993; Fiore et al. 1994; Wetter et al. 1995).

Therapists also use many behavioural methods for helping smokers quit. There are basically two categories of behavioural methods for stopping smoking: aversion strategies and self-management strategies. Each of these includes several techniques

(Kamarck & Lichtenstein 1985; Lichtenstein & Mermelstein 1984; Sarafino 1996). **Aversion strategies** involve the use of unpleasant stimuli to discourage behaviour — in this case, smoking. Therapists have tried three main types of unpleasant stimuli: electric shock, imagined negative scenes and cigarette smoke itself. When *electric shock* is used in aversion methods, the level of shock is usually predetermined by increasing it from a low level until the person feels that it is uncomfortable or somewhat painful. The shock is then paired with smoking situations. Using *imagined negative scenes* involves having the person think about a sequence of events, such as getting ready to smoke but becoming nauseated and vomiting. Cigarette smoke can be made into an unpleasant stimulus in several ways. One way, called *satiation*, has the person double or triple his or her usual smoking rate at home for some period of time. Using cigarette smoke as an aversion strategy for controlling smoking appears to be more effective than imagined scenes or electric shock (Kamarck & Lichtenstein 1985; Lichtenstein & Mermelstein 1984). For some smokers, aversion strategies may be useful as a first step in a treatment program for quitting.

Self-management strategies involve techniques that are designed to help people gain control over environmental conditions that sustain an undesirable behaviour such as smoking (N. T. Blaney 1985; Lichtenstein & Mermelstein 1984; Sarafino 1996). These strategies are based on the recognition that efforts to change behaviour need to address the *behaviour itself* and its *antecedents* and *consequences*. Figure 7.3 describes four of the many self-management techniques therapists use to help people stop smoking. Each of these self-management methods is useful in stopping smoking, but they are most effective when used together, rather than separately (Sarafino 1996). A recent addition to these techniques that shows great promise involves a *scheduled reduction* in the number of cigarettes smoked. The program begins by having the person smoke the usual number of cigarettes, but they must be smoked at specified regular intervals, such as on the half-hour during waking hours. Then the schedule is changed to fewer and fewer cigarettes with longer and longer intervals. In a test of this technique, all smokers used a self-management program (Cinciripini et al. 1995). Of those who used the scheduled reduction method, 44 per cent were still abstaining a year later; of those who quit 'cold turkey,' only 22 per cent were still abstinent. Another technique similar to scheduled reduction is **nicotine fading** (Foxx & Brown 1979), which involves getting the smoker to switch to cigarette brands of progressively lower nicotine content, while self-monitoring nicotine intake, in order to reduce total nicotine to complete abstinence over a number of weeks. In a study by Lando and McGovern (1985), which used nicotine fading either alone or in combination with other treatments, initial rates of abstinence were high but had declined by 12 months to 44 per cent when used with aversion strategies, and 26 per cent when used alone.

Several other therapy techniques have been tested, sometimes receiving a great deal of media attention. But research has not demonstrated that they are clearly more effective than control conditions (N.T. Blaney 1985; Glasgow & Lichtenstein 1987; Hunt & Matarazzo 1982). These techniques include *hypnosis*, *systematic desensitisation* and *Restricted Environmental Stimulation Therapy* (REST). In the REST technique, the smoker lies on a bed for a 24-hour period in a very dark and quiet chamber, with no objects or stimulation available, but is allowed to eat, drink and use the toilet freely (Suedfeld & Ikard 1974; Suedfeld 1990).

Research has shown that some of the drug methods, aversion strategies and self-management strategies are useful in controlling smoking, but none is highly effective *alone* (USDHHS 1989). As a result, they are often combined in *multidimensional approaches* to improve their effectiveness (Lando 1993; Shiffman 1993). For instance, studies have found that programs combining behavioural methods with the nicotine patch or nicotine gum are far more effective than using either approach alone (Baillie et al. 1994; Cinciripini et al. 1996; Laforge et al. 1995; Mattick & Baillie 1992). Regardless of the particular treatment techniques a program uses, it is more likely to succeed in stopping smoking if it includes three features. First, using biochemical analyses to verify self-reports of smoking and demonstrating these verification procedures at the *beginning* of treatment enhances the success of a program (Glynn, Gruder & Jegerski 1986). Second, a brief daily telephone call to the smokers improves their compliance with certain procedures, such as self-monitoring (McConnell, Biglan & Severson 1984). Third, physician involvement helps: people are more likely to decide to quit smoking and stick with it if they are advised to stop by their *doctor*, receive a prescription for nicotine, are shown on an apparatus how impaired their respiratory system is and have been diagnosed with a serious smoking-related disease (Jones 1991; Ockene et al. 1991, 1992, 1994; Risser & Belcher 1990).

Figure 7.3 Some self-management techniques for stopping smoking

- *Self-monitoring* is a procedure in which people record information pertaining to their problem behaviour, such as how often they smoked and the circumstances, place and time of each instance. To encourage self-monitoring, a pencil and paper can be kept with the smokers' cigarettes. Although this technique by itself can produce a temporary decrease in smoking, its utility is mainly in gathering information to be used in other techniques.
- *Stimulus control* procedures address the antecedents by altering elements of the environment that serve as cues and lead a person to perform the problem behaviour. Many smokers report that they regularly have (and '*need* to have') a cigarette in certain situations, such as after meals, or with coffee or alcohol, or when talking on the phone, or while sitting in a favourite chair watching TV. Elements of these environments can be altered in many ways, for example by removing smoking cues such as ashtrays and matches or by restricting the time spent watching TV or sitting at the table after meals. Stimulus control procedures by themselves are moderately effective in reducing smoking and are very useful when combined with other techniques.
- *Response substitution* involves replacing a problem behaviour with an alternative response, particularly one that is incompatible with or not likely to be performed at the same time as the problem behaviour. A smoker who 'has to have a cigarette with coffee after breakfast' could skip coffee and take a shower right after breakfast. People are not likely to smoke in the shower (although some smokers do!).
- *Behavioural contracting* is a technique whereby certain conditions and consequences regarding the problem behaviour are spelled out in a contract. Behavioural contracts usually indicate the conditions under which the behaviour may or may not occur and specify what reinforcing and punishing consequences will be applied and when. Contracts for quitting smoking often have the person deposit a substantial sum of money, which is then meted out if he or she meets certain goals. This technique seems to be effective in controlling smoking, but only while the contingencies are in effect.

Succeeding at quitting and abstaining for good

Quitting smoking is one thing — *staying* quit is another. As Mark Twain noted: 'To cease smoking is the easiest thing I ever did; I ought to know because I've done it a thousand times' (Grunberg & Bowen 1985). The methods we have considered work well in helping people stop smoking, but preventing backsliding is a major problem.

Regardless of how smokers quit, their likelihood of **relapse** — that is, returning to the full-blown pattern of behaviour — is very high in the first weeks and months after stopping. Most people who quit smoking start again within a year — estimates of relapse rates vary from 50 to 80 per cent, depending on many factors, including the methods used in quitting, how heavily the person smoked, and characteristics of the individual and his or her environment (Curry & McBride 1994). Withdrawal symptoms probably contribute strongly to immediate relapses, but these symptoms decline sharply in the first week or so after stopping (Gritz, Carr & Marcus 1991; Killen & Fortman 1994). Smokers who are trying to quit need to be reassured that their cravings and negative feelings will diminish greatly in less than a month. What other factors lead people to return to smoking?

One important factor in smoking relapse is *stress*: people who experience high levels of stress are more likely to start smoking again than those who experience less stress (Caplan, Cobb & French 1975; Lichtenstein et al. 1986; Shiffman et al. 1996). Ex-smokers who go back to smoking often report that acute episodes of anxiety or frustration at work or at home led to their relapse (Shiffman 1986). Sheldon Cohen and Edward Lichtenstein (1990) examined the role of stress in relapse longitudinally among smokers who had decided to quit. The subjects were interviewed before quitting and at one, three and six months after their quit date regarding their recent stress levels and smoking status, with biochemical verification. Those subjects who remained continuously abstinent over the full six months reported less and less stress at each interview, but those who relapsed early reported high levels of stress throughout. Some evidence also suggested that the abstinent subjects' reduced stress not only helped them succeed but may have resulted partly from succeeding, such as by increasing their feelings of self-efficacy and self-esteem. People who get treatment for stopping smoking need to receive training in ways to cope with stress without relying on smoking as a coping strategy (Shadel & Mermelstein 1993).

Another factor in smoking relapse is *social support*, which can operate in at least two ways. First, high levels of positive social support can prevent individuals from backsliding by buffering them against stress, as we saw in chapter 4. Second, social support can directly prevent relapse if people in the ex-smoker's social network encourage the person not to smoke (Colletti & Brownell 1983; Nides et al. 1995). Encouragement can come from the person's family, friends and co-workers, as well as from buddy systems in self-help support groups. Research has shown that abstinence is much higher when social support is combined with relapse prevention training in minimal assistance and community-based interventions (Mattick & Baillie 1992). But not all social contacts help prevent a relapse. Some social situations often encourage a relapse, particularly when the ex-smoker is in a restaurant or bar (Shiffman 1986). Unfortunately, many people who quit smoking do not have the kind of support they need, and may even be explicitly *discouraged* from abstinence by others offering them cigarettes or expressing doubt that they will remain abstinent (Sorensen, Pechacek & Pallonen 1986).

People's beliefs and attributions about themselves can also affect whether they return to smoking. Research has shown that people with high levels of *self-efficacy* for quitting and remaining abstinent are less likely to relapse than individuals with less self-efficacy (Curry & McBride 1994; Kavanagh et al. 1993; Stuart, Borland & McMurray 1994). Maintaining a sense of self-efficacy for remaining abstinent is not always easy. Psychologists G. Alan Marlatt and Judith Gordon (1980) have proposed that for many individuals who quit a behaviour, experiencing a *lapse* — an instance or episode of backsliding — can destroy their confidence in remaining abstinent and precipitate a full relapse. This is called the **abstinence-violation effect**. Because these people are committed to total abstinence, they tend to feel guilty about any lapse, even with just one cigarette, for example, and see their violation as a sign of a personal failure. They might think, for instance, 'I don't have any willpower at all and I cannot change.' Although some studies testing this proposal with people who experienced lapses in quitting smoking have supported this proposal, other research has not (Baer et al. 1989; Curry, Marlatt & Gordon 1987; Shiffman et al. 1996). Still, research has found that relapses can be reduced in two ways: (1) by training people to cope with lapses and maintain self-efficacy, and (2) by providing 'booster' sessions or contacts (Curry & McBride 1994). Booster sessions have incorporated cognitive-behavioural skills training with relapse prevention techniques, social support, weight control, cue exposure and conditioning procedures, or the addition of pharmacological treatments (Mermelstein, Karnatz & Reichmann 1992). Carefully conducted contacts, even by phone, can reduce relapses substantially by providing counselling on dealing with difficult situations that could lead to lapses (Zhu et al. 1996).

An interesting thing happens to smoker's beliefs when they relapse: they tend to lower their perceptions of the health risks of smoking. A study of people who relapsed after completing a treatment program to stop smoking found that they reported strong beliefs that smoking could harm their health when they entered the program, but after they relapsed these beliefs decreased (Gibbons, McGovern & Lando 1991). Why? They probably used cognitive processes, such as motivated reasoning or denial, to cope with the fact that their attempt to quit smoking failed. This finding is important because it means relapsers may not be ready to retry quitting until their beliefs change back again. Many smokers deny or minimise the health risks of smoking, thereby decreasing the likelihood that they will try to quit (Lee 1989; Strecher, Kreuter & Kobrin 1995).

Some people who go back to smoking claim they did so because they were *gaining weight* (Perkins 1994). Smokers tend to weigh less than non-smokers, and when individuals stop smoking, most — but not all — do tend to gain several kilograms over the next few years (Grunberg & Bowen 1985; Williamson et al. 1991). There are two reasons why this is so (Klesges, Benowitz & Meyers 1991). First, ex-smokers often increase their caloric intake, sometimes by eating more fats and sweet-tasting carbohydrates. Second, the amount of energy they expend in metabolism declines, for at least a short time after quitting. Thus both behavioural and physiological factors contribute to the changes in weight that ex-smokers experience. To prevent weight gain, many ex-smokers may need to control their diets, get more exercise and perhaps use a nicotine supplement. Research has shown that ex-smokers who used nicotine gum during the weeks after quitting gained much less weight than controls who used a placebo gum (Doherty et al. 1996; Perkins 1994).

The factors that lead an ex-smoker to smoke again are very powerful; controlling them will be difficult. Some efforts to do this with behavioural methods have been tried, but have had mixed success (Brandon, Zelman & Baker 1987; Glasgow & Lichtenstein 1987; Hall et al. 1984). As you might expect, these programs have been more successful with people who had been lighter smokers than with heavier smokers — the ones who are likely to need help the most. Combining behavioural and pharmacological methods to prevent relapse appears promising (Klesges, Benowitz & Meyers 1991).

Alcohol use and abuse

People's use of alcoholic beverages has a very long history, beginning before the eras of ancient Egypt, Greece and Rome, when using wine and beer was very common. Its popularity continued through the centuries and around the world — except in cultures that strongly prohibit its use, as in Islamic nations. Colonial Australians were influenced by the heavy drinking patterns back home in England. Powell (1988), addressing the influence of England in the seventeenth and eighteenth centuries on colonial drinking in Australia, wrote that:

> gin drinking was the only way out of the dreariness, hardship and insecurity of the lives of the poor ... Many convicts who came to Australia in its colonial days came out of such a milieu and brought their drinking habits with them. The harsh life of the penal settlements was no doubt seen by many as simply another degraded, poverty ridden spot, worsened by its 16 000 miles of separation from friends and family. It is small wonder that many used alcohol to soften the harsh environment. (p. 5)

Australia has long had a reputation for being a nation of heavy drinkers. Comparison of existing records on colonial consumption of alcohol (mostly rum) with alcohol consumption back in England and in America indicates that the early settlers were drinking less (Butlin 1983; Dingle 1978, 1980). The only exception was the alcohol intake for the 1830s, when Australians were drinking heavily. Drinking declined in the next decade only to rise with the gold rush of the 1850s. The first attempts at prohibition centred on the banning of hotels on the goldfields (Powell 1988). But the diggers simply returned to town to do their drinking in the many taverns and sly grog shops that were established. In the 1870s temperance workers attributed poverty in the cities to alcohol. While they had previously advocated temperance or abstinence, the focus became prohibition of the sale of alcohol. Minor success in prohibition came in the form of banning the sale of liquor on Sundays and later, in 1916, in the legal enforcement of a 6 o'clock closing time for hotels in the eastern states (Powell 1988). These changes, however, did not persist over time. The Anti-Drink Movement in Australia had relatively little influence on attitudes to alcohol and drinking behaviour. People today believe alcohol has both good and bad effects.

Who drinks, and how much?

The casualness of young people's attitudes to drinking is reflected in anecdotal evidence offered by high-school students boasting of 'big nights out' or 'getting plastered'. Drinking contests are held at university, with both men and women participating. Are there differences in the drinking patterns and behaviour of different groups within Australian society?

Age, gender and alcohol use

People's experience with drinking alcoholic beverages is influenced by age and gender in most societies. In Australia, drinking typically begins before leaving high school. In a large study that assessed the drinking behaviour of more than 20 000 Australian teenagers, it was found that over 90 per cent of 17-year-olds had tried alcohol, with 50 per cent of them using alcohol on a regular basis (Hill et al. 1987). Experimentation with alcohol begins around age 16 for males and age $17\frac{1}{2}$ for females. About one quarter of this age group can be classified as regular heavy drinkers (Makkai & McAllister 1998). As with tobacco use, female adolescents between 14 and 19 years have heavier drinking patterns than males. Twenty-six per cent of female adolescents in this age group are heavy drinkers, while only 15 per cent of males drink heavily (Makkai & McAllister 1998). Findings from the Women's Health Australia study (Jonas, Dobson & Brown 2000) indicate that patterns of alcohol consumption for women between the ages of 18 and 23 are influenced by sociodemographic factors such as marital status and socioeconomic status. For example, heavy drinking was more likely among women who were single, without domestic responsibilities, living away from home and supported by parents. Binge-drinking was common across socioeconomic groups, although women from higher status backgrounds tended to have a drinking pattern characterised by low intake levels most of the time, with weekly binge drinking (Jonas, Dobson & Brown 2000). Often an individual's early experience with alcohol occurs in the home with the parents present, such as at a special occasion. But most teenage drinking occurs in different circumstances, and typically in the presence of friends (Wilks & Callan 1990). Even though it is illegal for most high-school students to purchase alcohol and to drink without parental supervision, they do anyway.

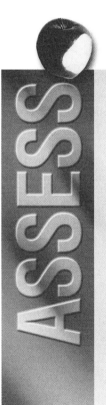

Assess yourself
WHAT'S TRUE ABOUT DRINKING?

Put a check mark in the space preceding each of the following statements you think is true.

_____ Alcohol is a stimulant that energises the body.

_____ Having a few drinks enhances people's performance during sex.

_____ After drinking heavily, people usually sober up a lot when they need to, such as to drive home.

_____ Most people drive better after having a few beers to relax them.

_____ Drinking coffee, taking a cold shower, and getting fresh air help someone who is drunk to sober up.

_____ People are more likely to get drunk if they switch drinks, such as from wine to beer, during an evening rather than sticking with the same kind of drink.

_____ Five 12-ounce (340 mL) glasses of beer won't make someone as tipsy as four mixed drinks, such as highballs.

_____ People seldom get drunk if they have a full meal before drinking heavily.

_____ People can cure a hangover by any of several methods.

_____ Most people with drinking problems are either 'skid row bums' or over 50 years of age.

Which statements did you think were true? They are wrong — all of the statements are false.

Source: Based on *Drinking Myths*, distributed by the US Jaycees.

Throughout adulthood and old age most people tend to show consistency in their drinking behaviour, although variations occur in alcohol consumption for different sociodemographic groups over time. National Drug Strategy surveys have indicated that alcohol consumption for Australians has declined over the last decade (ABS 1998; AIHW 2000; Makkai & McAllister 1998). This decline has been most notable in the frequency of weekly drinking (four to seven days a week) for those under 30 years of age, although there has been a comparable increase in drinking by this age group on one to three days a month (Makkai & McAllister 1998).

Sociocultural differences in using alcohol

Alcohol use varies widely across cultures around the world: people in Norway drink very little, and the French and Italians consume a great deal of alcohol, mainly wine, which they commonly have with meals (Criqui & Ringel 1994). In Australia, drinking is more pronounced in Australian-born persons and migrants from the United Kingdom and Ireland. Only a small proportion of Asian migrants consume alcohol excessively (AIHW 1998).

Differences in alcohol use occur between Aboriginal people and non-Aboriginal Australians. Aboriginal people are more likely than other Australians to drink at unsafe levels (AIHW 1998; Perkins et al. 1994). In a cross-sectional survey of urban Aboriginals (Perkins et al. 1994), 65 per cent of males and 50 per cent of females aged between 25 and 39 years were current alcohol drinkers. Of these 74 per cent were drinking at levels considered harmful to health (that is, more than 40 grams of alcohol per day for women, and more than 60 grams of alcohol per day for men). The incidence of harmful drinking is even more problematic in remote Aboriginal communities, where 92 per cent of drinkers were drinking at unsafe levels (Hunter, Hall & Spargo 1991).

Unsafe drinking patterns are also found in indigenous adolescents. Data from the 1996 study of secondary schools in New South Wales (Forero et al. 1999) indicated that 59 per cent of Aboriginal boys, compared with 33 per cent of non-Aboriginal boys, reported drinking at hazardous levels, while 44 per cent of Aboriginal girls and 34 per cent or non-Aboriginal girls reported hazardous drinking. Indigenous children (younger than 12 years), however, are no more likely than their non-indigenous peers to have tried alcohol, with some research indicating less experimentation with alcohol among indigenous children (Gray et al. 1997; Dunne et al. 2000).

Cross-cultural data on adolescent attitudes towards drinking may help explain differences in actual drinking and later adult consumption of alcohol. Research by Wilks and Callan (1990) and Wilks, Callan and Forsyth (1985) found that teenage drinking in Australia, the United States and New Guinea was determined more by feelings of happiness, enjoyment, sociability and relaxation associated with drinking, than by the taste of alcohol. Australian and American teenagers identified physical side effects of excessive drinking, such as addiction, vomiting, suffering a hangover and risk of motor vehicle accidents, as being disadvantages of drinking. Papua New Guinea teenagers, on the other hand, were more concerned with financial and social costs associated with drinking. These social costs included family problems, arguments and fighting.

Problem drinking

More than 60 per cent of Australian men and women aged over 18 years drink alcohol at least occasionally (AIHW 1998; Makkai & McAllister 1998). Most of these people are light-to-moderate drinkers, consuming fewer than, say, 60 drinks a month. Drinking patterns have declined over the past decade for both males and females, although this has occurred largely for those drinking moderately — that is, on one to three days per week. Many people drink much more heavily, but not all of these drinkers meet the criteria for substance abuse we described earlier. The proportion of frequent drinkers, or those who drink on four to seven days in a week, has declined since the late 1980s. About 37 per cent of Australian males and 19 per cent of females can be classified as frequent drinkers (Makkai & McAllister 1998). Some heavy drinkers are psychologically dependent on having, say, three drinks late at night to help them sleep, but their social-and occupational functioning are not seriously impaired. Of those individuals who develop problems associated with drinking, most — but not all — do so within about five years of starting to drink regularly (Sarason & Sarason 1984).

How many drinkers meet the criteria for substance abuse? Estimates indicate that 5 per cent of women and 13 per cent of men in Australia are heavy drinkers. National Drug Strategy surveys (Makkai & McAllister 1998) have indicated that the proportion of persons drinking heavily has increased over time. In 1995 72 per cent of drinkers reported alcohol consumption above the daily recommended levels for males and females. People who abuse alcohol drink heavily on a regular basis, are psychologically dependent on it, and suffer social and occupational impairments. These people are called **problem drinkers**. They often get drunk, frequently drink alone, regularly drink during the day or go to work intoxicated, drive under the influence and so on. Of adult problem drinkers, males outnumber females by a ratio of about 2 to 1, but alcohol abuse develops most commonly between the ages of 18 and 29 for both sexes (McCrady 1988; Makkai & McAllister 1998). More than half of those who abuse alcohol are physically dependent on it or addicted to it, and therefore are classified as **alcoholics**. These people have developed a very high tolerance for alcohol, often suffer blackout periods or substantial memory losses, and experience delirium tremens, the withdrawal syndrome commonly seen when alcoholics stop drinking. The symptoms of withdrawal often include intense anxiety, tremors and frightening hallucinations. Although alcoholics often drink the equivalent of a fifth of whisky (about 700 mL) a day, 230 mL can sometimes be sufficient to produce addiction in humans (Davidson 1985).

Who abuses alcohol? Many people have an image of the 'typical' alcoholic as a scruffy looking, unemployed derelict with no family or friends. But this image is valid for only a small minority of people who abuse alcohol (Mayer 1983; McCrady 1988). Most problem drinkers are married, living with their families and employed. Many women who are problem drinkers are homemakers, and a large proportion of alcoholic women are married to men who drink heavily. Although individuals from lower socio-economic groups — especially homeless people — are at greater risk than the more advantaged for abusing alcohol, large numbers of problem drinkers come from higher socioeconomic groups and hold high-status jobs. Problem drinking is very rare in childhood; its prevalence increases in adolescence, rises sharply in early adulthood and gradually declines thereafter (Makkai & McAllister 1998). Alcohol abuse is a major social problem that affects substantial numbers of people from almost all segments of many societies around the world.

Why people use and abuse alcohol

In examining why people use and abuse alcohol, we need to consider why individuals start to drink in the first place. The chief reasons for starting to drink involve social and cultural factors (Bandura 1986; Jessor 1984). Children and adolescents perceive through watching others that drinking is 'fun' — people who are drinking are often boisterous, laughing and, perhaps, celebrating. These people are typically family members, friends and celebrities on TV or in movies — all of whom are powerful models. Through social learning processes, such as by watching TV shows and advertisements, children and adolescents acquire *expectancies* about the positive effects of alcohol (Grube & Wallack 1994; Oei, Lim & Young 1991). These expectancies can be in regard to alcohol reducing social anxiety or making people feel more relaxed. Research has shown that men and women expect alcohol to have more positive effects in regard to social assertiveness, tension reduction and reducing social anxiety for those of their own gender, than for the opposite sex. Alcohol was perceived by both males and females to enhance sexual response in women more than in men, while physical arousal and aggression was perceived as being greater in men as a result of drinking (Edgar & Knight 1994). Teenagers also perceive that drinking is 'sociable' and 'grown up', two things they generally want very much to be. As a result, when teenagers are offered a drink by their parents or friends, they are likely to see this as a very positive opportunity.

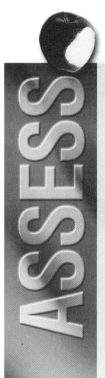

Assess yourself
DO YOU ABUSE ALCOHOL?

Ask yourself the following questions about your drinking.

- Do you usually have more than 14 drinks a week (assume a 'drink' is one mixed drink, 700 mL of beer or the equivalent)?
- Do you often think about how or when you are going to drink again?
- Is your job or academic performance suffering by your drinking?
- Has your health declined since you started drinking a lot?
- Do family or friends mention your drinking to you?

- Do you sometimes stop and start drinking to 'test' yourself?
- Have you been stopped for drink driving in the past year?

If you answered 'yes' to the first question, consider changing your drinking pattern. If you answered 'yes' to any additional questions, consult your university's counselling centre for advice or help.

Sources: Based on TSC (1992); and USDHHS (1995).

Adolescents continue drinking partly for the same reasons they started, but these factors intensify, and new ones come into play. For one thing, the role of peers increases. Although teenagers usually begin drinking under their parents' supervision, drinking at home tends to remain at about the same level throughout adolescence, while drinking with peers at parties or in cars increases steadily. In a study of adolescent views on risky and illegal alcohol use (Wilks 1992), peer group pressure was identified as a significant influence on drinking. Reasons for drinking that reflected peer influence included 'being able to boast about drinking to their friends', 'wanting to be part of the group', 'being pushed into drinking by other young people' and 'wanting to look grown up'. In late adolescence and early adulthood, drinkers drink frequently and almost always socially, with friends at parties or in bars. The social aspect is important in two ways (McCarty 1985; NIAAA 1993). First, in social drinking, modelling processes affect the behaviour — for example, people tend to adjust their drinking rates to match those of their companions. Second, drinking socially creates a subjective norm in individuals that the behaviour is appropriate and desirable.

Operant conditioning is another process by which people continue or increase their drinking behaviour through either positive or negative reinforcement (Davidson 1985; NIAAA 1993). Individuals may receive *positive* reinforcement for drinking if they like the taste of a drink or the feeling they get from it, or if they think that they succeeded in business deals or social relationships as a consequence of drinking. Having reinforcing experiences with drinking increases individuals' expectancies for desirable consequences when deciding to drink in the future (Adesso 1985). In the case of *negative* reinforcement — that is, the reduction of an unpleasant situation — people often use alcohol to reduce stress (Cappell & Greeley 1987; Young, Oei & Knight 1990). Research has shown that people drink more when they experience higher levels, rather than lower levels, of stress (Baer et al. 1987). Also, individuals drink to suppress their negative thoughts about themselves (Hull, Young & Jouriles 1986). But the effects of alcohol on people's anxiety and tension are not so simple: Although drinkers report that alcohol reduces tension and improves their mood, it seems to do so only with the first few drinks they consume in a series; after people consume many drinks, their anxiety and depression levels usually increase (Adesso 1985; Davidson 1985; Hull & Bond 1986). *Antecedent cues* associated with alcohol, such as the sight of beer being poured from the tap, or the smell of whisky, can elicit cravings for alcohol. Desire for alcohol has been found to be greater in heavy drinkers than light drinkers (Greeley et al. 1993) exposed to alcohol-related cues, and in those persons with negative affect or depression (Greeley, Swift & Heather 1992).

Why can most people drink in moderation, but others become problem drinkers? Part of the answer lies in psychosocial differences between these people. Compared with individuals who do not abuse alcohol, those who do are more likely to perceive fewer negative consequences for drinking (Hansen, Raynor & Wolkenstein 1991). They also tend to experience higher levels of stress and live in environments that encourage drinking. But a complete answer also includes biological factors (Zucker & Gomberg 1986). Dozens of twin and adoption studies, as well as research with animals, have clearly demonstrated a genetic influence in the development of drinking problems (Ciraulo & Renner 1991; Schuckit 1985). Twin studies in general have found that if one member of a same-sex twin pair is alcoholic, the risk of the other member being alcoholic is twice as great if the twins are identical rather than fraternal. Assessing the genetic contributions to behaviour is difficult, although some work has been done in this area. The Australian NHMRC twin panel survey on 3000 adult twins found genetic factors to account for 58 per cent of the variation in female alcohol consumption and 45 per cent of the variation in male drinking. The contribution of genetic factors to problem drinking was more variable, explaining from 8 to 44 per cent of the variation in female drinking, and between 10 and 50 per cent of drinking in males (Heath & Martin 1994). The results of adoption studies indicate that adopted children of alcoholics are about four times more likely to become problem drinkers than other adoptees, irrespective of the drinking habits of their adoptive parents. But the interplay of genetic and psychosocial factors seems to be very complex, and their relative impact depends on the person's gender and the timing and severity of alcohol abuse. For instance, heredity plays a much stronger role when the abuse begins before age 25 than after (Kranzler & Anton 1994).

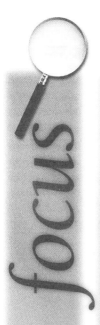

Focus on research
How does heredity lead to alcohol abuse?

It's one thing to know that heredity affects the development of alcohol abuse — as twin and adoption studies have shown — and another thing to know *how* it does. One way to understand how involves comparing individuals who are genetically at *high risk* for becoming alcoholic with those who are at *low risk*, where risk is determined by whether they have close relatives who abuse alcohol.

In these studies, the high-risk and low-risk subjects are matched on the basis of important variables, such as age, amount of alcohol consumed per week, race and amount of education. A critical feature of these studies is that the subjects are tested during the late adolescent or early adulthood years, *before* any of them actually develops a drinking problem. In the research, the subjects receive either an alcoholic drink or a placebo and are then tested for their reaction to the drink. The alcoholic drink is a pretty strong one — the equivalent of a few drinks — and the placebo looks, smells and tastes like the alcoholic drink. The subjects in these studies have been males because the reactions of females to alcohol may be affected by their menstrual cycles or birth control pills.

What kinds of reactions to alcohol have been studied in these subjects, and what was found? Marc Schuckit (1985) examined the subjective feeling of intoxication, as rated by the subjects an hour or more after taking the drink. Of the individuals who had the alcoholic drink, those in the high-risk group reported less intoxication than those in the low-risk group, and both of these groups reported far higher intoxication levels than those who drank the placebo. David Newlin and James Thomson (1991) used a somewhat different approach. They administered alcohol to each high- and low-risk subject on three separate days and took physiological measures, such as heart rate and skin conductance (GSR). On a fourth day the subjects got a placebo. The results revealed that the physiological reactions to alcohol were stronger among the high-risk than the low-risk subjects, and these differences increased across the tests with alcohol.

What do these findings suggest regarding how heredity may lead to alcohol abuse? Schuckit's findings suggest that people who are genetically prone to becoming problem drinkers may have an impaired ability to perceive alcohol's effects. As a result, they fail to notice the symptoms of drunkenness early enough to stop drinking. The physiological differences in Newlin and Thomson's study suggest a role for reinforcement: perhaps high-risk individuals find alcohol more rewarding each time they drink, but low-risk people do not. Other research has found that heavy drinkers develop heightened physiological reactions and positive feelings to alcohol-related stimuli, such as seeing or smelling liquor, especially when alcohol is available (Turkkan, McCaul & Stitzer 1989). Genetic factors seem to combine with operant and classical conditioning processes in the development of drinking problems.

Drinking and health

Drinking too much is associated with a wide range of health hazards for the drinker and for people he or she may harm. Drinkers can harm others in several ways. Pregnant women who drink more than two drinks a day place their babies at substantial risk for health problems, such as being born with low birth weight or *foetal alcohol syndrome*, which can involve serious cognitive and physical defects (Cooper 1987; NIAAA 1993). And drinking lesser amounts during pregnancy has been associated with impaired learning ability in the child. The safest advice to pregnant women is *not to drink at all*.

Drinking also increases the chance that individuals will harm themselves and others through accidents of various types, from unintentionally firing a gun to having a mishap while driving a car, boating or skiing (Smith & Kraus 1988). Consuming alcohol impairs cognitive, perceptual and motor performance for several hours, particularly the first two or three hours after drinks are consumed. The degree of impairment individuals experience can vary widely from one person to the next and depends on the rate of drinking and the person's weight. Figure 7.4 gives the *average* impairment for driving — but for some people, one or two drinks may be too many to drive safely.

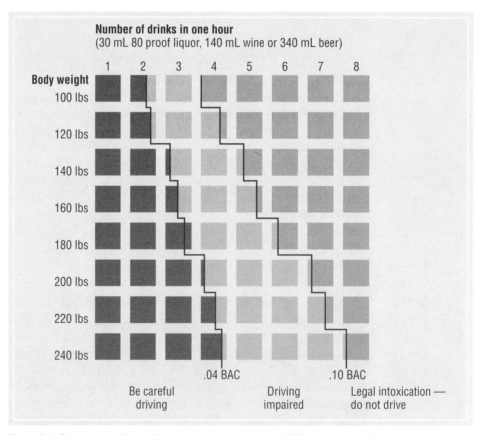

Figure 7.4 The average effects of blood alcohol concentration (BAC) on driving. Although alcohol varies from one person to the next, two drinks (the equivalent of two 140 mL glasses of wine) in a one-hour period will make most adults' driving unsafe.

Source: Reproduced courtesy of CMI Inc.; www.alcoholtest.com.

Many people have misconceptions about the effects of alcohol, believing that drinking on a full stomach prevents drunkenness, or thinking, 'I'll be OK as soon as I get behind the wheel,' for example. One study had sober college students estimate the effects of alcohol in a variety of drinking scenarios (Jaccard & Turrisi 1987). The subjects' judgements revealed several misconceptions about alcohol: for instance, they underestimated the impact alcohol has two or three hours after drinking; thought that later drinks in a series have less impact than the first couple; and downplayed the effects of beer relative to wine, and wine relative to mixed drinks. Although beer contains a smaller percentage of alcohol than other liquors, many people seem to interpret this to mean that 'beer does not make you as drunk as hard liquor,' which is false. Getting drunk just takes a greater volume of beer than straight hard liquor.

Long-term heavy drinkers place themselves at risk for developing several health problems (NIAAA 1993). One of the main risks is for a disease of the liver called *cirrhosis*. Heavy drinking over a long period is one of several conditions that can cause liver cells to die off and be replaced by permanent, nonfunctional scar tissue. When this scar tissue becomes extensive, the liver is less able to cleanse the blood and regulate its composition. Cirrhosis causes close to one thousand deaths each year. Heavy drinking also presents other health risks: it has been linked to the development of some forms of *cancer*, *high blood pressure*, and *heart* and *brain damage* (AIHW 1998). The brain damage many alcoholics develop can impair their perceptual and memory functions (Goldman 1983; Parsons 1986). These functions may recover gradually after the person stops drinking, but some impairments may persist for years or never disappear. As you might expect, long-term alcoholics who continue to drink die much earlier than non-alcoholics. But if they quit, their mortality risk approaches that of non-alcoholics in several years (Bullock, Reed & Grant 1992).

Some people believe that drinking in moderation — having, say, a drink or two a day — is *good* for their health, and they may be right. Several large-scale longitudinal studies, following many thousands of people across many years, have found that people who drink light or moderate amounts of alcohol each month have lower morbidity and mortality rates than individuals who drink heavily or who do not drink at all (Friedman & Kimball 1986; Gordon & Doyle 1987; Gordon & Kannel 1984; Rimm et al. 1991). Does moderate drinking cause better health? We cannot be sure because of the quasi-experimental nature of these studies. If it does, the greatest benefit may be in reducing coronary heart disease, particularly if the beverage is wine (Criqui & Ringel 1994). Although the reason alcohol may protect people from heart disease is not yet clear, there is evidence supporting two possibilities. First, alcohol affects the body's response to stress, reducing cardiovascular and endocrine (for example catecholamine production) reactions (Levenson 1986). Second, alcohol appears to alter levels of substances in the blood that protect the blood vessels from cholesterol (Facchini, Chen & Reaven 1994; Gaziano et al. 1993) Still, we do not know enough about the effects of alcohol to recommend its light use for heart attack prevention.

Preventing alcohol abuse

Individuals and agencies concerned with public health around the world have tried many different approaches to preventing alcohol abuse. The most common methods have been of three types: public policy and legal approaches, health promotion and education, and early intervention approaches.

Public policy and legal approaches for preventing alcohol abuse are designed to reduce per capita consumption of alcohol by creating barriers to drinking (Ashley &

Rankin 1988; Mattick & Jarvis 1994). These approaches include limiting the number of outlets where alcoholic beverages can be bought and restricting the times when they are on sale. These two methods do not seem to be very effective in reducing drinking. A more effective method is to prohibit underage individuals from buying or consuming alcohol. This method reduces alcohol consumption and related automobile accidents among individuals in the late adolescent and early adulthood years. One of the most effective methods for reducing per capita alcohol consumption and preventing alcohol-related health problems is to increase the price of alcoholic beverages through taxation (Hawks & Lenton 1995).

Health promotion and education approaches for preventing alcohol abuse provide information and training to help people avoid drinking heavily. Most of these programs have been directed at children and adolescents in schools. More recent programs have demonstrated that *social influence* methods, like those we considered for preventing smoking, can be effective in reducing the amount of drinking among adolescents, and the effects may last two or three years (Kivlahan et al. 1990; Klepp, Kelder & Perry 1995).

Early intervention approaches for preventing alcohol abuse focus on detecting the beginning stages of heavy drinking and providing information and help to reverse the individual's pattern of drinking (Ashley & Rankin 1988; Mattick & Jarvis 1994; Heather 1989b). These efforts have been directed mainly at three populations: drink drivers, employees and medical patients. Efforts with drink drivers have been disappointing — several very different approaches have been tested and shown to be successful *only* with people who are relatively *light* drinkers, not with heavy drinkers (McGuire 1982). Indeed, heavy drinkers who receive interventions often have *worse* subsequent records of alcohol-related accidents and driving violations than heavy drinkers who receive no treatment.

For early intervention approaches with drinking employees and medical patients, however, the picture is brighter (Ashley & Rankin 1988; Engstrom 1984). If the drinking problem is detected early, successful intervention may simply involve providing information and advice, and the person may be able to reduce his or her drinking pattern to one of moderation (Ashley & Rankin 1988; NIAAA 1993). If the problem is detected after addiction has set in, the treatment must be more intensive, and the person may not be able to return to drinking at all. Many employers and unions in the United States provide *employee assistance programs* (EAPs) to help individuals who have personal problems, such as with drinking or stress (USDHHS 1990). An EAP can be helpful, but employees are usually not asked to use one until their problems are severe enough to affect their work, and may not use them at all if they worry that counsellors will leak information back to their bosses. The work site should be a good place for preventing alcohol abuse because most individuals who abuse alcohol have jobs, and drinking is often related to stresses on the job (Mayer 1983). Unfortunately, wellness programs at work sites rarely include specific efforts to prevent employees from beginning to drink heavily (Nathan 1985).

An example of an early intervention with medical patients that has been effective is the Scottish DRAMS (Drink Reasonably and Moderately with Self-control) Scheme. Patients who are suspected of having a drinking problem are given a medical questionnaire to complete on the medical and social consequences of their drinking. They are then screened for the presence of alcohol in the blood using either GGT (liver enzyme gamma-glutamyl transferase) or MCV (mean cellular volume) indicators and blood alcohol concentration. This is followed by assessment of readiness to change drinking behaviour. Drinkers at the *action* stage of Prochaska and DiClemente's change process are then asked to complete a drinking diary. Medical results are discussed in conjunction with the drinking diary and medical questionnaire. The patient is then introduced to a self-help booklet and given advice in developing a plan of action to reduce drinking. Further consultations are arranged to monitor drinking behaviour and blood tests conducted as part of the review process. Reduced drinking is then maintained with self-help information on identification of high-risk situations leading to relapse, and instruction is given on coping skills and the use of cognitive restructuring to change maladaptive alcohol-related beliefs and expectancies (Heather 1987).

Treatments for alcohol abuse

In psychology and medicine, the term *spontaneous remission* refers to the disappearance of symptoms or problems without the benefit of formal treatment. Many people who abuse alcohol stop or markedly reduce their drinking on their own, without treatment. What proportion of people who abuse alcohol recover on their own? The best estimates available are based on data from a small number of studies of treatment effectiveness in which some problem drinkers were randomly assigned to control groups that received no treatment. Using the data on the control subjects, William Miller and Reid Hester (1980) calculated that spontaneous remission — stopping or markedly reducing drinking — occurs in about 19 per cent of alcohol abuse cases. Compared with drinkers who do not quit on their own, those who do generally report having had social support from a spouse and having changed the way they weighed the pros and cons of drinking — for example realising 'I was sick and tired of it, really weary of it' (Sobel et al. 1993).

Alcohol abusers who quit drinking on their own and those who seek treatment often have an important thing in common: They want to change. We saw in chapter 6 that the *stages of change model* is useful in describing people's readiness to modify health-related behaviours. A critical transition occurs when the person's stage of readiness moves from *contemplation*, or thinking about changing, to *preparation* and *action*. According to psychologist William Miller (1989a), this transition is like a door that opens for a period of time and closes if the alcohol abuser doesn't use it in that time; using it can be encouraged in several ways, such as:

- giving the person clear advice about why and how to change
- removing important barriers for change
- introducing external consequences, such as rewards for changing or real threats (for example of being fired) if no change occurs
- offering help and showing a helping attitude.

These and other approaches can be used by family members, friends, co-workers, doctors or therapists to increase the person's motivation for change. Such encouragement forms the basis of **motivational interviewing** (Miller 1983). By getting the alcohol abuser to reflect on the negative consequences of his or her drinking, and discussing options for change of drinking patterns, the individual is encouraged towards increased motivation and a readiness to enter the *action* stage of change. Research has shown that when persons with drinking problems receive motivational interviewing in addition to standard treatment, they have higher abstinence rates (Bien, Miller & Boroughs 1993).

Because of the physical dependence alcoholics have when they enter treatment, the first step in their recovery is **detoxification** — the drying-out process of getting an addicted person safely through the period of withdrawal from a substance. This is an essential step for all addicted individuals before treatment can proceed. Because withdrawal symptoms can be very severe, sometimes even causing death, detoxification often takes place in hospitals under medical supervision, using medication to control the symptoms (Ciraulo & Renner 1991; Miller & Hester 1985). Improved assessment procedures and detoxification methods have reduced the need for direct medical supervision during alcohol withdrawal. It is now possible to identify those alcoholics who are likely to need medical supervision and those who are not. About half of alcoholics who seek treatment can undergo detoxification at home if they receive careful assistance and support from trained individuals.

Where should treatment occur, and what should be the goals and criteria for success?

In designing a treatment program, one of the many decisions the treatment team needs to make is whether it should be carried out in a residential setting or on an outpatient basis. Is residential treatment more effective than nonresidential treatment? Most evidence indicates that it is not (Mattick & Jarvis 1994). Problem drinkers can usually receive all or most of their treatment as outpatients. Treatment need not be intensive for improvements to drinking patterns to occur (Emrick 1975). Minimal or brief interventions can be as effective as intensive treatment (Orford & Edwards 1977; Heather 1989a) for drinkers with low levels of alcohol dependence. Although abstinence rates do not appear to differ for intensive compared with brief interventions, there is some indication that extended treatment may reduce the amount of harm caused by drinking.

Ideally, treatment should 'cure' the person's drinking problem forever, but at what point can the team expect that their assessments of the success of treatment are likely to reflect durable effects? On this issue, there is considerable agreement among researchers: they generally recommend and use a minimum follow-up interval of 12–18 months to determine the success of treatment (Emrick & Hansen 1983; Nathan 1986). Many programs today also attempt to verify self-reports of drinking behaviour through other sources — through reports by the ex-drinker's spouse or through blood or breath tests for instance — and measure other outcomes of treatment, such as physical health, employment status and legal problems encountered.

Another decision the treatment team needs to make is whether the program should aim to have all of its problem drinkers become *permanently abstinent* or whether some can return gradually to *controlled drinking*. This distinction generated a bitter controversy in the 1980s (Marlatt 1983; Peele 1984). Research findings had indicated earlier that some problem drinkers — including alcoholics — can learn to drink in moderation after first becoming abstinent (Armor, Polich & Stambul 1978; Davies 1962; Polich, Armor & Braiker 1981; Sobel & Sobel 1976, 1978). Other researchers strongly attacked some of this research and the idea that people who abuse alcohol may be able to control their drinking (Block 1976; Pendery, Maltzman & West 1982). Although the controversy is not completely resolved, it does appear that *some* problem drinkers can learn through treatment to drink in moderation (Miller & Hester 1980; Peele 1984). Problem drinkers who have the best prospects for controlled drinking:

- are relatively young
- are socially stable — that is, married and/or employed
- have had a relatively brief history of alcohol abuse
- have *not* suffered severe withdrawal symptoms while becoming abstinent
- prefer trying to drink in moderation, and have *not* made a personal commitment to abstinence as a goal.

In other words, individuals who have the best chances of succeeding in controlled drinking are those who have the least resemblance to chronic alcoholics. For long-term alcoholics today, pursuing the goal of controlled drinking is unrealistic and probably not in their best interests (Nathan 1986; Sandberg & Marlatt 1991).

Alcoholics Anonymous

Alcoholics Anonymous (AA) is a widely known self-help program that was founded in the 1930s by people with drinking problems (Bean-Bayog 1991; McCrady & Irvine 1989). The program now has thousands of chapters throughout the United States, Australia and other countries, and has set up organisations to help alcoholics' families, such as *Alateen* for their adolescent children and *Alanon* for adults in the family. The AA philosophy includes two basic views. First, people who abuse alcohol are alcoholics and remain alcoholics for life, even if they never take another drink. Second, taking one drink after becoming abstinent can be enough to set off an alcoholic binge and, therefore, must be avoided. As a result, AA is committed to the goal of permanent and total abstinence, and their approach is aimed at helping their members resist even one drink.

Because the AA philosophy has its roots in evangelical Protestantism, the program emphasises the individual's needs for spiritual awakening, public confession and contrition (McCrady & Irvine 1989). This philosophy can be seen in the Twelve Steps AA uses to help drinkers quit — for example, one step is, 'Admitted to God, to ourselves, and to another human being the exact nature of our wrongs.' Members attend frequent AA meetings, which use the Twelve Steps to promote frank discussions about the members' experiences with alcohol and difficulties resisting drinking. An important feature of the AA approach is that its members develop friendships with other ex-drinkers and get encouragement from each other and from knowing individuals who have succeeded.

Does AA work, and is it more effective than other approaches for helping drinkers quit? AA claims a very high rate of success: for example, one AA report claimed that 75 per cent of those 'who really tried' became abstinent (Miller & Hester 1980). But AA's overall effectiveness is actually unknown because its membership is anonymous and the organisation does not keep systematic information about people who attend. One way to compare the AA program with other approaches would be to assign a pool of problem drinkers to different programs randomly, as one experiment did (Brandsma, Maultsby & Welsh 1980). The subjects — most of whom had been referred by the courts because of their drinking problems — were assigned to either an AA program, one of three other treatment programs or a control group. The results revealed greater improvement among those who received treatment than those who did not, and the subjects in the AA program showed somewhat less improvement than those in other treatments. Other studies have produced mixed findings regarding the effectiveness of AA (McCrady & Irvine 1989). It may be, however, that AA is the best approach for certain types of problem drinkers, particularly those who need an authoritarian structure and the intense social support of other problem drinkers (Miller & Hester 1980). AA is being used more and more as an approach to prevent relapse after other forms of treatment (NIAAA 1993).

Insight therapy

Many approaches to psychotherapy are designed to help the person achieve *insight* — an understanding of the roots of his or her problem. The rationale for these approaches is that insight is necessary for the person to work through and solve the problem (Davison & Neale 1994). Although the nature of psychotherapy can vary widely and depends on the theoretical orientation of the therapist, most types of *insight therapy* involve some form of counselling and have similar goals for treating people with drinking problems. These goals include helping drinkers to accept that they need help, believe that they are worthwhile individuals, understand the factors that led them to drink heavily and cope effectively with these factors. Insight-oriented psychotherapy can be conducted with individual clients or with groups, and it appears to be modestly effective in treating drinking problems (Miller & Hester 1980).

Behavioural and cognitive methods

Drinking excessively and smoking cigarettes heavily have a great deal in common — these behaviours can lead to addiction and they are difficult to quit. As a result, variations of the methods we considered in the section on treatment for stopping smoking may apply to stopping drinking, too.

Aversion strategies — using unpleasant stimuli to discourage behaviour — have been applied as treatments for alcohol abuse. One aversion strategy involves pairing drinking with electric shock, but this method has not been very successful in stopping people's problem drinking (Miller & Hester 1980). A much more effective aversion strategy has been to have the person take an **emetic drug**, such as *emetine*, that induces nausea when alcohol is consumed. In a typical half-hour session, the person first receives an injection of emetine and then repeatedly drinks an alcoholic beverage, each time quickly becoming nauseated and vomiting (Miller & Hester 1980). The person undergoes several of these sessions, typically as an inpatient in a hospital, and then receives booster sessions periodically after discharge. A study of hundreds of problem drinkers who received emetine therapy revealed that 63 per cent of the men and women remained abstinent during the 12 months after treatment, and half of these individuals remained abstinent for the next two years (Wiens & Menustik 1983). Other studies using emetine therapy have also demonstrated high rates of success (Miller & Hester 1980).

Because *self-management strategies* are useful in helping people stop smoking, you might expect them to aid in quitting drinking — and they do (Hester & Miller 1989; Lang & Marlatt 1982). Successful treatment programs have used:

- self-monitoring to help problem drinkers determine the situations that elicit and maintain drinking behaviour
- stimulus control procedures to change or eliminate environmental cues that promote drinking, for example by socialising with people who don't drink
- response substitution, such as finding someone to talk to instead of drinking when upset
- behavioural contracting to help structure a set of rewards for abstinence and punishment for drinking.

The problem drinker's family can play an important role in self-management. Research has found that training family members, such as the alcoholic's spouse, in these strategies enables them to help in the drinker's self-management efforts, rather than undermining these efforts (Sisson & Azrin 1986).

Other methods seem to be useful in helping people quit drinking. For example, social skills training has been used to teach alcohol-refusal and assertiveness in high-risk interpersonal situations (Mattick & Jarvis 1994). Problem drinkers have also been trained in *stress management* techniques (Stockwell & Town 1989). This approach has value because feelings of anxiety and tension increase people's drinking behaviour. Cognitive restructuring has also been used to alter alcohol-related beliefs and expectancies (Oei, Lim & Young 1991). Another method involves *counteracting classical conditioning* that occurs with long-term drug use: stimuli associated with drinking, such as seeing the liquor bottle, gain the ability to produce internal conditioned responses like those that happen when the person is actually drinking. To reduce these internal reactions to conditioned stimuli, therapists have had problem drinkers repeatedly experience alcohol-related stimuli, such as holding a beer can, while not allowing them to drink. This approach has had some success by itself and in combination with other behavioural methods (Blakey & Baker 1980; Drummond & Glautier 1994; Monti et al. 1993).

In a meta-analysis that compared different types of treatment for problem drinking, cognitive behavioural approaches that involved cognitive restructuring and social skills training were found to have superior outcomes in relation to reduced drinking and abstinence (Oei, Lim & Young 1991).

Chemical therapies

Drugs are sometimes prescribed as a component of treatment for alcohol abuse. One approach uses an emetic drug called *disulfiram* (brand name Antabuse), which the person needs to take each day orally (Ciraulo & Renner 1991; Schuckit 1996). In addition to producing nausea if the person drinks, it has some important side effects that can preclude its use — it causes drowsiness, raises blood pressure, and has physiological effects that make it inappropriate for people with heart and liver diseases. For those who can use it, disulfiram can be an effective therapy, but getting them to take the drug consistently is often a problem. Behavioural principles help explain the effects of disulfiram on abstinence. The nausea effects of the drug lead to aversion to drinking due to classical conditioning processes. Under an operant conditioning model, disulfiram also acts as a powerful punishment for drinking. While alcohol is not being used, extinction of conditioned craving responses to drinking-associated cues may also occur (Heather 1989b). Several other chemicals appear promising for treating alcohol abuse, but their utility has not been sufficiently demonstrated (Schuckit 1996).

Treatment success and the relapse problem

Many different techniques can be effective in helping people overcome drinking problems. Which ones should be used? One consideration is cost: some of the most effective methods are among the least expensive to implement (Holder et al. 1991). Another concern is to *match* the techniques with the needs of the person (Glasser 1980; Miller 1989b). Doing this requires two steps: (1) assessing the person's drinking problem, readiness to change, and beliefs and personality, and (2) negotiating with the person the goals of treatment and the amount and type of help to use. Treatment programs that combine appropriate techniques generally offer the strongest promise for success, at least in the first year or two after treatment begins (Costello et al. 1980; Moos & Finney 1983).

Who succeeds when treated for alcohol abuse? Generally speaking, problem drinkers who function the best at the start of treatment, those with an internal locus of control, and those drinkers with a high level of social stability are the most likely to succeed (Heather 1989a). Thus,

> high socioeconomic status, a stable marriage or relationship, a steady and supportive employment milieu, higher education (12 years or more), a stable residential setting, and no criminal record (or few convictions) have all been related to a good prognosis irrespective of the type of treatment employed. (Caddy & Block, 1985, p. 353)

But many people drop out of treatment for alcohol abuse — and of those who complete a program, less than a majority maintain their improvement in drinking behaviour beyond the first year or so. This seems to be the case regardless of the treatment characteristics, even when the more successful multidimensional approaches are used (Costello et al. 1980; Nathan 1986).

The problem of *relapse* is at least as severe in efforts to stop drinking as it is in quitting smoking. Many of the more successful treatment approaches for alcohol abuse produce very high rates of success initially, but these rates decline sharply by the end of the first year and again during the next two years (Nathan 1986). Studies of problem drinkers who relapsed have found that the circumstances preceding the relapse generally involve *negative emotional states*, such as depression or anxiety, *interpersonal conflict*, such as arguments with family members or co-workers, and *social pressure* to drink (Abrams et al. 1986; Hodgins, el-Guebaly & Armstrong 1995; Sandberg & Marlatt 1991). Alcoholics often use these circumstances to justify a lapse, saying for instance, 'With all these hassles, I *deserve* a couple of drinks.' One way to help prevent relapses involves training in *social and problem-solving skills* to resist the urge to return to drinking in highly tempting situations, such as in a restaurant with friends who have drinks (Chaney 1989; Chaney, O'Leary & Marlatt 1978). Coping skills appear to have an interactive effect with outcome expectancies and self-efficacy in increasing the likelihood of relapse (Allsop & Sanders 1989). An alcoholic who has poor coping skills for dealing with high-risk situations, and who lacks confidence in his or her ability to remain sober, is more likely to have outcome expectancies that equate one drink with continued drinking after a lapse. Such beliefs are challenged through cognitive restructuring in treatment, while making salient the negative outcome expectancies of returning to heavy drinking. In addition, social support systems, like those in AA programs, are likely to help ex-drinkers avoid relapse (Colletti & Brownell 1983). Discovering effective methods of preventing relapse among problem drinkers has become a major focus of research.

Drug use and abuse

The word 'drug' can refer to a wide variety of substances, including prescription and non-prescription medicine, that people may take into their bodies. We will limit the term *drug* to mean psychoactive substances other than nicotine and alcohol that can cause physical or psychological dependence. Like smoking and drinking, the use of drugs has a long history — for example, the Chinese evidently used marijuana 27 centuries B.C. In the United States, addiction to narcotics was widespread among people of all ages in the nineteenth century. Many 'patent medicines' in those days contained opium and were sold without government regulation. As a result, large numbers of people became addicted at early ages (Kett 1977). Laws were enacted in the early 1900s against the use of narcotics in America.

Who uses drugs, and why

Drug use has become a serious problem in many countries of the world, especially in North America and Europe. Drug usage in Australia is much lower, at around 2 to 3 per cent of the population for most drugs other than marijuana (Makkai & McAllister 1998). Some individuals are more likely than others to use drugs. We'll look first at which segments of society are more likely to use drugs, and then we'll consider why.

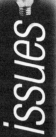

Highlight on issues

issues

Types and effects of drugs

'Oh, I feel so light, like a feather,' said Dolores, after taking several hits from a 'joint'. That lightness of feeling is a common effect people get from smoking a marijuana cigarette. Each drug has its own set of general psychological and physiological effects (Ciraulo & Shader 1991; Schuster & Kilbey 1992; Winger, Hofmann & Woods 1992). Some drugs are highly addictive, and others have little potential for producing physical dependence. Drugs are usually classified into four categories: stimulants, depressants, hallucinogens and narcotics.

Stimulants are chemicals that produce physiological and psychological arousal, keeping the user awake and making the world seem to race by. This category of drugs includes *amphetamines*, *caffeine* and *cocaine*, which can be inhaled, injected or smoked ('crack'). Chronic use of stimulants can produce mental confusion, exhaustion and weight loss — and can lead to psychological dependence. Physical dependence on amphetamines, cocaine or caffeine can develop; the withdrawal symptoms often are subtle but are still very influential on behaviour.

Depressants decrease arousal and increase relaxation. People use these drugs to reduce anxiety and induce sleep. Depressants include various *tranquillisers* (such as Valium) and *barbiturates*, which are commonly called 'downers'. Excessive and chronic use of depressants interferes with motor and emotional stability and produces psychological dependence. Addiction can develop with long-term use of depressants and can occur rapidly for barbiturates.

Hallucinogens produce perceptual distortions, such as when the body or mind feels light. The most commonly used drug of this type is *marijuana*, which people use for the relaxation and intoxication it causes. Other hallucinogens, such as *mescaline*, LSD (lysergic acid diethylamine) and PCP (phencyclidine), often produce a feeling of exhilaration. Hallucinogens have a relatively low potential for causing physical dependence, but chronic use of these drugs can lead to psychological dependence.

Narcotics or *opiates* are sedatives that relieve pain. In many people, but not all, they produce a euphoric and relaxed feeling. The narcotics include *morphine*, *codeine* and *heroin*. These drugs, especially heroin, generally cause intense physical *and* psychological dependence when used in large doses continually.

The effects of drugs can vary. The same dose of a drug may produce quite different reactions in different people and in the same person on different occasions (Bardo & Risner 1985). Why? Physiological processes, such as metabolism and absorption by tissues, vary from one person to the next and within each individual over time. Partly because very young people and the elderly have lower rates of metabolism than others do, they tend to experience relatively strong reactions to drugs. Stress can also influence the effects of a drug. Being under stress causes physiological changes that may increase a drug's impact.

Age, gender and sociocultural differences in drug use

We have seen that smoking and drinking are more likely to begin in adolescence than at any other time in the life span. This developmental pattern is true for using most drugs, too. Two types of drugs that are exceptions to this pattern are tranquillisers and barbiturates: Using these drugs commonly begins in adulthood, often with prescriptions from doctors (AMA 1989; Ciraulo & Shader 1991; Davison & Neale 1994).

One of the most popular drugs in Australia is marijuana. Three out of every 10 Australian adults have smoked marijuana at some stage in their life. Of those Australians who have smoked marijuana in the last 12 months, 37 per cent reported that they smoked marijuana once a week or more. Its use sometimes begins before the tenth grade — about 18 per cent of Australian teenagers try it before the age of 15 (Makkai & McAllister 1998). In a survey of 1270 high-school students in years 7, 10 and 11 in the metropolitan area of Sydney (Rob, Reynolds & Finlayson 1990), marijuana use was reported by 4.2 per cent of 12-year-olds (grade 7), while 26.5 per cent of 15-year-olds (year 10) and 26.7 per cent of year 11 students had used the drug in the week prior to the survey. More recently, the 1998 National Drug Strategy Household Survey found that 35 per cent of 14- to 19-year-olds have used marijuana in the past 12 months (Reid, Lynskey & Copeland 2000). While 45 per cent had experimented with the drug at least once during their lifetime, they did not necessarily progress to become regular users. Teenagers' use of most other drugs tends to begin somewhat later and is much less prevalent — for instance, only 1 per cent of Australian adults reported having used cocaine in the previous 12 months in the 1985–95 National Drug Strategy surveys, and most of these persons were in their twenties (Makkai & McAllister 1998). Illicit use of drugs like marijuana has increased since 1990, especially in adolescents (AIHW 2000; Makkai & McAllister 1998). These changes have coincided with adolescents' beliefs about whether drugs are harmful, rather than changes in drug availability (Johnston, O'Malley & Bachman 1995). Drug use is far more prevalent in males than females at virtually all adolescent and adult ages and for almost all drug types (Makkai & McAllister 1998). For example, the highest prevalence of marijuana use is by males at 20 to 29 years of age. Adolescents who use tobacco and alcohol frequently are more likely to use illicit drugs (Heaven 1996; Reid, Lynskey & Copeland 2000). Those adolescents applying for drug treatment are more inclined to be poly-substance users, with alcohol, cannabis and heroin being used heavily (Spooner, Mattick & Noffs 2000). The likelihood that individuals will progress from a less serious drug, such as marijuana, to a more serious drug, such as cocaine, is related to how heavily the earlier drug was used (Kandel & Faust 1975; Newcomb & Bentler 1986). Heavy users of a less serious drug are more likely to begin using more serious drugs than light users are.

Why adolescents use drugs

Why do teens try marijuana and other drugs? They do so for many of the same reasons that they start to drink or smoke cigarettes (Hansen et al. 1987; Stein, Newcomb & Bentler 1987). Two of the strongest factors in determining initial and early stages of drug use are availability and social learning. Teenagers see peers and important adults, such as parents and celebrities, model behaviours and attitudes that promote drug use. Studies have shown that adolescents are more likely to use marijuana and other drugs if their parents and friends use mood-altering substances such as alcohol and marijuana (Brook, Whiteman & Gordon 1983; Jessor & Jessor 1977; Stein, Newcomb & Bentler 1987). Teenagers' marijuana use seems to be affected more by their friends' than their parents' substance use, and the first introduction of most youths to marijuana is through a friend (Kandel 1974).

After people start using drugs, they tend to continue if they like the experience — that is, if the drug makes them 'feel good' or helps them feel *better* than they felt before taking it (Barrett 1985). Many people claim that taking drugs reduces their anxiety and tension. In other words, drugs have reinforcing effects. Then, with continued use, drug-related stimuli become conditioned to the drug's effects and can elicit physiological reactions like those the drug itself produces (Caggiula et al. 1992; Childress 1996). Because people often use drugs in the presence of friends and other peers, social pressure and encouragement also tend to maintain and increase drug use.

Why do some individuals progress from drug use to *drug abuse*? Personality traits seem to affect whether people abuse drugs. Compared with individuals who use drugs occasionally, those who go on to abuse drugs tend to be *more* rebellious, impulsive, accepting of illegal behaviour and oriented towards sensation seeking; and they tend to be *less* socially conforming and less committed to a religion (Brook et al. 1986; Cox 1985; Newcomb, Maddahian & Bentler 1986; Stein, Newcomb & Bentler 1987). Other risk factors identified include poorer school performance, school absenteeism, early sexual experimentation, and alcohol and cigarette use (Heaven 1996). Factors in the adolescent's home environment also appear to influence drug use. In the study by Rob, Reynolds & Finlayson (1990) reported earlier, marijuana users were twice as likely as non-users to come from broken homes, or from families with poorer family relationships and to have mothers who worked full-time because of marital break-up.

Drug use and health

The effects of drug use and abuse on people's health are not as well documented as those of drinking and cigarette smoking. This is because drug use became widespread only since the early 1960s, it is still much less prevalent than drinking and smoking, and many drug users are unwilling to admit to researchers that they use drugs — a criminal offense — for fear of being prosecuted. Nevertheless, some health effects are known. For example, drugs taken by women during pregnancy cross the placenta and may harm the foetus; and babies born to addicted mothers are likely to be addicted, too (Cook, Petersen & Moore 1990). Also, smoking marijuana damages the user's lungs (Bloom et al. 1987). Furthermore, drug use is implicated in automobile accidents (Jessor 1984).

The health effects of cocaine are becoming increasingly clear, particularly with regard to the cardiovascular system (Altman 1988; Rowbotham & Lowenstein 1990). Taking cocaine causes the person's blood vessels to constrict, heart rate to speed up, and blood pressure to increase suddenly. It can also trigger cardiac arrhythmia. These events can cause a stroke or myocardial infarction. Sometimes damage to the heart muscle can occur without pain or other clear symptoms and leave streaks of permanent, nonfunctional cells that cause the heart to beat irregularly. Any of these cardiovascular conditions can lead to death. Cocaine also produces harmful conditions in other parts of the body: It can destroy cells in the liver, cause brain seizures and damage cells in the nose when it is sniffed.

Preventing and stopping drug abuse

Two public health approaches can be used to prevent teenage drug abuse. One way is directed at children and adolescents through educational programs and campaigns in the schools and mass media. Children and adolescents can be taught how to resist starting to use drugs, using programs based on the *social influence* and *life skills training* methods we considered in preventing smoking. These programs have effectively reduced the likelihood of using drugs, such as marijuana, in many individuals (Botvin et al. 1990; Botvin & Wills 1985). The second approach is directed at getting the parents more actively involved in supervising their children. A prospective study showed that children of parents who provide little monitoring, rules and supervision are four times more likely to try drugs in the future than children with actively involved parents (Chilcoat, Dishion & Anthony 1995).

Drug abuse involves entrenched behaviours that are difficult to stop, particularly if physical dependence has developed. Most of the approaches that have been tried for treating drug abuse are similar to those we considered for stopping drinking. The outcomes of research on treating drug abuse seem to point to two conclusions (Bardo & Risner 1985; Schuster & Kilbey 1992; Tims, Fletcher & Hubbard 1991). First, the more promising treatment approaches include behavioural and cognitive methods, such as self-management techniques. Second, for cases of narcotic addiction, effective treatment programs also use chemical agents to block the euphoric effects of heroin, morphine or codeine. The most widely used agent is called **methadone**, a chemical that has physiological effects that are similar to those of opiates, except for two things: (1) it does not produce euphoria and (2) when it is taken regularly, it prevents euphoria from occurring if the person then takes an opiate (O'Brien 1996). Methadone is usually taken orally. Having a narcotics addict take methadone — or a similar agent, *levoalpha acetylmethadyl* (LAAM) — regularly as a substitute for the opiate is called *methadone maintenance*. Research has shown that treatment combining methadone and psychological treatment is far more effective than methadone alone (McClellan et al. 1993).

Although methadone maintenance can be very effective in reducing the addict's craving for opiates, preventing withdrawal symptoms and enabling the person to function in society, it also has some drawbacks (Callahan 1980; Sarason & Sarason 1984). For one thing, methadone is a form of narcotic, too — and the person can become physically dependent on it. Taking methadone may also lead to weight gain and increased alcohol use, and sometimes produces involuntary muscle jerking. One other problem with methadone is that it does not stop addicts from using other drugs, such as cocaine, which is a non-narcotic. But this problem seems to have been solved: programs often stipulate that before addicts get their next dose of methadone, they must submit to a urine test, which must show no evidence of drug taking. This approach is very effective in stopping methadone users from using non-narcotic drugs (Callahan 1980).

In our discussions of stopping smoking and drinking, we noted that relapse is a persistent and important problem. It is also a problem in stopping drug abuse, such as of marijuana (Stephens, Roffman & Simpson 1994). But methadone maintenance approaches have reduced the relapse rates for ex-opiate users. To prevent relapse with regard to all the substances we have considered in this chapter, programs for quitting will need to (1) enhance substance abusers' motivation to quit; (2) develop ways to match individuals to particular methods that are most likely to succeed for them; (3) teach them critical skills early in the program for avoiding relapse; and (4) have an aftercare program that involves continued monitoring of their behaviour, provides helpful social support and helps them adjust to a general lifestyle change (Brownell et al. 1986; Sandberg & Marlatt 1991).

Other solutions to aspects of the drug problem in Australia have been debated in recent years. These include having trials of medically prescribed heroin to minimise the harm associated with heroin (Gaughwin 2000), and trialling supervised injecting rooms to reduce fatal overdosing in drug addicts (Bammer 2000). A safe injecting room was opened recently in Sydney, although it is too soon to judge its success. It has been argued that providing supervised injecting rooms would reduce the number of persons injecting in public places, and further reduce the risk to the community of discarded needles and syringes (Bammer 2000). Arguments against these trials have centred on sending the 'wrong message' to young people about illegal drug use, and concern that drug use would escalate as a result of the trials.

Summary

People's use of tobacco, alcohol or drugs can affect their health, particularly if the substance is abused. Addiction is a condition in which individuals have become psychologically and physically dependent on the substance. People who are physically dependent on a substance have developed a tolerance for it and suffer withdrawal symptoms when they abruptly stop using it. Substance abuse exists when a person has shown a clear pattern of pathological use for at least a month with resulting problems in social and occupational functioning.

Smoking tobacco in Australia reached its greatest popularity in the mid-1960s, and then declined after the United States Surgeon General released a report describing its harmful health effects. Most people who become cigarette smokers begin the habit in adolescence. Although a larger percentage of men than women smoke, this gap has decreased in recent years. People in Australia are more likely to smoke if they are from lower rather than higher socioeconomic groups. Psychosocial factors influence whether individuals will start to smoke.

Whether people go on to smoke on a regular basis is determined by biopsychosocial factors. The likelihood of individuals becoming regular smokers increases if they have peer and adult models of smoking, experience peer pressure to smoke, and find that smoking helps them relax and experience less tension. Cigarette smoke contains tars, carbon monoxide and nicotine, a chemical that appears to produce physical dependence. Established smokers continue to smoke for at least two reasons: (1) the nicotine regulation model proposes that they smoke to maintain a certain level of nicotine in their bodies and avoid withdrawal, and (2) the biobehavioural model proposes that they smoke to regulate their performance and mood. Research has shown that heredity also plays a role in people's becoming smokers. Smoking reduces the person's life expectancy and increases the risk of lung cancer, other cancers, cardiovascular disease and chronic obstructive pulmonary disease. Breathing second-hand smoke is called passive smoking and is also harmful to one's health.

Programs to prevent smoking attempt to address relevant psychosocial factors by providing information and teaching important social skills. These programs teach children and adolescents about the immediate and long-term consequences of smoking, the ways modelling and peer pressure influence their tendency to smoke, and the ways they can resist these forces. Some programs also teach general social, cognitive and coping skills. Once people become regular smokers, many of them — even those who are heavy smokers — are able to quit on their own, but many others are not. For those who have trouble stopping, therapists use several approaches that help. These approaches include having the smoker take nicotine directly, using aversion strategies, and having the smoker learn and apply self-management strategies, such as self-monitoring and behavioural contracting. Combining effective methods in a multi-dimensional approach improves treatment success. Many people who quit eventually return to smoking. Relapse can result if the person experiences high levels of stress, has little helpful social support, or if there is an abstinence-violation effect, feelings of low self-efficacy or an increase in body weight.

Colonial Australians brought their heavy drinking patterns with them from England. Although Australia has a reputation as a drinking nation, early Australians were not drinking more than their American or British counterparts. The 1830s was a period of particularly heavy drinking, although Prohibition during the gold rush of the 1850s and later in the early 1900s changed drinking patterns of Australians. Most Australian adults drink at least occasionally. Many of those who drink abuse alcohol and are classified as problem drinkers. About half of the problem drinkers are physically dependent on alcohol and are classified as alcoholics. People who are addicted to alcohol suffer withdrawal symptoms called delirium tremens when they quit drinking. Psychosocial factors — such as modelling, social pressure and reinforcement — have a very powerful influence on drinking. Heredity plays an important role in the development of alcohol abuse.

Heavy drinking is related to a variety of health problems, including foetal alcohol syndrome in babies of drinking mothers, automobile accidents and such diseases as cirrhosis of the liver, cancer, high blood pressure and brain damage. The most promising programs for preventing alcohol abuse involve public policy and legal approaches, health promotion and education approaches, and early intervention approaches. For people who become problem drinkers, the first step in their recovery is detoxification. Treatment approaches for stopping drinking include Alcoholics Anonymous, insight therapy, a variety of behavioural and cognitive methods, and using emetic drugs. Minimal interventions have been found to be as effective as intensive treatment for those drinkers with low levels of alcohol dependence.

Many people use and abuse drugs that can be classified as stimulants, depressants, hallucinogens and narcotics. Drugs differ in their potential for producing physical and psychological dependence. Drug abuse is related to a number of psychosocial factors, such as modelling, social pressure, reinforcement and personality traits. Drug usage among adolescents is associated with frequent alcohol use and cigarette smoking. The health effects of drug use and abuse are becoming increasingly clear. For example, using cocaine produces cardiovascular reactions that can cause a potentially fatal myocardial infarction. Prevention efforts today focus on social influence methods, like those used in preventing smoking and drinking. The most effective programs for treating drug abuse involve behavioural and cognitive methods; treatments for narcotic addiction often use drugs, such as methadone, that block the euphoric effects of opiates. Relapse is a critical problem in treatment programs for all of the substances discussed in this chapter.

Key terms

abstinence-violation effect	detoxification	nicotine fading	self-management strategies
addiction	emetic drug	nicotine regulation model	stimulants
alcoholics	hallucinogens	passive smoking	substance abuse
aversion strategies	methadone	physical dependence	tars
biobehavioural model	motivational interviewing	problem drinkers	tolerance
carbon monoxide	narcotics	psychological dependence	withdrawal
depressants	nicotine	relapse	

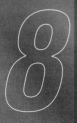

Improving nutrition, weight control and diet, physical activity and safety

Prologue

'Let's share something with each other,' said the health expert to the members of a community work-shop. 'What excuses do we find ourselves using for not eating more healthily, not exercising regularly and not behaving in other ways that promote health, such as reducing alcohol consumption or quitting smoking? I'll start it off,' she continued, 'by confessing that I sometimes skip exercising because I run out of time. What excuses do you use?' The answers came quickly:

'I never seem to have the energy to exercise.'

'My wife sprained her ankle jogging, and I know lots of other people who've injured themselves exercising.'

'I don't have the time to prepare healthy meals.'

'My grandparents ate high-fat diets and lived past 85.'

'My kids hate vegetables and my husband insists on having meat for dinner.'

'I enjoy one or two beers with my mates. What's wrong with that?'

'Smoking calms me down.'

'If I didn't smoke, I'd get fat.'

'I've had my habits for so long — it's hard to change.'

People cite many reasons for not leading more healthy lifestyles. Some of the obstacles they describe can be overcome fairly easily, but others are more difficult. In most cases, people could find ways to overcome obstacles to healthy behaviour if they believed it was important and were motivated to do so. As we noted previously in the health belief model, changing existing habits is very difficult. Many of the barriers that impede change are real for the individual involved. If a parent says they do not have time to prepare healthy meals, what does it mean? It could be that they are so tied up in caring for children, or having to fit in meal preparation along with holding down a full-time job, that they find it impossible to juggle the time they have. To take time out to prepare good meals may have a low priority, and it will take effort and energy to re-set priorities, or to do less of one or more of another, for what reward?

In this chapter, we discuss how nutrition, weight control, exercise and safety measures are impor-tant to people's health. We also examine what people do and do not do in these areas of their life-styles, as well as why they behave as they do and how they can change unhealthy behaviours. As we study these lifestyle factors, we will consider important questions and problems people have in leading healthy lives. Which foods are healthy, and which are not? What determines the preferences people have for different foods, such as sweets? Why do overweight individuals have such a hard time losing weight and keeping it off? What kinds of exercise benefit health? What hazards exist in our environments, and how can we protect ourselves from them?

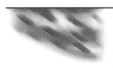

Nutrition

'You are what you eat,' as the saying goes. This saying has at least two meanings. The most common meaning is that the quality of your diet can determine how you look, act and feel. Another meaning is that

> food and the human body are made up of the same classes of chemicals: water, carbohydrates, fats, proteins, vitamins, and minerals . . . Each of these classes makes identifiable contributions to the metabolic processes of all cells in the body. (Greenfield, 1985, pp. 293–4)

In this section, we will examine aspects of both meanings, beginning with the components of food and their importance in metabolic processes.

Components of food

Healthy diets provide optimal amounts of all essential nutrients for the body's metabolic needs. In addition to water, food contains five types of chemical components that provide specific nutrients for body functioning (Greenfield 1985; Holum 1994; USDA 1995). The five types of components and their roles in metabolism are as follows:

1. *Carbohydrates* include simple and complex sugars that constitute major sources of energy for the body. Simple sugars include *glucose*, which is found in foods made of animal products, and *fructose*, which is found in fruits and honey. Diets may also provide more complex sugars, such as *sucrose* (table sugar), *lactose* in milk products, and *starch* in many plants.

2. *Lipids* or 'fats' also provide energy for the body. Lipids include saturated and polyunsaturated fats, as well as cholesterol.

3. *Proteins* are important mainly in the body's synthesis of new cell material. They are composed of organic molecules called *amino acids*; about half of the 20 or so known amino acids are essential for body development and functioning and must be provided by our diet.

4. *Vitamins* are organic chemicals that regulate metabolism and functions of the body. They are used in converting nutrients to energy, producing hormones, and breaking down waste products and toxins. Some vitamins (A, D, E and K) are *fat-soluble* — they dissolve in fats and are stored in the body's fatty tissue. The remaining vitamins (B and C) are *water-soluble* — the body stores very little of these vitamins and excretes excess quantities as waste.

5. *Minerals* are inorganic substances, such as calcium, phosphorus, potassium, sodium, iron, iodine and zinc, each of which is important in body development and functioning. For example, calcium and phosphorus are components of bones and teeth, potassium and sodium are involved in nerve transmission and iron is important in transporting oxygen in the blood.

Food also contains *fibre*, which is not considered a nutrient because it is not used in metabolism but is still needed in the process of digestion.

People can get all the nutrients and fibre they need by eating diets that consist of a variety of foods from five basic groups: grains, fruits, vegetables, milk products, and meats and fish, as shown in figure 8.1. Breads and cereals made of whole grains have more fibre than those made of grains that are 'enriched' or 'fortified' with nutrients. Most people who eat healthily do not need to supplement their diets with vitamins and other nutrients — one carrot, for instance, provides enough vitamin A to last 4 days. Women who are pregnant have greater needs of all nutrients; although most of the extra nutrients can come from adjustments in their diets, they should also take recommended supplements, such as of iron (Hegsted 1984; St. Jeor, Sutnick & Scott 1988). And women who have a specific, detectable gene may need to take folic acid, a B vitamin, to prevent their babies from developing a severe birth defect called *spina bifida* (Whitehead et al. 1995). Some people who take supplements have an attitude of 'the more the better'. But it is possible to overdo taking some nutrients, leading to a form of 'poisoning' if they accumulate in the body. For example, too much of vitamins A and D can pose serious health hazards to the liver and kidneys, respectively. The value of taking moderate doses of vitamin C or E daily is still controversial (CU 1994b).

Unprocessed foods are generally more healthy than processed foods, which often contain additives that benefit the food industry more than the consumer. These additives include: *preservatives* that lengthen the shelf life of the food, *emulsifiers* to enable oil and water to mix, *thickeners* and *stabilisers* that improve or maintain the texture of foods, and *flavour enhancers* that heighten the natural taste of foods (Klockenbrink 1987). Although most additives are not dangerous to people's health, some cause allergic reactions or may be carcinogenic. Some additives are known to be harmful to specific groups of individuals; for example, the flavour enhancer disodium guanylate should be avoided by people who have gout. Children may be especially vulnerable to the effects of additives because their body systems are still forming and maturing rapidly and, kilo-for-kilo, they eat more than adults.

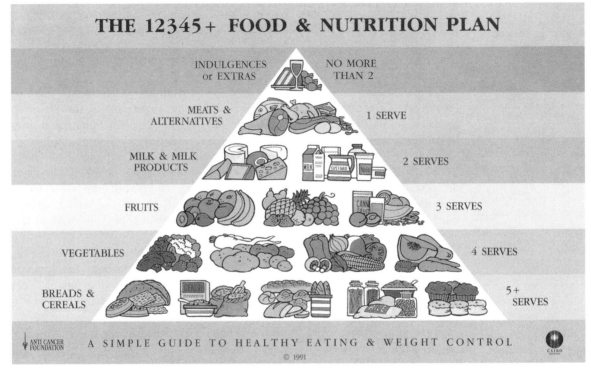

Figure 8.1 Food and Nutrition Plan. A diagram indicating the relative number of servings of different classes of foods a healthy diet should contain each day (CSIRO Human Nutrition & Anti-Cancer Foundation of SA 2001; www.dhn.csiro.au/12345fdplan.html). Smaller amounts are recommended for foods in the upper levels than for those in the lower levels of the pyramid.

What people eat

Australian eating patterns over time

Since the early days of settlement the eating patterns of Australians have been influenced mostly by British dietary patterns within different social strata. Vast differences existed in food consumed by rural peasants compared with the affluent classes in seventeenth- and eighteenth-century England (Clements 1986). The diet of rural people consisted of cereal gruels and soups based on peas, roots and green leaves with the occasional addition of a piece of salted pork. For the upper classes, it was quite common to feast on several courses of game, garden vegetables, bread and cakes made from locally produced cereals, beer and cider. The First Fleet at Sydney Cove in 1788 subsisted on provisions of flour, biscuit, oatmeal, rice, peas, cheese, butter, salted beef, pork and vinegar (Wahlqvist 1988). These provisions were rationed among the convicts and overseers over the next two years. Malnutrition and scurvy were common. In the first years of settlement, problems were encountered in establishing agriculture and maintaining livestock, but by 1813 settlers enjoyed a varied diet of mutton, wheat, potatoes, fruit and vegetables, milk, butter, cheese, tea and sugar (Clements 1986). With the growth of cities the working, middle and upper classes emerged. Red meat was consumed by all three groups, with the working classes cultivating vegetable gardens. Differences in eating patterns centred mainly on the variety of food consumed, with the upper classes able to afford extra delicacies (Clements 1986). Since the second half of the nineteenth century Australians have had one of the highest intakes of red meat in the world. The quantity of meat consumed is understandable when one considers the energy requirements of work like timber logging, cane cutting and shearing. As Clements (1986) notes, it was not uncommon for meat to be eaten three times a day.

> On the larger sheep stations and among the urban elite, breakfast consisted of four to six mutton chops, often with bacon and eggs, short cakes and oatmeal, the last named in households of Scottish origin; lunch and dinner were more substantial with two or three joints, invariably roasted, and four or five vegetables, ... dinner was distinguished from lunch by having several varieties of desserts compared with one at lunch. (p. 36)

These dietary patterns continued for the most part with the exception of the Depression and the war years. Fruit and vegetables were not eaten to the same extent as meat, a trend that appears to have remained to the present day (AIHW 1998, 2000). The influx of migrants to Australia after World War II led to the adoption of foods of these cultural groups. Today the diet of Australians reflects the multicultural nature of this country. Some noticeable trends in the eating patterns of Australians over the past thirty years include an increase in the consumption of poultry, lamb and pork in preference to mutton, increased use of convenience and fast foods, a change to vegetable oils for cooking and low-fat spreads, a decrease in bread consumption, an increase in use of low-fat milk and other dairy products, and increased consumption of wine and coffee in preference to beer and tea (Wahlqvist 1988).

The Australian diet compared with those of other countries

Diets vary across cultural groups (Criqui & Ringel 1994). For instance, Danes consume 60 per cent more animal fat than Australians, who consume twice as much as Israelis and Japanese. And Italians and Spaniards consume 40 per cent more vegetables than Finnish and Australian people. For most of the twentieth century, Australian diets showed a fairly consistent trend: people consumed more and more sugar, animal fats and animal proteins, while consuming less and less fibre (Clements 1986). Their consumption of vegetables, fruits and cereals declined while that of meats and sugary foods, such as soft drinks and processed goods, increased. The way food is prepared also changed and affected people's diets. Consider the potato, for example: a baked or boiled potato by itself has few calories and almost no fat, but when french-fried or made into potato chips, its calorie and fat content skyrockets. Australians' increased use of processed and fast foods has contributed to the changes in their diets.

How healthy are people's diets in Australia today? One dimension of this question involves their consumption of sugars and animal fats, which is far too high (AIHW 1998). Nutritionists and others concerned with people's health have been recommending that Australians reduce these components in their diets. Are Australians beginning to follow these recommendations? Yes, in some ways (AIHW 1998). Since 1980 people's consumption of red meats has declined, and they're eating more fish and poultry, cereals and grains, and fruits and vegetables. But they've also increased their intake of sugars and soft drinks. There are marked differences, however, in the nutrient intakes of different sociodemographic groups in Australia. For example, fat consumption is lower in older males and in males of higher occupational status. Those who have lower fat intakes tend to consume more fibre, refined and natural sugars, and alcohol (Baghurst, Baghurst & Record 1994). Levels of dietary cholesterol are higher in lower occupational groups. Persons of lower socioeconomic status are also less likely to follow dietary guidelines such as not adding salt to meals, removing the skin from cooked chicken, not adding sugar to drinks and cereal, and leaving the peel on fruits (Turrell & Najman 1995). The nutrient intake of Australian males is also different from that of females. Males tend to consume more fat; more women than men eat fruit and vegetables. Most Australians at all ages consume sufficient amounts of the essential nutrients (Baghurst, Baghurst & Record 1990). However, women and the elderly may not be consuming sufficiently high levels of calcium, iron, magnesium and vitamin B_6 — and supplements of these nutrients may be warranted.

Why do people eat what they eat? Diets are determined by biopsychosocial factors (Logue 1991; Rozin 1989; Rozin & Fallon 1981). Most people around the world — even newborn babies — like sweet tastes and avoid bitter tastes. These preferences appear to be inborn. Other evidence indicates that brain chemicals can lead people to eat fatty foods and activate their brain pleasure centres when they do (Azar 1994). But people also acquire food preferences as a result of their individual and social experiences (Birch 1989; Rozin 1989; Schutz & Diaz-Knauf 1989). Children receive certain foods, but not others, depending on cultural and economic conditions — and simply being exposed to a food may increase their liking of it. They also observe in person and through TV commercials how other people respond to a food and tend to become more attracted to it if they see others eat it and like it. Through social experiences, people can develop ideas about foods they have never even tried. Suppose you saw TV commercials for two new chocolate sweets, one with 'a special fruit filling' and the other filled with cockroaches. How would you feel about trying these products? Yet, cockroaches are a great delicacy in some cultures.

Enormous numbers of children around the world simply do not have nutritious diets available to them for proper growth and development. A study of the average heights of children in different parts of the world revealed that the smallest children tend to live in highly impoverished areas, and the tallest in wealthier locations (Meredith 1978). For example, children in the Netherlands, a prosperous, well-fed and healthy nation, were found to be nearly 20 per cent taller than children in rural India and Thailand, where poverty, famine and disease have been common. The study also found contrasts between children from rich and poor families living in the same area: in Hong Kong, for instance, upper-class Chinese children were taller than their lower-class counterparts. But these same upper-class Chinese were shorter than upper-class children living in the Netherlands. Such regional and social class differences in bodily growth are due to many variables, including genetics, nutrition and disease.

What eating behaviours are practised among young Australians? In a study of 791 North Queensland children aged 12 to 14 years (Nowak & Speare 1996), girls were found to have better knowledge of good eating practices, to eat more fruit and vegetables, and fewer high-fat and high-sugar foods than boys. Core cereal foods such as wholemeal bread, rice and pasta were eaten by more boys than girls. Only one quarter of the students surveyed had reported food intakes in line with the dietary recommendations for calcium intake, core cereal foods and fruits/vegetables. These findings are consistent with studies in other states that report adolescent eating patterns well below the recommended dietary intake of core food groups (DCSH 1986; Magery & Boulton 1995; Jenner & Miller 1991). Dietary differences between girls and boys may be influenced by social ideals of the male macho image, and feminine thinness as portrayed by fashion and the media.

Nutrition and health

Australian mass media announce almost daily that many people eat diets that are not as healthy as they should be. Some individuals have responded by using foods and substances sold at health food stores. Although some of these products — such as whole grains — are clearly beneficial, many supplements and other products are of dubious worth (CU 1994c, 1995a). Some people attempt to improve their diets by becoming *vegetarians*. There are degrees of vegetarianism, ranging from simply avoiding red meats to strictly using only plant foods and no animal products whatsoever. When people avoid all animal products, they must plan very carefully to ensure that their diets, and especially their children's, contain a balance of proteins and sufficient amounts of essential vitamins and minerals (Dwyer 1991). The most common dietary culprits in many nations of the world are those associated with the development of atherosclerosis, hypertension, diabetes and cancer.

Diet and atherosclerosis

Cholesterol is the main dietary factor in atherosclerosis, the deposit of fatty plaques in our blood vessels. These fatty plaques narrow the coronary blood vessels and restrict the blood flow to the heart muscle, increasing the likelihood of a heart attack. As we saw in chapter 2, cholesterol is a fatty substance. Our bodies produce most of the cholesterol in blood, and our diets provide the remainder. Whether cholesterol forms plaques in our blood vessels depends on the presence of different types of cholesterol-carrying proteins called **lipoproteins**. There are three types of lipoproteins: **Low-density lipoprotein** (LDL) and **very-low-density lipoprotein** (VLDL) are associated with *increased* cholesterol deposits, but **high-density lipoprotein** (HDL) is associated with *decreased* likelihood of plaque build-up (AHA 1994; Cooper 1988). Cholesterol carried by LDL and VLDL is often called 'bad cholesterol' because it travels *towards* the body cells, whereas cholesterol carried by HDL is 'good cholesterol' because it travels *away* from the cells to be processed or removed by the liver.

How much cholesterol in the blood is too much? Normal levels of cholesterol increase with age in adulthood. The Risk Factor Prevalence Study, the most recent national study of blood cholesterol, conducted by the National Heart Foundation in 1989, indicated that more than 47 per cent of Australian men, and 39 per cent of Australian women between the ages of 20 and 69 years (or approximately 4.5 million persons) had cholesterol levels over 5.5 mmol/L (Bennett & Magnus 1994). Total cholesterol levels have decreased over time for males between the ages of 25 and 34 years, while for older men the HDL cholesterol levels have increased (Bennett & Magnus 1994). For women, total cholesterol, HDL and LDL cholesterol have fallen, especially in older age groups (Bennett & Magnus 1994). A prospective study followed the health of more than 350 000 middle-aged Americans for six years and found that, within any age group, the higher the subjects' cholesterol levels at the start of the study, the greater their risk of death from heart disease or stroke (Stamler et al. 1986). The risk for individuals with cholesterol levels above 245 mg or 6.3 mmol/L was 3.4 times as high as for those with levels below 180 or 4.6 mmol/L. Experts agree that long-term high levels of cholesterol in the blood can lead to heart disease and stroke, and the general rule of thumb is that people with total serum cholesterol levels of 6.5 mmol/L or more are at high risk (NHMRC 1991; Owen et al. 1990). But there are two limitations to this rule. First, cholesterol levels of people over age 70 are not related to heart disease morbidity or mortality (Krumholz et al. 1994). Second, the rule doesn't take the 'good' and 'bad' types of cholesterol into account, which is important to do because the greater the amount of HDL in one's total serum cholesterol, the lower the risk of cardiovascular disease (Cooper 1988; Gordon et al. 1989). For example, a 50-year-old man with 6.4 mmol/L of total cholesterol, 1.8 mmol/L of which is HDL, is likely to be at low risk.

People's cholesterol levels are determined partly by heredity and partly by their life-styles (Hopkins 1992; Rona et al. 1985). Some evidence suggests that smoking ciga-rettes may increase LDL and decrease HDL levels (Muscat et al. 1991). Diet is an important factor: some foods, such as eggs, many milk products and fatty meats, con-tain very high concentrations of cholesterol. Australians have been reducing their intake of cholesterol recently, but still consume far too much (Bennet & Magnus 1994). The National Heart Foundation of Australia (1987) has set a desirable level of below 5.5 mmol/L for blood cholesterol. Children after the preschool years should follow diets like those recommended for adults. Those children whose parents or grandparents had heart disease at early ages should have their cholesterol levels and diets assessed. Atherosclerosis can begin in childhood, and children need to develop good eating habits early so that they do not have entrenched habits to overcome later (Cooper 1988; DISC 1995). If changes in patients' diets do not lower high-cholesterol levels enough, physicians may also prescribe medication.

Does lowering serum cholesterol reduce cardiovascular illness? Yes. Studies have demonstrated that large reductions in serum cholesterol, produced with combined dietary and drug treatment, retard and often *reverse* the development of atherosclerosis (Superko & Krauss 1994). Other research found that heart disease patients who underwent a surgical procedure that rerouted the small intestine, which greatly low-ered cholesterol absorption into the blood, showed less progression of their disease and fewer heart attacks during a 10-year follow-up than similar patients who did not have the procedure (Buchwald et al. 1990). But there may be a caution about other health effects of lowering people's cholesterol. Although current evidence is incon-sistent and inconclusive, some studies have found that markedly reduced serum chol-esterol is associated with reduced longevity (Atrens 1994) and with non-illness deaths, such as from accidents, suicide and violence (Muldoon & Manuck 1992; Muldoon, Manuck & Matthews 1990). It may be that lowering cholesterol increases some people's recklessness or aggressiveness. But a study found that the hostility and depression levels of middle-aged men and women who participated in a five-year cholesterol-lowering program decreased by the end of the program (Weidner et al. 1992).

Is mortality from heart disease associated with the amount of saturated fat in the diet? Research by Keys (1970, 1980) found that over a 10-year period death from heart disease was positively associated with dietary fat in seven countries. Yet in another, larger-scale study of 37 countries (Pickard 1986), death from heart disease was not found to be related to any dietary variables. Other evidence against saturated fat as a risk factor for heart disease comes from the lack of a consistent relationship between dietary fat intake and death from heart disease over the past 40 years (Atrens 1994). Prior to 1970 a positive association was found between death from heart disease and dietary fat intake in the English-speaking countries of Australia, Canada and the United States. After 1970 the steady increases in fat intake in these countries show no associated relationship to the observed decline in death from heart disease (Atrens 1994; FAO 1993). This anomaly in findings could be explained by changes having occurred in other risk factors related to heart disease, for example smoking or physical activity. The decline in heart disease might also be explained by a greater awareness of the effects of stress on cardiac functioning, combined with psychological interventions to help manage stress, such as relaxation training, and interventions to change Type A behaviour patterns.

Diet and hypertension

Ten per cent of Australian adults are hypertensive, having blood pressures at or exceeding 160 systolic/95 diastolic (AIHW 1998). Although medication can lower blood pressure, the first methods doctors advise usually involve lifestyle changes, especially losing weight and restricting certain foods in the patient's diet. People who are at risk for developing hypertension can effectively reduce their risk by making such changes (Stamler et al. 1989).

Of all the substances in people's diets that could affect blood pressure, *sodium* — such as in salt (sodium chloride) — may play the strongest role. Studies have shown that consuming high levels of sodium increases blood pressure and people's reactivity in stressful situations (Denton et al. 1995; Falkner & Light 1986; Kaplan 1986). A tea-spoon of salt contains about 2000 mg of sodium, and between 1100 and 3300 mg a day is considered safe and adequate (Zamula 1987). But the average Australian probably consumes 7000 mg of sodium daily, some of which comes from adding salt to foods. The rest comes mainly from eating foods that already contain high levels of sodium, as do many processed meats, potato chips and cereals, for example. Because sodium can elevate blood pressure, doctors often place hypertensive patients on low-sodium diets. Although some people are more sensitive to the effects of sodium than others (Sullivan 1991), the evidence is now very clear that reducing dietary sodium lowers blood pressure in hypertensives and normotensives alike (Law, Frost & Wald 1991).

Caffeine is another dietary substance that can affect blood pressure. Most of the caffeine people consume generally comes from drinking caffeinated coffee, strong tea and cola beverages. Caffeine increases people's reactivity to stress and raises their blood pressure at least temporarily (France & Ditto 1988; Green & Suls 1996; James 1993; Lovallo et al. 1991, 1996).

Does caffeine consumption lead to hypertension and coronary heart disease? One study followed the health of more than 1900 men for 19 years and found that subjects who drank six or more cups of coffee a day had much higher mortality rates from coronary heart disease than those who drank less (LeGrady et al. 1987). But other studies have found opposing results (Grobbee et al. 1990; Salvaggio et al. 1990). And a meta-analysis of several studies found no link between the amount of caffeine consumption and heart disease (Kawachi, Colditz & Stone 1994). Habitual coffee drinkers do not appear to be at greater risk of cardiovascular disease.

Diet and cancer

Diets high in fat and low in fibre are associated with the development of cancer, particularly cancer of the colon (ACS 1996; Bristol et al. 1985) and prostate gland (Giovanucci et al. 1993; Wang et al. 1995). The diets of most Australians do not conform to the recommendations of the Australian Cancer Society. Surveys have found that Australians were far more likely to eat foods that pose a higher risk of cancer — such as red meats, bacon and lunch meats — than to eat foods that pose a lower risk, such as fruits, certain vegetables and high-fibre breads and cereals (AIHW 1998).

Other possible cancer-protective components of diets are vitamins A, C and E. Many fruits and vegetables are rich in *beta-carotene*, which the body converts to vitamin A; and they are also good sources of vitamins C and E. Early studies yielded results suggesting that these vitamins may protect people from cancers, but more recent research has produced opposing results (Byers et al. 1987; Greenberg et al. 1994). On the basis of the early findings, some people began to supplement their diets with these vitamins. Nutritionists recommend against doing this with vitamin A because it builds up in the body, and it is too easy to overdose.

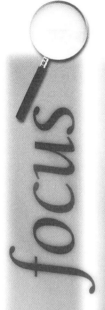

Focus on research
Interventions to reduce cholesterol intake

Most people can lower their cholesterol intake markedly if they will modify their eating habits, sometimes by making very simple changes. For example, a person whose cholesterol intake averages 400 mg per day can lower this amount to 251 mg by substituting low-cholesterol foods, such as cereals, for just four eggs per week — an egg contains about 260 mg of cholesterol. Other ways to reduce cholesterol intake include reducing the amounts and changing the types of meats in the diet, broiling or baking foods instead of frying, using low-cholesterol vegetable fats for cooking, and using low-fat dairy products. Most cereals, breads, fruits, nuts, and vegetables contain little or no cholesterol. But people should be wary of some processed foods that do not specify the kind of vegetable oil they use — these products often contain *saturated* fats (coconut or palm oils) rather than the more expensive polyunsaturated fats, such as corn or soybean oils. Oils that derive from certain plants, such as olives, consist of *monounsaturated* fats that contain no cholesterol and appear to *lower* serum LDL, but not HDL, cholesterol (Brody 1993; Cooper 1988).

Because most Americans and Australians consume too much cholesterol, researchers have tested intervention programs to help people lower their intake levels. One of these programs conducted in the United States was part of the Multiple Risk Factor Intervention Trial (MRFIT) and was designed to modify the diets of thousands of men over a period of six years (Caggiula et al. 1981; Dolecek et al. 1986; Gorder et al. 1986). The subjects were between 35 and 57 years of age at the start of the study and were at risk of coronary heart disease because of high serum cholesterol levels, high blood pressure and cigarette smoking. Before they entered the study, they had already made self-initiated changes to reduce saturated fats in their diets. The subjects were randomly assigned to two groups, so that half of the men participated in the intervention program and the remainder were simply referred to their physicians as a 'usual care' control group. All the subjects returned periodically for medical examinations and to report the diets they consumed during the prior 24 hours. The men in the intervention received counselling on an individual basis each year, when they and 'their homemakers' participated in group meetings that provided information about the benefits of and methods for modifying their diets.

The MRFIT program was successful in modifying the men's diets substantially and lowering their serum cholesterol levels. The men who most needed to modify their diets tended to do so and achieved the greatest gains.

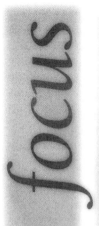

But because these improvements fell short of the program's goals and guidelines of the American Heart Association, other researchers have tried to find more successful approaches by comparing the effectiveness of different methods. One study compared three methods with male and female adult volunteers from the general population — that is, they were *not* selected for being at high risk for health problems (Foreyt et al. 1979). The subjects were randomly assigned to three conditions: One group simply received a *booklet* describing a low-cholesterol diet program; another group attended a series of *nutrition education* classes; and a third group received a *behavioural/education* program that combined the nutrition education classes with self-management training. Serum cholesterol levels were assessed at the start of the study and after three, six and 12 months. The results indicated that the behavioural/education program was the most effective approach, but that a follow-up program may be needed to maintain improved diets. The success of this approach is especially impressive because the subjects did not have very high serum cholesterol levels to begin with.

Another large-scale intervention to reduce cholesterol and cardiovascular mortality was the Helsinki Heart Study (Frick et al. 1987). This intervention used a biomedical approach to modify HDL in 4081 middle-aged men (40 to 55 years), and monitored their health status over five years. An intensive screening procedure was used to ensure that the males were free from any coronary symptoms at the start of the study, and did not differ on other risk factors such as Type A behaviour, smoking and alcohol consumption. Those males at risk of coronary disease because of high levels of blood lipids were then randomly allocated to receive either the drug Gemfibrozil or a placebo. Results indicated that Genfibrozil was effective in reducing serum total cholesterol, LDL cholesterol, non-HDL cholesterol and triglycerides while increasing HDL cholesterol, which is protective against heart disease. The Helsinki Heart Study reported a 26 per cent lower mortality from coronary heart disease in the treatment group compared with the placebo group. However, there were more deaths overall in the Genfibrozil group.

Interventions to reduce high serum cholesterol levels need to involve behavioural and educational programs for the patient, training and cooperation by other members of the patient's household, support groups, and a long-term follow-up program (Carmody et al. 1982). They also need to address the reasons people do not change their diets, such as their low self-efficacy or readiness for change, strong taste preferences for high-fat foods and difficulties obtaining low-fat foods when not eating at home (McCann et al. 1995, 1996; Terry, Oakland & Ankeny 1991).

What people include in their diets is clearly related to their risk of developing several major chronic diseases. Other dietary problems that affect health arise from consuming too many calories: Experimental research with animals has shown that reducing calorie intake by 30 per cent from standard nutritious diets decreases metabolism, slows the ageing process and increases longevity (Lane et al. 1996). Eating too much food can be unhealthy, as we are about to see.

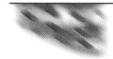

Weight control and diet

People in many cultures around the world are very 'weight conscious'. In Australia, individuals often start being concerned about their weight in childhood, particularly if they are overweight and are teased and excluded from social groups (Abraham &

Llewellyn-Jones 1992). When children reach the teenage years, many become greatly preoccupied with their physical appearance and would like to change how they look (Conger & Petersen 1984). They frequently express concerns about skin problems and wanting to have a better figure or more athletic body, to be taller or shorter, and to be the 'right' weight. People with less-than-ideal bodies are often thought of as lazy and self-indulgent, and many of them wish or strive for bodies they are biologically unable to achieve (Brownell 1991).

Being the 'wrong' weight often affects people's self-esteem, (Ben-Tovim & Walker 1991). An American study of overweight 10- to 16-year-olds found that the girls' self-esteem declined sharply and consistently through those years, but the boys' self-esteem only declined during the early years (Mendelson & White 1985). Perhaps as overweight boys get older, some degree of bulk is considered 'manly'.

Australian adolescents, although less overweight than American adolescents, never-theless are just as concerned about their weight and shape (Nowak & Crawford 1998). In a Melbourne study (Paxton et al. 1991), 71 per cent of girls and 33 per cent of boys reported that they would like to be thinner, compared with 37 per cent of boys and only 8 per cent of girls who wanted to gain weight. Similar findings were reported in a North Queensland study (Nowak, Speare & Crawford 1996), where twice as many girls (52 per cent) as boys (27 per cent) wanted to lose weight, whereas twice as many boys (20 per cent) as girls (8 per cent) wanted to gain weight. Almost half the girls and a quarter of the boys had tried to lose weight in the previous year, indicating that concern with thinness is well established by the age of 12 in Australian adolescents. Among those attempting to lose weight, unacceptable methods such as diuretics, laxatives, weight loss pills, weight loss powders or vomiting had been used by about 10 per cent of adolescents.

Australian adolescent females appear to have greater body image disturbance and dissatisfaction than males (Maude et al. 1993). A substantial number of normal weight females consider themselves overweight, while underweight females perceive them-selves as being an appropriate weight. Adolescent males, on the other hand, consider themselves a good weight, even when they are over the normal weight range. Male and female adolescents have been found to differ in their weight-related eating behaviour (Nowak 1998). Boys attempting to lose weight tend to reduce their sweet foods and snack intake while increasing healthy foods such as fruit, yoghurt and low-fat milk. Girls who are trying to lose weight tend to skip meals like breakfast and lunch, and consume less milk, bread, meat, sweets and fatty foods. For girls, some reduction in meals, snacks, core cereals, dairy foods and sweet, but not savoury, fatty foods persisted after the weight loss.

The greater concern among females than males about their weight — especially about being overweight — continues in adulthood (Kenny & Adams 1994). *Whether* individuals do anything about their weight and *what* they do can have important implications for their health.

Overweight and obesity

No matter how fit we are, our bodies have some fat — and they should. Having fat only becomes a problem when we have too much. The question is: How much is too much? Determining how much fat a person's body has is not as easy as it may seem. Bulk or stockiness alone can be misleading, since some stocky people simply have larger skeletal frames than other people do, or their bodies are more muscular. As a result, precise assessment of overweight is done with either the *body mass index* (BMI) or complex methods for accurately measuring the amount of body fat an individual has (Perri, Nezu & Viegener 1992). To calculate your BMI, you divide your weight in kilograms by your height in centimetres squared. Most people have BMIs in the 20s (Abraham & Llewellyn-Jones 1992).

A more common and simple approach for assessing whether someone is overly fat is based on data regarding *desirable weights* of men and women, determined through studies of mortality rates. A standard chart of desirable weights is presented in table 8.1. The table provides the healthy weight range according to height. For example, a person who is 173 cm tall (without shoes) has a desirable weight range of 59–74 kg, including an allowance for clothing. People are classified as **overweight** if their weight exceeds this range by 10–20 per cent, and **obese** if they are more than 20 per cent over that range (or a BMI greater than 27) (AMA 1989; Perri, Nezu & Viegener 1992; Himes & Dietz 1994). If the man in our example weighed 82 kg (with clothes), he would be overweight; if he weighed 89 or more, he would be obese.

Table 8.1   Healthy weights for men and women (over 18 years)

Height (no shoes)		Healthy weight range
cm	ft ins	kg
140	4' 7"	39–49
142	4' 8"	40–50
145	4' 9"	42–52
148	4' 10"	44–55
150	4' 11"	45–56
152	5' 0"	46–58
155	5' 1"	48–60
158	5' 2"	50–62
160	5' 3"	51–64
162	5' 4"	52–66
165	5' 5"	54–68
168	5' 6"	56–71
170	5' 7"	58–72
173	5' 8"	59–74
175	5' 9"	61–76
178	5' 10"	63–79
180	5' 11"	65–81
183	6' 0"	66–83
185	6' 1"	68–85
188	6' 2"	71–88
190	6' 3"	72–90
193	6' 4"	74–92
195	6' 5"	77–95
198	6' 6"	78–98
200	6' 7"	80–100

Based on weights with least risk of disease or death from heart disease, diabetes, stroke and cancer.

Based on Body Mass Index 20–25. BMI calculated as $\dfrac{\text{Weight (kg)}}{\text{Height (m)}^2}$

Source: Borushek (2001).

Why people become overly fat

Obesity has increased since 1980 for both Australian males and females, in particular those aged between 25 and 64 years (AIHW 2000). Two out of three Australian males (64 per cent) and about half the adult females (49 per cent) are overweight or obese. This represents about 7.4 million adult Australians (AIHW 2000). The prevalence of overly fat people varies with nationality, sociocultural factors, gender and age. In Australia, the percentage of women who are overweight is higher for indigenous and Torres Strait Islander groups (AIHW 1998). Age changes in weight also depend on gender. Among men, the prevalence rate of being too heavy increases until about age 50; among women, the prevalence rate increases into old age (Millar & Stephens 1987; AIHW 1998). And research has revealed a disturbing trend: among children and the population as a whole in Australia, the percentage who are overly fat has increased substantially during the past few decades (AIHW 1998, Gortmaker et al. 1987; Zaldivar 1993).

People add fat to their bodies because they consume more calories than they burn up through metabolism. If there are 3500 calories in half a kilogram of stored fat in the body (Borushek 1986), then to work off half a kilogram of stored fat, a person would have to reduce their food intake by 500 calories a day for a week. If the person's weekly calorie expenditure is usually 2500, then additional exercise of over 180 minutes of brisk walking per week will usually ensure this. Approximately 300 calories are used up per one hour of brisk walking (Borushek 1986). The body stores excess calories as fat in *adipose tissue*, which consists of cells that vary in number and size (Logue 1991). According to researcher Margaret Straw, the

> growth of adipose tissue throughout childhood and adolescence involves both an increase in cell size and in cell number. Thereafter, it appears that growth in adipose tissue is initially associated with an increase in cell size; if cell size becomes excessive, new adipose tissue is generated through an increase in the number of cells. (1983, p. 223)

A major reason why adults tend to gain weight as they get older is that metabolism and physical activity decline with age (Smith 1984). To maintain their younger weight levels, people need to exercise and take in fewer calories as they get older. Both biological and psychosocial factors affect weight control.

Biological factors in weight control

Because the metabolic rates of individuals can differ greatly, some thin people consume many more calories than some heavy people do and still stay slim. Fat tissue is less metabolically active than lean tissue, 'so fatness itself can directly lower metabolic rate if fat tissue begins to replace lean tissue' (Rodin 1981, p. 362). This may be one of the reasons why many individuals who have become obese no longer overeat, as they did while they were gaining weight. Not all heavy people eat a great deal — indeed, studies have found that obese and normal-weight individuals do not differ in the amount or type of food they report having consumed recently, such as in the past 24 hours (Braitman, Adlin & Stanton 1985; Shah & Jeffery 1991). It is possible, however, that heavy and normal-weight people differ in the accuracy of their reports. Studies of dietary intake with adult subjects have found that under-reporting is very common and is more likely among heavy than normal-weight individuals, females than males, and people with little education (Klesges, Eck & Ray 1995; Lichtman et al. 1992).

Many people believe individuals become obese because of glandular problems. Although malfunctioning endocrine glands can cause extreme weight gains, this occurs in only a small percentage of obese people (Robinson & Lawler 1977). Are other biological processes important in the development of obesity? Yes — heredity clearly plays a role (Epstein & Cluss 1986). Researchers have identified a defective gene in animals that disrupts the balance between metabolism and energy intake (Barina 1995; Lee et al. 1996; Zhang et al. 1994). Human twin studies have shown that identical twins reared apart or together are much more alike in their degree of obesity than are same-sex fraternal twins (Allison et al. 1994; Stunkard, Foch & Hrubec 1986). Adoption studies have found that children's being overweight is much more strongly related to the weight of their biological parents than to that of their adoptive parents (Price et al. 1987; Stunkard et al. 1986). Relationships have also been noted between the fatness of parents in general and that of their offspring. About 7 per cent of the offspring of normal-weight parents are obese. But among families with one obese parent, 40 per cent of the children are likely to be obese; and if both parents are obese, the figure may jump to 80 per cent (Mayer 1975, 1980). These parent–child similarities may not be the result only of genetic factors — for instance, children learn many of their eating habits and food preferences from their parents.

How does heredity affect our weight? Part of the answer seems to be described in **set-point theory**, which proposes that each person's body has a certain or 'set' weight that it strives to maintain (Bennett & Gurin 1982; Keesey 1986; Keesey & Powley 1975). The body tries to maintain its weight near the set-point by means of a thermostat-like physiological mechanism. When a person's weight departs from the set-point, the body takes corrective measures, such as by increasing or decreasing metabolism. If body weight has a set-point, people whose caloric intake is either drastically reduced or increased for a few months should show rapid corresponding weight changes initially, but their weight should then show slower changes and reach a limit. Studies have found that these predictions are correct and that people quickly return to their original weight when they can eat what they want again (Keys et al. 1950; Leibel, Rosenbaum & Hirsch 1995; Sims 1974, 1976).

The mechanism controlling the set-point seems to involve the hypothalamus (Keesey 1986; Keesey & Powley 1975). Research with animals has shown that damage to specific parts of the hypothalamus causes weight to change and eventually level off, suggesting that a new set-point has been established. If the damage is in the *lateral* region of the hypothalamus, the new set-point is for a lower weight; damage to the *ventromedial* region leads to obesity. One way the hypothalamus might regulate body weight is by monitoring some aspect of fat cells. One study, for instance, found that after obese people lost weight, they began to produce large amounts of an enzyme that makes it easier to store fat in cells and gain weight (Kern et al. 1990). Moreover, the more obese the people were before losing weight, the more of this enzyme they produced. It may be that the loss of fat in cells triggers the hypothalamus to initiate enzyme production to maintain the set-point.

Another way the hypothalamus may affect the process of weight control is by regulating the level of insulin in the person's blood (Keesey & Powley 1975). **Insulin** is a hormone, produced by the pancreas, that speeds the conversion of sugar (glucose) to fat and promotes the storage of fat in adipose tissue (Rodin 1981, 1985). Obese individuals tend to have high serum levels of insulin — a condition called *hyperinsulinemia*. Elevations in serum insulin levels increase the person's sensations of hunger, perceived pleasantness of sweet tastes and food consumption. Taken together, these findings indicate that weight gain results from a biopsychosocial process in which physiological factors interact with psychological and environmental factors (Rodin 1985).

It seems likely that the setting and function of the set-point in regulating a person's weight depend on the number and size of fat cells in the body. Psychologist Kelly Brownell (1986b) has suggested that people whose weights are above the set-point may be able to reduce fairly readily until the fat cells reach their lower limit in *size*. The body weight at which this level is reached would depend on the *number* of fat cells in the body. Since the number of fat cells increases mainly in childhood and adolescence, the diets of individuals during that time in the life span are likely to be very important. Obese children between two and 10 years of age have fat cells that are as large as those of adults (Knittle et al. 1981). As these children gain weight, they do so mainly by adding fat cells. Fat cell size for normal-weight children does not reach adult levels until age 12, and the number of their fat cells does not increase very much between two and 10 years of age.

Evidence indicates that the number of fat cells can increase, but *not* decrease (Brownell 1982). Individuals who develop too many fat cells — a condition called *fat-cell hyperplasia* — may be doomed to a difficult struggle against a high set-point for the rest of their lives. When fat-cell-hyperplastic adults try to lose weight, their fat cells shrink and

> send out metabolic signals similar to those during food deprivation. As a result, bodily mechanisms respond as though the person were starving, resulting in, among other things, an increase in hunger and a decrease in basal metabolism so that energy stores (i.e., fat) are maintained more efficiently. (Buck 1988, p. 467)

This suggests that the diets children eat may be critical in determining whether they become overly fat. It may be possible to help prevent obesity by encouraging children to exercise, eat in moderation and consume nutritious diets that do not lead to hyperplasia (Brownell 1986b). Once the person's set-point becomes established, however, changing it appears to be very difficult, although not impossible. Sustained effort and change in diet and exercise are required. Eating behaviour is learned behaviour, and therefore can be unlearned through the application of psychological principles. Individuals can be taught to identify antecedent cues to eating (e.g. having a biscuit with coffee), eliminating the conditioned association between the stimulus cue and eating, and substituting more appropriate food choices, which are then reinforced.

Psychosocial factors in weight control

Psychosocial factors are also involved in weight control. For one thing, many people claim to eat more when they are anxious or upset, and evidence indicates that stress can induce eating (Arnow, Kenardy & Agras 1992; Logue 1991). Emotional states (positive or negative) can trigger overeating of non-nutritional food if it is made salient (i.e. is in view and tempting) (Andrews & Jones 1990). Other research has shown that when women perceive the ideal weight to be different from how they feel about their bodies most of the time, they are more likely to restrain their eating (Tiggemann 1996). Feeling fat as a measure of body-image dissatisfaction, as opposed to actually being overweight, is associated with depressed affect and low self-esteem (Tiggemann 1996). Lifestyle is important, too. People who regularly drink a lot of alcohol tend to gain weight for two reasons: drinking adds calories to the diet and reduces the body's disposal of fat (Suter, Schutz & Jequier 1992; Tremblay et al. 1995). Watching television can affect weight control, too, by decreasing people's physical activity and by presenting mainly low-nutrient, sweet foods in shows and commercials (Gortmaker, Dietz & Cheung 1990; Story & Faulkner 1990). Watching television can also decrease the rate at which the body burns calories. A study compared obese and normal-weight children's metabolic rates while they simply rested and while they watched the show 'The Wonder Years' (Klesges et al. 1992). During the show, the children's metabolic rates dropped to *below* their resting rates — 12 per cent below for the normal-weight and 16 per cent below for the obese subjects.

Another psychosocial factor in weight control is the person's sensitivity to food-related cues in the environment: obese people are more sensitive than non-obese people to certain cues (Schachter 1971). For example, they eat more than normal-weight people when food tastes good, but eat less than normal-weight individuals when it tastes bad. This stronger responsiveness to food cues suggests that obese individuals may be more susceptible than non-obese people to, say, the influence of a sales pitch when deciding whether to have a dessert. A study tested this possibility in a restaurant by having the waitress describe or display a dessert to her diners (Herman, Olmstead & Polivy 1983). The results showed that obese diners were more influenced by the description or display of the dessert than non-obese diners were. Because of this susceptibility to food-related cues, obese children may have difficulty controlling their eating at home. Studies examining family behaviours at mealtimes have shown that parents give more encouragement for eating and offer food more often to heavier children than to slimmer ones (Baranowski & Nader 1985).

For many people, keeping their weight at a desired level is a struggle in which they constantly worry about what they eat and try to resist eating what they want. These people have been described as *restrained* eaters (Herman & Mack 1975; Herman & Polivy 1980; Ruderman 1986). At the other end of the spectrum are *unrestrained* eaters, who eat freely as the desire strikes them. This distinction forms the basis of **restraint theory**, which proposes that restrained eaters tend to develop abnormal eating patterns marked by vacillating between inhibited consumption, such as dieting, and overindulgence. According to this theory, the inhibited eating behaviour of restrained eaters often becomes temporarily 'disinhibited', or released, by certain events, and this produces a bout of overeating.

Research has supported the idea of disinhibition by comparing the behaviour of individuals assessed as restrained or unrestrained eaters on the basis of their responses to a questionnaire (Ruderman 1986; Weber, Klesges & Klesges 1988). One type of event that appears to disinhibit restrained eaters is the perception that they have already violated their diet, as might happen at a dinner party that begins with a fattening first course. After eating this course, restrained eaters may think, 'I've blown it now — I might as well eat what I want.' Dieting is an all-or-none thing for them, and simply *anticipating* violating their diet may sometimes be enough to lead restrained eaters to give up trying to inhibit their eating for the moment. Psychologists refer to this loss of control over eating as *disinhibition* (Polivy & Herman 1985). Experimental studies have compared the eating behaviour of restrained and unrestrained eaters, after being required to consume a high-calorie preload, or snack (e.g. a bowl of potato crisps). Unrestrained eaters, given such a preload, typically reduce their consumption in the subsequent taste task, while restrained eaters experience disinhibition and counter-regulate their eating, consuming more than if they had not had the preload (Touyz & Beaumont 1985; Wardle 1990). Some research (Seddon & Berry 1996) has found that watching advertisements with stereotypical images of slim, attractive women has the same disinhibitory effect for restrained eaters. Another type of event that leads restrained eaters to overindulge is experiencing negative emotional states, such as anxiety or depression. Last, social influence through modelling can affect the food consumption of both restrained and unrestrained eaters.

It is tempting to think that obese people are simply unrestrained eaters, but we currently have little evidence that obese and non-obese individuals differ in their food consumption. A very different view comes from nutrition researcher Barbara Rolls (1995), who presented evidence that people who are obese or are normal-weight, restrained eaters share an insensitivity to the fat content of food. When yoghurts that were secretly spiked with different amounts of fat were given to subjects to eat before lunch, male and female *normal-weight, unrestrained* eaters ate *less* at lunch if the yoghurt contained a lot of fat. But men and women who were *obese* or *normal-weight, restrained* eaters did not adjust their intake at lunch to compensate for the amount of fat in their yoghurt. And for the obese individuals, being restrained or unrestrained eaters had no effect. But the relationship between these effects and the development of obesity is still unclear.

Being overweight and health

In a study of overweight and normal-weight men and women, subjects were asked to rate their own health on a 10-point scale, where 1 equalled the 'worst health' and 10 equalled the 'best health' they could imagine (Laffrey 1986). The ratings of the overweight and normal-weight individuals were about the same, averaging in the mid-7s. Are overweight and normal-weight people equally healthy?

To answer this question, we need to consider two factors, one of which is the *degree of being overweight*. Research has clearly demonstrated that obesity is associated with high cholesterol levels and the development of hypertension, coronary heart disease and diabetes (AHA 1994; Chan et al. 1994; Jeffery 1991, 1992; Manson et al. 1990, 1995). The greater the severity of obesity, the greater the person's risk of developing and dying from heart disease and diabetes. Thus, a person whose weight exceeds the desirable weight by 50 per cent has a much greater risk of heart disease and diabetes morbidity and mortality than someone whose weight is 20 per cent over. But the risk of dying from these diseases for someone whose weight is less than, say, 10% over the desirable weight is almost as low as for someone at the desirable weight. One thing to keep in mind, however, is that people of ideal weight are not necessarily at low risk themselves — recall from the previous chapter that individuals who smoke cigarettes tend to weigh less than those who do not.

The second factor in assessing the health risks of being heavy involves the *distribution of fat* on the body. Whereas heavy men tend to have much of their fat concentrated in the abdominal region, heavy women have more of their fat on the thighs, hips and buttocks (Brownell 1986a). Since men have a higher prevalence of cardiovascular disorders than women, these and other health problems may be related to having bodies that are 'rounded in the middle.' The results of a study of over 30 000 women support this possibility (Hartz, Rupley & Rimm 1984). Subjects whose *ratio of waist to hip girth* — that is, their waist measurements compared to their hip measurements — was large had a higher incidence of hypertension and diabetes than those whose ratio was small. Other studies with women and with men have also found higher rates of hypertension, diabetes, coronary heart disease and mortality among people with higher, rather than lower, ratios of waist to hip girth (Folsom et al. 1993; Gillum 1987a, 1987b; Welin et al. 1987). The reasons for the influence of fat distribution on health are not clear.

Preventing obesity

Being obese presents disadvantages to the person's health and social relationships in childhood and adulthood (Bray 1984; Brownell 1986b). Is it true, as many people believe, that children tend to outgrow weight problems, or that they will find it easy to lose weight when they are interested in dating? Probably neither belief is true for most children (Brownell 1986b; Woodall & Epstein 1983). Losing weight after becoming obese is not easy at any age, and this is one reason why it is important to try to prevent people becoming overweight.

Preventing obesity should begin in childhood (Brownell 1986b; Woodall & Epstein 1983). Beginning fairly early is important for two reasons. First, obesity in childhood is likely to continue into adult life (Serdula et al. 1993). As figure 8.2 depicts, this likelihood depends on the age of the child — although only 14 per cent of obese infants become obese adults, 70 per cent of obese 10- to 13-year-olds do. Few normal-weight children become obese adults. Another reason to begin early is to prevent the excess development of fat cells, which occurs in childhood and adolescence. Obese adults who were fat in childhood have the double burden of dealing with bigger fat cells and more of them.

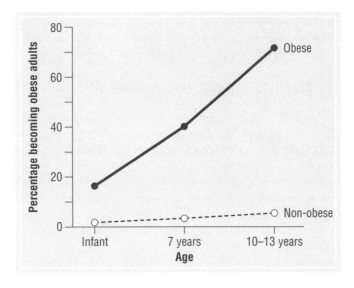

Figure 8.2 Percentage of obese and non-obese children who eventually become obese adults, as a function of age when weight status is assessed.

Source: Data from Epstein, reported in Brownell (1986b, p. 313).

Most children will not require special preventive efforts to control their weight. Those who will need these efforts are likely either to have a family history of obesity or to have become overweight already (Woodall & Epstein 1983). Efforts to help control their weight need to focus on improving the diets and physical activity of the children, and should include their families in the program (Brezinka 1992; Flodmark et al. 1993). Health and physical education programs in schools provide excellent opportunities to promote healthy eating and exercise habits. Studies have shown, for example, that children who receive instruction on healthy diets begin to bring more healthy lunches to school and throw fewer healthy foods away (McBride & Browne 1993; Striegel-Moore & Rodin 1985; Wadden & Brownell 1984). Children who are at risk of becoming obese on the basis of family history or current overweight can be identified and given special attention and training in dietary and exercise behaviour (Brownell 1986b). School programs for preventing obesity are most effective when they include a variety of training methods, involve cafeteria and educational facilities and staff, and enlist the cooperation of the parents (Striegel-Moore & Rodin 1985).

Parents provide almost all the food that comes into the house and most of the food their children eat. They also model and encourage eating and physical activity patterns. Nutritionists and other researchers have identified several ways parents can help their children avoid becoming overly fat (Striegel-Moore & Rodin 1985; Suitor & Hunter 1980).

- Encourage regular physical activity and restrict TV watching.
- Don't use unhealthy food rewards for eating a nonpreferred food (e.g., 'You may have dessert if you eat your peas'); use praise as the reward instead.
- Decrease buying high-cholesterol and sugary foods of all kinds — have less of them in the house.
- Use fruits, nuts and other healthy foods as regular desserts, and reserve rich cakes and other less healthy desserts for special occasions or once-a-week treats.
- Make sure the child eats a healthy breakfast (with few eggs) each day and does not have high-calorie snacks at night. Calories consumed early in the day tend to be used as fuel; metabolism generally decreases later in the day, and calories consumed at night often become fat.
- Monitor the child's weight on a regular basis and compare it against a chart of desirable weights. Consult a pediatrician about the diet periodically.

Childhood is probably the ideal time to establish activity and dietary habits to prevent individuals from becoming overly fat. Parents, schools and the mass media can play important roles in helping people control their weight.

Dieting and treatments to lose weight

Many millions of people around the world are dieting on any given day of the year, especially in the spring when they are getting ready to bare their bodies in the summer. Some individuals try to lose weight because they are concerned about the health risks of being overly fat: losing weight does in fact improve blood pressure and levels of lipids and lipoproteins (Datillo & Kris-Etherton 1992; Linden & Chambers 1994). But many people are motivated by how they look and what others think of them.

By Australian tastes, fatness is considered unattractive, particularly for females — and this confers important disadvantages for heavy people in social situations, such as dating. There is also a social stigma to being fat because many people *blame* heavy individuals for their condition, believing they simply lack willpower. Experiments by William DeJong (1980) had high-school girls rate whether they thought they would like girls they did not know. The subjects gave lower ratings for an obese girl than for a normal-weight girl unless the obese girl described an acceptable reason for her weight, such as a 'thyroid condition', or indicated that she had recently lost a good deal of weight. The social aspects of overweight can be distressing to those who see themselves as being too heavy, and this often motivates them to try to lose weight.

Most people try to reduce their weight on their own by 'going on a diet', and about half of them increase their physical activity, too (Bennett 1991; Serdula et al. 1994). Does this approach work? Losing weight and keeping it off is difficult for most people. Individuals are more likely to succeed if they have a high degree of self-efficacy or confidence that they can do it, and if they have constructive social support from their families and others in their social network (Colletti & Brownell 1983; Edell et al. 1987). Those with high self-efficacy and response efficacy, or the expectancy that the dietary changes are useful in eliminating health risk, are more likely to follow a low-fat diet to prevent, for instance, coronary heart disease (Plotnikoff & Higginbotham 1995). Many people go on frequent diets, losing, say, 10 per cent of their weight and gaining it right back. Kelly Brownell (1988) has described repeated cycles of substantial weight loss and gain as *yo-yo dieting*. Although early evidence suggested that people who diet repeatedly have a harder time losing weight in the future, a review of current evidence indicates that they do not (Wing 1992). Still, the best approach to dieting involves losing weight gradually and making permanent lifestyle changes that the dieter and his or her family can accept and maintain.

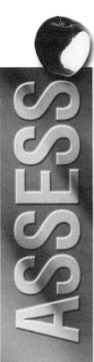

Assess yourself

HOW DO YOU SCORE ON EATING EFFICACY?

Perceptions of self-efficacy with regard to eating may be an important influence on dieting weight loss success. Rate the likelihood that you would have difficulty controlling your overeating in each of the situations below using the following scale.

1	2	3	4	5	6	7
No difficulty controlling eating		Moderate difficulty controlling eating			Most difficulty in controlling eating	

1. ____ Overeating after work or school
2. ____ Overeating when you feel restless
3. ____ Overeating around holiday time
4. ____ Overeating when you feel upset
5. ____ Overeating when tense
6. ____ Overeating with friends
7. ____ Overeating when preparing food
8. ____ Overeating when irritable
9. ____ Overeating as part of a social occasion dealing with food, as at a restaurant or dinner party
10. ____ Overeating with family members
11. ____ Overeating when annoyed
12. ____ Overeating when angry
13. ____ Overeating when you are angry at yourself
14. ____ Overeating when depressed
15. ____ Overeating when you feel impatient
16. ____ Overeating when you want to sit back and enjoy some food
17. ____ Overeating after an argument
18. ____ Overeating when you feel frustrated
19. ____ Overeating when tempting food is in front of you
20. ____ Overeating when you want to cheer up
21. ____ Overeating when there is a lot of food available to you (the refrigerator is full)
22. ____ Overeating when you feel overly sensitive
23. ____ Overating when nervous
24. ____ Overeating when hungry
25. ____ Overating when anxious or worried.

Now add up your score across the items. Higher scores indicate less self-efficacy for eating.

Source: Glynn & Ruderman (1986).

Overweight and obese people are likely to have a great deal of difficulty making, and sticking to, the lifestyle changes needed to lose weight, but it appears that many of them can do it successfully. In the previous chapter we examined a study by Stanley Schachter (1982) of people who stopped smoking on their own. That study also investigated whether people who had a history of being overweight (at least 15 per cent above the desirable weight) were successful in reducing on their own. Many of them succeeded, reducing to the desirable weight or within 10 per cent of it and maintaining the lower weight over many years. But a later study replicated Schachter's procedure and found that some succeeded in losing weight, but most did not (Rzewnicki & Forgays 1987).

Although many people can lose weight on their own and keep it off, others feel they need help. Probably all of those who seek help have tried to reduce on their own at some time — perhaps numerous times — and either failed to reduce or could not maintain the new weight. What kinds of help do people seek, and what works?

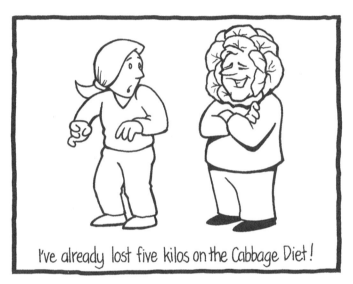

I've already lost five kilos on the Cabbage Diet!

Commercial and 'fad diet' plans

One kind of help millions of people try is the latest 'miracle diet', which is often 'guaranteed' to work in a short time. There never seems to be a shortage of these 'crash' *fad diets* — many of which are not only ineffective, but are nutritionally unsound and often produce unpleasant and unhealthy side effects (Beck et al. 1990; Warshaw 1992). Some of these fad diets prescribe a strict dietary regimen with virtually no deviations permitted — the 'Scarsdale Diet' outlined a specific breakfast, for example, that the dieter was to eat each day. Other fad diets have people eat a single type of food, such as only fruit, as in the 'Beverly Hills Diet'. Several commercial plans sell low-calorie liquid or solid replacements for part or all of the person's diet, but provide little or no help in maintaining weight loss later. Little evidence exists for the success they claim (Rosenthal 1992). No crash diet is a substitute for adopting a healthy lifestyle of exercise and moderately sized, balanced meals.

Exercise

Some people think that exercising is self-defeating when they try to control their weight because they associate exercising with large appetites (Suitor & Hunter 1980). They have heard, for instance, that some rugby league players eat enormous meals. But these players generally have huge bodies and they are trying to maintain their weight, not lose weight. For some positions in rugby, bulk is a great advantage.

Physical activity is an important component in controlling weight. One of its benefits is that it increases metabolism, thereby helping the body to burn off an increased number of calories. Unfortunately, dieters often fail to exercise as part of reducing because they notice that it takes a lot of exercise to use up a few hundred calories — for instance, they would have to jog about half an hour to burn off the

400 or so calories in a milkshake. But studies of dieting obese individuals have revealed a variety of benefits of exercise in weight control, and these advantages seem to accumulate over time. The main benefit of exercise in the first couple of months of weight reduction is that it focuses the reduction mostly on body fat, while preserving lean tissue (Hill et al. 1987). Over the next several months, combining exercise with reduced caloric intake leads to greater weight losses than dieting alone (Epstein et al. 1985). Thereafter, compared with dieters who do not exercise, those who do exercise are better able to maintain their reduced weight, probably because their improved fitness makes being physically active increasingly easy for them (Epstein et al. 1988).

Behavioural techniques

People who try to lose weight usually find that changing their eating patterns is very hard to do. Why? A major reason is that they don't know how to gain control over environmental conditions — antecedents and consequences — that maintain their eating patterns. Psychological interventions using behavioural techniques have been developed to help dieters gain the control they need. Richard Stuart (1967) conducted a pioneering study of the utility of behavioural techniques, such as self-monitoring and stimulus control, in helping several obese women lose weight over a 12-month period. The results were quite impressive: Each of the eight women who stayed with the program lost weight fairly consistently throughout the year, losing from 12 to 21 kilos.

The dramatic success of Stuart's program prompted dozens of other researchers to study the usefulness of behavioural techniques in weight control. The outcome of these studies suggests the following conclusions (Haddock et al. 1994; Perri, Nezu & Viegener 1992; Wilson 1984): First, behavioural techniques are generally helpful in losing weight, but they do not work with all people. Second, behavioural programs have very low dropout rates, and people who complete a program lose an average of about 10 per cent of their original weight in the first four months. Third, the more individuals weigh at the start of treatment and the longer the program, the more weight they lose. Fourth, behavioural methods are more effective in helping people lose weight than any other approach, except certain medical treatments. Fifth, a clear majority of individuals who complete a behavioural program for weight control maintain their lower weight for at least a year. Although most studies of behavioural programs have used adult subjects, research has shown that these techniques are also effective with children of various ages (Haddock et al. 1994).

What techniques do behavioural programs for weight loss use? Although the specific techniques vary somewhat from one program to the next, they typically include the following components (Perri, Nezu & Viegener 1992; Stunkard & Berthold 1985; Wilson 1984):

- *nutrition and exercise counselling*
- *self-monitoring* by keeping careful records of the foods eaten, when, where, with whom and under what circumstances
- *stimulus control* techniques, such as shopping for food with a list, storing food out of sight and eating at home in only one room
- *altering the act of eating* — for example by chewing the food very thoroughly before swallowing, and putting utensils down on the table between mouthfuls.
- *behavioural contracting*, or setting up a system of rewards for sticking to the diet.

Some programs have found that having dieters use portable computers to plan and monitor their physical activity and calorie intake enhances weight loss and subsequent lifestyle maintainance (Agras 1987; Burnett, Taylor & Agras 1985). One behavioural approach that does *not* work and has for the most part been abandoned for treating weight problems involves using aversive strategies, such as pairing eating certain foods with unpleasant stimuli (Straw 1983).

Behavioural programs have also been used with cognitive approaches. In a method called *cognitive restructuring*, dieters learn how to counter pessimistic thoughts they have about dieting and their self-efficacy. For example, a person who thinks, 'Everyone in my family has a weight problem. It's in my genes,' would learn to counter this thought with, 'That just makes it harder, not impossible. If I stick with this program, I will succeed' (Stunkard 1987). Another method, called *problem-solving training*, is designed to teach people strategies to help them deal with everyday difficulties they encounter in sticking to their diets (Perri, Nezu & Viegener 1992). Individuals often have difficulty sticking to a diet at family celebrations, when eating at restaurants, and when under stress, for instance. The skills learned in problem-solving training enable people to find solutions to these difficulties. Overweight people who can generate these kinds of solutions tend to lose more weight and have fewer lapses than others do (Drapkin, Wing & Shiffman 1995).

Last, family-based behavioural programs have been highly effective in helping obese children and their parents lose weight together over a 10-year period (Epstein et al. 1995). The interventions were most successful when they focused on weight loss in both the parents and children, included exercise in the program, and had the children and parents reward each other for diet and exercise behaviour. Other research has also shown that rewarding overweight individuals for *not* engaging in sedentary activities, such as watching TV or playing computer games, is very helpful in promoting weight loss (Epstein, Valoski, Vara et al. 1995).

Self-help groups and work-site weight-loss programs

Although there are dozens of self-help organisations for weight control, *Weight Watchers* is the most widely known of these groups, with hundreds of thousands of people attending each week (Brownell 1986a). The Weight Watchers approach uses several behavioural techniques, such as self-monitoring, along with nutritional information and group meetings for social support. *Gut Busters* is an Australian weight loss initiative aimed at middle aged men in particular. Another Australian initiative is *Lighten Up*, a community-based weight management program that uses educational, skill development, self-help and environmental strategies to help people lose weight (Harvey et al. 1998). Both programs have been successful in helping people lose weight. Different self-help organisations have their own mix of methods to help people lose weight (Chesney 1984; Perri, Nezu & Viegener 1992). In the US, *Take Off Pounds Sensibly* (TOPS), for example, uses few behavioural techniques even though research has demonstrated that the program might be more effective if it did. *Overeaters Anonymous* uses an approach like that of Alcoholics Anonymous. Unfortunately, very little research has been done to evaluate the success of self-help groups because they have been 'notoriously unwilling to permit external evaluation' of their effectiveness (Brownell 1986a, p. 525). But evidence so far suggests that dropout rates for self-help groups are extremely high — for instance, assessments of attrition rates in some groups revealed that over 50 per cent of the members dropped out in the first six weeks alone (Stunkard 1987).

Work-site weight-loss programs have been introduced and evaluated in a variety of businesses and industries. These programs generally used behavioural techniques, but were not very successful (Foreyt & Leavesley 1991). High dropout rates and small weight losses have been common, suggesting that inadequate motivation is a major problem. Evidence indicates that these problems can be reduced by two approaches: gearing the program to the workers' stages of readiness to change, and providing incentives for participation (Gomel et al. 1993). An example of using incentives comes from three successful *weight-loss competitions* introduced in different businesses and industries in the United States (Brownell et al. 1984). In one competition, for instance, the presidents of banks issued challenges to each other's bank for a weight loss contest over a three-month period. All participating employees from each bank made up a team, with each participant having a reasonable weight-loss goal. The prize for the team that achieved the greatest percentage of its weight loss goal was a pool of money to which each participant contributed $5. The only program they received to help them reduce was a series of weekly manuals that gave information about such factors as nutrition, exercise, self-monitoring, stimulus control and reinforcement. The outcome for the three competitions was impressive: Only one of the 213 overweight or obese individuals dropped out of the contest, and the average weight loss was 5.4 kilos — about half a kilo a week. A follow-up of the bank employees six months later showed that the overweight and obese individuals kept off 80 per cent of the weight they lost in the competition. Clearly, addressing the *motivation* of dieters is a useful approach.

Medically supervised approaches

Some approaches for losing weight involve medical procedures or require supervision of a physician. One approach that requires medical supervision uses prescribed drugs that suppress one's appetite. At one time, *amphetamines* seemed to be useful because they suppress appetite and increase metabolism. They have since been abandoned because they produce psychological and, perhaps, physical dependence. Preferred diet drugs today include two appetite suppressants: *fenfluramine* and *phentermine*, which do not seem to cause dependence and have tolerable side effects, such as dry mouth. These drugs are sometimes used in combination, commonly called 'fen-phen', but they may be contraindicated for people with certain medical or psychological conditions, such as depression (CU 1996b; Perri, Nezu & Viegener 1992). Appetite suppressants are very effective, and the resulting weight loss is maintained as long as the person continues taking the drug. These drugs should be used only by people who are *obese*, some of whom may need to take them indefinitely (Stallone & Stunkard 1991). Unfortunately, commercial diet plans have already begun making these drugs available for non-obese individuals.

Another medical approach to losing weight involves placing the patient on a *very-low-calorie diet* (VLCD) regimen. VLCDs contain fewer than 800 calories per day — and often have only 500 or so (Agras 1987; Perri, Nezu & Viegener 1992; Wilson 1984). A VLCD can be unsafe to use if it is deficient in protein and potassium, but 'protein sparing' VLCDs are safe if the patients do not have certain medical conditions, such as heart disease, and their health is monitored regularly. Although VLCDs produce rapid and substantial weight losses, they have unpleasant side effects, such as constipation and fatigue. Furthermore, relapse rates are high in the months following VLCDs. A study of obese patients revealed large weight losses during VLCD treatment, but most subjects regained the lost weight in the subsequent three years (Wadden, Stunkard & Liebschutz 1988). Some of the patients who relapsed sought additional treatment, which again helped. The characteristics of obese persons in clinics may explain the poor prognosis for weight loss treatments. Compared with obese individuals in the general population, those seeking treatment are more likely to be binge eaters, be more overweight and have more psychological problems (Brownell & Rodin 1994). VLCDs are appropriate mainly for otherwise healthy obese patients who are more than 20 kilos overweight, have failed to control their weight with behavioural techniques, and whose obesity poses an unusually high health risk (Agras 1987).

The most drastic medical approaches for losing weight involve surgery, particularly to the stomach or intestines. In one surgical approach called *gastric restriction*, the size of the stomach is reduced by literally stapling part of it up; a less commonly used method is to remove part of the intestines to reduce the amount of nutrients absorbed from the digestive system. Although these approaches effectively reduce weight, they entail some surgical risk and may produce unpleasant side effects — for example, some patients who have undergone gastric restriction surgery experience nausea, vomiting and abdominal pain after eating. As a result, these methods are recommended only for patients who are more than 100 per cent overweight and have failed to lose weight by less drastic means (Perri, Nezu & Viegener 1992; Stunkard, Stinnett & Smoller 1986). The surgical procedure called *liposuction*, in which adipose tissue is torn from the body and sucked out with a tube, is not really a weight reduction method — its function is strictly cosmetic (Henig 1988). It is used for removing only a few kilos of fat from a specific region of the body, such as the thighs or abdomen, and it entails risks during the procedure and may have unpleasant after-effects.

We have considered methods for losing weight that range from adjusting one's diet and exercising to using surgical procedures. Choosing the most appropriate approaches to use requires *matching* the methods to people's weight problems and characteristics, such as their metabolic function, dieting history and financial resources. Psychologists Kelly Brownell and Thomas Wadden (1991) have outlined a series of steps that can be used for matching individuals to weight control approaches. For example, someone who is 10 per cent overweight might be advised to use a structured self-dieting approach or a work-site program, but someone who is 100 per cent overweight would probably need to use medically supervised approaches.

Relapse after weight loss

The problem of relapse after completing treatment to lose weight is similar to that which many people experience after receiving treatment to quit smoking, drinking or using drugs (Brownell et al. 1986). The reasons for relapse are similar, too: they often relate to certain types of situations, such as being upset (Grilo, Shiffman & Wing 1989; Jeffery, French & Schmid 1990). Although many individuals who lose weight in behavioural programs maintain their lower weight for at least a year without follow-up treatment programs, many others do not. But when we interpret weight gain in the years after dieters have reduced, we need to keep in mind that people tend to gain weight as they get older — $\frac{1}{2}$ or 1 kilo a year in middle-aged Australians, on average. A fair assessment of a weight loss program's success should also take into account *the weight dieters didn't gain* that other people do (Perri, Nezu & Viegener 1992).

Michael Perri and his colleagues (1988) demonstrated that follow-up treatment programs can be effective in reducing the relapse problem in weight control. In this study, obese men and women lost an average of 5.7 kilos in a behavioural program for dietary and exercise behaviours. The subjects were then randomly assigned to different follow-up treatment conditions that were balanced for degree of the subjects' over-weight. Assessments 18 months later revealed that the average weight losses the subjects maintained was 4.8 kilos for those who received follow-up treatment and only 1.6 kilos for those who received no follow-up treatment. Analysis of the follow-up treatments revealed two critical components in their success: (1) frequent therapist meetings to deal with specific problems individuals were having in maintaining their weight and (2) social influences of other members of a treatment group. These findings are very encouraging and suggest that many obese individuals who have lost weight would benefit from having continued meetings with therapists, relapse 'hot lines' to call and support groups.

Most people who lose weight do not use effective ways to maintain the loss. If you wanted to lose weight and keep it off, what methods could you use? Here are some.

- When losing the weight, use behavioural techniques — such as self-monitoring and stimulus control — to diet and increase exercise. Choose a reasonable final weight goal, and plan to lose weight *gradually*, such as half a kilo a week or less. Weigh yourself each time you exercise.
- Reduce the fat content of your diet by substituting other foods, particularly carbo-hydrates, which gram-for-gram have fewer calories and turn into body fat less readily.
- After reaching your weight goal, continue your lifestyle changes by using behav-ioural methods, such as keeping diet and exercise records, avoiding situations that prompt lapses, and rewarding good behaviour.
- Recognise that maintaining your lower weight requires that the lifestyle changes be *permanent*. Occasional lapses are not a problem as long as you get back on track as soon as possible.
- Join a self-help or support group, especially if you find that you have too many lapses.

Anorexia and bulimia

Although overeating is a very common weight control problem with psychosocial relationships, it is not considered to be a psychiatric disorder. In contrast, two rela-tively unusual eating problems — *anorexia nervosa* and *bulimia nervosa* — are included as psychiatric disorders in the *Diagnostic and Statistical Manual of Mental Disorders* (DSM-IV) of the American Psychiatric Association (1994). People with these two dis-orders use extreme ways to keep their weight down. Anorexia is illustrated in the following case study of a 19-year-old, 160 cm tall student named Frances who had been 9 kilos overweight six years earlier. She

> weighed 83 lbs [38 kilos] upon admission [to therapy]. She reported eating very little food each day (estimated to be less than 500 kcal). She exercised for at least 3 hours each day by attending aerobics classes and running. When she did consume a normal meal, she purged it via self-induced vomiting. . . . She never binged (i.e., ate large quantities of food). She was obsessed with fears of weight gain. (Williamson, Cubic & Fuller 1992, p. 367)

When she was younger, she had been teased by peers and repeatedly criticised by her mother for being overweight. As Frances's case shows, **anorexia nervosa** is an eating disorder that involves a drastic reduction in food intake and an unhealthy loss of weight. This disorder is characterised by a weight loss of at least 25 per cent, efforts to maintain body weight 15 per cent below the normal weight for one's age and height, and an intense fear of becoming fat, which continues despite the extreme loss of weight (Abraham & Llewellyn-Jones 1992; Logue 1991). The starvation in anorexia may be so extreme as to cause or contribute to the person's death — for instance by causing extremely low blood pressure, heart damage or cardiac arrhythmias (due to low body levels of electrolytes, such as sodium or potassium).

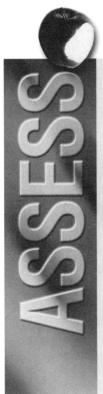

Assess yourself
YOUR WEIGHT CONTROL PATTERNS

For each of the following questions, put a check mark in the preceding space if your answer is 'yes'.

_____ Do you watch your calorie intake more carefully than anyone else you know?

_____ Do you weigh less than the 'desirable weight' range for your height and frame given in table 8.1 on page 317?

_____ Do you think gaining a few kilos during a holiday season would be a terrible thing?

_____ Have you ever eaten so much so quickly that you felt like you had lost control of your eating?

_____ If yes, has this happened more than about 10 times in the past year?

_____ Have you ever eaten a lot and then tried to 'purge' the food by using laxatives, diuretics or self-induced vomiting?

_____ If yes, has this happened more than about 10 times in the past year?

_____ Have you felt a lot of emotional distress in recent months?

_____ Do you often eat fewer than two meals a day?

_____ Do you regularly exercise more than 10 hours a week to lose weight?

How many 'yes' answers did you give? A high number suggests that you may have an eating disorder. If your number is from 3 to 5, you may want to consider getting professional help, especially if your situation seems to be getting worse; 6 or more, you should seek help right away. You can find help through your university counselling office or by contacting professional organisations, such as the Australian Psychological Society and the College of Clinical Pyschologists, for contact details of eating disorder clinics and practitioners in your area.

Sources: Based on material in Brownell (1989); Davison & Neale (1994); Logue (1991).

It is difficult to know how prevalent eating disorders are. A study that compared women's medical records with returned surveys on eating disorders to the researchers found that many of those who did not return the survey did in fact have eating disorders (Beglin & Fairburn 1992). And so, existing prevalence data are likely to be underestimates. Anorexia nervosa occurs 10 or 15 times more frequently in females than males; its incidence increases during the adolescent years and probably declines in early adulthood (Hoek et al. 1995; Levey, McDermott & Lee 1989; Patton 1992; Polivy & Thomsen 1988; Werry 1986). Studies in North America and Europe have found that it afflicts about one in every 250 adolescent girls, is more prevalent in upper-class than lower-class individuals, and appears to have become more prevalent since the 1960s (Hoek et al. 1995; Lacey & Birtchnell 1986; Polivy & Thomsen 1988). Anorexia is especially common among dance students, models and athletes who feel pressured to control their weight (French & Jeffery 1994; Levey, McDermott & Lee 1989).

Bulimia nervosa is an eating disorder that is characterised by recurrent episodes of *binge eating*, generally followed by *purging* by self-induced vomiting, laxative use or other means to prevent gaining weight (Abraham & Llewellyn-Jones 1992; Logue 1991; Weeda-Mannak 1990). This disorder can cause a wide range of medical problems, including inflammation of the digestive tract and cardiac problems, such as arrhythmias resulting from low levels of electrolytes. Bulimic individuals are aware that their eating pattern is abnormal, are fearful of having lost control of their eating, and tend to be depressed and self-critical after a bulimic episode.

Bulimia was not recognised as a distinct syndrome until the late 1970s. As a result, less is known about this disorder than about anorexia (Agras 1987). Bulimia is far more prevalent among females than males and is more likely to occur in adolescence and early adulthood than at other times in the life span. Findings from studies of university students suggest that this disorder is more prevalent than anorexia nervosa, afflicting perhaps 1 to 3 per cent of female adolescents (Agras 1987; Logue 1991; Weeda-Mannak 1990). Many individuals exhibit some bulimic behaviours, such as purging, but are not classified as bulimics because they engage in these behaviours infrequently.

Why people become anorexics and bulimics

What causes the eccentric eating habits of anorexia and bulimia? The answer is still unclear, and researchers have suggested biological, psychological and cultural factors that may be involved. There is evidence for genetic and physiological links to these disorders, but it is quite limited. For example, studies have examined the occurrence of anorexia and bulimia in twins and found that these disorders are far more likely to appear in *both* twin members if they are identical twins rather than fraternal twins (Holland, Sicotte & Treasure 1988; Kendler et al. 1991; Walters & Kendler 1995). Other research findings indicate that the hypothalamus of anorexics may function abnormally (Gold et al. 1986).

Cultural factors may provide the answer to two obvious questions about these eating disorders: Why is the prevalence of anorexia and bulimia so much greater among females, and why has it increased in recent years? Beauty plays a central role in the sex-role stereotype of women in many cultures, and Western cultures have witnessed recent changes in their ideals about female beauty (Polivy & Thomsen 1988; Striegel-Moore, Silberstein & Rodin 1986). These changes are evident in the body proportions of models and actresses. Years ago, the 'ideally beautiful woman' had a figure that was more rounded, with larger bust and hip measurements. After 1960 or so, the ideal figure of a woman became much thinner, and the social pressures on women to be slender increased. As we saw earlier, females are more likely than males to wish they were thinner and to diet. Research on Australian university students found that even the most overweight males are more satisfied with their bodies than the most underweight females (Kenny & Adams 1994). Compared with overweight males, females of different weight ranges scored higher on the Eating Disorders Inventory (Garner & Olmsted 1984), a diagnostic screening instrument, particularly on the sub-scales of drive for thinness, bulimia, body dissatisfaction and ineffectiveness. Gender differences begin to show up by age 11 or so (Cohen, Brownell & Felix 1990; Kenny & Adams 1994; Nowak 1998). In social interactions with other children, parents and teachers, girls more than boys are given the message: thin is better (Attie & Brooks-Gunn 1987). Once the message is clear they reach puberty, when girls add an average of over 9 kilos of fat to their bodies while boys add muscle. This is a no-win situation for adolescent girls. How do they deal with it?

When adolescents — especially females — start trying to control their weight, they typically adjust their diets in a normal manner. But the methods they use sometimes become more extreme, involving occasional fasting or purging. A study of more than 1700 15-year-old male and female high-school students in the United States, for instance, revealed that about 13 per cent of them had engaged in some form of purging behaviour, with the rate for females being twice as high as that for males (Killen et al. 1986). Most of these purging behaviours occurred infrequently — on a monthly basis or less. Weight loss behaviours in Australian adolescents are comparable to those of their American peers. In a study of Victorian high-school students (Maude et al. 1993), 47 per cent of girls and 28 per cent of boys reported using an extreme weight loss method at least occasionally, the most common methods being fasting and crash dieting. Weekly use of an extreme weight loss method was reported by 10 per cent of both girls and boys. Girls engaged in more weight loss behaviours, including vomiting, than did boys. The results of prospective studies indicate that individuals who become anorexic and bulimic typically start out dieting normally but have relatively strong concerns about their weight, and then begin using more extreme methods (French & Jeffery 1994; Killen et al. 1994; Patton 1992). Those dieters who go on to develop an eating disorder tend to have neurotic and depressive symptoms not present in dieters who do not develop an eating disorder (Patton 1992). While Aboriginal and Torres Strait Islander girls tend to be heavier than white girls of the same age (Wang, Hoy & McDonald 2000), they do not appear to be as concerned about weight, which may explain the lower rates of eating disorders in these groups. Dieters with strong weight concerns may come to rely more and more on fasting and purging because these methods keep weight off. Because bulimics are restrained eaters, they may binge as a result of becoming disinhibited by events, such as feelings of anxiety (Polivy & Thomsen 1988).

Body size overestimations are particularly pronounced among anorexics and bulimics. Among anorexics, for example, the idea that they are overweight persists long after they have become slim. When they are reduced to skin and bones, anorexics still claim to be 'too fat' and greatly overestimate their size (Askevold 1975; Crisp & Kalucy 1974). Other experimental research (Freeman et al. 1991) which used a computerised infra-red monitor to track eye movements, found that when shown a picture of themselves, dieting disordered patients focus on those parts of their body with which they are most dissatisfied, while normal patients scan the whole body. This would seem to indicate that anorexics and bulimics process body shape information differently from non-eating-disordered persons.

Treatments for anorexia and bulimia

Because anorexia nervosa involves a severe and health-threatening underweight condition, the first priority in treating this disorder when there is extreme weight loss is to restore the person's body weight and nutrition to as near normal as possible (Abraham

& Llewellyn-Jones 1992). This is often done in a hospital setting. Several approaches that include behavioural techniques and drug therapy are effective for putting weight on (Agras 1987; Logue 1991; Williamson, Cubic & Fuller 1992). But keeping the weight on is difficult; about half of previously treated anorexics continue to have eating problems and often show other social and emotional difficulties, such as depression. Australian research (Jones, Halford & Dooley 1993) that has examined long-term outcomes of anorexia nervosa found that two-thirds of treated anorexics, when contacted 5.7 years later, showed clinical improvement, although the majority had higher than normal scores on anorexic symptomatology, social maladjustment, anxiety and hostility. The other third exhibited distorted attitudes towards eating, overconcern about their body shape, poor social functioning, anxiety, hostility, depression and external locus of control. In addition to psychopathology, weight-recovered anorexic patients may engage in a wide range of behaviours such as bingeing, vomiting and excessive exercise (Windauer et al. 1993) typically associated with anorexia.

Treatment for anorexia needs to include cognitive methods to alter irrational thinking, such as the person's distorted body image, and follow-up efforts should address any continued desire to restrict food intake, and various interpersonal and job-related problems. Frequently, issues of control over self are involved in eating disorders (Bruch 1973). An important component of treatment is to recognise such issues, and enable the person to begin to take control over parts of his or her life, in addition to the eating, while taking control away from parents and others, who inhibit the person's sense of control over his or her destiny. This involves listening to anorexic patients, treating them with dignity, and encouraging them to take greater control of their lives.

Treatments for bulimia nervosa are especially effective when they combine behavioural and cognitive approaches with *antidepressant drugs* that elevate the person's mood (Agras & McCann 1987; Agras et al. 1992). Behavioural and cognitive techniques — such as self-monitoring, reinforcement, relaxation training and cognitive restructuring — focus on reducing binging and purging behaviours (Agras 1987; Wilson & Smith 1987).

Is treatment more successful for bulimia than for anorexia? Cognitive behaviour therapy has been found to be more effective than behavioural therapy alone, or interpersonal psychotherapy (Fairburn et al. 1991). In a meta-analytic comparison of 12 different treatments for bulimia, cognitive behaviour therapy had superior outcomes to other forms of therapy (family, inpatient, systemic), psychoeducation or pharmacological treatments (Whitbread & McGown 1994). But the few studies that have assessed the long-term success of bulimia treatments have found fairly high relapse rates (Weeda-Mannak 1990). One study with female bulimic patients compared treatments using behavioural methods only or both behavioural and cognitive methods with a control condition that used only self-monitoring (Thackwray et al. 1993). Follow-up assessments six months later revealed no bingeing or purging in 69 per cent of the women who received the cognitive behavioural treatment, 38 per cent of those with the behavioural treatment, and 15 per cent of the controls. This outcome is encouraging, but would be more so if there had been an independent source to confirm the subjects' reports of bingeing and purging.

We have discussed the problems people have in controlling their weight through adjustments in their diets. We have also seen that exercise can play an important role in reducing body fat and, thereby, can enhance people's health. The next section examines exercise as a means of becoming fit and keeping well.

Physical activity

A fitness boom seems to have occurred in many Western cultures. For instance, bicyclists and joggers today can be seen on roads and paths in suburbs, and fitness centres seem to have sprung up everywhere. In the past decade, walking has increased in popularity (AIHW 2000). However, most Australian adults' lifestyles still include very little or irregular physical activity (Australian Sports Commission 1999; Brown & Bauman 2000). The 1997 Active Australia National Physical Activity Survey found that only 50 per cent of men and 49 per cent of women between the ages of 18 and 75 engage in regular physical activity (ASC 1999). We've all heard that exercise is healthy. We will see why in this section.

The health effects of exercise

If you asked fitness-conscious people why they exercise, they would probably give a variety of reasons: 'Exercising helps me keep my weight down,' 'I like it when I'm in shape — and so does my boyfriend,' 'It helps me unwind and relieves my tension,' 'Being in shape keeps me sharp on my job,' 'I don't get sick as often when I'm fit,' and 'It makes people's hearts stronger, so they live longer.' These answers describe several psychosocial and physical health benefits of exercising and are, for the most part, correct.

Three psychosocial benefits of exercise have been studied extensively. First, research has shown that engaging in regular vigorous exercise is associated with lower feelings of *stress* and anxiety, as we discussed in chapter 5. Second, people who get involved in fitness programs report that their *work performance* and attitudes improve — they make fewer errors, for instance (Folkins & Sime 1981) or concentration improves (Moore 1993). Third, participating in regular exercise is linked to enhanced *self-concepts* of individuals, especially children (Dishman 1986; Folkins & Sime 1981). These enhancements in the self-concept may occur because individuals who exercise are better able to control their weight, maintain an attractive appearance, and engage successfully in physical activities and sports — all of which help these people to feel heightened self-esteem and to receive the many social advantages that accrue with being fit.

As a result, psychological wellbeing and positive mood increase (Moore 1993; Dua & Hargreaves 1992). But most studies of psychosocial benefits from exercise have used correlational or retrospective methods, making it difficult to determine cause–effect relationships, and some evidence suggests that part of the self-reported benefits may have resulted from a placebo effect of the subjects' expecting that psychosocial benefits would occur (Byrne & Byrne 1993; Desharnais et al. 1993).

Of the many physiological effects that physical activity produces, one effect is especially intriguing: vigorous exercise seems to increase the body's production of *endorphins*, which are morphine-like chemical substances. Studies have shown that endorphin levels in the blood are higher after exercise than before (Carr et al. 1981). Some researchers claim that the euphoric 'runner's high' that many individuals feel after a very vigorous aerobic workout results from high levels of endorphins reaching the brain. These researchers have also proposed that these higher endorphin levels may be responsible for decreases in both the stress and sensations of pain many people feel during or after vigorous exercise. Spirduso & Gilliam-MacRae (1991) found that compared to non-exercisers, regular aerobic exercisers have lower levels of chronic stress, react less strongly to stressors and recover more efficiently from stressors.

Exercise can enhance many aspects of people's physical fitness throughout the life span. In the early childhood years, aerobic exercise improves agility and cardiovascular function (Alpert et al. 1990). At the other end of the life span, older adults generally show a gradual decline in their physical work capacity — as reflected in their muscle flexibility, strength and endurance (Buchner et al. 1992). This decline occurs partly because many individuals get less exercise as they get older. An 18-year longitudinal study examined the physical work capacity of men who were over 50 years of age at the start of the study and who engaged in aerobic exercise regularly (Kasch, Wallace & Van Camp 1985). The work capacity of these men decreased only slightly across the 18 years, whereas individuals in the general population tend to show a 1 to 2 per cent decrease per year. Also, the percentage of body fat and resting blood pressure of these men did not show the increases that usually occur during these years. This and other evidence clearly indicates that engaging in aerobic exercise curbs the usual decline in fitness that people experience as they get older (Buchner et al. 1992).

The physical benefits people gain from vigorous and regular exercise are reflected not only in their improved work capacity but also in their enhanced health and longevity (Lee, Hsieh & Paffenbarger 1995; Rodriguez et al. 1994). The main health benefits achieved through exercise relate to preventing cardiovascular problems and some forms of cancer (ACS 1996; AHA 1994; Blair et al. 1992). Many studies have demonstrated that individuals who regularly engage in vigorous physical activity are less likely to develop and die from coronary heart disease (CHD) than those who lead relatively sedentary lives (Powell et al. 1987). Although, for ethical reasons, no experimental research has been done in which human subjects were randomly assigned to exercise and nonexercise conditions, research with animals, and prospective studies with humans, indicate that the link between physical activity and reduced risk of CHD seems to be causal.

How does engaging in regular vigorous activity protect individuals against CHD? The role of exercise in reducing blood pressure is especially clear. Studies have shown that children and adults who are physically active have lower systolic and diastolic blood pressure than those who are not (Haskell 1984; Hofman et al. 1987; Panico et al. 1987). Furthermore, prospective studies have found that people who are physically fit and active are less likely to develop hypertension than less-fit and inactive people (Blair et al. 1992). The evidence regarding whether exercising by itself can decrease blood pressure in hypertensive patients was inconsistent in early studies (Siegel & Blumenthal 1991). But more recent experimental research has shown that exercise lowers blood pressure in both hypertensive and normotensive people (Arroll & Beaglehole 1992; Braith et al. 1994; Kokkinos et al. 1995; Pescatello et al. 1991). Exercise may also prevent CHD in two other ways: by reducing the occurrence of arrhythmic heartbeats and by decreasing LDL while increasing HDL serum cholesterol. Some evidence supports each of these possibilities (Blair et al. 1992).

The risk of developing cancer has been linked to low physical activity; the evidence is fairly strong for colon cancer and more modest for other cancers, such as of the breast and prostate (Blair et al. 1992). Although the reason for this link is unclear, part of it may involve the beneficial effect of both immediate and long-term exercise on the immune system (Boutcher 1991). One study tested healthy, physically active 24- to 35-year-olds and 65- to 79-year-olds for the effects of a vigorous exercise session on immune function (Fiatarone et al. 1989). Natural killer cell number and function were similar in both age groups before the session and increased substantially in both groups in response to the exercise.

Not all effects of exercise are beneficial — there can be hazards as well. One hazard occurs when people jog or bicycle in traffic, of course, risking a collision. But the most common problems that arise involve injury to bones or muscles from other kinds of accidents and from overstraining the body (Haskell 1985). Sports-related injuries cost Australia over one billion dollars each year (Kirkby 1995). Many injuries happen to people who do not exercise regularly or are beginners. The main dangers to these people come from overtaxing their bodies and from unsafe exercise conditions, such as having improper shoes. Exercising too long in very hot weather can lead to heat exhaustion — with symptoms of dizziness, rapid and weak pulse, and headache — or a more severe condition called heatstroke, which can be fatal.

Highlight on issues

Types and amounts of healthy exercise

All physical activities — even just fidgeting — use energy and burn calories. *Exercise* is a special class of physical activity in which people exert their bodies in a structured and repetitive way for the sake of health or body development. There are several types of exercise, each with its own form of activity and physical goals. Let's see what these types of exercise are and what pattern of activities experts recommend to benefit most people's health.

Isotonics, isometrics and isokinetics

Isotonic, isometric and isokinetic exercise differ in the types of activities and their effects. **Isotonic exercise** refers to a type of activity that builds strength *and* endurance by the person's moving a heavy object, exerting most of the muscle force in one direction. This type of exercise includes weight-lifting and many calisthenics. In doing push-ups, for example, most of the exertion occurs in raising the body.

Isometric exercise mainly builds strength rather than endurance, since the individual exerts muscle force against an *immovable* object. An example of an isometric exercise is the 'chair lift': The person sits in a standard unupholstered chair, grasps the sides of the seat with both hands, and pulls upward, straining the arm muscles. The pulling doesn't move the seat. **Isokinetic exercise** builds strength *and* endurance by the person's exerting muscle force in more than one direction in the course of moving an object. An example would be in exerting substantial force to push foward and to pull it back. Isokinetic exercise typically requires special equipment, such as Nautilus machines.

Aerobics

The word *aerobic* literally means 'with oxygen'. What does oxygen have to do with exercise? When we exert ourselves in physical activity, the energy for it comes from the metabolic process of burning fatty acids and glucose in the presence of oxygen. Continuous exertion at high intensity over many minutes requires a great deal of oxygen. Being 'in shape' means the person consumes a high *volume of oxygen* (VO_2) per heartbeat during physical exertion.

The term **aerobic exercise** refers to energetic physical activity that requires high levels of oxygen over an extended number of minutes — say, half an hour. Aerobic activities generally involve rhythmical actions that move the body over a distance or against gravity — as occurs in fast dancing, jogging, bicycling, swimming or certain calisthenics. Performing aerobic activity with sufficient intensity and duration on a regular basis increases the body's ability to extract oxygen from the blood and burn fatty acids and glucose efficiently.

An ideal exercise program for health

How much and what kinds of exercise are best for fitness? To answer this question, we need to recognise that any specific program depends on the individual's age, current health and physical capacity, goals, interests and opportunities, such as whether facilities or partners are available (Haskell 1985; Ribisl 1984). Almost all individuals need to begin with a moderate *starter program* and progress in a gradual manner towards fitness, and people who are elderly or less fit should progress more slowly than others. Starting gradually avoids muscle soreness and injury and allows the body to adapt to increasing demands, such as in the use of oxygen. Heavy exercise without sufficient oxygen simply causes the muscles to fatigue.

An ideal exercise program would involve about three hours of exercise a week divided into three to five sessions, each having three phases (Blair et al. 1992; Haskell 1985; Ribisl 1984):

1. *Warm-up.* Each session should start with two types of warm-up activities: (1) stretching and flexibility exercises for various major muscle groups, such as of the neck, back, shoulders, abdomen and legs, and (2) strength and endurance exercises, such as sit-ups, push-ups and pull-ups.
2. *Aerobics.* The next 20–40 minutes involves rhythmical exercise of large muscle groups, performed vigorously enough to raise the heart (pulse) rate to a moderately high target range. The easiest way to estimate the target range for an adult is to use a formula based on the person's age: The *minimum* heart rate is 160 pulse beats per minute minus the person's age; the *maximum* is 200 minus age (La Place 1984). Thus, 30-year-olds would maintain their heart rate between 130 and 170 beats per minute during aerobics.
3. *Cool-down.* The last few minutes of exercise should taper off in intensity to return the body to its normal state. These exercises can include calisthenics or walking.

Although these recommendations seem fairly rigid, there is room for flexibility. For instance, people who exercise at the upper end of their target range can use fewer or shorter exercise periods each week (Simons-Morton et al. 1988). Also, because of the variety of possible exercises that can be performed during each phase, individuals can tailor the program to their goals and interests. They can vary the aerobics they do, jogging on one day, skipping rope on another, playing football on another, and so on. If they want to firm their abdomens, they can focus on appropriate activities during the warm-up and cool-down phases.

Is the ideal necessary to benefit health?

Not all people can or will get the ideal amount and type of physical activity. Can they benefit from less? Absolutely, and the activity needn't be 'exercise'. Individuals can get substantial health and fitness benefits from just 30 minutes of daily moderate activity — such as walking briskly, taking a leisurely bicycle ride, or gardening — and this activity can occur in, say, 10-minute periods rather than all at once (Blair et al. 1992). The closer to the ideal type and amount of activity one gets, the greater the benefits. But the most important thing for maintaining health is *not* to have an almost completely sedentary lifestyle.

An infrequent but extremely serious hazard of exercise is in precipitating cardiac arrest. A study of autopsy reports for individuals who had died in association with exercising revealed that almost all these people died of cardiac arrest, and most of them had cardiovascular problems that existed prior to the attack (Northcote, Flannigan & Ballantyne 1986). Most of these problems could have been detected by medical screening, and the deaths of these people might have been avoided through medical counselling. Special exercise programs and recommendations are available for individuals who have specific health problems, such as diabetes and CHD (Ribisl 1984).

Another health hazard that relates to exercising is people's use of *anabolic steroids* — male hormones that build tissue — to increase muscle size and strength. Many more males than females use steroids, and most users are elite athletes who want to enhance their performance (Strauss & Yesalis 1991). Using steroids over an extended period has several negative health effects. It raises LDL and lowers HDL serum cholesterol, and is related to liver and kidney tumors and to heart attacks and strokes. It also has a permanent masculinising effect in women, increasing facial hair and lowering the voice, for instance. In males, it increases acne and balding and decreases the size and firmness of testes, at least temporarily. And adolescents who use steroids often share needles with others, putting each other at risk for HIV infection, and tend to use other drugs, too (DuRant et al. 1993). Tentative evidence suggests that continued steroid use may lead to psychological and physical dependence (Brower et al. 1990).

Exercise can be addictive. The positive aspects of exercise addiction include (1) regular physical activity, (2) increased self-confidence, self-awareness, mental alertness and physical wellbeing, (3) intrinsic satisfaction, (4) acceptance of self and (5) an experience of euphoria while engaging in the physical activity (Glasser 1976). The negative aspects of exercise addiction include compulsive exercising, or engaging in exercise as a way of dealing with hidden feelings of inadequacy or to gain approval from others. Compared with non-addicted exercisers, male and female exercise addicts have been found to be more restless and stressed prior to the exercise, to experience a high degree of positive affect after engaging in physical activity, are more depressed, anxious and angry if a workout is missed, and tend to ignore physical discomfort (Anshel 1991).

Conclusions regarding the health effects of exercise are fairly clear. Practising vigorous exercise on a regular basis is psychologically and physically healthy, particularly for preventing heart disease. People who begin exercise programs should guard against overtaxing their bodies, exercise under safe conditions with proper skills, and have periodic medical examinations to determine whether any underlying risks exist. Although more people exercise today than was the case years ago, most adults in technologically advanced countries probably do not get enough regular and energetic physical activity to gain substantial health benefits.

Who gets enough physical activity, who does not — and why

Physical activity varies across cultures. Probably most people around the world have lifestyles that provide regular, vigorous and sustained activity naturally, without actually doing exercises. They commute to work by bicycle, for instance, or have jobs that involve energetic work, as farmers, labourers and homemakers often do. These people can get very healthy amounts of physical activity if it occurs in at least three episodes a week, totalling about three hours (Blair et al. 1992). But most people in Australia and probably most other industrialised nations have relatively sedentary life circumstances. And many individuals who could be physically active in their normal lifestyles choose not to be — they may take rest breaks rather than sustaining an activity or opt to use a machine instead of doing a task manually. The high levels of physical activity people have in childhood decline sharply in adolescence (Meredith & Dwyer 1991). Because little is known about people's everyday physical activities, we will focus our discussion on factors associated with doing and not doing exercises.

Many factors influence whether individuals exercise. In Australia, men exercise more than women (AIHW 1998; Lee 1991). In addition, people who exercise tend to be young and well-educated adults, members of upper socioeconomic groups and individuals who have participated in exercise in the past (Stephens & Caspersen 1994). People who do *not* exercise tend to be blue-collar workers, older and at relatively high risk for developing CHD, such as by being overweight or smoking cigarettes. From the standpoint of performing health-protective behaviour, those whose health would benefit most from physical activity seem to be the most resistant to starting or maintaining an exercise program. Quitting smoking may help: A study of smokers found that those who quit were more likely to start exercising than those who didn't (Perkins et al. 1993). Exercise may even facilitate quitting in smokers, as cigarette cravings have been reported to be lower in smokers in an exercise intervention, compared with controls (Grove, Wilkinsen & Dawson 1993).

Whether people exercise is also related to social influences in their lives and to their beliefs. Social influences on exercise behaviour involve modelling, encouragement and reinforcement by peers and family. Studies have found that adults who exercise tend to have spouses who encourage them to do so, and children and adolescents who exercise or engage in sports tend to have friends or family who also do so (Dishman, Sallis & Orenstein 1985; Gottlieb & Baker 1986; Sallis et al. 1988). People's beliefs can influence exercising in at least two ways. First, individuals with high self-efficacy regarding their ability to exercise are more likely to do so than those with low self-efficacy (Clark et al. 1995; Wilcox & Storandt 1996). Second, people's perceived susceptibility to illness, one of the components of the health belief model, can spur them to exercise. This was demonstrated in research in which subjects received information describing their level of fitness or indicating they might be susceptible to health problems that could be prevented through exercise (Godin et al. 1987; Wurtele & Maddux 1987). Compared with subjects who did not get such information, those who did were more likely to start exercising.

When individuals are asked why they don't exercise, the most common reason they give is that they cannot find the time (Dishman 1991; Godin et al. 1992). Actually, of course, people generally do have the time but choose to use it in other ways. People also report not exercising because they have no convenient place to do it or because the weather or other environmental conditions make it unpleasant or impossible. Another factor is age — as adults get older, most of them

> gradually disengage from participating in physical activities due less, it appears, to decrements in physiological functioning ability than to cultural and psychosocial factors which persuade them that vigorous exercise is not appropriate for the elderly. Sedentary social role models, distorted body image, exaggerated notions of risk, expectations of disapproval, fear of failure, misinformation, and limited previous involvement in physical activities all conspire to limit the elderly's desire to be active. (Vertinsky & Auman 1988, p. 16)

These forces against exercise are particularly strong among many of today's elderly women, whose past sex-role experiences have taught them that men are more socially and physically suited to vigorous activity than females. Although both male and female older people tend to underrate their physical capabilities and exaggerate their health risks in performing energetic exercise after middle age, women are especially prone to these beliefs (Vertinsky & Auman 1988; Woods & Birren 1984). Health care workers and organisations for the elderly have many opportunities to dispel incorrect beliefs about health risks, change sex-role stereotypes regarding exercise and encourage older individuals to develop more active lifestyles.

Promoting physical activity

A person who spends time watching youngsters play is likely to have the impression that children are innately very active — running, jumping and climbing — and that they do not need to be encouraged to exercise, as older individuals do. Although children are generally more active than adults, and about three-fifths of schoolchildren and adolescents get healthy levels of exercise throughout the year, many other children are not active enough (Simons-Morton et al. 1988). People of all ages could benefit from school, park and work-site recreation programs and facilities to promote exercise.

Researchers have outlined several strategies that are important in promoting exercise behaviour. Figure 8.3 groups these strategies into several categories. Note that it is possible to promote physical activity by giving rewards for increased exercising *and* for decreased sedentary behaviour (Epstein, Saelens & O'Brien 1995). One other factor that is important in people's starting and sticking with an exercise routine is their *readiness* to do so, in terms of the stages of change model that we discussed in chapter 6. Research has shown that people who are at the contemplation stage — that is, those who are considering the change seriously — are more likely to start exercising and to exercise vigorously once they do than are people at the precontemplation stage (Armstrong et al. 1992; Marcus & Simkin 1994; Vita & Owen 1995). In regard to physical activity, 13 per cent of Australians could be classified as belonging to the precontemplation stage of change, 10 per cent to the contemplation stage, 16 per cent are preparing to exercise regularly, 23 per cent are currently active, and 38 per cent are in the maintenance stage (Booth et al. 1993).

The promotion of physical activity can also occur in general practice. In a study of general practitioners in the city of Perth, Australia (Bull et al. 1995), 93 per cent of doctors enquired about the current level of physical activity when seeing patients with symptoms of conditions that could benefit from exercise. However, physical activity was not usually discussed as part of routine practice with new patients, and information on their physical activity was recorded by only 20 per cent of doctors. The benefits of exercise were discussed by 60 per cent of doctors, while advice about specific programs occurred less frequently. Although doctors believed that the promotion of physical exercise during patient consultations was desirable, lack of time, insufficient educational resources and the preference of patients for drug treatment were cited as barriers to the promotion of physical activity.

To obtain the full health benefits of physical activity, people need to continue doing exercises or being very active in their normal lifestyles throughout their lives. Few people in industrialised societies achieve this ideal. Of those individuals who are already exercising regularly at any given time, about half will quit in the coming year (Dishman, Sallis & Orenstein 1985). Although the strategies we have just examined improve people's adherence to exercise programs, the dropout and relapse rates are too high even in well-designed and supervised programs introduced for students in university and for employees at their work sites (Bélisle, Roskies & Lévesque 1987; Oldridge 1984).

Safety and harm reduction

Unsafe conditions threaten people's health in virtually all environments, such as in traffic, at home, on the job and at the beach. These conditions produce huge numbers of illnesses, injuries and deaths each year. In most cases, these health problems could have been avoided if the victim or other people had used reasonable safety precautions. Sometimes people don't know how to prevent injury — as is often the case for elderly individuals who become injured when they fall — but safety training can reduce these injuries (Tinetti et al. 1994). Let's see what is known about the hazards people face and how to help people live safer lives.

Figure 8.3 Strategies to promote exercising

- *Pre-assessment.* Before people begin an exercise program, they need to determine their purposes for exercising and the benefits they can expect. They should also assess their health status, preferably through a medical checkup.
- *Exercise selection.* The exercises included in the program should be tailored to meet the health needs of the individual and his or her interests and purposes, such as firming up certain parts of the body. People are more likely to stick with the program if it includes exercises that they enjoy doing.
- *Exercise conditions.* Before people start an exercise program, they should determine when and where they will exercise and arrange to get any equipment they will need. Some people seem to adhere to a program if they pick a fixed time for exercising and refuse to schedule anything else at that time; others can be more flexible and still make sure to exercise about every other day. The exercise conditions should be safe and convenient.

- *Goals.* Most people adhere to a program more closely if they write out a specific sequence of goals and consequences for exercise behaviour in a behavioural contract. The goals should be graduated, beginning at a modest level. They should also be measurable — as body weight or number of push-ups would be — rather than vague, such as 'to feel good'.
- *Consequences.* Some individuals may need tangible reinforcers to maintain their exercise behaviour in the early stages of the program. After these people get in shape, many will find that the enjoyment of exercise and the physical benefits are sufficient rewards.
- *Social influence.* People are more likely to start and stick with an exercise program if these efforts have the support and encouragement of family and friends. Exercising with a partner or in groups sometimes enhances people's motivation to continue in a program.
- *Record keeping.* People can enhance their motivation to exercise by keeping records of their weight and performance. Seeing on paper how far they have progressed can be very reinforcing.

Sources: Dishman, Sallis & Orenstein (1985); Oldridge (1984); Ribisl (1984); Serfass & Gerberich (1984).

Accidents

Injury accounts for 6 per cent of all deaths in Australia (AIHW 2000). In 1998 there were 7946 deaths due to injury or poisoning. In 1996, suicide accounted for 32 per cent of injury deaths and traffic fatalities accounted for 29 per cent; other types of injury accounted for 39 per cent (AIHW 1998). Included in the last category, in order of most lives claimed, are falls, fires, machinery accidents, poisoning, homicide and drowning. Accidental injury peaks within three age groups — for children younger than five years, young adults and older persons (AIHW 1998). The nature of the injury differs, so that for very young children drowning and traffic accidents are the main causes of death, while for young adults it is motor vehicle accidents, and for the elderly, injury associated with falls. Males have higher rates of injury than females. Injury-related mortality is higher among indigenous people. The cost of injury to the Australian health care system in 1993–94 has been estimated at around

$2.6 billion (AIHW: Mathers & Penm 1999). Many occupations place workers at risk of injury because of exposure to dangerous chemicals or dangerous situations involving machinery. The industries with the highest mortality rates include mining; construction; agriculture, forestry and fishing; plant, machinery and transport; and electrical occupations (AIHW: Harrison & Cripps 1994).

Data from the Australian Institute of Health and Welfare reveal that accidental injury is:

- the fourth most frequent cause of death in the Australian population as a whole
- the leading cause of death in Australian children between the ages of one and 15
- the second leading cause of death in males between the ages of 25 and 45 (AIHW 1998, 2000).

Another way to see the relative impact of injury versus disease on life is to estimate the years of life lost by the victims of these causes of death. We could, for instance, use the age of 65 as a standard, subtract the age of death of each person who dies earlier, and then total all the years lost to injuries separately from those lost to disease. Accidental injury accounts for around 118 000 potential years of life lost in Australia (AIHW 1998, 2000).

How can accidental injuries be prevented? Road traffic fatalities in Australia have been reduced through a number of measures such as the introduction of compulsory seatbelt use, random breath testing, electronic speed cameras, improved road conditions and programs that teach safer driving (Brindle 1992). Legislative change has been effective in reducing death and injury to cyclists. In Victoria, the number of cyclists killed or admitted to hospital was reduced by 23 per cent in the year following introduction of a law requiring the wearing of helmets when riding bicycles (Cameron et al. 1994).

Another strategy that has been used to reduce the incidence of death and injury due to motor vehicle accidents is the use of drink-driving rehabilitation programs, since alcohol is implicated in many road accidents. In 1996 in New South Wales, it was estimated that alcohol was involved in 18 per cent of road fatalities (Roads & Traffic Authority 1998). In South Australia, between 1985 and 1992, 38 per cent of killed drivers and 30 per cent of injured drivers had a blood alcohol concentration (BAC) of 0.08 g/100 mL or higher (Holubowycz, Kloeden & McLean 1994). In Australia, there are two types of *drink-driving rehabilitation programs* — road traffic safety programs and health therapeutic programs (Sanson-Fisher et al. 1990). Road traffic safety rehabilitation programs are offered to convicted drink-drivers in the hope of reducing the likelihood of drink-driving in the future. Therapeutic programs are aimed at persons with alcohol-related problems, with the assumption that treatment for such problems will reduce the incidence of drink-driving. Rehabilitation programs use a number of approaches — among them education about the effects of drinking, attitude change and skills training. Some of the skills taught include monitoring the effects of alcohol on driving, learning to identify circumstances that lead to drink-driving, and modifying such behaviour (Sanson-Fisher et al. 1990). While rehabilitation interventions have had some effect in averting drink-driving, this is an area where health psychologists can provide more needed services.

Reduction of injuries within the workplace has been the concern of occupational health and safety organisations and industrial relations bodies such as employers, unions and government. Regulatory practices have been in effect since the mid-1980s. *Worksafe Australia* is responsible for occupational health policy and safety performance standards. It monitors work-related injury at a national level through its compilations of workers' compensation data (AIHW: Harrison & Cripps 1994).

Environmental hazards

Some people believe that they don't need to wear sunscreen unless they are fair-skinned. Others believe that the ultraviolet radiation from the sun is only harmful in tropical regions of Australia, and others value a tan more than sun protection. Ever since the French fashion designer Coco Chanel made tanning fashionable, people in many parts of the world have come to believe tans are attractive and healthy. This belief develops by early adolescence (Broadstock, Borland & Gason 1992).

Today we know that excessive exposure to the sun's ultraviolet rays makes the skin age and can cause skin cancers, particularly in people who are fair skinned and burn easily (Harrison et al. 1994). Keep in mind that sunlamps and sunbeds have the same effect, and the more exposure to them, the greater the chance of getting cancer (Westerdahl et al. 1994). Although most cases of skin cancer can be easily treated and cured, others cannot, especially if they are discovered late (Armstrong & English 1996). Dermatologists and other health care practitioners recognise that most people will not stay out of the sun and that many strive for a 'healthy' and attractive tan. As a result, these practitioners recommend that most people use sunscreens with a Sun Protection Factor (SPF) of 15+. Australians have been increasing their use of sunscreens since 1980.

Another strategy that has been used in Australia is to publish and broadcast via the media the daily UV index issued by the Bureau of Meteorology. The UV numerical index ranges from 0 to 20, and indicates the 'estimated solar erythemal irradiance incident on a horizontal surface at the surface of the earth' (ICNIRP 1995). Research indicates that although around 90 per cent of Queensland residents know of the UV index, only one-third of them reported that their behaviour was influenced by the forecasts. While more men than women were aware of the UV levels forecast, more women reported having altered their outdoor behaviour because of the index (Alberink et al. 2000).

Community health education and school-based programs have also been used in skin cancer prevention. In chapter 6, we introduced the Slip! Slop! Slap! campaign, and the SunSmart program, which attempted to increase knowledge about skin cancer risk and the harmful effects of ultraviolet radiation. Other programs, like *Kidskin*, have been developed for young children (Milne et al. 1999). *Kidskin* teaches children how to reduce exposure to the sun, through sun-protective measures. Parents of children in schools that received the *Kidskin* intervention reported greater use by their child of sun protection measures such as wearing protective clothing, seeking shade and reducing time spent outdoors in the middle of the day. These effects, however, may not translate to longer-term behaviour. After two years of intervention, there were no differences between intervention and control children in the use of hats or sunscreen (Milne et al. 2000).

Ultraviolet radiation is only one of many environmental hazards people need to guard against. Many harmful chemicals and gases can be found in people's households, work sites and general communities. Figure 8.4 describes some of these hazards. People who work with hazardous materials need to know what the substances are, what dangers they pose and how to use them safely. Employers have a duty of care to notify and train employees regarding the safe use of hazardous materials. Local governments should provide information about the exposure of residents to hazardous materials. If people know that a danger exists, they can try to take protective action (for example by drinking bottled water), become involved in community change, and notify their physician so that appropriate tests can be done periodically as secondary prevention (Winett, King & Altman 1989).

People are becoming increasingly concerned about the chemicals and gases that pervade our lives. They should be vigilant — but they should also be aware of three things: First, not every chemical or gas is harmful. Second, exposure to toxic or carcinogenic substances poses little risk when the contact is infrequent and the dosage is small (Ames & Gold 1990; Cohen & Ellwein 1990). Third, some harmful substances may have benefits that outweigh their dangers. For example, chlorinating water has all but erased many of the waterborne infections that once threatened enormous numbers of lives. But chlorinated water often has very small amounts of the carcinogen *chloroform* in it. Given these circumstances, the benefits of chlorination appear to outweigh the risks. Future environmental challenges at a global level include depletion of the ozone layer, climatic change and acid rain. The NHMRC has outlined some potential health effects of long-term climate change, which are listed in figure 8.5.

Figure 8.4 Some hazardous chemicals and gases that can occur in households, work sites and communities

Household hazards

People's homes contain various chemicals, such as pesticides and cleaning solvents, that are health hazards if they are accessible to children or used without adequate ventilation. Two other hazards are:

- *Lead* poisoning, which presents a serious health problem for developing embryos and children, and can damage their nervous system and impair intelligence and hearing (Harvey 1984). Children may ingest lead in many ways, such as by mouthing objects painted with lead-based paints, drinking water from a plumbing system with poorly soldered lead joints, or drinking acidic beverages from lead-glazed ceramics. Pregnant women who ingest leaded water or beverages may pass the substance on to their developing babies.
- *Radon*, a radioactive gas that can lead to lung cancer with long-term exposure. Breathing air with moderately high levels of radon for many hours each day presents the same cancer risk as smoking one or two packs of cigarettes a day.

Work-site hazards

Millions of people have jobs that can bring them into contact with hazardous substances, some of which are toxic or carcinogenic (Anderson 1982; Baker 1988; Clever & Omenn 1988; Levy 1985).

- *Asbestos* is a substance that has been used in buildings and equipment as a fire retardant. People who have regular contact with it risk developing lung cancer.
- *Benzine* exposure at high levels and over time is linked to bone marrow cancer; *vinyl chloride*, with liver cancer; aromatic amines, with bladder cancer; and *cadmium*, with prostate cancer.

Community hazards

The air, water and ground have become polluted with harmful chemicals and gases in communities around the world. This pollution can harm people directly or by getting into the foods they eat.

- *Chemical waste* from industry and other sources can contain toxic substances, such as cyanide, benzine and lead (Holusha 1991). The accidental, massive release of cyanide gas at a Union Carbide plant in Bhopal, India, killed thousands of people.
- *Radiation* gets into the environment from nuclear power, hospital, military and industrial sources. Exposure at high levels or for extended periods causes cancer, as seen after the massive radiation release in 1986 at the Soviet nuclear power plant in Chernobyl (Kolata 1992a).

This chapter has provided an overview of many studies relating to issues of improving general health and wellbeing. Weight control, appropriate levels of exercise and a quality diet are essential and ought to be pursued. Keeping oneself and loved ones safe in the home, at school, at work and at play are such important goals and aspirations that it is difficult to understand why a substantial proportion of the population engages in behaviours that are detrimental to health and wellbeing, as we saw for instance in the numbers of adults who drive with a BAC in excess of 0.05 g/100 mL. Health psychologists have a role in understanding the complexities of behaviour, and the dynamics that underpin health and safety.

Figure 8.5 Potential health effects of long-term climate change

• Increases in skin cancer and ocular damage due to increased exposure to ultraviolet radiation as depletion of the ozone layer progresses, and cloud density and precipitation decrease	• Adverse effects on health and welfare resulting from the economic consequences of climate change. There may also be positive aspects as employment grows in renewable energy technology industries and value-added export markets are created.
• Increasing exposure to allergens and resultant respiratory effects	• Introduction or reintroduction of exotic communicable diseases
• Increases in waterborne disease	• Reduction of the community's economic and social wellbeing due to international environmental degradation and population migration
• Higher incidence of heat stress, particularly among vulnerable groups such as the elderly, the frail and workers	• Changes in agricultural productivity, with consequent socioeconomic and sociocultural effects
• Increases in the transmission of vector-borne diseases	
• Injury, social dislocation and post-traumatic psychological problems resulting from more frequent natural disasters	

Source: Nutbeam et al. (1993). Derived from NHMRC (1991).

Summary

In addition to water, food contains five types of chemical components: carbohydrates, lipids or 'fats', proteins, vitamins and minerals. People can get all the nutrients and fibre they need by eating diets that include grains, fruits, vegetables, milk products, and meats and fish. Until recently, the trend in Australian diets was towards consuming more and more sugar, animal fats, and animal proteins, while consuming less and less fibre. People's food preferences are determined by biological and psychosocial factors.

Diet is associated with the development of atherosclerosis, hypertension and cancer. Cholesterol is the main dietary culprit in atherosclerosis. Whether plaques form in our blood vessels depends on the presence of three types of lipoproteins: low-density lipoprotein, very-low-density lipoprotein and high-density lipoprotein. People's serum cholesterol levels are determined by genetic factors and by the foods they eat. Although Australians have been reducing their intake of cholesterol recently, they still consume far too much. Intervention programs can be effective in helping people reduce dietary cholesterol substantially. High blood pressure can result from consuming too much sodium. Diets high in fat and low in fibre increase people's risk of cancer, especially cancer of the colon.

Many people are very conscious of and concerned about their weight. Most concerns among Australians are with being too fat rather than too thin, particularly among females. One method for determining whether individuals are too heavy is to compare their weights against the desirable weights given in standard tables. People are classified as overweight if their weight exceeds their desirable weight by 10 per cent; they are considered obese if their weight is more than 20 per cent above the desirable weight. People become fat because they consume more calories than they burn up through metabolism. The excess calories are stored as fat in adipose tissue, which contains cells that can increase in size and number, especially in childhood and adolescence. Heredity plays a role in weight control, probably by affecting the set-point for body weight. Psychosocial factors also affect weight control. Restraint theory proposes that individuals who struggle constantly to keep their weight down develop abnormal eating patterns of inhibition and disinhibition.

Obesity is associated with the development of hypertension, coronary heart disease and diabetes. These health risks depend on two obesity factors: the amount and location of fat tissue. The risks increase as the degree of obesity increases and when fat is concentrated in the abdominal region, rather than mostly in the thighs, hips and buttocks. Prevention of obesity should begin in childhood to avoid fat-cell hyperplasia. Schools and parents can play important roles in this effort.

Most heavy people try to reduce their weight on their own by going on a diet. Although overweight and obese individuals are likely to have difficulty adopting lifestyles that maintain a lower weight, many of them can do it successfully. Heavy people who are not able to lose weight on their own often seek help through fad diets, exercise programs, behavioural techniques, self-help groups and work-site weight-loss programs. Behavioural programs are more effective than other approaches. In relatively extreme cases, drastic procedures with medical supervision may be warranted; these procedures include placing the patient on a very-low-calorie diet, using appetite-suppressing drugs or performing surgery. Although most people who lose weight in behavioural programs keep most of that weight off, others do not. Obese individuals who complete behavioural programs are less likely to relapse if the programs include frequent follow-up meetings with weight-control therapists and social influences of other members in a treatment group.

Anorexia nervosa is an eating disorder that results in an unhealthy and extreme loss of weight. Bulimia nervosa is an eating disorder that involves recurrent episodes of binge eating and purging. Both of these disorders occur mainly in adolescence and early adulthood and are much more prevalent in females than in males. Treatment for anorexia is more difficult and less successful than that for bulimia.

More people are exercising today than were years ago. Three types of exercise are isotonic, isometric and isokinetic. Aerobic exercise refers to energetic physical activity that involves rhythmical movement of large muscle groups and requires high levels of oxygen over a period of half an hour or so. A healthy program of exercise includes a warm-up phase, an aerobic exercise phase, and a cool-down phase. Engaging regularly in vigorous exercise reduces stress, improves work performance and enhances the person's self-concept. It also increases people's life span and protects them against coronary heart disease, partly because it reduces blood pressure. People who exercise tend to be young and well-educated adults from the upper social classes. Individuals whose health would benefit most from physical activity seem to be the most resistant to starting and maintaining exercising.

Thousands of people die each year in accidents involving traffic mishaps, falls, drownings, fires, poisonings and firearms. The death rates for motor vehicle accidents increase dramatically during adolescence. There are many environmental hazards that people need to guard against. These include excessive exposure to sunlight and harmful chemicals and gases.

Key terms

aerobic exercise	insulin	lipoproteins	restraint theory
anorexia nervosa	isokinetic exercise	low-density lipoprotein	set-point theory
bulimia nervosa	isometric exercise	obese	very-low-density lipoprotein
high-density lipoprotein	isotonic exercise	overweight	

4

Becoming ill and getting medical treatment

9 Using health services

Prologue

Jo's life had just undergone major changes — she had been promoted by her employer and relocated to a new town with her two children. Then she noticed that a mole had developed on her shoulder. Uncertain whether the mole was a sign of something serious, and harried by her current pressures, she decided to wait before doing anything about it. Then, soon after she found a new family doctor, her youngest child became ill with the flu. Jo made an appointment for 10-year-old Mary with Dr Armstrong and thought, 'If I get a chance, I'll mention the mole to the doctor when we go, and have him look at it.' But she wondered if he would be like their last doctor, who would sweep into the examining room, hurriedly ask very specific short-answer questions, dominate the conversation and rush on to the next patient.

Fortunately, Dr Armstrong was not like their last doctor. He started the visit by chatting a little with Mary to learn more about her and to establish a friendly relationship. Then he asked her about her health problem, did some physical tests, and discussed with her and Jo what they needed to do to treat the illness. At the end of that discussion, he switched the focus to Jo, asking about her job and general life situation to assess possible risk factors. When he asked, 'How has your health been recently?' she anxiously told him about the mole, which he inspected. He told her that it looked harmless — as most moles are. He added, 'People who have a mole should inspect it periodically, once a month or so. If it changes colour, bleeds, grows or changes in any other way, please have me examine it without delay. Some moles develop into a skin cancer called melanoma, which can be treated effectively if we catch it early. I'll give you some information about moles before you leave.'

Jo left the office very much relieved that the doctor had examined the mole and pronounced it harmless. She also noted that if the mole had been the beginnings of melanoma, they would have caught it early. She felt secure in having found a competent and caring doctor whom she and her children could talk to easily and trust.

With this chapter, our main focus in this book begins to *shift from primary to secondary prevention* efforts. Most health care systems engage chiefly in secondary and tertiary care, providing treatment to stop or reverse a problem or to retard damage it might cause and rehabilitate the person. In this chapter we will see that the relationship formed between the patient and the health care *practitioner* — or health professional — can influence the actions they take in primary, secondary and tertiary prevention. The importance of this relationship will become clear as we discuss the kinds of health services available to people, how patients decide when to use these services and why some patients use health services effectively whereas others do not. As we examine these topics, you will find answers to questions you may have about people's use of health services. How do people decide they are sick and may need medical attention? Why do some individuals seek health care more readily than others? How can patients influence their health care? Do people follow medical advice — and if not, why don't they comply?

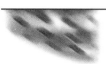

Types of health services

Systems of medical care delivery and management are complex in most societies, particularly in industrialised nations like Australia, where the medical system consists of an enormous variety of health services. To see the complex nature of health care systems, we will consider the specialised functions of health care workers, compare office-based and inpatient treatment, and contrast the Australian medical system with systems in other countries.

Specialised functions of practitioners

Medical care systems are staffed by health care workers who differ greatly in their roles and specialties. The Australian system, for instance, employs just over half a million professionals (AIHW 2000), including physicians of many types — general practitioners, paediatricians, cardiologists, neurosurgeons, dermatologists, gynaecologists, psychiatrists and so on — as well as nurses, dentists, optometrists, respiratory therapists, physical therapists, medical social workers and dietitians, to name only a small number. Each type of practitioner provides a different kind of health service, using specialised knowledge and skills.

Because each of these services involves an enormous amount of knowledge and skill that grows and changes very rapidly, individual practitioners cannot perform the services of several specialties simultaneously with a high degree of skill. The advantage in organising the health care system into specialties is that patients can receive the greatest expertise available for each aspect of the treatment of each health problem. But this great advantage is not without drawbacks. For instance, the many professionals who provide care for a particular individual do not always communicate with each other effectively, so that the physician in charge of the treatment may not have a full picture of the person's condition or progress. Also, because many practitioners work with a patient very briefly — performing just a few medical tests for example — the contact these practitioners have with patients is often impersonal.

Office-based and in-patient treatment

When we get sick and seek professional treatment, the first place we usually go is to our family doctor at his or her office. This practitioner can either treat the illness, refer us to a specialist for treatment or arrange for hospitalisation.

People with serious illnesses who require medical attention either on a continuous basis or with complex equipment or procedures generally receive treatment as in-patients in hospitals and nursing homes. *Hospitals* are the most complex medical facilities in medical care systems, employing highly sophisticated equipment and skilled practitioners from almost all specialty areas. As a result, they can provide a wide variety of services, ranging from emergency care, to diagnostic testing, to curative treatment, to rehabilitation and social services. Many hospitals also offer health promotion facilities, such as quit smoking and weight loss programs. Some hospitals have specialised missions, such as in providing care for children or for certain health problems — cancer, eye diseases or orthopaedic problems for instance.

Nursing homes and hostels have become integrated to provide residential aged care facilities for individuals who need relatively long-term medical and personal care, particularly if the patients or their families cannot provide this care (AIHW 2000). The large majority of patients in nursing homes are handicapped or frail, elderly individuals who often need help in day-to-day activities such as dressing and bathing themselves. In 1998 there were 85.6 residential aged care places per 1000 persons aged 70 and over in Australia (AIHW 2000). On any given day, nursing homes serve many more individuals than hospitals do. This is because there are more aged care facilities in comparison to hospitals, and patients stay there for fairly long periods of time. Some nursing homes are designed and staffed to provide skilled nursing and rehabilitative services, whereas others focus mainly on individuals who require lesser degrees of health-related care and services. Although most Australian nursing homes provide high-quality care, some others do not and have attracted media attention for having unsanitary conditions, abusing patients and failing to follow doctors' instructions for giving drugs.

People with serious health problems have been relying less and less on in-patient services in recent years, using *out-patient* or *home and community health care* instead. In Australia, hospital admissions increased during the 1970s, declined somewhat during the 1980s and then increased again in 1991. Part of this increase reflects the increase in the number of same-day admissions that are included in the statistical calculation. The number of day surgeries has doubled since 1987 (AIHW 1996, 2000). The shift away from in-patient care has occurred because of the fast-rising costs of hospital and nursing home services and because technological advances have made it possible to maintain medical treatment with out-patients. An example of a widely used techno-logical device that provides treatment on an out-patient basis is the *pacemaker*, which sends electrical pulses to regulate heartbeat. Many individuals with pacemakers can even transmit electrocardiograms by telephone to their doctors' offices. Another device is a pocket-size pump that can deliver precise amounts of medication on a specific schedule. Clients who use home care usually begin their treatment on an in-patient basis, but are then discharged into the care of a home health care service.

Out-patient care offers some advantages over in-patient care. For one thing, home care is likely to be less expensive. Also, people usually prefer being at home, and can often return to work or school while receiving out-patient treatment. But for some patients — particularly the elderly — home health care can present problems if they lack needed help from family or friends and do not have means of transportation to make periodic visits to their doctors (Shanas & Maddox 1985).

The Australian health care system

When most Australians get sick and need treatment, medical costs are covered either by Medicare, the national health insurance scheme, or by private health insurance. Medicare is financed in part by a levy on taxable income, the remaining expenditure being met by general revenue. No levy is paid by those on very low incomes, while a surcharge of 1 per cent is paid by high income earners who do not have private health insurance. The surcharge was imposed to encourage high income earners to take out private health insurance (AIHW 2000).

About 33 per cent of Australians have private health insurance (AIHW 2000). Since the introduction of Medicare in 1984, the percentage of Australians with private health insurance had declined to around 30.5 per cent in June 1998. While initiatives such as the Private Health Insurance Incentive Scheme (PHIIS), with its reduced premiums, and more recently the 30 per cent tax rebate on premiums, have increased the numbers of persons with private health insurance, this increase has been minimal. Low-income Australians are less likely to have private health insurance (Lairson, Hindson & Hauquitz 1995).

Medicare allows for free in-patient care at public hospitals and free medical services from doctors who bulk bill. Of course, Australians can choose to consult a private practitioner on a fee-for-service basis. In such cases, the rebate is 85 per cent of the scheduled fee, the gap between the rebate and fee schedule being paid by the patient. Some practitioners have argued that bulk billing leads to overservicing and superficial care (Douglas & Saltman 1991). Also, access to free medical care may lead to patients consulting a number of bulk-billing practices for acute problems. While this may not appear problematic at first, there is the danger that health outcomes are compromised by the lack of complete medical records for the patient over time, and practitioner responsibility towards patients may also be diminished when continuity of care from the same doctor does not exist (Buetow 1995).

Australians receive medical care that is among the very finest in the world. But the health care system has some flaws — namely, the rising cost of health care, the long waiting time for some elective surgery and the unequal distribution of medical services in rural areas.

Comparison of the Australian health care system with those in other countries

How does the Australian health care system compare with those of other countries? In the United States, health care funding and service provision lie in the private sector, with government assistance for those unable to afford private health care being provided through one of two insurance programs: Medicare for the elderly and Medicaid for low-income earners. Most Americans pay for medical costs with the health insurance their employers provide. Approximately 15 per cent of Americans do not have private health insurance (USBC 1995), and this percentage has been increasing among Hispanics and blacks.

Several decades ago, office-based medical treatment in the United States was given only by private-practice practitioners who charged a fee for each service. Recently, however, managed-care programs have become widely available and now provide medical care for about one in five insured Americans (CU 1996a; Miller & Luft 1994; USDHHS 1995). The most common of these programs is the health-maintenance organisation (HMO), which charges an annual fee that members or their employers pay. Members are entitled to use the services of any affiliated physician or hospital with little or no additional charges. Another type of managed-care plan — called the preferred provider organisation (PPO) — is very similar to some HMOs. Each PPO consists of a network of affiliated doctors and hospitals who have agreed to discount their usual charges. The PPO's members may go to any affiliated physician or hospital.

Is the medical care provided by HMOs as good as that given by private doctors? An overview of findings from research comparing fee-for-service insurance plans with HMOs indicates that patients in HMOs:

• are less likely to be admitted to a hospital, and when admitted, are likely to leave sooner
• use more preventive examinations and procedures
• receive procedures and tests that are less costly, but their medical care is comparable otherwise
• report being somewhat less satisfied with the care they received but much more satisfied with the costs to them (Miller & Luft 1994).

The US health care system is highly specialised, but it is the most expensive in terms of costs per citizen. The percentage of the gross domestic product that is spent on health care in the United States is 13.9 per cent compared with 8.3 per cent in Australia (AIHW 2000). Expenditure on health, however, is higher in Australia compared with New Zealand (7.6 per cent) and the United Kingdom (6.8 per cent) (Taylor & Salkeld 1996; AIHW 2000). Other problems with the US health care system include its inaccessibility to those with inadequate or no insurance, the unequal distribution of care even among those who are insured, and the complexity of managed care alternatives (Wenneker, Weissman & Epstein 1990).

Australia is not alone in its national health insurance scheme. Canada, Japan and most European countries have adopted health care systems that incorporate national health insurance programs for all of their citizens (Schmidt & Dlugosch 1991). In the United Kingdom, the government plays a major role in the funding and provision of services through the National Health Service. Only 10 per cent of health costs in the United Kingdom are met by the private sector, although there has been a shift in recent years towards privatisation (Pollock 1995).

The health care systems with national health insurance programs have unique structures and are financed differently. For instance, some systems provide insurance through the government, but others require employers to provide it; in some systems most physicians are employed by the government, but in others most doctors are privately employed.

Containment of health care costs has been an issue in many countries, including Australia. Because costs have been increasing steadily in most countries, efforts are being made around the world, such as in Germany, Canada and France (Atkinson 1994; Swardson 1995; Whitney 1996), to slow these increases. One strategy adopted in Australia is *casemix*, a type of managed care we encountered in a different form in the US health system. **Casemix** works on diseases being classified into Diagnostic Related Groupings (DRG), the cure of which is costed. Such a procedure allows health expenditure, the bulk of which is directed to hospitals, to be made in terms of the cost of treating certain diseases, rather than on retrospective bed-day subsidies. Also, as government health budgets shrink, some Australian private hospitals are entering into contracts with medical practitioners to provide particular medical care for a pre-negotiated remuneration package.

In any health care system, a critical step in seeking medical attention is finding a regular doctor to contact when we are sick. He or she can either cure our illness or help us find other help within the system. Now, suppose someone who has a regular doctor develops some symptoms — say, nausea and a 40° fever. Will the person go to the doctor? An important step in using health services involves deciding when we are sick enough to require medical attention in the first place. This is the topic of the next section.

Perceiving and interpreting symptoms

If you came down with a case of strep throat as a child, chances are the symptoms you experienced were obvious to you and your parents. You had a very sore throat, fever and headache, for instance. Your doctor asked about your symptoms, took your temperature and did some tests, then prescribed a curative course of action. From experiences of this type, you learned that symptoms accompany illness — and when they go away, you are well again. You also learned that certain symptoms reliably signal certain illnesses, and that some symptoms are more serious than others. As an adult, you decide whether to visit your physician on the basis of the symptoms you perceive and what they mean to you.

Perceiving symptoms

Perceiving symptoms of illness is more complicated than it may seem. It is true that we perceive internal states on the basis of physical sensations, and we are more likely to notice strong sensations than weak ones. But we do not assess our internal states very accurately. For example, people's estimates of their own heart rate and degree of nasal congestion correlate poorly with physiological measures of these states (Pennebaker 1983; Skelton & Pennebaker 1982). Symptom perception in asthma is likewise often inaccurate, with reported breathlessness not being confirmed by changes in lung function (Rietveld & Prins 1998). Individuals also have trouble perceiving external symptoms, such as whether a mole-like skin lesion is melanoma (Miles & Meehan 1995). Partly because of people's low degree of accuracy in assessing signs of illness, the point at which people recognise a symptom can differ from one individual to the next and within the same person from one time to the next. Furthermore, people do not always notice a symptom — even a strong one — when it is there, and sometimes they may perceive a symptom that has no actual physical basis. Let's see what factors affect our perception of symptoms.

Individual differences

'He's such a big baby; he notices every little ache and pain,' you may have heard someone say. Why do some individuals report more symptoms than others? One reason is that some people simply *have* more symptoms than others, of course. Another possibility is that people could differ in the sensations they experience from the same symptom, such as a specific intensity of a painful stimulus. But research has cast doubt on this possibility. For instance, studies testing large numbers of normal individuals with stimuli of different temperatures have found that people seem to have a uniform threshold at which heat becomes painful — 'almost all persons begin to feel pain when the tissue temperature rises to a level between 44°C and 46°C' (Guyton 1985, p. 302). On the other hand, individuals differ in the degree of pain they will tolerate before doing something about it, such as taking medication (Karoly 1985; Melzack & Wall 1982). And there is some indication that female chronic pain patients may react differently to pain, reporting higher levels of pain than male patients (Robinson et al. 1998).

The extent to which illness symptoms will be perceived appears to be determined by coping style. Some people are vigilant to cues that their health is at threat. This coping style has been labelled as *monitoring*. Others prefer to engage in cognitive avoidance, ignoring any symptoms of ill health. These are the 'blunters'. Research by van Zuuren and Dooper (1999) found that the monitoring coping style is associated with health behaviours performed for the purpose of detecting disease. Monitors would be more likely to be aware of changes to their bodily functioning.

Some individuals seem to pay more attention to their internal states than others do (Pennebaker 1983). They show a heightened awareness of or sensitivity to their body sensations. As a result, these people notice changes more quickly than individuals who tend to focus their attention on external happenings. But this does not mean internally focused individuals are more *accurate* in their perceptions of internal changes — indeed, research has found that they are more likely than externally focused people to overestimate changes in their bodily functions, such as heart rate (Pennebaker 1983). Other research has shown that among patients who seek medical treatment for symptoms, those who are internally focused tend to have less severe illnesses and perceive their recovery as slower than those who pay less attention to their internal states (Miller, Brody & Summerton 1987). These findings suggest that many internally focused individuals may pay *too much* attention to their internal states and, in so doing, magnify departures from normal bodily sensations.

Competing environmental stimuli

You may have heard anecdotes about athletes who were unaware of a major injury they had suffered during a competition until after the sporting event was over — *then* it hurt! The extent to which people pay attention to internal stimuli at any given time depends partly on the nature or degree of environmental stimuli that are present at that time.

When the environment contains a great deal of sensory information or is highly exciting, people become less likely to notice internal sensations. James Pennebaker

(1983) has described several findings from research that are consistent with this view. For example:

> people are far more likely to report a variety of physical symptoms and sensations when the external environment is boring or lacking in information than when they must be attentive to the environment. ... Similarly, individuals are more likely to notice itching or tickling sensations in their throats and emit coughs during boring parts of movies than during interesting portions. (p. 191)

Also, people who hold boring jobs or live alone tend to report more physical symptoms and use more aspirin and sleeping pills than those who hold interesting jobs or live with other people.

Psychosocial influences

Because people are not very accurate in assessing their actual internal physical states, their perception of body sensations can be heavily influenced by cognitive, social and emotional factors (Johns & Littlejohn 1999; Skelton & Pennebaker 1982). One way researchers have demonstrated the role of cognitive factors in symptom perception is in the effects of *placebos*, which are inert substances or sham treatments (Melzack & Wall 1982; Roberts 1995). For example, people who receive a placebo 'drug' to reduce their pain, not knowing the drug is inert, often report that it relieves their symptoms or sensations.

Positive placebo suggestion (e.g. messages about the beneficial effects of a painful stimulus) have also been found to increase pain tolerance. In an experimental study by Staats, Hekmat and Staats (1998), subjects provided with positive placebo suggestion had a higher pain tolerance for ice-water hand immersion than those given negative placebo suggestion or no suggestion. Such findings have implications not only for how symptoms will be perceived, but also in helping patients cope with invasive or painful medical procedures by altering cognitive appraisals of body sensations.

Emotional and cognitive factors appear to contribute to inaccurate symptom perception in asthma. Airway obstruction is often not attended to by adults and children, while breathlessness may be reported in the absence of reduced lung function (Rietveld, Prins & Kolk 1996; Rubinfeld & Pain 1977). Negative emotional states such as anxiety and distress have been associated with inaccurate perceptions of asthmatic symptoms (Hudgel, Cooperson & Kinsman 1982). Rietveld and Prins (1998) have suggested that if the person is distressed or anxious, selective attention to symptoms may occur if previous asthma attacks have been associated with similar emotional states. During negative emotional states, ambiguous symptoms are more likely to be interpreted as an asthma attack.

> ...the cognitive compensation for the often ambiguous sensory information associated with pathophysiology is characterised by integration of external, situational information in the symptom perceptual process and by interpretation of information in congruence with illness-schemas. There are two reciprocal mechanisms responsible for a false interpretation of sensations and symptoms, resulting in either overperception or underperception of pathophysiology. The eventual verbal expression of symptoms is subjected to high-order cognitions. Hence, the process of biased symptom perception may operate from the stimulus-level to high-order reasoning, and the latter may either facilitate or interfere with the results of unconscious perceptual processes. ... emotional factors may constitute alternative or complementary explanations for inaccuracies in symptom perception. (Rietveld & Prins 1998, p. 168)

The combined roles of cognitive, social and emotional factors in symptom perception can be seen in two interesting phenomena. The first is called *medical student's disease*. As medical students learn about the symptoms of various diseases, more than two-thirds of them come to believe incorrectly that they have contracted one of these illnesses at one time or another (Mechanic 1972). The second phenomenon, called *mass psychogenic illness*, involves widespread symptom perception among a large group of individuals, even though tests indicate that their symptoms have no medical basis either in their bodies or in the environment, such as from toxic substances. Michael Colligan and his associates (1979) have described a case of mass psychogenic illness that began one summer morning at an electronics plant in a Midwestern US city. A female production worker became faint, and another female worker who came to her aid also fainted. Soon, many other workers began reporting dizziness, headache, nausea and difficulty breathing; 20 workers were taken to the hospital; and the building was evacuated. Two similar episodes occurred days later after the plant reopened. Medical and environmental tests after each episode revealed no abnormalities that could account for the symptoms the workers experienced.

A more recent case of mass psychogenic illness involved exposure to toxic gas at a high school in Tennessee. Soon after a teacher noticed an odour, she developed headache, nausea, shortness of breath and dizziness. Many students and teachers developed similar symptoms so the school was evacuated. Toxic fumes were found at the outbreak of the symptoms, and floor drain traps were discovered to be ineffective in keeping gas out of the classroom where symptoms first developed. However, as many other teachers and students from other classrooms developed similar symptoms, this would seem to suggest mass psychogenic illness (Jones et al. 2000).

Why do such phenomena occur? Researchers have described several reasons (Colligan et al. 1979; Mechanic 1972, 1980; Skelton & Pennebaker 1982). The symptoms perceived by individuals with medical student's disease and mass psychogenic illness often involve common physiological sensations, such as headache or dizziness, that are vague and highly subjective in nature. Cognitive factors come into play when the person exaggerates these sensations and attaches to them more importance than they warrant. Modelling is a social factor that undoubtedly contributes to the contagion in mass psychogenic illness; and the symptoms experienced in medical student's disease often seem to be modelled after those of a patient the students have seen. An important emotional factor in these phenomena is stress — that is, medical student's disease and mass psychogenic illness tend to occur when people have been experiencing high levels of anxiety, heavy workloads or disturbing interpersonal conflicts. In some cases, stress may cause or exaggerate the sensations individuals perceive, as when nausea or headache are the symptoms the person notices. Research has shown that people report heightened symptoms when they experience negative emotional states, particularly anxiety (Leventhal et al. 1996; Watson & Pennebaker 1989), and these negative emotions may be interpreted as actual symptoms of a chronic disease (Rainville et al. 1992).

Sociocultural differences

People in different cultures seem to differ in their perceptions of and reactions to illness symptoms, such as pain. For instance, individuals display much more distress and disability to painful symptoms in some cultures than in others (Young & Zane 1995). These differences may result from cultural norms for reinforcing stoical versus distressed and disabled behaviours when in pain. One study compared the behavioural and emotional functioning of individuals with long-term low back pain conditions in six different countries (Sanders et al. 1992). American pain patients reported the greatest overall impairment, such as of their work and social activities. Italians and New Zealanders reported the second largest impairments, followed by Japanese, Colombian and Mexican pain patients. These cultural differences did not result from differences in the severity or duration of the subjects' pain conditions.

In summary, people's perception of a symptom depends on the strength of the underlying physical sensation, their tendency to pay attention to their internal states, the degree to which external stimuli compete for their attention, stress and usual coping style (topics covered in chapters 3 to 5), and a variety of cognitive, social and emotional processes. We encountered some of these cognitive processes in the health belief model discussed in chapter 6. What individuals do when they perceive symptoms is the topic of the next section.

Interpreting and responding to symptoms

Psychiatrist George Engel (1980) described the case of a 55-year-old man whom he called Mr Glover, who suffered his second heart attack six months after his first. He was at work, alone at his desk, when

> he began to experience general unease and discomfort and then during the next minutes growing 'pressure' over his mid-anterior chest and an aching sensation down the left arm to the elbow. The similarity of those symptoms to those of his heart attack six months earlier immediately came to mind ... but he dismissed this in favour of 'fatigue,' 'gas,' 'muscle strain,' and, finally, 'emotional tension.' But the negation itself, '*not* another heart attack,' leaves no doubt that the idea 'heart attack' was very much in his mind despite his apparent denial. Behaviourally, he alternated between sitting quietly to 'let it pass,' pacing about the office 'to work it off,' and taking Alka-Seltzer. (p. 539)

When Mr Glover's boss noticed his strange behaviour and sick appearance, she convinced him to let her take him to the hospital.

People's prior experiences affect their interpretation of and response to the symptoms they perceive. The knowledge individuals extract from their experiences plays an important role in their decisions about what the symptoms reflect and whether they warrant professional attention. Probably most often, this knowledge helps people make appropriate judgements. A study found, for instance, that one of the strongest factors in mothers' correct decisions to seek medical care for their children is prior experience — that is, whether the child or a relative had a similar problem in the past (Turk et al. 1985). But sometimes people's prior experiences and expectations can lead them to incorrect interpretations of their symptoms. For example, many elderly individuals assume tiredness and weakness are symptoms of old age rather than signs of illness (Leventhal & Prohaska 1986; Prohaska et al. 1987). And people who notice symptoms while under long-term, intense stress may attribute the symptoms to their stress reaction (Cameron, Leventhal & Leventhal 1995). Although these interpretations may sometimes be correct, they may also lead people to ignore symptoms that do, in fact, need treatment.

In the case of Mr Glover, his prior experience did not help him interpret and respond to the symptoms appropriately. His reaction to the classic heart attack symptoms he was having was governed by emotion, probably elicited by his earlier attack. Although fear can motivate a person towards health-protective behaviour, it can also motivate maladaptive avoidance behaviour. As we saw in chapter 6, *conflict theory* proposes that stress can interfere with rational decision making (Janis 1984; Janis & Mann 1977). In Mr Glover's case, he perceived severe risks in both seeking and not seeking medical care. He tried to deny the meaning of the symptoms, but that didn't seem to work, and the real meaning was still on his mind. As conflict theory predicts in these circumstances, he used a *hypervigilant* coping pattern: He believed he was fast running out of time and began to search frantically for a solution, as when he tried sitting quietly, pacing and taking Alka-Seltzer.

Mr Glover finally decided to go to the hospital after his boss persuaded him that his symptoms needed treatment. Before people decide to seek medical attention for their symptoms, they typically get advice from friends, relatives or co-workers (Croyle & Barger 1993; Sanders 1982). These advisers form a **lay referral system**, an informal network of non-practitioners who provide their own information and interpretations regarding the person's symptoms (Freidson 1961). People in the lay referral system provide information or advice when the person requests it, or even if he or she simply looks sick or mentions the symptoms. Close family or friends are generally the first people consulted for lay referral, and they might:

- help interpret a symptom — such as, 'Jim and his sister Lyn both had rashes like that. They were just allergic to a new soap their mother had bought.'
- give advice about seeking medical attention — as in, 'Mary had a dizzy spell like the one you just had, and it was a mild stroke. You'd better call your doctor.'
- recommend a remedy — such as, 'A little chicken soup, some aspirin and bed rest, and you'll be fine in no time.'
- recommend consulting another lay referral person — as in, 'Pat had the same problem. You should give him a call.'

Stage in the life span also contributes to choice of lay advice for a problem. For instance, Australian adolescents are more likely to seek advice for a health problem from parents and peers before seeing the family doctor (Praeger & Liebenberg 1994). As adolescents get older, advice is sought from peers before discussing the health problem with family members. Professional help seeking was determined by the nature of the problem (Boldero & Fallon 1995).

Although the lay referral system often provides good advice, laypersons are, of course, far more likely than practitioners to recommend actions that worsen the condition or delay the person's use of appropriate and needed treatment (Sanders 1982).

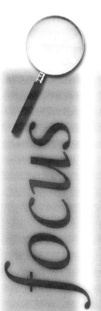

Focus on research
People's ideas about illness

Do you believe that disease is caused by germs, that all diseases have noticeable symptoms or that we are cured when the symptoms disappear? From our direct experiences and the things we read and hear about illnesses throughout our lives, we develop ideas and expectations about disease. Some of these ideas are correct, and some of them are not. We use this information to construct *cognitive representations* or **commonsense models** of different illnesses (Croyle & Barger 1993; Lau & Hartman

1983; Leventhal, Leventhal & Contrada 1997). These models can affect our health-related behaviour and seem to involve four basic components of how people think about disease:

1. *Illness identity* consists of the name and symptoms of the disease. American college students know a good deal about the symptoms of various common diseases, such as mumps, flu and ulcers (Bishop & Converse 1986).

(continued)

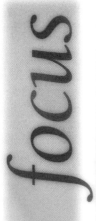

2. *Causes and underlying pathology* are concerned with ideas about how one gets the disease and what physiological events occur with it. 'I got a cold because a girl sneezed her germs in my face,' someone might say. Or a cancer patient might think, 'I got it from microwave ovens.' Some of these ideas may be correct, but others are not.

3. *Time line* involves prognosis ideas, such as how long the disease takes to appear and how long it lasts. A letter to an American newspaper columnist, Ann Landers (1992), provides an example: A person who developed severe symptoms of salmonella 30 minutes after eating chicken on an aircraft believed the airline chicken caused the illness, not knowing that salmonella symptoms take more than 24 hours to appear.

4. *Consequences* involve ideas about the expected effects and outcome of an illness. Many people mistakenly believe, for instance, that the diagnosis of breast cancer is a death sentence, that the disease is always painful and that the woman must lose the breast.

Although is it not yet clear that people use all of these dimensions for all illnesses, they appear to use many types of information and sources to develop their commonsense models. One type of information people seem to use in judging the seriousness of an illness is its *prevalence*. John Jemmott and his colleagues have reported a series of studies showing that people tend to believe rare diseases are more serious than common ones (Jemmott, Croyle & Ditto 1988; Jemmott, Ditto & Croyle 1986). In the first of these studies, the researchers recruited college students for a 'Health Awareness Project' and had the subjects fill out questionnaires about their health and undergo several medical tests, such as for blood pressure and eyesight.

One of these tests was false — it was called the 'Thioamine Acetylase Saliva Reaction Test' and purportedly assessed an enzyme deficiency that could lead to a disorder of the pancreas. Each subject was shown the results of the test, indicating that he or she had the deficiency, and told either that the deficiency was rare or that it was prevalent. Such a procedure would be considered unethical today and would not be passed by an ethics review committee because of the unnecessary distress caused to research participants as a result of a false diagnosis and misleading information about disease risk. The subjects then completed a questionnaire that included items asking them to rate the seriousness of various diseases, including 'thioamine acetylase deficiency.' (The subjects were then debriefed immediately so they would understand that they were not ill, the disease was fictitious, and the test results were fabricated.) Those subjects who were led to believe that the deficiency was rare rated the disease as being more serious than those who were told the deficiency was prevalent.

Commonsense models of illness are important because people with incorrect ideas may fail to adopt healthy behaviours to prevent illness, seek treatment when symptoms occur or follow their physician's recommendations after a disease is diagnosed.

Using and misusing health services

The pharmacist is often the first health professional people consult when they have a health problem. A customer might ask, 'My hands get these red patches that peel, and hand creams don't do any good. Do you have anything that will help?' When pharmacists suggest an over-the-counter remedy, they usually recommend that the person see a doctor if it doesn't work. Many Australians who become ill use unconventional therapies, such as massage or herbal methods, either instead of or in addition to medical care, usually without telling their doctors.

A South Australian study of 3004 respondents (MacLennan, Wilson & Taylor 1996) found that 48.5 per cent had used alternative medicines and 20.3 per cent had consulted an alternative therapist. Alternative medicines such as vitamins, herbal medicines, mineral supplements and homoeopathic medicines were more likely to be used by females, those aged between 15 and 34, the better educated and employed respondents. Chiropractors were the most commonly consulted alternative practitioners, although naturopaths, iridologists and reflexologists were also consulted. The user profile for alternative therapists was similar to that for alternative medicine use, although country residents were more likely to consult an alternative therapist. Undoubtedly, the use of alternative health care is much higher for Australia as a whole than for South Australia alone.

Most prospective patients clearly try hard to avoid contacting their doctor. Australians visit their doctor on average about 5.4 times a year (AIHW 2000). What are the most frequent *acute* and *chronic* conditions discussed in these contacts? The acute conditions are flu, common cold, fractures or dislocations, sprains or strains, wounds and ear infections; the chronic conditions are hypertension, orthopaedic problems, arthritis, diabetes, asthma and heart disease. Of course, these illnesses are not evenly distributed over the Australian population — and as you might expect, some segments of the population who become ill are more likely to use health services than are others.

Who uses health services?

Public health researchers have outlined several demographic and sociocultural factors that are related to the use of health services in Australia. Let's look at these factors.

Age and gender

One factor in using health services is *age*. In general, young children and the elderly contact their doctor more often each year than adolescents and young adults do (AIHW 1998). Young children visit doctors for general checkups and vaccinations, and they develop a variety of infectious childhood diseases. As we saw in chapter 2, children's immune systems are relatively weak at birth but develop rapidly in the early years. Children are relatively high users of medical services, but it is parents who make the choices for them. While physical health status is the most important determiner of health care use in Australian children, a study by Ward and Pratt (1996) found that the number of doctor visits for children was associated with three factors — the mother's use of health services, how much stress the mother was experiencing, and a problematic relationship between a distressed mother and her child. Doctor contacts decline in late childhood and remain relatively infrequent in early adulthood, but increase in the middle-age and elderly years as the incidence of chronic diseases rises.

Figure 9.1 depicts how doctor's visits vary with the patient's *gender*. Women have a higher rate of doctor contacts than men (AIHW 2000). This gender difference does not exist in childhood but begins to appear during adolescence. Much of the gender difference in doctor contacts in early adulthood certainly results from the medical care women require when they become pregnant. But even when visits to the doctor for pregnancy and childbirth are not counted, women still use medical services more than men. The reasons for this difference in use of medical care are unclear, but researchers have offered several possible explanations (Verbrugge 1985). One obvious explanation is that women may simply develop more illnesses that require medical attention. Although men are more likely than women to develop fatal chronic diseases, women show higher rates of medical drug use and illness from acute conditions, such as respiratory infections, and from non-fatal chronic diseases, such as arthritis and migraine headache. Another explanation is that men are more hesitant than women to admit having symptoms and to seek medical care for the symptoms they experience. This difference in responding to symptoms probably reflects sex-role stereotypes; that is, Australian society encourages men more than women to ignore pain and to be tough and independent. Yet another explanation for the higher rate of medical usage by women could be that as women are primarily responsible for taking children to doctors, they may receive a 'vicarious consultation' — that is, they may discuss personal health problems with the doctor while the child is being treated.

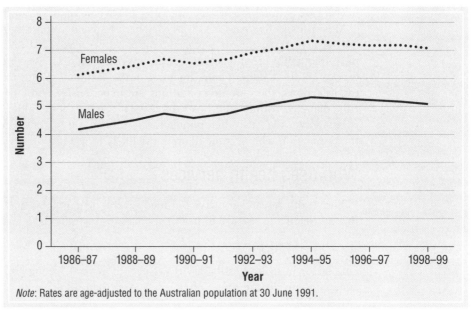

Figure 9.1 Average number of doctor consultations per year (1986–87 to 1998–99) for males and females

Source: AIHW (2000, figure 5.14).

Sociocultural factors in using health services

Are certain groups within Australian society disadvantaged in terms of access to medical care? For instance, are those from higher socioeconomic backgrounds, as determined by occupational status and educational attainment, more likely to obtain the required medical treatment when ill? Health service use indicates that Australians with lower levels of education are not disadvantaged in terms of access to care, although low-occupation families may be disadvantaged for some services (Wiggers, Sanson-Fisher & Halpin 1995). Those with lower education make greater use of medical and general practitioner services, while the occupationally disadvantaged have a higher use of allied and alternative health services.

Differential usage between socioeconomic groups is apparent for dental care and specialist services. Indigenous Australians and low-income families are far more likely to use medical providers who bulk-bill and hospital emergency rooms for medical care. This is probably because disadvantaged people are less likely to have regular doctors (Flack et al. 1995). The gap between social groups in utilisation of health services in Australia has narrowed since 1984 with the introduction of Medicare, the national health insurance scheme. Medicare is most likely responsible for the increase in doctor visits that occurred between 1988 and 1995 (AIHW 1996).

Despite the help Medicare provides in offsetting the cost of medical treatment for socially disadvantaged groups, these people may be required to make co-payments when the medical provider does not directly bill the service to the Health Insurance Commission (HIC). Co-payments or additional costs by the patient are also likely for specialist services. Poor people tend to become sick more often and require longer hospital stays (Penn et al. 1995) Unlike higher-income groups who can afford private health insurance, they are more likely to receive public hospital care. Low-income people's lack of knowledge about preventive care and preventive services, probably contributes to their high illness rates.

The expense of medical care is not the only reason for the gap between social and cultural groups in using certain private and specialist health services (Flack et al. 1995; Penn et al. 1995; Young & Zane 1995). First, individuals from lower socio-economic groups tend to perceive themselves as being less susceptible to illness than do more advantaged groups. As a result, low-income people are less likely to seek out preventive care. Second, people with low incomes and from minority groups are less likely to have regular sources of health care than others are. Often this situation develops because low-income areas of cities and rural regions are unable to attract doctors to provide health services there. In addition, people in the lower classes and from minority groups may feel less welcomed by, and trustful of, the health care system than other individuals. Third, language may serve as a barrier to health care for immigrants if they do not speak English and no translators are available (Dolman et al. 1996). These and many other factors tend to reduce the likelihood that low-income individuals will use health services for preventive care and when they are ill.

Why people use, don't use and delay using health services

Health psychologists and others who study health care have discovered many factors that influence whether and when individuals are likely to seek medical care. Some of these factors involve people's ideas and beliefs about treating illness.

Ideas, beliefs and using health services

An ailing man who was considering whether to seek treatment thought, 'Remember how the medicine Kevin's doctor gave him made him sicker? I don't trust doctors.' Some-times patients develop health problems as a *result* of medical treatment, and these problems are called **iatrogenic conditions**. The condition can result either from a practitioner's error or as a normal side effect or risk of the treatment, as may occur when people undergo surgery or begin to take a new medication. In Kevin's case, the medic-ation he received caused an allergic reaction. Positive and negative stories we hear about the treatment patients receive may influence our decisions to use medical services.

Not trusting practitioners is one reason many people fail to seek the care they need, and we can consider two issues of trust. First, individuals may avoid getting care because they worry about the confidentiality of information they disclose to, or that is discovered by, their practitioners. For instance, a study found that most American adolescents have health concerns they want to keep private from their parents, and one-fourth said they would forgo treatment if their parents could find out about it (Cheng et al. 1993). Second, minority group members have heard stories, some of which are true, of discriminatory practices and atrocities carried out by medical personnel against them (Dula 1994).

Many people in various parts of the world, including industrialised nations, choose to seek *alternative medicine* or *folk medicine* treatments when they are ill instead of, or in addition to, getting medical care (Belluck 1996; CU 1994b; Landrine & Klonoff 1992; Vecchio 1994). Because these treatment approaches are so varied and have little in common with each other, we may simply define them as treatments that seem inconsistent with the biomedical model and so far have little or no scientific evidence for their effectiveness. These treatments include using herbs to treat hypertension, hypnosis to treat broken bones, acupuncture to treat depression, and seaweed extract or copper bracelets to treat arthritis. Some alternative or folk treatment methods probably do have value, but others clearly do not. Many people who use alternative or folk approaches learned to do so through their religious or cultural backgrounds. Nevertheless, huge industries are being built around tea-tree oil and the growing of herbs. Moreover, many universities in Australia have programs to train naturopaths.

Social and emotional factors and seeking medical care

Social and emotional factors can play important roles in people's decisions about seeking treatment for their symptoms. Let's see how by first examining the role of emotions.

Earlier we considered the case of Mr Glover, who delayed medical treatment for clear symptoms of a heart attack. Strong emotional reactions to symptoms sometimes impede people's use of health services. Individuals may perceive a disease to be so serious that they are reluctant to seek medical attention for their symptoms because of the extreme anxiety and fear their perceptions generate. As a result, the threat these individuals perceive does not increase their likelihood of using health services, but may decrease it. Interviews with hundreds of adults, for instance, revealed that people perceive cancer as an extremely painful disease, and 18 per cent of these people said they might be reluctant to seek medical care for cancer symptoms because of their fear of the physical pain they associate with the disease and its treatment (Levin, Cleeland & Dar 1985). Expectations of pain probably also play a strong role in people's fear of dental care (Gatchel 1980). People may also avoid medical care if they fear embarrassment, such as when adults have problems of bladder control.

Social factors influence people's tendencies to seek medical care for their symptoms. For example, many men believe getting medical care is a sign of weakness, violating their social role for being strong. But social factors can also encourage people to seek care, such as through the process of lay referral. According to sociologist Irving Zola (1973), three types of 'social triggers' can prompt people to seek treatment. One of these social triggers is *perceived interference* of the symptoms with individuals' interpersonal relations or activities. For example, a man with an ulcer experienced pain when he consumed certain foods and beverages, such as beer. One day after one of these painful episodes, he decided to seek treatment, saying, 'If you can't drink beer with friends, what the hell' (Zola 1973, p. 684). Similarly, symptoms that interfere with work may spur a person to seek care. An *interpersonal crisis* can also serve as a trigger, particularly if the person uses medical treatment as a means of resolving or escaping the crisis. Zola described an example of a woman who was having serious problems with her relatives while she was on vacation. She decided to enter a hospital and have a benign cyst removed so that her relatives would 'stop bothering' her. The third type of social trigger is called *sanctioning*, in which someone asks or insists that an ill person have his or her symptoms treated. For instance, a man who had been having problems with his vision for a while finally went to a doctor after his wife prodded him to do so. Sometimes overt prodding isn't even necessary — sick individuals who simply believe significant others want them to seek treatment are more likely to do so than those who believe others think they should wait (Timko 1987).

Stages in delaying medical care

When symptoms of a potentially serious illness develop, seeking treatment promptly is imperative. **Treatment delay** refers to the time that elapses between when a person first notices a symptom and when he or she enters medical care. In medical emergencies, such as severe injury or a heart attack, people often seek help in a matter of minutes or hours, as Mr Glover did. Some drugs for treating heart attacks can prevent myocardial damage if administered within, say, an hour or so after the attack begins. What determines how long people wait?

On the basis of extensive interviews with patients at a clinic, Martin Safer and his colleagues discovered that treatment delay occurs as a sequence of three stages (Safer et al. 1979). As figure 9.2 illustrates, the three stages are:

1. *appraisal delay*: the time a person takes to interpret a symptom as an indication of illness
2. *illness delay*: the time taken between recognising one is ill and deciding to seek medical attention
3. *utilisation delay*: the time after deciding to seek medical care until actually going in to use that health service.

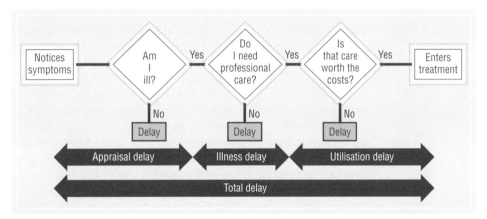

Figure 9.2 Treatment delay is conceptualised as having three stages: appraisal delay, illness delay and utilisation delay.

Source: Safer et al. (1979, figure 1).

The researchers also assessed the patients' reasons for delaying treatment and found that different factors were important for different stages of delay. During the *appraisal delay* stage, the sensory experience of a symptom had the greatest impact on delay — for instance, patients recognised a symptom as an indication of illness more quickly if they experienced severe pain or bleeding than if they did not.

In the *illness delay* stage, thoughts about the symptom had the greatest impact. Thus, individuals decided to seek medical attention more quickly if (1) the symptom was new than if it had been experienced many times before and if (2) they spent little time thinking about the symptom and its implications than if they spent a lot of time doing so. During the *utilisation delay* stage, perceptions of benefits and barriers were important — delay was shortest for those people who were less concerned about the cost of treatment, had severe pain and felt that their symptoms could be cured. In addition, the researchers found that having a major non-illness problem or life event, such as a marriage or divorce, was an important factor that increased the *total* treatment delay.

How long did these people wait before going in for medical care after first noticing a symptom? For half of these patients, treatment delay was about a week or less, but many of the others waited two months or more. Some of these people may have delayed a long time because they were not experiencing pain. As we just discussed, *not having pain* is a major factor in delaying. This factor is potentially very important because pain is *not* a major symptom of many very serious diseases, such as hypertension and diabetes. Pain is also not one of the main warning signs of cancer, which include a change in bowel or bladder habits, obvious change in a wart or mole, and a lump in the breast or other tissue (ACS 1989). Most people who notice a warning sign of cancer wait at least a month before visiting a doctor, and between 35 and 50 per cent delay for more than three months (Antonovsky & Hartman 1974). People need to know what the symptoms of serious diseases are and realise that some illnesses do not have the signs people often rely on in deciding whether to seek medical care.

Misusing health services

In a sense, delaying medical care is a *misuse* of health services, but a more obvious misuse is *overuse* — that is, using health services repeatedly when there is no need. People in the general population commonly refer to patients who overuse medical care as 'hypochondriacs' and think these people are either malingering or imagining symptoms, so that the illness is 'all in their heads.' But this common view is inaccurate. Although some individuals do imagine symptoms and some malinger to get various benefits of the sick role, *hypochondriacs* tend to interpret real but benign bodily sensations as symptoms of illness — deciding, for example, that their gastric pains are signs of a serious disease rather than the results of eating spicy foods (Barsky & Klerman 1983; Skelton & Pennebaker 1982). They may also amplify minor sensations, such as muscle soreness or twinges, and perceive them as very painful. Because of these characteristics, psychologists and psychiatrists use the term **hypochondriasis** to refer to the tendency for individuals to worry excessively about their own health, monitor their bodily sensations closely, make frequent unfounded medical complaints and believe they are ill despite reassurances by physicians that they are not (Barsky & Klerman 1983; Costa & McCrae 1985; Kellner 1985, 1987; Skelton & Pennebaker 1982).

Paul Costa and Robert McCrae (1980, 1985) have demonstrated an important link between hypochondriasis and emotional maladjustment, or *neuroticism*, which they defined as

> a broad dimension of normal personality that encompasses a variety of specific traits, including self-consciousness, inability to inhibit cravings, and vulnerability to stress as well as the tendency to experience anxiety, hostility, and depression. (1985, p. 21)

These researchers tested about 1000 normal adults, using two self-report scales: (1) the Cornell Medical Index to assess the subjects' 'somatic complaints', or medical conditions or symptoms, and (2) the Emotional Stability Scale to measure neuroticism. The subjects were in generally good health and ranged in age from under 20 to over 90. Analysis of the questionnaire responses showed that somatic complaints increased with neuroticism — individuals who scored high on neuroticism reported two to three times as many somatic complaints as those who scored low on neuroticism. Recent research has confirmed the relationship between neuroticism and physical symptom reports (Williams & Wiebe 2000). Additionally, negative emotions appear to mediate the relationship between neuroticism and symptom reporting, so that when individuals are experiencing negative emotional states such as depression, minor symptoms are intensified and perceived as indicating serious illness.

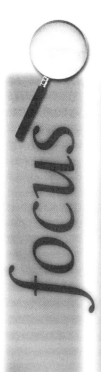

Focus on research
Neuroticism and symptom presentation

In an experimental study by Ellington and Wiebe (1999), psychology students varying in neuroticism role-played an imagined health condition of either low severity (strep throat) or high severity (acute appendicitis) to a confederate medical student supposedly learning interviewing skills.

As indicated in the figure, participants high on neuroticism presented more psychosocial concerns when describing the more serious medical condition of appendicitis compared with strep throat. Their account of the condition was more detailed, and information was presented in an emotionally laden manner. Participants low on neuroticism did not discuss psychosocial concerns when the medical condition was severe.

In a further study, family practice doctors evaluated a subsample of the videotaped roleplays to assess whether their attitudes and medical decisions would be influenced by the symptom presentations of those high on neuroticism. While doctors were able to perceive appendicitis symptoms as more severe than the step throat symptoms of low-neuroticism participants, they were unable to distinguish the severity of symptoms for the two conditions reported by high-neuroticism participants. The doctors indicated that they would be more likely to prescribe psychiatric medication, schedule follow-up appointments and make referrals to mental health professionals for the high-neuroticism participants. The investigators concluded that the symptom presentation style of high-neuroticism patients might mislead doctors to focus on psychological symptoms rather than organic symptoms.

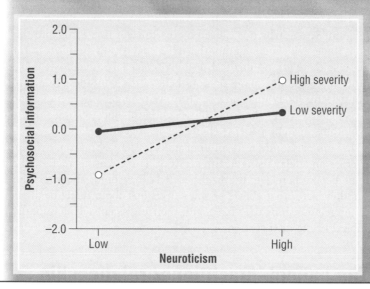

Figure 9.3
Psychosocial information presented as a function of neuroticism and severity of condition

Source: Ellington and Wiebe (1999, figure 1).

Do these findings mean that neuroticism causes more complaints, or that having many illnesses causes neuroticism? Although either causal direction is possible, some of the clearest research findings so far suggest that 'neuroticism appears to lead to complaints' (Costa & McCrae 1985, p. 23). A prospective study, for example, assessed hypochondriasis in several hundred patients who had suffered episodes of chest pain — or *angina* — with minimal or no coronary disease (Wielgosz et al. 1984). The absence of coronary disease was determined by a test called a *coronary angiography*, which measures whether the coronary arteries are constricted. A year later, each person was interviewed regarding his or her health and asked about the frequency and severity of chest pain during the preceding six weeks. The researchers evaluated the relationship between the patients' recent pain and several factors, such as the severity of pain they had experienced in their initial episodes. But the factor that was most predictive of continued pain was hypochondriasis: Patients who were greatly preoccupied with personal somatic complaints after the initial episodes reported far more continued and unimproved pain a year later than those who were not so hypochondriacal. Other researchers have found similar links between angina and sensitivity to body sensations (Davies et al. 1993).

Many people believe hypochondriasis increases in old age. Costa and McCrae (1980, 1985) have presented evidence that this belief is incorrect. For one thing, neuroticism does not increase with age. Second, although older individuals have more somatic complaints and use health services more than younger adults do, the greater somatic complaints of the elderly are mainly related to *real* problems — sensory, cardiovascular and genitourinary conditions, which are known to increase in old age. If elderly people were prone to hypochondriasis, we would expect them to report more complaints with regard to other body systems, too. But they do not. This indicates that the elderly use health services more than younger individuals simply because they are less healthy. The proportion of people who are hypochondriacs appears to be no higher in old age than in earlier adult periods.

One other issue should be discussed: Sometimes people may have real health problems that medical technology cannot yet confirm. A clear and increasingly frequent example is a condition called *chronic fatigue syndrome* (CFS). The main symptom of CFS is persistent or frequently occurring severe fatigue for a period of several months, but other symptoms can include frequent infections and headaches (CU 1990; Stone et al. 1994). Not long ago doctors thought that this condition was an extended form of mononucleosis, which is caused by the Epstein-Barr virus, but this idea has been ruled out. Some evidence suggests that CFS may result from an immune system disorder. Because there are no medical tests to detect CFS, diagnosis is based on ruling out all other diseases, and many doctors believe the condition is 'all in the patients' heads'. But it seems likely that these doctors are wrong. Some evidence now suggests that CFS is associated with subnormal blood pressure, and treating this condition reduces CFS symptoms in some patients (Bou-Holaigah et al. 1995).

To summarise, there is an enormous variety of reasons why people use, don't use, overuse and delay using health services. These reasons include the nature of the symptoms people perceive, the health beliefs they hold, and social and emotional factors. Another factor that affects people's decisions about using health services is the quality of the relationships they have with their physicians. This important relationship is the subject of the next section.

The patient–practitioner relationship

A woman who had been receiving treatment for cancer at a clinic on a regular basis began to procrastinate about going in for periodic examinations and care. When her family asked why she had not gone in on schedule, she replied, 'They gave me a new doctor, and he's not very nice. He treats me like a number, and I feel uncomfortable talking to him — he talks down to me when I ask him questions.' Many patients have stories about negative experiences with practitioners, and these experiences can lead people to delay or stop getting the medical attention they need. These stories often involve the practitioner's hurried manner, insensitivity, lack of responsiveness, failure to explain the medical problem or the treatment, or unwillingness to involve the client in planning the treatment. Problems like these are likely to be aggravated if the client and practitioner have very different cultural backgrounds (Young & Zane 1995).

Patient preferences for participation in medical care

When people visit their doctor about health problems, do they just want to be 'cured' or do they also want to know about the illnesses and how to treat them? How involved do they want to be in decisions and activities in their treatment? Doctors often misjudge their patients' answers to these kinds of questions (Daltroy 1993). Correctly judging the amount and type of participation people prefer can be important — patient–practitioner relationships depend to some extent on the compatibility between what the patient wants and what the practitioner provides.

People differ in the participation they want in their medical care. Although almost all patients want to know what their illnesses are and how to treat them, some want more details about the illnesses, self-administration of treatment and involvement in decisions than others do (Beutow 1995; Krantz, Baum & Wideman 1980). Research has discovered some interesting things about clients' participation preferences. For one thing, elderly individuals are more likely than younger adults to want health professionals to make health-related decisions for them (Woodward & Wallston 1987). Cancer patients who are high on the coping style of 'monitoring' prefer to be involved in medical treatment decisions (Ong et al. 1999). Providing the amount and type of participation individuals want enhances their adjustment to and satisfaction with medical treatment (Auerbach, Martelli & Mercuri 1983; Martelli et al. 1987). And patients who report that they usually want or take an active role in their treatment tend to adjust to their recovery periods better and recover faster than those who prefer an inactive role (Brody et al. 1989; Mahler & Kulik 1991).

Just as people differ in the information and involvement they want regarding their health, practitioners differ in the participation they are inclined to provide. For instance, research has shown that some doctors are more inclined than others to share their authority and decision making even among colleagues (Eisenberg, Kitz & Webber 1983). What happens in the patient–practitioner relationship when the person wants a different level of participation from what the practitioner is willing to give? A large-scale survey by Marie Haug and Bebe Lavin (1981) had patients and doctors describe their own attitudes and behaviour regarding the participation of clients in health care. The subjects' responses suggested three conclusions. First, although both the patients and the physicians expressed the attitude that clients should participate in activities and decisions pertaining to their health, neither the patients nor the physicians behaved in this way very often. Second, when the person wants a high level of participation but the practitioner wants to take total responsibility, conflict can be expected. As a result, the client either finds or is told to find another doctor. Third, when a patient wants the doctor to take charge but the doctor wants the person to participate, both may feel uncomfortable. This may lead to the doctor taking charge or the client finding a 'take charge' physician.

These findings indicate that a mismatch between the patient's and the practitioner's ideas about participation can impair their relationship. The results of other research indicate that mismatches of this type can increase the stress people experience during unpleasant medical procedures (Auerbach, Martelli & Mercuri 1983; Miller & Mangan 1983). In deciding how much information and involvement to provide each client, practitioners clearly need to assess and consider how much the person wants.

The practitioner's behaviour and style

Imagine this test: You recently completed medical training and have just started working in a bulk-billing clinic as a general practitioner. Your next patient this morning is waiting in an examination room, which you are preparing to enter. Your task will be to decide whether this client has one or more of the more than 1300 disease entities known to medicine (Mentzer & Snyder 1982). Or maybe the person has no physical problem at all. You have 20 minutes.

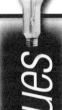

Highlight on issues

Fighting for your life

Not all victims of serious diseases who are getting medical care receive the most effective treatments available (Kolata 1992b). Although this situation sometimes occurs because a doctor is overworked or not competent, it's more likely to result from physicians' difficulty keeping up with rapid advances in medical knowledge and their reluctance to switch from a procedure that works reasonably well to one that may work better. What can people do to get the best possible treatment?

Patients and people close to them can join the fight for their lives by taking an active interest in their illnesses and health care (CU 1995b; Laszlo 1987; Paulson 1988). Let's consider a hypothetical case of a man named Mick who has a life-threatening illness, cancer. Once he receives the diagnosis, he and his family can swing into action. They can:

- get information about the disease and the usual courses of treatment. Information about cancer is readily available on the Internet and in books they can purchase in bookstores or consult through public, university and medical school libraries.
- make a list of questions to ask for each meeting with doctors working on his case. If possible, Mick should have a relative or friend accompany him to discussions with doctors concerning treatment options. One of them should take notes during the meeting, and they should ask to know all possible treatment options and determine what each

treatment involves, what the risks are, and the likelihood of success. Be sure all uncertainties have been cleared up before leaving each meeting.
- broaden their sources of information. The Australian Cancer Society has toll-free phone numbers to call for publications and information about cancer support groups, treatment methods, treatment centres, and oncologists — that is, doctors who specialise in treating various forms of cancer. At least one of the specialists Mick consults regarding treatment options should be a qualified medical oncologist, preferably one at a major university or teaching hospital. Many people consult only the original doctor on their case, and this is a mistake.
- use reputable information sources to find out about very new medical procedures (and even some risky experimental ones). Even though many newer approaches may provide the most effective treatment, not all doctors know about them or feel comfortable about recommending them. Individuals who have other serious illnesses can join the fight for their lives in similar ways. When patients and people close to them take an active interest in their health care, they can play an informed role in discussions and negotiations with their doctors towards making decisions. Patients who do this can be satisfied that they are getting the best treatment available and feel a sense of efficacy in themselves and in their doctors.

Diagnosing and treating health problems are difficult tasks, which different doctors undertake with their own behaviours and styles of interacting with patients. Patrick Byrne and Barrie Long (1976) identified different styles of interacting by analysing about 2500 tape-recorded medical consultations with doctors in several countries, including England, Ireland, Australia and Holland. Each doctor tended to use a consistent style for all clients being treated. Most of the styles were classified as **doctor-centred**, in which the doctor asked questions that required only brief answers — generally 'yes' or 'no' — and focused mainly on the first problem the person mentioned. These doctors tended to ignore attempts by a patient to discuss other problems he or she might have had. Doctor-centred physicians seemed to be intent on establishing a link between the initial problem and some organic disorder, without being sidetracked. In contrast, physicians who used the opposite, **patient-centred** style took less controlling roles. They tended to ask open-ended questions, such as 'Can you describe the situations when the pain occurs?', that allow a patient to relate more information and introduce new facts that may be pertinent. They also tended to avoid using medical jargon and to allow clients to participate in some of the decision making.

The patient–practitioner relationship depends on the ability of the two participants to communicate with each other. But doctors sometimes impede communication by using *medical jargon* or technical terms. For example, telling hypertensive patients to 'reduce sodium intake' is an accurate recommendation, but will they know what it means? Some people will know exactly what sodium is, others won't have any idea, and others will think it only means table salt, not realising that there are other sources of dietary sodium. Studies have found that most patients, particularly those with limited education, fail to understand many of the terms their doctors use — such terms as 'mucus', 'sutures' and 'glucose', for instance (DiMatteo & DiNicola 1982). These terms are used by doctors even when they do not expect their patients to understand them (McKinlay 1975). Although jargon is useful for accuracy and for communicating among medical professionals, practitioners who use medical and technical terms in talking with clients without explaining the terms or checking comprehension can create confusion, incorrect ideas and dissatisfaction in them.

Why would doctors use terms with a patient when they do not expect the person to understand? Sometimes they may do this 'out of habit' — that is, the terms are so familiar to them that they forget the client is less medically sophisticated. Or they may feel — perhaps in a patronising way — that the person 'doesn't need to know'. Other reasons for using jargon may involve their perceptions of what would benefit the patient or the medical staff (DiMatteo & DiNicola 1982; McKinlay 1975). How might using jargon benefit the client? Sometimes doctors may feel that the person is better off not knowing exactly what the disease or its treatment may entail; knowing may produce too much stress or interfere with treatment, they may think. And how may using jargon with a patient benefit the medical staff? For one thing, using medical terms without explanations keeps interactions between the client and practitioners short. Jargon is often used by health care professionals as a 'blocking mechanism' to keep interaction at a superficial level (Wilkinson 1991). It may also reduce the chances that the client will react emotionally to the information, ask questions about the treatment or discover if errors have been made. Finally, using 'big words' the client does not understand elevates the status of practitioners.

First and foremost, people prefer to have a practitioner they think is competent. But there are other factors that are important in the patient–practitioner relationship, too — especially the *sensitivity, warmth* and *concern* the person perceives in the practitioner's behaviour. Studies have demonstrated that most people prefer and evaluate highly dentists and doctors who seem friendly and interested in them as individuals, show empathy for their feelings, project a feeling of reassurance, and present a calm and competent image (Corah et al. 1988; DiMatteo et al. 1985; Sanchez-Menegay, Hudes & Cummings 1992). In contrast, practitioners who seem emotionally neutral are often evaluated less positively, perhaps because they appear detached and unconcerned. People assess these characteristics not just by the words the practitioner uses, but by his or her body language — facial expressions, eye contact, and body positions (DiMatteo 1985; DiMatteo, Friedman & Taranta 1979; Thompson 1984). Australian research has found that health care professionals are typically low in their demonstration of empathy when communicating with patients (Reynolds & Scott 2000).

The behaviour and style of practitioners can have important implications for them and their patients. Research has shown that people tend to express greater satisfaction with doctors who give them a chance to talk, take the time to listen, give clear explanations about illnesses and treatments, and project a feeling of concern and reassurance than for doctors who do not (Roter 1989; Williams, Weinman & Dale 1998). The greater satisfaction these patients feel may translate into a higher likelihood that they will keep appointments with their doctors. A study found that physicians who were more sensitive to others' emotions had fewer cancellations of appointments that were not rescheduled than doctors who were less sensitive (DiMatteo, Hays & Prince 1986).

Do doctors and patients have different views about what constitutes a good medical consultation? This was the question Helen Winefield and associates (Winefield & Murrell 1991, 1992) were interested in studying in their research on Australian general practice consultations. They examined the speech patterns of doctors and patients during the consultation and linked such patterns to both doctor and patient satisfaction with the consultation. In the diagnostic stage of the consultation, doctors were most satisfied when they asked open questions that elicited information from the patient to help with diagnosis. Patient satisfaction in the diagnostic stage was associated with the doctor asking specific questions about symptoms and providing evaluative feedback about their actions. In the prescriptive stage, doctors were most satisfied when they gave information about treatment, while patients preferred consultations where they were able to express their attitudes towards the recommended treatment or explore feelings about their medical condition.

Recent research has found that satisfaction with patient-centred communication during medical consultations may depend on individual characteristics of the patient (Graugaard & Finset 2000) and doctor–patient congruence in preferences for type of communication (Krupat et al. 2000). Patients with high trait anxiety are more satisfied and feel more comfortable with doctor-centred communication, whereas those with low trait anxiety prefer a more patient-centred physician style. When the individual orientations of patients and doctors match (i.e., both prefer doctor-centred or patient-centred communications), satisfaction with the consultation is likely to be higher.

The patient's behaviour and style

It takes two to tango, as the saying goes. Although the practitioner's behaviour plays an important role in the relationship he or she forms with a patient, the client's behaviour and style are important, too. Doctors reported in a survey, for instance, that patients sometimes do things that can be very troubling or unsettling for a doctor (Smith & Zimny 1988). Some of these behaviours include:

• expressing criticism or anger towards the doctor
• ignoring or not listening to what the doctor is trying to say

- insisting on laboratory tests, medications or procedures the doctor thinks are unnecessary
- requesting that the doctor certify something, such as a disability, that he or she thinks is untrue
- making sexually suggestive remarks or behaviours towards the doctor.

Assess yourself

DO YOU KNOW WHAT MEDICAL TERMS MEAN?

The following 10 medical terms were used in McKinlay's (1975) study of patients' understanding of medical jargon, which is described in the text. Match the terms with the definitions given below: In the space preceding each term, place the number for the corresponding definition.

____ antibiotic   ____ mucus

____ breech   ____ protein

____ enamel   ____ purgative

____ glucose   ____ suture

____ membrane   ____ umbilicus

1. The rump or back part.
2. A small scar on the abdomen; the navel.
3. A substance that makes up plant and animal tissue.
4. A simple sugar that the body manufactures from ingested food.
5. A joining together of separated tissue or bone, or a device to achieve this joining.
6. A sheet of tissue that covers or lines a body organ.
7. An agent that works against bacterial infections.
8. A hard, glossy coating or surface.
9. A substance or procedure that causes a cleansing of a body organ, as occurs in a bowel movement.
10. A secretion of body tissues.

Check your answers against the key below. Did you get them all correct? Would you have known as many of the definitions if they weren't given? Would your friends — especially those who have not gone to university — know the terms?

Answers, in order:

7, 1, 8, 4, 6, 10, 3, 9, 5, 2

If behaviours such as these lead to a breakdown in the relationship between patient and practitioner, the quality of the medical care the client receives may suffer.

The potential for people to bring malpractice suits against practitioners has also affected their relationship, making doctors wary of patients and less satisfied with their careers (Kolata 1990). These suits are stressful, emotionally devastating, and vindictive experiences for clients and physicians alike, regardless of who wins. Many practitioners in rural areas of Australia will not deliver babies because of the high cost of insurance premiums against malpractice suits. Patients who have poor relationships with their doctors are more likely to file malpractice suits than those who do not. These suits usually claim incompetence or negligence in the physician's treatment, but they sometimes allege that the doctor did not communicate important information to the client.

Do patients do things that impair patient–practitioner communication? Yes. For one thing, they may not give signs of any distress they are feeling about their conditions or treatment (Roter & Ewart 1992). Sometimes clients also describe their symptoms in ways that impair communication. As an example, two women who had developed the same condition, *hyperopia* (farsightedness), went to their doctors for medical care (Zola 1973). In response to the practitioner's question, 'What seems to be the trouble?' one client simply said, 'I can't see to thread a needle or read the paper.' The other patient answered, 'I have a constant headache and my eyes seem to get all red and burny.' Each patient's manner or focus in describing her problem was different, and neither expanded the description with significant facts when asked if she had anything to add.

Why do patients describe their symptoms for the same health problem so differently? One reason may lie in the way they perceive or interpret different symptoms. As we saw earlier, people differ in the attention they pay to internal states and the degree to which they associate different sensations with health problems. Also, individuals form different commonsense models of illness. When reporting symptoms to a doctor, people may describe only or mainly those problems they think are important, based on their own notions (Bishop & Converse 1986). Last, clients may try either to emphasise or to downplay a symptom they believe may reflect a serious illness. For example, hypochondriacs may try to maximise the physician's attention to a sensation they are worried about, whereas other patients may describe a worrisome symptom very casually or offhandedly in the hope that the doctor will agree that 'it's nothing'.

Another communication problem can occur in medical situations when patients cannot describe their symptoms in terms the doctor can clearly understand. This often occurs when the person either is very young or lacks a good command of the doctor's primary language. Since World War II Australia has had large numbers of immigrants from many parts of the world who do not speak English well. Their English descriptions of their problems are likely to be inaccurate and incomplete. They are also unlikely to understand fully what their illnesses are or what they need to do to treat them.

Several things can be done to improve communication between patients and practitioners. Doctors' interviewing skills can be enhanced with training programs that teach how and when to summarise information, ask questions and check for comprehension (Roter & Hall 1989). Interaction is more than interviewing skills and giving advice. It is also about the ability of doctors to listen effectively and display empathy in communication. Some research has indicated that interventions aimed at training patients in communication skills has been effective in increasing information-seeking in patients, rephrasing to check comprehension of a medication regimen and information recall (McGee & Cegala 1998). Researchers have also found that a simple approach can improve clients' communication: While patients wait for their visits, have them fill out a form that has them list any questions they have and encourages them to ask questions when they see the doctor (Thompson, Nanni & Schwankovsky 1990). It may also be helpful for patients to fill out pain charts and symptom checklists, indicating the intensity of felt pain and symptoms.

One thing to keep in mind with respect to the way patient–practitioner relationships develop is that practitioners don't always get feedback regarding their work. For example, although a patient may visit the doctor again if symptoms persist or if the illness is serious or long term, doctors cannot be certain that *not* hearing from a person means a diagnosis was correct or the treatment was effective. And as we are about to see, practitioners usually cannot be sure to what extent a client is following the medical *regimen* — the treatment program or lifestyle change — they recommended.

Compliance: adhering to medical advice

'Now don't tell the doctor, but I don't always take my medicine when I'm supposed to,' Kylie whispered to a friend in her doctor's waiting room. People don't always *adhere to*, or *comply with*, their practitioner's advice. **Adherence** and **compliance** are terms that refer to the degree to which patients carry out the behaviours and treatments their practitioners recommend. Most researchers have used these terms interchangeably, and we will, too. But *adherence* is a more satisfactory term because the dictionary definition of the word *compliance* — 'giving in to a request or demand' or 'acquiescence' — suggests that the practitioner uses an authoritarian style and that the person obeys reluctantly (DiMatteo & DiNicola 1982; Turk & Meichenbaum 1991). The remainder of this chapter examines the extent to which clients fail to follow medical advice, why they do and do not comply, and what can be done to increase their adherence.

Extent of the non-adherence problem

How widespread is the problem of non-compliance? Answering this question is actually more difficult than it may seem (Cluss & Epstein 1985; Turk & Meichenbaum 1991). First of all, failures to adhere may occur for many different types of medical advice — for instance, patients may fail to take their medication as directed, not show up for recommended appointments, skip or stop doing rehabilitation exercises, or 'cheat a little' in following specific diet or other lifestyle changes advised by practitioners. Second, people can violate each of these types of advice in many different ways. In failing to take their medication as directed, for example, they might omit some doses, use a drug for the wrong reasons, take medication in the wrong amount or at the wrong time, or discontinue the drug before the prescribed course of therapy ends. Some conditions like diabetes require multiple disease management behaviours such as adherence to a specified diet and exercise, urine testing and insulin injections. The patient may comply with some regime behaviours but not others. Finally, there is the problem of determining whether a person has or has not complied. What is the most accurate and practical way to assess compliance?

Researchers assess patient adherence to medical recommendations in several different ways, and each way has advantages and disadvantages (Cluss & Epstein 1985; DiMatteo & DiNicola 1982; Ley 1988; Turk & Meichenbaum 1991). One of the easiest approaches for measuring compliance is to *ask a practitioner* who works with the client to estimate it. As it turns out, however, practitioners do not really know; they generally overestimate their patients' compliance and are poor at estimating which clients adhere better than others. Another simple approach is to *ask the patient*. But people tend to over-report their adherence, perhaps because they know they should 'follow the doctor's orders'. Some research (Steele, Jackson & Gutmann 1990) has found that when doctors used an 'information intensive' questioning style to ask about adherence to medication (i.e. patients are asked specific questions about when and how they took the medication, and any changes that had occurred), they were 80 per cent more successful in predicting actual adherence than if an indirect questioning style was used where it was assumed that the medication had been taken. Assessing adherence by asking either the doctor or the patient are very subjective methods and open to various forms of bias, including lying and wishful thinking. As a result, researchers who use these approaches today usually supplement them with reports of family members or medical personnel and with other methods that are more objective. Figure 9.4 describes three relatively objective approaches for assessing adherence to using medication.

Figure 9.4 Objective methods for assessing adherence to using medication

- *Pill or quantity accounting*, in which the remaining medication is measured, such as by counting the number of pills left. This is compared against the quantity that should be left at that point in treatment if the patient has been following the directions correctly. Of course, this method does not reveal whether the person used the medication at the right times, and patients who expect an accounting and want to conceal their non-compliance can discard some of the contents.
- *Medication-recording dispensers* contain mechanical or electromechanical recording devices that can count and record the time when the dispenser is used. Although this approach is expensive to implement, it assesses compliance accurately as long as the patient does not deliberately create a ruse. If patients know about the device and want to avoid taking the medicine, they can operate the dispenser at the right time and discard the drug.
- *Biochemical tests*, such as of the patient's blood or urine. This approach can assess whether medication was used recently, but usually cannot determine how much or when, and it can be very time-consuming and expensive to implement.

Despite the complexities in assessing adherence, we can provide some general answers to the question we started with: How widespread is the problem of non-compliance? Speaking in very broad terms, the average rate of non-compliance to medical advice is about 40 per cent — that is, *two of every five patients fail to adhere* reasonably closely to their regimens (DiMatteo 1985). Conversely, the overall rate of *adherence* is about 60 per cent. Adherence varies considerably, depending on the type of medical advice, the duration of the recommended regimen, and whether its purpose is to prevent an illness from occurring or to treat or cure an illness that has developed. An overview of the findings of research on compliance indicates the following conclusions (Cluss & Epstein 1985; Daltroy et al. 1991; McColl, Hart & Chung 1996).

- The average adherence rate for taking medicine to treat acute illnesses with short-term treatment regimens is about 78 per cent; for chronic illnesses with long-term regimens, the rate drops to about 54 per cent.
- The average adherence rate for taking medicine to prevent illness is roughly 60 per cent for both short-term and long-term regimens.
- Patients' adherence to scheduled appointments with a practitioner is much higher if the client initiated the appointment than if the practitioner did.
- Adherence to recommended changes in lifestyle, such as stopping smoking or altering one's diet, is generally quite variable and often very low.
- Patients are more likely to adhere to long-term medication if they understand the purpose of the treatment.

But keep in mind two things about these conclusions. First, the percentages given may *overestimate* compliance. This is because studies

> generally include in their sample only those patients who are willing to participate in a research project. It is reasonable to assume that this subgroup of volunteers may be different in motivational or other characteristics, making them more likely to comply as a group than others who are not willing to participate. (Cluss & Epstein 1985, p. 410)

Second, the rates we cited do not reflect the range of non-adherence by patients: some adhere exactly to a medical regimen, others do not comply at all, and probably most comply to some degree.

Why patients do and do not adhere to medical advice

We have seen that practitioners do not generally know how well their clients adhere to medical advice. What do physicians think when they learn their patients have not followed their advice? They are concerned about the effects of non-adherence on the person's health, of course, and they tend to place most of the 'blame' on the patients — their 'uncooperative' personalities, inability to understand the advice or difficult life situations (Levinson et al. 1993). But studies have shown that both the practitioners and their patients influence adherence (Dunbar-Jacob et al. 1998; Ley 1988; Myers & Midence 1998). Researchers have studied dozens of factors to determine their relationship to adherence. We'll begin with the role of characteristics of the regimen and illness.

Medical treatments and illness characteristics

The medical treatments practitioners advise can differ in many ways, such as in their complexity, duration, cost, side effects and the degree to which they require changes in the patient's habits. Let's see whether and how each of these factors relates to compliance.

Some treatments require clients to change *long-standing habits* — for example, to begin and maintain exercising regularly, reduce the calories or certain components in their diets, stop smoking cigarettes or cut down on drinking alcoholic beverages. We have seen in previous chapters that these changes can be very difficult for people to make. Recommendations by doctors can induce many patients to make changes in such habits, particularly if the individuals are at high risk for serious illness (Dolecek et al. 1986; Pederson 1982). But studies have consistently found that people are much less likely to adhere to medical advice for changes in personal habits than to advice for taking medication (Haynes 1976).

Some treatments are more *complex* than others — such as by requiring the person to take two or more drugs, each with its own special instructions: 'Take one of these pills after meals, and two of these other pills at bedtime, and one of these other pills every eight hours.' As you might expect, the greater the number of drugs and the more complex the medication schedule and dosage, the greater the likelihood the person will make an error, thereby failing to adhere to the regimen (Haynes 1976; Kirscht & Rosenstock 1979). Regimens also become difficult if they have the patient do a variety of complicated tasks — as, for example, individuals suffering from chronic *kidney disease* must do (Cameron 1986; Finn & Alcorn 1986; NKF 1990; Swigonski 1987). Many of these patients must:

- undergo *haemodialysis*, in which the blood is shunted from an artery to a filtering apparatus and returned to a vein. This procedure generally takes four to six hours three times a week, during which time the person may either sleep or engage in a sedentary activity, such as reading.
- take large quantities of medication and vitamins — sometimes involving dozens of pills a day — while also strictly limiting fluid intake.
- severely restrict their dietary intake of *sodium*, mainly salt; *potassium* and *phosphorus*, which are found in many fruits and vegetables; and *protein*, especially meats and dairy products.

In general, the more a client is required to do, and the greater the number of prescribed medications, the more likely compliance will suffer (Gilbert, Luszcz & Owen 1993).

The emotional state of the patient may interact with type of regimen to affect adherence. For example, in a study by Carney et al. (1998), patients with heart disease who had frequent angina were less likely to adhere to a daily regimen of aspirin than patients with asymptomatic heart disease who did not experience chest pain. Non-adherence in the angina patients was linked with higher levels of depression and feelings of helplessness. Those patients with asymptomatic heart disease were less depressed because they were less aware of somatic sensations, and adhered more. Other research has found that compliance in heart transplantation patients depends on psychological distress immediately after the surgery (Dew 1994).

Many people believe the duration, expense and side effects of a medical treatment are major factors in whether people adhere to their practitioner's advice. Studies have confirmed the role of *duration* — compliance tends to decline over time (Parrish 1986; Varni & Babani 1986). Short-term treatments are usually prescribed for acute illnesses and show beneficial effects fairly quickly and dramatically, but long-term regimens usually apply to chronic health problems and have slower and less obvious beneficial effects. Do the *expense* and *side effects* of treatment also affect adherence? The evidence regarding these factors is not very consistent (DiMatteo & DiNicola 1982; Haynes 1976). Some studies have found that the expense and side effects of treatment seem to distinguish between patients who comply and those who do not, but other studies have not confirmed these findings. It may be that the sick-role behaviours of most people are not strongly affected by these factors — for these individuals, the treatment expense may not prevent them from adhering because they have sufficient incomes to pay for medication, or they have insurance to cover the costs of care, or they feel the benefits of the treatment are essential despite the cost. Similarly, most drugs do not have noticeable or worrisome side effects. But what happens, for instance, when individuals cannot afford their medicine, or its side effects do become a problem? Some patients may reduce the dosage of the drug or discontinue using it entirely. The expense and side effects of treatment can impair adherence for some individuals.

Many people also think patients who have health problems that could disable them or threaten their lives are more likely to adhere to their treatment regimens than individuals who have less serious illnesses. But whether this idea is correct seems to depend on whose perspective of the severity of the health problem we consider — the patient's or the practitioner's. When illness severity is judged by *doctors*, clients with serious illnesses are no more likely to adhere than those with milder health problems (Becker & Rosenstock 1984; Haynes 1976). Perhaps this is because many very serious health problems, such as hypertension and atherosclerosis, have no symptoms that worry people greatly or interfere with their functioning; on the other hand, many less serious illnesses do have such symptoms. In contrast, when illness severity is judged by *patients* who have the health problem, adherence increases with severity. Those clients who perceive their illness as relatively serious generally show better adherence to their treatment regimens than those who perceive their illness to be less severe (Becker & Rosenstock 1984).

Age, gender and sociocultural factors

Most early studies of adherence found little or no association between compliance in general and clients' specific personal and demographic characteristics, such as their age, gender, social class, race and religion (Haynes 1976). This lack of a relationship between sociodemographic patient characteristics and medication adherence was confirmed in the more recent Medical Outcomes Study, which examined long-term adherence for more than 8000 patients (Stewart & Ware 1992). Does this mean these factors are never linked to compliance? Probably not. For one thing, although each of these factors is not *by itself* strongly related to adherence, when they are *joined* — for example gender plus age plus social class — their combination shows a stronger association to compliance (Korsch, Fine & Negrete 1978). What's more, some of these factors may be related to adherence in some circumstances but not others.

Consider the factor of *age*, which seems to affect adherence in different ways, depending on the ages of the subjects and types of illness.

- For childhood cancer patients, problems in adherence to specific care procedures, such as using antibiotics correctly, were greater for younger than for older children (Manne et al. 1993). Although these procedures were mainly controlled by the parents, the child's age made a difference.
- Among child and adolescent diabetics, adolescents showed less adherence to their special diets than children did (Johnson et al. 1992).
- For 35- to 84-year-old hypertensive individuals, adherence to taking medications was poorest for those over 75 and highest for 65- to 74-year-olds, with other ages falling in between (Morrell et al. 1995).
- Elderly Australian women (aged 83 years and over) who had been hospitalised after fracture, joint replacement or falls were unlikely to comply with wearing an external hip protector because of the effort involved, appearance, cost and unfamiliarity with the protectors (Cameron & Quine 1994).

Children become increasingly responsible for their own medical treatment as they get older (La Greca & Stone 1985). Adolescents may be less likely than individuals from other age groups to comply with long-term treatments that single them out or make them different from peers. Medical adherence in the elderly can be affected by a number of factors. The elderly are more likely to suffer from a number of chronic conditions that require complex management procedures for which they may have little understanding. Hearing and eyesight problems may cause them to misunderstand the doctor's instructions. The elderly may underuse or stop using medication that causes unpleasant side effects such as dizziness, drowsiness or constipation. Emotional problems such as depression may lead to non-adherence in the elderly. The packaging of some medications involving blister packs or safety seals may make adherence difficult for those with manual dexterity problems. Adherence may also be hindered if the elderly person does not have a supportive network of family or friends (McElnay & McCallion 1998; Murdaugh 1998).

The effects of gender on adherence may depend on specific circumstances, and aspects of treatment. For instance, girls adhere more to diet and urine testing in diabetes management (Harkavy et al. 1983; Lorenz, Christensen & Pichert 1985), while boys are more compliant on exercising and injection regularity (Johnson et al. 1990). Women's concerns about controlling their weight appear to interfere with their using medication to control their blood sugar (Polonsky et al. 1994).

Sociocultural influences can also determine adherence. For instance, occupational status has been found to predict non-adherence with an exercise program for cardiac rehabilitation patients (Tooth, McKenna & Colquhoun 1993). Blue-collar workers were less likely to comply with a home-based walking program and held less positive expectations regarding the benefits of exercise. Non-adherence may have been influenced by beliefs, associated with blue-collar work, that physical labour is sufficient activity for rehabilitation. Some cultural groups may have beliefs or customs that undermine adherence. Indigenous people have a high incidence of heart disease, diabetes and alcohol abuse. Yet implementing lifestyle behaviour changes can be problematic when working with indigenous people who value personal autonomy and subscribe to a pervasive belief in the right of others to conduct themselves as they wish. There are strong disincentives to interfere in other peoples' business' (Brady 1995, p. 1491).

Psychosocial aspects of the patient

The seriousness of an illness and the costs of its treatment can affect compliance, depending on the point of view of the patient. Perceived seriousness and perceived costs and benefits are two psychosocial factors that should have a familiar ring by now — we have examined them before as components in the *health belief model*. The components of the health belief model are just as important in explaining why people do and do not adhere to medical advice as they are in explaining other health-related behaviours, such as whether people are likely to adopt health behaviours or use health services (Becker 1979; Becker & Rosenstock 1984; Rosenstock & Kirscht 1979). Thus, a patient who feels threatened by an illness and believes the benefits of the recommended regimen outweigh the barriers is likely to adhere to his or her practitioner's advice. But individuals who do not feel threatened by the health problem or assess that the barriers of the regimen outweigh the benefits are unlikely to comply.

Patients who hold negative beliefs about their prescribed medication, such as that dependence is dangerous, or that there may be side effects, are less likely to comply with medical recommendations (Horne and Weinman 1999). Adherence may be improved when patients discuss medical beliefs with practitioners. For example, practitioners who have explored barriers to cervical cancer screening during consultations with at-risk women, have been successful in getting these women to consent to a Pap smear (Ward et al. 1991). But whether compliance is higher for preventive diagnostic screening than for treatment regimens requires further study.

Earlier we saw that individuals develop commonsense models of illness. These cognitive representations of illness can be either correct or incorrect. Lay notions of illness can affect medical adherence. For example, behavioural management of non-insulin-dependent diabetes through diet has been found to be better for patients whose illness models implicated former dietary practices and being overweight in the development of their current medical condition (Schoenberg, Amey & Coward 1998).

Some researchers have pointed out that noncompliance is often *deliberate* and based on *valid reasons*, regardless of whether the reasons are medically sound (Horne 1998; Kaplan & Simon 1990; Turk & Meichenbaum 1991). This is called **rational non-adherence**. How can non-adherence to medical advice be rational? Patients may be acting rationally when they fail to take medication as directed because they:
- have reason to believe the medication isn't helping
- feel that its side effects are very unpleasant, worrisome or seriously reducing the quality of their lives
- are confused about when to take it, or how much
- don't have the money to buy the next refill
- want to 'see if the illness is still there' when they withdraw the medication.

These are not unreasonable reasons — and sometimes the clients may be medically correct in not adhering, such as when they experience serious or unexpected side effects. A study of arthritis patients found that most instances of non-adherence were for unintentional reasons, such as forgetting; the most common *intentional* reasons for not taking medication were the side effects and the cost (Lorish, Richards & Brown 1989).

Patients' adherence to medical advice is often affected by cognitive and emotional factors operating at the time they receive the recommendations. Patients generally forget much of what the doctor tells them (Ley 1988, 1989). Instructions and advice are more likely to be forgotten than is other information. Those patients with greater medical knowledge recall more information, although more intelligent patients do not remember more than less intelligent patients. Information is more likely to be remembered when it is presented early in the consultation, if the information is perceived by the patient as important, and the number of statements to be recalled is small. Patients often interpret information in terms of their model of illness. For example, if a patient with high blood pressure has a belief that hypertension can be cured with a short course of treatment, long-term compliance is unlikely to occur. Anxious patients tend to recall more information than those less anxious, and older patients remember just as much as younger patients. For people to comply with a treatment regimen, they must be cognitively and emotionally able to understand and remember what they are to do. The directions they receive are often complex and given at a time when they may not be listening as carefully as they should. Even when health information is given in writing, most adult patients may not understand it if it is written much above the fifth grade reading level (Estey, Musseau & Keehn 1994).

Personal beliefs and expectancies of patients also affect adherence to medical advice in the management of chronic conditions. One cognitive factor that appears to determine treatment adherence is self-efficacy, or the patient's belief in his or her ability to maintain behaviour change. In a study by Kavanaugh, Gooley and Wilson (1993) self-efficacy expectations of diabetic adults were found to predict adherence to diabetes management involving exercise and dieting regimens, even after controlling for the effects of glycaemic control and type of diabetes. Blood glucose levels at post-test confirmed adherence to the diabetes management plan. Other research (Florian & Elad 1998) has shown that mothers' sense of empowerment, which has parallels with the concept of self-efficacy, can contribute to better metabolic control in adolescent children with insulin-dependent diabetes.

Personality traits of patients do not appear to be linked to medical adherence (Bosley, Fosbury & Cochrane 1995; Dunbar-Jacob et al. 1998), although there is some evidence that psychological states such as anxiety, depression and optimism may determine certain types of adherence. Hypertensive patients with high anxiety have been reported to adhere less to medication than those low on anxiety (Nelson et al. 1978). Exercise adherence for older adults is greater for those who are less anxious (Emery, Hauck & Blumenthal 1992). Mixed results have been found for depression and adherence. Some studies have reported greater adherence for depressed persons (Heiby, Onorato & Sato 1985), while others have reported less adherence (Graveley & Oseasohn 1991). Dispositional optimism has been linked to compliance with medical follow-up recommendations (Friedman et al. 1995).

One psychosocial factor that is associated with adherence is *social support*. Generally speaking, people who feel they receive the comfort, caring and help they need from other individuals or groups are more likely to follow medical advice than clients who have less social support (DiMatteo & DiNicola 1982). This support can come from the patient's family, friends or support groups, such as the many organisations to help people deal with specific illnesses. The support patients receive seems to be most beneficial to regimen adherence when it specifically involves help and encouragement in caring for the health problem (Carmody et al. 1982; Stanton 1987). But social relationships can sometimes lead to non-compliance. Mary Swigonski (1987) studied kidney disease patients whose complex treatment regimen included restricting fluid intake and found that the more social support the individuals had, the greater the likelihood of non-adherence for fluids. As she pointed out, social gatherings often occur with food and beverages present — in meetings for lunch, dinner, drinks or just a cup of coffee, for instance. Engaging in many social activities like these makes it difficult for patients to restrict their fluid consumption.

Patient–practitioner interactions

The word 'doctor' comes from the Latin *docere*, which means 'to teach'. Two features of good teaching involve explaining information in a clear and organised fashion, and assessing whether the learner has learned or understands. Some medical practitioners are good teachers; others are not. Doctors do not always make sure the patient understands what they have said. Successful communication in patient–practitioner interactions is essential if the client is to adhere to the advice (Noble 1998).

Communicating with patients

If your doctor told you to 'take two tablets twice a day', would you take four tablets during the day, two in the morning and two at night, or only one in the morning and one at night? Or what if your doctor told you to 'take one tablet every six hours'? Does that mean you should wake up in the middle of each night to take one? Or would it be okay simply to take four tablets a day, equally spaced during your waking hours? Would you ask? Sometimes the information people get from practitioners is not very clear. You might argue that the advice *was* clear: every six hours, on the dot. But practitioners need to anticipate unspoken questions — saying, for instance, 'You'll need to wake up to take one because the infection may recur if the medicine wears off.' If practitioners don't do this, patients usually answer these questions for themselves, often incorrectly.

Many people leave their doctors' offices not knowing how to follow their treatment regimens. Bonnie Svarstad (1976) reported the results of research in which she interviewed patients at a community health centre and checked their medication containers after they visited their doctors. She also recorded the verbal interactions between the doctors and their clients. The results of this research demonstrated four things. First, the patients' knowledge about their treatment was seriously deficient — for example, half of the clients did not know how long they should continue taking their medication, and about one-fifth of them did not know the purpose of or how often to take the prescribed drugs. Second, an important reason for the patients' poor knowledge was that the doctors often did not provide the needed information. For most of the prescriptions, for example, the doctors failed to give explicit instructions on how regularly or how often to use the medication. For that matter, some of the drugs were never discussed at all during the visit. Third, the clients asked very few questions during the visits. Fourth, the more explicit the doctors' directions, the more the people complied, which Svarstad measured by pill counts at the patients' homes about a week later.

Other research has indicated that doctor–patient communication may contribute to failure to return for follow-up consultations as well as diminished understanding of health status. In a study by McColl, Hart & Chung (1996) about one in five clients who were treated at an Adelaide sexually transmitted disease (STD) clinic did not realise that they needed to return to the clinic to obtain test results, did not know which infection they had been treated for and assumed that they had been cleared for an STD because they had not heard from the clinic. It appears that the lack of clarity in communication is no less common in the area of notification of Pap test results (Schofield et al. 1994). If abnormal results are not adequately communicated to women, adherence with follow-up recommendations is unlikely.

A person's adherence to medical advice depends on the practitioner's communicating information. Good communication takes time and is much more likely to occur when the practitioner's style is more patient-centred than doctor-centred.

Adherence and the patient–practitioner relationship

As we have seen, people generally prefer medical care that involves a patient-centred style. Research has shown that individuals who have good relationships with their physicians are more satisfied with their medical care, and are more likely to adhere to the medical advice they receive (Ley 1988; Wensing, Grol & Smits 1994; Winefield, Murrell & Clifford 1995).

Barbara Korsch and her colleagues have examined the link between patients' satisfaction with medical care and compliance (Francis, Korsch & Morris 1969; Freemon et al. 1971; Korsch, Gozzi & Francis 1968). The research methodology involved tape-recording several hundred paediatric consultations at a walk-in clinic and then interviewing the mothers immediately after they left the doctor's office. Although most of the mothers reported being at least moderately satisfied with the visits, nearly one-fifth of the mothers said they did not receive clear statements of what was wrong with their children, and about half did not know what caused the illnesses. The most common complaint of the mothers was that the doctor did not seem to respond warmly or sympathetically to their anxiety about their children. One mother, for instance, felt the doctor did not pay attention to her concern that the convulsions her child experienced might damage his brain.

This research also assessed whether compliance was related to the mothers' satisfaction with their visits. A week or two after the medical consultation, the researchers visited the mothers to determine their adherence to the recommended regimens. This assessment was done through the mothers' reports and, when possible, through pill counts or contacts with the pharmacy. The results revealed that those mothers who were very satisfied with the physician's warmth, concern and communication of information were three times more likely to adhere closely to the regimens than those who were dissatisfied. It may be that doctors who succeed in fostering compliance are those who use patient-centred styles.

To summarise, the reasons why patients do and do not adhere to medical advice include some factors that are associated mainly with the clients, some with the practitioners and some with the way these people interrelate. While reading this material, you may have thought, 'Couldn't many of the circumstances that lead to non-adherence be changed to enhance compliance?' The next section examines this question.

Increasing patient adherence

Implicit in our interest in enhancing adherence is the assumption that doing so is important — that it would benefit the person's health. How important is adherence to the patient's health? If it is very important, should health care workers aim for each client to comply perfectly to his or her regimen, or would a lesser degree of adherence be acceptable? We will address these questions briefly before considering ways to increase compliance.

Non-adherence and health outcomes

By not adhering to regimens recommended by their physicians, people increase their risk of developing health problems they don't already have or of prolonging or worsening their current illnesses. Estimates suggest that 20 per cent of hospital admissions probably result from patients' non-adherence to medication regimens (Ley 1982). A study found that heart attack patients who adhered poorly to taking prescribed medication were nearly three times more likely to die in the next year than those who adhered fairly closely (Gallagher, Viscoli & Horwitz 1993).

But failing to follow a practitioner's orders exactly is not always detrimental to the client's health. One reason is that some treatments are harmful and have side effects that produce iatrogenic conditions. Patients should notify their physicians when a treatment causes problems. Another reason is that doctors sometimes prescribe unnecessary drugs or other procedures with non-medical goals in mind, such as to avoid risking malpractice suits. Of course, in the great majority of cases, the doctor's recommendations are correct and are in the client's best interests. Yet even when medically sound advice is given, some people who follow their doctors' orders closely show little benefit from the treatment, whereas other individuals who are much less compliant show substantial improvements in their health (Cluss & Epstein 1985; Hayes et al. 1994).

The importance of following medical advice closely seems to depend on the particular health problem and the treatment prescribed. For hypertensive patients, for instance, consuming 80 per cent of the medication prescribed to reduce their blood pressure is probably the minimum level of compliance needed to treat hypertension effectively. For other health problems, however, 'an 80 per cent rate of compliance may be unnecessary' (Epstein & Cluss 1982, p. 952). And so, following the usual regimen of penicillin for treating rheumatic fever at only a 50 per cent rate may be sufficiently effective. Unhealthy non-compliance might therefore be defined as 'the point below which the desired preventive or therapeutic result is unlikely to be achieved with the medication prescribed' (Parrish 1986, p. 456). Unfortunately, however, compliance cutoff points still need to be established for individual illnesses and treatments.

Although more research is needed to determine compliance cutoff points, two things should be clear. First, *perfect* adherence may not be necessary in many cases. Second, the current adherence levels of clients are very far from perfect and need to be improved.

Methods for enhancing compliance

Probably most physicians in the past who have dealt with the compliance problem at all did so after the fact. Rather than trying to prevent non-compliance, they tried to correct it if and when they learned about it. How did they try to correct it? A study examined this question and found that the first step doctors used when a patient failed to adhere was to give a 'thorough explanation of the regimen and repeat it so that the patient understands' (Davis 1966). As we have seen, explaining the regimen and making sure the person understands can prevent non-compliance in the first place.

Getting practitioners to improve their *style of communicating* with patients is not necessarily difficult to accomplish. In one study, for instance, researchers designed a brief program to instruct doctors about the kinds of reasons hypertensive people have for not adhering to their regimens and about ways to detect and improve low compliance (Inui, Yourtee & Williamson 1976). About half of the doctors at a hospital clinic received the instructional program, and the remainder served as controls. Compared with the control doctors, the physicians who received the program subsequently spent more time giving information during patient visits — and, more importantly, their clients showed more knowledge about their regimens and illnesses, greater adherence in taking medications and better blood pressure control. Often such changes in doctor behaviour last indefinitely (Roter & Hall 1989).

Because patients often misunderstand or forget medical recommendations, practitioners are also learning specific *techniques for presenting medical information*. Several methods are particularly effective (Ley 1982; Myers & Midence 1998; Parrish 1986; Rosenstock 1985). These methods include:

- simplifying verbal instructions by using clear and straightforward language and sentences
- using specific and concrete statements — such as, 'You should walk one kilometre a day for the first week, and two kilometres after that,' instead of, 'You should get daily exercise.'
- breaking down a complicated or long-term regimen into smaller segments. The patient might begin the regimen by doing only part of it and then adding to it later; or the regimen might involve a series of smaller goals that the client believes he or she can achieve

- emphasising key information by stating why it is important and offering it early in the presentation
- using simple, written instructions
- having the patient repeat instructions or state them in his or her own words.

These techniques appear to be more effective in improving compliance with short-term regimens than with long-term regimens (Haynes 1982).

Another approach that appears to promote adherence at least for short-term regimens is to have the person state explicitly that he or she will comply. An experiment by James Kulik and Patricia Carlino (1987) demonstrated this in a paediatric setting with the parents of children who were suffering from acute infections. The researchers randomly assigned the subjects to two groups. Parents in the experimental group were simply asked by the doctor, 'Will you promise me you'll give all the doses?' and all agreed; parents in the control condition were not asked for this commitment. When the patients returned for a follow-up visit about 10 days later, their recovery was medically evaluated and compliance was assessed both by interviewing the parents and by analysing the children's urine. Compared with the control group, those in the experimental condition showed higher compliance rates and greater recovery from their illnesses.

Social and motivational forces in a patient's life can have important effects on adherence, particularly when the regimen is long term or requires lifestyle changes. One approach that makes use of social and motivational factors is for the practitioner or client to recruit constructive sources of *social support* (Jenkins 1979; Peck & King 1985; Rosenstock 1985). Family and friends who are committed to the regimen can promote compliance by having positive attitudes about the treatment activities and making sure they occur. Individuals who receive encouragement, praise, reminders, and assistance in carrying out the regimen are more likely to comply than those who do not. Effective social support can also come from self-help groups, patient groups and organisations established to help with specific health problems. These groups can give information and assistance, provide a sense of comfort and belongingness, and bolster the person's sense of esteem. Practitioners can help patients make contact with appropriate groups.

Several *behavioural methods* are also effective in enhancing patients' motivation to adhere to their treatment regimens (DiMatteo & DiNicola 1982; Epstein & Cluss 1982; Haynes 1982; Jenkins 1979). These methods include:
- *tailoring the regimen*, in which activities in the treatment are designed to be compatible with the patient's habits and rituals. For example, taking a pill at home at breakfast or while preparing for bed is easier to do and remember for most people than taking it in the middle of the day.
- *providing prompts and reminders*, which serve as cues to perform recommended activities. These cues can include reminder phone calls for appointments or notes posted at home that remind the client to exercise. Innovative drug packaging can also help — for instance, some drugs today come in dispensers with dated compartments or built-in reminder alarms.
- *self-monitoring*, in which the patient keeps a written record of regimen activities, such as the foods eaten each day
- *behavioural contracting*, whereby the practitioner and client negotiate a series of treatment activities and goals in writing and specify rewards the patient will receive for succeeding.

A major advantage of these methods is that the client can become actively involved in their design and execution (Turk & Meichenbaum 1991). Furthermore, the patient can carry them out alone or with the aid of the practitioner, family or friends.

The procedures we have examined for increasing patient compliance often involve the practitioner in much more constructive interactions with the person than just giving brief instructions. Although some of these methods are easy to incorporate into existing ways of interacting with clients, others are complicated and time-consuming to arrange and involve skills that are outside the expertise of most medical workers. When people have treatment regimens that are difficult for them to adhere to, the skills of health care workers who are trained in psychological principles may be needed to enhance the patients' treatment compliance and, thereby, their health.

Summary

Health care systems for the delivery and management of medical care are complex, involving professionals with a wide variety of specialised functions who provide in-patient and office-based treatment. In-patient treatment for people with serious illnesses occurs in hospitals; nursing homes provide care primarily for elderly individuals who need long-term medical and personal care. Australia has a mixed health care system funded by the public and private sectors. Not all countries have health care systems that provide insurance for their citizens. Australia is fortunate to have a national insurance scheme that provides universal access to medical care. Unlike Australia, the United States has managed care alternatives such as health maintenance organisations and preferred provider organisations. These two office-based treatment approaches appear to provide similar types and quality of service and were devised as cost-cutting alternatives. Casemix, a type of managed care, was adopted in Australia to curtail hospital costs. It works on diseases being classified into diagnostic related groups, the cure of which is costed.

People decide they are sick and in need of medical attention mainly on the basis of the symptoms they perceive. The point at which people notice a symptom differs from one individual to the next and within the same person from one time to another. Some people seem to pay closer attention to their internal states than others and are, therefore, more likely to notice changes in physical sensations and to perceive these sensations as symptoms. People are less likely to notice internal sensations when the environment contains a great deal of sensory information or is very exciting than when it has few external stimuli to compete for their attention. Because people generally do not assess their internal states very accurately, psychosocial factors can have a strong influence on the perception of symptoms and may produce two interesting phenomena: medical student's disease and mass psychogenic illness. People's health-related behaviours are influenced by commonsense models they develop of different illnesses. A commonsense model consists of information about the illness identity and its causes and underlying pathology, time line and consequences.

Many factors affect how individuals interpret and respond to the symptoms they perceive. The knowledge people extract from their experience with symptoms generally helps them to make appropriate decisions about seeking medical attention. Sometimes people's prior experiences and their emotions, such as intense fear or anxiety, can lead them to interpret their symptoms incorrectly and delay seeking care. Before individuals decide to seek medical attention, they typically get advice from their lay referral system, which consists of relatives, friends and co-workers.

Certain demographic characteristics are associated with the use of health services. Young children and the elderly use health services more than adolescents and young adults do, and women use more medical drugs and have higher rates of illness from acute and non-fatal chronic illnesses than men do. When economically disadvantaged Australians are sick, they are less likely to contact private doctors at their offices and more likely to use medical providers who bulk-bill and hospital emergency services, probably because they do not have a regular doctor. This class difference is especially troubling because individuals from the lower classes have higher rates of health problems and poorer health habits than those from higher classes.

People's health beliefs and ideas about iatrogenic conditions may affect whether they decide to seek medical care. Treatment delay appears to involve three stages — appraisal delay, illness delay and utilisation delay — each of which is affected by different factors. Many individuals wait several months before seeking attention for symptoms of serious illnesses, such as cancer. In contrast, some people overuse health services. Hypochondriasis involves the tendency for a person to interpret real but benign bodily sensations as symptoms of illness despite reassurances by a doctor that they are harmless. Studies have shown that hypochondriasis is linked to emotional maladjustment, but it is not more common in old age than at other ages.

People generally express high levels of satisfaction with the care they receive from doctors who communicate with a patient-centred rather than a doctor-centred style. There is some indication that satisfaction with the consultation may depend on personality characteristics of patients, along with congruence between doctors and patients in preferences for communication. Patient-centred doctors tend to ask open-ended questions, avoid using medical jargon or technical terms, and allow clients to participate in some of the decision making regarding the treatment of their illness. These doctors are also likely to project feelings of concern and reassurance and to give clear explanations about illnesses and treatments. Of course, patients vary in their behaviours and styles, too, and may impair communication with their doctors because of the manners or focuses they use in describing their symptoms.

Patient compliance with or adherence to medical advice varies greatly, and non-compliance is very common. About two of every five clients fail to adhere reasonably closely to the medical regimens their doctors prescribe. Individuals tend to be less compliant for long-term regimens to treat chronic diseases than for short-term regimens to treat acute illnesses, and they are particularly unlikely to comply with recommendations to change long-standing habits. Also, the more complicated the regimen, the more likely adherence will suffer. Adherence is affected by various psychosocial factors, including rational non-adherence decisions and the patient's health beliefs, social support, and cognitive and emotional conditions when receiving medical advice. Many people leave their physicians' offices not knowing how to follow the prescribed regimens. Patients tend to adhere closely to their regimens when their practitioners are warm and caring, give them opportunities to talk, and explain their illnesses and treatments clearly. A variety of behavioural and communication-enhancing methods can help to improve people's adherence to medical advice.

Key terms

adherence	compliance	iatrogenic conditions	rational non-adherence
casemix	doctor-centred	lay referral system	treatment delay
commonsense models	hypochondriasis	patient-centred	

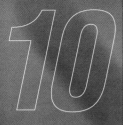

10

In the hospital: the setting, procedures and effects on patients

Prologue

'I had a fast-growing conviction that a hospital was no place for a person who was seriously ill,' a patient once wrote. This patient developed and recovered from a typically incurable and fatal crippling disease. The symptoms he experienced began with a fever and general achiness — the kinds of sensations we usually associate with minor illnesses. Within a week, however, his condition worsened, and he began to have difficulty moving his neck, legs, arms and hands. He was soon hospitalised for the diagnostic tests that pinpointed his disease.

What experiences led to this patient's negative view of hospitals? He described one example.

> I was astounded when four technicians from four different departments took four separate and substantial blood samples on the same day. That the hospital didn't take the trouble to coordinate the tests, using one blood specimen, seemed to me inexplicable and irresponsible. When the technicians came the second day to fill their containers with blood for processing in separate laboratories, I turned them away and had a sign posted on my door saying that I would give just one specimen every three days and that I expected the different departments to draw from it for their individual needs. (Cousins 1985, pp. 55–6)

He also criticised other hospital practices, such as waking patients from sleep to carry out regular routines. In his view, sleep in the hospital is an 'uncommon blessing' that should not be interrupted casually.

Few people enjoy being hospitalised, even under the best of circumstances. Although many people probably have more positive feelings about their hospital experiences than this patient had, some have even worse impressions. We have all heard stories of mistakes being made or other situations that produced more serious health problems than those with which the patient was admitted to the hospital. This chapter focuses on the experience of being hospitalised. First we examine the hospital — its history, setting and procedures — as well as the roles and points of view of the hospital staff. Then we consider what being hospitalised is like from the perspective of patients, and what can be done to assess and provide help for their psychological needs. As we study these topics, we will consider important questions that are of great concern to patients, their families and practitioners. For instance, hospital personnel have difficult jobs — what impact does this have on them? How do people adjust to being hospitalised? What special needs do children have as patients, and how can hospitals and parents help? How can practitioners reduce the stress individuals experience with unpleasant, painful and surgical procedures?

The hospital — its history, setting and procedures

Hospitals in industrialised countries around the world are typically large institutions with separate wards or buildings for different kinds of health problems and treatment procedures. These institutions have changed in their long history, and so have people's attitudes about them. People in Australia today are more likely than people years ago to view hospitals as places to go to get well rather than to die, even though most are in hospitals when they die. Let's see how hospitals began and evolved.

How the hospital evolved

Special places to care for the ill did not always exist. One of the earliest examples of this approach can be seen in the ancient Greeks' establishment of temples where sick people would pray and receive cures or advice from the god Aesculapius (Anderson &

Gevitz 1983). But the idea of having special facilities to house and treat the sick probably began with the Roman military, who established separate barracks for their ill and disabled soldiers.

The first institutions established to care for the sick were associated with Christian monasteries and had a broad charitable purpose — that of helping the less fortunate members of society. As a result, these facilities housed not only sick people, but also orphans, the poor and even travellers who needed lodging. One of the earliest of these hospitals, the Hôtel-Dieu of Lyons in present-day France, was established in A.D. 542 (Anderson & Gevitz 1983). The charitable purposes of hospitals in Western Europe continued with little change until the eighteenth and nineteenth centuries, when these institutions became more specialised in two ways.

> First, the conventional approach of lumping all types of dependents into the same facility was gradually discarded as hospitals became repositories for the poor sick. Not all of the medically incapacitated were admitted, though — only the 'worthy poor,' i.e., those lower class individuals adjudged by administrators and sponsors to be potentially useful citizens capable of making a contribution to the commonweal. Others, namely the aged, the very young, the physically handicapped, and the mentally deficient ... were confined to abysmally kept poorhouses, irrespective of whether they were in need of medical attention. The second change was that hospitals became more medically specialised. Wards were established for different illness categories. ... By keeping patients with the same or seemingly related ailments together, one could readily make far more detailed comparisons and thus advance learning. (Anderson & Gevitz 1983, p. 307)

Similar approaches to those used in Britain were used for the care of the sick in the penal colony of New South Wales. A hospital was erected when the colony was established in 1788 (*Australian Encyclopaedia* 1996). In 1796 a new general hospital was built for prisoners, Crown employees, servants and free settlers. This hospital was replaced in 1816 by a larger establishment and came to be known as the 'rum hospital', because the contractors received a three-year monopoly over the importation of rum into the colony. The Sydney Infirmary, a voluntary hospital, was established within the General Hospital in the 1840s and later changed its name to the 'Sydney Hospital' (Cumpston 1989).

Up until the final transportation of convicts, hospitals were associated with filth, disease and immorality since they were places where medical care was administered mostly to convicts. Sick people from well-to-do families were treated within their own homes. It was not until the sanitary reform of the 1860s that Australian public hospitals became associated with middle-class respectability as places for the administering of medical and nursing care (Bashford 1994). Private acute hospitals in Australia date back to the 1840s. Such hospitals were funded by public donations and were established for upper-class people who did not wish to be treated in public hospitals where the facilities and medical care were for the most part rudimentary. The Australian armed forces have maintained their own system of medical and hospital establishments since the first military hospital of 1797 (*Australian Encyclopaedia* 1996).

Australian hospitals in the early twentieth century gained a much more positive reputation and attracted patients from all social classes. In 1997–98 about 5.5 million people were admitted to the nation's hospitals (AIHW 2000). Sixty-seven per cent of these admissions (3 747 532 persons) were to public acute hospitals, 32 per cent (1 792 976 persons) to private acute hospitals and 0.4 per cent (22 566 persons) to public psychiatric hospitals (AIHW 2000). Of the admissions for 1997–98 about 2.5 million were day-only admissions, usually for diagnostic procedures (AIHW 2000). When psychiatric hospitals are excluded, the average length of stay for non-same-day patients was 3.8 days across public and private hospitals. More of the patients admitted to public hospitals were children aged under five years. Across private and public hospitals, patients were admitted mostly for diseases of the digestive system, childbirth and complications of pregnancy, diseases of the circulatory system, asthma, injury and poisoning, or cancer. In 1998 there were 734 public acute hospitals, 317 private acute hospitals, and 24 public psychiatric hospitals in Australia (AIHW 1999a). Other private facilities included 175 private free-standing day hospital centres (AIHW 2000). Repatriation General Hospitals, which offer care to veterans and their dependants, have been integrated into the public hospital system in most States or have become privatised. Over the past decade, public hospital beds have declined from 4.1 to 2.8 per 1000 persons, while private hospital beds have remained constant at around 1.3 beds per 1000 (AIHW 1999d; AIHW 2000).

Hospitals today involve a wider variety of functions than ever before. They provide services to in-patients and out-patients to cure disease and repair injury, prevent illness, conduct diagnostic tests, and aid people's rehabilitation and life situations after being discharged. They are also involved in conducting research and teaching current and future medical personnel. To carry out these complex and varied functions, hospitals require organised hierarchies of personnel with specific roles and lines of authority, as we are about to see.

The organisation and functioning of hospitals

The Australian public hospital structure usually begins with an honorary board of directors or management committee that has responsibility for the governance and management of the hospital. This involves determining the hospital's objectives and how best to meet them, managing finances and appointing executives. In hospitals where there is no such board, the central hospital authority, usually a Health Department, assumes managerial functions. With the recent restructuring of the public hospital system, Area Health Boards have assumed responsibility for both community health services and public hospital services within a designated geographical area. For example, in Queensland, boards that were responsible for groups of hospitals within a district were replaced with Regional Health Authorities concerned with integration of health services, strategic planning and policy development (*Australian Encyclopaedia* 1996; Grant 1985).

At the next level of organisational structure within the hospital is the chief executive officer (CEO), sometimes referred to as the Manager or Hospital Secretary, who is directly answerable to the board. The CEO, who may not have a medical qualification, is in charge of hospital staff involved in the various functions of hospital care — provision of medical services, nursing patients and business/hotel services. In larger hospitals the top level of management may include a team composed of the CEO, the Director of Medical Services (or Medical Superintendent), the Director of Nursing and a Director of Administrative Services. In psychiatric hospitals, the CEO is usually a psychiatrist and is designated as the medical superintendent. The hospital administrators are mainly in charge of the day-to-day business of the institution, such as in purchasing equipment and supplies, keeping records and accounts, and providing food and maintenance services. These functions often affect the medical care patients receive (*Australian Encyclopaedia* 1996; Grant 1985).

The medical staff are responsible for patient care and therefore have the most direct impact on the health of the patients. Many of these attending physicians are employed in private practice and are paid by the hospital in a fee-for-service arrangement. Some of the larger hospitals have salaried medical staff such as interns, residents, registrars, staff specialists, and heads of radiology and pathology. Teaching hospitals typically offer conjoint appointments where the doctor is both a specialist within the hospital and a member of the teaching staff in the university medical school (*Australian Encyclopaedia* 1996; Grant 1985).

Nurses form the next rung in the hierarchy of medical staff in hospitals. Although many physicians think of nurses as their assistants, nurses are actually salaried employees of the hospitals who have two functions: caring for patients and managing the wards (Aiken 1983). Because the former function is medical and the latter is administrative, nurses may receive directives from physicians and administrators. Sometimes the orders nurses receive from these two sources are incompatible and cause conflict, such as when a physician orders an action that the administration has banned as a cost-cutting measure. Whose directives should the nurse follow? The answer isn't always clear. Nurses also experience conflicts and difficulties from the discrepancy between their high level of training and low involvement in medical decision making (Aiken 1983, Easterbrook 1987). Nurses are, of course, as important as doctors to a patient's recovery; they spend more time with the person, often explaining medical regimens and procedures when physicians do not.

The medical staff also includes a great variety of allied health workers, such as physical therapists, respiratory therapists, laboratory technicians, pharmacists' assistants and dietitians (Ginzberg 1983). These workers often have less authority than nurses. At the bottom of the medical staff hierarchy are orderlies and other workers whose roles require less advanced skills than those of the allied health workers.

Roles, goals and communication

Picture this scene: As the ambulance crew wheels the victim of a motor vehicle accident into the emergency room, the medical staff swings into action. Their specific actions and roles are dictated by the presenting health problems of the patient and would be different if the person had suffered serious burns in a fire or experienced symptoms of a heart attack, for instance. Quick assessments and decisions need to be made regarding tests to perform, medications to administer and procedures to apply to control the damage, stabilise the person's body functions and set the stage for recovery. Nurses and orderlies know the usual procedures for patients with the presenting problems and begin to perform their roles without specific instruction — for example, a nurse may prepare to take a blood sample and an orderly may wheel a piece of equipment into place. The doctor is, of course, in charge and either conducts needed actions directly or orders others to do them. The health psychologist may be called upon in the rehabilitation of the cardiac patient, or in helping the victim of a motor vehicle accident adjust to his or her injury or disability. Support may be provided to the accident patient's family who are in a state of shock. Or the health psychologist may help the spouse of a terminally ill patient cope with impending loss. The role of the health psychologist in the modern general hospital is expanding in recognition of the important contribution that can be made by psychologists in the diagnosis and treatment of psychological aspects of physical illness, injury and disability.

Assess yourself
WHO'S WHO IN PHYSICIAN CARE

Coordinating patient care

Years ago, the typical hospital patient received services from a small team of doctors and nurses who worked side by side in close communication throughout the person's stay (Benoliel 1977). This situation rarely exists today. Instead, assessment and treatment procedures for a hospitalised person involve a wide array of personnel who have different specialisations and carry out their roles separately, often with little contact with each other and with the patient. The danger in the current approach is that the patient's care can become *fragmented*, or uncoordinated, with seemingly no-one in charge. Hospitals attempt to minimise this danger by giving a particular staff position — usually a nursing position — responsibility for coordinating the care of each patient in a ward (Aiken 1983; Benoliel 1977; Kneut 1982). But *direct* communication — say, between the patient's doctor and physical therapist — is best. It uses more of a team approach, leaves less opportunity for errors, and provides important information and feedback to each team member.

Health hazards in hospitals

Communication among medical personnel is also important because hospitals contain many health hazards for personnel and patients. These hazards include chemicals that are used in treatment and various other hospital procedures (Clever & Omenn 1988). One substance, called *ethylene oxide*, for example, is widely used as a sterilising agent for medical supplies and equipment. Long-term high-level exposure to this chemical has been linked with the development of several forms of cancer. Hospitals need to maintain good channels of communication to protect their workers from high exposure to such chemicals when equipment is malfunctioning or improperly designed. Hospitals also need to protect patients from unsafe exposure to various substances used in their treatment.

Another hazard in hospitals is the potential exposure of personnel and patients to disease-causing micro-organisms (Clever & LeGuyader 1995). As we saw earlier, hospitals prior to the twentieth century were places where infection spread quickly and widely, and patients often died of diseases they did not have when they entered. Although the spreading of infection in hospitals has been greatly reduced, it has not been eliminated.

In Australia, the monitoring of **nosocomial infection**, an infection that a patient contracts while in the hospital setting, has been a recent initiative. Some data exist on wound infection rates and hospital-acquired bacteraemias although all hospitals are not included in the estimation of these figures (Ansari et al. 1994). While the percentage of all patients who acquire and die from a nosocomial infection is unknown at this stage, contaminated wound infection appears to be higher in Tasmanian, ACT and Queensland hospitals (with percentage rates of 5.0, 4.9 and 4.5). To combat this problem, national guidelines for hospital infection control have been developed and widely adopted. According to these guidelines, each hospital should have a central sterile supply department (CSSD) to ensure adequate infection control and quality standards. In 1994 the Australian Standard, a code of practice, was introduced for the cleaning, disinfecting and sterilising of medical and surgical equipment.

Hospitals have attempted to reduce nosocomial infections by establishing regulations regarding such issues as when medical workers must wash their hands or wear masks. But hospital personnel sometimes break these rules, and doctors may be the worst offenders. In an American study of hundreds of hospitals, Bertram Raven and Robert Haley (1982) surveyed about 8000 nurses (ICNs), and epidemiologists to determine whether medical workers adhere to infection control regulations and what is done when they do not. The reports of nurses and epidemiologists agreed that hospital workers showed very good compliance with the rules, but doctors were considerably less likely to comply than were nurses and laboratory technicians. To find out how the ICNs would handle violations of the rules by doctors, nurses and technicians, the ICNs were also asked how often they would 'say something to a staff member' who violated infection control rules, such as by entering a strict isolation area without putting on a mask or by discarding an unprotected syringe in a waste basket. Their responses indicated that ICNs usually correct nurses and technicians, but they are much less likely to correct doctors.

Although nosocomial infection continues to be a serious problem in hospitals, role relationships among medical personnel seem to impair the communication needed to reduce the spread of disease. In general, personnel feel much less comfortable giving advice or corrective feedback to an individual whose status is higher than their own than to someone whose status is equal to or lower than theirs. Hospitals need to find constructive ways to enable a staff member at a lower level of the medical staff hierarchy to give feedback to individuals at higher levels regarding their non-adherence to infection control regulations.

The funding of medical services

The costs of medical services have probably always been high and continue to be high. In 1997–98 public acute hospitals cost $12 836 million to operate. The Commonwealth government provided about two-thirds of the funds to meet total health expenditure, while the remainder of the funds came from State governments, health insurance funds and service users (AIHW 2000, 1999a).

The past 50 years have seen a number of programs introduced to help contain medical costs in Australia (Brooks 1999; Grant 1985). The *Hospital Benefits Act* of 1945 allowed the Commonwealth to enter into agreements with the States to subsidise hospital beds. In 1952 a contributory health benefits scheme was introduced as part of the voluntary health insurance scheme, whereby the Commonwealth continued to pay a bed-day subsidy for all patients but made an additional contribution for patients who had hospital insurance cover. The States were asked to reintroduce charges for all public ward patients. Queensland was the only State where public patients did not pay hospital fees because of pre-existing legislation. New agreements between the States and the federal government were made with the introduction of Medibank in 1975. The federal government paid 50 per cent of public hospital operating costs; charges were abolished, as was means testing for the poor. In 1981 the States were given greater autonomy in terms of health expenditure through 'identified health grants' from the Commonwealth. Once again, with the exception of Queensland, free hospitalisation was eliminated. In 1984 universal access to free public hospital care was introduced through the Medicare program. Medicare grants were provided by the Commonwealth, in addition to the identified health grants, to help meet increased medical costs to the States. The remaining revenue for public hospitals today comes mostly from patients with private health insurance. Australians who choose to be private patients in public hospitals, can have most of the hospital accommodation and nursing charges met by private insurance, while the Medicare benefit subsidises part of the cost of doctors' charges. For private patients in hospitals, the Medicare benefit for medical services is 75 per cent of the Medicare Benefits Schedule fee.

Operating costs in public hospitals have decreased somewhat with the adoption of casemix funding in some States (AIHW 2000). With casemix funding, patients are classified into a **'diagnostic related group'** depending on the medical condition being treated. Each DRG receives a fixed funding allocation irrespective of length of stay and hospital treatment. The funding allocation reflects the average cost of treating individuals in the corresponding diagnostic related group, based on past recovery rates for similar people. If the patient's condition does not respond to the treatment as readily as expected and requires extra care, the hospital usually bears the cost beyond the funding allocation. But if the patient's condition responds better than expected, the hospital keeps the excess payment.

Managed care as an alternative to funding medical services has been debated within both Australia and the United States. While managed care may reduce medical costs, concern has centred on a number of issues — most importantly, the right of patients to receive optimal care and full entitlement of covered benefits, and the right of doctors to determine patient care without approval from health plans.

Concern about the spiralling costs of medical care has led to changes in hospital procedures. How have hospital procedures changed? Although some institutions in Australia, such as nursing homes, focus on treating patients who require long-term care, the great majority of hospitals were established to treat people quickly and discharge them in good health (Grant 1985). Most hospitals keep patients for an average of less than two weeks, and are classified as acute hospitals. The rate at which acute hospitals admit and discharge patients has increased within the past decade from 168 to 201 per 1000 persons (AIHW 1999a). The average length of stay during this period has decreased from 5.2 to 4.4 days. These decreases reflect three important changes. First, people are having more same-day surgery, and procedures done on an outpatient basis. In 1997–98 same-day surgery accounted for 43 per cent of public acute hospital separations (i.e. discharged patients). Second, medical procedures are becoming increasingly efficient. For example, new surgical methods for correcting orthopaedic injuries entail little or no cutting of healthy tissue, so that recovery time and pain are greatly diminished. And emergency room diagnoses are being made more quickly with the aid of new, accurate tests, such as for heart attacks (Puleo et al. 1994). Third, patients are being released at earlier stages of recovery, so that a larger part of their recovery time is spent at home while receiving care as out-patients. Although there is some concern that people are being released too quickly from hospitals, for the most part patients have not been harmed (Kahn, Keeler et al. 1990; Kahn, Rogers et al. 1990; Lave 1989; Rogers et al. 1990).

People typically prefer being released from the hospital as early as possible. Being hospitalised is in many ways a negative experience — financially, physically, socially and emotionally. The next section considers the impact on the patient of being hospitalised.

Being hospitalised

Although being sick is unpleasant and being seriously ill is worse, being hospitalised adds many other negative aspects to a person's sick-role experience: It drastically disrupts the individual's lifestyle, involves a high degree of dependency on others and presents many events that can be extremely distressing. The unpleasantness may begin at admission, such as when an admitting nurse at a public hospital assumes that the patient does not have private health insurance. Part of the unpleasantness of being hospitalised relates to the interactions between the patient and the hospital staff.

Relations with the hospital staff

Imagine that you have just been admitted to a hospital. How should you behave towards the staff if you don't get the care or information you want? Patients typically enter the hospital with a clear social role — that of being dependent for their very lives on the medical staff, who have most of the knowledge, authority and power in their relationship (CU 1995b; Rodin & Janis 1979; Taylor 1979). The patient is a stranger in the hospital community and is likely to be unfamiliar with its structure, procedures and terminology. These conditions often make the person feel uneasy in an already worrisome situation.

Anxiety is probably the most common and pervasive emotion of hospitalised people (Newman 1984a). If their health problems have not yet been identified, they worry about what the problems are, what the outcomes will be and how the illnesses will influence their lives. If the diagnoses have been made, they worry about many other matters, such as what the treatment will be like and the degree to which it will be successful. Many of the worries patients have stem from uncertainties that result from a lack of information. Although the lack of information may occur because tests have not yet been completed, frequently it occurs because no-one has taken the time to inform the person (CU 1995b). One hospital patient, for example, gave the following description of experiences with a doctor.

> He'll say well, we'll talk about it next time. And next time he'll talk fast, he out-talks you — and rushes out of the room and then when he's out of the room you think, well, I was supposed to ask him what he's going to do about my medicine ... you run in the hall and he has disappeared that fast. (Tagliacozzo & Mauksch 1972, p. 177)

Hospitals are busy places, but the limited time of medical personnel is only one reason for their failure to provide the information patients may need. Practitioners sometimes withhold information or disguise it with jargon because they expect the person will misunderstand it or be alarmed by it (McKinlay 1975).

Many patients react to not being informed by their doctors by gathering information from other patients, asking orderlies and nurses, and eavesdropping. As one patient put it:

> Well, I ask the nurses about the blood pressure and if they don't tell me, I go to my chart and look at it. It's six of one and half-a-dozen of the other. When the doctor comes by, I listen to him. I get some information from him when he's speaking about me to the students, although he doesn't know he's giving it to me. (McKinlay 1975, p. 9)

People are resourceful, but the information they receive in these indirect ways may be incorrect or misleading. If so, the beliefs these individuals develop may impair compliance with the advice of the medical staff or lead to unnecessary emotional suffering. Thus, withholding information may produce, rather than prevent, misunderstandings and alarm in patients.

Another common characteristic of the way practitioners interact with patients is called **depersonalisation**, or treating the patient as though he or she were either not present or not a person. Sociologist Erving Goffman referred to this characteristic as 'non-person treatment' and described the practitioner's behaviour in the following way.

> The patient is greeted with what passes as civility, and said farewell to in the same fashion, with everything in between going on as if the patient weren't there as a person at all, but only as a possession someone has left behind. (1961, pp. 341–2)

An example of depersonalisation in Australian hospitals is staff referring to the patient by their illness or operation (e.g. the cholecystectomy in room 2). Why do practitioners treat patients as non-persons? One reason, according to Goffman (1961), is that practitioners want to distance themselves from the fact that the body they are treating belongs to a thinking and worried person — a person who can observe what is going on, ask questions and behave in ways that can interfere with their work. He compared this situation to that of a mechanic who repairs a car or appliance in a shop without the owner present. The implication of Goffman's view is that medical workers try to save themselves and the patient a lot of trouble, awkwardness and anxiety by acting as if the person had dropped off the defective body at the hospital for repair and would pick it up when it was ready.

There are also many emotional factors that lead hospital workers to treat patients in a depersonalised manner. Hospital jobs can be very hectic, particularly when many emergencies punctuate the day. Furthermore, practitioners' jobs entail heavy responsibilities and, sometimes, risks to their own health, as when they work with hazardous chemicals or patients with serious contagious illnesses (Clever & Omenn 1988; O'Donnell et al. 1987). Quite literally, the activities and decisions of hospital workers have life-or-death implications for their patients and themselves. These features can create high levels of stress, which may lead workers to give less personalised care. Sometimes practitioners who are under prolonged stress may even begin to blame patients for their health problems, thinking, for instance, 'You wouldn't have this illness if you had taken care of yourself and not smoked' (Maslach & Jackson 1982). Last, practitioners need ways to protect themselves emotionally when a patient takes a turn for the worse or dies (Benoliel 1977; Kneut 1982). The death of a patient can be a crushing experience. Depersonalisation probably helps practitioners be relatively detached and less emotionally affected when death occurs.

Some hospitals in Australia and other countries are changing the look and feel of their wards. Wards have rooms with home-like furnishings and libraries with medical and health information, and the staff work as a team with a nurse-coordinator for each patient.

Sick-role behaviour in the hospital

Relations between patients and practitioners in the hospital are affected not only by the behaviour of the medical staff, but by the patient's behaviour, too. A hospital presents an unfamiliar and strange environment that requires psychological and social adjustments that most patients have difficulty making. They must get used to a lack of privacy, strict rules and time schedules, having their activities restricted, having little control over events around them, and being dependent on others. Pain is a common feature of many medical conditions, and many patients have to cope with post-operative pain. Some research (Calderone 1990) has found gender differences in the type of medication that is requested by patients who have undergone the same surgery. Male patients requested more pain-killers, while female patients requested more sedative medication. The psychosocial transition to the sick role is dependent on a number of individual, interpersonal and institutional factors. How are patients supposed to behave in the hospital?

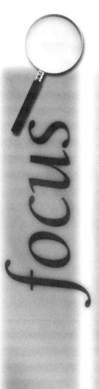

Focus on research
Burnout among health care professionals

Hour after hour, day after day, people who work with people who are suffering and distressed must cope with the stress these encounters produce. All jobs have stressful conditions of some kind, such as heavy work loads, deadlines and interpersonal conflicts. But workers in certain professions — for example police work, social work and health care — have the added emotional burden of working continuously in emotionally charged situations that involve feelings of anxiety, fear, embarrassment and hostility. This burden makes the risk of 'burnout' greater in these professions than in most others. **Burnout** is a state of psychosocial and physical exhaustion that results from chronic exposure to high levels of stress with little personal control (Baron 1986; McKnight & Glass 1995; Parker & Kulik 1995). Workers who experience burnout tend to show low levels of job satisfaction and high levels of absenteeism, job turnover, and alcohol and drug abuse.

What psychological characteristics contribute to burnout in workers? Christina Maslach and Susan Jackson (1982) have developed the Maslach Burnout Inventory (MBI) and used it in research with health care workers. This treatment assesses three psychosocial components of burnout. These are:

1. *emotional exhaustion* — the feeling of being drained of emotional resources and being unable to help others on a psychological level. People who feel this way are likely to agree with the MBI item, 'Working with people all day is really a strain for me.'

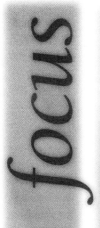

2. *depersonalisation* — a lack of personal regard for others, as shown by treating people as objects, having little concern for and sensitivity to their needs, and developing callous attitudes towards them. Workers with this characteristic tend to agree with the statement, 'I worry that this job is hardening me emotionally.'

3. *perceived inadequacy of professional accomplishment* — the feeling of falling short of personal expectations for work performance. Workers who feel this way are likely to *disagree* with the MBI item. 'I feel I'm positively influencing other people's lives through my work.'

Maslach and Jackson administered the MBI to a large sample of workers in a variety of helping professions and to separate samples of nurses and physicians.

This research produced several important findings. First, the nurses, physicians, and workers in various helping professions reported fairly similar, high levels of emotional exhaustion. Second, differences were found among occupations for the two other components of burnout: the nurses showed the lowest degree of depersonalisation and the doctors reported the least dissatisfaction with their sense of accomplishment in their work. The researchers suggested that the low degree of depersonalisation among nurses may reflect a sex difference in empathy toward people since the females consistently showed less depersonalisation than the males in the helping professions sample, and almost all the nurses but few of the doctors were females. The relatively high sense of accomplishment among doctors may be the result of such factors as their high pay and status in the medical staff hierarchy. Finally, Maslach and Jackson found that the more time health care workers spent in direct care of patients, the greater was their risk of emotional exhaustion. For instance, doctors who spent almost all their time in direct care reported greater emotional exhaustion than those who spent some of their time in teaching or administrative duties.

What can hospitals do to help health care workers avoid or cope with burnout? We can describe two ways (Baron 1986; Maslach & Jackson 1982; Orpen 1991). First, hospitals can provide opportunities for workers to mix direct care for patients and other tasks in their daily activities whenever possible. Second, hospitals can help establish support groups for their health care workers. Meetings of these groups can provide opportunities for workers to share the difficulties they are experiencing and help each other cope.

When patients enter the hospital, they have ideas about how they should behave. Judith Lorber (1975) studied these ideas and the sick-role behaviour of more than 100 patients who entered a hospital for elective surgery. The large majority of these subjects were over 40 years of age; they were selected to represent people having surgeries ranging from routine to very serious. Lorber interviewed the patients when they began and ended their hospital stays, asking them to indicate their degree of agreement or disagreement with several statements, such as: 'The best thing to do in the hospital is to keep quiet and do what you're told,' 'I cooperate best as a patient when I know the reason for what I have to do,' and 'When I'm sick, I expect to be pampered and catered to.' The subjects' responses to such items indicated whether they thought patients should be *active* or *passive*. Subjects' agreement with the first of these items and disagreement with the second two, for example, would indicate that they believe patients should be passive, or 'conforming'. One finding of this study was that patients who had passive beliefs when they entered were less likely than those with active beliefs to argue with the staff and complain about minor discomforts.

Another purpose of this study was to examine the reactions of the medical staff to the patients' sick-role behaviours. At the end of each patient's stay, the medical staff rated the individual as a 'good patient', 'average patient', or 'problem patient'. They were also asked to provide verbal descriptions of the patient's behaviour and their reactions when the behaviour occurred. In general, the individuals rated as *good patients* were those who behaved passively, being cooperative, uncomplaining and stoical; those rated as *problem patients* were seen as uncooperative, constantly complaining, overemotional and dependent. One example of a problem patient was a 74-year-old man who had had his gall bladder removed and had had postoperative psychological and medical complications. He

> was labelled a problem patient by the surgeon, resident, intern, and day staff nurse. In the questionnaire, the resident said the patient's uncooperativeness made it difficult to perform routine procedures on him. The surgeon wrote that the patient was 'lachrymose, combative, and generally impossible' … the surgeon added that the patient had called him names, lied, and generally carried on. (Lorber 1975, p. 218)

Patients may be labelled as problem patients when they do not conform to the wishes of the health care staff or submit to hospital routines and practices for valid reasons. A disclosure from a patient illustrates this point.

> my midwife and consulting doctor did not require routine urine testing for my antenatal care, yet before my chart would be sent to the doctor for my appointment I was required to provide one. Staff would become frustrated with me when I refused to provide one on the basis that it was unnecessary to my care.

Often hospital routines and practices are for 'routine's sake' and efficiency, rather than for the welfare of the patient. Labelling patients as 'problem patients' implies inappropriate blame for 'misbehaviour'.

An important consequence of poor patient–practitioner relationships is that the patient is less likely to adhere to medical recommendations, as we saw in chapter 9. But the opposite behaviour of patients — being overly passive or too considerate — can present problems, too. One very sick person 'didn't want to bother' the nurses, even when she should have. As a result, the nurses' routines were disrupted by having to check on her status very frequently to make sure she was all right. Patients who are too passive in the hospital may fail to take active roles in their recovery, thereby limiting their rehabilitation (Taylor 1979). Ideal relationships between patients and practitioners foster mutual involvement in the treatment process.

Often patients' severe medical conditions make their difficult behaviour understandable, so the staff in Lorber's study distinguished between two types of problem patients. One type consists of individuals who are very seriously ill, having severe complications or poor prognoses. Although these patients show problem behaviours and require a lot of attention, the staff often forgives their behaviour because of their medical conditions. The second type consists of people who are not seriously ill but take up more time and attention than is warranted by their conditions — they frequently argue, complain or fail to cooperate with the staff. Why do patients who are not seriously ill behave so disruptively? One possibility is that this behaviour is their reaction to being angry at their loss of freedoms and control (Taylor 1979). For instance, a patient may not be allowed to walk for a while because of a leg injury, or watch television late because it would disturb other patients, or have visitors at certain times because their presence might make the work of the medical staff more difficult. People's angry responses to being controlled or believing their freedom is threatened are called **reactance** (Brehm 1966).

Psychologist Shelley Taylor has described how hospital patients sometimes show reactance in their

> petty acts of mutiny such as making passes at nurses, drinking in one's room, smoking against medical advice, and wandering up and down the halls. Such minor incidents tend to irritate nursing and custodial staff, but rarely do any damage. However, petty acts of mutiny can turn into self-sabotage, such as failing to take medications which are essential to recovery, or engaging in acts which have potentially fatal consequences. Coupled with these mutinous acts against the hospital routine and treatment regimen are frequent demands upon the staff for attention, treatment, and medication, and frequent complaints regarding the quality of same. (1979, p. 172)

How does the hospital staff deal with problem patients? In many cases, hospital workers respond in a pleasant manner — for example by providing reassurance or explanations (Lorber 1975). In other cases, the response is not so positive. Staff members sometimes scold patients, or begin to ignore their problem behaviour, or respond less quickly to their calls for attention. In addition, hospital personnel often deal with problem patients by administering sedatives and, in highly problematic cases, even by arranging for premature discharge.

Fortunately, the large majority of patients are not problem patients (Lorber 1975). Most hospitalised people try to be considerate, recognising that medical workers have difficult jobs. One patient compared being in a hospital with being at a hotel.

> If it is a hotel you won't hesitate to pick up a phone or to complain; in a hospital you think twice about it — you figure maybe they are busy or shorthanded. ... It's a much more human thing, the hospital ... it's more personal. (Tagliacozzo & Mauksch 1972, p. 175)

Others behave as 'good patients' because they are wary of the consequences of being disliked by the staff. These people do not want to appear to be 'troublemakers,' by being too demanding or too dependent. They may think an angered staff may 'refuse to answer your bell' or 'refuse to make your bed', for instance. As a result, these patients may anxiously watch the clock when their medication does not arrive on time, rather than reminding the nurse (Tagliacozzo & Mauksch 1972).

The sick-role behaviour of hospitalised individuals is affected by many factors in addition to the seriousness of their illnesses, their ideas about how they should behave and their reactions to their restricted freedoms. As we have seen, social interactions in a medical setting involve a 'two-way street' in which both the patient's and the practitioner's behaviour are important. Patients respond differently to medical staff who grumble or frown when asked to do something than to staff who carry out requests cheerfully and seem to want to help (Tagliacozzo & Mauksch 1972). Finally, sick-role behaviour depends on how well patients cope with their medical conditions and the medical treatment procedures they experience in the hospital.

Patient satisfaction

If you have been admitted to a hospital recently you may have evaluated your stay in terms of the success of the operation, the amount of pain you had, or the friendliness of the nursing staff and their readiness to assist you. Perhaps you would have preferred to see the attending surgeon a little more often to ask about the medical procedure or concerns that you had. You may not have thought that the food was as good as that from home. Or perhaps you welcomed the tea and biscuits as a way of breaking the long days lying in a hospital bed. You may have compared your hospital experience with those of visiting family and friends. Do patients have similar views on what they expect from their hospitalisation, and what aspects of hospitalisation lead to patient satisfaction with the care received?

Hardy, West and Hill (1996) sought to answer this question by investigating hundreds of patients in the United Kingdom. They distinguished between proximal (factors within the individual) and organisational components of patient satisfaction. The factors within the individual relating to patient satisfaction were the overall process of care in the hospital, improvement in and understanding of health, and psychological wellbeing. Of the organisational variables, attentiveness of medical and nursing staff was the best predictor of overall satisfaction. Information received from doctors and nurses; the attitudes of secondary staff such as cleaners, pathology nurses and X-ray staff; and initial experiences on arrival at the hospital all affected understanding of the medical condition and improvement in physical health. Psychological wellbeing of patients was influenced by the provision of medical information, the admission procedures, involvement of the patient in the treatment, ward cleanliness and the attitudes of ancillary staff.

Emotional adjustment in the hospital

Imagine that you are 31 years old and have been diagnosed with breast cancer. You are waiting in your hospital room for a mastectomy procedure. You do not wish to lose a breast at such a young age, but without the surgery you will die. Following the surgery you will have to have radiotherapy for five weeks, and chemotherapy for the next six months in a four-week cycle, which will leave you weak and nauseated for days at a time. You have been told that the chemotherapy could make you infertile, and even bring on early menopause. This was the real experience of Jane McGrath, wife of Australian test cricketer Glen McGrath, which is described in their book *A Love for Life* (McGrath & McGrath 2000). Being hospitalised with a serious illness or injury produces enormous stress and anxiety.

Hospitalised people must cope with their emotions, and they tend to adjust gradually. For example, most surgical patients experience anxiety levels that are especially high when they are admitted, remain quite high prior to the operation, and then decline steadily during the week or two after surgery (Newman 1984a). But sometimes the anxiety levels of patients increase with time. Ben-Zur et al. (2000) reported high anxiety levels and negative moods in patients up to 20 months after their coronary artery bypass graft surgery, which they linked to ineffective emotion-focused coping strategies. Depression in the first weeks after surgery has been associated with poorer physical recovery, diminished mental health and reduced activity in coronary bypass patients at three months' follow-up (Morris 1999). And there is some indication that pre-operative anxiety is associated with greater psychological distress, more physical symptoms and longer recovery (Grossi et al. 1998: de Groot et al. 1997).

The way a patient adjusts to his or her health problem and treatment in the hospital depends on a wide variety of factors, such as the person's age or gender and characteristics of the illness or injury (Moos 1982). For instance, young adults often have more difficulty coping with serious illnesses than older individuals do. A study of older patients who had undergone knee-replacement surgery found that those who had a sense of purpose in life tended to recover faster, and showed better mental health (Smith & Zautra 2000). Also, men tend to be more distressed than women by illnesses that reduce their vigour and physical abilities, but women often have an especially difficult time adjusting to facial injuries or losing a breast.

Coping processes in hospital patients

Coping style can affect how patients adjust to hospitalisation and how they respond to surgery (Kessler 1999). How would you try to cope with the stress and anxiety of being hospitalised? You can get an indication of the answer by turning back to page 172 in chapter 5, where you assessed your tendency to use coping processes to achieve two main goals: to alter the problem causing the stress and to regulate the emotional response to the problem. Some of the situations that produce stress in hospital can be altered by the patient's taking action, such as by asking for medication to reduce pain or by reading information about the health problem. Because these actions can reduce the demands of the stressor or expand the person's resources for dealing with it, they are examples of *problem-focused coping*. There is some indication that problem-focused coping facilitates recovery at least in coronary bypass patients, and that coping may interact with personal factors such as optimism and Type B personality to speed recovery (Khalid & Sial 1998).

Patients in hospital experience many stressors they believe they cannot change. In some cases these beliefs are correct, as when a person whose spinal cord was severed in an accident must cope with not being able to walk. But in other cases they are incorrect, as when a patient does not realise that it may be possible to use another medication if the current one produces discomfort or other side effects. People who believe they can do nothing to change a stressor usually try to cope with their emotions and the situation by using methods classified as *emotion-focused coping*. Patients may try to regulate their emotions by denying unpleasant facts, performing distracting activities or seeking social support for example. Research has consistently shown that social support aids people's recovery from and adjustment to illness (Elizur & Hitsh 1999; Kulik & Mahler 1989; Schwarzer & Schroeder 1997).

The type of coping patients use may depend on the nature of the medical treatment or the type of surgery being performed. In a study by Koutsosimou, McDonald and Davey (1996), patients who had undergone surgery following a traffic accident reported more emotion-focused coping than other surgical patients, with the exception of gynaecological surgery patients. Accident patients also reported less use of task-oriented and avoidance coping strategies than all other groups except general surgery patients. Accident surgery patients may engage in more emotion-focused coping in an attempt to deal with unanticipated trauma and pain. Also, accident patients have less time to prepare psychologically for surgery as they may have little forewarning of the surgery.

Cognitive processes in coping

One cognitive process many patients engage in after becoming ill or injured is attributing *blame* — trying to answer the question, 'Who's at fault for my condition?' They often grapple with this issue while in hospital. Some people blame mainly themselves, others blame someone else, and others attribute their conditions to luck or God's will.

Does the way people attribute blame affect their success in coping with their conditions? We might expect, for instance, that people who blame themselves would have intense feelings of guilt and self-recrimination and, therefore, have more difficulty adjusting to their condition than those who blame someone else. On the other hand, blaming someone else may induce intense feelings of anger and bitterness, which would impair adjustment.

Research has examined this issue and found that the more blame for a traumatic event that individuals attribute to themselves or other people, the poorer their adjustment tends to be (Downey, Silver & Wortman 1990). The findings of several other studies suggest that poor adjustment may be more strongly related to blaming others than to self-blame (Bulman & Wortman 1977; Kiecolt-Glaser & Williams 1987; Taylor, Lichtman & Wood 1984). Although it is unclear why adjustment is so difficult when patients blame someone else, the reason may be that these people feel an added sense of injustice if the person they blame did not suffer severe consequences, too. These feelings are reflected in such statements as, 'I'm paralysed, but the driver only broke his leg,' or, 'I can't walk now, but the guy who shot me is now walking free' (Bulman & Wortman 1977, p. 360).

Another cognitive process that patients engage in involves the assessment of their personal control. Patients enter the hospital with the expectation of losing some degree of personal control, either from the effects of the illness itself or from being dependent on the actions of the medical staff. Hospital environments encourage patients to believe their involvement in the treatment process is irrelevant — that they are *helpless*. Patients often express this feeling, saying, 'When you are really sick, you are at the mercy of the hospital staff,' or, 'Trying to change things is futile and won't get you anywhere' (Tagliacozzo & Mauksch 1972). Those people who feel this way are likely to behave like 'good patients' (Taylor 1979). Some patients enter the hospital feeling quite helpless right from the start, but others try to exert control and fail. Through repeated failures in exerting control, many people learn to be helpless in the hospital, eventually making no effort to initiate changes when control is actually possible. One study, for instance, found that patients' helplessness and feelings of depression increased with time in hospital, even as their health improved (Raps et al. 1982). Yet recent research has indicated that some patients do not wish to exercise control over their medical treatment, preferring to leave control to medical professionals (Peerbhoy et al. 1998).

The connections among 'good patient' behaviour, helplessness and depression can be seen in the case of a 50-year-old divorced man who had suffered burns over 40 per cent of his body. When he returned to the hospital six months later for a follow-up visit, his hands were still stiff, and he was having many psychological problems. He had moved in with his very supportive daughter and son-in-law

> in hopes that he would be able to take care of repair work that needed doing around the house. When it became clear that he was not able to do any of these things to his satisfaction, he became increasingly depressed. . . . On reviewing his case it turned out that he had indeed been a very 'good' patient, quiet and cooperative. He never asked any questions about the details or the implications of his illness. (Steiner & Clark 1977, p. 139)

This case is consistent with Taylor's (1979, p. 171) view that 'the so-called "good patient" is often actually in a state of helplessness,' which may eventually lead to feelings of depression.

Helping patients cope

Suppose you were having surgery with *full anaesthesia*. Would it make any difference to your recovery if *during surgery* someone said to you, 'How quickly you recover from your operation depends on you,' and gave suggestions of things you should do to speed recovery? Perhaps. An experiment demonstrated that anaesthetised patients who received this kind of information recovered more quickly and had fewer complications than control patients who got no suggestions during their operations (Evans & Richardson 1988). These results and those of other studies indicate that people hear and understand at least broad meanings while anaesthetised, even though they cannot say what they heard (Bennett 1989). This is important for two reasons: (1) medical staff often make negative or disparaging remarks during surgery, and (2) it may be possible to help surgical patients cope by giving them constructive suggestions while they are anaesthetised.

An effective way to help hospitalised people cope is to provide psychological counselling during their stays. Walter Gruen (1975) gave brief counselling sessions to heart attack patients almost every day during the three weeks or so that they were in the hospital. Compared with a control group, the subjects who received the counselling spent fewer days in intensive care and in the hospital, had fewer heart complications and less psychological depression during their stays, and showed fewer signs of anxiety problems when contacted about four months after discharge.

Gruen's (1975) research was extended in Australia by Oldenburg, Andrews and Perkins (1985), who compared the long-term effects of two types of in-hospital intervention for coronary patients against no psychological treatment. Patients either received an intensive intervention of behavioural counselling, relaxation and education or a basic intervention of relaxation and education. The control group received standard medical and nursing care. Compared with the control group, the two intervention groups showed less anxiety, less Type A behaviour and better psychological functioning during the intervention and at 12 months. The control group patients had higher rates of smoking and alcohol consumption at 12 months' follow-up. Differences were also noted between the groups on health care dependence. The control group had a greater use of medication, more hospital admissions and more visits to the doctor.

A circumstance in the hospital that may help a patient adjust to his or her illness and impending treatment is sharing a room with a person who is recovering after undergoing a similar medical procedure. James Kulik and Heike Mahler (1987a) conducted an experiment with 46- to 69-year-old male patients who were scheduled for coronary bypass surgery. Upon admission, each subject was assigned a room-mate, based on room availability, for the two days prior to surgery. About half of them shared rooms with men who were also awaiting operations, and the remaining subjects shared rooms with patients who had already had operations and were recovering. Assessments were made of the subjects' anxiety the evening before their surgeries, physical activity during the week after the operation and speed of recovery. The results showed that compared with the subjects who had pre-operative room-mates, those with room-mates who had already undergone surgery were far less anxious before their operation, engaged in much more physical activity after surgery and were able to leave the hospital an average of 1.4 days sooner.

Although patients entering a hospital for surgery typically prefer having room-mates who are already recovering from surgery, honouring such requests would be logistically very difficult (Kulik & Mahler 1987a). In addition, we don't yet know *why* the type of room-mate affects patients' adjustment. The findings of subsequent research suggest that having two pre-surgery patients share a room may increase the anxiety of both individuals by some form of 'emotional contagion' (Kulik, Moore & Mahler 1993).

Helping the patient's family cope

Patients are not the only people who may need help coping with a medical condition, treatment or surgery. Family members and significant others may require supportive counselling to facilitate acceptance of a medical diagnosis and adjustment to the patient's condition. Partners may have to care for the patient upon discharge, helping the person to make lifestyle behaviour changes. Caregivers may spend much of their time watching for symptoms, fearing relapse in the patient. Caring for an ill member of the family can affect the caregiver's health and emotional state (Schultz et al. 1995). Some research, for instance, has found that depression in carers of patients who have undergone heart surgery is related to physical health and role strain (Coker 1998). The carer's social activities may also decline (Braithwaite 1990). Social support in carers of coronary patients has been found to moderate depression. Supportive interventions for families and carers of patients with specific conditions can facilitate adjustment (Brannon & Feist 1992; Kiecolt-Glaser, Dyer & Shuttleworth 1988).

Preparing patients for stressful medical procedures

Preparing people psychologically for surgery has important implications for their recovery: The more anxiety patients feel before surgery, the more difficult their adjustment and recovery are likely to be after surgery. People with high pre-operative anxiety tend to report more pain, use more medication for pain, stay in the hospital longer, and report more anxiety and depression during their recovery than patients with less pre-operative fear (Anderson & Masur 1983; Johnson 1983). What can psychologists do to reduce the stress people experience in conjunction with medical procedures?

Psychological preparation for surgery

Although several methods seem to be useful in helping people cope with impending surgery, the most effective of these approaches are those that enhance patients' sense of *control* over the situation or the recovery process (Anderson & Masur 1983; Mathews & Ridgeway 1984; Thompson 1981). These approaches are generally designed to give the person one or more of the following types of control:

- *behavioural control* — being able to reduce discomfort or promote recovery during or after the medical procedure by performing certain actions, such as special breathing or coughing exercises
- *cognitive control* — knowing how to focus on the benefits of the medical procedure and not its unpleasant aspects
- *informational control* — gaining knowledge about the events and/or sensations to expect during or after the medical procedure.

Patients can acquire the knowledge for these types of control in many ways, such as through discussion with practitioners, reading, listening to tape recordings, or watching film or video recordings.

An example of an approach to enhance *cognitive control* comes from an experiment with individuals who were in the hospital to undergo major *elective* surgeries that typically have favourable prognoses (Langer, Janis & Wolfer 1975). The researchers assigned the subjects to groups on a random basis, but also tried to equate the groups for several characteristics, such as age, sex and seriousness of the operation. One of the groups received training in cognitive control that pointed out how paying attention to negative aspects of an experience increases stress and taught them to focus on the positive aspects of their impending surgery when feeling distressed by the surgical experience. A comparison group spent an equal amount of time with a psychologist, but they engaged in only general conversation about the hospital experience. The records and nurses' ratings on the surgical ward revealed important benefits of training in cognitive control: The patients who received this training showed greater reductions in pre-operative stress behaviour, less post-operative stress, and fewer requests for medication after surgery than the comparison subjects.

Several other studies have demonstrated beneficial effects of enhancing surgical patients' *informational* and *behavioural control* (Anderson 1987; Andrew 1970; Johnson et al. 1978; Johnston & Vögele 1993). One experiment was conducted by Erling Anderson with 60 adult male cardiac patients who were scheduled for coronary bypass surgery. The researcher randomly assigned the subjects to three groups. One group had a general conversation with the researcher and received the *standard preparation* of the hospital, in which the patient and a nurse discussed two pamphlets that outlined the procedures related to the upcoming surgery. A second group received the standard preparation plus training to enhance *informational control*, which delivered procedural and sensory information in two ways: (1) the subjects watched a videotape called 'Living Proof', which presents interviews with recovered bypass patients and follows a patient from admission through various pre-operative tests and exercises, preparation for surgery, recovery and discharge; and (2) they were given an audiotape, describing sensations they might experience, that they could play in their rooms. The third group received training in both *informational and behavioural control*. These subjects had the same pre-operative training as the informational control group but were also taught how to perform various behaviours, such as coughing exercises and ways to turn in bed, that they would need to do after the operation.

Anderson (1987) used a variety of measures to assess the effects of these methods of psychological preparation on the patients' adjustment and recovery. For example, the patients filled out a questionnaire (the State–Trait Anxiety Inventory) to measure their distress at three times: when they were admitted, the evening before surgery and one week after the operation. As figure 10.1 on the following page depicts, the subjects' anxiety levels in the three groups were almost identical on admission but then diverged after the different preparation methods were conducted. Both types of psychological preparation reduced the patients' anxiety substantially before and after the operation. Assessments were also made of the subjects' use of pain medication and length of stay in the hospital, but the three groups did not differ on these measures. Finally, the patients' blood pressures were monitored closely because dangerous levels of acute hypertension occur very commonly during the first 12 hours following bypass surgery. For this critical measure, psychological preparation had a very beneficial effect. Of the patients who received the standard preparation, 75 per cent developed acute hypertension and required medication to dilate their blood vessels. In contrast, only 45 per cent of subjects in the informational control group and 40 per cent of those in the informational and behavioural control group had episodes of acute hypertension.

Since this earlier research, many studies have compared the benefits of different types of preparation for patients undergoing a range of surgical procedures. In a meta-analysis of 38 studies on the benefits of psychological preparation for surgery, Johnston and Voegele (1993) found that procedural information and behavioural instructions had the most effect on negative mood, pain and medication, recovery time, length of stay, physical symptoms and satisfaction.

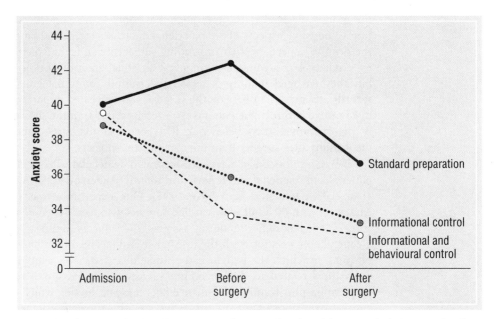

Figure 10.1 Anxiety levels of cardiac surgery patients as a function of the psychological preparation they received. Anxiety was measured by the State–Trait Anxiety Inventory at three times: on admission, the evening before surgery and one week after the operation.

Source: Adapted from Anderson (1987, figure 1).

The studies we have examined clearly demonstrate the value of psychological preparations that increase patients' sense of control when awaiting operations. One thing to keep in mind about providing information to people about medical procedures is that unclear information can lead to misconceptions and anxiety and do more harm than good (Wallace 1986). Patients need to receive straightforward and clear materials and instructions, and they need to discuss this information with medical and psychological staff. Of course, surgery is only one of many types of stressful medical procedures that may occur in the hospital, and patients often dread experiencing each of them.

Psychological preparations for non-surgical procedures.

How would you like to be awake while a physician inserts a thin, hollow tube called a *catheter* into one of your blood vessels, gently threads it towards your heart, and then injects dye through the catheter? This is a procedure called *cardiac catheterisation*, which is used with people who show signs of cardiovascular disorders, such as damage to a major blood vessel or heart valve. The dye enables practitioners to see the damage with the aid of X-ray or other radiological devices. By using this procedure, physicians can determine whether to recommend other medical procedures, such as bypass or open-heart surgery. A patient undergoing cardiac catheterisation receives tranquillising medication and a local anaesthetic for the area where the tube enters the body. This procedure is typically not painful, but it is quite unpleasant and produces strange and frightening sensations, such as 'hot flashes' when dye is injected into the heart.

How might patients and hospital staff benefit by the use of psychological preparations for people undergoing cardiac catheterisation? Preparing them for unpleasant medical procedures should help to reduce patients' anxiety and disruptive behaviour during the procedures, for example, as well as their general level of stress prior to surgery. Philip Kendall and his associates (1979) examined the effects of psychological preparation for cardiac catheterisation on the anxiety experienced by male patients, about two-thirds of whom had undergone the procedure at least a year earlier. The subjects were randomly assigned to four groups. One group received training in *cognitive control* methods from a therapist, learning how to recognise signs of their own anxiety and ways to cope when these signs occur. Another group received preparation to enhance their *informational control*, learning about the procedures and sensations to expect through printed materials and discussions with therapists. Two other groups served as comparison (control) conditions. Analyses of the patients' self-reports and of hospital staff ratings showed that both the cognitive and the informational control preparations effectively reduced patients' anxiety; subjects who received these preparations experienced less anxiety than those in the two comparison groups before and during catheterisation.

As you may have surmised, the catheterisation procedure requires that the patient be inactive. There are no actions the person can take to make the process occur more smoothly or pleasantly — that is, the patient has little or no behavioural control. This is true of many but not all aversive medical procedures. One medical procedure in which patients can perform useful actions is called an *endoscopy*, which is used in diagnosing ulcers and other disorders of the digestive tract. The most aversive aspect of an endoscopic examination is that a long, flexible fibre-optic tube, about a centimetre in diameter, must be passed through the patient's mouth and down to the stomach and intestine. This tube remains in the digestive tract, transmitting images of the lining, for about 15 to 30 minutes. During this procedure, the person is awake, but has received tranquillising medication, and the throat has been swabbed with a local anaesthetic.

In an experiment with patients who had never undergone an endoscopy before, Jean Johnson and Howard Leventhal (1974) provided psychological preparation to enhance the behavioural and informational control the subjects could use during the procedure. Training for behavioural control included teaching the subjects helpful ways to breathe and swallow while the throat is swabbed and the tube is inserted. Instructions for informational control involved descriptions of the procedures and sensations the subjects could expect during the examination. Some patients received instruction for either behavioural control or informational control, some had both types of preparation, and others served as a comparison group, receiving no psychological preparation. All patients, however, received a standard explanation of the endoscopic procedure from a physician. The researchers found that subjects in the comparison group tended to show more emotional behaviour and gagging during the procedure than those who received psychological preparation, particularly if this preparation included instruction for both informational and behavioural control.

In summary, psychological preparation can enhance patients' sense of control and their adjustment to non-surgical medical procedures. Generally speaking, when these procedures offer little opportunity for the person to take helpful action, psychological preparation to promote informational and cognitive control may be especially effective. But when patients will undergo procedures in which they can take direct action to facilitate the process and reduce their own discomfort, preparation should usually include approaches to enhance behavioural control.

Coping styles and psychological preparation

People use many different styles in coping with stress, as we discussed in chapter 5. When faced with stressful medical procedures, for instance, some individuals tend to cope by using *avoidance* strategies to minimise the impact of the situation. They may deny that a threat exists; refuse to seek or attend to threatening information, perhaps saying, 'I don't want to know'; or suppress unpleasant thoughts. In contrast, other individuals tend to use *attention* or 'vigilant' strategies, seeking detailed information about the situation (Newman 1984a). Some research has found that avoidant coping is not adaptive, for instance in adjusting to low back pain (Ugolini 1999). Other studies have found that patients who use avoidance strategies often show better emotional adjustment to medical procedures such as blood donation or dental surgery than those who use attention strategies (Kaloupek, White & Wong 1984). Elderly patients who are avoidant copers have been found to have shorter hospital stays, less psychological distress and better recovery than those who are vigilant copers (Sgandurra et al. 1998). Also, there is some indication that avoidance can be beneficial to adjustment among patients with cancer. Sherliker and Steptoe (2000) found that patients with advanced metastatic cancer who were participating in a clinical trial of new anti-cancer drugs were able to maintain a positive mood by ignoring their condition. How do people who use avoidance strategies react to psychological preparations that enhance their control?

Researchers have examined this question by using approaches to enhance informational control with patients who were classified as using avoidance or attention styles. One of these studies was conducted by Suzanne Miller and Charles Mangan (1983) with women who were scheduled to undergo an unpleasant but painless diagnostic test for gynaecological cancer. The subjects were classified as using avoidance or attention styles on the basis of their responses in a questionnaire. By random assignment, half of the avoidance subjects (called 'blunters') and the attention subjects ('monitors') received extensive information regarding the procedures and sensations they would experience during the examination; the remaining subjects got very little information about the examination. Measures of the patients' distress were taken at three times: before receiving the information, after getting the information but before the examination, and after the examination. Figure 10.2 presents the results of this research, using the patients' pulse rates as the measure of distress. These findings indicate that monitors who receive very little information and blunters who receive extensive information react negatively to the amount of information they receive, as shown by their continued high pulse rates after the examination.

More recent research has indicated that low-monitoring patients may benefit from certain types of surgery preparation. Miro and Raich (1999) compared high versus low monitors on three types of preparation for surgery. One group of patients received sensory and procedural information. Another group received relaxation training and the third group acted as a control. Low monitors who received relaxation training experienced less surgical pain, and were more active at follow-up, compared with low-monitoring control patients.

Other research has confirmed these findings and shown that psychological preparation for medical procedures is most effective when its content is matched to the needs of the person (Carpenter, Gatchel & Hasegawa 1994; Litt, Nye & Shafer 1995; Ludwick-Rosenthal & Neufeld 1993). In addition, the number of times people see the information seems to affect the amount of stress they experience. In one study, patients awaiting endoscopic examinations filled out a questionnaire that assessed their coping styles and then watched a videotape that showed the procedures and sensations they could expect during their own endoscopies (Shipley et al. 1978). Some subjects watched the informational tape only once, and others viewed it three times. A comparison group watched an irrelevant tape. Measures of the patients' anxiety during their endoscopies included heart rate and questionnaire assessments by the patients and practitioners after the examinations. The study found that *avoidance copers* who saw the informational tape only once experienced more anxiety than those who saw it three times and those who watched the irrelevant tape. Of the *attention copers*, those who watched the irrelevant tape experienced the most anxiety, and those who viewed the informational tape three times had the least anxiety.

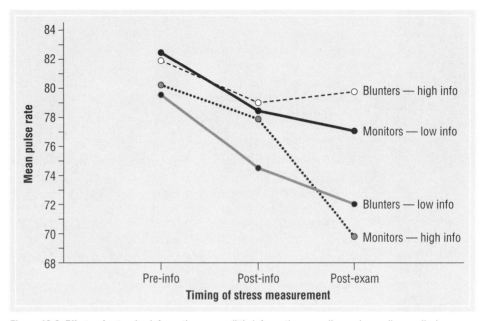

Figure 10.2 Effects of extensive information versus little information regarding an impending medical examination on the stress experienced by patients who use avoidance coping strategies ('blunters') or attention strategies ('monitors'). Pulse rate, the measure of stress, was taken for each subject three times: before receiving the information, after the information and after the examination. High pulse rate indicates more distress.

Source: Miller & Mangan (1983, figure 7).

Highlight on issues

issues

Lamaze training as a method of psychological preparation for a medical procedure

During much of the twentieth century, Australians generally accepted two ideas about childbirth: (1) the mother will experience intense and prolonged pain unless she is given tranquillising and pain-reducing drugs, and (2) the use of drugs is best for the mother and her baby. But these beliefs have changed since the 1960s for two reasons. First, research has shown that drugs given to the mother during childbirth pass through the placenta and can harm the baby, for instance by impairing the newborn's spontaneous breathing (Bowes et al. 1970). Second, anthropologists have reported that women in cultures where childbirth is regarded as an easy and open process most often have shorter and less complicated labours than women in cultures where birth is regarded as fearful and private (Mead & Newton 1967).

(*continued*)

Could it be that part of the difficulty many mothers have in childbirth is the result of the inadequate psychological preparation they receive?

Because of these considerations, many prospective mothers opt for antenatal preparation involving 'natural childbirth' methods, such as **Lamaze training**. Natural childbirth methods generally involve three components: preparation, participation and minimal medication (Parfitt 1977). Birth is essentially a process in which the muscles of the uterus contract in a rhythmical pattern to push the baby out. A fearful woman is likely to tighten her muscles, which then act against the natural muscular contractions and make labour more painful. A main purpose of natural childbirth methods is to prepare the woman to be more relaxed and better able to control her breathing and muscular activity to help in the process at each stage.

In addition to the social support women in Lamaze training get from the baby's father and the people in the training meetings, the method is designed to enhance the mother's sense of control. Lamaze training includes features that promote:

- *informational control*, such as by providing descriptions of the physiological processes in birth and the procedures and sensations to expect during labour and delivery
- *behavioural control*, for example through instruction and practice in muscle relaxation and special breathing techniques
- *cognitive control*, such as by teaching the woman to stare at an object in the room or to concentrate on images or phrases during the childbirth process.

Most Australian obstetricians today recommend antenatal preparation classes, which teach the expectant mother how to relax and breathe to facilitate coping with the delivery, minimise pain and reduce fear.

Is Lamaze preparation beneficial? Although the results of studies suggest that it is, the evidence is not yet very clear (Wideman & Singer 1984). Research has found, for instance, that women who receive Lamaze training use less pain-killing medication during delivery and are less anxious about the birth procedure than those who do not; but these studies have used quasi-experimental designs and self-report methods. Part of the difficulty in interpreting these findings is that women who choose natural childbirth are different from those who do not — for example, they tend to be from higher social classes and report lower anxiety levels even before receiving the training.

The view that childbirth is a natural event has led some Australian women to consider other natural birth options, such as the *Leboyer* method (Leboyer 1977), where the infant is handled gently to minimise fear and pain. In the Leboyer birth the infant is welcomed into a quiet, warm, dark environment, given time to recover from the birth, allowed to begin to breathe in its own time, gently massaged and placed into a warm bath. The mother bonds with the infant immediately after birth. The father is present at the birth, providing emotional support to the mother in labour, and significant family members can also be present. Women who choose to have a Leboyer birth in hospital have been found to have lower rates of induced labour, forceps delivery and Caesarean section (Lumley & Astbury 1980). Infants delivered by the Leboyer method appear less distressed, and have been reported to be easy to care for (Lumley & Astbury 1980). Birth centres combine many of the features discussed above. For example, birth centres provide antenatal education and childbirth preparation, a place for birth that incorporates elements of the Leboyer technique while having access to medical emergency treatment, family access to the birth, and postnatal care.

The benefits of psychological preparations for medical procedures seem to depend on the patients' coping styles, and it may be that different preparations are more helpful for people using avoidance strategies than for those using attention strategies. Although being exposed to information about impending medical procedures more than once appears to help all patients, it may be particularly beneficial to those who tend to cope by using avoidance strategies.

When the hospitalised patient is a child

About half a million patients admitted to acute hospitals in Australia each year are under the age of 15 years (AIHW 1999a). This represents about 10 per cent of all hospital admissions. We have seen that adults become distressed by pain and illness, think hospitals are big and frightening places, and become anxious when undergoing unpleasant or painful medical procedures. So do children, but their level of psychosocial development may make some aspects of the hospital experience particularly difficult for them. For one thing, children are less able than adults to influence and understand what is happening to them. Children at young ages may also feel abandoned or unloved by being without their families, and some may even believe that they were put in the hospital as punishment for misbehaviour. What special adjustments do children need to make when they are hospitalised, and how well do they cope? Answers to these questions depend partly on the child's age.

Hospitalisation in the early years of childhood

The experience of being hospitalised is distressing for children of all ages, but the reasons for their distress tend to change as they get older (Mabe, Treiber & Riley 1991; McClowry & McLeod 1990; Sarafino 1986). For toddlers and preschool children — who are rarely inactive when healthy — a hospital experience that involves being immobilised can be very stressful. These children may protest loudly and struggle against medically necessary devices that restrain their movement (Smith & Autman 1985). But the most salient source of stress of young children in the hospital is being separated from their parents.

Separation distress is the normal reaction of being upset and crying that young children exhibit when they are separated from their parents, particularly in unfamiliar surroundings (Ainsworth 1973, 1979). Late in the first year of life, most infants begin showing this reaction, even in everyday short separations of a few minutes or hours. As figure 10.3 illustrates, the tendency of children to show distress in situations of short-term separation peaks at roughly 15 months of age. This is true of children from a wide variety of cultures around the world. After that age, the percentage of children showing distress with short-term separations declines universally (Super 1981). But hospitalisation can involve prolonged periods of separation, with little parent–child contact for days, weeks or longer. How well do toddlers and preschool-age children cope with long-term separation?

Prolonged separation produces dramatic and, perhaps, long-lasting reactions in young children. During hospitalisation, children's conduct often regresses sharply, reverting to forms of behaviour they may have used at younger ages. Thus, they may become less sociable and start wetting the bed and having temper tantrums again (Peterson & Mori 1988; Ramsey 1982). John Bowlby (1969, 1973) has described the behavioural and psychological consequences that unfold during the first weeks of prolonged separation. The initial reaction is one of *protest*, in which the child displays excessive crying, calling and searching for his or her parents, typically the mother. Following this period, the child reacts with *despair*, usually reflected in reduced activity, withdrawal and apparent hopelessness. Finally, if separation from the parents is quite long or permanent, such as if they died, the child enters the final period of *detachment*. The child's behaviour is 'back to normal'; but if the parents return, the child seems to reject them, no longer seeking interaction or contact with them.

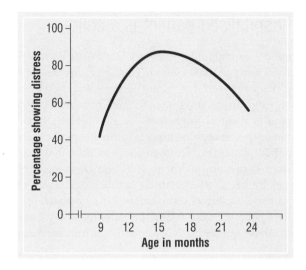

Figure 10.3 Children's tendency to exhibit separation distress when tested with short-term separations at different ages. The graph represents approximate percentages at each age, averaged across cultures — for example, the reaction occurs in about 90 per cent of American working-class infants and 70–80 per cent of Guatemalan babies at 15 months (Super 1981).

Source: Sarafino & Armstrong (1986, figure 5.3).

After a prolonged or difficult stay in the hospital, young children often display anxious behaviour at home. They may continue their regressive behaviours, begin having nightmares, or become very clinging and unwilling to let their mothers out of their sight. One child named Sara, for instance, had attended preschool and was becoming quite independent for her age before having a difficult hospital experience that included receiving 22 injections in just two days. After she returned home, she was highly anxious. Her mother reported:

> She follows me everywhere! I can't even go to the bathroom alone. She wakes up screaming five or six times at night, shaking and crying, 'The nurses are giving me shots! I can't run away! They're tying me down' ... and when I approach her, she backs away and shakes like a hurt puppy! (Ramsey 1982, p. 332)

Sara's hospital experience was very traumatic. Subsequently, she seemed to be afraid that if she was separated from her mother, she would again be left alone and unprotected.

Preschoolers do not yet think very logically and, as a result, may have many misconceptions about their health problems and why things happen in the hospital (Carson, Gravey & Council 1992; Eiser 1985; Ramsey 1982; Smith & Autman 1985). They may, for example, believe their illnesses or the treatments they receive are punishments for having been bad. These ideas probably come from two sources: (1) young children's general belief that breaking rules leads to inevitable punishment, and (2) adults' statements that link disobedience with getting sick or injured — such as, 'You'll catch cold if you don't wear your coat,' 'You'll fall and hurt yourself if you climb trees' or 'You'll get an upset stomach if you eat too many lollies.' Some adults even threaten children with going to the doctor or having an operation if they continue to disobey (Eiser 1985). In the hospital, young children sometimes become worried by seeing other patients with disfigurements, such as an amputation or extensive scars. These children may think one of these conditions may happen to themselves in the hospital. As a result, many young children have greater difficulty coping with medical procedures and adjusting to hospitalisation (Manne et al. 1993; Carson, Gravley & Council 1992).

Hospitalised school-age children

Advances in school-age children's psychosocial development enable them to cope with some aspects of hospitalisation better than younger patients can. For instance, although prolonged separation from their parents can be difficult for older children, they can usually tolerate it more easily than preschoolers can. The cognitive ability of school-age children progresses rapidly, but they sometimes retain earlier misconceptions about their illnesses or develop new ones. An older child's incorrect ideas can be seen in a nursing student's report about a 10-year-old haemophiliac patient.

> When I asked him what happened when he bled, he said, 'Oh . . . there's a hemophiliac bug eating his way in and out of my blood vessels, and that's what makes me bleed.' And when asked what caused his disease, he answered, 'Well, it's 'cause I ate too much candy after my mom told me not to.' (Ramsey 1982, pp. 335–6)

Clearly, the idea that illness is a punishment can continue long after early childhood.

Four aspects of hospitalisation seem to become increasingly difficult for children as they get older (Ramsey 1982; Smith & Autman 1985). One aspect relates to their feelings of personal control. As children get older and their greater cognitive and social abilities strengthen their sense of control, the limited independence and influence they experience in the hospital may become very irritating and distressing. Second, the increased cognitive abilities of school-age children allow them to think about and worry about the outcomes of their illness or treatment, such as whether they will be physically harmed or even die. Third, being away from friends and schoolmates can lead to feelings of loneliness, boredom, and concern about losing friends or status in their social groups. Fourth, as children get older — particularly when they are entering puberty — they tend to become more embarrassed by exposing their bodies to strangers or needing help with 'private' activities, such as toileting.

Helping children cope with being hospitalised

Studies conducted in industrialised nations in the 1950s revealed that most children who were hospitalised were very poorly prepared for the experience (Eiser 1985). Perhaps three-quarters of them, for instance, either were told nothing about why they were there, or received only vague reasons, or learned why by overhearing others' conversations. This situation has changed since then, and children today are much better prepared for stays in the hospital (La Greca & Stone 1985), although there is still room for improvement. As recently as 1995 a survey of Victorian hospitals found that only four hospitals offered formal preparation programs for children and their families. While 90 per cent of hospitals offered informal hospital preparation, this related mostly to procedural information in the form of brochures, hospital tours and visits to schools by hospital staff (Whelan & Kirkby 1995).

Ideally, psychological preparation should begin before the child enters the hospital, if possible. Research has shown that children cope better with medical procedures if their parents give them information about their illnesses and treatment and try to allay their fears than if the parents do not (Kirkby & Whelan 1996; Melamed 1993;

Melamed & Bush 1985). Parents can help their child cope with an impending hospital stay in several ways (Sarafino 1986). They can:

- explain the reason for the stay and what it will be like
- give the child opportunities to ask questions, answering them carefully and in a way he or she can understand
- read with the child a children's book that describes a child's hospital experience
- take the child to the hospital and explain some of the hospital routines, such as what to do about going to the bathroom and how he or she will be woken in the morning and have breakfast in bed
- describe when the parents will be with the child
- maintain a calm and confident manner, thereby conveying the message that there is no need to be very frightened.

Parents who appear highly agitated and anxious about their child's welfare before medical treatment seem to transmit their fear and be unable to allay their child's anxiety effectively. Studies have found that children with highly anxious parents do not cope as well with medical procedures as those with parents who are relatively calm (Bush et al. 1986; Fosson, Martin & Haley 1990; Mabe, Treiber & Riley 1991; Melamed & Bush 1985). Children of anxious parents tend to be less cooperative with medical staff and show increased anxiety (Fosson, Martin & Haley 1990; Mabe, Treiber & Riley 1991). However, parental behaviours alone do not account for poor adjustment to hospitalisation by children. In addition to parent behaviours, the temperament of the child seems to determine how well the child responds to medical procedures. Non-involvement by mothers the day before surgery has been found to increase distress during anaesthetic induction only in those children previously rated as having a temperament of 'adapting poorly to change' (Lumley et al. 1990). Similarly, maternal distraction was associated with less distress in children only if they tended to withdraw from stressors rather than having a less avoidant response style.

When the child is admitted to hospital, one or both of the parents (or another very familiar adult) should accompany and remain with the child at least until he or she is settled in. Many parents stay much longer, taking advantage of opportunities hospitals provide today for a parent to 'room in' with the child, especially when the patient is very young or very seriously ill (Olivet 1982).

In the United States, most paediatric hospitals also provide psychological preparation for their patients (Melamed & Bush 1985). This is the preferred situation and one that Australian hospitals should adopt. Research has shown that paediatric counselling (incorporating procedural information, sensory information and coping skills) prior to surgery can have beneficial effects in terms of reducing anxiety and fear in children and parents. Therapeutic play techniques such as use of puppets, dramatic play and art can be used to assess whether children have understood what will happen to them during surgery, and whether further preparation is required (Abbott 1990).

What kinds of psychological preparation do hospitals provide? Basically, four approaches have been used, all of which are designed to furnish information to the parents and/or the child (Eiser 1985). One approach simply involves distributing leaflets to the parents to share with the child. The leaflets contain information about hospital routines and medical procedures the child is likely to experience. In another approach, hospital personnel discuss the routines and procedures with the parents and child. Often this is done at home, before admission. The third method involves using puppets in a play activity to demonstrate medical procedures, such as surgery or cardiac catheterisation. This approach may be especially appropriate for preschoolers and younger school-age children. These three methods are probably the approaches most commonly used by hospitals to help children cope with medical procedures (La Greca & Stone 1985).

The fourth approach uses a video or film presentation. This method was evaluated in an experiment by Barbara Melamed and Lawrence Siegel (1975) with 4- to 12-year-old children who were in the hospital for elective surgery, such as for hernias or tonsillectomies. The researchers assigned the children to two groups, matching the subjects for age, sex, race and type of operation. One group saw a film that was relevant to having surgery, and the other group saw a film about a boy who goes on a nature trip in the country. The relevant film, entitled *Ethan Has an Operation*, portrays the hospital experience of a seven-year-old boy,

> showing various events that most children encounter when hospitalised for elective surgery from the time of admission to time of discharge including the child's orientation to the hospital ward and medical personnel such as the surgeon and anaesthesiologist; having a blood test and exposure to standard hospital equipment; separation from the mother; and scenes in the operating and recovery rooms. In addition to explanations of the hospital procedures provided by the medical staff, various scenes are narrated by the child, who describes his feelings and concerns. (Melamed & Siegel 1975, p. 514)

Although Ethan exhibits visible apprehension initially, he overcomes his fear and has the operation without serious distress.

To assess the emotional adjustment of the children in the two groups the evening before surgery and at a follow-up visit about three weeks after the operation, the researchers used three types of measures: the children's hand sweating, questionnaire self-reports of fear and ratings of their emotional behaviour by trained observers. The results with all three measures revealed that the children who saw the film about Ethan's operation experienced less anxiety before and after surgery than those who saw the irrelevant film. Several studies have found similar benefits in reducing children's medical fears with video presentations (Eiser 1985; Miller & Green 1984). What's more, video preparations for surgery are cost-effective: A study of children in the hospital for elective surgery found that those who received video preparation recovered more quickly than those who did not. The savings from being released from the hospital sooner amounted to several times the cost of providing the preparation (Pinto & Hollandsworth 1989).

Although most children benefit from information about impending medical procedures presented by any of the methods we have considered, not all children do — and some are actually made *more* anxious by the preparation. Studies have shown that the effects of the preparation depend on its timing and on the child's age, coping style and previous medical experience (Dahlquist et al. 1986; Melamed & Bush 1985; Melamed, Dearborn & Hermecz 1983; Miller & Green 1984). More specifically, children younger than age seven or so seem to profit from information presented shortly before the medical procedure, whereas older children are more likely to benefit from information presented several days before. Young children more than older ones may be made more anxious by information if they have had prior difficult experiences with medical procedures (Carson, Council & Gravley 1991). Also, some evidence indicates that children who tend to use avoidance strategies to cope with stressful events probably derive less benefit from information about medical procedures than those who use attention strategies.

Hospitals and medical workers usually try to make a child's stay as pleasant as they can. Paediatric nurses, for instance, receive training in the special needs of children and ways to introduce tests and equipment in a non-threatening manner (Ramsey 1982). When preparing to take the child's blood pressure with a sphygmomanometer, for example, the nurse might demonstrate its use on someone else and say, 'When I squeeze this ball, the thing on the arm just becomes tight, like a belt. It doesn't hurt — it just gets tight. . . . Now when I'm done, I make it get loose and take it off.' Often when a young child undergoes stressful procedures, such as drawing blood, a parent is present. Although most techniques parents use to help reduce the child's distress don't work very well, one that does involves distracting attention from the procedure — for instance by saying, 'Look at this nice picture' (Manne et al. 1992, 1994). But distraction is beneficial in coping with only certain phases of medical procedures, namely during the anticipatory phase. Children respond with less distress during painful procedures if parents encourage focused breathing rather than distracting the child (Blount, Sturges & Powers 1990). Hospital paediatric wards also arrange for children to play together when possible and try to have entertainment, such as a clown show, for their patients. For most hospitalised children who have positive health outcomes today, the stress of their hospital experience tends to be temporary and does not seem to produce serious long-term emotional problems (Thompson & Vernon 1993).

People of all ages can have difficulty coping with hospitalisation and medical procedures. Some of the patients' concerns may relate to factors outside the hospital, for example their family (Peterson, Beck & Rowell 1992). Parents of young children may worry about their children's safety while they are hospitalised. If undergoing major surgery, parents may worry that the surgery will not be successful, or that they may die. Patients may also worry that their medical conditions may interfere with work and providing for their families. Older patients may be concerned about post-operative pain and the possibility of incapacitation. Research has found that when patients are provided with the opportunity to discuss their concerns, receive sensory and procedural information about what to expect, and are taught how they can facilitate recuperation, they experience less anxiety, use less pain medication, recover faster and are discharged earlier (Schmitt & Wooldridge 1973). Psychological interventions can help promote positive emotional adjustment among patients and reduce the psychological problems that may be associated with their medical conditions.

How health psychologists assist hospitalised patients

Some patients in hospitals have illnesses that result partly from psychosocial factors, such as Type A behaviour or alcohol abuse, and some individuals develop psychosocial problems because of their illnesses, hospitalisations or treatment regimens. In the former case, health psychologists are interested in correcting the factors that produced the disease to help these patients recover and prevent recurrences of their illnesses. In the latter case, health psychologists try to help clients cope with their illnesses, treatment regimens, possible disabilities or deformities, and, for terminal conditions, with impending death. The potential importance of the help psychologists provide can be seen in research findings on psychological depression in cardiovascular disease patients: Compared with patients who are not depressed, those who are very depressed are much more likely to develop subsequent cardiac problems (Morris 1999).

The number of psychologists working in hospitals in Australia and their role in treatment programs for patients have expanded greatly since the 1980s (Owen & Oldenburg 1992). Psychologists:

- consult with patients' specialists, such as cardiologists, neurologists and paediatricians, to provide diagnostic and counselling services
- assess clients' needs for, and provide, psychological preparation to cope with surgery and other stressful procedures
- help patients adhere to medication and treatment regimens in the hospital
- provide behavioural programs for improving clients' self-care skills and compliance with medical and lifestyle regimens after discharge
- assist in rehabilitation processes, such as by promoting adherence to physical therapy, helping family members adjust to a patient's condition, and helping clients decide on new careers, if needed.

Let's look at how health psychologists assist patients, beginning with determining who needs and wants help.

Initial steps in helping

Patients who need psychological help generally don't request it themselves — the request usually comes from a doctor or nurse who has noticed signs of a psychological, social or intellectual problem (Huszti & Walker 1991). This is not an ideal situation, since most medical staff are not trained to identify signs of distress or behavioural problems. A study found that doctors are not very good at recognising emotional problems in their clients — they tend to judge that such problems exist if they think the patient has a severe medical illness and is dissatisfied with the present treatment (Jones, Mabe & Riley 1989). A brief training seminar does not improve their judgements (Deshields et al. 1995).

After the psychologist receives the request to see a patient, he or she then consults the person who made the request and reviews the client's medical record. The next step involves interviewing the patient and/or relevant family members to arrive at an impression of what the problem is and its history and status (Sweet 1991). Sometimes the resulting impression is sufficient for the psychologist to decide how to help, but frequently more information is needed and can be obtained by administering psychological tests.

Tests for psychological assessment of medical patients

Psychologists have developed hundreds of instruments to assess a wide variety of psychological characteristics of people. *Measures in Health Psychology: A User's Portfolio* (Johnston, Wright & Weinman 1995) is a compendium of measures in health psychology, some of which are specific to medical settings, patient conditions and psychological aspects of illness. Some of these scales are Skevington's (1990) Beliefs about Pain Control Questionnaire; Rosentiel and Keefe's (1983) Pain Coping Strategies Questionnaire; Zigmond and Snaith's (1983) Hospital Anxiety and Depression Scale; Felton and Revenson's (1984) Acceptance of Illness Scale; Marteau's (1990) Attitudes towards Doctors and Medicine Scale; Wolf, Putnam, James and Stiles' (1978) Medical Interview Satisfaction Scale; and Partridge and Johnston's (1989) Recovery Locus of Control Scale.

The tests the psychologist administers depend on the type of illness or problem the patient seems to have (Derogatis et al. 1995; Sweet 1991). For example, patients with serious head injuries and behavioural signs of neurological problems are especially likely to be assessed with tests of intelligence, academic skills, and specific perceptual and motor functions. Clients who will need to change existing or planned careers may be tested for vocational interests and abilities. Some of the most widely used instruments employed to test hospital patients assess their psychosocial needs and problems (Piotrowski & Lubin 1990).

Specialised tests for medical patients

In recent years, psychologists have developed new tests that are specifically designed to assess psychological characteristics associated with physical illness. These tests include instruments such as the Coping with Surgical Stress Scale (Krohne et al. 2000) and other measures we considered in chapters 3 and 4, which assess people's stress and their Type A and Type B behaviour patterns — two characteristics that are frequently associated with heart disease. As we saw in chapter 5, psychological methods can be applied effectively to reduce people's stress and modify their Type A behaviour, thereby lowering their risk of heart attack. We turn now to a discussion of other psychological tests that were designed specifically for medical populations.

The **Millon Behavioral Health Inventory** (MBHI) is a self-report questionnaire that was developed to assess specific psychosocial factors and decision-making issues that are known to be relevant for medical patients (Green 1985; Millon, Green & Meagher 1982). It consists of 150 true/false items that provide health care workers with information regarding the client's:

- *basic coping style*, or the way the person tends to approach difficult life situations and interact with other people.
- *psychogenic attitude*, which includes assessments of the patient's experience of stress, tendency towards helplessness and hopelessness, social support and hypochondriacal tendencies.

The MBHI also attempts to assess the client's reaction to his or her illness and predict difficulties with the treatment regimen. Although the MBHI is being used in a variety of medical settings, such as in pain treatment centres and cancer units, and it should prove to be a valuable tool, more research is needed to establish its utility. Some evidence for its usefulness in medical settings has been found (Gatchel et al. 1986).

The **Psychosocial Adjustment to Illness Scale** (PAIS) is another psychological test designed specifically for use with medical patients (Derogatis 1977, 1986). The PAIS consists of just 46 items, and the person responds to each item on a four-point scale, such as 'not at all,' 'mildly', 'moderately', or 'markedly'. This test is available in two forms — one that patients can fill out on their own and one that is administered by an interviewer. It was designed to assess seven psychosocial characteristics of the client's life, each of which has been associated with adjustment to medical illness. Figure 10.4 outlines these characteristics. The results of several studies appear to confirm the ability of the PAIS to measure adjustment problems accurately in patients with a variety of serious illnesses, such as kidney disease, hypertension and cancer (Derogatis 1986).

In summary, psychologists have begun to develop instruments specifically for the purpose of assessing the psychological needs and problems of medical patients. These tests, and those yet to be developed, offer considerable promise for aiding health psychologists and other health care workers in promoting the health and adjustment of their patients.

Figure 10.4 Patients' psychosocial characteristics assessed by the Psychosocial Adjustment to Illness Scale (PAIS)

- *Health care orientation* — the nature of the patient's attitudes about health care in general, views regarding health care professionals, and expectancies about his or her health problem and its treatment
- *Vocational environment* — the impact of the health problem on such issues as the person's vocational performance and satisfaction
- *Domestic environment* — difficulties the health problem will present for the client and his or her family in the home environment

- *Sexual relationships* — modifications in sexual activity as a result of the health problem.
- *Extended family relationships* — disruptions in relationships between the patient and family members outside of his or her immediate family
- *Social environment* — the impact of the health problem on the client's socialising and leisure-time activities
- *Psychological distress* — the effect of the health problem on such factors as the patient's self-esteem and feelings of depression, anxiety and hostility.

Promoting patients' health and adjustment

Once health psychologists determine the nature and extent of the client's difficulty, they decide which specific therapeutic techniques should be applied to address it. As we have seen in previous chapters, behavioural and cognitive methods have been applied with some degree of success — sometimes with great success — in a wide variety of primary, secondary and tertiary prevention efforts. These techniques are useful in helping people improve their eating and exercise habits, stop smoking and curb their drinking, and reduce the stress and other negative emotional states they experience (Parker 1995; Sarafino 1996; Turk & Salovey 1995). Psychoeducational interventions with a supportive counselling component (Oldenburg, Andrews & Perkins 1985) have likewise been effective in helping patients make the required lifestyle changes. Psychological functioning of patients and recovery can be enhanced through provision of social support (Elizur & Hirsh 1999). Also, as we saw in chapter 9, adherence to treatment is more likely when the patient has a supportive network of family and friends.

Many hospitalised people develop severe psychosocial problems, particularly if their illnesses or injuries continue to be life-threatening or leave them disfigured or handicapped. These individuals and their families often need help to overcome feelings of depression and counselling to anticipate and plan for the difficulties they are likely to experience. As nurse-educator Catherine Norris has noted:

> When someone says, 'I never really got over my operation,' it means that that person has not accomplished the formidable tasks of convalescence. These include reassessment of one's goals in life, reintegration of a changed body image, working out feelings about dependence and independence, and coping with heightened emotional reactions and role failure, as well as making physical adaptations. (1990, p. 47)

Several psychological approaches are helpful in dealing with patients' psychosocial problems. These approaches often involve group-discussion and cognitive-behavioural therapy to identify, examine and replace negative thought patterns with more constructive ones (Davison & Neale 1994; Turk & Salovey 1995).

The approaches health psychologists currently use in promoting patients' health and adjustment sometimes have important limitations, particularly in their continued effectiveness over long periods of time and in preventing relapse, such as in health-related lifestyle changes. Health psychologists are working to enhance their effectiveness in helping clients by improving the techniques they use, but they must also continue to develop stronger relationships with medical professionals, such as by expanding their knowledge of the language and rules of hospital settings (Huszti & Walker 1991). More and more, medical and psychological staff are working together to improve these relationships for the benefit of their patients.

Summary

The huge hospitals of today evolved from institutions in Europe that were established to give help to people with various needs — the sick, the poor, orphans and even travellers who needed lodging. Many of the hospitals in colonial Australia administered care mostly to convicts and the poor. Well-to-do individuals received better care at home. In the early twentieth century, hospitals gained a much better reputation and began to attract patients from all social classes.

The hospital medical staff has a typical hierarchy of authority with physicians at the top, followed by nurses and various allied health workers. Years ago, patients received care from hospital personnel who worked together as a team. Today, the great variety of hospital personnel with different specialisations function more separately, which can lead to fragmented health care. Good communication among hospital personnel not only improves the treatment patients receive but can help protect patients and health care workers from potential hazards in the hospital, such as from toxic substances and nosocomial infection. A number of medical schemes have been introduced by various federal governments since 1945. Medicare allows all eligible Australian citizens access to free medical care and treatment in public hospitals. While the demand for hospitalised care has increased over time, this has not been accompanied by a substantial increase in the availability of hospital beds, and length of stay has likewise decreased.

Being hospitalised is unpleasant because of the disruptions it produces in the patients' lifestyles, the high degree of dependency patients have on others, the experience of aversive medical procedures, and the many worries patients have about their conditions, treatment and futures. Many of these worries develop because patients do not always receive the information they need. Also, sometimes the treatment people receive is characterised by depersonalisation, which may result from practitioners wanting to be efficient in handling heavy work loads or to protect themselves emotionally when patients' conditions worsen. Working in emotionally charged situations can lead to burnout among health care professionals, especially those who spend almost all of their time providing direct care to clients.

Some patients enter hospital with the idea that the sick role involves being passive. These people are generally described by hospital staff as 'good patients', being relatively cooperative, uncomplaining and stoical. Other clients believe they should be more active in their sick-role behaviour. Some of these people are described as 'problem patients', showing little cooperation, voicing many complaints, and being very dependent and emotional. When problem patients are very seriously ill, their difficult behaviour is usually understandable to the medical staff. But other problem patients take up more time and attention than their conditions seem to warrant, and may display angry reactance behaviour in response to having their freedoms or control curtailed. Patients and practitioners contribute to the relationship they develop with each other in the hospital. Patient satisfaction with the hospitalisation experience appears to depend on three factors — the overall process of care; improvement in, and understanding of health; and psychological wellbeing.

Patients engage in problem-focused and emotion-focused coping techniques to adjust to the stress and anxiety they experience in hospital. Some of their anxiety stems from their impending surgery and from non-surgical medical procedures, such as cardiac catheterisation and endoscopy. High levels of anxiety before surgery, for instance, appear to impair people's physical recovery after the operation. Reducing the anxiety connected with medical procedures can be accomplished through methods of psychological preparation that provide clients with behavioural, cognitive and informational control. Lamaze training for childbirth seems to provide these kinds of preparation.

Although most patients benefit from methods of psychological preparation that enhance control, some benefit more than others. One factor that seems to affect the success of these methods is whether the patient's coping style tends towards avoidance rather than attention strategies. Children's separation distress in the hospital can be reduced if parents visit often or room in. Children can also benefit from psychological preparation for medical procedures, but the success of providing children with information depends on its timing and on their ages, coping styles and previous medical experience.

The role of psychologists in the overall treatment effort for hospitalised people has increased in recent years, particularly in preparing clients for surgery and other medical procedures, helping them adjust to their medical conditions, and enhancing their adherence to treatment regimens after discharge. To identify the needs and problems of patients, psychologists use personality tests and instruments developed specifically for use with medical clients, such as the Millon Behavioral Health Inventory and the Psychosocial Adjustment to Illness Scale.

Key terms

burnout	Lamaze training	nosocomial infection	reactance
depersonalisation	Millon Behavioral Health Inventory	Psychosocial Adjustment to Illness Scale	separation distress
diagnostic related group			

PART 5

Physical symptoms: pain and discomfort

11 The nature and symptoms of pain

Prologue

'Wouldn't it be wonderful never to experience pain,' many people have thought when they or others they have known were suffering. Pain hurts, and people typically dislike it and try to avoid it. But being able to sense pain is critical to our survival — without it, how would we know when we are injured? We could have a sprained ankle or an ulcer, for instance, without realising it, and not seek treatment. And how would we know we are about to be injured, such as when we approach a hot flame without seeing it? Pain serves as a signal to take protective action.

Are there people who do not feel pain? Yes — several disorders can reduce or eliminate the ability to sense pain. People with a condition called *congenital insensitivity to pain*, which is present from birth, may report only a 'tingling' or 'itching' sensation when seriously injured. A young woman with this disorder

> seemed normal in every way, except that she had never felt pain. As a child she had bitten off the tip of her tongue while chewing food, and had suffered third-degree burns after kneeling on a hot radiator to look out of a window. When examined by a psychologist ... in the laboratory, she reported that she did not feel pain when noxious stimuli were presented. She felt no pain when parts of her body were subjected to strong electric shock, to hot water at temperatures that usually produce reports of burning pain, or to a prolonged ice-bath. Equally astonishing was the fact that she showed no changes in blood pressure, heart rate, or respiration when these stimuli were presented. Furthermore, she could not remember ever sneezing or coughing, the gag reflex could be elicited only with great difficulty, and the cornea reflexes (to protect the eyes) were absent. (Melzack, quoted in Bakal 1979, p. 141)

This disorder contributed to her death at the age of 29. People with congenital insensitivity to pain often die young because injuries or illnesses, such as acute appendicitis, go unnoticed (Chapman 1984; Manfredi et al. 1981).

Health psychologists study pain because it influences whether individuals seek and comply with medical treatment and because being in pain can be very stressful, particularly when it is intense or enduring. In this chapter we examine the nature and symptoms of pain, and the effects it has on its victims when it is severe. As we consider these topics, you will find answers to questions you may have about pain. What is pain, and what is the physical basis for it? Can people feel pain when there is no underlying physical disorder? Do psychosocial factors affect our experience of pain? Since pain is a subjective experience, how do psychologists assess how much pain a person feels?

What is pain?

Pain is the sensory and emotional experience of discomfort, which is usually associated with actual or threatened tissue damage or irritation (Sanders 1985). Virtually all people experience pain and at all ages — from the pains of birth for mother and baby, to those of colic and teething in infancy, to those of injury and illness in childhood and adulthood. Some pain becomes chronic, as with arthritis, problems of the lower back, migraine headache or cancer.

People's experience with pain is important for several reasons. For one thing, no medical complaint is more common than pain. According to researcher Paul Karoly, pain is the 'most pervasive symptom in medical practice, the most frequently stated "cause" of disability, and the single most compelling force underlying an individual's choice to seek or avoid medical care' (1985, p. 461). As we saw in chapter 9, people are more likely to seek medical treatment without delay if they feel pain. Also, severe and prolonged pain can come to dominate the lives of its victims, impairing their general functioning, ability to work, social relationships and emotional adjustment. Last, pain has enormous social and economic effects on all societies of the world. Headaches were the most commonly reported illness condition in the most recent National Health Survey in Australia (ABS 1996b), and back pain is Australia's greatest cause of workers' compensation claims and work time lost each year (Ganora 1986). It has been estimated that the economic costs of severe pain, including lost productivity, welfare payments and compensation, are potentially the highest for any health problem, costing Australia $30 billion per year (Presley & Cousins 1992).

The qualities and dimensions of pain

Our sensations of pain can be quite varied and have many different qualities. We might describe some pains as 'sharp' and others as 'dull', for example — and sharp pains can have either a stabbing or a pricking feel. Some pains involve a burning sensation; others have a cramping, itching or aching feel. Some pains are throbbing, or constant, or shooting, or pervasive, or localised. Often the feelings we experience depend on the kinds of irritation or damage that has occurred and its location. For instance, when damage occurs deep within the body, individuals usually report feeling a 'dull' or 'aching' pain; but damage produced by a brief noxious event to the skin is often described as 'sharp' (McClintic 1985; Schiffman 1976).

The painful conditions people experience also differ according to the origin of the pain and the duration of the conditions. We will consider two dimensions that describe these differences, beginning with the degree to which the origin of the pain can be traced to existing tissue damage.

Organic versus psychogenic pain

People who suffer physical injuries, such as a serious burn, experience pain that is clearly related to tissue damage. When discomfort is caused mainly by tissue damage, it is described as *organic pain*. For other pains, no tissue damage appears to exist — at least, medical examinations fail to find an organic basis. The discomfort involved in these pains seems to result primarily from psychological processes. For this reason, this type of discomfort is described as *psychogenic pain*. Extreme examples of psychogenic pain are sometimes seen in the hallucinations of psychotic individuals: I once talked with a schizophrenic man who claimed — and *really* looked like — he was 'feeling' the stings from being 'shot by enemy agents with ray guns'.

Not long ago, researchers considered organic and psychogenic pain to be separate entities, with psychogenic pain not involving 'real' sensations. As pain researcher Donald Bakal has noted, a practitioner's reference to pain as 'psychogenic'

> was taken to mean 'due to psychological causes,' which implied that the patient was 'imagining' his pain or that it was not really pain simply because an organic basis could not be found. Psychogenic pain is not experienced differently, however, from that arising from physical disease or injury. Psychogenic and organic pain both hurt. (1979, p. 167)

Researchers now recognise that virtually all pain experiences involve an interplay of both physiological and psychological factors. As a result, the dimension of pain involving organic and psychogenic causes is viewed as a continuum rather than a dichotomy. Different pain experiences simply involve different mixtures of organic and psychogenic factors. A mixture of these factors seems clear in, for example, cases of migraine, the pain of which results from distended cranial arteries, which can be triggered by a variety of factors, the most common being stress (Martin 1993). But some pain patients experience chronic discomfort for which no physical basis can be detected. Psychiatrists call this condition *pain disorder* (classified within *somatoform disorders*) and often assume the origin is mainly psychogenic (Davison & Neale 1994). Keep in mind, however, that failing to find a physical basis for someone's pain does not necessarily mean there is none. Unfortunately, many health care workers still think pain that has no demonstrated physical basis is purely psychogenic, and their patients struggle to prove that 'the pain isn't just in my head, Doc' (Karoly 1985).

Acute versus chronic pain

Experiencing pain either continuously or frequently over a period of many months or years is different from having occasional and isolated short-term bouts with pain. The length of experience an individual has had with a painful condition is an important dimension in describing his or her pain.

Most of the painful conditions people experience are temporary — the pain arrives and then subsides in a matter of minutes, days or even weeks, often with the aid of pain-killers or other treatments prescribed by a doctor. If a similar painful condition occurs in the future, it is not connected in a direct way to the earlier experience. This is the case for most everyday headaches, for instance, and for the pain typically produced by such conditions as toothaches, muscle strains, accidental wounds and surgery.

Acute pain refers to the discomfort people experience with temporary painful conditions that last less than six months or so (Chapman 1991; Turk, Meichenbaum & Genest 1983). Patients with acute pain often have higher than normal levels of anxiety while the pain exists, but their distress subsides as their condition improves and their pain decreases (Fordyce & Steger 1979).

When a painful condition lasts for more than a few months, patients continue to have high levels of anxiety and tend to develop feelings of hopelessness and helplessness because various medical treatments have failed to alleviate their condition. Pain can come to dominate their lives. This is what often happens when pain becomes *chronic*.

> Pain patients frequently say that they could stand their pain much better if they could only get a good night's sleep. . . . They feel worn down, worn out, exhausted. They find themselves getting more and more irritable with their families, they have fewer and fewer friends, and fewer and fewer interests. Gradually, as time goes by, the boundaries of their world seem to shrink. They become more and more preoccupied with their pain, less and less interested in the world around them. Their world begins to center around home, doctor's office, and pharmacy. (Sternbach, quoted in Bakal 1979, p. 165)

People's experience of pain is very different when the condition is chronic than when it is acute. Furthermore, many chronic sufferers leave their jobs for emotional and physical reasons and must live on reduced incomes at the same time that their medical bills are piling up.

People's experience with chronic pain also depends on two factors: (1) whether the underlying condition is *benign* or is *malignant* and worsening, and (2) whether the discomfort exists *continuously* or occurs in frequent and intense *episodes*. Using these factors, Dennis Turk, Donald Meichenbaum and Myles Genest (1983) have described three types of chronic pain.

1. **Chronic/recurrent pain** stems from benign causes and is characterised by repeated and intense episodes of pain separated by periods without pain. Two examples of chronic/recurrent pain are migraine headaches and tension-type headaches; another example is *myofascial pain*, a syndrome that typically involves shooting or radiating, but dull, pain in the muscles and connective tissue of the head and neck, and sometimes the back (Hare & Milano 1985; Turk, Meichenbaum & Genest 1983).

2. **Chronic/intractable/benign pain** refers to discomfort that is typically present all of the time, with varying levels of intensity, and is not related to an underlying malignant condition. Chronic low back pain often follows this pattern.

3. **Chronic/progressive pain** is characterised by continuous discomfort, is associated with a malignant condition and becomes increasingly intense as the underlying condition worsens. Two of the most prominent malignant conditions that frequently produce chronic/progressive pain are rheumatoid arthritis and cancer.

As we shall see later in this chapter and in the next one, the type of pain people experience influences their psychosocial adjustment and the treatment they receive to control their discomfort.

Perceiving pain

Of the several perceptual senses the human body uses, the sense of pain has three important and unique properties (Chapman 1984; Melzack & Wall 1982). First, although nerve fibres in the body sense and send signals of tissue damage, the receptor cells for pain are different from those of other perceptual systems, such as vision. Whereas the visual system contains specific receptor cells that transmit only messages about a particular type of stimulation — light — there are no *specific* receptor cells in the body that transmit *only* information about pain. Second, the body senses pain in response to many types of noxious stimuli, such as physical pressure, lacerations, and intense heat or cold. Third, the perception of pain almost always includes a strong emotional component. As we are about to see, perceiving pain involves a complex interplay of physiological and psychological processes.

The physiology of pain perception

To describe the physiology of perceiving pain, we will trace the bodily reaction to tissue damage, as when the body receives a cut or burn. The noxious stimulation instantly triggers chemical activity at the site of injury, releasing chemicals called **algogenic substances** that exist naturally in the tissue (Chapman 1984). These chemicals — which include *serotonin*, *histamine* and *bradykinin* — function to promote immune system activity, cause inflammation at the injured site and activate endings of nerve fibres in the damaged region, signalling injury.

The signal of injury is transmitted by afferent neurons of the peripheral nervous system to the spinal cord, which carries the signal to the brain. The afferent nerve endings in a damaged region of the body that respond to pain stimuli and signal injury are called **nociceptors** (AMA 1989; Chapman 1984; Tortora & Grabowski 1993). These fibres

> have no special structure for detecting injury; they are simply free nerve endings. They may be found in skin, blood vessels, subcutaneous tissue, muscle, ... joints, and other structures. When activated, these end organs, like other receptors, generate impulses that are transmitted along peripheral fibres to the central nervous system. (Chapman 1984, p. 1261)

There are several types of afferent peripheral fibres, and pain signals are carried by only two types: A-delta and C fibres. *A-delta fibres* are coated with myelin, a fatty substance that enables neurons to transmit impulses very quickly. These fibres are associated with sharp, well-localised and distinct pain experiences. *C fibres* transmit impulses more slowly — because they are not coated with myelin — and seem to be involved in experiences of diffuse dull, burning or aching pain sensations (Bakal 1979; Chapman 1984; Melzack & Wall 1982).

Signals from A-delta and C fibres follow different paths when they reach the brain (Bloom, Lazerson & Hofstadter 1985; Guyton 1985). A-delta signals, which reflect sharp pain, pass through specific areas of the thalamus on their way to motor and sensory areas of the cerebral cortex (refer back to figures 2.3 and 2.4 on pages 47 and 48). This suggests that signals of sharp pain receive special attention in our sensory awareness, probably so that we can respond to them quickly. On the other hand, C fibre signals, which reflect burning or aching pain, terminate mainly in the brainstem and lower portions of the forebrain, such as the limbic system, thalamus and hypothalamus. The remaining C fibre impulses spread to many areas of the brain by connecting with a diffuse network of neurons. Signals of dull pain are less likely to command our immediate attention than those of sharp pain, but are more likely to affect our mood, general emotional state and motivation.

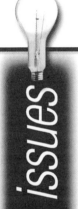

Highlight on issues

Acute pain in burn patients

Almost every day we hear or read about people being seriously burned, such as in a fire or through scalding. Each year in Australia, 66 000 people, including more than 10 000 children under 15 years of age, suffer from burns and scalds (ABS 1996b). A significant proportion of these individuals receive burns that are serious enough to require hospitalisation, and these people suffer acute pain both from their injuries and from the treatment procedures that must be performed.

Medical workers describe the severity of a burn on the basis of its location and with two measures of its damage (Pillitteri 1981). One measure estimates the amount of skin *area* affected in terms of the percentage of the body surface burned; the other assesses the *depth* of the burn, expressed in three 'degrees':

1. *First-degree burns* involve damage restricted to the epidermis, or outermost layer of skin. The skin turns red, but does not blister — as, for example, in most cases of sunburn.

2. *Second-degree burns* are those that include damage to the dermis, the layer below the epidermis. These burns are quite painful, often form blisters, and can result from scalding and fire.

3. *Third-degree burns* destroy the epidermis and dermis down to the underlying layer of fat, and may extend to the muscle and bone. These burns usually result from fire. Because the nerve endings are generally damaged in third-degree burns, there is generally no pain sensation in these regions initially.

Practitioners assess the depth of a burn by its appearance and the sensitivity of the region to pain.

Hospital treatment for patients with severe burns progresses through three phases (Wernick 1983; Winters 1985). The first few days after the burn is called the *emergency phase*, during which medical staff assess the severity of the burn and work to maintain the patient's body functions and defences, such as in preventing infection and keeping a balance of fluids and electrolytes. The acute phase extends from the end of the emergency phase until the burned area is covered with new skin. This process can take from several days to several months, depending on the severity of the burn. The pain is constant during most or all of this phase, particularly when nerve endings begin to regenerate in third-degree burns. Suffering is generally

> greatest during 'tankings,' in which the patient is lowered on a stretcher into a large tub. The old dressings are removed and the patient is gently scrubbed to remove encrusted medication. Debridement, which is usually necessary during the early weeks of hospitalization, involves the vigorous cutting away of dead tissue in burned areas. The process, which may last for more than an hour and involve several people working on different parts of the body simultaneously, ends when fresh medication and new dressings are applied. (Wernick 1983, p. 196)

These and many other painful medical procedures occur very frequently, and burn patients must also do exercises for physical or occupational therapy. Last, the *rehabilitation phase* begins at about the time of discharge from the hospital and continues until the scar tissue has matured. Although the pain has now subsided, itching in the healed area (which should not be scratched) can be a source of discomfort, as can using devices and doing exercises to prevent scarring and contractures (skin shrinkage that can restrict the person's range of motion).

Analgesic medication is the main approach for controlling acute pain in the hospital (Kanner 1986). But psychological approaches can also help burn patients cope with their pain so that they need less medication. Robert Wernick (1983) used a program of psychological preparation with adult severe-burn patients. This preparation was designed to enhance the patients' sense of informational, behavioural and cognitive control over their discomfort, especially with regard to the tanking and debridement procedures. Although these patients were not specifically asked to reduce their use of drugs, they subsequently requested much less medication than patients in a comparison (control) group who received the standard hospital preparation. Similar preparation methods have also been successful with children (Tarnowski, Rasnake & Drabman 1987).

So far, the description we have given of physiological reactions to tissue damage makes it seem as though the process of perceiving pain is rather straightforward. But it actually isn't. One phenomenon that complicates the picture is that pains originating from internal organs are often perceived as coming from other parts of the body, usually near the surface of the skin. This is called **referred pain** (AMA 1989; Melzack & Wall 1982; McClintic 1985). The pain people experience in a heart attack provides one of the most widely known examples of this phenomenon: the pain is referred to the shoulders, the pectoral area of the chest and the arms. Other examples of referred pain include:

- pain perceived to be in the shoulder that results from inflammation of the diaphragm
- pain in the upper-middle abdomen during the first stages of appendicitis (the appendix is deep in the lower right side)
- pain in the ear or in the wrong area of the mouth that results from a toothache.

Referred pain results when sensory impulses from an internal organ and the skin use the same pathway in the spinal cord (AMA 1989; Tortora & Grabowski 1993). Because people are more familiar with sensations from the skin than from internal organs, they tend to perceive the spinal cord impulses as coming from the skin. Another issue that complicates our understanding of pain perception is that people feel pains that have no apparent physical basis, as the next section discusses.

Pain without apparent physical basis

Some pains people experience are quite mysterious, since they occur for no apparent 'reason' — for instance, no noxious stimulus is present. Most of these pain experiences belong to one of three syndromes: neuralgia, causalgia or phantom limb pain. These syndromes often begin with tissue damage, such as from an injury, but the pain (1) persists long after healing is complete, (2) may spread and increase in intensity, and (3) may become stronger than the pain experienced with the initial damage (AMA 1989; Melzack & Wall 1982).

Neuralgia is an extremely painful syndrome in which the patient experiences recurrent episodes of intense shooting or stabbing pain along the course of a nerve (AMA 1989; Chapman 1984; Melzack & Wall 1982). In one form of this syndrome called *trigeminal neuralgia*, excruciating spasms of pain occur along the trigeminal nerve that projects throughout the face. Episodes of neuralgia occur very suddenly and without any apparent cause. Curiously, attacks of neuralgia can be provoked more readily by innocuous stimuli than by noxious ones. For instance, drawing a cotton ball across the skin can trigger an attack, but a pin prick does not.

Another mysterious pain syndrome is *causalgia*, which is characterised by recurrent episodes of severe burning pain (AMA 1989; Melzack & Wall 1982; Weisenberg 1977). A patient with causalgia might report, for instance, that the pain feels 'like my arm is pressed against a hot stove'. In this syndrome, the pain feels as though it originates in a region of the body where the patient had at some earlier time been seriously wounded, such as by a gunshot or stabbing. Curiously, only a small minority of severely wounded patients develop causalgia — but for those who do, the pain persists long after the wound has healed and damaged nerves have regenerated. Episodes of causalgia often occur spontaneously and

> may take minutes or hours to subside, but may occur repeatedly each day for years after the injury. The frequency and intensity of the spontaneous pain-attacks may increase over the years, and the pain may even spread to distant areas of the body. (Melzack, quoted in Bakal 1979, p. 142)

Like neuralgia, attacks of causalgia can be triggered by minor stimuli, such as a gentle touch or a puff of air.

Phantom limb pain is an especially puzzling phenomenon because the patient — an amputee or someone whose peripheral nervous system is irreparably damaged — feels pain in a limb that either is no longer there or has no functioning nerves (AMA 1989; Chapman 1984; Melzack & Wall 1982). After an amputation, for instance, most patients claim to have sensations of their limb still being there — such as by feeling it 'move' — and most of these individuals report feeling pain, too (Katz & Melzack 1990). Phantom limb pain generally persists for months or years, can be quite severe and sometimes resembles the pain produced by the injury that required the amputation. Although the pain tends to decrease over time, it sometimes gets worse (Bakal 1979). Individuals with phantom limb pain may experience either recurrent or continuous pain and may describe it as shooting, burning or cramping. For example, many patients who feel pain in a phantom hand report sensing that the hand is tightly clenched and its fingernails are digging into the palm.

Why do people feel pain when no noxious stimulation is present? Perhaps the answer relates to the neural damage that precedes the development of causalgia and phantom limb pain — and perhaps even neuralgia involves neural damage, albeit of a less obvious nature, such as from infection (Hare & Milano 1985). But then why is it that the large majority of patients who suffer obvious neural damage do not develop these curious pain syndromes? Although the puzzle is far from being solved, the explanation will almost surely involve both physiological and psychological factors.

The role of the 'meaning' of pain

Some people evidently like pain — at least under some, usually sexual, circumstances — and are described as *masochists*. For them, the meaning of pain seems to be different from what it is for most people. Some psychologists believe individuals may come to like pain through classical conditioning — that is, by participating in or viewing activities that associate pain with pleasure in a sexual context (Wincze 1977). Most of the evidence for the view that the meaning of pain can change by its association with pleasure comes from research with animals. For example, Ivan Pavlov (1927) demonstrated that dogs' negative reaction to aversive stimuli, such as electric shocks or skin pricks, changed if the stimuli repeatedly preceded presentation of food. Eventually, the dogs would try to approach the aversive stimuli, which now signalled that food, not danger, was coming.

Physician Henry Beecher (1956) described a dramatic example of how the meaning of pain affects people's experience of it. During World War II he had examined soldiers who had recently been very seriously wounded and were in a field hospital for treatment. Of these men, only 49 per cent claimed to be in 'moderate' or 'severe' pain and only 32 per cent requested medication when asked if they 'wanted something to relieve it'. Some years later, Beecher conducted a similar examination — this time with civilian men who had just undergone surgery. Although the surgical wounds were in the same body regions as those of the soldiers, the soldiers' wounds had been more extensive. Nevertheless, 75 per cent of the civilians claimed to be in 'moderate' or 'severe' pain and 83 per cent requested medication. (The pain-killers used for the soldiers and civilians were narcotics.)

Why did the soldiers — who had more extensive wounds — perceive less pain than the civilians? Beecher described the meaning the injuries had for the soldiers.

> the men studied had been subjected to almost uninterrupted fire for weeks. Notable in this group of soldiers was their optimistic, even cheerful, state of mind. ... They thought the war was over for them and that they would soon be well enough to be sent home. It is not difficult to understand their relief on being delivered from this area of danger. The battlefield wound marked the end of disaster for them. (1956, p. 1069)

For the civilian surgical patients, however, the wound marked the *start* of a personal disaster and their condition represented a major disruption in their lives.

We discussed in chapter 9 how people's perceptions of body sensations are influenced by cognitive, social and emotional factors — for instance, they are less likely to notice pain when they are distracted by competing environmental stimuli, such as while participating in competitive sports. Psychological factors play an important role in perceiving pain, and theories of pain need to take these factors into account.

Theories of pain

You have probably seen demonstrations in which hypnotised people were instructed that they would not feel pain — they were then pricked by a pin and did not react. When people under hypnosis do not react to noxious stimulation, do they still perceive the pain — only 'it doesn't matter' to them? Similarly, do patients who seem relaxed while under the influence of pain-killers actually perceive their pain? Some theories of pain would answer 'yes' to these questions (Karoly 1985). Let's look at two of these theories as we begin to examine how to explain pain perception.

Early theories of pain

In the early 1900s the dominant theories of pain took a very mechanistic view of pain perception, proposing that if a receptor is activated by an appropriate stimulus, the signal travels to the spinal cord and then the brain, and sensation results (Melzack & Wall 1965, 1982; Schneider & Tarshis 1975; Weisenberg 1977). *Specificity theory* argued, for example, that the body has a separate sensory system for perceiving pain — just as it does for hearing and vision — and this system contains its own special receptors for detecting pain stimuli, its own peripheral nerves and pathway to the brain, and its own area of the brain for processing pain signals. But this structure is not correct.

Another view of pain, called *pattern theory*, proposed that there is no separate system for perceiving pain, and the receptors for pain are shared with other senses, such as of touch. According to this view, people feel pain when certain patterns of neural activity occur, such as when appropriate types of activity reach excessively high levels in the brain. These patterns occur only with intense stimulation. Because strong and mild stimuli of the same sense modality produce different patterns of neural activity, being hit hard feels painful, but being caressed does not.

None of the early theories adequately explained pain perception (Melzack & Wall 1982). Pattern theory has been criticised because it requires that the stimuli triggering pain must be intense. Thus, it cannot account for the fact that innocuous stimuli can trigger episodes of causalgia and neuralgia. Perhaps the most serious problem with the early theories is that they do not attempt to explain why the experience of pain is affected by psychological factors, such as the person's ideas about the meaning of pain, beliefs about the likelihood of pain, and attention to (or distraction from) noxious events. Partly because these theories overlook the role of psychological factors, they incorrectly predict that a person must feel just as much pain when hypnotised as when not hypnotised, even though he or she does not show it. Research findings indicate that people who are instructed not to feel pain actually do feel less pain when deeply hypnotised than when in the normal waking state (Hilgard & Hilgard 1983).

The gate-control theory of pain

In the 1960s Ronald Melzack and Patrick Wall (1965, 1982) introduced the **gate-control theory** of pain perception. This theory integrated useful conceptions from earlier theories and improved on them in several ways, particularly by describing a physiological mechanism by which psychological factors can affect people's experience of pain. As a result, the gate-control theory can account for many phenomena in pain perception that have vexed earlier theorists. For instance, it does not have to predict that hypnotised people must feel noxious stimulation (Karoly 1985).

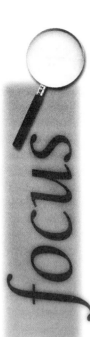

Focus on research
Inducing pain in laboratory research

To conduct an experiment dealing with pain, researchers sometimes need to create a physically painful situation for human subjects. How can they accomplish this in a standard way without harming the subjects? Several approaches have been used safely; two of the more common methods are the *cold-pressor procedure* and the *muscle-ischaemia procedure* (Turk; Meichenbaum & Genest 1983). Let's look at these two methods and research that has used them.

The cold-pressor procedure

The cold-pressor procedure basically involves immersing the subject's hand and forearm in ice water for a few minutes. A special apparatus is used, like the one illustrated in figure 11.1, so that the researcher can maintain a standard procedure across all subjects. The apparatus consists of an armrest mounted on an ice chest filled with water, which is maintained at a temperature of 2°C (35.6°F). Water at this temperature produces a continuous pain that subjects describe as 'aching' or 'crushing'. A pump circulates the water to prevent it from warming in local areas around the arm.

Before using the apparatus, the subject's arm is immersed in a bucket of room-temperature water for one minute. The researcher also explains the cold-pressor procedure, solicits questions and indicates that some temporary discolouration of the arm is common. When the procedure is over and the subject's arm is removed from the apparatus, the researcher notes that the discomfort will decrease rapidly but that it sometimes increases first for a short while (Turk, Meichenbaum & Genest 1983). When using this procedure, the subject's pain may be assessed in several ways, such as by self-ratings or by the length of time he or she is willing to endure the discomfort.

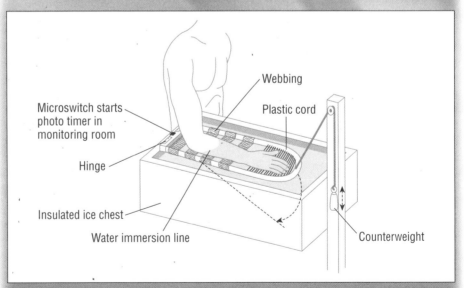

Figure 11.1 Apparatus for the cold-pressor procedure

(*continued*)

An experiment by Michel Girodo and Douglas Wood (1979) used the cold-pressor procedure to examine the role of coping methods on pain perception. The subjects were randomly assigned to several conditions, with each subject undergoing the cold-pressor procedure twice. Before the second procedure, subjects in different groups received different types of training for coping with pain. We will focus on two groups. One group was trained to cope by making positive *self-statements*; they were taught a list of 20 statements, such as, 'No matter how cold it gets, I can handle it,' and 'It's not the worst thing that can happen.' For the other group, training involved the same self-statements, but they also received an *explanation* of how using these statements can enhance their personal control and help them cope with the pain. Immediately after each cold-pressor procedure, the subjects rated their experience of pain on an 11-point scale, ranging from 'no pain felt' to 'worst pain ever felt'. Comparing data from the first and the second procedure revealed that the pain ratings *decreased* for subjects who received the explanation for making the statements and *increased* for those who did not receive the explanation. These results suggest that people's experience of pain may be affected by their beliefs about the purpose of using self-statements.

The muscle-ischaemia procedure

The condition of *ischaemia* — or insufficient blood flow — is an important stimulus for the experience of pain when circulation is blocked in internal organs (AMA 1989). The pain people experience in a heart attack, for instance, results from poor blood flow in the blood vessels to the heart muscle.

The muscle-ischaemia procedure for inducing pain involves reducing blood flow to the muscles of the arm. This is accomplished by wrapping the cuff of a sphygmomanometer (blood pressure testing device) around the arm, inflating it and maintaining the pressure at a high level — 240 mm Hg (Turk, Meichenbaum & Genest 1983). This pressure produces pain without causing damage and can be applied safely for 50 minutes or so. Before the procedure begins, the arm is raised over the subject's head for one minute to drain excess venous blood. The researcher also informs the subject that the procedure is safe and harmless, but that it is uncomfortable and may produce temporary numbness, throbbing, changes in arm temperature, and discolouration of the arm and hand. When the cuff is being removed, the researcher informs the subject that the discomfort will continue for a short while before subsiding. The subject then raises the arm over his or her head (sometimes with the aid of the other arm) to allow blood flow to return gradually and comfortably — a process taking three to five minutes. As with the cold-pressor procedure, measures of muscle-ischaemia pain can include self-ratings and endurance.

Another way to measure muscle-ischaemia pain involves a modification to the procedure we described; that is, the cuff is inflated only to the point at which the subject first reports discomfort. This approach provides an assessment of the individual's pain *threshold*. Researchers used this approach to examine the effects of laughter and relaxation experiences on people's discomfort thresholds (Cogan et al. 1987). In this case, the researchers randomly assigned subjects to four conditions, each involving a different type of experience immediately preceding assessment of discomfort. The *laughter* group listened to a comedy recording by Lily Tomlin, and every subject did in fact laugh out loud; the *relaxation* group listened to a tape designed to induce progressive muscle relaxation; the *narrative* group listened to a tape of a lecture on ethics and sociology; and a control group did not listen to any recording.

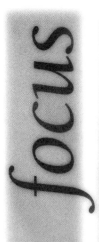

The pain thresholds, or cuff pressures at which subjects reported discomfort, were more than 50 per cent higher for individuals in the laughter and relaxation groups than for those in the narrative and control groups.

Using muscle-ischaemia, cold-pressor and other procedures to induce pain, researchers have found almost no correlation in the thresholds for different types of pain *within* individuals (Janal et al. 1994). This conclusion suggests that most people cannot be characterised as 'stoical' or 'sensitive' to pain in general.

Pain research and ethical standards

When conducting any kind of research with human subjects, psychologists in Australia are obliged to follow the ethical codes of any institutions involved — for example, universities and hospitals, the National Health and Medical Research Council, and the Australian Psychological Society (APS). Some of the guidelines are especially pertinent for research with aversive stimuli. For example, the APS Code of Ethics states that when the research necessarily involves participants in physical or mental stress, the psychologist must inform participants concerning the procedures to be used, and the physical and psychological effects to be expected. No research procedures likely to cause severe distress are permitted under any circumstances. The Code also states that if unexpected stress reactions of significance occur, the psychologist has the responsibility immediately to alleviate such reactions and to terminate the investigation.

If the subjects are children, researchers should also obtain consent for each child's participation from an appropriate guardian, usually a parent.

The gating mechanism

At the heart of the gate-control theory is a neural 'gate' that can be opened or closed to varying degrees, thereby modulating incoming pain signals before they reach the brain. The theory proposes that the *gating mechanism* is located in the spinal cord — more specifically, in the *substantia gelatinosa* of the *dorsal horns*, which are part of the *grey matter* that runs the length of the core of the spinal cord. Figure 11.2 depicts how the gate-control process works. You can see in both diagrams of the figure that signals of noxious stimulation enter the gating mechanism (substantia gelatinosa) of the spinal cord from small-diameter *pain fibres*, A-delta and C fibres. After these signals pass through the gating mechanism, they activate *transmission cells*, which send impulses to the brain. When the output of signals from the transmission cells reaches a critical level, the person perceives pain; the greater the output beyond this level, the greater the pain intensity.

The two diagrams in the figure illustrate how the gating mechanism controls the output of impulses by the transmission cells. When pain signals enter the spinal cord and the gate is open, the transmission cells send impulses freely; but to the extent that the gate is closed, the output of the transmission cells is inhibited. What controls the opening and closing of the gate? The gate-control theory proposes that three factors are involved. These are:

1. *the amount of activity in the pain fibres.* Activity in these fibres tends to open the gate. The stronger the noxious stimulation, the more active the pain fibres.
2. *the amount of activity in other peripheral fibres* — that is, those fibres that carry information about harmless stimuli or mild irritation, such as touching, rubbing or lightly scratching the skin. These are large-diameter fibres called *A-beta fibres*.

Activity in A-beta fibres tends to close the gate, inhibiting the perception of pain when noxious stimulation exists. This would explain why gently massaging or applying heat to sore muscles decreases the pain.

3. *messages that descend from the brain.* Neurons in the brainstem and cortex have efferent pathways to the spinal cord, and the impulses they send can open or close the gate. The effects of some brain processes, such as those in anxiety or excitement, probably have a general impact, opening or closing the gate for *all* inputs from *any* areas of the body. But the impact of other brain processes may be very specific, applying only to some inputs from certain parts of the body. The idea that brain impulses influence the gating mechanism helps to explain why people who are hypnotised or distracted by competing environmental stimuli may not notice the pain of an injury.

The theory proposes that the gating mechanism responds to the combined effects of these three factors. As Melzack and Wall have stated, 'The degree to which the gate increases or decreases sensory transmission is determined by the relative activity in large-diameter (A-beta) and small-diameter (A-delta and C) fibres and by descending influences from the brain' (1982, p. 222). Figure 11.3 presents a wide variety of conditions in people's lives that seem to open or close the gate. For instance, anxiety and boredom are conditions that tend to open the gate, and positive emotions and distraction tend to close it.

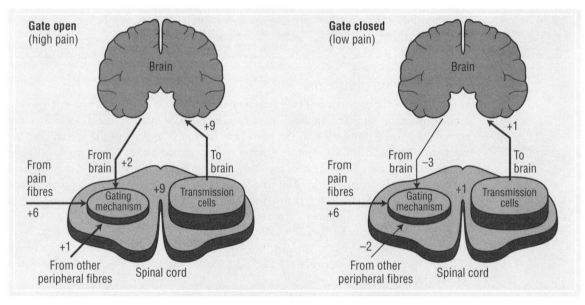

Figure 11.2 Two diagrams to illustrate gate-control theory predictions when strong pain signals arrive from *pain fibres* (A-delta and C) at the spinal cord, along with signals from other *peripheral fibres* (A-beta) and the *brain.* The diagram on the left depicts what conditions might exist when the gate is *open* and the person feels strong pain; the one on the right shows a scenario when the gate is *closed* and the person feels little pain. The thick arrows indicate 'stimulation' conditions that tend to open the gate and send pain signals through, and the thin ones indicate the opposite, 'inhibition' effect. The numbers that accompany each arrow represent hypothetical values for the degrees of pain *stimulation* (positive numbers) or *inhibition* (negative numbers). Pain signals enter the spinal cord and pass through a gating mechanism before activating transmission cells, which send impulses to the brain.

Source: From information in Melzack & Wall (1965, 1982).

Figure 11.3 Conditions that can open or close the pain gate

Conditions that open the gate	Conditions that close the gate

• Physical conditions
  Extent of the injury
  Inappropriate activity level
• Emotional conditions
  Anxiety or worry
  Tension
  Depression
• Mental conditions
  Focusing on the pain
  Boredom; little involvement in life activities
	• Physical conditions
	  Medication
	  Counterstimulation (e.g. heat or massage)
	• Emotional conditions
	  Positive emotions (e.g. happiness or optimism)
	  Relaxation
	  Rest
	• Mental conditions
	  Intense concentration or distraction
	  Involvement and interest in life activities

Source: Based on material by Karol et al., cited in Turk, Meichenbaum & Genest (1983).

Evidence on the gate-control theory

The gate-control theory has stimulated a great deal of research and has received strong support from the findings of many, but not all, of these studies (Melzack & Wall 1982; Winters 1985). One study, for instance, confirmed the prediction from gate-control theory that impulses from the brain can inhibit the perception of pain. David Reynolds (1969) conducted this study with rats as subjects. He first implanted an electrode in the midbrain portion of each rat's brainstem, varying the exact location from one rat to the next. Then he made sure they could feel pain by applying a clamp to their tails — and all reacted. Several days later, he tested whether stimulation through the electrode would block pain. While providing continuous, mild electrical stimulation, he again applied the clamp. Although most of the subjects did show a pain reaction, those with electrodes in a particular region of the midbrain — the **periaqueductal grey area of the brainstem** — did not. The electrical stimulation had produced a state of not being able to feel pain, or *analgesia*, in these rats. Then Reynolds used these few rats for a dramatic demonstration: He performed abdominal surgery on them while they were awake and with only the analgesia produced through electrode stimulation. Subsequent studies by other researchers have confirmed that stimulation to the periaqueductal grey area can induce analgesia in animals and in humans. Moreover, they have determined that morphine works as a pain-killer by activating the brainstem to send impulses down the spinal cord (Chapman 1984; Melzack & Wall 1982; Winters 1985).

Other research findings have contradicted some details of the theory. But, as one reviewer has noted:

> Regardless of the specific wiring diagrams involved, the gate-control theory of pain has been the most influential and important current theory of pain perception. It ties together many of the puzzling aspects of pain perception and control. It has had profound influence on pain research and the clinical control of pain. It has generated new interest in pain perception, stimulating a multidisciplinary view of pain for research and treatment. It has been able to demonstrate the tremendous importance of psychological variables. (Weisenberg 1977, p. 1012).

The gate-control theory clearly takes a biopsychosocial perspective in explaining how people perceive pain. You will see many features of this theory as you read the material in the next section.

Biopsychosocial aspects of pain

Why does electrical stimulation to the periaqueductal grey area of the brainstem produce analgesia? The search for an answer to this question played an important part in major discoveries about the neurochemical bases of pain. We will begin this section by examining some of these discoveries and seeing that the neurochemical substances that underlie acute pain are linked to psychosocial processes. Then we will consider how psychosocial factors are related to the experience of chronic pain.

Neurochemical transmission and inhibition of pain

The phenomenon whereby stimulation to the brainstem produces insensitivity to pain has been given the name **stimulation-produced analgesia** (SPA). To understand how SPA occurs, we need to see how transmission cells are activated to send pain signals to the brain. This activation is triggered by a neurotransmitter called *substance P* that is secreted by small-diameter pain fibres and crosses the synapse to the transmission cells (Chapman 1984; Tortora & Grabowski 1993). SPA occurs when another chemical blocks the pain fibres' release of substance P. Let's see how this happens and what this other chemical is.

What stimulating the periaqueductal grey area does

Electrical stimulation to the periaqueductal grey area starts a neurochemical chain reaction that seems to take the course shown in figure 11.4. The impulse travels down the brainstem to the spinal cord, where the neurotransmitter *serotonin* activates nerve cells called 'inhibitory interneurons'. Impulses in these interneurons then cause the release of the neurotransmitter *endorphin* at the synapse with pain fibres; endorphin inhibits these fibres from releasing substance P (Tortora & Grabowski 1993; Winters 1985). Endorphin is a chemical belonging to a class of opiate-like substances called **endogenous opioids** that the body produces naturally; *enkephalin* is another of these chemicals. (*Endogenous* means 'developing from within', and *oid* is a suffix meaning 'resembling'.) Endogenous opioids and opiates (morphine and heroin) appear to function in much the same way in reducing pain (Snyder 1977; Winters 1985). Many neurons in the central nervous system have receptors that are sensitive to both opiates and opioids, and allow these chemicals to bind to them.

How opiates and opioids work

Researchers have studied the action of opiates and endogenous opioids by using the drug *naloxone*, which acts in opposition to opiates and opioids and prevents them from working as pain-killers (Bloom, Lazerson & Hofstadter 1985; Winters 1985). In fact, doctors administer naloxone to counteract the effects of heroin in addicts who have taken an overdose of the narcotic. In studying the action of opioids, researchers have examined whether these chemicals are involved in the phenomenon of SPA and found that naloxone blocks the analgesic effects of electrical stimulation to the periaqueductal grey area. One study, for instance, found that when animals received naloxone prior to brainstem stimulation, they continued to feel pain — they felt a noxious stimulus and reacted strongly. But if they did not receive naloxone, analgesia occurred, and they did not react to the noxious stimulus (Akil, Mayer & Liebeskind 1976). Furthermore, research with humans found that injecting naloxone in patients who have undergone tooth extractions increases their pain (Levine, Gordon & Fields 1978). These findings indicate that endogenous opioids are involved in producing SPA.

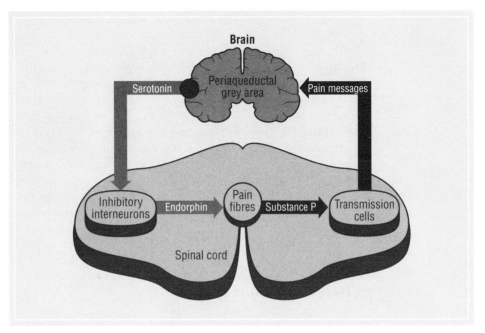

Figure 11.4 The chain of activity involved in SPA. Stimulation to the periaqueductal grey area of the brain starts a sequence of electrochemical reactions, eventually leading to inhibition (shown by shaded arrows) of the pain fibres' release of substance P, thereby reducing pain messages from the transmission cells to the brain.

The human body evidently contains its own natural pain-killing substances, but the mechanisms by which they reduce pain are more complicated than they once appeared. For one thing, studies have found that naloxone does not always block SPA; the effect of naloxone may depend on exactly where the electrode delivers stimulation in the periaqueductal grey area (Cannon et al. 1982). As Melzack and Wall have noted:

> It soon became apparent that there was not one but several descending control systems, and that some are sensitive to naloxone and others are not. Furthermore, a host of non-opioid transmitters — such as noradrenalin, acetylcholine and dopamine — are also involved in analgesia. ... The role of endorphins and enkephalins — despite their undoubted existence — is becoming more hazy. They play a role in pain and analgesia, but the nature of that role is poorly understood. It is possible that they are involved in sudden stress or sudden injury to prevent the animal or person from being overwhelmed by pain, but there is little evidence that they play a role beyond that. (1982, p. 174)

Part of the reason for questioning the extent to which endogenous opioids influence pain is that research on these chemicals has focused mainly on their role in momentary pain that generally lasts only seconds or minutes. Some research findings suggest that neurotransmitters may have different effects for momentary pain than for pain lasting for an hour or more (Melzack & Wall 1982).

Furthermore, when morphine is given to control pain, tolerance to the drug occurs quickly for momentary pain but does *not* seem to occur for longer-lasting acute pain and for chronic severe pain, such as that experienced by some cancer patients. These patients, for example, 'show little evidence of tolerance to morphine,' so that 'the same dose maintains its effectiveness' during months or years of use (Melzack & Wall 1982, p. 176). Just why these differences in tolerance occur is unclear.

Although researchers do not have a full understanding of the mechanisms by which endogenous opioids work, it seems clear that having internal pain-relieving chemicals serves an adaptive function. It enables people to regulate the pain they experience to some extent so that they can attend to other matters, such as taking immediate action to survive serious injuries. Pain activates this analgesic system (Winters 1985). But most of the time, high levels of endogenous opioid activity are not needed and would be maladaptive since chronic analgesia would undermine the value of pain as a warning signal. And people can use cognitive coping processes, such as diverting our attention, to supplement our use of endogenous opiods (Bruehl et al. 1996). Perhaps because pain and emotions are closely linked, studies have found that psychological stress can trigger endogenous opioid activity (Bloom, Lazerson & Hofstadter 1985; Winters 1985). The release of endogenous opioids in times of stress may help to explain how injured athletes in competition and soldiers on the battlefield continue to function with little or no perception of pain. The connection between stress, coping and opioid activity points up the interplay between biological and psychosocial factors in people's experience of pain.

Personal and social experiences and pain

Imagine this scene: Little Stevie is a year old and is in the paediatrician's office to receive a standard immunisation shot, as he has done before. As the physician approaches with the needle, Stevie starts to cry and tries to kick the doctor. He is reacting in anticipation of pain — something he learned through *classical conditioning* when he received vaccinations before.

Learning and pain

We learn to associate pain with antecedent cues and its consequences, especially if the pain is severe and repeated, as it usually is with chronic pain (Martin, Milech & Nathan 1993). Many individuals who suffer from migraine headaches, for example, often can tell when headaches are on the way because they experience symptoms, such as dizziness, that precede the pain. These symptoms become conditioned stimuli that tend to produce distress, a conditioned response, and may heighten the perception of pain when it arrives. Also, words or concepts that describe the pain people have experienced can become conditioned stimuli and produce conditioned responses. A study demonstrated this with migraine sufferers and non-sufferers by measuring their physiological arousal in response to pain-related words, such as 'throbbing', 'sickening', 'stabbing', 'scalding' and 'itching' (Jamner & Tursky 1987). The migraine sufferers displayed much stronger physiological reactions to these words — especially the words that described their own experience with migraine pain — than the non-sufferers did. And the results of other research indicate that people who suffer from chronic pain, such as headaches, show lower thresholds for pain stimuli than others do (Ukestad & Wittrock 1996). Perhaps they learn to notice and react more strongly to low levels of pain.

Highlight on issues

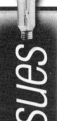

Placebos and pain

You have probably heard of doctors prescribing a medicine that actually consisted of 'sugar pills' when they could not find a physical cause for a patient's complaints or did not know of any medication that would help. You may also have heard that this treatment sometimes works — the patient claims the symptoms are reduced. An inert substance or procedure that produces an effect is called a *placebo*. Studies have shown that placebos can often be effective in treating a wide variety of ailments, including coughs, nausea and hypertension, at least on a temporary basis (Agras 1984; Roberts 1995; Sobel 1990).

Placebos can also be effective in treating pain (Melzack & Wall 1982). They do not always work, but they seem to produce substantial relief in about half as many patients as do real drugs, such as aspirin or morphine. The effect of placebos depends on the patient's belief that they will work — for instance, they are more effective:

- with large doses — such as more capsules or larger ones — than with smaller doses
- when injected than when taken orally
- when the practitioner indicates explicitly and strongly that they will work.

Unfortunately, however, the effectiveness of placebos in treating pain tends to decline with repeated use.

Why do placebos reduce pain? One explanation is that the patient's expectation that the treatment will work triggers the release of endogenous opioids in the body, thereby inhibiting the transmission of pain signals (Fields & Levine 1984). An experiment with dental patients who had had impacted wisdom teeth removed found evidence that this is the case (Levine, Gordon & Fields 1978). Patients who volunteered to participate in the study all received nitrous oxide anaesthetic at the start of surgery, an injection two hours later, and another injection three hours after that. The subjects were told the substance in each injection might increase, decrease or have no effect on the pain. These injections contained either naloxone or a placebo and were randomly assigned, using the following pattern: one group of subjects got the placebo as their first injection and naloxone as their second; another group got naloxone first and the placebo second; and a third group received placebos for both. The researchers used a double-blind procedure so that neither the subject nor the practitioner knew which substance was injected.

To determine the effects of these treatments, the researchers had the subjects rate the intensity of their pain several times during the study. The results revealed two important findings: First, the patients reported much more pain when given naloxone than when given the placebo. Second, of the subjects who got the placebo first and then naloxone, those who reported pain relief with the placebo reported increased pain with the naloxone, but those who did not respond to the placebo showed no change in their pain with the naloxone. Because the effects of naloxone occurred mainly among subjects who had gotten relief from the placebo, these findings suggest that placebos relieve pain by activating endogenous opioids. The role of opioids in the placebo effect of relieving pain has been confirmed by other researchers, using the cold-pressor procedure to induce pain (Bandura et al. 1987).

The effects of placebos are fascinating and important, but they also present major ethical dilemmas for practitioners. Is it appropriate to use placebo drugs or procedures to treat symptoms and illnesses — and if so, when and under what circumstances?

Learning also influences the way people behave when they are in pain. People in pain behave in characteristic ways — they may moan, grimace or limp, for instance. These actions are called **pain behaviours**, and they can be classified into four types (Turk, Wack & Kerns 1985). These are:

- *facial/audible expression of distress*, as when people clench their teeth, moan or grimace
- *distorted ambulation or posture*, such as moving in a guarded or protective fashion, stooping while walking, or rubbing or holding the painful area
- *negative affect*, such as being irritable
- *avoidance of activity*, as when people lie down frequently during the day, stay home from work, or refrain from motor or strenuous behaviour.

Pain behaviours are a part of the sick role, and sometimes people in pain begin to exaggerate these behaviours because, they think, 'No one believes me' (Hendler 1984). Regardless of why the behaviours start, they are often strengthened or maintained by reinforcement in *operant conditioning*, as Wilbert Fordyce has pointed out (1976; Fordyce & Steger 1979). When pain persists and becomes chronic, these behaviours often become part of the person's habits and lifestyle. People with entrenched patterns of pain behaviour usually feel powerless to change.

How are pain behaviours reinforced? Although being sick or in pain is unpleasant, it sometimes has benefits, or 'secondary gains'. Someone who is in pain may be relieved of certain chores around the house or of going to work, for instance. Also, when an individual has a painful condition that flares up in certain circumstances, such as when lifting heavy objects, he or she may begin to avoid these activities. In both of these situations, pain behaviour is reinforced if the person does not like doing these activities in the first place — thus, getting out of doing them is rewarding. Another way pain behaviour and other sick-role behaviours may be reinforced is if the person receives disability payments. Studies conducted with injured or ill patients who either do or do not get disability compensation have shown that those who *do* receive payments tend to remain hospitalised longer, take longer to return to work, and report more chronic pain and less success from pain treatments (Block, Kremer & Gaylor 1980b; Chapman 1991; Rohling, Binder & Langhinrichsen-Rohling 1995; Schrader et al. 1996). Part of these differences probably reflects a willingness of those receiving compensation to take more time to recover and try to prevent a relapse. Many patients with disability compensation show substantial emotional and behavioural improvements from pain rehabilitation programs (Trabin, Rader & Cummings 1987).

Social processes and pain

People who suffer with pain also receive attention, care and affection from family and friends, which provide social reinforcement for pain behaviour. Researchers have demonstrated this relationship with both child and adult patients. Karen Gil and her colleagues (1988) conducted a study of parents' reactions to the pain behaviour of their children who suffered from a chronic skin disorder that causes severe itching. Practitioners discourage scratching the itch since it can cause peeling and infection. The researchers videotaped the behaviour of each child and his or her parent in the child's hospital room. As you might expect, the parents paid attention to the scratching, perhaps because of the harm it can do. But what effect did the attention have? An analysis of the children's behaviours revealed that parent attention appeared to *increase* scratching, rather than decrease it. The results also indicated that paying attention to the children when they were *not* scratching seemed to reduce their scratching behaviour.

Research has also examined how the reactions of spouses affect their husbands' or wives' pain behaviour. One study used questionnaire reports by pain patients and their spouses to assess how the patients' behaviours were related to their spouses' being solicitous — that is, reacting to pain behaviours by giving attention and care (Flor, Kerns & Turk 1987). Higher levels of solicitousness by the spouse were associated with patients showing more pain behaviour and less activity, such as in visiting friends or going shopping. In another study, patients with chronic pain reported their perceptions of their spouses' solicitousness regarding their pain behaviour (Block, Kremer & Gaylor 1980a). The patients were also interviewed individually in two meetings in which they were aware of being observed through a one-way mirror and who was observing. In one interview, the observer was the patient's spouse; in the other, the observer was identified as a hospital employee. All patients were asked to describe their pain in each interview. The interesting finding was that the degree of pain they reported varied, depending on two factors: (1) whether the spouse or the employee was observing and (2) whether the patient thought the spouse was solicitous. Patients who felt their spouses were solicitous reported *more* pain when their spouses watched than when the employee did. In contrast, patients who felt their spouses were not solicitous reported *less* pain when their spouses watched than when the employee did.

The findings of research on parents' and spouses' reactions to chronic pain behaviour illustrate the impact of each family member's behaviour on the behaviour of others within the family system (Flor, Kerns & Turk 1987; Gil et al. 1987; Kerns & Weiss 1994). Showing care and concern when people are in pain is, of course, important and constructive. But when family members are highly solicitous to pain behaviour without encouraging other behaviours, particularly those that allow the patient to become increasingly active, they are likely to promote sick-role behaviour. This situation may then develop into a vicious circle of solicitousness leading to more pain behaviour, which elicits more solicitousness, and so on. The patient's diminished activity may also lead to physical deterioration, such as through muscle atrophy, and lead to progressively more pain and less activity. These social processes in the family system of pain patients are gradual and insidious — they tend to increase the patients' dependency and decrease their self-efficacy and self-esteem.

Gender, sociocultural factors and pain

Studies have found gender and sociocultural differences in the experience of pain. For instance, men and women in surveys report having different types of and reactions to pain. More women than men report having had migraine headaches and pain conditions of the lower back and the pelvic area, and more women report that pain interfered with their daily activities (Lester, Lefebvre & Keefe 1994; Lipton, Silberstein & Stewart 1994). Surveys of adults in different countries who suffer from chronic low back pain revealed greater work and social impairments among Americans, followed by Italians and New Zealanders, and then by Japanese, Colombian and Mexican individuals (Sanders et al. 1992). Even within countries, marked sociocultural differences have been found, such as in an Australian study that reported highly significant differences between Australians of Anglo-Saxon origin and Australians of European origin (e.g. Greeks, Italians and Yugoslavians) in terms of family attitudes towards chronic pain, attitudes towards psychological treatment, and even response to psychological treatment (Elton & Stanley 1982). The reasons for these gender and sociocultural differences are not clear, but they may include differences in the social support and financial consequences these people receive for being sick.

Emotions, coping processes and pain

People in chronic pain experience high levels of anger, fear and sadness (Fernandez & Milburn 1994). Pain and emotion are intimately linked, and cognitive processes mediate this link. In a study of these relationships, Gerry Kent (1985) had dental patients fill out a brief dental anxiety scale while waiting for their appointments. Then they rated the pain they expected in their visits. After the appointment, the patients rated the pain they actually experienced, and rated it again by mail three months later. The results revealed that anxiety played a role in their expectations of pain and in their memories of it three months later. The patients with high dental anxiety expected *and* later remembered four times as much pain as they experienced. In contrast, the low-anxiety patients expected and remembered less than twice as much pain as they experienced. These findings suggest that high-anxiety patients' memories of pain are determined more by what they expect than by what they feel.

Does emotion affect pain?

A study of emotion and pain compared the anxiety and stress levels of children who suffered from migraine headache with those of their best friends, and then had the migraine sufferers keep diaries of their headaches over the next four months. Although the scores on tests of anxiety and stress were about the same for the two groups and were within the normal range, migraine sufferers with high levels of anxiety had more frequent and severe headaches than those with lower anxiety (Cooper et al. 1987). Other investigations using self-report methods have found that migraine and tension-type headaches tend to occur after periods of heightened stress and that Type A individuals have more frequent chronic headaches than others do (DeBenedittis, Lorenzetti & Pieri 1990; Köhler & Haimerl 1990; Woods et al. 1984). These studies clearly indicate that stress and headache are related. Has any research shown that stress causes headaches?

Convincing evidence that stress can cause headaches comes from a series of studies by Paul Martin and colleagues at the University of Western Australia, in which they investigated whether commonly reported headache triggers such as stress, visual disturbance, noise and hunger can indeed bring on headaches (Martin & Teoh 1999; Martin & Todd 2001; Martin & Seneviratne 1997). These studies included adult subjects who suffered from migraine and tension-type headache, and matched non-headache control subjects. Experimental sessions were divided into four phases: *adaptation* (seven minutes); *baseline* (seven minutes); *challenge* (33 minutes); and *recovery* (seven minutes). During the three shorter phases of the session, subjects were instructed to relax. The effects of stress were evaluated by contrasting two conditions during the challenge phase of the study. In one condition, stress was induced by instructing subjects to try to solve a series of 100 anagrams, some of which were difficult to solve and some of which had no solution. Stress levels were further increased by giving subjects feedback at the end of each block of 10 anagrams that usually suggested that their performance was below average, and this feedback was given regardless of actual performance. The other condition used in the challenge phase was a control condition in which subjects were instructed to relax. A manipulation check confirmed that subjects found the 'stress' condition more stressful than the control condition.

In all three studies, the introduction of the stress condition was associated with a significant increase in rated headache activity, and the increase significantly differed from the change associated with the control condition. At an individual level, in one study, 93 per cent of subjects indicated that a headache began or got worse in response to the stress condition, compared with 36 per cent of subjects indicating that a headache began or got worse in response to the control condition (Martin & Seneviratne 1997). Headaches arose in response to stress for both sufferers of migraine and tension-type headache. These are important findings that indicate that stress can cause headaches.

Stress is also related to other kinds of pain, but whether stress causes the pain is still in question. Research has demonstrated, for instance, that people who suffer from recurrent low back pain report chronically higher levels of anxiety and tension than pain-free control subjects do, but these mood states do not worsen during 24 hours or so preceding pain attacks (Feuerstein, Carter & Papciak 1987). What is clear, however, is that pain is very stressful and that many people with chronic pain consider their discomfort — the actual pain and the physical limitations it produces — to be the most prominent stressor in their lives (Turner, Clancy & Vitaliano 1987).

Coping with pain

Part of the stress that chronic pain patients experience stems from their common belief that they have little personal control over their pain, aside from avoiding activities they believe can trigger an attack or make it worse. As a result, they tend to deal with their stress by using emotion-focused coping strategies. That is, rather than trying to alter the problem itself, they try to regulate their emotional responses to it. Some of the more common coping methods that chronic pain patients use include hoping or praying the pain will get better some day, telling themselves they can be brave and carry on despite their discomfort, and diverting their attention, such as by counting numbers or running a song through their heads (Keefe & Dolan 1986; Rosenstiel & Keefe 1983). These approaches are not very effective in reducing chronic pain.

How effectively do people cope with pain? One way researchers have tried to answer this question involves assessing pain patients' emotional adjustment with psychological tests, particularly the **Minnesota Multiphasic Personality Inventory (MMPI)**. This test contains several scales, three of which are especially relevant for medical patients. These three scales assess: *hypochondriasis*, the tendency towards being preoccupied with physical symptoms and health; *depression*, feelings of unhappiness, pessimism and hopelessness; and *hysteria*, the tendency to cope with problems by developing physical symptoms and using avoidance methods, such as denial. Because the MMPI is given and scored in a standardised manner and the test has been administered to large samples of people, norms exist that allow psychologists to compare an individual's scores on the different scales with those of the general population. For instance, a score of 70 or above on any scale occurs in less than 5 per cent of the population and is considered extreme and clinically significant (Anastasi 1982). Psychologists generally refer to hypochondriasis, depression and hysteria as the *neurotic triad* because psychiatric patients with neurotic disorders often have high scores on these three scales.

Studies carried out using the MMPI with pain patients have found some fairly consistent outcomes (Cox, Chapman & Black 1978; Rappaport et al. 1987; Rosen et al. 1987). These outcomes lead to three conclusions. First, individuals who suffer from various types of chronic pain, such as severe headache and low back pain, show a characteristic MMPI profile that includes extremely high scores on all three of the neurotic triad scales. But their scores on the remaining MMPI scales tend to be well within the normal range, as figure 11.5 illustrates. Second, this pattern of response appears to hold true whether or not their pain has a known organic source. In other words, individuals whose pain might be classified by a doctor as psychogenic tend to show similar problems of adjustment on the MMPI as those whose pain has a clear organic basis. Third, individuals with acute pain, such as patients recovering from injuries, sometimes have moderately elevated scores on the neurotic triad scales, but these scores and those for the remaining MMPI scales are generally well within the normal range. These findings make sense and reflect the differential psychological impact of pain that patients expect will end soon versus pain that they fear will never end. Keep in mind also that people with chronic/recurrent pain conditions show worse psychological symptoms during pain episodes than during pain-free periods (Holroyd et al. 1993).

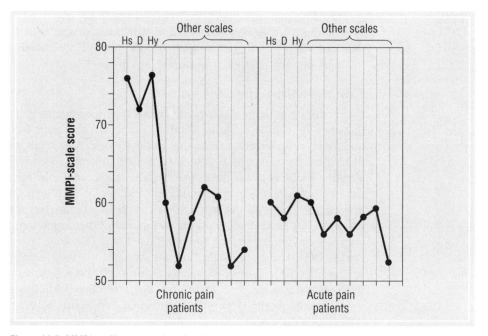

Figure 11.5 MMPI profiles comparing chronic pain and acute pain patients: Chronic pain patients typically show abnormally high scores (70 or above) on the 'neurotic triad' scales (Hs = hypochondriasis, D = depression, Hy = hysteria), but not on the seven other MMPI scales.

Sources: These data were averaged across mean scores presented in two studies (Cox, Chapman & Black 1978; Rosen et al. 1987).

It is clear that being in frequent, severe discomfort is related to having high scores on the MMPI neurotic triad scales, but does chronic pain cause maladjustment? One school of thought is that the causal sequence may be the other way around — that is, that some individuals have 'pain-prone' personalities that predispose them to experience chronic pain (Blumer & Heilbronn 1982). According to this view, chronic pain may be a symptom of a psychological disorder, such as depression, that preceded the pain syndrome. But most current evidence points in the other direction — indicating, for instance, that people in chronic pain become depressed because of the stress they experience without being able to change their situations (Anderson et al. 1985; Turk & Holzman 1986). They develop a sense of helplessness, which leads to depression. As Melzack and Wall have noted, one line of evidence of pain leading to depression

derives from studies of patients who are eventually relieved of their pain. ... In one study, it was found that patients who had pain of more than six months' duration — due to spinal injuries, post-herpetic neuralgia and other problems — showed significant decreases in several indices of psychological disturbance when their pain was abolished by successful surgery. (1982, p. 49)

Of course, this does not mean psychological factors cannot lead to physical pain — as we have seen, stress can cause headaches. One study examined this issue prospectively for eight years and found evidence for both causal directions: people who are depressed are somewhat more likely than others to develop a chronic pain condition in the future, and people with chronic pain are much more likely than others to become depressed (Magni et al. 1994). Thus, pain and maladjustment involve interacting processes, with each feeding on the other over time, but chronic pain is more likely to lead to maladjustment than the other way around. Also keep in mind that not all patients with severe chronic pain become maladjusted — some adapt to their conditions much better than others do (Klapow et al. 1993; Linton et al. 1994).

To summarise, the process by which people perceive pain involves a complex chain of physiological and neurochemical events. These events can be affected by a variety of psychosocial processes, such as people's beliefs about whether a drug will reduce their discomfort. Pain also affects and can be influenced by people's learning, cognition, social experiences and stress. Although people can indicate through their behaviour that they are feeling pain, the pain they perceive is actually a private and subjective experience. How can researchers and clinicians who work with patients who have painful symptoms assess the level and type of pain these individuals perceive? We turn now to answering this question.

Assessing people's pain

Researchers and clinicians have developed a variety of techniques for assessing people's pain. Although virtually all these methods can be applied both in research and in treating pain patients, some techniques are used more often in research, whereas others are used mostly to supplement a detailed medical history in clinical practice. In either setting, it is advisable to use two or more different measurement techniques to enhance the accuracy of the assessment (Bradley 1994). We will organise our discussion of techniques for measuring people's pain by classifying them into three distinct groups: self-report methods, behavioural assessment approaches and psychophysiological measures.

Self-report methods

Perhaps the most obvious approach to measuring people's pain is to ask them to describe their discomfort, either in their own words or by filling out a rating scale or questionnaire. In treating a patient's pain, health care workers ask where the pain is, what it feels like, how strong it is and when it tends to occur. With chronic pain patients, medical and psychological professionals often incorporate this kind of questioning within the structure of a clinical interview.

Interview methods in assessing pain

To treat chronic pain effectively, professionals need more information than just a description of the pain. Interviews with the patient and key others, such as family members and co-workers, provide a rich source of background information in the early phases of treatment (Chapman 1991; Karoly 1985; Turk, Meichenbaum & Genest 1983). These discussions ordinarily focus on such issues as:

- the history of the pain problem, including when it started, how it progressed and what approaches have been used for controlling it

- the patient's emotional adjustment, currently and before the pain syndrome began
- the patient's lifestyle — recreational interests, exercise patterns, diet, and so on — before the pain condition began
- the pain syndrome's impact on the patient's current lifestyle, interpersonal relations and work
- the social context of pain episodes, such as events in the family before an attack and how family members respond when the pain occurs
- factors that seem to trigger attacks or make them worse
- how the patient typically tries to cope with the pain.

The information obtained in these interviews can also be supplemented by having the patient and key others fill out questionnaires (Turk, Meichenbaum & Genest 1983).

Pain rating scales and diaries

One of the most direct, simple and commonly used ways to assess pain is to have individuals rate some aspect of their discomfort on a scale (Chapman et al. 1985; Jensen et al. 1989; Karoly 1985). This approach is used very often to measure how strong the pain is, and three different types of scales for rating pain intensity are illustrated in figure 11.6. One type is the *visual analogue scale*, which has people rate their pain by marking a point on a line that has labels only at each end. This type of scale is very easy for people to use and can be used with children as young as five years of age (Karoly 1985). The *box scale* has individuals choose one number from a series of numbers that represent levels of pain within a specified range. The *verbal rating scale* has people describe their pain by choosing a word or phrase from several that are given.

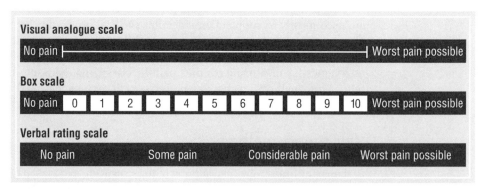

Figure 11.6 The visual analogue, box and verbal rating scales. Example instructions are as follows: *visual analogue scale* — 'Mark a point on the line to show how strong your pain is'; *box scale* — 'Rate the level of your pain by circling one number on the scale, where 0 means "no pain" and 10 means "worst pain possible"'; *verbal rating scale* — 'Circle the one phrase that best describes your pain.' The labels and number of choices on a scale can be different from those shown here.

Because rating scales are so easy and quick to use, people can rate their pain frequently. Averaging these ratings across time gives a more accurate picture of the pain the person generally experiences than individual ratings do (Jensen & McFarland 1993). Repeated ratings can also reveal how the pain changed over time, such as during everyday activities or during the course of an experiment. As an example, Dennis Turk and his colleagues have described how this approach can be used with chronic pain patients (Turk, Meichenbaum & Genest 1983). Each hour of a day, the patients rate their pain on index cards, which have separate scales for each hour.

They do this for, say, two weeks, also indicating whenever they take pain medication. Before starting this procedure, they learn what to say if someone sees them filling out the card and asks what they are doing, ways to remind themselves to do each hourly rating and what to do if they forget. One use of repeated ratings is in showing the ebb and flow of pain intensity that patients often experience. For instance, one patient's wife

> believed that her husband was experiencing incapacitating and severe pain every waking hour of his life. This belief contributed to her preventing him from participating in any but the simplest chores around the house. Their social life had deteriorated, and the couple had grown increasingly depressed over the course of four years. Upon hearing that her husband experienced only moderate pain most of the time, that he indeed felt capable of various tasks, and that he actually resented his wife's efforts at pampering him, she was helped to alter her behaviour. (Turk, Meichenbaum & Genest 1983, pp. 218–9)

Repeated ratings during each day may also reveal patterns in the timing of severe pain. Is the pain most severe in the evening, or on certain days? If so, are there aspects of the environment that may be responsible and, perhaps, changeable?

Pain ratings can also be used in a *pain diary*, which is a detailed record of a person's pain experiences. As figure 11.7 illustrates, the pain diary a patient keeps would include pain ratings and information about the time and circumstances of pain episodes, any medications taken and comments about each episode.

PAIN DIARY for _____ Phil _____

Date: ___ 3-5-01 ___   Did you change your medication today? If yes, describe _____ No _____

Pain Rating Scale: No pain | 0 | 1 | 2 | 3 | 4 | 5 | Unbearable pain

Time	Pain rating and body location	Activity at start of pain	What medicine did you take, and how much?	Pain rating after 1 or 2 hours	Comments and other problems
8.30 pm	4/lower back	Leaned over to turn on bath water	Aspirin (2)	3-helped a little	Could stand up and walk better
11.00 pm	2/lower back, dull ache	Lying flat on back in bed	Ibuprofen (Brufen) (2)	1-helped	Couldn't sleep at first; got to sleep by 1.00

Figure 11.7 A pain diary. The chronic pain patient keeps a daily record of important information about pain episodes.

Pain questionnaires

Pain is only partly described by the intensity of the discomfort people feel — the experience of pain has many qualities and dimensions. Ronald Melzack began to recognise the multidimensional nature of pain through his interactions with pain patients. He described in an interview how this realisation emerged from talks he had with a woman who suffered from phantom limb pain. She

> would describe burning pains that were like a red-hot poker being shoved through her toes and her ankle. She would cry out from the pain in her legs. Of course, there were no legs. Well, that made me realise the utter subjectivity of pain — no objective physical measure is very likely to capture that. ... I began to write down the words she used to describe her pain. I realised that the words describing the *emotional-motivational* component of her pain — 'exhausting, sickening, terrifying, punishing' — were very different from those for the *sensory* component — 'shooting, scalding, splitting, cramping'. Later I came to see there was also an *evaluative* component, such as 'it's unbearable' or 'it's annoying'. I wrote down the words other patients used, too, but I didn't know what to do with them. (Warga 1987, p. 53, italics added)

Melzack determined that pain involves three broad dimensions — *affective* (emotional-motivational), *sensory* and *evaluative* — by conducting a study in which subjects sorted over 100 pain-related words into separate groups of their own making (Melzack & Torgerson 1971).

Melzack's research also indicated that each of the three dimensions consisted of sub-classes. For instance, the sensory dimension included a subclass with the words 'hot', 'burning', 'scalding' and 'searing' — words relating to temperature. Notice that these four words connote increasingly hot temperatures, with searing being the hottest. Similarly, the affective dimension included a subclass of three words relating to fear: 'fearful', 'frightful', 'terrifying'. Then, by determining the degree of pain reflected by each word, Melzack (1975), a professor at McGill University in Montreal, was able to construct an instrument to measure pain. This test is called the **McGill Pain Questionnaire** (MPQ), which you filled out in the Assess Yourself exercise.

Part 2 of the MPQ presents a list of descriptive words, separated into a total of 20 subclasses. The test instructs the person to select from each subclass the best word to describe his or her pain. Each word in each class has an assigned value based on the degree of pain it reflects. Let's look, for instance, at subclass 7, which ranges from 'hot' to 'searing'. Selecting 'searing' would contribute the highest number of points from this subclass to the person's pain score ('hot' would contribute the lowest number). The sum of these points across the 20 subclasses is called the *pain rating index*. Part 4 of the MPQ contains a series of verbal rating scales; the one that rates 'your pain right now' yields a separate score called the *present pain intensity*.

The MPQ appears to have many strengths as an instrument for assessing chronic pain, both for research and for clinical purposes. For one thing, research has generally confirmed that the experience of pain is multidimensional, involving between two and four dimensions (Brennan, Barrett & Garretson 1987). Also, individuals with similar pain syndromes tend to choose the same patterns of words to describe their pain. But people suffering from very different types of pain — for example toothache, arthritis, cancer and phantom limb pain — choose different patterns of words in the MPQ to describe their different pain experiences (Melzack & Wall 1982). The main limitation of the MPQ is that it requires a fairly strong English vocabulary (Chapman et al. 1985; Karoly 1985). For instance, it includes a few words, such as 'taut' and 'lancinating', that many people may not know. Moreover, sometimes respondents must make very fine distinctions between words, as with 'throbbing', 'beating' and 'pounding'. Even if an interviewer is present to define the words, the MPQ may be of limited use with people who have poor English skills and children under about 12 years of age.

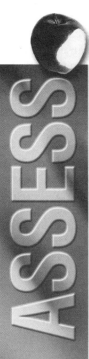

Assess yourself
DESCRIBING YOUR PAIN

Use the questionnaire in figure 11.8 to assess an acute or chronic pain you have experienced. Try to choose a painful condition that you either currently have, had recently or remember vividly from the past. If the pain you assess is not current, answer the questions as if it is. Do this now.

Figure 11.8 The McGill Pain Questionnaire

Source: Melzack (1975).

Ronald Melzack (1975) developed this questionnaire and described its scoring system, which is too complex to explain here. You can get a sense of the pain you assessed in two ways: (1) Review the answers you chose — for instance, questions 2 and 3 of Part 4 tell you its range of intensity. (2) Refer back to your answers as you read the description of the McGill Pain Questionnaire in the text.

Part 1.   Where is your pain?
Please mark on the drawing below, the areas where you feel pain. Put E if external, or I if internal, near the areas which you mark. Put EI if both external and internal.

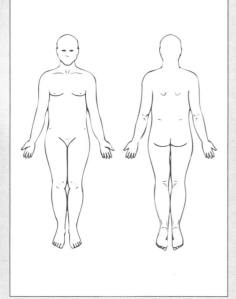

Part 2.   What does your pain feel like?
Some of the words below describe your present pain. Circle ONLY those words that best describe it. Leave out any category that is not suitable. Use only a single word in each appropriate category — the one that applies best.

1	2	3	4
Flickering	Jumping	Pricking	Sharp
Quivering	Flashing	Boring	Cutting
Pulsing	Shooting	Drilling	Lacerating
Throbbing		Stabbing	
Beating		Lancinating	
Pounding			

5	6	7	8
Pinching	Tugging	Hot	Tingling
Pressing	Pulling	Burning	Itchy
Gnawing	Wrenching	Scalding	Smarting
Cramping		Searing	Stinging
Crushing			

9	10	11	12
Dull	Tender	Tiring	Sickening
Sore	Taut	Exhausting	Suffocating
Hurting	Rasping		
Aching	Splitting		
Heavy			

13	14	15	16
Fearful	Punishing	Wretched	Annoying
Frightful	Gruelling	Blinding	Troublesome
Terrifying	Cruel		Miserable
	Vicious		Unbearable
	Killing		

17	18	19	20
Spreading	Tight	Cool	Nagging
Radiating	Numb	Cold	Nauseating
Penetrating	Drawing	Freezing	Dreadful
Piercing	Squeezing		Torturing
	Tearing		

Part 3.   How does your pain change with time?
1. Which word or words would you use to describe the *pattern* of your pain?

1	2	3
Continuous	Rhythmic	Brief
Steady	Periodic	Momentary
Constant	Intermittent	Transient

2. What kind of things *relieve* your pain?

3. What kind of things *increase* your pain?

Part 4.   How strong is your pain?
People agree that the following 5 words represent pain of increasing intensity. They are:

1	2	3	4	5
Mild	Discomforting	Distressing	Horrible	Excruciating

To answer each question below, write the number of the most appropriate word in the space beside the question.
1. Which word describes your pain right now?   _____
2. Which word describes it at its worst?   _____
3. Which word describes it when it is least?   _____
4. Which word describes the worst toothache you ever had?   _____
5. Which word describes the worst headache you ever had?   _____
6. Which word describes the worst stomach-ache you ever had?   _____

The MPQ is the best-known and most widely used pain questionnaire today. Researchers have developed other pain questionnaires, but they have not been very thoroughly studied yet. One of the more promising ones is the *West Haven–Yale Multidimensional Pain Inventory* (Kerns, Turk & Rudy 1985). Other questionnaires have been developed for specific pain syndromes, such as the Psychological Assessment of Headache Questionnaire (Martin 1993).

Behavioural assessment approaches

Because people tend to exhibit pain behaviours when they are in discomfort, it should be possible to assess their pain by observing their behaviour. A person with intense pain is likely to behave differently from someone with moderate pain. An individual with headache pain tends to behave differently from a person with low back pain. And a chronic pain sufferer is likely to have somewhat different patterns of pain behaviour if the pain is recurrent than if it is intractable. Psychologists have developed procedures for assessing pain behaviour in two types of situations: in *everyday activities* and in *structured clinical sessions*.

Assessing pain behaviour in structured clinical sessions

Procedures are available whereby health care workers can assess the pain behaviour of patients in structured clinical sessions. These sessions are usually conducted in hospital settings and are structured by the specific pain behaviours to be assessed and the tasks the patient is asked to perform. One approach of this kind has been developed into a pain assessment instrument — the *UAB Pain Behaviour Scale* — for use by nurses during their standard routines, such as in early-morning rounds (Richards et al. 1982). The nurse has the patient perform several activities and rates each of 10 behaviours, such as the patient's mobility and use of medication, on a three-point scale: 'none', 'occasional' and 'frequent'. These ratings are converted into numerical values and summed for a total score.

Some studies using structured clinical sessions have focused on assessing discomfort in patients suffering from low back pain (Follick, Ahern & Aberger 1985; Keefe & Block 1982; Kleinke & Spangler 1988; Öhlund et al. 1994). Each investigation had patients perform a standard set of activities. In the study by Chris Kleinke and Arthur Spangler, for example, the patients were asked to walk, pick up an object on the floor, remove their shoes while sitting and perform several exercises, such as trunk rotations, toe touching and sit-ups. The patients in each investigation were videotaped, and trained assessors rated their performance for several pain behaviours, such as guarded movement, rubbing the pain area, grimacing and sighing. These studies have shown that pain behaviours can be assessed easily and reliably and that behavioural assessments correlate well with patients' self-ratings of pain.

Assessing pain behaviour in everyday activities

How does the pain patient behave in everyday activities, especially at home? Does the person spend much of his or her time in bed, complain of discomfort a lot, seek help frequently in moving or walk with a limp most of the time? How much of these behaviours does the person exhibit? These are the kinds of behavioural assessments that can be made regarding the everyday activities of a patient.

Family members or key others in the patient's life are usually the best people to make these everyday assessments of pain behaviour. These people must, of course, be willing to help and be trained to make careful observations and keep accurate records.

Pain researcher Wilbert Fordyce (1976) has recommended a procedure whereby the assessor — the client's spouse — compiles a list of five to ten behaviours that generally signal when the patient is in pain. Then the spouse receives training in watching for these behaviours and keeping track of the amount of time the patient exhibits them. Finally, the spouse is trained to monitor how people, including the assessor, react to the client's pain behaviour. This procedure is useful not only in assessing the patient's pain experiences but in determining their impact on his or her life and the social context that may maintain pain behaviours.

Several modifications or supplements to Fordyce's procedure have been described by other researchers (Turk, Meichenbaum & Genest 1983). For example, the assessor — usually the patient's spouse — may fill out a rating scale periodically to measure the intensity of the pain, as reflected by the client's behaviour. Also, the spouse may keep a pain diary about the patient's severe pain episodes, recording the date and time, as well as where the episode occurred, such as in the car or at home in bed. Then the spouse describes what he or she:

• noticed as behaviours that suggested the patient was in pain
• thought and felt during the episode
• did in order to help, along with a rating of the action's effectiveness, ranging on a scale from 'did not help at all' to 'seemed to stop the pain completely'.

These supplemental procedures provide additional data that can be of value in dealing with interpersonal issues that influence the pain experience.

Psychophysiological measures

Another approach for assessing pain involves taking measurements of physiological activity, since pain has both sensory and emotional components that can produce changes in bodily functions. *Psychophysiology* is the study of mental or emotional processes as reflected by changes they produce in physiological activity (Lykken 1987).

One psychophysiological measure researchers have used for assessing pain uses an apparatus called an *electromyograph* (EMG) to measure the electrical activity in muscles, which reflects their tension. Because *muscle tension* is associated with various pain states, such as headaches and low back pain, we might expect EMG recordings to be different between pain patients and pain-free controls. Studies have compared EMG recordings of headache and low back pain patients while *not* in pain with recordings of pain-free subjects and have generally not confirmed this expectation (Blanchard & Andrasik 1985; Chapman et al. 1985). But the findings of other research suggest that differences between pain patients and controls may exist when the subjects' muscles are active (Chapman et al. 1985). Whether EMG patterns differ between headache and headache-free periods is debatable, as some studies have found elevated EMG associated with headaches (e.g. Haynes et al. 1975), while others have found evidence of headaches being associated with relaxation, perhaps as a rebound following stress (e.g. Martin & Mathews 1978). More research is needed, however, to verify that EMG measurements provide a useful measure of pain.

Researchers have also attempted to assess people's pain with measures of *autonomic activity*, such as of heart rate and skin conductance. A study by John Dowling (1983) used these two measures of autonomic activity on college students before, during and after they underwent a cold-pressor procedure. Before the procedure, measurements of skin conductance and heart rate were taken during a *warning* period, as the subjects awaited a signal to immerse the hand in the ice-cold water; after the procedure, measurements were taken during a *resting* period, when the subjects knew they would not experience further pain. The results showed that autonomic activity during *both* the warning period and immersion correlated moderately with the length of time the subjects left their hands in the water. Finding that pain tolerance correlated with autonomic activity during the warning period is interesting and illustrates a limitation to this measure of pain — that is, changes in autonomic activity readily occur in the absence of the sensation of pain. Although some measures of autonomic activity may be useful in assessing the emotional component of pain, they are not likely to be useful beyond that role (Chapman et al. 1985).

The last psychophysiological measure of pain we will consider involves the electrical activity of the brain, as measured by the *electroencephalograph* (EEG). When a person's sensory system detects a stimulus, such as a clicking sound from earphones, the signal to the brain produces a change in EEG voltage. Electrical changes produced by stimuli are called evoked potentials and show up in EEG recordings as sharp surges or peaks in the graph. Research has demonstrated that pain stimuli produce *evoked potentials* that vary in magnitude — the amplitudes of the surges increase with the intensity of the stimuli, decrease when subjects take analgesics, and correlate with people's subjective reports of pain (Chapman et al. 1985).

Even though psychophysiological measures provide objective assessments of bodily changes that occur in response to pain, these changes may also be affected by other factors, such as attention, diet and stress. In clinical situations, measures of muscle tension, autonomic activity and evoked potential are probably best used as supplements to self-report and behavioural assessment approaches (Chapman et al. 1985).

Pain in children

We have focused in this chapter mainly on the experience of pain by adults, and we have mentioned many different types of discomfort and pain syndromes. Virtually every pain condition we have considered is experienced by children, too (Goodman & McGrath 1991; Lavigne, Schulein & Hahn 1986b). Children suffer acute pain from illnesses and injury, often being victims of burns and fractures for instance. They also experience pain associated with chronic diseases, such as arthritis and cancer, and suffer from a wide range of painful conditions that do not have known physical bases — conditions such as recurrent abdominal pain, causalgia, and migraine and tension-type headache. Indeed, some children suffer from a curious painful condition — unique to their age group — that involves pain deep in the arms or legs but not near a joint. The condition is sometimes called 'growing pains', which may be a misnomer because it is most prevalent among eight- to 12-year-olds, a time when growth is relatively slow for children (Lavigne, Schulein & Hahn 1986b).

Much less is known about the pain people experience in childhood than at other times in their lives (Bush 1987; Jeans 1983). In fact, there is still some controversy about the age at which children begin to feel pain strongly, with some practitioners believing that infants under about three months of age feel relatively little pain. This belief derives from (1) the knowledge that babies' nervous systems are very immaturely developed and (2) the results of early studies, which found, for instance, that newborns did not pull an arm or leg away when the limb was pricked with a pin. Because of the belief that very young infants are insensitive to pain, doctors in the past often performed surgery on babies using only a mild anaesthetic or muscle relaxant. Minor operations, such as circumcision, were commonly done on infants with little or no anaesthesia. But this situation changed rapidly in the 1980s as a result of new research. Let's see what is known today about pain in children.

Pain and children's sensory and cognitive development

Although the issue of whether babies are as sensitive as adults to pain is not yet resolved, one thing is clear: newborn babies feel pain. The fact that they typically cry when slapped on the rump if they do not start to breathe after birth certainly suggests that they feel pain. Is clearer evidence available?

Better evidence that young babies perceive pain comes from studies with newborns as they underwent noxious medical procedures, such as when the foot is pierced to draw a blood sample. One of these studies found that babies' reactions to the noxious stimulus included a 'pain' facial expression: They had their eyes squeezed, brows contracted, tongue taut and mouth open (Grunau & Craig 1987). This pattern is comparable to the expression adults display when in pain. Another study found that the pattern of newborns' crying varied with the intensity of the noxious procedure they experienced (Porter, Miller & Marshall 1986). Highly noxious procedures elicited cries with certain characteristics, such as relatively high-pitched peak tones, that adults judged as indicating 'urgency'. If newborns feel pain, why didn't the babies in the early research withdraw their limbs when pricked by a pin? The answer probably has to do with the pain behaviour measured: withdrawing the limb requires that the subjects coordinate sensory events with their motor responses — a cognitive operation that babies do poorly during their first weeks of life.

One difficulty young children have in expressing their experience of pain is that their language abilities are very limited. Toddlers may know the word 'hurt', but they do not usually have many other words to describe their pain (McGrath 1987; Mills 1989). Instead of telling adults of their pain, they may display other pain behaviours, such as crying, rubbing the affected area or clenching their jaws. Mary Ellen Jeans (1983) interviewed five- to 13-year-old children to determine their knowledge about pain. When asked to describe pain, the five-year-olds used only an average of five different adjectives in their descriptions. But the children's use of different adjectives increased with age, with the 13-year-olds using an average of 26. The strategies the children gave for coping with pain also changed as they got older. Children under age 10 reported physical strategies, such as rubbing the painful area, almost exclusively. In contrast, the 13-year-olds cited more varied strategies, and 35 per cent of their descriptions reflected psychological coping strategies, such as distracting their attention.

Assessing pain in children

When a patient has symptoms that include pain, the doctor usually needs to know its location, intensity, quality, duration and temporal patterning. This information helps in making an accurate diagnosis. But children's ability to provide this information is quite limited, especially if they are young.

Although researchers are currently working to develop questionnaires and other self-report procedures to assess children's pain, doctors today must rely mainly on interviews and behavioural assessment approaches (Bush 1987; Lavigne, Schulein & Hahn 1986a; McGrath 1987). Effectively interviewing children requires a great deal of skill in developing rapport with them, asking the right questions in ways they can understand and knowing what their answers mean. Behavioural assessment approaches probably provide the most valuable source of information about the pain younger children experience. The most obvious of these approaches simply involves having the parents report pain behaviours they have observed. Other behavioural assessments involve structured clinical sessions in which health care workers rate or record the occurrence of pain behaviour.

What kinds of self-report methods for assessing children's pain are researchers developing? Much of the research has been directed at finding effective ways for children to describe the intensity of their pain (Lavigne, Schulein & Hahn 1986a; McGrath 1987). It appears that children as young as five years of age can understand and use visual analogue scales correctly and reliably. They can also use verbal rating scales if the choices are labelled in ways they can understand, such as with faces indicating graded degrees of distress. But more research is needed to determine how accurately the ratings children give reflect their actual pain. Last, two pain questionnaires have been developed: one is the Pediatric Pain Questionnaire (Varni & Thompson 1986) and the other is the Children's Comprehensive Pain Questionnaire (McGrath 1987). Both instruments are designed to measure multiple dimensions of the pain experiences of children from about 4 years of age to adolescence. Adults may help the children fill out portions of the questionnaires when they lack needed reading skills.

Children's pain experiences are undoubtedly affected by a wide variety of psychosocial factors, particularly the social environment in which pain occurs (Bush 1987). Parents serve as models and agents of reinforcement for the pain behaviour of their children. But little is known about the personality and family characteristics of children that may contribute to the intensity and frequency of their pain. The vast majority of studies on pain have focused on adult subjects, not on children, and the studies conducted with children have generally produced unclear results because they were often poorly designed and carried out (Jeans 1983; Lavigne, Schulein & Hahn 1986b). In addition, researchers need to overcome the difficulties in assessing children's pain so that they can do the kind of high-quality research that is needed.

Summary

Although pain is typically unpleasant, it is critical for our survival because it warns us of actual or threatened tissue damage. It is the most frequent medical complaint of patients and the most commonly stated reason for disability. Pain includes both sensory and emotional components, and it has many different qualities. Sometimes pain feels sharp, and other times it's dull; sometimes it's localised, and other times it's pervasive; sometimes it has a burning sensation, and other times it has a cramping or aching feeling.

Pain experiences also vary along a continuum, ranging from those that are mostly organic in origin to those that are mostly psychogenic. Virtually all pain experiences involve an interplay of both physiological and psychological processes, but the mixture of organic and psychogenic factors varies. Most painful experiences involve acute pain, which eventually disappears. They may last just a moment or as long as a few months, as with a very serious burn. Other pain conditions last for more than a few months, and are described as chronic. Long-lasting pain can be classified as chronic/recurrent, chronic/intractable/benign and chronic/progressive pain.

The body's tissues contain algogenic substances that are released at the site where an injury occurs, thereby activating nociceptors, which are afferent-free nerve endings. Pain signals are carried towards the central nervous system by two types of afferent peripheral fibres: (1) A-delta fibres carry signals of sharp and well-localised pain rapidly through the thalamus to motor and sensory areas of the cortex. These signals probably receive special attention in our sensory awareness, permitting a quick response. (2) C fibres carry information about dull and diffuse pain. These signals travel relatively slowly and terminate mainly in the brainstem and lower portions of the forebrain.

The process of pain perception involves three curious and fascinating types of phenomena. The first type is called referred pain, whereby pain originating from internal organs is perceived as coming from other parts of the body. The second type involves pain with no apparent physical basis. Neuralgia, causalgia and phantom limb pain are syndromes that involve intense pain even though no noxious stimulus is present. In the third type of phenomenon, the meaning of pain affects people's experience of it. Individuals for whom pain means a personal disaster is almost over and better things are coming seem to perceive less pain than do individuals with similar wounds who believe the personal disaster is just beginning.

The gate-control theory of pain proposes that neural signals of pain pass through a gate that can modulate the signals before they reach the brain. The degree to which the gate is open or closed depends on three factors: the amount of activity in the pain fibres, the amount of activity in other peripheral fibres, and messages that descend from the brain. This theory allows for the influence of psychological factors in pain perception. The phenomenon of stimulation-produced analgesia supports this theory, demonstrating that stimulation to the periaqueductal grey area of the brainstem can block the sensation of noxious stimulation elsewhere in the body. The findings of research with a drug called naloxone indicate that this phenomenon depends on the action of endogenous opioids — a class of neurochemicals that includes endorphin and enkephalin. The effect of placebos in reducing pain also depends on opioids.

Psychological processes play an important role in the experience of pain. People in pain generally display pain behaviours, such as moaning, guarded movement or avoidance of activity. These behaviours are often reinforced — for instance when they result in the person being relieved of doing disliked activities or receiving special attention, care and affection. Pain and stress are intimately linked: Pain is stressful, and stress can produce pain — at least headache pain. People often have difficult times coping with chronic pain, which can lead to psychological maladjustment.

A person's pain can be assessed in several ways. Self-report methods include interviews, rating scales and pain questionnaires. The McGill Pain Questionnaire assesses three dimensions of pain: affective, sensory and evaluative. Behavioural assessment approaches can measure pain in the person's everyday activities and in structured clinical sessions. Psychophysiological measures of pain assess muscle tension, autonomic activity and evoked potentials of the brain. Children can perceive pain when they are born, but assessing pain in children is extremely difficult because of their limited language development.

Key terms

acute pain	chronic/recurrent pain	Minnesota Multiphasic Personality Inventory (MMPI)	pain behaviours
algogenic substances	endogenous opioids		periaqueductal grey area of the brainstem
chronic/intractable/benign pain	gate-control theory	nociceptors	
chronic/progressive pain	McGill Pain Questionnaire	pain	referred pain
			stimulation-produced analgesia

12 Managing and controlling clinical pain

Prologue

'Ouch! My foot hurts,' the little girl cried as she tried to walk. The nurse responded quickly, saying, 'I'm sorry it hurts. Show me where it hurts .... Let's get some exercise some other time.' This 3-year-old girl was a patient who had had a difficult life. She was in her tenth month of hospitalisation after receiving second- and third-degree burns to her legs and buttocks from having been immersed in scaldingly hot water. There was some evidence that the burn had been deliberately inflicted, and that she was a victim of child abuse.

After all these months this little girl's discomfort was not over. She still needed physiotherapy and operations for plastic surgery, and she still had to wear uncomfortable knee-extension splints to prevent contractures. But her therapy was not going well. What had become clear was that the hospital staff were inadvertently reinforcing her pain behaviour by comforting her and allowing her to avoid disliked activities. James Varni and Karen Thompson have described how this situation was not in the child's long-term best interests, having disrupted her physical, social and emotional rehabilitation.

> Physical therapy was essentially terminated because of the patient's interfering pain behaviors. Two patterns emerged when the patient was placed in her bedroom in the crib with knee extension splints on. First, the child would struggle until she had removed the splints, resulting in further contractures and the need for additional plastic surgery. Second, if she failed to remove the splints, her crying would intensify to the point of screaming. At times she would fall asleep, exhausted, and continue sobbing well into the naptime hour. Other times, she would continue screaming until, in consideration of the other children, the nursing staff would remove her to a separate room for the remainder of the hour. (1986, p. 382)

Her rehabilitation and interactions with adults and other children were being limited because of her behaviour, and she was clearly not coping with her situation in constructive ways.

What can be done to help patients who, like this girl, have developed chronic pain behaviours that interfere with their rehabilitation? We will examine in this chapter how she was helped and what methods are effective in reversing chronic pain behaviours. We will also discuss a variety of techniques and programs for treating and helping patients control the pain experience. As we study these issues, we will try to answer other questions you may have about dealing with pain. Do effective treatments for acute pain also work with chronic pain? What role do drugs have in treating pain, and how can patients decrease drug use? Do such methods as hypnosis and acupuncture really work in reducing pain? What are pain clinics, and are they effective in treating pain?

Clinical pain

Not all of our pain experiences receive professional treatment, and not all of them require it. The term **clinical pain** refers to any pain that receives or requires professional treatment. The pain may be either acute or chronic and may result from known or unknown causes (Sanders 1985). Clinical pain calls for treatment in and of itself, and not only because it may be a symptom of a progressive disease, such as arthritis or cancer. Relieving pain is important for humanitarian reasons, of course — and doing so also produces medical and psychosocial benefits for the patient (Chapman 1984). Let's look at medical and psychosocial issues that are associated with controlling clinical pain, beginning with acute pain.

Acute clinical pain

By using techniques to prevent or relieve acute pain, practitioners make medical procedures go more smoothly, reduce patients' stress and anxiety, and help them recover more quickly. Much of the acute pain people experience in today's world has little survival value (Chapman 1984). What survival value would there be in feeling the pain as a dentist drills a tooth or a surgeon removes an appendix? How would people's survival be enhanced by feeling the intense pain that accompanies normal healing while resting in a hospital during the days after surgery?

When competent medical care is available, these pains are not useful. Yet during recovery after surgery in the United States, 30 per cent of patients experience mild pain, 30 per cent have moderate pain, and 40 per cent suffer severe or very severe pain (Chapman 1984). The level of pain varies, depending on the type of surgery involved and a wide variety of psychosocial factors, such as the patients' past medical experiences, anxiety prior to the operations and knowledge about the sensations they can expect. Post-operative pain that is not adequately reduced can cause abnormal physiological reactions that can lead to medical complications and even death. For instance, inadequately relieved pain and muscle spasms that may arise from abdominal and chest surgery can prevent patients from breathing deeply and coughing, thereby allowing bacterial infections to take hold in the lungs and cause pneumonia (Chapman 1984).

In the past decade, Acute Pain Service units have been established in many hospitals in Australia and other countries, usually staffed by a specialist anaesthetist and specialist nurse, in collaboration with surgeons and ward nursing staff (Cousins 2000). Treatment by such units has been reported to achieve highly effective pain relief in more than 90 per cent of patients (NHMRC 1999). And yet many patients with post-operative pain and many more with other forms of severe acute pain are not offered such services (Cousins 2000).

Chronic clinical pain

When pain persists and becomes chronic, patients begin to perceive its nature differently. Although in the acute phase the pain was very aversive, the patients expected it to end and did not see it as a permanent part of their lives. As the pain persists, patients tend to become discouraged and angry and are likely to seek the opinions of many other doctors. This can be constructive. But when this is not successful, and as patients come to see less and less connection between their discomfort and any known or treatable disorder, increasing hopelessness and despair may lead them to resort to consulting quacks (Chapman 1984).

The transition from acute to chronic pain is a critical time when many of these patients tend to develop pervasive feelings of helplessness (Keefe 1982). The neurotic triad — hypochondriasis, depression and hysteria — often becomes a dominant aspect of their personalities, especially if the pain is severe and disabling (Bradley & Van der Heide 1984; Rosen et al. 1987). These changes typically parallel alterations in the patients' lifestyles, employment status and family lives, as the following letter from a wife to her husband's therapist reflects.

perhaps if I could explain my husband's attitudes it might help you understand his problems. ... The questionnaire you gave him to complete and send back became a tremendous ordeal for him. Why, I'll never know, because the questions were simple, but in the state of mind he is in, everything gets to be a chore. ... Since his back operation five years ago he has become increasingly impatient and progressively slower with no ambition at all to even try to help himself. He had made himself an invalid and it has become very difficult for me or my family to tolerate his constant complaining. He blames me, blames our two sons, who he says don't help him around the house when in fact he does little or nothing to help himself. He does exactly the same things day after day with projects he starts and never completes and always because of his health. . . . To dwell on his illness is what he wants and only that he will do, believe me. He needs psychiatry of some kind. (Flor & Turk 1985, p. 268)

A study of people who had suffered for years with severe chronic/recurrent and chronic/intractable/benign pain found that about half had considered suicide because of their conditions (Hitchcock, Ferrell & McCaffery 1994). Chronic pain often creates a broad array of long-term psychosocial problems and impaired interrelationships, which distinguish its victims from those of acute pain (Weir et al. 1994).

Individuals who receive treatment for their pain after it has progressed and become chronic tend to exhibit certain physical and psychosocial symptoms that characterise a 'chronic pain syndrome'. According to psychologist Steven Sanders (1985), these symptoms include:

- associated tissue damage or irritation, which may be minor or major
- persistent pain complaints and other pain behaviours, such as grimacing or guarded movement, when in discomfort
- disrupted daily activity patterns, characterised either by a general reduction or by recurrent large fluctuations
- disrupted social, marital, employment and recreational activities
- excessive use of drugs or repeated use of surgical procedures to relieve pain
- disturbed sleep patterns
- increased anxiety and depression.

Chronic pain patients usually exhibit the first two symptoms and at least one of the remaining ones. Generally speaking, the more symptoms the patient presents, the greater the impact the pain has had and the greater the maladjustment it has produced.

Because of the differences between acute pain and chronic pain in their duration and the effects they have on their victims, these conditions usually require different treatment methods. Health care professionals need to distinguish between acute and chronic pain conditions and provide the most appropriate pain relief techniques for the patient's needs. Failing to do so can make the condition worse (Chapman 1984). Keeping this caution in mind, we will turn our attention for the remainder of this chapter to the wide variety of medical, psychological and physical techniques available to help control patients' pain.

Medical treatments for pain

A few centuries ago, peasants in Western cultures commonly treated pain by piercing the affected area of the body with a 'vigorous' twig of a tree, believing that the twig would absorb the pain from the body (Turk, Meichenbaum & Genest 1983). Then, to prevent anyone from getting the pain from that twig, they buried it deep in the ground. Other early practices for controlling pain were not so far-fetched, but they were crudely applied, even by physicians. In nineteenth-century Australia, alcoholic beverages and 'medicines' laced with opium were readily available. Many people used these substances to alleviate pain, and doctors commonly employed them as anaesthetics for surgery before the mid-1800s, when ether was introduced. Today when patients suffer from pain, doctors try to reduce the discomfort in two ways — chemically and surgically.

Surgical methods for treating pain

Treating chronic pain with surgical methods is a relatively radical approach, and some surgical procedures are more useful than others. In some procedures, the surgery removes or disconnects portions of the peripheral nervous system or the spinal cord, thereby preventing pain signals from reaching the brain. These are extreme procedures — and if they are successful, they produce numbness and, sometimes, paralysis in the region of the body served by the affected nerves. But these procedures seldom provide long-term relief from the pain, which is often replaced after some days or months by pain and other sensations that are worse than the original condition (Hare & Milano 1985; Melzack & Wall 1982). Because of the poor prospects of permanent relief and the risks involved in these surgical procedures, they are rarely used today.

Other surgical procedures for relieving pain do not remove or disconnect nerve fibres and are much more successful. One example is the *synovectomy*, a technique whereby a surgeon removes membranes that become inflamed in arthritic joints (AMA 1989; Anderson et al. 1985). Another example is *spinal fusion*, a procedure that joins two or more adjacent vertebrae to treat severe back pain (AMA 1989). Using surgical procedures to treat back pain has become very common in the United States, but there is little evidence that they produce better long-term pain reduction than nonsurgical methods, and they are used at a far lower rate in other developed countries, including Australia, where the rate is less than half the American rate (Cherkin et al. 1994; Volinn, Turczyn & Loeser 1994). Surgical procedures for chronic skeletal pain conditions are most appropriate when the person is severely disabled and non-surgical treatment methods have failed. Doctors and patients usually prefer other medical approaches, such as chemical methods.

Chemical methods for treating pain

Although medical research has led to many advances in treating pain since the 1800s, this progress has been slow. The field of medicine has been much more concerned with developing methods for curing disease than with reducing pain (Melzack & Wall 1982). In a recent editorial in the *Medical Journal of Australia*, Michael Cousins, the director of the Pain Management and Research Centre at the University of Sydney, argued that relief of severe pain is a basic human right (Cousins 2000). Cousins advocated two strategies for the relief of acute pain that have emerged in the last five to ten years. The first was a 'multimodal analgesic strategy' involving the combined use of different analgesics, and the second was to consider using more aggressive, and possibly pre-emptive, approaches to management of early post-operative pain to reduce the likelihood of chronic pain developing. Let's look at the use of chemical methods for treating acute and chronic pain.

Using chemicals for acute pain

Many pharmaceuticals are very effective for relieving acute pain, such as after surgery. Doctors choose the specific drug and dosage by considering many factors, such as how intense the pain is and its location and cause. Do practitioners use these chemicals effectively, giving as much pain relief as they safely can? The degree to which they do depends on characteristics of the drug, the patients, and sociocultural factors. Medical workers and patients generally prefer not to use narcotic drugs, mainly because of the possibility of addiction. In some countries, such as in Latin America, using narcotics for pain relief is extremely rare (DePalma 1996). Other cultures have become much more accepting of narcotic pain control.

The management of acute pain in most institutions has changed very little in the past 40 years and 50 per cent to 70 per cent of patients still receive insufficient analgesia (Ferrante & Covino 1990). Those who receive too little pain relief tend to be children and minority group members, even when compared with other patients with the same medical condition (Bush 1987; Cleeland et al. 1994; Ng et al. 1996; Schechter, Allen & Hanson 1986). For instance, when the patient is a child, practitioners tend to administer pain-killing medication less frequently, give doses below the recommended level and discontinue medication earlier, especially if the drug is a narcotic. The reasons for these age and sociocultural differences are unclear. In the case of children, it may be that practitioners believe children feel less pain than adults or are more likely to become addicted to a drug (Bush, Holmbeck & Cockrell 1989). Or children may simply request less medication, perhaps because they dislike injections or taking pills more than adults do. Similar reasons may explain the differences among minority group members.

The conventional ways for administering pain-killing chemicals involve giving injections or pills, and these are given under one of two arrangements: a prescribed schedule or 'as needed' (called PRN for the Latin *pro re nata*) by the patient. But two other methods are available today (Chapman 1984; Kanner 1986; Melzack & Wall 1982). In one of these methods — called an *epidural block* — practitioners inject narcotics or local anaesthetics epidurally, that is, near the membrane that surrounds the spinal cord. These chemicals then prevent pain signals from being transmitted to the brain. The second technique is called *patient-controlled analgesia*. This procedure allows the patient to determine how much pain-killer, such as morphine, he or she needs, and get it without delay. The patient simply pushes a button to activate a computerised pump that dispenses a preset dose of the chemical through a needle that remains inserted continuously. Practitioners monitor the patient's use of the drug and set limits on the rate and amount of its use.

Do patients abuse the opportunity to control their use of narcotics for pain control? Current evidence suggests that the risk of abuse is low for most patients, at least under certain circumstances. A study by Marc Citron and his colleagues (1986) examined this issue with hospitalised men with severe cancer pain. They were placed on a patient-controlled analgesia procedure for a little over two days, on average. A doctor preset for each patient the dosage of morphine the pump would deliver and a lockout time — that is, the interval after a dose when no more morphine would be available. The average lockout time was about 30 minutes. The results revealed that the patients' rate of morphine use *declined* over time rather than increased, being used far more heavily in the first few hours than it was later. During the first four hours, the subjects took about one dose per hour, on average, consuming morphine at a rate of 4 milligrams an hour. But their use dropped sharply after the initial high use — for the remainder of the two days, their rate of morphine use was less than 40 per cent of the earlier rate. These patients were free to take much more medication, but they did not. Similar results have been found with male and female adolescent patients following surgery (Tyler 1990). But there is a caution in using patient-controlled analgesia with patients who are relatively young, have high levels of anxiety or have low levels of social support: They tend to use more of the drug than other acute pain patients do (Gil et al. 1990).

Using chemicals for chronic pain

Many health care practitioners have long advocated using narcotics for the relief of severe pain in cancer patients, and narcotic analgesics are commonly prescribed when these patients are dying (Foley 1985). In some cases of cancer, severe pain becomes chronic and is associated with progression of the disease. Despite guidelines to treat clinical pain more aggressively, a large percentage of Australian cancer patients receive inadequate analgesic drugs. Why? Part of the reason is that cancer patients — especially older, less educated ones — often fear they will become addicted if the drug is a narcotic and believe that 'good' patients don't complain (Ward et al. 1993). Practitioners need to discuss these issues with their patients and correct misconceptions.

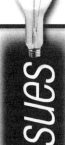

Highlight on issues

issues

Types of pain-relieving chemicals

The most common medical approaches for treating pain today involve the use of various chemicals, some of which are used mainly in hospitals. There are four types of chemicals for treating pain.

1. *Peripherally active analgesics* make up one type of pain-relieving chemical (Aronoff, Wagner & Spangle 1986). As the name implies, these drugs reduce pain by their action in the peripheral nervous system, such as by inhibiting the synthesis of neurochemicals that sensitise nociceptors to algogenic substances released at the site of tissue damage. These analgesics include *aspirin*, *paracetamol* (brand names Disprin and Panadol), and *ibuprofen* (Brufen and Nurofen). Aspirin was first manufactured in the late 1800s and is by far the best-known and most widely used drug in this class, with many hundreds of millions taken by Australians each year. Aspirin is a remarkable drug, being a very effective analgesic for mild-to-moderate pain, while also reducing fever and inflammation. Using aspirin on an occasional basis has no adverse effects, but heavy use can cause irritation of the stomach lining. Peripherally acting analgesics provide substantial pain relief for a wide variety of pain conditions, especially arthritis and other conditions that involve inflammation (Anderson et al. 1985; Kanner 1986).

2. *Centrally acting analgesics* are narcotics that act by binding to opiate receptors in the central nervous system (Aronoff, Wagner & Spangler 1986). These narcotics are either derived directly from the opium poppy — as are codeine and morphine — or they are synthetic substances, such as heroin (not manufactured in Australia for medical purposes), methadone, and the brand name drugs Anamorf and Physeptone. Narcotics are highly effective in reducing severe pain, and they are far more potent when administered by injection than orally (Kanner 1986; Winters 1985). The chief reservation doctors and patients have in using narcotics for pain relief is the potential these drugs have for producing tolerance, in which the individual requires increasingly large doses, and for causing addiction. Some patients fear becoming or being thought of as junkies, and may fail to take prescribed pain-killing drugs for that reason. There is some controversy about the risks of narcotic tolerance and addiction in pain patients (compare, for example, Aronoff, Wagner & Spangler 1986 and Melzack & Wall 1982).

3. *Local anaesthetics*, such as novocaine, lignocaine, and bupivacaine, make up the third category of chemicals for relieving pain (AMA 1989; Melzack & Wall 1982; Winters 1985). Although local anaesthetics can be applied topically, they are much more potent when injected at the site where the pain originates, as a dentist does before drilling or pulling a tooth. These chemicals work by blocking nerve cells in the region from generating impulses — and they often continue to relieve pain for hours or days after the chemical action has worn off (Hare & Milano 1985). Long-term use of currently available local anaesthetics is not recommended because of their serious side effects (Melzack & Wall 1982).

4. *Indirectly acting drugs* affect non-pain conditions, such as emotions, that produce or contribute to pain. These drugs include sedatives, tranquillisers, and antidepressants (Aronoff, Wagner & Spangler 1986; Foley 1985). *Sedatives*, such as barbiturates, and *tranquillisers*, such as diazepam (Valium), are depressants — they depress bodily functions by decreasing the transmission of impulses throughout the central nervous system. Although pain patients often claim sedatives and tranquillisers help them, there is no clear evidence that these drugs alleviate pain as much as they reduce anxiety and help patients sleep. The danger with using depressants for pain relief is that chronic use can produce psychological and physical dependence. Drugs classed as *antidepressants* reduce psychological depression, and some may also relieve pain.

Because of the terminal nature of cancer, practitioners generally view the options for pain relief in these patients differently from the options for those who have other types of chronic pain. Research has shown that narcotics are effective in treating a variety of chronic pain conditions (Jadad et al. 1992). For example, researchers tested the utility of drug therapy, combining methadone and an antidepressant, over a two-year period for men and women patients with severe phantom limb pain (Urban et al. 1986). The subjects reported having had the pain syndrome for an average of five years, being in pain almost constantly, having limited their lifestyles because of it, and having used a wide variety of treatments for pain relief in the past, including narcotics. They began the drug therapy as hospital in-patients, reported at discharge that their pain had been reduced by about two-thirds, and maintained this level of pain reduction throughout the next two years with very low daily doses of each drug.

These findings are very important and indicate that narcotics in low doses can provide effective pain relief without requiring progressively larger doses or leading to addiction. Because of a growing body of similar findings, Australian practitioners are using narcotics more than in the past for patients who are severely disabled by their chronic pain conditions, such as severe back injury. But increases in using narcotics for chronic pain are occurring cautiously for at least three reasons. First, the findings we have described need to be confirmed with a greater variety of subjects and types of pain conditions. Despite the low risk that drug abuse appears to have for most pain patients, it probably poses a high risk for *some* patients. Second, studies need to determine specifically how patients' lives and functioning are altered by taking daily doses of narcotics. Third, researchers need to find out why tolerance and addiction to narcotics are less likely when they are taken for pain relief. Is it because the doses are so small, for instance, or that the practitioners monitor and set limits on the drug use? Or is it that the patients believe they may lose their pain-killers if they use them too much?

Although future research findings may lead to a wider application of narcotics for pain sufferers — particularly some who suffer disabling chronic/intractable/benign pain — it seems unlikely that these drugs will prove to be a valuable component of treatment for the vast majority of chronic pain patients. And even though the widely used non-narcotic chemicals we described earlier can help in relieving chronic pain, health care professionals often prefer not to rely on them for long-term pain control for two reasons. First, drugs often have undesirable side effects and can lead to psychological and, sometimes, physical dependence. Second, chemical methods are usually not sufficient for controlling pain by themselves. Other approaches are also needed — as physician Ronald Kanner has noted, 'There is no *single* answer to pain' (1986, p. 2113).

The need for other approaches in helping pain patients can be seen in the findings of research on three issues. First, studies of coping patterns have found that chronic headache patients tend to use maladaptive ways of coping with everyday stressors more than do non-headache control subjects (Mosley et al. 1990). Second, arthritis patients with high feelings of helplessness before drug treatment begins report poorer treatment success in reducing pain and disability than do comparable low-helplessness patients (Nicassio et al. 1993). Third, *placebo* drugs seem to affect patients' reports of pain. Research has investigated the effectiveness of various drugs — analgesics, tranquillisers and chemicals that constrict blood vessels — in treating migraine and tension-type headache, using double-blind procedures and giving some subjects placebos (Andrasik, Blake & McCarran 1986; Feuerstein & Gainer 1982). These studies have shown that although many headache patients claim to experience substantial relief when taking one drug or another, so do many who take the placebo. Because placebo effects result from psychological processes, we might expect that treatments using psychological methods might also relieve pain. As we saw in chapter 11 when considering the gate-control theory of pain, separating physiological and psychosocial aspects of a person's pain experience is artificial.

Because psychosocial factors are so important in people's experience of chronic pain, many medical practitioners treat pain patients by joining forces with psychologists and other health care professionals, such as social workers, physiotherapists and occupational therapists. When introducing a team approach to chronic pain patients, doctors need to describe the rationale for it and the functions each professional can provide. As psychologists Roy Cameron and Larry Shepel have noted, for instance,

> pain patients might balk at the suggestion that they see a psychologist. They typically believe, generally quite correctly, that their problems have a physical basis. Hence, the relevance of a psychological consultation may not be evident to the patient. The meaning of the referral also may be unclear. The patient may infer that the physician making the referral believes the problem to be somehow less than real, or believes the patient to be seriously maladjusted psychologically. Patients who interpret the referral this way are likely to be guarded with the psychologist. (1986, p. 242)

The doctor should state clearly that (1) he or she realises the patient is 'obviously living in a great deal of pain,' (2) patients can help themselves control their pain by working with these other professionals, and (3) the doctor will be an active part of the team.

To summarise, medical treatments of pain focus mainly on using chemical approaches to reduce discomfort. For chronic pain patients, these approaches can be enhanced when combined with pain control methods that other health care professions provide. Doctors usually want to minimise the use of medication by their patients, especially when drugs would be taken on a long-term basis. Reducing the patient's drug consumption is one of the goals in using other methods of pain control with pain patients.

Behavioural and cognitive methods for treating pain

Gate-control theory changed the way many health care workers conceptualise pain by proposing that pain can be controlled not only by biochemical methods that alter sensory input directly, but by modifying motivational and cognitive processes, too. This more complex view of pain provided the rationale for psychologists to develop techniques to help patients (1) *cope more effectively* with the pain and other stressors they experience and (2) *reduce their reliance on drugs* for pain control. Some of the methods psychologists developed involve behavioural and cognitive techniques, and we will examine three of these approaches in this section. The first approach focuses on changing patients' pain behaviour through techniques of operant conditioning.

The operant approach

At the start of this chapter, we described the case of a three-year-old girl whose rehabilitation after suffering severe burns months earlier was hampered by her pattern of pain behaviours. The help therapists provided was successful. It used an *operant approach*, in which therapists apply operant conditioning techniques to modify patients' behaviour.

The approach the therapists used in changing this girl's behaviour involved extinction procedures for her pain behaviour and reinforcement for appropriate, or 'well', behaviour (Varni et al. 1986; Varni & Thompson 1986). Initial observations of the child's social environment revealed that her pain behaviours — crying, complaining of pain, resisting the nurse's efforts to put her splints on and so forth — were maintained by the hospital staff giving attention to those behaviours and allowing her to avoid uncomfortable or disliked activities, such as physiotherapy. To change this situation, the therapists instructed the hospital staff to:

- ignore the pain behaviours they paid attention to in the past
- provide rewards for compliant behaviour — telling her, for instance, 'If you don't cry while I put your splints on, you can have some cookies when I'm finished,' or, 'If you do this exercise, we can play a game.'
- praise her if she helps in putting on the splints, sleeps through naptime, goes for a period of time without complaining or does an exercise.

Changing the consequences of her behaviour in these ways had a dramatic effect: her pain behaviours decreased sharply, and she began to comply with requests to do exercises, make positive comments about her accomplishments and assist in putting on her splints.

The operant approach to treating pain can be adapted for use with individuals of all ages, in hospitals and at home — and elements of the operant approach can be introduced before pain behaviour becomes chronic. But treatment programs using this approach are usually applied to patients whose chronic pain has already produced serious difficulties in their lives. These programs typically have two main goals: The first is to reduce the patient's reliance on medication. This can be achieved with the patient's approval, using a technique described by Wilbert Fordyce (1976). One feature of this technique is that the medication is given on a fixed schedule, such as every four hours, rather than whenever the patient requests it. This makes receiving the pain-killer independent of requesting it, thereby eliminating any reinforcing effect the drug may have on that pain behaviour. In addition, the medication is mixed with a flavoured syrup to mask its taste. Then, over a period of several weeks, the dosage of medication in this 'pain cocktail' is gradually reduced until the syrup contains little or no drugs.

The second goal of the operant approach is to reduce the disability that generally accompanies chronic pain conditions. This is accomplished by altering the consequences for behaviour so that they promote 'well' behaviour and discourage pain behaviour, as we just saw in the program with the young burn patient. The chief feature of this approach is that the therapist trains people in the patient's social environment to monitor and keep a record of pain behaviours, try not to reinforce them and systematically reward physical activity. The reinforcers may be of any kind — attention, praise and smiles, sweets, money or the opportunity to watch TV for example — and may be formalised within a behavioural contract (Fordyce 1976; Roberts 1986). The therapist periodically reviews the record of pain behaviour to determine whether changes in the program are needed.

Is the operant approach effective? Studies have shown that operant techniques can successfully increase patients' activity levels and decrease medication use (Bradley 1983; Groenman et al. 1990; Roberts 1986; Turk, Rudy & Sorkin 1992). Although these findings are promising, some reservations should be mentioned. First, most of the studies have not included control groups, so that it is difficult to know whether changes in the patients' behaviour in these studies resulted specifically from the operant methods or from other factors, such as simply being in a hospital. Second, not all chronic pain patients are likely to benefit from the operant approach. For one thing, the goals of this approach seem more appropriate for patients with chronic/recurrent or chronic/intractable/benign pain than for those with chronic/progressive pain, such as in cancer patients. Also, patients are less likely to show behavioural improvements if they or people in their social environment are unwilling to participate and if they receive disability compensation (Fordyce 1976). Despite these reservations, it seems clear that the operant approach can be a very useful component in treatment programs for many acute and chronic pain patients.

Relaxation and biofeedback

Many people experience chronic episodes of pain that result from underlying physiological processes, and these processes are often triggered by stress. If these patients could control their stress or the physiological processes that cause pain, they should be able to decrease the frequency or intensity of discomfort they experience. Headache provides a good example of the way stress and physiological arousal may influence pain. The classic model of migraine is a two-stage process, with intra- and extracranial vasoconstriction during the pre-headache or prodromal phase followed by a rebound phenomenon of intra- and extracranial vasodilation during the headache phase. The classic view of tension-type headache is that it arises from sustained contraction of skeletal muscles in the region of the head and neck. Research over the last three decades has lent some support to the classic model of migraine but cast doubt on the classic model of tension-type headache, with some evidence suggesting that both types of headache are due to vascular rather than muscular mechanisms (see Martin 1998 for a review of the evidence). Whatever the precise nature of the physiological mechanisms of headaches, numerous studies have shown that stress is the most common, but certainly not the only, trigger of both migraine and tension-type headache.

Figure 12.1 shows a simplified 'functional' model of chronic headaches in which factors such as stress, referred to as 'immediate' antecedents, trigger headaches through activating physiological mechanisms. Extra boxes are included in the model, however, because the pathological processes are complicated. For example, if a headache sufferer responds to a stress-triggered headache by worrying about the impact of having a headache on completing the day's work and by becoming distressed, then this completes a stress–headache–stress vicious cycle, as denoted by the feedback loop in the figure. If the 'setting' factor for the headache is a dysfunctional marriage — that is, the most common source of stress for a particular headache sufferer lies in marital difficulties — and headaches lead to irritability which in turn results in arguments between the headache sufferer and her or his spouse, then the reaction to the headaches, or consequence of the headaches, can feed back to the setting factor of the dysfunctional marriage, resulting in further deterioration in the relationship.

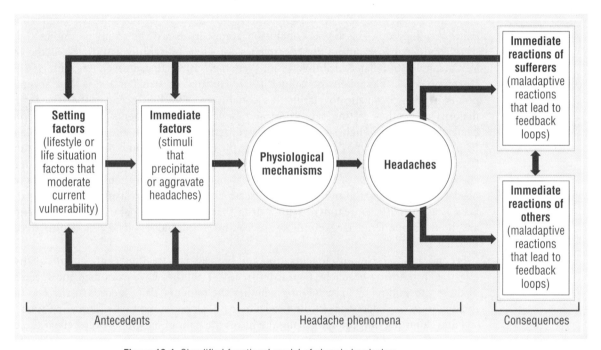

Figure 12.1 Simplified functional model of chronic headaches

Source: Adapted from Martin (1993).

Because of the connection of stress and physiological processes in producing pain, therapists have applied the methods of progressive muscle relaxation and biofeedback in helping patients control their pain. These treatments are usually conducted in weekly sessions that span about two or three months (see, for example, Blanchard et al. 1986). We saw in chapter 5 that patients using the technique of *progressive muscle relaxation* focus their attention on specific muscle groups while alternately tightening and relaxing these muscles. Patients who receive training in relaxation to control pain are urged to use this technique to reduce feelings of stress, particularly if they feel pain episodes coming on. Figure 12.1 shows why reducing stress might be effective in controlling headache pain.

In *biofeedback* procedures, patients learn to exert voluntary control over a bodily function, such as heart rate, by monitoring its status with information, usually from electronic devices. Of the many physiological processes people can learn to control through biofeedback, two have received particular attention in the treatment of pain. One of these processes focuses on muscle activity and is used for tension-type headaches. Patients learn to control the tension of specific muscle groups — such as those in the scalp and neck — by receiving biofeedback from an electromyograph (EMG) device, which measures electrical activity in the muscles. The other process is used for migraine headaches by focusing on the constriction and dilation of arteries — such as those in the head — which can be measured indirectly on the basis of the temperature of the skin in the region of the target blood vessels. Patients learn to control arterial dilation through temperature biofeedback — as the arteries dilate and contain more blood, the region becomes warmer. Therapists urge patients who learn to control muscle tension or arterial dilation to practise this skill at home and use it when they feel pain episodes beginning — doing so greatly improves treatment success (Gauthier, Côté & French 1994).

Do progressive muscle relaxation and biofeedback procedures help in relieving pain? Yes, they do. This broad conclusion comes from reviews of many studies that were conducted to examine the effectiveness of these procedures (Andrasik, Blake & McCarran 1986; Belar & Kibrick 1986; Blanchard 1987; Bogaards & ter Kuile 1994; Chapman 1991; Feuerstein & Gainer 1982; Holroyd & Penzien 1985). But several points need to be made to clarify this conclusion. The first point is that the large majority of studies testing relaxation and biofeedback treatments have focused on headache pain. Although some studies have demonstrated that these treatments can help alleviate other types of pain, such as arthritic, phantom limb and low back pain (Bradley 1983; Bradley et al. 1987; Flor & Birbaumer 1993), current knowledge about the effectiveness of these procedures is based mainly on their ability to relieve headache pain. For migraine headache, treatment combining relaxation and biofeedback is as effective as treatment with a drug that prevents arterial dilation, and using all three components is even more successful (Holroyd et al. 1995; Holroyd & Penzien 1990).

Second, progressive muscle relaxation and biofeedback treatments are about equally effective in relieving headache pain (Martin 1998). Studies have examined the success of these procedures by (1) assessing whether the patients' daily records at the end of treatment showed decreases in the headache pain, as measured by its frequency, intensity and duration, and (2) comparing the headache pain of patients who received these treatments with those who were in control groups. In one type of control group, the subjects receive no training but monitor their headache pain with daily records; in another type of control condition, subjects keep records and receive a placebo treatment, such as by taking sham medication or by receiving biofeedback sessions that give false feedback about changes in the subjects' bodily functions. Generally speaking, treatment with relaxation or biofeedback is about twice as effective in relieving pain as placebo conditions, which are more effective than just monitoring headache pain. Figure 12.2 depicts these effects for tension-type headache sufferers, averaged across subjects in many studies.

Third, the graph in figure 12.2 suggests that tension-type headache sufferers get slightly more pain relief with biofeedback than with progressive muscle relaxation treatment, and that they seem to gain even more relief when these treatments are combined. This may be the case and may be important for clinical purposes, but these differences are not reliable because patients vary greatly in the amount of benefit they get from these treatments. For instance, among subjects who received relaxation treatment only, the percentage by which their pain improved ranged from 17 per cent to 94 per cent; among those who had the combined treatment, improvements ranged from 29 per cent to 88 per cent (Holroyd & Penzien 1985). This variability is important, for it reflects that some pain patients seem to gain relatively little relief with these treatments (Blanchard & Andrasik 1985; Holroyd & Penzien 1985). In addition, biofeedback treatment is relatively expensive to conduct, and the likelihood of improvement beyond just using relaxation for many pain conditions may not justify its expense (Turk, Meichenbaum & Berman 1979). However, it may be possible to predict who will benefit most from biofeedback treatment. Tentative evidence suggests, for example, that most children are good candidates for biofeedback treatment (Keefe & Gil 1985).

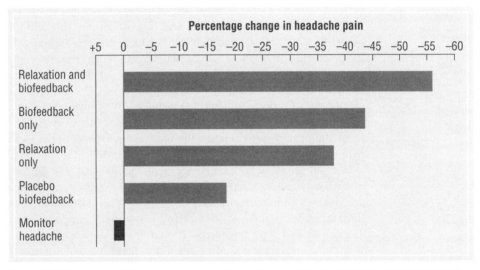

Figure 12.2 Percentage of change in headache pain, pre-treatment to post-treatment, across many studies with patients suffering from chronic tension-type headaches. Treatments consisted of EMG biofeedback, or relaxation, or EMG biofeedback and relaxation combined. Control conditions consisted of placebo biofeedback or simply monitoring headache pain.

Source: Data from Holroyd & Penzien (1985, table IV).

Fourth, although progressive muscle relaxation and biofeedback treatment result in decreases in headaches, it is not clear how they achieve their effects. EMG feedback training does not seem to achieve its beneficial effects by training patients to reduce their muscle tension, as teaching them to increase their muscle tension works equally well (Andrask & Holroyd 1980)! These findings are consistent with the evidence discussed earlier suggesting that tension-type headaches are not caused by excessive muscle tension as originally believed. Similarly, thermal biofeedback designed to train patients to cool their hands works as well as the conventional approach of training them to warm their hands (Gauthier et al. 1981). If biofeedback training is superior to placebo control procedures but does not work by learned control of the targeted physiological mechanisms, how does it achieve its beneficial effects? A number of researchers have responded to this question by suggesting that the critical changes are cognitive rather than physiological (Holroyd et al. 1984; Mizener, Thomas & Billings 1988). In essence, the argument is that as patients perceive themselves as succeeding at the biofeedback task, they begin to view their headaches as being more controllable, and themselves as more capable of influencing their headaches. These cognitive changes lead to new and more persistent efforts to cope with headache-related stresses, and subsequent reduction in headaches.

Progressive muscle relaxation and biofeedback techniques are very helpful in controlling the discomfort many chronic pain patients experience, but these treatments do not provide all the pain relief most patients need. Because chronic pain involves a complex interplay of sensory and psychosocial factors, therapists generally use these techniques along with several other approaches, especially cognitive therapies that address the thought patterns that occur when people experience pain.

Cognitive techniques

What do people think about when they experience pain? In an acute pain situation, some people focus on the ordeal and how uncomfortable and miserable they are, but others do not (Turk & Rudy 1986). For example, researchers asked children and adolescents what they think about when getting an injection at their dentist's office (Brown et al. 1986). More than 80 per cent of the subjects reported thoughts that focused on negative emotions and pain, such as, 'This hurts, I hate shots,' 'I'm scared,' and 'My heart is pounding and I feel shaky.' One-fourth of the subjects had thoughts of escaping or avoiding the situation, as in, 'I want to run away.' These types of thoughts focus the person's attention on the unpleasant aspects of the experience and make the pain worse (Keefe et al. 1994; Turk & Rudy 1986).

Not all people who experience acute pain focus on the ordeal and discomfort; many use cognitive strategies to modify their experience. For instance, by 10 years of age, many children report that they try to cope with pain in a dental situation by thinking about something else or by reassuring themselves by saying such things as, 'It's not so bad,' or, 'Be brave' (Brown et al. 1986). Even though children's coping skills tend to improve as they get older, many patients in adulthood still exaggerate the fearful aspects of the painful medical procedures they experience (Chaves & Brown 1987).

How do people cope with chronic pain? Some approaches they use involve *active coping*, in which they try to keep functioning by ignoring their pain or keeping busy with an interesting activity. Other approaches involve *passive coping*, such as taking to bed or curtailing social activities. For many chronic pain patients, a vicious circle develops in which passive coping leads to feelings of helplessness and depression, which leads to more passive coping, and so on (Smith & Wallston 1992). Family and friends influence people's coping patterns by reinforcing some behaviours, but not others (Menefee et al. 1996). The way chronic pain patients cope also depends on the way in which they view their condition (Williams & Keefe 1991). Those who believe that their pain will last a very long time and that they and their doctors don't know what causes their pain tend to cope poorly, thinking the worst about their conditions and feeling that active coping strategies will not work. On the other hand, patients who believe that they understand the nature of their pain and that their condition will improve over time tend to use active coping strategies. Those who cope well are more likely to return to work despite their pain (Linton & Buer 1995).

To help people cope effectively with pain, medical and psychological practitioners need to assess and address their patients' beliefs. Cognitive techniques for treating pain involve active coping strategies, and many of these methods are, in fact, quite effective in helping people cope with pain. These techniques can be classified into three basic types: *distraction*, *imagery* and *redefinition* (Fernandez 1986; McCaul & Malott 1984). We will examine these methods and consider their usefulness for people with acute and chronic pain.

Focus on research
How durable are the effects of relaxation and biofeedback treatments for pain?

After a patient completes the treatment for chronic pain, how long do the effects of the treatment last? Do the effects wear off in a few weeks or months? This is an issue of great importance in health psychology: As we saw in earlier chapters, psychological interventions do not always last, such as in cases of alcohol abuse, and relapse often occurs. Edward Blanchard, Frank Andrasik and their associates have addressed this issue by conducting a five-year follow-up investigation on chronic headache patients who completed training either for progressive muscle relaxation or for both relaxation and biofeedback (Blanchard et al. 1986; Blanchard, Andrasik et al. 1987; Blanchard, Appelbaum et al. 1987).

The subjects in this research were adult patients who had suffered an average of 18 years either from muscle-contraction (tension-type) headache or from 'vascular' headache, which includes both migraine and combined (migraine plus tension-type) headache. All patients received relaxation training in ten sessions, spanning eight weeks. Those patients whose headache pain had not improved by at least 60 per cent were offered additional treatment with biofeedback. All subjects had an audiotape to guide their practice of relaxation, and the vascular patients who received training in temperature biofeedback were given a temperature-monitoring device to use at home. The subjects kept daily 'headache diaries' with four ratings each day of their

headache pain. Psychological assessment before the treatment and again a few months after treatment revealed that the subjects' feeling of depression and anxiety decreased substantially (Blanchard et al. 1986).

Of the subjects who completed the treatment and continued to be available for the study, the researchers attempted to follow only those whose headache pain had been improved by at least 50 per cent at the end of treatment. During the first six months after treatment, these 38 subjects continued to keep their daily headache diaries, were interviewed by a therapist monthly, and received treatment booster sessions at these interviews if they desired them. Thereafter, each patient who continued in the study met with a therapist yearly and was paid for participating.

A major difficulty in doing longitudinal research is that the number of original subjects who are available and willing to participate declines over time. At the time of the last annual follow-up, only 21 patients (9 muscle-contraction and 12 vascular) could be located and agreed to participate. To assess the treatment's continued success, the researchers used the ratings these subjects made during each of seven four-week periods: as pre-treatment, post-treatment and years 1 through 5 in the follow-up. As figure 12.3 shows, the treatment effects were quite durable for the patients who continued in the study.

(continued)

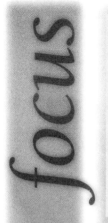

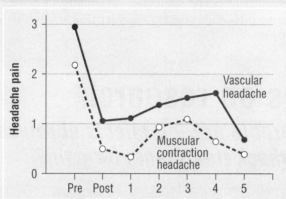

Figure 12.3 Averaged ratings of headache pain for muscle-contraction (tension-type) and vascular (migraine and combined) headache patients who successfully completed treatment and continued to participate in the follow-up. The graphs depict these ratings at pre-treatment, post-treatment and follow-up years 1 through 5.

Source: Data from Blanchard, Appelbaum et al. (1987, table 1).

What about the 17 patients who did not continue through the five-year follow-up — were their treatments durable? Although there is no way of knowing for sure, there is reason to believe they were (Blanchard, Andrasik et al. 1987; Blanchard, Appelbaum et al. 1987). Most of these patients simply could not be located, but five were contacted and did not indicate that they were having pain problems when they declined to partici-pate. Moreover, most of those who dropped out during the five years had reported very suc-cessful pain relief in the last follow-up they had completed, which suggests that they dropped out for reasons other than a relapse in pain. The results of several other follow-up studies show that treating chronic headache with relaxation training or thermal biofeedback leads to reductions in headaches that are maintained for at least three to six years, but improvements achieved via EMG biofeedback training seem to progressively deteriorate after 12 months, although not back to pre-treatment levels (Blanchard 1987; Sorbi, Tellegen & Du Long 1989).

Distraction

At your dentist's office, do the examination rooms have colourful pictures or large windows with nice views on all the walls a patient can see while in the dental chair? My dentist's rooms do, and I use the pictures and windows to distract my attention when I feel the need. **Distraction** is the technique of focusing on a non-painful stimulus in the immediate environment to divert our attention from discomfort (Fernandez 1986). We can be distracted from pain in many ways, such as by looking at a picture, listening to someone's voice, singing a song, counting ceiling tiles, playing a video game or doing mathematics problems.

Not all distraction attempts are likely to work in relieving pain. Research on acute pain has shown that these strategies are more effective if the pain is mild or moderate than if it is strong (McCaul & Malott 1984). Does the amount of attention the distrac-tion task attracts affect how well it works? Evidence from a series of experiments using the cold-pressor procedure and different distraction tasks indicates that it does not (McCaul, Monson & Maki 1992). The subjects were college students. The distraction tasks all involved watching a computer screen that presented numbers, but the sub-jects with the least complex task (which the researchers called the control group) simply watched the screen, whereas the subjects with the most complex task had to use the numbers in a complicated activity. The results revealed that the complexity of the task did not influence the pain distress ratings the subjects made while their hands were in the cold water.

An important factor in whether a distraction technique relieves pain is whether it seems credible to the person. A study demonstrated this by having college students undergo the cold-pressor procedure while listening to distracting stimuli through earphones (Melzack, Weisz & Sprague 1963). During the cold-pressor test, the subjects in one condition listened to a clearly noticeable sound, such as music, after having been told that they could control its volume and that dentists had found that loud sound helps reduce pain. Subjects in another condition got similar instructions, but they tried to listen for a low-intensity 'hum' that really didn't exist. The subjects who heard the noticeable sound kept their hands in the cold water longer than those who listened for the hum.

Why was the nonexistent hum less effective than the sound in helping the subjects tolerate pain? Since there was no sound, the subjects probably didn't believe the technique would work. Because of the role that credibility can play in using distraction methods, therapists may need to help patients understand how these techniques can work. One therapist described the following approach for doing this.

> First, I ask the patient to be aware of the sensations in his thighs as he sits in his chair. I note that those sensations are real, and they have a physical basis, but they are not normally experienced because other things occupy his attention. Then I suggest that he think of a TV set: he could block out the channel 9 signal by tuning in channel 11; the channel 9 signal is still there, but not being tuned in. I suggest that while his pain signals are real, he can learn to 'tune them out. . . .' A number of pain patients have reported that they frequently think of the TV metaphor when experiencing pain and take appropriate action to 'tune out.' (Cameron, quoted in Turk, Meichenbaum & Genest 1983, p. 284)

By providing plausible explanations for a recommended technique, therapists can increase its effectiveness and the likelihood that the patient will use it.

Distraction strategies are especially useful for reducing acute pain, such as that experienced in some medical or dental procedures, but they can also provide relief for chronic pain patients in some circumstances. Singing a song or staring intently at a stimulus can divert the person's attention for a short while — and this may be a great help, for instance for an arthritis sufferer who experiences heightened pain when climbing stairs. People who want to use distraction for moderate levels of continuous pain may get longer-lasting relief by engaging in an extended engrossing activity, such as watching a movie or reading a book.

Imagery

Sometimes when children are about to receive injections, their parents will say something like, 'It'll be easier if you think about something nice, like the fun things we did at the park.' **Non-pain imagery** — sometimes called *guided imagery* — is a strategy whereby the person tries to alleviate discomfort by conjuring up a mental scene that is unrelated to or incompatible with the pain (Fernandez 1986). The most common type of imagery people use involves scenes that are pleasant to them — they think of 'something nice'. This scene might involve being at the beach or in the country, for instance. Therapists usually encourage, or 'guide', the person to include aspects of a variety of senses: vision, hearing, taste, smell and touch. As an example, the scene at the beach could include the sight and smell of the ocean water, the sound of the waves and the warm, grainy feel of the sand. Other types of imagery for controlling pain are not necessarily pleasant — they can involve such themes as having an argument with someone or replacing the feeling of pain with another sensation, such as a tingling feeling. The person generally tries to keep the imagined event in mind as long as possible.

The imagery technique is in many ways like distraction. The main difference is that imagery is based on the person's imagination rather than on real objects or events in the environment. As a result, individuals who use imagery do not have to depend on the environment to provide a suitably distracting stimulus. They can develop one or more scenes that work reliably, which they 'carry' around in their heads. They can then call one of these scenes up for pain relief whenever they need it. Imagery seems to work best when it attracts high levels of the person's attention or involvement, and it is likely to work better with mild or moderate pain than with strong pain (McCaul & Malott 1984; Turk, Meichenbaum & Genest 1983). Although imagery clearly helps in reducing acute pain, the extent of this technique's usefulness with longer-lasting pain episodes is unclear. One limitation with using imagery in pain control is that some individuals are less adept in imagining scenes than others (Melzack & Wall 1982).

Redefinition

The third type of cognitive strategy for reducing discomfort is **pain redefinition**, in which the person substitutes constructive or realistic thoughts about the pain experience for ones that arouse feelings of threat or harm (Fernandez 1986; McCaul & Malott 1984). Therapists can help people redefine their pain experiences in several ways. For one thing, providing information about the sensations to expect in medical procedures can reduce the pain patients experience when undergoing these procedures (Anderson & Masur 1983). Since many patients have misconceptions or exaggerated expectations about the discomfort they will feel, providing realistic information helps them redefine the experiences before they occur.

Another approach that can be helpful in redefining pain experiences involves engaging in an internal dialogue, using positive self-statements. There are basically two kinds of self-statements for controlling pain (Fernandez 1986): *Coping statements* emphasise the person's ability to tolerate the discomfort, as when people say to themselves, 'It hurts, but you're in control,' or, 'Be brave — you can take it.' *Reinterpretative statements* are designed to negate the unpleasant aspects of the discomfort, as when people think, 'It's not so bad,' 'It's not the worst thing that could happen,' or, 'It hurts, but think of the benefits of this experience.' This last statement can be particularly appropriate when undergoing painful medical procedures.

A third approach for redefining pain experiences involves helping the patients see that some of their beliefs are illogical and are making the discomfort worse. We see how this process can work in the following dialogue between a therapist and 'Mrs D', a 56-year-old patient who worried that her chronic/recurrent head pain was actually caused by a tumour, which repeated neurological tests had failed to reveal. The therapist suggested that they examine those thoughts.

MRS D: Yes, I know they're not true but I cannot help it.

THERAPIST: You don't think you have control over your thoughts?

MRS D: Yes, they just come to me.

T: Well, let's come back to the idea that your thoughts are automatic. First, let's break down your flood of negative thoughts and look at each part separately. Do you really think that you have a tumor?

MRS D: I don't know. I guess not (pause) but it's hard not to worry about it. My head hurts so bad.

T: Yes, I know. So how do you convince yourself that you don't have a tumor or something else seriously wrong?

MRS D: Well, as you know I've been examined many times by the best neurologists around. They say I'm OK. Also, my pain always goes away and I've never had any other neurological problems. My only problem is the pain. But, it's hard to remember these facts when my pain is so awful.

T: It's much easier to be positive about your condition when you're not suffering. Nevertheless, rationally, you really are convinced that there's nothing seriously wrong.

MRS D: I guess so. If only I could remember that when my pain starts coming on.

T: So the goal of our work today could be to figure out a strategy to increase the likelihood that you'll remember the positive thoughts during a pain episode.

MRS D: Yes, that sounds good.

T: Let's start by generating a list of accurate statements about your pain. Then we can talk about ways you can cue yourself to remember the list when you begin to feel pain. You already mentioned a couple of beliefs about your pain; that is, that there's nothing seriously wrong, that the pain always goes away, and that, other than the pain, you feel pretty healthy. Can you think of other accurate and positive thoughts? (Holzman, Turk & Kerns 1986, pp. 45–6)

In this example, the therapist helped the patient examine the logic of her thought patterns and generate a list of ideas that she believed were incompatible with her irrational fears. They later rehearsed these beliefs so that she could use them as self-statements when pain episodes occurred.

The value of cognitive strategies in controlling pain

Studies have found that cognitive strategies are effective in reducing acute pain (Fernandez & Turk 1989; Manne et al. 1994). Distraction and imagery seem to be particularly useful with mild or moderate pain, and redefinition appears to be more effective with strong pain (McCaul & Malott 1984). How helpful are cognitive methods for treating chronic pain? The answer is likely to depend on many factors, such as the severity of the pain and the type of illness. But research has shown that treatments combining behavioural and cognitive methods are at least as effective as chemical methods in reducing chronic tension-type headaches (Holroyd et al. 1991). There is also some evidence that redefinition is more effective than distraction in relieving chronic pain. A study compared these two techniques in reducing the chronic pain of patients who were receiving physical rehabilitation for a variety of medical problems, including arthritis, amputation and spinal cord injury (Rybstein-Blinchik 1979). Although both techniques were effective, patients who received redefinition training reported less pain and exhibited less pain behaviour than those who were trained in distraction.

Because each type of cognitive strategy can be helpful in treating clinical pain, programs to help chronic pain sufferers control their pain generally combine different types of strategies. In one study, for instance, arthritis sufferers received a five-week pain control program that included training in distraction, imagery and redefinition (O'Leary et al. 1988). The program gave special emphasis to having the patients use these techniques in specific painful activities, such as carrying groceries, climbing stairs and mopping floors. A control group simply received a self-help book for arthritis sufferers. Assessments made just before and just after the program was conducted revealed that it was very effective. The control group showed little or no improvement during that time period. In contrast, the treated group reported having less pain, greater self-efficacy, less depression and improved sleep patterns.

Another study used a program that combined imagery, redefinition and progressive muscle relaxation training to treat chronic low back pain patients (Turner 1982). Some subjects received this program, others received a program of only relaxation training and a third group served as controls. Compared with the control subjects, the patients in both programs reported much less pain, depression and disability by the end of treatment — and these improvements were similar for the patients in both programs. A follow-up on the patients in the two programs more than 18 months later revealed that the benefits of the treatments were maintained, as measured by the subjects' ratings of pain and reports of health care use. But the patients who received the program combining cognitive strategies and relaxation also showed a marked improvement in their employment, working 60 per cent more hours per week than those who had the program of relaxation only.

To summarise, several behavioural and cognitive methods are effective in helping people control acute and chronic pain. These methods include operant techniques, progressive muscle relaxation and biofeedback, and the cognitive strategies of distraction, imagery and redefinition. Behavioural and cognitive methods seem to be most helpful when used in combination.

Hypnosis and insight-oriented psychotherapy

You may have noticed that the behavioural and cognitive methods we just described for relieving pain sound familiar — and they should. For the most part, they involve psychological procedures derived from the stress reduction techniques we considered in chapter 5. Because people's experiences of pain include an emotional component and are stressful, and because behavioural and cognitive methods are effective in reducing stress, psychologists have adapted these techniques to help people control their pain. Other psychological approaches have also been applied to relieve pain. These approaches include hypnosis and insight therapy.

Hypnosis as a treatment for pain

In the mid-1800s before ether was discovered, dramatic reports began to appear of doctors performing major surgery on individuals using hypnosis as the sole method of analgesia (Bakal 1979; Barber 1986). In one such case of a woman with breast cancer, a surgeon made an incision halfway across her chest and removed the tumour as well as several enlarged glands in her armpit. During the procedure, the woman conversed with the surgeon and showed no signs of feeling pain. Another doctor reported having done hundreds of major surgeries with hypnosis as the only analgesic, and argued that the patients experienced no pain. Were all of these operations painless? Probably not — although many patients *claimed* to feel no pain, some showed other pain behaviours, such as facial expressions, suggesting they were suppressing their agony (Bakal 1979). Nevertheless, hypnosis does appear to reduce the intensity of acute pain that some individuals experience (Hilgard & Hilgard 1983).

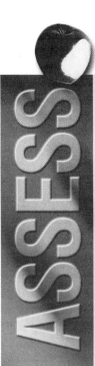

Assess yourself

WOULD BEHAVIOURAL OR COGNITIVE METHODS HELP *YOUR* PAIN?

Pain Self-management Checklist

<u>How often</u> have you used these pain self-management strategies (over the last month).
Indicate your answer by circling <u>one</u> of the numbers (0–4) beside each item.

Thinking back over the last month, how often have you done these?

	Never	Sometimes			Very often
1. If pain stops you doing something, do you ever work out other ways to do it? (Like, if you normally sit to do a task but find sitting is difficult owing to pain, have you worked out other ways to do it? Think of an example.)	0	1	2	3	4
2. Taking <u>regular</u> short breaks when engaging in activities, including sitting or standing, which stir up your pain (such as standing up for 5 minutes every 20 minutes).	0	1	2	3	4
3. Thinking that your doctors will find a cure for your pain?	0	1	2	3	4
4. Using pain-killers to allow you to do something you know will stir up your pain (like driving or standing too long, or carrying too much).	0	1	2	3	4
5. Taking more than the recommended dose of any drug related to your pain; or using alcohol for pain relief.	0	1	2	3	4
6. Taking a drug that only 'takes the edge off' your pain.	0	1	2	3	4
7. Having <u>one</u> or more long rest periods (more than 45 minutes) (lying or sitting) during the day (8:00 am to 8:00 pm).	0	1	2	3	4
8. Lying in bed at night worrying or getting stressed.	0	1	2	3	4
9. Because of pain, having others perform your normal household duties (like washing-up, cooking, vacuuming).	0	1	2	3	4
10. Doing an activity or task until it is completed, <u>regardless</u> of pain, and then resting.	0	1	2	3	4
11. Because of pain, using aids (like sticks, braces or collars).	0	1	2	3	4
12. Seeing a physiotherapist, doctor, chiropractor or other health care provider about your pain (in the last month).	0	1	2	3	4
13. Thinking that increased pain means you might have injured yourself (or made your injury worse).	0	1	2	3	4
14. Thinking that doctors have missed something, or that you need more investigations to explain your pain.	0	1	2	3	4
15. Thinking that pain relief is necessary before you can become more active generally.	0	1	2	3	4
16. When your pain gets worse, do you ever have upsetting thoughts (e.g., 'I can't go on; not again; why me?')	0	1	2	3	4
17. When your pain gets worse, do you ever take a tablet or have an injection?	0	1	2	3	4
18. Do you ever make comparisons between what you are like now and how you were before the onset of your pain?	0	1	2	3	4

Source: M. K. Nicholas, University of Sydney Pain Management & Research Centre, Royal North Shore Hospital. Copyright © 1999. Reproduced with permission.

How and why does hypnosis reduce pain? First of all, we should note that hypnosis is not effective for all people — in fact, it produces a high degree of analgesia in only a minority of individuals (Hilgard & Hilgard 1983; Melzack & Wall 1982). People vary in their ability to be hypnotised, and those who can be hypnotised very easily and deeply seem to gain more pain relief from hypnosis than those who are less hypnotically susceptible (DeBenedittis, Panerai & Villamira 1989; Spanos, Perlini & Robertson 1989). The mechanisms underlying the pain relief that some individuals get from hypnosis are not clear. Part of the mechanism may involve the deep relaxation people experience when hypnotised — as we saw earlier, relaxation can help relieve pain. Cognitive factors also seem to be involved (Barber 1986; Turk, Meichenbaum & Genest 1983). Hypnosis often produces states of heightened attention to internal images and inattention to environmental stimuli. For instance, while under hypnosis, people may experience 'positive' hallucinations, in which they perceive objects and events that are not really there, or 'negative' hallucinations, in which they fail to perceive things they ordinarily would. Because hypnosis may produce analgesia somewhat like placebos do, researchers have looked for neurophysiological mechanisms that may underlie hypnotic pain relief. Although research has apparently cast doubt on the role of endorphins, findings for other neurochemicals seem more promising (Barber 1986; DeBenedittis, Panerai & Villamira 1989).

Hypnosis has always been viewed as an odd phenomenon, and its role in pain relief has not changed that view. When it produces analgesia, it can do so very quickly and dramatically. Furthermore, patients who experience hypnotic analgesia sometimes do not even believe they were hypnotised, perhaps because they have unrealistic ideas about what it feels like to be hypnotised. One person, for example, underwent a normally painful dental procedure with only hypnosis as an anaesthetic. He claimed to the dentist that he was not hypnotised 'because I can't be hypnotised' and that the reason he did not feel pain was that 'you didn't do anything to me that would hurt' (Barber 1986).

In some cases these patients' claims that they were not hypnotised may actually be right. According to researcher Theodore Barber (1982), laboratory research on acute pain, induced by cold-pressor or muscle-ischaemia procedures, has produced the following conclusions.

- Hypnosis can reduce pain.
- When hypnotised, the people who gain the most pain relief from suggestions of analgesia tend to be those who are highly responsive to other suggestions, such as that their arm is becoming light.
- Whether under hypnosis or not, individuals who are told to try not to feel pain tend to use distraction and redefinition techniques.
- Contrary to the common myths about hypnosis, people usually show as much pain reduction using cognitive strategies, such as imagery and redefinition, as they do under hypnosis.

It may be that some patients who were supposedly hypnotised actually were not, and they may have applied cognitive strategies to reduce the pain.

Can hypnosis also help relieve chronic pain? Although some research has found support for the effectiveness of hypnosis in treating chronic headache, low back pain and cancer pain, almost all these studies either lacked appropriate control groups or simply provided descriptions of individual cases (Barber 1986; Melzack & Wall 1982). As a result, there is little clear evidence that hypnosis provides any better relief for chronic pain than a placebo drug or sham treatment would. The success of hypnosis with acute pain suggests that it might be effective with chronic pain, but better research is needed to demonstrate this clearly. Even if this research is eventually done and confirms its usefulness, hypnosis is likely to be most effective when used along with other therapy techniques, such as behavioural and cognitive methods, rather than as the sole treatment approach (Barber 1986).

Insight therapy for pain

Many approaches to psychotherapy involve helping individuals achieve insights into the roots of their problems. *Insight therapy* focuses on discovering these roots, especially when they involve underlying motivations. Of course, most psychotherapy approaches try to help clients understand why problem behaviours occur, but this understanding is the main focus in insight therapy, and changing clients' behaviour is secondary (Davison & Neale 1994). In the case of chronic pain patients, the insights often relate to the feelings these patients and their families have about the pain condition, the way they deal with pain behaviours, and the changes that have developed in the interpersonal relationships of these people. Insight therapy can be used in individual treatment and in groups.

One insight-oriented approach involves showing patients how their pain behaviour is part of 'pain games' they play with other people (Szasz, cited in Bakal 1979). In these games, individuals with chronic pain seem to take on roles in which they continually seek to confirm their identities as suffering persons, maintain their dependent lifestyles, and receive various secondary gains, such as attention and sympathy. These patients are probably not aware of what is actually happening in these games, and the purpose of this psychotherapeutic approach is to make them aware. The assumption is that once patients gain an insight into how their behaviour patterns are affecting their lives, they can give up the games if they want to and are shown how. Studies with chronic pain patients have found that treatment programs that include an insight-oriented component can successfully reduce pain, but the specific value of insight as part of the programs was not assessed (Turk, Meichenbaum & Genest 1983).

Conducting psychotherapy for chronic pain patients within a group format rather than individually has several advantages. Figure 12.4 describes some of these advantages in helping patients cope with their pain and disability. The pain group provides a forum for talking about their worst fears and conflicts to people who share these concerns and understand. Patients often say, 'I'm afraid the pain will get worse,' 'I was beginning to believe I was imagining the pain,' and 'I can't do things because of the pain, and I feel guilty, helpless, frustrated, and angry' (Hendler 1984). Patients in the group may answer, for instance, 'You hurt whether you go shopping or not; so the choice isn't between having pain or not, it's between whether you go shopping or stay home!' (Gentry & Owens 1986). These people can say things to each other that others could not, without seeming cruel. Group members can also correct each other's misconceptions, share their own ways for managing pain on a day-to-day basis, give each other hope and social support, and detect and confront each others' pain games.

Insight-oriented approaches can also help chronic pain patients and their families understand the problems they experience in their relationships within the family system (Flor & Turk 1985; Roy 1985). For instance, when a spouse suffers from chronic pain, both spouses experience feelings of frustration, anger, helplessness and guilt that they often do not communicate openly to each other. These feelings can result from changes in their roles, general style of communication and sexual relationship. The following excerpt shows how a therapist was able to help a pain patient, John Cox, and his wife gain insights about their feelings and behaviour. The three of them were discussing a pain episode John had had while he watched TV with his wife, and the therapist asked the wife how she reacted when she realised he was in pain:

MRS COX: I really felt sorry for John, but I didn't know what to do. I just tried to watch the show and not say anything to him. At those times I feel … so helpless.

T: Mr Cox, it sounds as if your wife tried to avoid talking about your pain. She sounds sort of helpless and frustrated … . How did you feel about her response?

MR COX: I think I got kind of mad at her because she seemed to be ignoring me, not really caring how I was feeling.

T: What do you think she should have done at that time?

MR COX: I don't really know.

T: Mr Cox, do you think there was anything she could have done to make you feel better?

MR COX: Not really.

T: … Perhaps at such times ignoring your pain may be the most she can do …

MR COX: Perhaps.

T: Perhaps?

MR COX: Well maybe she did know how I was feeling, but I felt upset that she didn't tell me. (Turk, Meichenbaum & Genest 1983, pp. 244–5)

Figure 12.4 Advantages of group psychotherapy over individual therapy in treating pain

1. *Efficiency*. Although each patient has unique problems, chronic pain sufferers also face common difficulties, such as depression and addiction to medication. As a result, they often need similar types of advice and information. Group meetings use the therapist's time more efficiently.
2. *Reduced isolation*. Chronic pain sufferers are typically isolated from extended social contact. This situation can lead to a sense of alienation, which involves feelings of being different from others and of anger and suspicion toward them. Group meetings can help to overcome these feelings.
3. *Credible feedback for patients*. Pain patients often resist feedback or advice from therapists, saying such things as, 'You don't know what it's like to live with pain 24 hours a day!' In their eyes, the type of feedback other patients can give may be more believable.
4. *A new reference group for patients*. Patients in a pain group develop new social networks of individuals whose experience is comparable to theirs and who can provide social pressure to conform to the realities and constructive 'rules' of living with pain and physical limitations.
5. *A different perspective for the therapist*. Watching the patient relate to other individuals in a group provides the therapist with certain kinds of information that may aid in identifying specific problems therapy should address, such as maladaptive coping styles.

Source: Based on Gentry & Owens (1986).

Insights such as these help family members understand each other's feelings and points of view, and this understanding can help to break down the long-standing confusion and conflicts that have developed over time. The resulting improvements in their relationships may then enable the therapist to get all or most of the family's cooperation in the treatment process.

In summary, hypnosis and insight-oriented approaches to psychotherapy offer promising techniques in the treatment of chronic pain. Although both approaches can probably enhance the success of pain control programs for many patients, there is currently little experimental research to confirm this belief. Thus far in our discussion of methods for reducing pain we have considered a variety of medical and psychological techniques. In the next section, we will see how physiotherapy and certain skin stimulation methods can also play important roles in controlling pain.

Physiotherapy and stimulation therapies for pain

Anthropologists and medical historians have noted that most, if not all, cultures in recorded history have learned that people can 'fight pain with pain' (Melzack & Wall 1982). One pain can cancel another — a brief or moderate pain can cancel a longer-lasting or stronger one. For example, you might reduce the pain of an injection by pressing your thumbnail into your forefinger as the shot is given. Reducing one pain by creating another is called **counter-irritation**. People in ancient cultures developed a counter-irritation procedure called *cupping* to relieve headaches, backaches and arthritic pain. In this procedure, one or more heated glass cups are inverted and pressed on the skin. As the air in the cup cools, it creates a vacuum, causing the skin to be bruised as it is drawn up into the cup. This method is still used in some parts of the world today (Melzack & Wall 1982).

The principle of counter-irritation is the basis for present-day stimulation therapies for reducing pain. After examining these pain control methods, we will discuss the important role other physical approaches can play in reducing pain.

Stimulation therapies

Why does counter-irritation relieve pain? One reason is that people actively distract their attention from the stronger pain to the milder one. Another explanation comes from gate-control theory. Recall that activity in the peripheral fibres that carry signals about mildly irritating stimuli tend to close the gate, thereby inhibiting the transmission cells from sending pain signals to the brain. Counter-irritation, such as massaging a sore muscle, activates these peripheral fibres, and this may close the gate and soothe the pain.

This gate-control view of how counter-irritation works led to the development of a pain control technique called **transcutaneous electrical nerve stimulation** (TENS). This technique involves placing electrodes on the skin near where the patient feels pain and stimulating that area with mild electric current, which is supplied by a small portable device. TENS can be effective in reducing acute muscular and post-operative pain in most patients (Chapman 1984; Hare & Milano 1985). In a dramatic example of its effectiveness, a nine-year-old boy began receiving TENS while still unconscious after kidney surgery. When he awoke, the hospital staff asked repeatedly if he felt pain in his belly, and he said, 'No, it doesn't hurt.' The startling thing about this example is that he did not even realise the surgery had already occurred — after the surgeon left the room, the boy talked

casually with the others in the room. When asked whether there was anything he feared, he began to cry and confessed his terror of the expected operation that would remove his kidney. His surprised nurse tried to reassure him that the surgery had already been done, and that there was nothing to worry about. He refused to believe her. 'But don't you remember?' she contended, 'That's why they put you to sleep this morning — so they could do the operation.' The little boy looked very threatened. 'It's not true!' he shouted,

'It's not true!' When asked why it couldn't be true, he asserted confidently, 'Because I haven't got any bandages.' We asked him to feel his belly, since his hands were outside of the bedclothes. When he did, an expression of astonishment came over his face. (Chapman 1984, p. 1265)

Now he claimed to feel pain and began to cry.

TENS has also been used in treating chronic pain, but its success has been mixed. When TENS does relieve discomfort for some chronic conditions, such as phantom limb pain, its effects are often short-lived (Bradley 1983; Hare & Milano 1985). But for patients with arthritis, TENS often produces substantial and long-lasting pain relief (Johnson 1984; Minor & Sanford 1993). Moreover, for other chronic pain conditions, such as certain forms of neuralgia, TENS sometimes produces long-lasting pain relief in patients who have gotten little or no relief from various other methods (Melzack & Wall 1982).

Another counter-irritation method that is used today for reducing pain is **acupuncture**, a technique in which fine metal needles are inserted under the skin at special locations and then twirled or electrically charged to create stimulation. Acupuncture has been used in China for at least the past 2000 years and was originally based on the idea that pain occurs when the life forces of yin and yang are out of balance (Bakal 1979; CU 1994a; Melzack & Wall 1982). Although most acupuncturists do not believe this rationale any longer, many, but not all, still determine the placement of the needles on the basis of charts that show hundreds of insertion points on the body. These acupuncturists believe that stimulation at several specific points relieves pain in associated parts of the body. On the nose and ear, for example, certain points are associated with the small intestine, whereas other points are associated with the kidney or heart or abdomen.

Does acupuncture work? Its ability to produce high levels of analgesia for acute pain in some individuals has been clearly and dramatically demonstrated — for instance, surgeons have performed major surgery on patients with only acupuncture anaesthesia. But research findings point to several conclusions about its effects and its limitations (Bakal 1979; Chapman 1984; Melzack & Wall 1982).

- Even in China, doctors perform only a small percentage (less than 10 per cent) of surgeries with acupuncture analgesia, and these operations are straightforward ones with little likelihood of complications. Patients must volunteer for the procedure, and then their doctors select appropriate candidates very carefully and make sure these patients are well indoctrinated.
- Acupuncture is rarely effective for surgical patients in Western cultures.
- Laboratory studies have shown that acupuncture produces only mild analgesia in most people.
- The degree of analgesia acupuncture produces depends on the intensity of the stimulation, and not on being applied at the exact points described on acupuncture charts.
- Pain patients who benefit most from acupuncture tend to be those who are also easily and deeply hypnotisable.

Acupuncture does *not* provide long-term relief for most chronic pain patients, but it is somewhat successful for pain conditions that involve tissue damage or tenderness (Carlsson & Sjölund 1994; Chapman 1984; Takeda & Wessel 1994).

It is tempting to conclude from these findings that acupuncture works simply through suggestion or distraction effects, but this seems unlikely because the technique also produces analgesia in animals, such as monkeys and mice (Melzack & Wall 1982).

Psychological factors cannot provide a full explanation. Perhaps gate-control theory can account for the effects of acupuncture: Stimulation through the needles may activate peripheral fibres that close the gate (Bakal 1979). Stimulation therapies can be useful in programs for treating pain, and so can several methods of physiotherapy.

Physiotherapy

Physiotherapy is an important rehabilitation component for many medical conditions — for instance, after injury or surgery patients perform exercises to enhance muscular strength and tissue flexibility to restore their range of motion. Physiotherapists have a variety of techniques they can incorporate into individualised treatment programs to help patients who suffer from acute and chronic pain conditions. Exercise is a common feature in these programs (Hare & Milano 1985; Wickersham 1984).

The therapist and patient generally plan the program together, setting daily or weekly goals that promote very gradual but steady progress. The progress is tailored to the patient's needs, being fast enough to promote a feeling of accomplishment but slow enough to prevent overexertion, reinjury or failure. In cases of acute injury, such as serious damage to the knee joint, the exercise program might span a year or two. The rationale for using exercise to control pain depends on the type of health problem the patient has — with arthritis, for instance, exercise helps by maintaining the flexibility of the joints and preventing them from becoming deformed (Minor & Sanford 1993; Wickersham 1984). Other approaches in physiotherapy, such as massage, traction, and applying heat or cold to the painful area of the body, seem to provide temporary pain relief (Tunks & Bellissimo 1991). The treatment people get from *chiropractors*, especially for neck and lower back pain, is not generally considered to be physiotherapy, but it also appears to relieve pain (Deyo et al. 1991).

Physiotherapy programs are widely used in treating two highly prevalent chronic pain conditions, arthritis and low back pain (Hare & Milano 1985; Minor & Sanford 1993; Wickersham 1984). For both of these conditions, exercise is probably the most important physiotherapy approach for achieving long-term pain relief. Research with low back pain patients, for instance, has shown that programs that gradually increase aerobic and back-strengthening exercise produce substantial improvements after the first month or two in patients' self-reports of pain and ability to perform physical activities, such as standing and lifting weights (Alaranta et al. 1994; Ashenberg et al. 1990; Manniche et al. 1988).

Sometimes physiotherapy is combined with behavioural methods in treating chronic pain to gain the benefits of each approach, and treatments for low back pain provide a good example again. A study by Richard Heinrich and his colleagues (1985) compared the benefits from physiotherapy with those of a program of behavioural and cognitive methods for adults with chronic low back pain. Both therapy programs met for 10 weeks for two hours each week. Assessments of pain and of physical and psychosocial functioning taken prior to, at the end of and six months after the program revealed two main findings. First, during the programs both groups experienced similar reductions in pain, which they maintained in the following months. Second, each group showed improvements that were specific to the programs they received: At the end of the programs and at follow-up, subjects in the physiotherapy group showed better physical functioning, and those in the behavioural/cognitive group showed better psychosocial adjustment. These findings suggest that chronic pain patients might benefit from receiving both types of treatment. Other research has found that low back pain patients show less pain behaviour, disability and self-reported pain with both physical and behavioural/cognitive therapy than with either approach alone (Turner et al. 1990).

In this chapter we have described many different types of treatment, including medical, psychological and physical therapies, and we have seen that each method can help to alleviate clinical pain. Some methods seem to be more effective than others, especially for particular types of pain conditions. Typically, no single approach is sufficient by itself. Therefore, specialists who provide treatment in pain clinics often apply several methods in combination.

Pain clinics

Before the 1970s, if a person's pain lingered, and his or her doctor could not determine its cause or find a remedy for the discomfort, that patient was left with virtually no reasonable treatment alternatives. In desperation, such people often tried extreme medical approaches that could lead to drug addiction or irreversible nerve damage, or they may have turned to charlatans. Although many people with chronic pain still use ill-conceived, desperate measures to gain relief from their discomfort, effective alternatives are available today, as we have seen. Effective pain control treatments can now be obtained through **pain clinics** (or *pain centres*), which are institutions or organisations that have been developed specifically for the treatment of chronic pain conditions.

The concept of having special institutions for treating pain originated with John Bonica, an anaesthesiologist who founded the first pain clinic at the University of Washington Medical School (Fordyce 1976; Melzack & Wall 1982). Soon other professionals followed suit, and today most large hospitals in Australia have a multi-disciplinary pain centre. The structure, methods and quality of pain clinics vary widely. Many pain clinics are private organisations, whereas others are affiliated with medical schools, university departments of behavioural medicine and hospitals; many provide in-patient treatment, while others focus on outpatient care; many incorporate a variety of treatment methods, whereas others provide basically one approach, such as acupuncture, hypnosis, biofeedback or TENS (Follick et al. 1985; Kanner 1986; Turk & Stacey 1997). Pain centres that have been accredited by the Commission on Accreditation of Rehabilitation Facilities in Tucson, Arizona, typically offer high-quality treatment (Chapman 1991).

Multidisciplinary programs

A theme that has appeared more than once in this chapter is that no single method for treating chronic pain is likely to succeed. In fact, one doctor has advised avoiding clinics that focus on applying a single approach, such as biofeedback or nerve block methods (Kanner 1986, p. 2113). *Multidisciplinary pain clinics* (or *centres*) — those that combine and integrate several effective approaches — are likely to succeed for the largest percentage of patients and provide the greatest pain relief for each individual. Clinics that have adopted multidisciplinary programs generally use assessment and treatment procedures for each patient that involve medical, psychosocial, physio-therapy, occupational therapy, and vocational factors and approaches (Follick et al. 1985; Turk & Stacey 1997).

Assessment procedures are used in determining the factors that are contributing to the patient's condition, identifying the specific problems to address in the program, and customising the program to match the needs of the patient (Chapman 1991; Turk & Stacey 1997). Although the goals and objectives of different multidisciplinary programs vary, they typically include:

- reducing the patient's experience of pain
- improving physical and lifestyle functioning
- decreasing or eliminating drug intake
- enhancing social support and family life
- reducing the patient's use of medical services.

Multidisciplinary programs generally integrate specific treatment components to achieve each goal (Follick et al. 1985). These programs include, for example, procedures to decrease the patient's reliance on medication and physical exercises to increase the person's strength, endurance, flexibility and range of motion. They provide counselling to improve family relationships and to enable the patient to find full-time employment when possible. And they offer a wide range of psychological services to reduce the experience of pain, decrease pain behaviour, and improve the patient's psychosocial adjustment to the pain condition.

Highlight on issues

issues

Physical activity and back pain

The spine has an intricate structure, with each of its many sections of bone, called *vertebrae*, being cushioned from adjacent sections by rubbery *disks* of connective tissue. Each vertebra is connected to adjacent ones by antler-shaped *facet joints* that enable the vertebrae to pivot against one another (Tortora & Grabowski 1993). But the spine depends on the muscles of the back and abdomen for support, without which it would just topple over. When all these muscles are strong and in good working order, they balance each other's action and keep the body's weight centred on the spine. But when these muscles are weak or the back muscles are under excessive or prolonged tension — sometimes owing to emotional stress — back problems tend to occur.

A 10-year longitudinal study of men and women found evidence suggesting that low back pain progresses over time through a vicious circle: Poor muscle function may lead to low back disorders, which lead to poorer muscle function, and so on (Leino, Aro & Hasan 1987).

Although back pain can arise from such conditions as arthritis and ruptured disks, this is not typical — medical examinations fail to find underlying physical causes in the large majority of back pain cases (Chapman 1984; Deyo et al. 1991). Most backaches seem to arise from muscle or ligament strains, lack of proper exercise, and normal wear and tear on facet joints. These problems tend to increase with age for many reasons — for instance, people's muscular conditioning usually declines as they get older, the effects of wear and tear accumulate, and the disks gradually dry out and provide less cushioning for the vertebrae. People whose jobs require frequent heavy lifting are more likely than other workers to develop low back pain (Kelsey & Hochberg 1988). Exercise can help to protect people from back problems, but such activities need to consist of *proper* exercises. People who do the wrong kinds of exercises do not get this protection, and those who overexert themselves can precipitate back pain.

(continued)

What kinds of physical activity can help protect against back problems? Proper exercise involves a program of back-strengthening and stretching activities, along with abdominal exercises. Many different exercises are available for these purposes; figure 12.5 presents a few easy ones. What should people do when they develop backaches? Medical advice in the past called for getting lots of bed rest and taking aspirin. But this advice has changed as a result of new research (Deyo et al. 1991; USDHHS 1994). Most backaches resolve themselves in a few days or weeks with or without medical attention. Doctors today recommend that the person *become active as soon as possible* — walking and exercising cautiously — even if it hurts a little. People with back pain should consult their doctor when the pain is:

- linked to a known injury, such as a fall
- severe enough to disable the sufferer and awaken him or her at night
- not relieved by changing position or lying down
- accompanied by nausea, fever, difficulty or pain in urinating, loss of bladder or bowel control, numbness or weakness in a leg or foot, or pain that shoots down the leg.

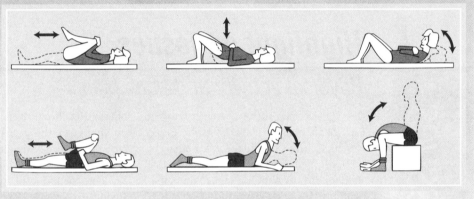

Figure 12.5 Six stretching and strengthening exercises to protect from low back pain

Evaluating the success of pain clinics

How effective are multidisciplinary pain clinics? To answer this question, we'll start by examining the procedures and results of two pain programs. Both programs were conducted by hospital-affiliated pain clinics, and the staff of both programs included doctors, psychologists, physiotherapists and occupational therapists. In contrast, one clinic was located in the United States and provided an in-patient program for intractable pain, while the other clinic was located in Australia and provided an out-patient program for chronic back pain.

The first of these programs took place at the Miller-Dwan Hospital Pain Control Center in Minnesota (Cinciripini & Floreen 1982). The program provided treatment for four weeks, with weekends off. The subjects were men and women who had suffered intractable pain from known injuries or diseases, such as arthritis, for at least a year and were unemployed because of their pain conditions. All subjects received the full program, which consisted of a medication reduction procedure, physiotherapy, relaxation and biofeedback training, self-monitoring, behavioural contracting, cognitive/behavioural group therapy, and family involvement and training. The researchers assessed the patients' behaviour and functioning at the start and at the end of the program, and in follow-ups six and 12 months after. By the end of this program, the patients' activity levels had increased and their pain experiences, pain behaviours, and drug use had decreased sharply — indeed, 90 per cent of the patients were now free of analgesic medication. The subjects who participated in the follow-up assessments reported that they continued to be active, and about half were employed. Moreover, their pain continued to diminish: before treatment their average pain rating was 4.6 on a 10-point scale, by the end of the program it was 2.2, and after a year it was 1.2.

The second program was conducted at the Essendon Campus of the Royal Melbourne Hospital (Flavell et al. 1996). The program consisted of two six-hour group sessions per week for six weeks, and promoted pain management rather than 'cure'. The subjects were men and women who had suffered from back pain for more than six months, and were consecutive referrals from a specialist in rehabilitation medicine over a two-and-a-half-year period. The treatment program consisted of exercise, hydrotherapy, training in safe 'manual-handling' techniques, and workshop work and relaxation sessions. Also, discussion and education sessions were held on medical issues, fitness, leisure, return to work and pain management. Subjects were assessed before the program, after the program and at three month follow-up with the West Haven–Yale Multidimensional Pain Inventory (WHYMPI — see chapter 11) and a four-minute walk test. At the completion of the program, the WHYMPI showed significant decreases in the amount that pain interfered with life, and significant increases in subject sense of control and activity level. However, severity of pain remained the same. All of these effects were maintained three months later.

Meta-analyses of dozens of studies have shown that people suffering with chronic pain who receive treatment at multidisciplinary pain centres report much less subsequent pain and are far more likely to return to work than individuals who have standard pain treatment (Cutler et al. 1994; Flor, Fydrich & Turk 1992). What's more, the cost of the treatment is only a small fraction of the medical and disability payments patients would receive for a year (Stieg & Turk 1988). Of course, not all pain patients benefit from this treatment, but most do. Programs that provide medical, psychosocial, physical and occupational therapy can improve chronic pain patients' psychosocial and physical functioning and reduce their pain, pain behaviour and drug use.

Summary

Pain that receives or requires professional attention is called clinical pain. Practitioners try to reduce acute clinical pain for humanitarian reasons and for practical reasons, such as to enable medical procedures to be carried out smoothly, reduce patients' stress, and help patients recover quickly and without complications. Relieving chronic pain is important because of the severe and pervasive impact it can have on almost every aspect of patients' lives. Although the medical treatment for pain may involve surgery if all other methods have failed, it usually involves pharmaceuticals selected from four types: peripherally acting analgesics; centrally acting analgesics; local anaesthetics; and indirectly acting drugs, such as sedatives, tranquillisers, and antidepressants. These chemical methods are used extensively for relieving acute pain, and they are sometimes administered by an epidural block or a patient-controlled analgesia technique. Health care professionals usually try not to rely on chemical methods for reducing chronic pain.

One of the main goals of behavioural and cognitive methods for treating chronic pain is to reduce the patient's drug consumption. The operant approach focuses on reducing pain behaviours through extinction procedures and increasing 'well' behaviour through reinforcement. Therapists apply methods of progressive muscle relaxation and biofeedback to reduce the stress and muscle tension that can cause or aggravate patients' pain experiences. Research mainly with headache patients has shown that relaxation and biofeedback training appear to produce effective and long-lasting pain relief. Cognitive techniques focus on changing thought patterns that increase the intensity or frequency of pain experiences. Distraction and non-pain imagery methods appear to be effective chiefly for mild or moderate acute pain or for brief episodes of heightened chronic pain. Pain redefinition can involve clarifying what a pain experience will be like, using positive self-statements, and correcting faulty beliefs and logic. Redefinition appears to be helpful in reducing strong pain and chronic pain.

Hypnosis seems to relieve pain only to the extent that the person can be deeply hypnotised, and it provides a high degree of analgesia in only a minority of individuals. In general, people can reduce their pain as effectively with cognitive strategies in the waking state as with hypnosis. Insight-oriented psychotherapies are designed to help people achieve an understanding of the roots of their problems. For pain patients, this may involve making them aware of what is happening in the pain games they play or of how others feel about their pain conditions. These insights can be achieved in pain groups or in individual and family therapy.

Counter-irritation is a procedure whereby a brief or moderate pain cancels a longer-lasting or stronger one. A pain control technique that is based on this procedure is called transcutaneous electrical nerve stimulation, in which mild electrical stimulation is applied to the skin at the painful region. This technique is effective for relieving acute pain and some types of chronic pain. Acupuncture is an ancient Asian procedure for reducing pain; it appears to produce high levels of analgesia for acute pain in some patients, but not in most. It does not seem to be very useful in treating chronic pain. Physiotherapy includes such approaches as exercise, massage, traction and the application of heat and cold to painful regions. These methods help to reduce pain and rehabilitate damaged or weakened tissue in muscles and joints. Proper exercise can protect individuals from low back pain.

Pain clinics are institutions developed specifically for treating chronic pain. Although some of these clinics focus on applying essentially one technique, such as hypnosis or biofeedback, the complex nature of chronic pain usually requires treatment approaches that integrate medical, psychosocial, physical and occupational therapy. Multidisciplinary pain clinics provide highly effective and long-lasting pain relief, while also rehabilitating their patients physically, psychologically, socially and vocationally.

Key terms

acupuncture	counter-irritation	non-pain imagery	pain redefinition
clinical pain	distraction	pain clinics	transcutaneous electrical nerve stimulation

PART

6

Chronic and life-threatening health problems

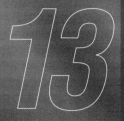

13 Serious and disabling chronic illnesses: causes, management and coping

Prologue

Most Australian kids like barbecues; Jeff certainly did. But with the barbecue came sauces and bread with added sugar and cakes for dessert and sugar-laden soft drinks. Jeff could not consume any of these. At the age of seven Jeff had been diagnosed with insulin-dependent diabetes mellitus (IDDM or Type 1 diabetes), and since then his life had been dominated by regular and frequent self-monitoring of blood sugar levels, twice-daily self-injections of insulin, and dietary restrictions and deprivations that were both onerous and limiting. Jeff knew that short of a miraculous medical discovery his life would never be free from this routine. At sixteen now, he wondered how he could achieve the full satisfaction of approaching adult life under the shadow of Type 1 diabetes. Could he maintain a complete social life where food and drink played such a pivotal part? Could he travel extensively when all of the paraphernalia of self-monitoring and self-injection had to go with him? Would he find a partner willing to share the life of someone with a chronic and potentially life-threatening condition? But right now, was it really worth being here at the school barbecue when everyone else was eating and drinking without restriction? Jeff sat on his own in the background and pondered what seemed to be a bleak future.

Different individuals react differently to developing a chronic illness. Their reactions depend on many factors, such as their coping skills and personalities, the social support they have, the nature and consequences of their illness, and the impact of the illness on their daily functioning. At the very least, having a chronic condition entails frequent impositions on the patients and their families. Chronically ill people may suffer periodic episodes of feeling poorly and need to have regular medical checkups, restrict their diets or other aspects of their lifestyles, or administer daily treatment, for instance. Many chronic conditions entail more than just impositions — they produce frequent pain or lead to disability or even death. Although the prospect of developing a chronic health problem is unappealing, most of us will develop at least one of these illnesses in our lifetime, and one of them, such as cancer or cardiovascular disease, will probably take our lives.

This chapter and the next focus mainly on *tertiary prevention* of chronic illness — to retard its progression, prevent disability and rehabilitate the person physically and psychologically. We examine how people react to and cope with chronic health problems and what can be done to help these people cope effectively. In contrast with the next chapter, which deals with illnesses that have high rates of mortality and with those processes relating to dying and death, the present chapter concentrates on health problems that are less likely to result in death but often lead to disability. This chapter begins by discussing people's reactions to having a chronic condition, then examines the experiences and needs of individuals living with various health problems, and ends by considering psychosocial interventions to enhance patients' long-term adaptation to their condition. These discussions address many questions that are of great concern to patients, to their families and friends, and probably to you. How do individuals react after their initial shock of learning that they have a chronic illness? What kinds of health problems usually involve the most difficult adjustments for people? How do patients' chronic conditions affect their families? What can families, friends and therapists do to help chronically ill people adapt effectively to their condition?

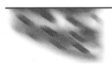

Adjusting to a chronic illness

'I felt like I'd been hit by a bus' — this is how many patients describe their first reaction upon learning that they have a disabling or life-threatening illness. Questions without immediate answers flash through their minds: Is the diagnosis right and, if so, what can we do about it? Will I be disabled, disfigured or in pain? Will I die? How soon will these consequences happen? What will happen to my family? Do I have adequate health cover and life insurance? Learning of a chronic health problem usually comes as a great shock, and this is often the first reaction individuals experience when the doctor tells them the diagnosis.

Initial reactions to having a chronic condition

By observing patients in rehabilitation and health settings, Franklin Shontz (1975) has described a sequence of reactions people tend to exhibit following the diagnosis of a serious illness. This sequence of reactions is:

- *shock* — an emergency response, marked by three characteristics: (1) being stunned or bewildered, (2) behaving in an automatic fashion, and (3) feeling a sense of detachment from the situation; that is, feeling like an observer rather than a participant in the events that occur. The shock may last only a short while or may continue for weeks; it occurs to some degree in any crisis situation people experience, and it is likely to be most pronounced when the crisis comes without warning.
- *encounter* — a phase that is marked by disorganised thinking and feelings of loss, grief, helplessness, despair and being overwhelmed by reality
- *retreat* — a phase in which people tend to use avoidance strategies, such as denying either the existence of the health problem or its implications. But then reality begins to intrude: the symptoms remain or get worse, additional diagnoses confirm the original one, and it becomes clear that adjustments need to be made.

Using retreat as a 'base of operation', patients tend to contact reality a little at a time until they reach some form of adjustment to the health problem and its implications.

Do all individuals react in the ways Shontz has described when they are diagnosed with a serious illness? No, but probably most do. For instance, when faced with a crisis, most people react with shock initially, but other individuals may be 'cool and collected', while others may be 'paralysed' with anxiety or may become 'hysterical' (Silver & Wortman 1980). In a large study of Australian survivors of myocardial infarction (Byrne & Whyte 1978; Byrne, Whyte & Lance 1979), it was reported that only about half of the cohort responded in what could be described as a psychologically adaptive manner. These patients expressed both anxiety and depression but in a manner and degree that was entirely consistent with the severe and life-threatening nature of their illness. Another 25 per cent reported excessive anxiety and/or depression — that is, an emotional response that was of clinical proportions and in need of professional management. The remaining 25 per cent manifested denial, which had the potential to interfere with treatment and rehabilitation by reducing compliance with management strategies. These maladaptive responses to heart attack were found to predict poorer outcomes, both medically and socially, than were evident in the majority of patients (Byrne 1987).

People who use denial and other avoidance strategies do so to control their emotional responses to a stressor, especially when they believe they can do nothing to change the situation (Croyle & Ditto 1990; Lazarus 1983). But the usefulness of this approach has limits. Although using avoidance strategies often provides psychological benefits early in the process of coping with health problems, excessive avoidance can soon become maladaptive to patients' physical and psychological wellbeing (Suls & Fletcher 1985). For example, when hospitalised people receive information about their conditions and future risk factors, those individuals who use avoidance strategies heavily gain less information about their conditions than those who use these strategies to a lesser degree (Shaw et al. 1985). Patients often need to make major decisions about their immediate treatment. How can they make these decisions rationally if they fail to take in the information practitioners present? Later they may need to take action to promote their recovery, reduce the likelihood of future health problems, and adjust their lifestyle, social relationships and means of employment. What factors influence how people cope with their health problems? The next section provides some answers to this question.

Influences on coping with a health crisis

Healthy people tend to take their health for granted. They expect to be able to carry out their daily activities and social roles from one day to the next without substantial disruptions due to illness. When a serious illness or injury occurs, their everyday life activities are disrupted. Regardless of whether the condition is temporary or chronic, the first phases in coping with it are similar. But there is an important difference: in contrast to the short-term disruptions that temporary illnesses cause, chronic health problems usually require that patients and their families make permanent behavioural, social and emotional adjustments.

When people learn that they have a serious chronic illness, the diagnosis quickly changes the way they view themselves and their lives. The plans they had for tomorrow and for the next days, weeks and years may be affected. Major plans and minor ones may change: Did they plan to go on a trip this weekend? They may change their minds now. Did they plan to complete a university degree or enter a specific career field, or get married and have children, or move to a new area when they retire? Some of these ideas for the future may evaporate after the diagnosis. As psychologists Frances Cohen and Richard Lazarus have noted, because the idea of

> being healthy, able, and having a normal physique is central to most people's image and evaluation, becoming ill can be a shock to a person's sense of security and to his or her self-image. Not only does it threaten the customary view of oneself, but it further underscores that one is indeed vulnerable ... and that one's life may be changed in major respects. As a result, adjustment to an illness or injury which is life-threatening or potentially disabling may require considerable coping effort. (1979, p. 218)

Potentially disabling or life-threatening conditions leave patients and their families with many uncertainties. Often no-one can tell for certain exactly what the course of the illness will be.

Why do some individuals cope differently from others after learning they have a chronic health problem? Rudolf Moos (1982; Moos & Schaefer 1986) has proposed the **crisis theory**, which describes a variety of factors that influence how people adjust during a crisis, such as having an illness. Figure 13.1 presents his conceptual model, showing that the outcome of the crisis — or the adjustment the person makes — depends on the coping process, which depends on three contributing influences: *illness-related* factors, *background and personal* factors, and *physical and social environmental* factors. We will look at these contributing influences, and then see how they affect the coping process the patient uses.

Illness-related factors

Some health problems present a greater threat to the person than others do — they may be more disabling, disfiguring, painful or life-threatening, for example. As you might expect, the greater the threats patients perceive for any of these factors, the more difficulty they are likely to have coping with their condition (Cohen & Lazarus 1979; Diamond 1983; Moos 1982). Being disfigured can be extremely difficult to adjust to, particularly when it involves the person's face. Individuals whose faces are badly scarred often withdraw from social encounters, sometimes completely. Their disfigurements are noticeable to anyone and usually cannot be hidden. Most people who see the disfigurement tend to react awkwardly and may even show feelings of revulsion. Even children react more negatively to people's facial disfigurements than to injuries to other parts of the body, such as when people are crippled or missing a limb (Richardson et al. 1961). In view of the substantial incidence of major physical trauma in Australia (Cameron et al. 1995), and in particular the trauma that occurs to children, this is an important area of concern.

Patients also have difficulty coping with illness-related factors that involve annoying or embarrassing changes in bodily functioning or that draw attention to their conditions (Bekkers et al. 1995; Diamond 1983; Norris 1990). People with some illnesses, for instance, may need artificial devices for excreting faecal or urinary wastes. These devices may be noticeable either visibly or by their odours, and many patients have exaggerated impressions of the social impact such devices have. Other chronically ill people must treat their conditions with ointments that may have odours or equipment that is visible or makes noise. Still others may experience periodic seizures or muscle spasms that can be embarrassing. Many people with chronic illnesses feel self-conscious about their health problems — or even stigmatised by them — and want to hide them from others (Scambler 1984).

Various other aspects of treatment regimens can make adjustment very difficult, too. Some treatments are painful or involve medications that produce serious side effects — either by leading to additional health problems or by interfering with the patient's daily functioning, such as by making the person immobile or drowsy. Other treatments may have schedules and require time commitments that make it difficult for the person to find or hold a job. Some treatments require patients and their families to make substantial changes in their lifestyles, which they might resent and fail to carry out. Each of these factors can impair people's adjustment to chronic health problems.

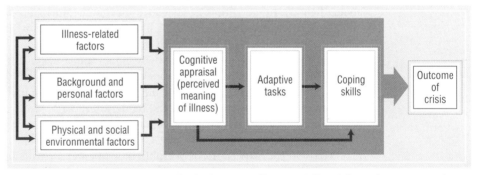

Figure 13.1 Crisis theory's three contributing influences (factors at left) and the coping process patients use in the first phases of adjusting psychologically to a serious illness

Source: Adapted from Moos (1982, figure 1).

Background and personal factors

People who cope well with chronic health problems have the psychological and behavioural resources to 'resolve the chronicity or "long-termness" of the situation, balance hope against despair, and find purpose and quality in life' (Diamond 1983, p. 683).

Often, these people have hardy or resilient personalities that allow them to see a good side in difficult situations (Pollock, Christian & Sands 1991). As an example, a 16-year-old boy named Ralfie, whose body had wasted away to 23 kilograms from a rare spinal-muscular disease, stated:

> When I take a bath and look at myself naked, I think, 'God Jesus.' I'm disappointed when it comes to my body, but when it comes to my inside, my personality, my sense of humor, I'm proud of the way I am. I think I'm a nicer person. The girls always tell me, 'You're very special. You're different than the other guys.' (Hurley 1987, p. 34)

People with chronic diseases who are like Ralfie can often find purpose and quality in their lives, maintain their self-esteem, and resist feeling helpless and hopeless.

The ways individuals cope with chronic health problems also depend on many other background and personal factors, such as their age, gender, social class, philosophical or religious commitments, emotional maturity and self-esteem (Moos & Schaefer 1986). With respect to gender differences, for instance, men are more likely than women to be 'threatened by the decreases in ambition, vigour, and physical prowess that often result from serious illness because, by comparison with women, they are confident in the stability of their physical abilities and bodily functioning' (Moos 1982, p. 132). Having a chronic illness often means that the individual must take on a dependent and passive role for a long period of time. For men, this can be especially difficult since it is inconsistent with the assertive and independent roles they generally occupy in most societies of the world.

The timing of a health problem in the person's life span also affects its impact on him or her. In the case of very young children, their limited cognitive abilities prevent them from understanding fully the nature of their illnesses, the treatments they must follow and the long-term implications of their conditions (Bibace & Walsh 1979; Burbach & Peterson 1986). Their concerns are likely to focus on any restrictions that are imposed on their lifestyles and activities, the frightening medical procedures they experience, and possible separations from their parents. As children get older and their comprehension improves, they may be able to participate in making some decisions about their treatment. Adolescents can understand information about their illnesses and treatment, but their needing to be like and feel accepted by their peers can lead to difficulties in coping with their health problems (La Greca & Stone 1985). Because of these motivations, adolescents may deny important aspects of their conditions and neglect their medical care to avoid appearing different from their friends.

In adulthood, too, the difficulties individuals have in coping with chronic health problems change with age (Mages & Mendelsohn 1979; Moos 1982). When people develop disabling or life-threatening illnesses or injuries in early adulthood, they tend to resent not having had the chance to develop their lives in the direction they planned — to get married, to have children or to enter a particular career. In contrast, middle-aged patients may have problems adjusting to the disruption of established roles and lifestyles and to being unable to finish tasks they have started, such as building up a business. In old age, people who develop chronic illnesses may resent not being able to enjoy the leisure they feel they earned in their lifetime of work and self-sacrifice.

Another personal factor that affects how people cope with chronic health problems is the set of beliefs they have about health and illness. Suppose an individual believes, for instance, that 'nothing is seriously wrong if you don't feel any pain'. This person is not likely to be very concerned when he or she develops a condition that has no clear symptoms, as happens with hypertension. People's beliefs are often wrong, and sometimes their misconceptions about the medical treatment or the effects of an illness can add to the difficulty they have adjusting to their health problems. The issue of coping with chronic illness extends to the effects that illness has on carers and on significant others in the patient's immediate environment. A recent Australian study carried out in Victoria examined the health and wellbeing of women family carers of those with chronic illness (Schofield et al. 1999). This study found that there was a strong association between the caring role and both poor health status and a poor sense of wellbeing, suggesting that the caring role has a distinctly negative impact on both the physical and mental health of the carers.

Physical and social environmental factors

Many physical and social features of our environments can affect the way we adjust to chronic health problems (Moos 1982). The physical aspects of a hospital environment, for instance, are usually very dull and confining for patients, thereby depressing their general morale and mood. Indeed, the physical environment of some parts of the hospital may be conspicuously frightening. The environment presented by many intensive and coronary care units, for example, with the profusion of mysterious technical equipment and the proximity to other dangerously ill people is likely to provide a chilling experience for many patients conscious enough to be aware of their physical setting. The environment may remind them in an unavoidable way of their own mortality and of the long period of recovery they must negotiate even if they do survive the acute illness event (Byrne 1987; Johnston 1997).

By contrast, the recent Australian trend towards birthing centres has provided an attractive alternative to many women who wish to have their babies in an environment free of the technical paraphernalia of traditional obstetric practice (Waldenstron & Lawson 1998). Birthing centres provide an environment closer to that of the home than the hospital, with non-hospital furnishings and decoration, and facilities for families to be present for the whole of the labour. They are, however, usually in close proximity to regular obstetric services so that if complications occur during the birth process women have access to all of the technical facilities they would have in a traditional obstetric unit.

Many patients have difficulty getting around their houses or performing self-help tasks, such as buttoning clothes or opening food containers, and lack special equipment or tools that can help them do these tasks and be more self-sufficient. These people's adjustment to their health problems can be impaired as long as these situations persist.

The patient's social environment functions as a system, with the behaviour of each person affecting the others (Kerns & Weiss 1994; Revenson 1994). The presence of social support, for example, generally helps patients and their families and friends cope with their illnesses. Individuals who live alone and have few friends or who have poor relationships with the people they live with tend to adjust poorly to chronic health conditions (Gentry & Kobasa 1984; Wallston et al. 1983). In a study of Australian patients hospitalised for stroke (Morris et al. 1991), the perceived inadequacy of social support, particularly from a spouse caregiver, was noticeably related to post-stroke depression. Moreover, the duration of the depressive illness varied systematically with the perceived inadequacy of social support; the poorer the support base the longer the duration of the depression. The authors noted the potential importance of this finding for the long-term management of stroke victims and underscored the value of adequate social support networks in the overall management of these patients.

But it is also true that sometimes people in a patient's social network may undermine effective coping by providing bad examples or poor advice (Suls 1982). The degree to which each member of the social system adjusts in constructive ways to the illness affects the adjustment of the others.

The primary source of social support for children and most adults who are ill typically comes from their immediate families (Cantor & Little 1985; Miller & Cafasso 1992). People in old age whose spouses are either deceased or unable to help are likely to receive support mainly from their children, but also from siblings, friends and neighbours. At almost any age, patients may join *support groups* for people with specific medical problems. These groups can provide informational and emotional support.

As figure 13.1 depicts, the three contributing influences are interrelated and can modify each other. The patient's social or cultural background, for instance, may affect the threat presented by the health problem and his or her access to special tools and equipment to promote self-sufficiency. These contributing factors combine to influence the coping process the person uses to deal with the crisis.

The coping process

Crisis theory proposes that coping begins with the patient's *cognitive appraisal* of the meaning or significance of the health problem to his or her life. The outcome of this appraisal leads the individual to formulate an array of *adaptive tasks* and to apply various *coping skills* to deal with these tasks. Let's see what these tasks and skills are.

The tasks and skills of coping

According to Moos (1982), people who are ill need to address two types of adaptive tasks in the coping process. These are:

- *tasks related to the illness or treatment*, which involve learning to (1) cope with the symptoms or disability the health problem causes, (2) adjust to the hospital environment and medical procedures needed to treat the problem, and (3) develop and maintain good relationships with their practitioners.
- *tasks related to general psychosocial functioning*, which involve striving to (1) control negative feelings and retain a positive outlook for the future, (2) maintain a satisfactory self-image and sense of competence, (3) preserve good relationships with family and friends, and (4) prepare for an uncertain future.

Achieving these goals can be very difficult for patients, particularly when their health problems may lead to disability, disfigurement or death. Still, many people with poor prognoses for their health manage to adapt successfully and make the most of their new life circumstances.

Crisis theory proposes that patients encounter these adaptive tasks in any health problem they experience. But the relative importance or salience of each task for each illness or injury depends on

> the nature of the disease, the personality of the individual involved, and the unique set of environmental circumstances. For the person suddenly rendered blind, the physical discomfort may be minor while the difficulty of restoring social relations can be overwhelming. ... A woman who has had a mastectomy may find that accepting her new self-image is her most significant task. Someone who is physically active, like a professional athlete or a construction worker, probably will experience more difficulty adjusting to a wheelchair than a person with a more sedentary occupation. (Moos 1982, p. 137)

Family members must make similar adjustments, and these individuals are critically important in helping patients achieve each goal. People are likely to adapt successfully to their chronic conditions if they have family members who participate actively in their treatment regimens, encourage them to be self-sufficient, and respond to their needs in a caring and sensitive manner.

What coping skills do patients and their families employ to deal with these adaptive tasks? Figure 13.2 describes several useful strategies that they commonly use. Each of these skills can help in achieving the goals of the various adaptive tasks and in leading to a positive outcome of the crisis. Is one approach best? Generally speaking, although moderate or temporary use of any specific skill can be beneficial, using any single skill exclusively may undermine the coping process (Moos 1982). Some coping skills may be more appropriate for dealing with some tasks than with others. As a result, people generally use these skills selectively, often in combination. For instance, seeking information may help patients deal with the symptoms, and setting reasonable goals may help them do exercises and reduce their incapacitation. Individuals who have adjusted successfully to each phase of the crises are ready to deal effectively with subsequent phases in their adjustment to their health problems.

Figure 13.2 Coping strategies for chronic health problems

- *Denying or minimising* the seriousness of the situation. As we have seen, this approach can be beneficial in the early phases of adjusting to a health problem. Patients may benefit from this approach by using it selectively to put aside their emotions temporarily, thereby saving them from feeling overwhelmed and giving them time to organise other personal coping resources. While denial may offer short-term relief, however, the longer-term harm may be significant. Patients continuing to deny a chronic illness may ignore medication advice, dietary and life-style change adivce, and other crucial aids to recovery.

- *Seeking information* about the health problem and treatment procedures.

- *Learning to provide one's own medical care* such as self-administering insulin injections. With this approach, patients gain a sense of control and personal effectiveness with respect to their conditions.

- *Setting concrete, limited goals* such as in exercising or in going to shows or social gatherings, and maintaining regular routines as much as possible. By doing this, patients and their families have things to look forward to and opportunities to achieve goals they consider meaningful.

- *Recruiting instrumental and emotional support* from family, friends and practitioners by expressing needs and feelings.

- *Considering possible future events* and stressful circumstances in order to know what lies ahead and to be prepared for unexpected difficulties.

- *Gaining a manageable perspective* on the health problem and its treatment by finding a long-term 'purpose' or 'meaning' for the experience. Patients often do this by applying religious beliefs or by recognising how they have been changed in positive ways by the experience.

Source: Based on Moos (1982).

Long-term adaptation to chronic health problems

Chronic disorders last for a very long time — and patients and their families need to adapt to the illnesses and whether they worsen, stay the same, or improve over time. The term **adaptation** refers to the process of making changes in order to adjust constructively to life's circumstances. For chronically ill individuals and their families, the adaptive changes they make can enhance their quality of life by promoting their effective physical, psychological and social functioning (Cohen & Lazarus 1983; Diamond 1983). What does 'quality of life' mean? **Quality of life** refers to the degree of excellence people appraise their lives to contain. People generally appraise excellence in terms of fulfilment or purpose, personal control, interpersonal relations, pleasant activities, personal and intellectual growth, and material possessions (Gill & Feinstein 1995). Cummins and his colleagues in Australia (Cummins et al. 1995; Gullone & Cummins 1999) have developed a valid and reliable, multi-dimensional instrument to assess quality of life in a broad range of populations. The *Comprehensive Quality of Life Scale* (ComQol) assesses seven independent domains of (a) material wellbeing, (b) health, (c) productivity, (d) intimacy, (e) safety, (f) place in community and (g) emotional wellbeing. The instrument has been successfully applied in a number of health and other human services settings to describe and quantify quality of life in those with a variety of both physical and psychological disorders.

Individuals who show effective long-term adaptation to chronic illness often have psychological resources that enable them to apply appropriate coping strategies to deal with the problems they face. When chronically ill people can expect to live for many years, they need to make many decisions, such as career selections, that involve examining their options based on realistic assessments of their conditions. People who continue to rely heavily on avoidance coping strategies, such as denial, are less likely to adapt effectively than those who use strategies that allow them to consider their situations more carefully and objectively (Suls & Fletcher 1985).

To summarise, most people tend to react to becoming seriously ill with shock, followed by a period of disorganised thinking and feelings of loss and helplessness. Avoidance strategies, such as denial, constitute one of several types of coping skills patients use to deal with the adaptive tasks they identify through the process of cognitive appraisal. The importance of each adaptive task depends on the person's personality, the physical and social environment, and the specific chronic health problem to which he or she must adjust.

Impacts of different chronic conditions

What is it like to live with a chronic health problem? To some extent, the answer depends on the illness. Beginning with this section, we will consider the impact of specific chronic medical conditions and treatments on patients and their families. The particular health problems we will examine were selected to illustrate disorders of different body systems and widely different adjustment difficulties. Some of these health problems tend to develop at much earlier ages than others; some require much more complex treatments than others; and some produce more pain and disability than others. Although the medical problems we will discuss in this chapter include some that can be life-threatening, none of these chronic conditions is among the most deadly ones people in Australia often develop — those of heart disease, cancer, stroke, and AIDS, which we will examine in the next chapter.

We will use a *life-span perspective* to order the health problems: Illnesses that generally begin in childhood will be presented first, and illnesses that usually begin in old age will be considered last. As we have seen, the impact of a health problem and the way people cope with it depend partly on the patient's age. We will start by considering the impact of asthma, a chronic respiratory disorder that generally begins in the early childhood years.

Asthma

We all experience respiratory disorders at one time or another. If we are fortunate, these disorders are limited to occasional bouts with winter colds and the flu. But many millions of people are not so fortunate — they suffer from various chronic respiratory problems. In some cases, these problems involve constant breathing impairments that vary in intensity from one day to the next. In other cases, the victims breathe normally most of the time but suffer recurrent episodes of impaired breathing. Some chronic respiratory illnesses, such as *emphysema*, result largely from environmental causes, such as cigarette smoking. Others do not. Some chronic respiratory disorders become severe enough to disable their victims and may even claim their lives. This can happen with *asthma*.

What is asthma?

Imagine being at home reading one evening and noticing that a slight whistling, wheezing sound starts to accompany each breath you take. Soon the sound becomes louder and your breathing becomes laboured. You try opening your mouth to breathe, but very little air goes in or out. When your chest begins to contract from the effort and your heart pounds rapidly, you are quite frightened and worry, 'Will my next gasp for air be my last?' This is what a major asthma attack is like. Victims of extreme attacks may begin to turn blue and look as if they are about to die, and some do die.

Asthma is a respiratory disorder involving recurrent episodes of impaired breathing when the airways become obstructed. This disease is very prevalent around the world, including in Australia. The National Health Survey conducted by the Australian Bureau of Statistics in 1995 (ABS 1995) revealed that 11 per cent of the total population suffered from asthma. This had increased from 8.5 per cent in 1989–90, suggesting either a change in the criteria for diagnosis of asthma or, perhaps more alarmingly, an increase in the environmental and other conditions underlying this serious and potentially life-threatening illness. Chronic obstructive pulmonary disease, a category of which asthma is a significant member, accounted for 4.8 per cent of all deaths in Australia in 1998 (ABS 1998), with annual Australian deaths explicitly from asthma numbering around 700. According to the Asthma Foundation of Victoria, asthma is the most common reason for childhood admission to hospital and it is the most common chronic condition of children and adolescents. Asthma typically declines from adolescence to adulthood, but both death and disability from asthma among adults remain significant contributors to Australia's health burden. The ABS data strongly linked prevalence of asthma with cigarette smoking. Asthma is clearly a major health problem. Let's see what causes asthma attacks.

The physiology, causes and effects of asthma

Asthma episodes typically begin when the immune system is activated to react in an allergic manner, producing antibodies that cause the bronchial tubes and other affected body tissues to release a chemical called *histamine*. This chemical causes irritation to those tissues. In an asthma attack, these events cause the bronchial tubes to become obstructed as their smooth muscles become inflamed, develop spasms and produce mucus (Busse 1990; Evans 1990). These events last perhaps an hour or two and can lead to tissue damage, thereby increasing the likelihood of more frequent and severe future attacks. For some asthmatics, airway inflammation becomes constant.

What causes asthma attacks? We do not have a full answer to this question, but we do know that attacks usually occur in the presence of certain conditions, called *triggers* (Evans 1990). Asthma triggers can include *personal factors*, such as having a respiratory infection or feelings of anger or anxiety; *environmental conditions*, such as air pollution, pollen or cold temperature; and *physical activities*, such as strenuous exercise (Janson-Bjerklie, Carrieri & Hudes 1986; Sarafino & Goldfedder 1995). The triggers that lead to attacks are different for different asthmatics, and some individuals have attacks only when two or more triggers occur at the same time (Evans 1990). The main triggers for many asthmatics are allergens — substances, such as pollens or moulds, that are known to cause allergic reactions. But other asthmatics do not have any known allergies, and other factors, such as physical exercise or cold air, are the main triggers for them. Tests for allergic reactions usually involve injecting a small amount of the allergen under the skin and checking to see if the skin in that area becomes inflamed.

Researchers demonstrated the important role of the immune system in the development of allergic reactions with a study involving transplanted bone marrow, the tissue that produces white blood cells (Agosti et al. 1988). The subjects were cancer patients who needed the transplants as part of their treatment. Each of the subjects and the donors was given skin tests with 17 allergen extracts — including house dust, cat hair, penicillin, mites and ragweed — before the transplant and one year after. In some of the pre-transplant tests, the donor showed a positive allergic reaction but the patient did not. When testing was done a year later, the subjects now showed reactions in 44.5 per cent of these tests. In other pre-transplant tests, neither the donor nor the patient showed an allergic reaction. This situation served as a control condition — and a year later the subjects showed reactions in only 3 per cent of these tests. These findings indicate that the bone marrow contains allergen-specific antibodies and that the donors' allergies were passed on to the patients. This research also produced evidence of asthma being transmitted from donors to people who previously had no history of asthma.

What causes the condition of asthma to develop? Twin studies and other genetic research have shown that heredity clearly plays a role in determining whether individuals develop asthma (Sarafino, Eastlack & McCarthy 1994). Research has also found evidence linking genetic factors to the severity of the condition and some of the specific triggers that are involved (Sarafino & Goldfedder 1995). Another factor that seems to be important is the person's history of respiratory infection: Individuals who contract serious viral infections in infancy or early childhood are more likely to develop asthma than individuals who do not (Li & O'Connell 1987; Sarafino & Dillon 1996). It may be that the infections damage the respiratory system, making it highly sensitive to certain triggering conditions.

Medical treatments for asthma

Medical approaches provide the cornerstone of treatment for asthma (Cluss & Fireman 1985; Evans 1990). Asthma treatments consist of three components, the first being to *avoid known triggers* of attacks. The second component involves medication. To treat an acute attack, patients mainly use *bronchodilators*, which open up constricted airways. To prevent attacks, patients can use *anti-inflammatories*, such as inhaled *corticosteroids* and *cromolyn*, which reduce bronchial inflammation or block the release of histamine and other chemicals that cause inflammation. Steroids that are inhaled in low doses have little risk of undesirable side effects, but those taken orally or in large doses can have serious side effects, such as rapid heartbeat and decreased bone density, and are usually reserved for people with severe asthma and used sparingly. Inhaled steroids are usually applied three or four times a day.

The third component of asthma treatments involves *exercise*. In the past, doctors advised many asthmatics to avoid exercise because it could induce an attack (Stockton 1988). But it now appears that the less these people exercise, the worse their condition gets. Many doctors today recommend treatments that carefully combine fitness training and the use of medication. Asthma's potential for producing disability and, sometimes, death makes it important that patients adhere to their treatments. Research has shown that individuals who comply with their treatments experience far fewer attacks and incidents of wheezing, for example (Cluss & Epstein 1985). But many asthmatics do not adhere closely, often failing to take medication to prevent attacks and using medication during an attack incorrectly (Cluss & Fireman 1985).

In the light of the seriousness of the illness, and of the potential threat to life of asthma attacks, compliance with treatments for asthma in Australia is not outstanding. A recent study in South Australia suggested that only 33 per cent of patients with doctor-diagnosed asthma possessed written action plans for use in the event of a serious attack (Ruffin et al. 1999). Moreover, this had declined from 42 per cent since a similar survey was conducted in 1995. Compliance with filling prescriptions for essential medication is as low as 70 per cent (Watts et al. 1997) and compliance with using medication, even when the prescription has been filled, is difficult to estimate, although it has been estimated at around 68 per cent in children (Smith, Seale & Shaw 1984). Less than half those asthmatics over the age of sixteen who were invited to participate in an education and compliance facilitation program agreed to do so (Abdulwadud et al. 1997) although attendance increased with age. In view of these obvious problems of compliance, and possibly of understanding, recent Australian work has focused on the effective use of videotape and picture book material to carry home the message to asthmatic children in the expectation that they will retain this into adulthood (Holzheimer, Mohay & Masters 1998).

Psychosocial factors in asthma

We saw in chapter 4 that psychosocial factors, including stress, can produce or aggravate an asthmatic episode. Many people with asthma report that the triggers of their attacks often involve their emotional states, such as being worried, angry or excited (Janson-Bjerklie, Carrieri & Hudes 1986). Experimental research has shown that emotional arousal, such as when watching an exciting movie, can trigger attacks in some children (Miller & Wood 1994). Studies have also found that *suggestion* can induce symptoms in some asthmatics. In one study, researchers had asthmatics inhale several doses of a placebo solution, with each succeeding dose labelled as containing an increasingly strong dose of an allergen (Luparello et al. 1968). Nearly half of the subjects developed symptoms, either as full asthmatic attacks or as spasms of the bronchial muscles. Another study confirmed this effect, finding that subjects who were told that the placebo solution they were inhaling was an irritant developed asthmatic symptoms (Butler & Steptoe 1986). But this research also showed that the asthmatic reaction could be negated if the subjects were first given another placebo that was described as a new asthma drug. In other words, the first suggestion blocked the second one.

Not all investigations using placebos and suggestion have succeeded in producing symptoms in asthmatics, but several have (Butler & Steptoe 1986; Cluss & Fireman 1985). Although there is little question that psychosocial factors can influence asthma attacks, we do not know how these factors work and which asthmatics are more affected by them. It is possible that psychosocial factors make asthmatics more sensitive to allergens or other conditions that trigger their attacks.

Asthma attacks are frightening for the patient and family alike, and frequent episodes are costly to the family and disrupt these people's lives and functioning (Cluss & Fireman 1985). Living with this disorder adds to the stress that asthmatics and their families experience, and studies have found that asthma is sometimes related to maladjustment in patients and their families (Werry 1986). This relationship probably involves two causal directions: (1) living with asthma sometimes leads to emotional problems, and (2) maladjustment in the family increases asthmatic episodes. Some asthmatics are chronically short of breath and have frequent attacks, and others have long attack-free periods. The psychosocial impact of asthma is likely to depend on how severe and disabling the condition is. One particular concern is that of quality of life in children with asthma. This is a frightening illness for children — one in which there may be significant limitations to lifestyle, whether necessary or only perceived. Davina French in Western Australia has worked with colleagues internationally to develop measures of quality of life in children with asthma in an attempt to quantify the impositions of this illness on young lifestyles (French, Christie & West 1994). This work has found wide acceptance in both the clinical and research arenas in monitoring the progress of asthmatic children through therapy and self-management (French & Carrol 1997). In the next section, we will examine what it is like to live with epilepsy, which is a disorder of the brain that produces recurrent seizures.

Epilepsy

Epilepsy is a condition marked by recurrent, sudden seizures that result from electrical disturbances of the cerebral cortex (Chelune 1987). Although the seizures epileptics may experience can vary greatly, the two most common types are the:

- *grand mal (or 'tonic-clonic') attack*, which is the most severe form and entails three phases. It begins with a very brief 'tonic' phase, in which the person loses consciousness and stops breathing temporarily. It then progresses to a longer 'clonic' phase that includes muscle spasms and twitching. In the last phase, the person relaxes and drifts into a comatose state until awakening. Sometimes before a grand mal attack epileptics experience an *aura*, which consists of unexplained sounds, smells or other sensations.
- *petit mal (or 'absence') attack*, which involves diminished consciousness, and in which the person stares blankly for a short while, perhaps only a few seconds, and may show slight facial twitching. When the spell ends, the person simply resumes whatever he or she was doing, sometimes not even being aware that the episode happened. Petit mal attacks occur mainly in childhood and usually disappear by adulthood.

Rates of true epilepsy are difficult to estimate since there are many undiagnosed cases and reports of episodic seizure activity for which epilepsy is not the real cause. Beran, Hall and Michelazzi (1985) suggested that a prevalence ratio of approximately 1 in 50 provided the best estimate of epilepsy rates in Australia when all other confounders had been taken account of, although other estimates suggest that between 1 in 80 and 1 in 200 Australians provide a closer guide to Australian rates of epilepsy. This illness strikes many children, and over and above the obvious medical and social costs involved, around 6.6 per 10 000 Australian children with epilepsy will die each year from the effects of the illness (Harvey, Nolan & Carlin 1993).

Although the condition can develop at any age, the great majority of epileptics experience their first seizures by 20 years of age (Seidenberg & Berent 1992). What causes epilepsy? Sometimes doctors find a specific neurological defect that is the cause of an epileptic's disorder, but usually they do not (Hauser & Hesdorffer 1990). Risk factors for developing epilepsy include a strong family history of the condition, severe head injury, infections of the central nervous system and stroke. Most people with epilepsy eventually become seizure-free for at least five years.

Medical treatments for epilepsy

Anticonvulsant drugs provide the main medical treatment for epilepsy (Sterman 1986). These medications do not work for all patients and may have undesirable side effects, such as drowsiness and, possibly, long-term cognitive impairments. Epileptics whose seizures result from clear neurological defects sometimes have the option of surgical treatment, particularly if they have frequent, severe attacks and medication does not work or the side effects are a problem. Neuropsychologists conduct tests to pinpoint the affected area of the brain and minimise cognitive and motor impairments the surgery might produce (DeAngelis 1990). After surgery, about 30 per cent of the patients no longer have seizures and 50 per cent experience markedly reduced attacks (Kaplan & Wyler 1983). But undergoing surgery without becoming seizure-free may lead to subsequent psychosocial difficulties, such as heightened anxiety and depression (Rose, Derry & McLachlan 1995).

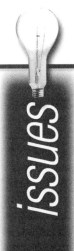

Highlight on issues

What to do for a seizure

The Epilepsy Foundation of Victoria (2000) recommends a simple set of steps to first aid during a seizure. First, the patient must be protected from hard objects, such as furniture, by removing these objects from the patient's field of reach. Second, the patient's head should be supported and they should be rolled onto their side. They should not be restrained and nothing should be put into their mouth. Consciousness usually returns in a few minutes and when this happens the patient should be reassured as to what has gone on. If the seizure lasts more than 10 minutes, if the patient remains unconscious or if this may be the person's first seizure, an ambulance should be called. It is important, the Foundation says, that whoever is giving first aid should remain calm, protect rather than restrain the patient, remain with them and reassure them.

Psychosocial factors in epilepsy

Because individuals who are having epileptic episodes lose control of their behaviour and 'act strange', their condition stigmatises them among people who do not understand it (Scambler 1984). This stigma is clear in the experience of a university student named Kurt when he witnessed a severe epileptic attack for the first time.

> In the centre of my college dining hall, a young man who worked in the kitchen had collapsed in a convulsion. Four students quickly piled on top of him. His arms and legs jerked violently and, in the process of trying to hold him down, the students seemed to be smothering him. The young man's face, twisted and red, made him appear to be in great pain and, somehow, inhuman. Yet I could see myself in his place — I had just found out that I had epilepsy.

I did not want to say anything, but I thought the four students, in their panic, might kill the young man. So I told the largest of them, who by then had a headlock on the kitchen worker, to let go. The student brushed off my concern and seemed irritated that I should bother him at such a time. I paused, then repeated my statement in louder tones. The student was angry. 'Look, kid, I'm a pre-med. I know what I'm doing. What makes you think you know so much?' I opened my mouth, but no words came out. Instead, I walked to a corner and leaned against a wall. As the young man's convulsions grew more violent, I whispered an apology to him and began to cry.

Just four weeks before, back home in Dallas, a neurologist had diagnosed my epilepsy. The doctor warned me — and so did members of my family soon afterward — that if I did not keep my epilepsy a secret, people would fear me and I would be subject to discrimination. (Eichenwald 1987, p. 30)

Not so many centuries ago, people believed that individuals with epilepsy were possessed by the devil, and many of its victims became social outcasts (Kaplan & Wyler 1983). Even today, epileptic attacks often arouse fear and horror in people who witness them.

Aside from the reactions their attacks produce in people, what other problems do epileptics face as a result of their illness? Restrictions on driving in those with epilepsy vary from one Australian State to another. Some States, such as Victoria, allow epileptics to hold driver's licences, but only if epileptic seizures are well under control. The Victorian Roads Authority (VicRoads) applies strict criteria in assessing this and driver's licences may be revoked if epilepsy becomes uncontrolled. If this happens, a stringent process of medical reassessment must take place in order for a licence to be restored. It is important, however, to carefully check the road traffic regulations relating to your own State or Territory in order to know what the law requires of epileptics who wish to hold driver's licences.

Epilepsy seems to be related to psychosocial processes in two ways. First, some evidence suggests that emotional arousal, such as anxiety, may increase the likelihood or severity of epileptic episodes (Goldstein 1990). Second, epileptics and their families sometimes adjust poorly to the disorder, especially if episodes are frequent and severe (Hauser & Hesdorffer 1990). Little research has been done on the psychosocial impact of epilepsy, but some evidence suggests that child epileptics suffer reduced self-esteem (Kerns & Curley 1985; Seidenberg & Berent 1992). Many of the adjustment problems that epileptics face can be reduced through counselling when the diagnosis is made and through the work of support groups.

Nervous system injuries

A woman named Leslie who suffered a *brain injury* in a car accident awoke after 17 days in a coma with, as she put it, the 'mentality of a cantankerous 13-year-old'. She remembers having bitten and pinched her physiotherapist and that when she awoke

I didn't know who I was, what happened to me. All of a sudden you wake up in this bed one day and these people are hurting you, bending your leg and such. And you think it's a dream or a nightmare of some kind. (Leonard 1990, p. 49)

This was the start of her long recovery. Many people suffer spinal cord injury in Australia each year. Estimates indicate that there are more than 25 new cases of severe spinal cord injury per million population annually in this country (Walsh 1988).

Young people are particularly at risk in this regard and vehicle accidents account for a significant proportion of new cases. Other factors, too, increase risk of severe spinal cord injury. Participation in rugby football poses a well-known risk for cervical spinal cord injury where the spine is injured close to the brain and therefore where the extent of resultant disability is greatest (Rotem et al. 1998). Those working in agricultural industries and especially with agricultural machinery also contribute in substantially higher proportions to overall spinal cord injury rates in Australia than do those in most city-based occupations (Young & Murphy 1998). Neuropsychologists and health psychologists play important roles in assessing these patients' impairments and helping them adapt to their conditions (Bleiberg, Ciulla & Katz 1991). In this section we will focus on the impact of having a spinal cord injury.

Prior to the 1940s, medical practitioners knew almost nothing about treating people who suffered a severe injury to the spinal cord (Hendrick 1985). In World War I, 80 per cent of the soldiers who received such injuries died within two weeks. People who survived severe spinal cord injuries had a poor prognosis for their future health, which was characterised by major health complications and a short life span. As a result, patients and practitioners had a defeatist attitude, and little attempt was made towards rehabilitation. In World War II, however, England established special medical units to develop and provide comprehensive care and rehabilitation techniques for people with spinal cord injuries. These medical units served as a model for others to be developed in countries around the world.

The prevalence, causes and physical effects of spinal cord injuries

The term **spinal cord injury** refers to neurological damage in the spine that results in the loss of motor control, sensation and reflexes in associated body areas. The damage may be caused by disease or by an injury that compresses, tears or severs the cord (Hendrick 1985). When the cord is badly torn or severed, the damage is permanent because little or no nerve tissue will regenerate; but if the cord is compressed or has an abrasion, some function may be recovered when the pressure is removed or healing occurs. As we saw in chapter 2, the degree to which the person's function is impaired depends on the amount of damage and its location. If the cord is completely severed in the neck region, *quadriplegia* results. If a lower portion is severed, *paraplegia* results. If the cord is not completely severed, partial function remains.

As we may deduce from the figures cited earlier, Australia has many thousands of people who live with the daily disability of spinal cord injury of one kind or another (paraplegia or quadriplegia). The great majority of Australians who receive spinal cord injuries are males, and most of them are between 10 and 30 years of age at the time. The most common cause is car and motorcycle accidents.

The physical effects patients experience after spinal cord injuries change over time and progress through two stages.

1. *Short-term effects.* The immediate physiological reaction is called 'spinal shock', which usually lasts between a few days and three months (Hendrick 1985; Nash & Smith 1982). In spinal shock, neural function is devastated either by the cord being severed or by inflammation at the site of lesser damage. The result is that the body cannot regulate blood pressure, temperature, respiration, and bladder and bowel function. Medical personnel must intervene to control these functions. Usually, the shorter the period of spinal shock, the better the prognosis of recovery.

2. *Long-term effects.* The full extent of spinal cord damage may not be clear for some time, and long-term predictions are difficult to make during the first six months or so (Hendrick 1985). If the cord is not severed, considerable functional recovery may

occur over a long period of time. If the cord is severed, some autonomic functions will recover, but other functions will not. People who survive severe damage to the higher regions of the cord are typically fully paralysed and unable to breathe without a respirator.

The initial care these patients receive typically focuses on their medical needs, with little or no attention to their psychological reactions (Brucker 1983). They receive very little information about their prognosis because it is so hard to predict, and the medical staff want to avoid the depression their speculations might produce. Once the condition of these individuals has stabilised, the process of rehabilitation begins. Almost all spinal cord injury patients enter rehabilitation expecting to regain total function and are not prepared to cope with the reality of permanent functional losses. A major goal for psychologists at this time is to help these people adjust to the demands and limitations of the rehabilitation process (Bleiberg, Ciulla & Katz 1991).

Physical rehabilitation

The process of physical rehabilitation for people with spinal cord injuries is geared towards helping them (1) regain as much physical function as the neurological damage will allow and (2) become as independent in their functioning as possible (Brucker 1983). This process focuses initially on training the patients to develop bladder and bowel control and on assisting them in moving paralysed limbs to maintain their range of motion (Hendrick 1985). Although many of these people will eventually be able to control their bladder functions, others will not and will need to use catheters or other devices. Hygienic bladder care is extremely important because a common cause of death in these patients after the spinal shock period is kidney failure from repeated infections (Hendrick 1985).

The next phase of rehabilitation extends the focus of physical therapy towards maintaining and improving the function of muscles over which the person has some control (Hendrick 1985). For example, quadriplegics receive special attention towards improving respiration; paraplegics do exercises to strengthen the upper body. When some neural connection to affected parts of the body remains, therapy with biofeedback to 're-educate' the muscles in those areas appears to help some, but not all, patients (Klose et al. 1993). The last phase of physical rehabilitation extends the therapy as much as possible to include activities of daily living. Those patients who have regained sufficient function learn how to perform self-care activities independently and to use devices to compensate for permanent physical losses. Some devices today are highly sophisticated and use computers, allowing paralysed individuals to turn on lights, answer the telephone and operate computer keyboards with voice commands.

Psychosocial aspects of spinal cord injury

People with spinal cord injuries face a long life ahead — an average of over 30 years after the injury (Brucker 1983). Their main challenge is to make the most of their remaining abilities and lead as full a life as possible. This can be very difficult for many with spinal cord injuries because they often suffer from chronic pain conditions as a complication of the injury and lack the resources to help them live and function independently (Mariano 1992; Tate, Maynard & Forchheimer 1993).

What can health care workers, family and friends do to help? A lot depends on the way they respond to the person's condition. John Adams and Erich Lindemann (1974) described and contrasted case studies of two young men, 17 and 18 years of age, who had suffered spinal cord injuries that rendered them quadriplegic. One adapted successfully, and the other did not. The patient who adapted well was able to accept the injury and abandon the part of his self-concept that was associated with his being a fine athlete. He then turned his energies towards academic pursuits and eventually became a history teacher. He also coached a local basketball team from his wheelchair. The other patient provides a striking contrast. He was never able to accept the injury or the permanence of his condition. He became extremely withdrawn and depressed — at one point he was spending 'much time in bed with the curtains drawn and frequently with the sheet over his head.' A few years later, he was readmitted to the hospital after taking an overdose of medication. At last contact, he was living at home, still clinging to the hope that he would walk again.

Why did these young men adapt so differently to their similar physical conditions? Adams and Lindemann noted the strikingly different ways these patients' families and friends responded to their condition. In the case of the patient who adapted well to his condition, his parents and friends also accepted his paralysis and provided an environment in which he could redefine his self-concept. For instance, his parents installed ramps in their home and widened doorways to accommodate a wheelchair. The other patient's family and friends were not able to accept his condition or provide the support he needed to help him adapt.

Family and friends can also help by providing social support without being overprotective and 'taking over' when the patient has difficulty performing self-help tasks. Having a disabled individual in the household increases the stress of all family members. They need to make many adjustments in daily living and, while doing so, must try not to make the person feel like a burden. If the patient is a husband or wife, his or her spouse faces very difficult adjustments (Hendrick 1985). Role changes occur immediately — at least for a while, and perhaps permanently. The healthy spouse, with or without the help of other family members, must suddenly take on full responsibility for providing the family's income, maintaining the household, caring for the children and caring for the disabled person. Sexual problems brought on by the patient's injury may become a major source of stress in the marital relationship.

Many people believe that all individuals who become paralysed below the waist lose all sexual function and interest. This belief is not correct (Alexander 1994; Brucker 1983; Hendrick 1985). Males usually lose their fertility. But although they initially lose the ability to have an erection, they often regain it to some degree. Females generally retain their fertility after paralysis, and about half become able to achieve orgasm. The most serious barriers to sexual function in people with spinal cord injuries appear to be psychosocial rather than physical. These patients and their sexual partners can overcome many of these barriers through counselling and education, such as in ways to position themselves during sex acts and to heighten the degree of stimulation they achieve.

Disabled people also experience many unpleasant thoughts about themselves, their future, their relations with other people in general, and physical barriers in society (Eisenberg 1984). They find that many places they once liked to go to are inaccessible by wheelchair, for example. Furthermore, people in general act strangely towards them — staring, or quickly averting their eyes, or behaving awkwardly or uncomfortably in their presence. These experiences tend to reduce the self-esteem of disabled people, many of whom have intense feelings of depression (Frank et al. 1987). Adapting to becoming disabled takes time, and a couple of years may pass before many individuals with spinal cord injuries report improvements in their adjustment and quality of life (Krause & Crewe 1991).

Of course many people with disabilities, and certainly those with spinal cord injury, are able to excel in a range of areas. This often requires herculean efforts on the part of many very talented and determined individuals but is perhaps epitomised in Australia by the Paralympics 2000, in which many of this country's best athletes competed with other disabled people from around the world in eighteen sporting events. Australian athletes with severe spinal cord injury took part in such events as wheelchair road racing and basketball, swimming and archery, and did so with great distinction.

Diabetes

'Too much of a good thing is wonderful,' the late actress Mae West once said. Although her rule might possibly apply for some good things, glucose in the blood is not one of them. The body needs glucose to fuel metabolic processes, but too much of it in the blood over a long period of time — a condition called *hyperglycaemia* — is the mark of *diabetes mellitus*. The body normally controls blood sugar levels with the hormone *insulin*, which the pancreas produces. In the disorder of diabetes, however, abnormal levels of glucose accumulate in the blood because the pancreas does not produce sufficient insulin (Kilo & Williamson 1987; Pohl, Gonder-Frederick & Cox 1984; May 1991).

Diabetes is among the most common chronic conditions in Australia. Rates of diabetes in Australia are somewhat difficult to estimate since many have the disease, at least in its early stages, without recognising it. For reasons not yet well understood, rates of Type I (insulin-dependent) diabetes in children are lower in the southern hemisphere than in northern climes, and Australia benefits from this geographic difference (Karvonen et al. 1993). Still, rates of diabetes in this country are sufficiently high to be of concern. More than 250 000 Australians suffer from diagnosed diabetes, of whom over 40 000 have Type I (insulin-dependent) diabetes. Some 7000 or more of these people are under the age of 25 years. An additional 225 000 or so are estimated to be undiagnosed diabetics. On the basis of these data, prevalence rates for diabetes in Australia are estimated at around 1.6 per cent for all ages and 2.1 per cent for those over 21 years; about 2.2 per cent of all Australian adults may also be diabetic and not know it (Welborn et al. 1989).

Regrettably, rates of Type II (non-insulin-dependent) diabetes among Australia's Aboriginal people are among the highest in the world (Daniel et al. 1999). This is largely related to the problem of obesity and poor diet among Aboriginal people (Gracey 1995). The effect of this is clearly evident in patterns of Aboriginal mortality, where diabetes-related conditions are a major cause of death (Veroni, Gracey & Rouse 1994). The imposition of a Western lifestyle on Aboriginal people has been very conspicuously counterproductive to their health, and one of the major challenges for health psychology in this country is to focus on ways in which poor health practices among indigenous people can be effectively altered.

The types and causes of diabetes

Diabetes is not a single disease — it occurs in two major patterns that require different kinds of treatment and may have somewhat different causes. The two forms of diabetes are:

- *Type I.* This form of diabetes typically develops in childhood or adolescence and accounts for only 5 to 10 per cent of diabetes cases. It is called **insulin-dependent diabetes mellitus** (IDDM) because cells of the pancreas that normally produce insulin have been disabled, and patients afflicted with Type I diabetes require insulin injections to prevent acute and very serious complications (Kilo & Williamson 1987; Pohl, Gonder-Frederick & Cox 1984). The main acute complication that occurs without insulin in Type I diabetes is called *ketoacidosis*, in which high levels of fatty acids in the blood lead to kidney malfunctions, thereby causing wastes to accumulate and poison the body. The symptoms of ketoacidosis generally begin with chronic thirst and urination, followed by an acute episode of nausea, vomiting, abdominal pain and laboured breathing. About one-third of new IDDM cases are diagnosed after these symptoms appear. If left untreated, ketoacidosis can lead to coma and death in a matter of days or weeks.

- *Type II*. The vast majority of diabetics have the second form of this disease, which is called **non-insulin-dependent diabetes mellitus** (NIDDM) because the pancreas does produce at least some insulin and treatment often does not require insulin injections. Most, but not all, people with NIDDM can manage their glucose levels without taking insulin by carefully following special diets and taking medication. Although NIDDM can develop at any age, it usually appears after the age of 40. This type of diabetes appears to have two *subtypes* that depend on the person's weight (Kilo & Williamson 1987; Wing, Nowalk & Guare 1988). Most NIDDM patients are very overweight and seem to produce substantial amounts of insulin — sometimes more than normal quantities — but their bodies seem to 'resist' the glucose-controlling action of insulin (Chan et al. 1994; Kohrt et al. 1993). In contrast, normal-weight NIDDM patients produce reduced levels of insulin. In either case, hyperglycaemia results.

What causes the pancreas to reduce its production of insulin? Although the causes are not well understood, twin studies have demonstrated that genetic factors are involved in both IDDM and NIDDM (Kilo & Williamson 1987; Pohl, Gonder-Frederick & Cox 1984; Wing, Nowalk & Guare 1988). The great majority of diabetics probably inherit some form of susceptibility to the effects of environmental conditions that could affect insulin production. In IDDM, one environmental condition seems to involve a viral infection that stimulates the immune system to attack pancreas cells (Conrad et al. 1994). For NIDDM, evidence exists for three possible conditions: diets high in fat and sugar, stress, and an overproduction of a protein that impairs the metabolism of sugars and carbohydrates (Maddux et al. 1995; Surwit 1993). At this time, however, the nature of people's susceptibility to diabetes and the environmental conditions involved are not clear.

Health implications of diabetes

Diabetes can be a direct cause of death and claims thousands of lives in Australia each year, largely through the process of cardiovascular disease. An upsetting aspect of these deaths is that many of them — perhaps one-third — result from acute complications, such as ketoacidosis, that 'are usually preventable by appropriate medical care' (Wing, Nowalk & Guare 1988, p. 246). Few diabetics die of acute complications if they follow the recommended medical regimens for controlling glucose levels (Santiago 1984).

But the deaths that are caused directly by diabetes constitute only part of the serious health effects of this disease (Crofford 1995; Kilo & Williamson 1987). Diabetes is implicated in the development of a variety of disabling health problems and contributes indirectly to many deaths each year. One health problem diabetes can lead to is *neuropathy*, or nerve disease. High blood glucose levels appear to cause chemical reactions that can destroy the myelin sheath that insulates nerve fibres. When this occurs in peripheral fibres, such as in the feet, the person may lose sensation in the affected area or have abnormal sensations, such as chronic pain. When the damage occurs in autonomic nerve fibres, the symptoms may include chronic dizziness, urinary incontinence and sexual impotence (in males).

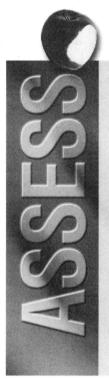

Assess yourself
Do you have diabetes?

About half of the people who have diabetes don't know it. To tell if you might have this disorder, put a check mark in the space preceding each of the following warning signs that are true for you.

_____ Very frequent urination

_____ Excessive thirst

_____ Often hungry, even after eating

_____ Unexplained large weight loss

_____ Chronically tired

_____ Occasional blurry vision

_____ Wounds heal very slowly

_____ Tingling or numbness in your feet

_____ Waist measurement greater than half your height

If you check three or more of these signs, see your doctor — one or two signs alone may not mean anything is wrong. But the more signs you checked, the greater the chance that you have diabetes.

(*Source:* Based on *Signs and Symptoms of Diabetes*, distributed by the American Diabetes Association.)

Diabetes can also lead to the development of other serious health problems. Physicians Charles Kilo and Joseph Williamson have noted that compared with individuals who are not diabetic, people who have diabetes are:
- 6.8 times more likely to become blind
- 11.3 times more likely to develop kidney disease
- 29.9 times more likely to get gangrene
- 4.6 times more likely to develop heart disease
- 5.4 times more likely to have a stroke (1987, p. 54).

The way diabetes contributes to these health problems is through its effects on the vascular system (Kilo & Williamson 1987; Wing, Nowalk & Guare 1988). High levels of glucose in the blood lead to a thickening of arterial walls as a result of atherosclerosis. This can occur in large blood vessels, such as those in the legs and near the heart, causing gangrene in a limb or heart disease. It can also occur in small blood vessels and capillaries, such as those in the eyes, kidneys and brain. Eye disease that results from diabetes can be treated effectively if caught early (Javitt et al. 1994).

The long-term health risks of diabetes are extremely serious, and patients and their families worry about them greatly (Holmes 1986; Wilkinson 1987). They worry about the possibilities of, for instance, dying prematurely, becoming blind, losing a limb if gangrene cannot be controlled, and being unable to perform sexually. Diabetics who are at greatest risk for these problems are those whose disease requires insulin in its treatment and starts in childhood, adolescence or early adulthood (Cameron 1986).

Medical treatments for diabetes

Ideally, the treatment for diabetes would enable the body to perform or simulate the normal biochemical activities for processing and maintaining normal levels of glucose. Medical treatments available today compensate for these differences, but they do not enable the body to function exactly as it normally does, such as in continuously monitoring the need for insulin and secreting this hormone in precisely needed bursts. Doctors generally prescribe somewhat different regimens for IDDM and NIDDM patients and tailor the treatment for individual needs (Kilo & Williamson 1987).

The main approach for treating diabetes entails a balancing act with medication, diet and regular exercise under medical supervision. Can diabetics reduce their long-term health risks by keeping their blood glucose levels within the normal range? Yes, these risks can be markedly reduced — with complications occurring much later and far less often — if diabetics receive intensive medical care and control their blood glucose levels by carefully following prescribed treatments (Crofford 1995; Santiago 1984; Wang, Lau & Chalmers 1993). But the *full extent* of the reduced risk is unclear because long-term complications of diabetes take many years or decades to develop, and many diabetics with good blood glucose control are not always able to keep their glucose levels consistently in the normal range. Treatments for diabetes today allow patients to have better control over their blood sugar than in the past, but these new methods are still not perfect. And many diabetics who have treatments that could provide good control over their blood glucose do not adhere to them closely.

Do diabetics adhere to their treatments?

Non-compliance with treatment is a major problem in managing diabetes. According to researchers who have reviewed studies on this issue, the most thorough survey of patients' adherence to diabetes treatments found that:
- 80 per cent of patients administered insulin in an unhygienic manner
- 58 per cent administered the wrong dose of insulin
- 77 per cent tested their glucose levels incorrectly or interpreted the results 'in a manner likely to be detrimental to their treatment'
- 75 per cent did not eat the prescribed foods
- 75 per cent did not eat with sufficient regularity (Wing et al. 1986, p. 78).

People with diabetes generally do *try* to adhere to their treatments, but they do not always succeed. One reason they fail may be that they rely on symptoms they perceive, such as dizziness or emotional states, in assessing their glucose levels (Cox et al. 1993; Diamond, Massey & Covey 1989). Although many diabetics can make crude estimates of their actual glucose levels on the basis of perceived symptoms, these judgements are usually not very accurate.

Research with IDDM patients, ranging from about 12 years of age to old age, found that they have more difficulty following dietary and exercise advice than the more 'medical' aspects of their treatments — testing their glucose levels and taking their insulin on time (Glasgow, McCaul & Schafer 1986, 1987). These patients' self-reports indicated they had complied fairly closely with their insulin and testing treatments. However, self-report data can be misleading. In two studies, for instance, researchers secretly inserted memory chips in blood glucose testing devices of adult and adolescent diabetics but also had the subjects keep records of their testing (Mazze et al. 1984; Wilson & Endres 1986). The results showed that many subjects' records were inaccurate — at least according to the memory chips' records. The records did *not* contain data for some tests the subjects had done and *did* contain data for tests that they did not actually perform.

Psychosocial factors and diabetes treatments

A 60-year-old diabetic named Beth had not been able to get her glucose levels under control (Holt 1995). Part of the problem was that she was mentally retarded but able to live on her own, and she didn't understand how to plan her diet. A domicillary-care nurse discovered an approach to help: They made up recipe cards for each meal, with pictures of its foods and a shopping list. Because there were cards for breakfast, lunch, dinner and snacks, Beth could choose the meal she wanted, shop for it and follow the recipe to make it. And she succeeded in doing so. Not understanding how to interpret glucose test results and adjust the treatment accordingly is a very common problem even among non-retarded diabetics (Patrick, Gill et al. 1994).

We saw in chapter 9 that compliance to medical recommendations generally tends to be low when the treatment is complex, must be followed for a long period of time, requires changes in the person's lifestyle and is designed to prevent rather than cure illness. Treatments for diabetes have all of these characteristics. In addition, psychosocial factors in patients' lives are related to compliance. Two of these factors are social support and self-efficacy. A study of NIDDM patients found that subjects' self-reports of adherence to dietary, exercise and glucose testing aspects of their treatment increased with their perceived social support (Wilson et al. 1986). But the role of social support is unclear because it was not related to actual glucose control, as measured by analysis of blood samples. Other research has shown that diabetics' self-efficacy for being able to follow diabetes treatment is related to their self-reports of subsequent adherence and their actual glucose control (Kavanaugh, Gooley & Wilson 1993; Skelly et al. 1995).

Stress impairs blood sugar control in many diabetics (Goetsch 1989; Gonder-Frederick et al. 1990; Moberg et al. 1994). When people are under stress, the adrenal glands release adrenalin and cortisol into the bloodstream (Surwit, Feinglos & Scovern 1983). Adrenalin causes the pancreas to decrease insulin production; *cortisol* causes the liver to increase glucose production and body tissues to decrease their use of glucose. These biochemical reactions to stress clearly worsen the glucose regulation problems of diabetics. What's more, stress can affect blood glucose levels indirectly by leading to non-adherence to diabetes treatments (Goldston et al. 1995).

People's everyday lives present many circumstances that make it difficult to adhere to diabetes treatments (Glasgow, McCaul & Schafer 1986). Diabetics may feel that testing their glucose levels at work or school is embarrassing, or forget to take their testing materials with them, or have difficulty getting up on weekend mornings to take their injections on time, or make mistakes in judgements about what they can eat, for example. Also, because some temporary weight gain tends to occur when diabetics get their glucose under control, many female patients, in an effort to control their weight, fail to take their insulin (Polonsky et al. 1994). Problems can also arise when dietary recommendations are incompatible with the food habits of patients in certain ethnic groups (Raymond & D'Eramo-Melkus 1993). Another problem is the frequent frustration diabetics feel when they 'didn't cheat', but their glucose control is off target for some other reason, such as their being under stress. And because diabetes is not itself a painful condition, patients may not always feel that following the treatment closely matters very much (Kilo & Williamson 1987).

One other psychosocial situation that can lead to non-compliance is when the patient and the doctor have different goals of treatment. A study demonstrated this by having doctors and the parents of diabetic children serve as subjects and asking them to assess hypothetical glucose test profiles (Marteau et al. 1987). The researchers presented the subjects with several different test results, including one each reflecting a normal glucose level, hypoglycaemia and three degrees of hyperglycaemia. The doctors were asked to pick the one profile they would be 'happiest to see' for a child at their clinic; the parents were asked to pick the one they would be 'happiest to see' for *their* own child. The results showed that the vast majority of doctors, but only about half of the parents, chose the profile reflecting the normal glucose level. More than a third of the parents chose either the mild or the moderate *hyperglycaemic* profile. This suggests that the main focus of doctors is on preventing long-term complications from developing. In comparison, parents seem to be more interested in preventing *hypoglycaemic* episodes and in promoting the day-to-day wellbeing and activity of their children. Not surprisingly, the children's actual glucose levels more closely matched the goals of their parents than those of doctors. Because much smaller deviations from normal blood sugar levels result in symptoms of hypoglycaemia than in those of hyperglycaemia, parents and diabetics may choose to err on the side of higher glucose levels (Varni & Babani 1986).

Highlight on issues

ISSUES

Self-managing diabetes

Managing diabetes requires several self-care activities that focus mainly on four components: self-monitoring of blood glucose, taking insulin or other medication, diet and exercise.

Self-monitoring blood glucose

Patients estimate the sugar content of their blood by testing either their urine or, more accurately, the blood itself (Gonder-Frederick et al. 1984; Kilo & Williamson 1987). To test the blood, a diabetic pricks his or her finger to get a drop of blood, puts the blood on a chemically treated strip of paper that changes colour in reaction to glucose, and wipes the blood off after a minute or so. The diabetic can then assess the sugar content either by comparing the colour on the strip visually against a colour chart or by inserting the strip into a small meter that displays a digital glucose reading. Although this procedure may sound simple, its accuracy depends on how precisely it is carried out. Waiting too long to wipe the blood off the strip or to assess the colour can change the reading. Treatments usually require NIDDM patients to

monitor blood glucose once a day and IDDM patients to do it four times: before each meal and at bedtime.

Taking insulin and oral medication

In the early 1920s a doctor named Frederick Banting devised a method that made it possible to extract insulin from the pancreas glands of slaughtered pigs and cattle. These animals are the chief sources of insulin for treating diabetes today. Over the years, refinements have been made to the insulin extracted, and forms of the hormone are available that last for different lengths of time. Most diabetics who need to take insulin inject it twice a day — morning and evening (Kilo & Williamson 1987; Pohl, Gonder-Frederick & Cox 1984; Wing, Nowalk & Guare 1988). But many diabetics need to take it more frequently to ensure better glucose control. Some diabetics are able to use a device called an insulin pump that can be implanted in the body and delivers small amounts of insulin continuously, with extra doses at mealtimes.

(continued)

One of the difficulties in using insulin is knowing how much to inject — taking too much may be as dangerous as taking too little. Using too much insulin can produce *hypoglycaemia*, the condition of having too little sugar in blood. Severe hypoglycaemia can cause insulin shock, in which the person lapses into a coma (Kilo & Williamson 1987). When hypoglycaemia is somewhat less severe, it can markedly impair cognitive and emotional functioning, making the person excited, irritable, confused and, sometimes, violent (Holmes 1986). Diabetics dread these episodes, and so do their families (Wilkinson 1987). Today's relatively precise methods for assessing blood glucose can help them reduce these episodes and adjust their insulin doses more accurately to keep glucose levels within the normal range. Adjusting doses can be a complicated task, and patients usually need careful training to do it correctly.

Many diabetics use drugs to control their blood glucose levels. Different types of chemicals work in different ways — for instance, some drugs increase insulin production in functioning pancreatic cells whereas others reduce the liver's production of glucose (Kilo & Williamson 1987). Doctors typically do periodic blood tests on these patients because these drugs sometimes become less effective in controlling glucose levels over time.

Diet and exercise

The diets doctors recommend for diabetics are designed to accomplish four things: (1) drastically reduce the intake of foods that contain sugar and some other carbohydrates that lead to high blood glucose levels, (2) reduce cholesterol consumption, (3) achieve and maintain a healthy body weight, and (4) maintain a balanced intake of nutrients (Kilo & Williamson 1987; Wing, Epstein & Nowalk 1984). People who must take insulin must also maintain consistency in the timing of their meals and, usually, in their calorie intake each day. Once they take their insulin, they generally need to eat within a range of time thereafter to prevent an episode of hypoglycaemia.

Because physical activity burns up glucose as fuel, exercise is an important component in the treatment of diabetes, too. Research has shown that engaging in physical activity after meals inhibits glucose production by the liver and increases glucose use by the muscles (Zinman 1984). Regular exercise also complements dietary efforts to reduce body weight and maintain overall fitness. But unplanned vigorous activity can cause an episode of hypoglycaemia. People with diabetes who engage in vigorous activity should eat a sufficient number of calories to last through the event or carry packets of medication to adjust their blood sugar quickly (Kilo & Williamson 1987).

Following a program to treat diabetes is difficult, but the risks of not doing so are very serious. It takes a good deal of planning, strong efforts to maintain the routine with only occasional departures, and the confidence of patients and their families that they can do it.

When the diabetic is a child or adolescent

Most parents of diabetic children cope well with the disease (Eiser 1985). Many family stressors remain, however, and stem from having to deal with occasional diabetic crises, take the child in for periodic medical examinations, give the glucose tests and injections, and make dietary adjustments, either by making special meals for the patient or by modifying the whole family's diet. Parents also worry more than their diabetic children about future health complications.

Diabetic children younger than, say, eight or 10 years of age have little knowledge or understanding about their conditions, possible long-term health problems, and why aspects of their treatments are necessary. They also do not see themselves as being very different from other children. As researcher Christine Eiser (1985) has noted, unlike children with other medical conditions, those with diabetes do not look different from other children and do not experience regular and painful medical procedures. The things that set diabetic children apart from others are their rigid eating patterns and dietary restrictions, their need to balance their intake of food carefully in relation to exercise, and, of course, the daily glucose monitoring and insulin injections. These are the kinds of things children dislike most about having diabetes (Eiser 1985). Most of these activities can be done at home or privately.

Maintaining the diabetes treatment regimen during childhood is essentially the parents' responsibility. When can children do some of the treatment activities on their own? Children's cognitive and motor abilities allow most of them to learn to select appropriate foods by eight years of age, give themselves injections by nine or 10, and perform glucose testing by 12 (Eiser 1985). Moreover, adolescent and pre-adolescent diabetics generally think children are able to manage their own diabetes care at around 12 years of age. Parents tend to agree — and as adolescence approaches they allow their children more and more responsibility for managing the diabetes treatment. But research has shown that the quality of diabetes care is often lower in adolescence than in the pre-adolescent years (Anderson et al. 1990; Bond, Aiken & Somerville 1992; Jacobson et al. 1987; Johnson et al. 1990). Compliance with glucose monitoring and diet declines with age in adolescence; blood sugar control also decreases, but non-adherence is probably not the only reason for decreased glucose control. Although the psychosocial immaturity of diabetics in early adolescence is probably responsible for many adherence problems, hormonal changes that occur during adolescence may make the task of controlling blood glucose more difficult (Eiser 1985).

By the time children with diabetes reach adolescence, they have the cognitive abilities to understand the disease and its long-term implications. Instead of feeling confident in their futures — as other teenagers do — they may see cloudy and vulnerable lives ahead, and feel angry and cheated (Holmes 1986). Teenagers' adherence to their diabetes treatments is relatively high among those who have high levels of self-esteem and social competence and have good relations with their parents (Hanson, Henggeler & Burghen 1987; Jacobson et al. 1987, 1994; Miller-Johnson et al. 1994). Teens who feel less sure of themselves may neglect their self-care activities partly because they may feel a greater need to avoid appearing different from their peers.

Arthritis

Before developing a severe case of arthritis, Ron had been active in sports for most of his 50 years of life, having played and coached high-school football and become an avid golfer and tennis player (McIlwain et al. 1991). In the past five years, playing golf and tennis became increasingly difficult because of pain in his knee and hip, and he eventually stopped playing completely. After two months of treatment with medication and exercise for this musculoskeletal disorder, he was able to resume these activities without severe pain.

Musculoskeletal disorders that affect the body's muscles, joints and connective tissues near the joints are called *rheumatic diseases* (Burg & Ingall 1985). Most cases of rheumatic disease are classified as **arthritis** — a category of more than 100 conditions that involve inflammation of the joints, pain, stiffness and, sometimes, swelling. Disorders of the bones and joints have probably always plagued humans and almost all other animals — archaeologists have found evidence of arthritis in the fossil bones of dinosaurs and prehistoric bears, for instance (Achterberg-Lawlis 1988). By far the most common arthritic condition is osteoarthritis, followed by rheumatoid arthritis and then gout.

The types and causes of arthritis

Osteoarthritis is a disease in which the joints degenerate, mainly as a result of wear and tear. People's risk of developing this condition increases with age and body weight and is associated with certain occupations in which particular joints are subjected to repeated heavy use (Kelsey & Hochberg 1988). For instance, weavers and cotton pickers often develop osteoarthritis of the hands, whereas ballet dancers tend to have the condition in their feet. *Gout* can affect any of the body's joints. In this disease, the body produces more uric acid than the kidneys can process, and the excess acid circulates in the blood and leaves crystalline deposits at the joints.

Rheumatoid arthritis is a disease that involves extreme inflammation of joint tissues and also affects the heart, blood vessels and lungs when it reaches advanced stages. It is potentially the most serious arthritic condition, being the most crippling and painful type. It often spreads to all of the body's joints. Although the mechanisms that lead to rheumatoid arthritis are unclear, they seem to involve an immune response that attacks the tissues and bones of the joints (AMA 1989; Benjamini & Leskowitz 1991). Some research has found evidence linking stress and rheumatoid arthritis, finding that patients reported that major stressful events often preceded the onset of the disease and its flare-ups (Achterberg-Lawlis 1988; Anderson et al. 1985).

Arthritis in its various forms strikes many Australians. The Arthritis Foundation of Western Australia (2000) estimates that about 2 million Australians, or around 13.4 per cent of the Australian population have arthritis; this involves around 7.5 per cent of the Australian work force. Arthritis affects the young as well as the old, and those who believe themselves to be physically fit as well as those whose levels of fitness are less than optimal. About 1 in 250 children suffer from juvenile chronic arthritis and around 10 per cent of 20-year-olds show signs of osteoarthritis, often linked to poor management of sporting injuries. Some 50 per cent of the population worry they might have arthritis but do not seek medical confirmation of this. The economic and other costs are substantial, the Foundation suggesting that arthritis costs the Australian community some $4.5 billion each year.

The effects and treatment of arthritis

Of the major chronic diseases that afflict people in Australia, arthritis is the leader each year in causing people to cut down on their usual activities, such as going to work. Any type of arthritis can disable its victims on a short-term or long-term basis. Elderly people are more likely to have functional limitations from osteoarthritis of the knee than from most other chronic illnesses (Guccione et al. 1994).

In the case of rheumatoid arthritis, some patients experience only mild episodes of inflammation and pain in a few joints; others, however, suffer intense pain in many joints, often showing the following progression.

- The lubricating fluid leaks out of the joints, usually in the knees, ankles, shoulders, elbows and wrists.
- Cartilage is destroyed and joint function is reduced.
- The conversion of organic matter into minerals for bones decreases near the joints.
- Bone erosions take place near the joints.
- Joints become dislocated and sometimes fused, producing deformities (Anderson et al. 1985).

Some of the people whose rheumatoid arthritis progresses to the later stages show associated damage to other organ systems, developing vascular or heart valve diseases for example.

What treatments can be used in managing the pain and functional impairment of arthritis? People with arthritis typically take some form of pain-relieving medication, especially aspirin and other drugs, such as ibuprofen, that reduce inflammation (Anderson et al. 1985; McIlwain et al. 1991). For relatively severe cases, two types of medication may be prescribed. *Steroids* are fast-acting drugs that tend to reduce inflammation, stiffness and swelling in a matter of hours. *Gold compounds* are salts that are soluble in liquid. Although most patients who are treated with gold get at least moderate relief, it usually takes weeks or months for them to notice improvements, and the action of this drug is not well understood. But using gold compounds and certain kinds of steroids for a long time can have serious side effects, such as gastrointestinal problems and kidney damage. In extreme cases when other medical approaches have not helped, surgeons replace affected joints with artificial ones.

Other approaches for managing arthritic pain and impairment involve maintaining proper body weight and, especially for people with gout, limiting certain foods and alcohol (McIlwain et al. 1991). Physiotherapy is very important and includes exercise, applying heat or cold, and using devices to prevent joint damage and assist patients in performing daily activities (Minor & Sanford 1993; Wickersham 1984). For example, a 58-year-old woman with rheumatoid arthritis whose hand pain and weakness made lifting heavy pots, opening jars and doing other household tasks difficult received the following physiotherapy components:

- *exercises* to increase hand strength and range of motion
- *splints*, which she wore on her left or right hand on alternating nights to reduce pain and swelling in her wrists and fingers
- *advice on devices* that can make daily activities easier, such as a cart to transport things, purses that hang from the shoulder instead of the hand, and handles with large diameters (Philips 1989).

Many arthritis sufferers supplement medical care with 'alternative medicine' methods, such as acupuncture and herbal therapy, especially if they are dissatisfied with medical procedures (Vecchio 1994).

Studies of compliance for medical treatments have shown that people with arthritis adhere closely to recommendations for the more powerful drugs, but not for milder ones, such as aspirin, and they adhere less closely with physiotherapy aspects of their treatments than with taking medication (Anderson et al. 1985). Many patients dislike physiotherapy, seeing its negative aspects, rather than its positive ones (Jensen & Lorish 1994). They feel, for instance, that exercising is boring and its value is not obvious.

Psychosocial factors in arthritis

Any chronic pain condition is distressing for the patients and their families, and the distress is worse if the pain is severe and frequent. If arthritic individuals are disabled by the pain, their condition produces a great deal of stress for them and their families.

People with severe rheumatoid arthritis experience at least some pain virtually every day, and on many days it is intense (Affleck et al. 1991). Research with adult arthritics has shown that those whose condition is severe are much more likely to feel helpless and seriously depressed than those with a milder condition (Anderson et al. 1985). One study, for instance, examined over 200 patients' disability and feelings of helplessness about their conditions over a one-year period (Nicassio et al. 1985). Their self-reports showed that their feelings of helplessness correlated with changes in their ability to perform daily activities, such as dressing, turning taps on and off, and getting in and out of a car. Other studies have found that the severity of a person's arthritic condition is related to feelings of helplessness, and that these feelings lead to maladjustment and depression (Nicassio et al. 1993; Parker et al. 1991; Smith & Wallston 1992; Smith, Peck & Ward 1990; Zautra et al. 1995).

Of course, not all individuals with severe arthritis experience serious emotional difficulties. Some people with severe arthritis feel a greater sense of personal control over their condition than others do, and this difference relates to their emotional adjustment. In a study examining this relationship, researchers interviewed adults with rheumatoid arthritis regarding their mood states and their perceptions of personal control over their illness (Affleck et al. 1987). These interviews revealed three main findings. First, the subjects generally thought their practitioners had greater control over the *course* of the disease than they did themselves. Second, of the patients who had relatively active symptoms, those who believed they could control their *daily symptoms* reported less mood disturbance than those who did not. Third, the subjects who saw themselves as *active partners* in decisions about their medical care and treatment showed better adjustment to their illness. These findings are also important because people with arthritis who understand their treatment and believe it can help are more likely to adhere closely to their medical treatments than those individuals who do not (Jette 1984).

What impact does the arthritis condition have on the psychological status of the patient's spouse? The severity of the disease by itself seems to have little impact. Spouses of arthritis patients seem to adapt similarly to different levels of disease severity — the feelings of distress or depression they report relate mainly to their perceptions of the quality of the marriage and of social support (Manne & Zautra 1990). But the impact of disease severity appears to depend on social support: as arthritis severity increases, spouses who perceive little social support in their lives report *more* depression, while spouses with high levels of social support report *less* depression (Revenson & Majerovitz 1991).

Alzheimer's disease

For a long time Martha, the wife of 75-year-old Alfred, denied her husband was sick, making excuses for his forgetful and odd behaviour. Then

> one evening, they were out dining with friends. During the meal, Alfred refused to remove his overcoat and wouldn't talk to anyone. Instead, he clanged his fork on his plate, put his napkin in his soup, and tried to eat his salad with his knife. When Martha whispered to him to put down his silverware, he yelled at her. She burst into tears. Finally, one of the male dinner guests led Alfred from the table, leaving a humiliated, mortified wife to confront a reality that could no longer be ignored: Alfred had Alzheimer's disease. (McCahon 1991, p. 44)

Dementia is a term that refers to a progressive loss of cognitive functions that often occurs in old age. By far the most common form of dementia is **Alzheimer's disease**, a brain disorder characterised by a deterioration of attention, memory and personality. Figure 13.3 illustrates the cognitive deficits of an Alzheimer victim. Alzheimer's disease is of increasing concern in Australia. Prevalence rates range from 0.72 per cent of the Australian population aged 60 to 64 years, through to 5.60 per cent in 75- to 79-year-olds, 11.11 per cent in 80- to 84-year-olds, and an alarming 23.60 per cent in those Australians 85 years and older (Jorm & Henderson 1993). Moreover, the projected prevalence of dementia in this country is expected to increase sharply over the coming 30 years (Jorm & Henderson 1993). While Alzheimer's disease is a condition that predominantly affects older people, it is not unknown for 40-year-olds to suffer from dementia. This may be the result of many possible causes, but the overall cost to the individual, the family and the community is very large indeed. The expected 10-year survival rate for those with Alzheimer's disease is around only 16 per cent.

The cognitive functions of people with Alzheimer's disease do not disappear all at once. Perhaps the most critical functions to go at first are *attention* and *memory*. Peter Vitaliano and his colleagues (1986) conducted a two-year follow-up study of Alzheimer victims with mild impairment and found that their main deficits initially were in their attentive and memory abilities. The extent of these deficits was strongly associated with the degree of their impairment two years later. As the disease progresses over several years, the effects of the disorder become more pronounced (Reichman 1990). Personality changes often emerge, with the victims becoming less spontaneous and more apathetic and withdrawn. Self-care deteriorates, and behaviour problems appear, as when these individuals wander and become lost. At some point, they may become frequently disoriented with regard to time, their location, and their identity. These declines develop faster if the patients suffer a severe loss of language or have a history of alcohol abuse or of neurological disorders, such as from a stroke or Parkinson's disease (Bracco et al. 1994; Teri, Hughes & Larson 1990).

The causes and treatment of Alzheimer's disease

What causes Alzheimer's disease? The most promising answer seems to involve a characteristic that differentiates the brains of Alzheimer victims from those of other elderly individuals: Alzheimer brains contain extensive *lesions*, consisting of gnarled and tangled nerve fibres and of a protein, called *beta-amyloid*, the body produces (Larson, Kukull & Katzman 1992; NIA 1995). Evidence now indicates that genetic defects may cause these large deposits to occur. For instance, one study examined stored tissue samples from many members of a family across three generations (Murrell et al. 1991). All members with the genetic defect also had Alzheimer's disease, and no member who did not have the defect had the disease. A likely gene involved in early onset of the disease has also been identified (Levy-Lahad et al. 1995). Two other findings are also important. First, one study found that people with the brain lesions that characterise the disease are far more likely to develop Alzheimer's symptoms if they have had strokes, even fairly mild ones, than if they have not (Snowdon et al. 1997). Second, research has found a link between the development of Alzheimer's disease and prior head injury (Larson, Kukull & Katzman 1992). It seems likely that this disease can result from several types of genetic defects and environmental factors.

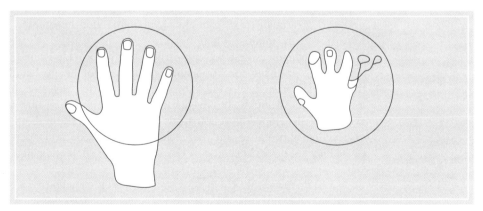

Figure 13.3 Illustration of cognitive deficits in Alzheimer's disease. A graphic artist with this disorder was asked to copy the drawing of a hand shown on the left. The hand he drew was much smaller and had distortions in spatial relationships, misplaced fingernails, and an incorrect number of fingers.

In Australia, diagnosis of Alzheimer's disease is usually made according to the criteria set out in DSM IV (APA 1994). These include multiple and progressive cognitive deficits involving memory, language (aphasia), motor functions (apraxia), identification and naming (agnosia), and executive functioning. It is important, in making such a diagnosis, to exclude identical cognitive dysfunction arising from other causes such as strokes, long-term alcohol or drug abuse, or a range of medical conditions that interfere with the overall metabolism of the brain. Jorm & Henderson (1993) have recommended the use of the Mini-Mental State Examination (Folstein, Folstein & McHugh 1975) as a convenient means of confirming diagnosis and of further quantifying the effects of Alzheimer's disease. Simpler, potentially accurate diagnostic methods are being developed that use brain scans and eye tests (Reiman et al. 1996; Scinto et al. 1994). No treatment exists yet to prevent or stop the progression of Alzheimer's disease.

Psychosocial effects of Alzheimer's disease

Most victims of Alzheimer's disease live at home and receive care from their spouses or adult children (Brown 1991; Gruetzner 1992). In the early stages of the disease, family members and others may be able to help maximise the person's functioning, for example by marking objects clearly and giving social support. But many families either don't know or deny that the person has Alzheimer's disease. As patients lose more and more of their cognitive function, their inability to do simple tasks and remember everyday things becomes very frustrating and often leads to feelings of helplessness, which may account for their high rates of depression (Migliorelli et al. 1995).

Alzheimer patients' behaviour becomes increasingly problematic as the disease progresses, producing great stress in the family. People with this disease may, for instance, accuse a family member of hiding things they cannot find, develop sleep disturbances and stay awake most of the night, get lost after wandering out of the house, lose control of their bowels and bladder, or become bedridden (Brown 1991; Gruetzner 1992). The demands in caring for Alzheimer patients can become physically and emotionally overwhelming, particularly when the caregivers are elderly spouses in failing health or grown children who have many career and family pressures of their own. The stress these caregivers experience is likely to affect their own health. Research comparing Alzheimer caregivers with control subjects found that the caregivers had lower immune function and reported more days of illness over the course of about a year (Kiecolt-Glaser et al. 1991). Those caregivers who reported lower levels of social support and greater distress from the dementia-related behaviours showed the greatest impairments in immune function.

In the Alzheimer's case we saw earlier, Martha provided care for Alfred at home for a few years until his condition got too difficult for her to handle. On the urging of their son, she placed Alfred in a nursing home but felt 'defeated, inadequate and guilty' for doing so. Although she loved her husband and visited him almost every day, she eventually developed psychological problems that showed up in her increasingly dishevelled appearance and her asking why Alfred didn't deteriorate faster. What caused *her* problems? Because of the awful future she anticipated for her and Alfred,

Martha desperately wanted to stay away, but didn't want her husband to miss her. For her, Alfred had died years ago. Having to accept that death daily was too much for her to bear. If only he would deteriorate to the point that he could no longer communicate or think, she could visit less often without feeling guilty. Staying away would give her some respite. (McCahon 1991, p. 46)

Alzheimer's patients survive an average of four to eight years after diagnosis (Jorm & Henderson 1993). Their families often feel that watching the person deteriorate over several years is unbearable — like watching an endless funeral. The slow deterioration, severe dementia-related behaviour problems and knowledge that it will only end when the patient dies generally makes Alzheimer's disease more difficult for families to adapt to than the other chronic illnesses we considered.

Braithwaite (1990) reported a significant Australian study of the impact of Alzheimer's disease and other chronic conditions of the elderly on those whose task it was to provide these people with their day-to-day care. These were typically family members, often themselves among the older age groups. The physical burden of such care influenced both the health and quality of life of these caregivers, but the emotional burden was often as difficult to bear. Families were forced to watch those they loved succumb to the gradual progression of disability, dependence and loss of contact with reality.

We have examined in this chapter what it is like to live with each of a wide variety of chronic health problems. Some of these disorders begin earlier in the life span than others, some are more visible to people than are others, some involve more difficult treatments than others, and some are more painful, disabling or life-threatening than others. Each of these differences is important in determining patients' and their families' adaptation to the health problems and the psychosocial help they may need from professionals.

Psychosocial interventions for people with chronic conditions

Before people actually experience specific chronic illnesses in their families, they usually have some ideas about how serious the health problems are. How do they feel about an illness after someone in the family develops it? Is it worse than they expected, or not as bad, or about the same? The answers to these questions should have a bearing on how well the family adjusts to health problems. One study had parents whose children had either diabetes, asthma, epilepsy or no chronic illness rate how serious each of the three health problems would be if their children were to develop it or had it now (Marteau & Johnston 1986). The ratings revealed two interesting findings: (1) the lowest ratings of seriousness the parents gave were for the health problems their own children had, and (2) parents whose children did not have chronic illnesses rated each of the health problems as being very serious. These findings indicate that parents who live with chronic illnesses in their children tend to have less negative views of the health problems than parents whose children do not have those illnesses. People are frightened by the prospects of health problems, but most families adjust fairly well if a child develops a chronic illness (Cadman et al. 1991).

As we have seen, not all people adjust well to chronic health conditions. The types of adjustment problems that commonly develop with chronic conditions are outlined in figure 13.4. The adjustment problems patients and their families experience depend on many factors, such as how visible, painful, disabling or life-threatening the illness is. Another factor is the patient's age (O'Dougherty & Brown 1990). Victims of chronic illness in the early childhood years may become excessively dependent on their parents if the parents are overprotective, such as by not allowing an epileptic child to play in a wading pool with careful supervision. In the later childhood and adolescent years, chronically ill individuals may experience school failure because of absences and peer criticism or rejection because of the illness. These circumstances can impair the development of friendships, self-confidence and self-esteem. Adults who develop a chronic condition may have difficulties if their illness leads them to stop working or change jobs, alter their parenting role, or change or stop their sexual relations.

Figure 13.4 Types of adjustment problems in chronic illness

- *Physical* — being unable to cope with disability or pain
- *Vocational* — having difficulty revising educational and career plans or finding a new job
- *Self-concept* — being unable to accept one's changed body image, self-esteem, and level of achievement or competence

- *Social* — having difficulty with losing enjoyable activities or finding new ones and coping with changed relationships with family, friends and sexual partners
- *Emotional* — experiencing high levels of denial, anxiety or depression
- *Compliance* — failing to adhere to the rehabilitation treatment

---

Ideally, intervention programs to help individuals with chronic health problems involve interdisciplinary teams of professionals — doctors, nurses, psychologists, physical and occupational therapists, vocational counsellors and social workers — working in an integrated manner towards the overall goals of rehabilitation (Bleiberg, Ciulla & Katz 1991). Psychologists contribute to this process by helping each client cope with the psychosocial implications of his or her medical condition and using behavioural and cognitive principles to enhance the person's participation in and adherence to the therapeutic regimen. We'll consider many useful psychosocial intervention approaches, most of which can be used either with individuals or in groups.

Education and support services

The first thing chronically ill people and their families need to help them adapt to a health problem is correct *information* about the disease and its prognosis and treatment. Part of the problem Martha had dealing with Alfred's Alzheimer's disease is that she was led to believe that he would 'be a vegetable' in a matter of months. But Alfred's deterioration went on for years, as it does for most Alzheimer victims. She needed better information and might also have benefited from community services for Alzheimer families. For instance, many Australian communities have *respite centres* where Alzheimer patients can get occasional day care and temporary overnight care, giving the family a break from the caregiving burden (Braithwaite 1990).

Effective systems of social support also enhance patients' and their families' adaptation to chronic health problems (Wallston et al. 1983). People with chronic medical conditions usually receive this support from family or friends, but it can also come from *support groups* that offer patients and/or family members information and opportunities to meet with people in similar circumstances. For example, support groups for Alzheimer families help by providing information, giving sensitive emotional support, and sharing members' own experiences and ways of dealing with everyday problems and difficult decisions, such as whether to place the patient in a nursing home (Gruetzner 1992; Kapust & Weintraub 1984). Individuals with specific health problems can get information about the availability of support groups in their geographical areas through their doctors, local community service agencies or the national organisations for the particular illnesses they have. Local newspapers often print announcements of support group meetings.

Training and education programs to promote correct self-care procedures are very important in helping patients and their families adapt to the illness. These programs can be provided by professionals in medical settings or by trained laypersons, such as in support groups.

Psychosocial factors are often involved in patients' failing to adhere to their medical treatments for managing chronic conditions. In chapter 9 we discussed a variety of methods that can enhance adherence. Some of these methods involve improving the way practitioners present information about the procedures and the importance of following the treatment. Other approaches use *behavioural methods*, such as tailoring the treatment to make it as compatible as possible with the person's habits, using prompts and reminders, having patients keep records of their self-care activities, and providing a system of rewards through the method of behavioural contracting. Promoting adherence to diabetes treatments provides a good example, and various behavioural approaches can help improve compliance with different aspects of the treatment (Goodall & Halford 1991; Wing et al. 1986). One study, for instance, used self-monitoring and behavioural contracting methods in an eight-week program to improve treatment adherence in three non-compliant 16- to 18-year-old IDDM patients: Kathy, Tom and Kim (Schafer, Glasgow & McCaul 1982). Both Kathy and Tom showed substantial improvements in their adherence and glucose control. Kim's self-care did not improve, probably because she came from a family with severe marital and family problems, and therapy had failed to resolve their conflicts. Family problems can have an overriding negative influence and undermine efforts to improve compliance with medical recommendations.

Another example of using behavioural methods, such as relaxation and conditioning programs, to enhance people's compliance with medical treatments involves the physical rehabilitation process for individuals with spinal cord injuries. Studies have demonstrated that reinforcement techniques are highly effective in improving these patients' performance of therapeutically beneficial behaviours (Brucker 1983). These behaviours include:

- increasing daily fluid intake to prevent urinary tract infections
- changing one's sitting or lying position frequently to reduce the occurrence of bed sores
- using orthopaedic devices to improve limb functioning
- performing exercises to increase strength and endurance.

One successful approach, for instance, involves praising the client for each measurable improvement, such as in arm strength, and periodically updating the person's graph that charts these improvements.

Relaxation and biofeedback

We have seen that stress and anxiety can aggravate some chronic conditions, such as by decreasing diabetics' ability to metabolise glucose and by triggering or worsening asthma attacks. As a result, psychologists use stress management techniques — especially *progressive muscle relaxation*, *biofeedback* and *systematic desensitisation* — to help patients control these psychosocial factors (Parker 1995).

Psychosocial intervention for asthma provides a good example of how stress management techniques can help. In using biofeedback with asthmatics, an apparatus gives feedback regarding airflow in breathing so that the asthma patient can learn to control the diameter of the bronchial airways. The purpose is to enable asthmatics to increase airflow when an attack begins. Relaxation approaches are used to help people with asthma reduce the role of tension in either initiating an attack or making it worse, such as if a victim begins to panic. In using systematic desensitisation, psychologists have asthmatics imagine or listen to increasingly fearful descriptions of asthma attacks while applying progressive muscle relaxation techniques. Studies have generally found that these approaches are effective and provide useful supplements to medical treatments for asthma (Sarafino 1997a). Psychologists have also been involved in developing self-management programs for asthmatics that include a variety of behavioural and counselling techniques to improve compliance, enhance self-esteem and reduce stress (Bauman 1993; Cluss & Fireman 1985). These programs are also very helpful.

Stress management approaches are useful with other chronic conditions, too. For instance, relaxation training can help diabetic patients manage their stress and their blood glucose levels (Surwit, Feinglos & Scovern 1983; Wing et al. 1986). People with epilepsy can benefit from both relaxation and biofeedback training. In using relaxation, epileptics are taught to recognise sensations and events that are associated with attacks and to apply relaxation techniques when those situations occur. In using biofeedback, epileptics receive intensive EEG feedback training to control their electrical brain activity (Goldstein 1990; Kaplan & Wyler 1983; Sterman 1986). Although not all individuals benefit from this approach, many do. Which patients are likely to benefit? One of the main problems in using biofeedback to reduce seizures is that there is no good way yet to determine in advance who will benefit from this approach and who will not. This is an important issue because the procedure is costly. Epileptics who receive biofeedback therapy usually require many hours of one-to-one training with a psychologist or other highly trained individual, using expensive equipment and computer analyses.

Cognitive approaches

An 18-year-old girl who was diagnosed as being diabetic entered group psychotherapy because she was having difficulty coping with her condition. As it turned out, she believed incorrectly that she now could not attend university, that she 'would constantly look drunk and crazy', and that no-one would want to be near her (Roback 1984). In therapy, she got information contradicting this belief and came to see that she could pursue her life goals much as she had planned before learning of her condition. *Cognitive approaches* in psychosocial intervention are designed to analyse and change incorrect beliefs and help individuals learn and use effective coping strategies (Davison & Neale 1994).

Many patients and their families experience strong feelings of helplessness, hopelessness and depression. In the case of Alzheimer's disease, research has found that elderly caregivers are two to five times more likely to suffer severe levels of depression than other elders (Neundorfer 1991). Their depression is related to the degree of stress or burden they perceive in their caregiving role, such as from the patient's memory and behavioural problems. One cognitive approach that can help people overcome depressive feelings is *cognitive restructuring*, whereby individuals or groups of patients discuss incorrect, stressful thoughts and beliefs and replace them with more constructive or realistic ones. This approach is very helpful in treating depression (Sarafino 1996).

Insight therapy

Insight therapy is designed to help people gain an understanding of the roots of their feelings and problems (Davison & Neale 1994). This approach is especially useful in helping patients deal with their anxieties and changes in their self-concepts or relationships with family and friends (Bleiberg, Ciulla & Katz 1991). As an example, one hospitalised quadriplegic man who became difficult to deal with each night revealed in group therapy that

> he found nighttime very frightening, because at night he felt particularly vulnerable and helpless. As a result, he worried excessively about himself and his future. This led to his making constant requests of the staff, which kept him distracted and reduced his anxiety. In the group, other patients further along in the adjustment process expressed having experienced similar feelings. Through this group experience, the patient learned that his feelings of fright and powerlessness were not unusual. ... After hearing other members express concerns similar to his own and receiving helpful feedback, this patient reported feeling more able to confront his disability and to solve the problems created by it. (Eisenberg 1984, p. 115)

Insight therapy has also been used in helping chronically ill people deal with sexual difficulties and understand the thoughts, needs and problems their friends and family members face.

Family therapy

Family therapy typically has the family meet as a group and draws on cognitive, behavioural and insight-oriented methods to examine and change patterns of interaction among family members (Davison & Neale 1994; Kerns 1995; Patterson & Garwick 1994). A family with a chronically ill member might meet to review household and medical-treatment responsibilities, discuss grievances and plan ways to alter daily routines. If the patient is a child, they may discuss, for instance:

- jealousies siblings may feel if the patient seems to be getting more or special attention
- activities the chronically ill person can engage in successfully to build his or her feelings of competence and self-esteem
- how to tell friends and relatives about the illness so they will understand what it is, the limitations it imposes on the patient, and what to do if an episode occurs
- how and when the ill person could take responsibility for or improve self-care.

Parents and their ill children often do not communicate about sharing responsibilities for the patients' care (Anderson et al. 1990). As a result, each person incorrectly assumes someone else is taking care of a task.

Sometimes a patient's *recovery* can present family problems. For example, a husband whose wife's epilepsy was greatly improved with surgery 'felt secure when his wife with epilepsy was dependent on him' but became uncomfortable when she was able to function on her own and take advantage of new opportunities (DeAngelis 1990). Family therapy can help to uncover and resolve anxieties that develop when the family dynamics and modes of interaction change in either a positive or a negative direction.

In summary, psychosocial intervention can apply a wide variety of approaches to address many different adjustment problems that chronically ill people and their families face. In most cases, using more than one approach provides the optimal help these people need.

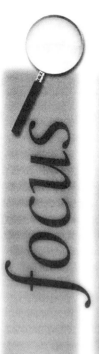

Focus on research
Cognitive/behavioural approaches in managing arthritis

Jerry Parker and his colleagues (1988) conducted a study to assess the effects of a program of cognitive and behavioural techniques in helping arthritis patients cope with their condition. The researchers randomly assigned 83 subjects from a Veterans Administration hospital to three groups. The *intervention* group received an intensive program of cognitive and behavioural techniques during a one-week stay at the hospital and subsequently met together periodically in support group sessions. The program consisted of training in pain redefinition and distraction techniques, awareness of pain behaviour, family dynamics and communication, and relaxation.

The two other groups received no psychosocial intervention. A *placebo* group received an intensive educational program of films and written materials on arthritis during a one-week stay, but no cognitive or behavioural methods were discussed. Because they also met subsequently in support groups, this group got as much time and attention as the intervention group did. The *control* group received the standard care for people with arthritis and were not asked to spend a week in the hospital or to attend support group meetings.

All subjects completed a wide variety of psychosocial measures and had their disease status evaluated by medical personnel at the start of the study and again after six and 12 months. At the last assessment, the intervention subjects were asked to rate the extent to which they continued to practise each of the techniques they were taught. Analysis of the data across the 12 months revealed three findings: First, the patients' disease status worsened, as one would expect for this disease. Second, the groups did not differ in their reports of pain and helplessness at six and 12 months. But third, those intervention subjects who reported a high degree of adherence to the cognitive/behavioural methods reported substantially less pain and helplessness than the placebo and control subjects. These results suggest that long-term *adherence* may be critical for chronically ill people to benefit from cognitive/behavioural interventions.

Summary

The initial reactions of individuals when diagnosed with chronic illnesses tend to follow three phases, beginning with shock, in which they are bewildered and behave in an automatic fashion. This phase is followed by an encounter reaction, characterised by feeling overwhelmed and helpless. The third phase involves a retreat reaction, in which people use avoidance coping strategies, such as denial, particularly if they believe they can do nothing to change the situation.

Crisis theory provides a model that describes how patients adjust to learning they have chronic health problems. According to this model, their adjustment depends on the coping processes they use, which, in turn, depend on illness-related, background and personal, and physical and social environmental factors. Patients begin the coping process with a cognitive appraisal of the meaning or significance of the health problem to their lives. This appraisal leads to their formulating adaptive tasks, such as adjusting to their symptoms or maintaining positive relations with family or friends, and applying various coping skills to deal with these tasks. These coping skills include denying or minimising the implications of their conditions, learning how to provide their own treatment, maintaining regular routines as well as possible, and discussing the future. Long-term adaptation to chronic health problems occurs when the patient and his or her family make adjustments that enhance the patient's quality of life by promoting effective physical, psychological and social functioning.

Some chronic conditions usually begin early in the life span, and asthma is one of them. Asthma is a respiratory disorder that produces periodic attacks in which the bronchial tubes become inflamed, constrict and develop spasms, resulting in extremely laboured breathing. Attacks are generally triggered by certain circumstances. For some asthmatics, the triggers are associated with allergies these individuals are known to have. Other asthma triggers include respiratory infections, weather conditions, air pollution and emotions, such as stress and anger. Although asthma is treated mainly with medication to prevent and combat attacks, exercise and stress management can also be useful.

Epilepsy is a disorder in which electrical disturbances in the brain produce seizures that vary in intensity. In grand mal attacks, the epileptic loses consciousness and exhibits muscle spasms. Sometimes specific neurological defects are identified as causing the disorder. Drugs provide the main form of treatment, but sometimes surgery and biofeedback are useful. Spinal cord injuries often occur in adolescence or early adulthood, are generally caused by accidents, and render the person paraplegic or quadriplegic. Intensive rehabilitation programs are geared towards helping these individuals regain as much physical function and independence as possible.

Other chronic health problems are more likely to begin in middle adulthood and old age than at other times in the life span. One of those chronic diseases is diabetes, in which the blood contains high levels of glucose. Some people with this disorder have insulin-dependent diabetes mellitus and must inject insulin daily to prevent very serious acute and long-term health complications. But the vast majority of diabetics have non-insulin-dependent diabetes mellitus, and most of them can use medication and diet to control their blood sugar.

Disorders that affect the joints and connective tissues are called rheumatic diseases. A class of rheumatic diseases that produces painful inflammation and stiffness of the joints is arthritis; the three most common types are osteoarthritis, rheumatoid arthritis and gout. Although each type can lead to disability, rheumatoid arthritis is usually the most crippling and painful of the three. Treatment is mainly through drugs, but also includes maintaining proper body weight and physical therapy.

Alzheimer's disease involves a progressive deterioration of the person's cognitive functions, beginning with attention and memory. Since there is no effective treatment for this disorder, therapy focuses on maximising the patient's functioning and helping the family cope.

Many chronically ill people and their families have difficulty adjusting to the health problem and its medical treatment. They can be helped with psychosocial intervention methods that involve education and support services, relaxation and biofeedback, cognitive approaches, insight therapy and family therapy.

Key terms

adaptation	asthma	insulin-dependent diabetes mellitus	quality of life
Alzheimer's disease	crisis theory		spinal cord injury
arthritis	epilepsy	non-insulin-dependent diabetes mellitus	

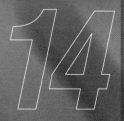

14 Heart disease, stroke, cancer and AIDS: causes, management and coping

Prologue

On most Saturday mornings during the winter months Ron played an impromptu social game of Australian Rules football with his mates. He was 45 years old and he thought he was invincible. After the game it was customary to sit in the tin shed by the side of the oval they called a club-house and have a beer and a cigarette. Of course, this was not the only time Ron indulged in a beer and a cigarette. He worked hard as a building site supervisor and smoked about 20 cigarettes a day; he also had several drinks after work each day and more on the weekends. This did not worry Ron. He was overweight, but not enormously so, and thought that his much-enjoyed Saturday episodes of football exertion indicated that he was very fit for his age. Ron had not had a medical checkup for some years. He considered himself to be a good provider for his family and would not have owned to a worry in the world. Three weeks ago, however, he was forced to admit to a worry, and a significant one at that. Just a few minutes into the football game, having just run the length of the field, he began to gasp for breath, he felt a vague nausea and he experienced a severe, oppressive pain in the left side of his chest. Ron was taken to the local hospital in a friend's car and, after several hours in the casualty department, he was admitted to the coronary care unit. He was discharged the next day with the good news — he had not suffered a heart attack. But the bad news was that he most probably was suffering from angina pectoris. He was scheduled for a complete cardiological examination, and that included another stint in hospital so that a coronary angiogram could be performed. This procedure was duly undertaken and Ron was informed by a rather sombre cardiologist that he was suffering from significant coronary artery disease and that his coronary circulation was compromised to the extent that he was at serious risk of myocardial infarction. He was advised that immediate coronary artery bypass graft surgery was indicated and that he could be admitted to hospital in two days' time for that surgery. Ron now sat in the hospital waiting area for his wife to collect him. He had to tell her of the outcome of his investigations and of the recommendations given to him by his cardiologist. He had to face the sudden realisation that his life was about to change in significant and perhaps frightening ways.

The death *rate* for heart disease has declined by more than half since 1960, but it is still the number one killer by far in Australia. Cancer is second. People know these are the leading causes of death — and for many patients and their families, being diagnosed with one of these diseases *means* death. AIDS also emerged in the 1980s as a killer, and public attention has focused on how it is spread, the large numbers of people infected with the virus, and the sharply increasing numbers of AIDS victims who die each year around the world. These high-mortality illnesses and others are the focus of this chapter.

Although many people react to having high-mortality chronic illnesses in positive and constructive ways, not all do. In this chapter we will examine how patients and their families react to and cope with health problems that have a high likelihood of taking their lives. We will also see the psychosocial adjustments these people make when the illnesses are terminal. As we study these difficult circumstances, we will consider many important issues and try to provide answers to questions you may have. What is it like to live with heart disease, stroke, cancer or AIDS? How do these illnesses affect the patient's functioning, and what treatments do they entail? What special problems exist when the victim is a child? What can be done to help terminally ill people and their loved ones cope?

Coping with and adapting to high-mortality illness

Many healthy individuals who want to estimate how much longer they are likely to live look up the statistical life expectancy for people their age and gender and probably adjust that figure on the basis of the longevity of other people in their families. But estimates of a person's life expectancy are very imprecise, and this is true even for people with health conditions that seriously threaten their lives. Public opinion aside, having a high-mortality disease — even cancer or AIDS — does not usually mean a person will die in a matter of a few weeks or months. Many cancer patients, for instance, survive for 10 or 20 years before the disease takes their lives, and some are totally cured. Still, no-one can tell for sure what the course of the disease will be, and these individuals and their families must adapt to this uncertainty.

Adapting while the prospects seem good

Since none of us knows for sure what lies ahead for us, we all live with some degree of uncertainty. But for patients with high-mortality illnesses, the uncertainty for them and their families is more real and urgent. Even though they may have good prospects for the future, either in the short run or more permanently, the diagnosis changes them.

Mortality is the main issue of concern to patients in the first few months of convalescence with a serious life-threatening illness. During this time, patients often show optimistic attitudes, hope they will be cured but begin to view their plans for the future more tentatively (Moos 1982; Weisman 1979). They also tend to switch from using mainly avoidance coping strategies to using active problem-focused approaches. As a patient's recovery progresses, he or she is able to return more and more to a regular routine, often gaining great satisfaction by once again being able to do simple household or self-help activities. Although convalescing individuals tend to be optimistic about their health, they are very watchful for symptoms and changes in their condition.

Having activities to occupy the day is important to convalescing people, particularly those with chronic high-mortality health problems. These activities give them some respite from thinking about their condition. Patients often try to isolate the disease from the rest of their lives by focusing on other things, such as preparing to do projects around the house or to return to work. Sometimes these plans and preparations can lead to problems, however, if patients overestimate what they can do. For example, a patient named Clay, who had suffered a serious stroke, described how he started making plans the day he left the hospital.

> That was a glorious day. I started planning all the things I could do with the incredible amount of free time I was going to have. Chores I put off, museums and galleries to visit, friends I had wanted to meet for lunch. It was not until several days later that I realized I simply couldn't do them. I didn't have the mental or physical strength, and I sank into depression. (Dahlberg 1977, p. 124)

Patients need to be encouraged to develop reasonable plans and to carry them out, especially with regard to going back to work or getting training to enter a new job, if necessary. Patients' efforts to isolate their diseases from the rest of their lives are likely to be even more effective when they finally resume most of their normal life activities.

Sometimes the helplessness that chronically ill people feel and the nurturing of their families lead to a cycle of continued dependence that persists when the patients are able to begin doing things for themselves. This was starting to happen with Clay after his stroke, and his wife realised it. As she described the situation:

> As time went on and he was gradually improving, I occasionally was concerned about his dependency on me, which seemed unnecessary. ... It can easily become a habit after the need no longer exists. Gradually, I started asking him to do certain things, leaving things

undone which were previously his domain, acting indecisively, and leaving decisions up to him. At first he was surprised, and then did what was needed. He gradually took over more and more, giving up his 'stroke personality.' (Dahlberg 1977, p. 128)

Gentle nudges by family members, like those from Clay's wife, can help patients become more self-sufficient, thereby making them feel useful and enhancing their self-esteem.

In the process of adapting to high-mortality illnesses over a long period of time, people make many important cognitive adjustments. By interviewing women who had had surgery for breast cancer a few years earlier, researchers found that these adjustments centre on three themes (Taylor 1983; Taylor, Lichtman & Wood 1984). First, seriously ill people often try to *find meaning* in their illness experiences, either by determining why the illnesses happened or by rethinking their attitudes and priorities. One woman said, for instance,

> I have much more enjoyment each day, each moment. I am not so worried about what is or isn't or what I wish I had. All those things you get entangled with don't seem to be part of my life right now. (Taylor 1983, p. 1163)

Second, many patients try to *gain a sense of control* over their illnesses, such as by engaging in activities that reduce the risk of their condition getting worse or increase their knowledge about their care. A man said of his wife:

> She got books, she got pamphlets, she studied, she talked to cancer patients, she found out everything that was happening to her, and she fought it. She went to war with it. She calls it taking in her covered wagons and surrounding it. (1983, p. 1164)

Third, they try to *restore their self-esteem*, often by comparing themselves with less fortunate people. In one example, a woman said:

> If I hadn't been married, I think this thing would have really gotten to me. I can't imagine dating or whatever knowing you have this thing and not knowing how to tell the man about it. (1983, p. 1166)

These cognitive adjustments seem to promote adaptation and probably help patients achieve or, in some cases, exceed their previous levels of psychosocial functioning.

Adapting in a recurrence or relapse

One thing that makes high-mortality diseases so dangerous is that the deadly medical conditions they produce have high rates of recurrence or relapse. Among stroke victims, for instance, 30 to 40 per cent develop another stroke within five years (Flinn, Dalsing & White 1986). The same may be said for coronary heart disease. Although mortality (death) rates from coronary heart disease have declined in Australia in the past two decades (AIHW 1999b), rates of recurrence among those who survive a myocardial infarction (or heart attack) are significantly higher than the population rate for primary heart attack. Patients correctly recognise their heightened vulnerability and worry about it, and so do their families.

A recurrence of the condition, or relapse, presents another crisis for patients and their families, which may be harder to cope with than the first (Moos 1982; Weisman

1979). They rightly perceive this event as a bad sign — it typically indicates that the prognosis is now worse than before, since additional damage has occurred. Patients focus again on the illness, being concerned about controlling its progression and forestalling a deterioration in their general functioning and quality of life. They undergo a new round of hospitalisation, medical procedures and, perhaps, surgery. In coping with setbacks in their condition, patients and their families go through the kinds of coping processes they experienced in the initial phases of their reaction to the original diagnosis. But they are likely to be less hopeful than they were before.

Living with any high-mortality disease can be stressful, but each disease creates a pattern of stresses that is unique. We turn now to considering how people adapt to living with specific high-mortality health problems, starting with heart disease.

Heart disease

Coronary heart disease refers to illnesses that result from the narrowing and blocking of the coronary arteries, which enmesh the heart and supply it with oxygen-rich blood. As we saw in chapter 2, blood vessels become narrowed as plaques build up in the condition called *atherosclerosis*. Blockage can occur if a clot of blood platelets develops and gets lodged in an artery, preventing blood flow.

If this blockage, technically called *occlusion*, is marked but incomplete, a build-up of certain chemicals in the heart muscle (the *myocardium*) resulting from oxygen deprivation to the muscle cells causes a condition called **angina pectoris**. This is the pain that Ron (in the introductory anecdote) experienced, although it can occur not just in the chest but also in the left arm and the jaw. It signals that the heart is being forced to work harder than its oxygen supply can sustain. If the occlusion is complete, however, muscle cells in the myocardium die within minutes of oxygen deprivation and the resulting condition is called **myocardial infarction** or 'heart attack'. This may result not just in severe chest pain but in other symptoms including nausea, sweating and loss of consciousness (these symptoms are listed in figure 14.1). Myocardial infarction is a very serious and potentially life-threatening condition.

The Australian Institute of Health and Welfare (1999) reported that in 1997 41 per cent of all deaths in Australia (52 641 people) were from cardiovascular disease, of which myocardial infarction accounted for a significant proportion. Every day of 1997 about 80 Australians died from coronary heart disease. Cardiovascular disease is quite clearly the single biggest killer of the Australian population. Regrettably, indigenous Australians have twice the death rate from cardiovascular disease as do white Australians. While this is a bleak picture, it must be remembered that cardiovascular disease is largely preventable by the adoption of sensible health behaviours. It is estimated (AIHW 1999c) that more than 80 per cent of the Australian population has at least one of the traditional risk factors for coronary heart disease (cigarette smoking, hypertension, obesity or a sedentary lifestyle). The application of even simple strategies of psychological intervention to these problems can achieve significant reductions in risk and contribute to the prevention of coronary heart disease.

The prognosis for a patient after a myocardial infarction depends on several factors, especially the extent of arterial damage and the condition of the heart's left ventricle (Langosch 1984). If the ventricle is functioning well, the survival rates after 10 years are 97 per cent when the damage involves one coronary blood vessel, 79 per cent when it involves two vessels, and 66 per cent for three vessels. But if ventricular functioning is impaired, these survival rates drop to 85 per cent, 58 per cent, and 40 per cent, respectively.

Who is at risk of heart disease, and why?

Several demographic, lifestyle and physiological characteristics are associated with developing heart disease.

Age, gender and sociocultural risk factors

The prevalence rates for heart disease increase as people get older, particularly after about 45 years of age. In the years prior to old age, far more men than women develop and die from heart disease (AIHW 1999c). However, although women are less likely than men to have heart attacks, they are more likely to die from them if they have them. As we mentioned earlier, indigenous Australians are considerably more likely to suffer a heart attack than are white Australians. The Australian Institute of Health and Welfare suggests that this difference is even more acute when indigenous Australians aged 25 to 64 are considered, among whom death rates from cardiovascular disease are seven times greater than for similar-aged Australian men and nine times greater than for similar-aged Australian women. The primary cause for this alarming imbalance, according to the National Heart Foundation, lies with differences in levels of basic risk factors. Indigenous Australians are far more likely than white Australians to smoke cigarettes, be obese and suffer from diabetes, and less likely to engage in leisure-time physical activity such as sport and exercise (AIHW 1999c).

Figure 14.1 Symptoms of a heart attack

Many victims delay going to hospital for hours because they don't know the symptoms of a heart attack. These are:
- uncomfortable pressure, fullness, squeezing or pain in the centre of the chest that lasts for more than a few minutes
- pain spreading to the shoulders, neck or arms

- chest discomfort with lightheadedness, fainting, sweating, nausea or shortness of breath.

Not all of these symptoms always happen in a heart attack — if some start to occur, the person should get medical care immediately. Prompt treatment can often prevent serious myocardial damage.

Source: AHA (1994, p. 18).

Lifestyle and biological risk factors

Part of the reason for age, sex and sociocultural differences in risk of heart disease lies in biological and lifestyle variations. For example, *hypertension* — the condition of having high blood pressure consistently over an extended period of time — is a major risk factor for heart disease (AIHW 1999c). In 1995 some 17 per cent of Australians were estimated to suffer from hypertension (AIHW 1999c). High blood pressure has no overt symptoms, but its presence indicates that the heart is working harder than normal. When this continues over a long period of time, the heart becomes *enlarged*. The more enlarged the heart becomes, the more difficulty it has meeting the demands of the body. High blood pressure also increases the development of atherosclerosis, causing blood vessels to become narrowed and less elastic. This increases the risk that a blood clot may become lodged in an artery and cause a myocardial infarction. Prevalence rates for hypertension increase with age and are higher in some indigenous Australian communities than they are for white Australians generally (AIHW 1999c).

Several other lifestyle and biological risk factors are important in heart disease. They include:

- family history of heart disease
- cigarette smoking
- high blood pressure
- high LDL and total cholesterol levels
- physical inactivity
- diabetes
- obesity
- stress.

People who stop smoking and reduce their cholesterol intake and blood pressure have half the risk of dying of heart disease (Jousilahti et al. 1995). In chapter 4 we saw that *stress* plays an important role in the development of heart disease, particularly through its connection to the Type A behaviour pattern and hypertension. Chronic stress, anger and hostility appear to contribute to people's high blood pressure (Byrne 2000).

Type A behaviour and heart disease

People who exhibit the Type A behaviour pattern tend to be highly hostile, competitive and impatient (Byrne 1996). When in stressful situations, Type A individuals — particularly those who experience frequent high levels of anger and hostility — often show high physiological *reactivity*, which includes increased blood pressure, catecholamine and corticosteroid levels (Smith 1992). Heart disease is associated with chronically high levels of hostility and of physiological reactivity.

Type A individuals chronically produce high levels of catecholamines and corticosteroids, especially when under stress (Pope & Smith 1991; Suarez et al. 1991). Chronic high levels of these hormones in the blood can damage the heart and blood vessels. Evidence now suggests that adrenalin (a catecholamine) increases the formation of platelet clots in the blood, which can block arteries and cause a heart attack (Markovitz & Matthews 1991). Although myocardial infarctions can happen at any time in any 24-hour day, they are most likely to occur on Mondays, at least for working people, and in the morning hours from 6 to 11 A.M., and least likely to occur during sleep at night (Muller et al. 1987; Somers et al. 1993; Willich et al. 1994). The increased risk in the morning hours probably occurs because dreaming shortly before waking and becoming active after waking increase blood pressure and catecholamines, which increase platelet clotting.

Medical treatment and rehabilitation of cardiac patients

Heart attack treatment follows a sequence from emergency care to a program of rehabilitation.

Initial treatment for heart attack

When heart attack victims enter the hospital, they receive emergency medical treatment to prevent or limit damage to the myocardium. Part of this treatment generally involves using *clot-dissolving medication* to free blocked arteries. Most patients are then placed in *coronary care units*, where medical staff can monitor their physiological functioning closely. The risk of another attack is high during the first few days. Medical assessments indicate whether certain other procedures are also needed. One procedure is called *balloon angioplasty*, in which a tiny balloon is inserted into the blocked artery and inflated to open the blood vessel. Another procedure, called *bypass surgery*, entails replacing the diseased section of artery with a healthy vessel taken from another part of the person's body.

As you might expect, most cardiac patients experience extremely high levels of anxiety in the first day or two of coronary care. Many of these people cope with this crisis through *denial*, and those who use denial tend to be less anxious in the first few days than those who do not (Byrne 1987). Regardless of whether cardiac patients use denial, their anxiety levels soon start to decline. After about the fourth day or so, the anxiety levels of those who do and do not use denial are about the same, but still higher than normal. These fairly high anxiety levels tend to persist for the remainder of their hospital stay (Byrne 1987). The cardiac patients who have the greatest difficulty coping are not necessarily the ones who are the most seriously ill — instead, they tend to be those who were experiencing distress and social problems before the heart attack.

Excessive anxiety, depression or denial can impair patients' recovery, and psychological intervention may be needed (Erdman 1990). For example, some patients may deny they had a heart attack and insist on leaving the hospital too early. Many patients anticipate psychosocial problems ahead, particularly in relation to their work. A program for rehabilitation generally begins after the first week, when heart attack patients are transferred to a general ward.

Rehabilitation of cardiac patients

Rehabilitation programs for heart attack patients are designed to promote recovery and reduce risk factors for having another attack (Erdman 1990). These programs provide patients with information on such topics as lifestyle changes and restrictions they should follow, medications to take and symptoms to expect. Many patients will experience recurrent angina pectoris episodes for many months or even years after discharge (Langosch 1984; Lavey & Winkle 1979). These episodes can be very frightening to them and their families. Sometimes the chest pain requires medical attention, but the patients do not seem to suffer tissue damage, and they often can simply take medication to control it. For some patients, the pain can be quite severe and even disabling (Lavey & Winkle 1979; Wielgosz et al. 1984). Medical tests often reveal no physical basis for the pain — that is, there is no substantial artery blockage or ventricle impairment — but the pain persists (Ketterer et al. 1996).

To reduce the likelihood of another infarction, most cardiac patients receive advice on lifestyle changes, such as to:
• quit smoking
• lose weight
• exercise
• reduce dietary fat and cholesterol
• reduce alcohol consumption.
It is clear from this list that these risk factors are essentially discretionary human behaviours; that is, they are behaviours acquired according to the same psychological rules and principles that govern the acquisition of the rich and complex entirety of human behaviours. As such, they are readily amenable to modification using a broad variety of psychological strategies that are well known to clinical and health psychologists (Byrne 1987). The notion that the recurrence of myocardial infarction is largely preventable is, therefore, quite central to the practice of clinical health psychology.

Because stress and hostility are linked to heart disease, these patients often receive training in stress management, too (Langosch 1984). Many heart attack victims who make healthy changes in their lifestyles and attitudes live longer than comparable people who have not had infarctions.

Some cardiac patients find it easy to adhere to their rehabilitation programs — but others do not, and may resent the restrictions their condition imposes. One person said of his doctor's advice:

> If he tells you that you cannot walk upstairs, he is telling you that you are weak, that you are no longer strong. He has taken something away from you — ah, your pride. You suddenly want to do what you are not supposed to do, what you have been doing all your life. . . . (Tagliacozzo & Mauksch 1972, p. 178)

Coronary patients with low self-efficacy for carrying out their medical treatments and who perceive little social support in their lives show less adherence to their treatments and slower recovery than those who have high levels of social support (Bastone & Kerns 1995; Fontana et al. 1989; Friis & Taff 1986).

Exercise is a very important aspect of rehabilitation programs for cardiac patients. A program of physical activity needs to be introduced gradually and tailored to each person's physical condition. It often begins in the hospital with supervised short-distance walking. In the following weeks the physical activities become more and more vigorous and long-lasting, and are likely to include long-distance walking, calisthenics, and often jogging, bicycling or swimming. Adhering to their exercise programs produces substantial physical and psychosocial benefits to these patients (Roviaro, Holmes & Holmsten 1984; Thompson & Thompson 1987). Patients who follow an exercise program show much greater improvements in a variety of physiological measures than do those who do not adhere to one — for example, they show lower resting heart rates, lower diastolic blood pressure while at rest, lower systolic blood pressure during exercise and greater treadmill endurance. Research has also shown that exercise reduces cardiac victims' risks of dying of a subsequent heart attack (O'Connor et al. 1989).

People with heart disease who adhere to their exercise programs show better psychosocial adjustment, too, as reflected in their self-concept, perceived health, sexual activity, and involvement in and enjoyment of active leisure activities. Unfortunately, about 50 per cent of cardiac patients who begin exercise programs discontinue them within the first six months (Dishman 1982; Dishman, Sallis & Orenstein 1985). People who drop out of exercise programs are likely to be those who smoke cigarettes, work in blue-collar occupations, and begin the programs with poorer cardiovascular function, higher body weight, more sedentary lifestyles, and greater anxiety and depression (Blumenthal et al. 1982; Dishman 1981; Oldridge & Spencer 1985). Compliance is likely to be higher if the rehabilitation program provides a special place, like a wellness centre, for the patients to do their exercising, instead of having them exercise on their own.

Cardiac patients may also have a difficult time making other lifestyle changes, particularly in their diets and in stopping smoking. Dietary changes to reduce fat and cholesterol are often hard to make because they have an impact on family life (Croog 1983). With respect to stopping smoking, studies have found that only perhaps 30 to 40 per cent of individuals who suffer myocardial infarctions quit or substantially reduce their smoking (Ockene et al. 1985; Rigotti et al. 1991), although this is not much different from cessation rates to be found in the general (non-cardiac) population (Byrne & Whyte 1987). Those who continue to smoke are in many ways like those who do not exercise. That is, compared to patients who quit, those who do not quit tend to be more anxious and from lower occupational and educational groups. Those who continue to smoke also tend to smoke heavily and have fewer negative attitudes about smoking.

The psychosocial impact of heart disease

'Is it okay for me to drive a car, do jobs around the house or lift heavy things?' heart attack patients often ask their doctors, fearing that overexertion could bring on new attacks (Erdman 1990). The extent of patients' disability is likely to affect how well they and their families adjust to their condition.

Being able to work has a special meaning to individuals who suffer from chronic health problems. People who have suffered heart attacks, for instance, often view returning to work as an important sign that they are recovering (Byrne 1987). A doctor's advice about returning to work depends on how severe the heart damage is. If the condition is not very severe, doctors have generally recommended that individuals return to work after about 60 days. But research has found that these patients can resume working about two weeks earlier without increasing their risk of another cardiac episode (Dennis et al. 1988). Doctors often advise people with heart disease to cut back on the amount of physical effort and stress they experience on the job. Following this advice may mean finding a new job, which may be difficult to do, particularly for people over age 50 or so. Patients who are near retirement age may simply leave the work force if they can. Nevertheless, most cardiac patients do go back to work, often with jobs that require less productivity or shorter hours than they previously had worked. A large study of return to work among Australian survivors of a first heart attack found that just over 70 per cent had returned to some kind of work, typically their old jobs, within three months of the attack. Less than 10 per cent took six months or longer (Byrne, Whyte & Butler 1981). Interestingly, there was no apparent relationship between return to work and the degree of physical effort involved in the job. Compared with individuals who do not return to work, those who do return tend to be younger, in better physical condition, better educated and employed in white-collar jobs. Delaying or failing to go back to work is often associated with having long-lasting emotional distress and depression (Byrne 1987).

Sometimes cardiac patients' work restrictions cause them to experience interpersonal problems with co-workers and heightened work stress. Sociologist Sydney Croog has described the case of a man who returned to his clerical job after a heart attack, but occasionally felt mild chest pain and shortness of breath. At first his co-workers were sympathetic and complied with his requests to lift heavy boxes for him. But after a while they started to resent these chores, as shown in this man's experience when asking

> a fellow worker to lift a box for him. The response comes, 'Why don't you go ahead and drop dead, you lazy son-of-a-bitch!'
>
> The solutions are limited for this 55-year-old man. Transferring to another department is not possible, as the company is a small one. Leaving for another job is not possible for many reasons. . . . So picking up the heavy boxes seems like the easiest solution — but for how long can he continue? What will be the eventual effects on his heart? (1983, pp. 300–301)

Going back to work usually contributes to the long-term wellbeing of a cardiac victim. But as this example illustrates, the work situation can also create problems that may impair the person's physical and psychosocial condition.

Cardiac illness and family relationships are closely interrelated. Studies have found that cardiac patients with strong social support recover faster and survive longer than those with less support (Berkman 1995; Reifman 1995). For many heart patients, family difficulties — such as quarrelling over financial or sexual problems — existed prior to the infarction, and these difficulties often become worse following heart attack (Croog & Fitzgerald 1978; Swan, Carmelli & Rosenman 1986). The illness adds to the original difficulties, such as by making the financial and sexual problems worse. What also seems to happen in these families is that a 'cycle of guilt and blame' tends to develop (Croog 1983). For example, a husband who suffers a myocardial infarction may blame his wife or children for his condition, and they may agree and feel guilty. But even when harmonious relations exist before the attack, the illness adds to the stress of all members of the family. One marital difficulty that may arise after a heart attack relates to sexual activity, which often never returns to the level that existed prior to the attack (Krantz & Deckel 1983; Michela 1987). Either or both spouses may fear that having sex could precipitate another attack, even though this risk is very low, especially if the patient exercises regularly (Muller et al. 1996). The marital satisfaction of both partners generally benefits by having little or no sex initially and then increasing its frequency gradually, with the advice of the patient's doctor (Michela 1987).

Families have an enormous impact on the process of cardiac rehabilitation: Patients adjust better, adhere more closely to their regimens and recover sooner if their efforts receive family encouragement (Kaplan & Toshima 1990; Krantz & Deckel 1983). But the danger exists that families will promote *cardiac invalidism*, in which people with heart disease become increasingly dependent and helpless. Research has shown that the beliefs a spouse has about the patient's physical capabilities can aid or retard rehabilitation. A study of this process examined the beliefs that wives held about their husbands' physical abilities several weeks after these men had suffered myocardial infarctions (Taylor et al., cited in Bandura 1986). Each wife evaluated her husband's cardiac and physical ability before and after one of three conditions: She either *observed* him perform vigorously on a treadmill, *participated* on the treadmill herself after watching him perform or was *uninvolved* in the treadmill situation. Analysis of the wives' evaluations revealed that the beliefs of the wives who were uninvolved in the treadmill situation or had simply observed their husbands' performance did not change — these wives continued to give low assessments of their husbands' physical abilities, even after receiving medical counselling to the contrary. In contrast, the wives who participated on the treadmill after watching their husbands perform raised their evaluations of their husbands' physical abilities. These results suggest that family members need to see and personally experience the physical feats the cardiac patient can perform. By doing so and receiving medical counselling, they can provide more effective encouragement for the person to become increasingly active.

What are the long-term emotional consequences of heart disease on people with heart conditions? Most cardiac patients experience higher than normal levels of anxiety and depression during the first weeks or months after their heart attacks, but their distress tends to decline during the next year or two (Carney et al. 1995; Byrne 1987). Most eventually adjust fairly well, especially if they have high levels of social support (Holahan et al. 1995). But if very high levels of anxiety and depression continue beyond a few months, these emotions become signs of poor adaptation and tend to be linked to decreased compliance with the cardiac regimen and deterioration in the person's physical condition. Coronary patients with severe anxiety or depression are much more likely to suffer subsequent cardiac problems such as arrhythmias or to die in the next several months than those who are less distressed (Carney et al. 1988; Frasure-Smith, Lespérance & Talajic 1993, 1995; Moser & Dracup 1996).

Psychosocial interventions for heart disease

Several types of interventions can enhance people's recovery from and long-term adaptation to having heart disease. Self-help and support groups, such as heart clubs, give coronary patients the opportunity to discuss and get advice about specific problems and stressors they face in their daily lives (Croog 1983). These groups provide helpful information and encourage cardiac victims to become active.

Interventions using technological devices can also benefit people's adjustment to their heart conditions. For instance, researchers equipped cardiac patients with electrocardiogram (ECG, or 'EKG') monitors that could transmit analyses of their heart function to a hospital nurse by telephone (Follick et al. 1988). The subjects called the nurse and transmitted the ECG analyses on a periodic schedule and whenever they felt certain symptoms. If an analysis indicated medical action was needed, the nurse dispatched a rescue squad and instructed the patient to take a drug. Compared with subjects who received the standard cardiac care, those with the ECG system were far less depressed during the next several months.

Can psychosocial interventions improve compliance with cardiac regimens? A study by Judith Ockene and her colleagues (1992) provided a cognitive/behavioural program to help coronary patients stop smoking. The program used manuals, tape recordings, and in-person and telephone counselling methods. A control group received only advice that they should quit. The program was effective in stopping people's smoking over the next 12 months, but only among those whose disease was relatively severe. The program did not affect the smoking of those individuals whose coronary damage was less severe, perhaps because they did not feel strongly threatened.

Other types of interventions involve *stress management* techniques. One Australian intervention program provided cardiac victims with information about their condition and treatment, training in relaxation to reduce stress, and counselling for their fears and anxieties while they were still in the hospital (Oldenburg, Perkins & Andrews 1985). Individuals who received this intervention showed far better psychosocial adjustment during the next year than those who received standard care. Another intervention found that stress management reduced the daily number of angina pectoris attacks by nearly 40 per cent compared with attacks of clients who received standard medical care (Bundy et al. 1994). Researchers have also used stress management techniques to modify patients' Type A behaviour and lower blood pressure. As we saw in chapter 5, these approaches can effectively reduce coronary risk (Friedman et al. 1986; Powell et al. 1984). Because of these benefits, training to help patients anticipate and manage stressful situations is an increasingly recommended component in cardiac rehabilitation programs (Langosch 1984).

Dean Ornish and his colleagues (1990) developed and tested a multicomponent intervention program of dietary, exercise and stress management approaches for cardiac rehabilitation. The patients who volunteered to participate were randomly assigned to receive either the program or standard medical care. The program had the people eat a mainly vegetarian diet, eliminate caffeine and restrict alcohol consumption, stop smoking, get moderate exercise regularly, meet regularly as support groups, and use stress management techniques, including relaxation and meditation. Medical assessments were made at the start of the study and at the end of a year. Comparisons of the two groups showed that the atherosclerosis and reports of chest pain worsened for the subjects who received standard medical care but improved for those in the intervention program. Although the results don't indicate which features of the program worked, they show that changes in lifestyle can unclog arteries. Other studies have not only confirmed these findings but found that intensive reduction of lifestyle risk factors reduces subsequent cardiac problems and hospitalisations (Gould et al. 1995; Haskell et al. 1994; Superko & Krauss 1994).

To summarise, recovery after a heart attack presents difficult physical and psychosocial challenges for patients and their families. Cardiac rehabilitation programs require individuals to adhere to programs of exercise, diet control, medication and stress management. These programs can reverse the disease process. The long-term impact of heart disease often involves emotional, vocational and marital problems that may require therapeutic interventions to enhance adaptation.

Stroke

Sitting at the breakfast table, Neil began to feel faint and weak, his vision dimmed, and the right side of his body became numb and tingly. As he realised he was having a stroke, he tried to say so, but the words would not come out. Soon he lost consciousness. As figure 14.2 shows, these are common symptoms of a **stroke** — a condition in which damage occurs in some area of the brain when the blood supply to that area is disrupted, depriving it of oxygen. According to the Australian Institute of Health and Welfare (1999), stroke accounted for around 9 per cent of all deaths in Australia in 1997. About 40 000 Australians each year will suffer a stroke, and about 25 per cent of these will die from the effects of the stroke within a month of the event. Moreover, stroke accounts for around 25 per cent of chronic disability in this country.

Causes, effects and rehabilitation of stroke

The disruption in blood supply that causes strokes occurs in two ways. In some cases, damage results from an *infarction* when the blood supply in a cerebral artery is sharply reduced or cut off, either when a blood clot (a *thrombus*) forms or a piece of plaque (an *embolus*) becomes lodged in that area of the artery. In other cases, damage results from a *haemorrhage*, in which a blood vessel ruptures and bleeds into the brain. A stroke caused by a haemorrhage generally occurs rapidly and causes the person to lose consciousness; most of the damage it produces happens in a few minutes. In contrast, a stroke caused by an infarction tends to occur more slowly, and the person is less likely to lose consciousness. Strokes from haemorrhages occur much less frequently but are much more likely to cause extensive damage and death than those from infarctions (Glick & Cerullo 1986).

Figure 14.2 Symptoms of stroke

Individuals who experience any of the following warning signs of a stroke should see a doctor immediately.	
• Sudden weakness or numbness of the face, arm or leg (typically on one side of the body)	• Loss of speech, or trouble talking or understanding speech
• Sudden dimness or loss of vision (usually in only one eye)	• Sudden, unexplained, severe headache
	• Unexplained dizziness, unsteadiness or sudden fall, especially if this occurs with any of the above symptoms.

Source: AHA (1994, p. 23).

Age, gender and sociocultural risk factors for stroke

The incidence of stroke is very low prior to the middle-age years and increases sharply after 55 years of age, doubling in each successive decade (AIHW 1999c). Rates of stroke in Australia are influenced by both age and sex. Clearly, older people are more likely to suffer a stroke than are younger people; around 50 per cent of all strokes are suffered by those 75 years of age and older (AIHW 1999c). Nonetheless, strokes do occur in younger people and cause significant disability. In younger age groups, strokes also bring about a considerable burden to the family through both economic and social loss. Stroke among younger people may be linked to a greater prevalence in several of the major risk factors (hypertension, cigarette smoking and obesity for example) than was the case in the past.

Stroke appears to be more common in women than in men, but the Australian Institute of Health and Welfare (1999c) suggests that this may be explained simply by the presence of a larger number of elderly women in the Australian population. Proportionately, rates of stroke are 30 per cent higher for men than they are for women.

While stroke is distributed across the whole of the Australian population, it is more likely to be seen among some groups than others. Australians who were born in Europe seem more prone to stroke than those born in Australia. Death from stroke is more likely among those from lower than from higher socioeconomic groups. Indigenous Australians suffer far higher rates of stroke than white Australians; stroke mortality is 1.7 times higher for indigenous Australian females than it is for white Australian females, and three times higher for indigenous Australian males than for white Australian males. Among younger age groups, this difference is even more alarming: indigenous Australians aged 25 to 64 years are eight times more likely to die from a stroke than are white Australians in the same age bracket (AIHW 1999c). Again, this tragic imbalance is most likely to reflect excessive levels of major risk factors such as hypertension, obesity, cigarette smoking and alcohol consumption among indigenous Australians.

Lifestyle and biological risk factors for stroke

Several lifestyle and biological factors can increase the risk of a person having a stroke, and some of them can be changed or treated. These risk factors are:
- high blood pressure
- cigarette smoking
- heart disease, diabetes and their risk factors, such as obesity and physical inactivity
- family history of stroke
- high red blood cell count, which makes the blood thicker and more likely to form clots
- 'mini-strokes', called *transient ischaemic attacks*, that may occur one or more times before a full stroke.

Many of the risk factors for stroke are the same as those for heart disease. As a result, people who have had strokes are usually asked to make similar lifestyle changes to those of people who have had heart attacks: lose weight, stop smoking, exercise, and reduce dietary fat and cholesterol.

The effects of strokes and rehabilitation

Strokes vary in severity. People who survive moderate or severe strokes generally suffer some degree of motor, sensory, cognitive or speech impairment as a result of brain damage. If enough cells are affected, the functions controlled by the damaged area of the brain can be severely disrupted. The extent and type of impairment stroke patients suffer and their medical treatment — drugs and surgery — can vary greatly, depending on the amount and location of damage (Caplan 1986). Getting immediate treatment is critical because clot-dissolving drugs can limit the damage from a stroke (Gorman 1996). The following discussion applies to strokes that produce at least moderately severe damage.

Although the initial deficits stroke victims experience can be permanent, these people often show considerable improvement over time. Medical treatment and physical, occupational and speech therapy can help patients regain some of the functions they lost. Some evidence suggests that younger stroke patients may show somewhat better recovery than older ones, and the functional impairments caused by haemorrhages are more easily overcome than those caused by infarction (Hier 1986). Haemorrhages often impair functioning partly by creating pressure on neurons. If that pressure is relieved by the blood being reabsorbed by the body, the person may gradually recover some of the lost functioning.

Stroke is one of the most disabling chronic illnesses (Guccione et al. 1994). The most common deficits stroke patients experience involve motor action (Gordon & Diller 1983; Newman 1984b). For these patients, some degree of paralysis occurs immediately, and the person usually cannot move the arm and leg on one side of the body. Which side becomes paralysed depends on which side of the brain is damaged: The left hemisphere of the brain controls movement of the right side of the body and the right hemisphere controls movement on the left side. As a result, the paralysis occurs on the side of the body opposite to the hemisphere that sustained damage in the stroke. Because of the paralysis, these patients often cannot walk, dress themselves or perform many usual self-help activities. After about six weeks of physical rehabilitation, about half of these patients can perform activities of daily living independently, and the great majority can get around on their own, although often with the aid of walking sticks or other devices (Gordon & Diller 1983). Biofeedback and physiotherapy methods are effective treatments for improving motor functioning in stroke victims (Moreland & Thompson 1994).

Other common deficits many stroke patients face involve cognitive functions — language, learning, memory and perception. The specific type of impairment they have depends on which side of the brain was damaged. In most people, the left hemisphere contains the areas that handle language processes, including speech and writing (Geschwind 1979). Thus, damage on the left side often causes language and learning deficits. A common language disorder in stroke patients is *aphasia*, which is marked by difficulty in understanding or using words. There are two kinds of aphasia: *receptive aphasia* refers to a difficulty in understanding verbal information; *expressive aphasia* involves a problem in producing language, even though the person can make the component sounds. For example, the individual may not be able to differentiate between two verbalised words, such as 'coal' and 'cold'. Or the patient may have difficulty remembering a sequence of things he or she is told to do — such as, 'Touch your right ear with your left hand, and touch your left eyebrow with your right hand.'

What deficits are associated with damage on the right side of the brain? The right hemisphere usually processes visual imagery, emotions and the perception of patterns, such as melodies (Geschwind 1979). As a result, visual disorders are common with right-brain damage (Gordon & Diller 1983). In one of these disorders, stroke patients fail to process information on the left side of the normal visual field — for example, they may fail to notice food on the left side of a tray, items on the left side of a menu, or a minus sign in an arithmetic task (see figure 14.3). This problem also impairs their ability to perceive distances correctly and causes them to bump into objects or door frames on the left side of the visual field, making them accident-prone. Sometimes patients with this disorder feel they are 'going crazy' when they hear someone speaking but cannot see the person because he or she is standing in the left side of the visual field. The discrepancy between what they are hearing and what they are seeing makes them wonder if they are hallucinating.

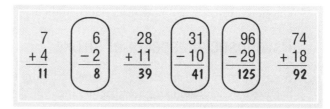

Figure 14.3 An illustration of arithmetic errors (circled items) a stroke patient with a visual disorder might make at the start of rehabilitation. In this case, the patient fails to scan to the left and assumes all of the problems involve addition. Rehabilitation can help patients overcome this deficit.

Like people in general, stroke patients with this visual disorder take for granted that what they see reflects the full size of their normal visual field. Because they think they see the whole field, they need to have their visual deficits clearly demonstrated. According to rehabilitation therapists Wayne Gordon and Leonard Diller, one effective approach involves placing paper money

> on the table in front of the patient. The large bills are purposely put on the impaired side. The patient is asked to pick up all of the money on the table. Naturally, a large sum of money remains on the table after the patient says that he or she has completed the task. Having the patient turn his or her head to see all the money that was left on the table is one way to begin to teach the patient that . . . this difficulty can be overcome by turning the head. (1983, p. 119)

Rehabilitation then proceeds by training the patients to use head turning automatically. A good way to start this training is to use an apparatus that has the patients track an object as it moves from the right to the left side of the visual field (Gordon & Diller 1983). Once patients master this task, they can begin training with paper and pencil tasks, such as learning to look for plus and minus signs in arithmetic problems.

The specific location of damage in the brain also can determine emotional disorders that stroke patients may show. Some studies have found associations between (1) specific left-hemisphere damage and patients' degree of depression and (2) specific right-hemisphere damage and patients' ability to interpret and express affect (Bleiberg 1986; Gordon & Diller 1983; Newman 1984b). An example of an emotional disorder some stroke patients have is called *pseudobulbar lability of affect*, which can occur in varying degrees.

> The essential features of the disorder are that the patient laughs or cries either on the basis of no provocation or minor provocation and that the patient is surprised and sometimes distressed by the discrepancy between how he feels and the emotions that he is displaying. In milder versions of the disorder, the emotional display is in the same direction as the patient's mood but simply is excessive given the intensity of the patient's mood. For example, the patient is thinking mildly sad thoughts that normally would not elicit tears and winds up in a state of wrenching sobbing. . . . In severer versions of the disorder, the

emotional display may be the opposite of the patient's inner mood. Thus, a patient's inner feelings of sadness may precipitate bouts of raucous laughter and a patient perceiving something as humorous and about to laugh may suddenly burst into tears. (Bleiberg 1986, p. 222)

In other emotional disorders, stroke patients may be unable to interpret other people's emotions correctly and may react oddly to them.

Psychosocial aspects of stroke

Recovery from a severe stroke is a long and arduous process. The initial physical and cognitive deficits are extremely frightening, but many patients are heartened by early gains in their functioning. Because of these gains, patients may become overly optimistic about the speed and degree of recovery to expect. Although patients with all chronic illnesses often rely on avoidance strategies to cope during the early phases of convalescence, denial seems to be more common among patients who have had strokes than those with heart disease or cancer (Krantz & Deckel 1983). Stroke patients who continue to deny their current or possible future limitations often retard their progress in rehabilitation.

When a stroke produces physical or cognitive deficits, the emotional adjustments can be very difficult. Stroke patients are very prone to depression (Bleiberg 1986; Krantz & Deckel 1983; Newman 1984b). Sometimes the brain damage itself can cause depression, as we mentioned earlier. But in all stroke cases that involve long-term impairment, psychosocial factors affect the success of patients' adaptation. As patients see the gains in recovery slowing down and begin to realise the extent of their impairment, feelings of hopelessness and helplessness may develop, leading to depression. Although stroke usually afflicts individuals who are beyond retirement age, many of its victims are employed when the illness occurs and suffer impairments that prevent them from returning to work. The results of follow-up studies suggest that less than half of stroke patients eventually resume working, but the rate of return tends to be higher among younger patients (Krantz & Deckel 1983; Newman 1984b). Some stroke victims who do not return to work are old enough to take advantage of early retirement opportunities, but others must leave the work force under less favourable circumstances, which can be financially and emotionally trying.

The impairments produced by stroke have important social effects on patients and their families, particularly when the patients are severely paralysed or have aphasia (Evans et al. 1992; Newman 1984b). Some families adjust to the patient's condition reasonably well, as in the following case.

> Mrs M. had always taken charge of bookkeeping and running the family. When her husband had a stroke, she adapted very well to his aphasia, inventing ways to communicate with him. When he developed cancer five years later, she helped him keep track of his medications by putting them in little cups at the beginning of the day, with coded instructions on how many to take and when to take them. In this way, Mr M., who worried that he hadn't taken his medication, could keep track of it when she wasn't there. (Gervasio 1986, p. 115)

But other families do not adjust well to the changing role relationships, and marital harmony often declines. In addition, the social contacts and leisure activities with friends also drop off for both the stroke patient and his or her spouse (Newman

1984b). Although the decrease in social and leisure activities increases with the extent of the victim's impairment, it is often substantial even when the person has made a good recovery. Family therapy and support groups can help stroke patients and their families adapt, but these approaches often need to address practical problems, such as not having transportation, before trying to resolve interpersonal problems (Evans et al. 1992; Krantz & Deckel 1983).

In summary, stroke is a high-mortality illness that involves neurological damage as a result of a disruption of blood flow to the brain. Survivors of stroke often suffer substantial physical and cognitive impairments, but medical treatment and physical, occupational and speech therapy can help these people regain many of their lost abilities. The more severe the remaining deficits after rehabilitation, the more likely patients are to experience psychosocial problems.

Cancer

Cancer is probably the disease many people fear most — the word 'cancer' itself scares many people, and they often overestimate the deaths that cancer causes (Burish et al. 1987). Receiving mammogram results indicating possible breast cancer can leave some women with high levels of anxiety months after further tests discount the suspicion (Lerman et al. 1991). But the distress from false-positive cancer tests is not very severe or long-lasting for most patients (Wardle et al. 1993).

Most practitioners recognise how people feel about cancer and are reluctant to discuss the disease and its effects with their patients. In a study some years ago of cancer victims who had begun radiation treatment, most reported that their doctors had not told them they had cancer (Peck 1972). Some even claimed their doctors said the condition was benign — such as a wart — but 80 per cent of the subjects said they knew it was cancer anyway. Doctors today are far more likely than in the past to share the bad news about serious medical conditions with their patients, but some probably still withhold distressing information about patients' diagnoses and prognoses (P. H. Blaney 1985; Laszlo 1987; Shuchman & Wilkes 1989).

The prevalence and types of cancer

A basic characteristic of life and growth is that body cells reproduce in an orderly and controlled fashion. Scientists know what the normal pattern of tissue growth looks like (Guyton 1985). Irregularities in this process can cause unrestricted cell growth, usually forming a tumour called a *neoplasm* (Tortora & Grabowski 1993). Although we know little about the process that maintains the proper number of different types of cells in the body, researchers have discovered an enzyme that exists mainly in tumour cells and may cause these cells to overproduce (Counter et al. 1994). Some neoplasms are harmless, or benign, but others are malignant.

Cancer is a disease of the cells and is characterised by unrestricted cell proliferation that usually forms a malignant neoplasm. Although there are more than 200 varieties of cancer, the great majority of cancers are of four types (Nelson 1989; Tortora & Grabowski 1993; Williams 1990). These four types are:

- *carcinomas*, which are malignant neoplasms of the skin cells and cells lining many body organs, such as the digestive, respiratory and reproductive tracts. About 85 per cent of human cancers are carcinomas.

- *lymphomas*, or cancers of the lymphatic system
- *sarcomas*, which are malignant neoplasms of the muscle, bone or connective tissue
- *leukaemias*, or cancers of the blood-forming organs, such as the bone marrow, that lead to an extreme proliferation of white blood cells.

An important characteristic of cancer cells is that they do not adhere to each other as strongly as normal cells do (Laszlo 1987; Williams 1990). As a result, they may separate and spread to other parts of the body through the blood or lymph systems. This migration is called *metastasis*, and the new neoplasms are known as *metastases*.

Cancer comes immediately after cardiovascular disease as the second most common cause of death in Australia. Around 345 000 new cases of cancer overall are diagnosed in Australia each year (AIHW 1999b). Many of these are non-melanocytic (benign) skin cancers, but even excluding these lesions, more than 77 000 new cases of malignant cancer were diagnosed in 1996 and in the same year more than 34 000 Australians died from cancer (AIHW 1999b). Less than half of all diagnosed cancers are eventually fatal, however, and rates of complete cure, or at least of substantial slowing of growth, are increasing yearly with advances in the medical treatment of cancers of most types. Moreover, the application of intervention strategies in health psychology to the prevention of cancer risk by targeting behavioural risk factors is making gains in the overall incidence of cancers in Australia. Nevertheless, as will be clear from the types of cancers noted above, cancer may afflict many locations and systems in the human body.

The sites, effects and causes of cancer

What are the physical effects of cancer, and how does it kill? Cancer progresses by spreading to different sites, and its growth at each site interferes with normal development and functioning. As the disease progresses, it also produces pain, often because the tumour creates pressure on normal tissue and nerves or blocks the flow of body fluids (Melzack & Wall 1982). Substantial pain afflicts 40 per cent of cancer victims in intermediate stages of the disease and 70 to 90 per cent of those with advanced cancer (Foley 1985; Greenwald, Bonica & Bergner 1987; Ward et al. 1993). The disease leads to death in direct and indirect ways. In the direct route, the cancer spreads over time to a vital organ, such as the brain, liver or lungs; it then competes for and takes most of the nutrients the organ tissues need to survive, thereby causing the organ to fail. Cancer kills indirectly in two ways: the disease itself weakens the victims, and both the disease and the treatment can impair the patient's appetite and ability to fight infection (Laszlo 1987).

Prognosis and causes of cancer

The prognosis for cancer depends on how early it is detected and its location (Battista & Grover 1988; Laszlo 1987; Williams 1990). Locations of the most common cancers vary according to country, and this in turn reflects variations in levels of risk factors (cigarette smoking, diet and the like) and environmental conditions (levels of ultraviolet radiation for example). In Australia in recent times, cancer of the prostate was the most common cancer in men (23.5 per cent of all male cancers) followed by colorectal cancer (14.2 per cent), cancer of the lung (12.2 per cent) and melanoma or malignant skin cancer (10.1 per cent). For women, cancer of the breast was most prevalent (27.5 per cent of all female cancers) followed by colorectal cancer (14.1 per cent), melanoma (9.9 per cent) and cancer of the lung (6.9 per cent). Cancer of the female sexual organs (uterus, ovary and cervix) accounted for a collective 9.7 per cent. Thus, while the most common cancer in each case attaches to a sexually unique part of the body (prostate in men and breast in women), there is also a good deal of commonality, with colorectal cancer attacking men and women essentially equally (AIHW 1999b). A more detailed breakdown of recent rates of various cancers in Australia, presented for males and females separately, can be seen in table 14.1.

Table 14.1   Most frequently occurring cancers in males and females in Australia, 1997

Type	New cases	%	Deaths	%
Colorectal	11 245	14.1	4678	13.8
Breast	10 166	12.8	2612	7.7
Prostate	9 725	12.2	2449	7.2
Melanoma	8 366	10.5	910	2.7
Lung	7 819	9.8	6683	19.7
Unknown site	3 169	4.0	2255	6.6
NHL*	3 137	3.9	1540	4.5
Bladder	2 681	3.4	807	2.4
Kidney	2 047	2.6	796	2.3
Stomach	1 919	2.4	1244	3.7

* Non-Hodgkin's Lymphoma
Source: AIHW (1999b).

We have seen in earlier chapters that cancer is caused by the interplay of genetic and environmental factors, and that stress can promote the development and progression of the disease. Environmental factors include smoking tobacco, diet, ultraviolet radiation, and household and work-site chemical hazards, among others. Some research has also found a link between certain viral infections and the development of some cancers, such as in the cervix and in the liver (Laszlo 1987; Williams 1990). In cervical cancer, viral transmission probably occurs during intercourse. Because not all women who are exposed to the viruses develop cancer, it seems likely that the effects of the infections depend on or combine with genetic and environmental factors to produce the disease.

Age, gender and sociocultural factors in cancer

The risk of developing cancer typically increases with age, especially from the middle-age years onward. For all types of cancer combined, incidence rates for the disease quadruple from 40 to 80 years of age (Mor et al. 1985). Australian data (AIHW 1999b) suggest that the effects of age on risk of cancer must be looked at in relation to the nature and location of the cancer itself. Although more than 70 per cent of all cancer deaths occur in those over 65 years of age, and although the incidence of lung cancer and melanoma increase progressively with age, cancer of the cervix peaks at middle age and then remains constant into the older age groups, while cancer of the testis peaks relatively early and then actually declines with age. There are also national differences in cancer prevalence — for instance, lung cancer is far more common in England than in Nigeria, and stomach cancer is far more common in Japan than in Uganda (AMA 1989). Rates of cancer in Australia are not dissimilar to those evident in other Westernised, developed countries. Aggregated rates are close to those of Canada and the United States but a little higher than those in the UK and Japan. Australian males have relatively low rates of lung cancer compared with many other countries. This advantage is not shared by Australian females (which, incidentally, may relate to the observation that females have higher rates of cigarette smoking than do males in this country). Australia also has high overall rates of colorectal cancer seen from an international perspective. Conversely, cancer of the stomach does not figure anywhere near so prominently in Australians as it does among those from many other countries (AIHW 1999b).

Diagnosing and treating cancer

People can increase the likelihood of early rather than late detection of certain cancers by knowing the warning signs of cancer and having or doing regular examinations, which are listed in figure 14.5.

Diagnosing cancer can involve three medical procedures (Laszlo 1987; Nguyen et al. 1994). First, *blood* or *urine* tests are useful for suggesting the presence of cancer by revealing telltale signs, such as unusual levels of certain hormones or enzymes. Second, *radiological imaging*, through X-ray and other techniques, allows doctors to see the structure of internal organs and whether a tumour exists. Third, the doctor does a *biopsy* by taking out a small piece of suspicious tissue and having it analysed. Even when the tissue is deep within the abdomen, it can generally be removed with minor surgical procedures and a local anaesthetic.

Figure 14.4 Common cancer sites

- *Skin cancer.* The vast majority of these cancers are *basal cell* and *squamous cell carcinomas*, and cure is almost assured with early detection. But about 5 per cent of skin cancers are *melanomas*, which form in the pigment-carrying skin cells and are more serious because they metastasise quickly. Still, more than 85 per cent of melanoma patients survive at least five years.
- *Prostate cancer.* Although prostate cancer can be detected in its early stages, when five-year survival rates exceed 98 per cent, these rates are unclear because the disease usually becomes evident after the men are over 70 years of age.
- *Breast cancer.* Early detection permits over 95 per cent of breast cancer patients to survive at least five years.

- *Lung cancer.* The 5-year survival rate is only 13 per cent overall, but it is three times as high if the disease is discovered while still localised. In lung cancer, neoplasms tend to metastasise while still small and, for this reason, they generally have already spread by the time they are discovered.
- *Colorectal cancer.* These cancers can be detected early — and if they are, over 90 per cent of the patients survive at least five years.
- *Uterine and cervical cancer.* Neoplasms of the uterus or cervix of the female reproductive system can be either *invasive*, or precancerous *carcinomas in situ*, which are discovered very early with Pap tests and are usually fully curable. For invasive cases detected early, the five-year survival rate is 91 per cent for cervical and 83 per cent for uterine cancer.

Source: ACS (1996).

The ideal goal of cancer treatment is to cure the disease — to free the person from it forever. This ideal is possible when all the neoplasms are found and eliminated (Guyton 1985; Laszlo 1987). If not all of the cancer was eliminated, the patient's symptoms may disappear for a time — or 'go into remission' — only to return at a later date. Sometimes doctors can be reasonably certain that all of the cancer was removed, but often they cannot be sure. This is why they use the individual's survival for at least five years as a gauge of a treatment's success. There are basically three types of treatment for cancer — surgery, radiation and chemotherapy — which may be used singly or in combination. When choosing the treatment components, patients and practitioners consider many factors, such as the size and site of the neoplasm, whether it has metastasised and how the treatment will affect the patient's quality of life. One factor that seems to affect the treatment choice, sometimes inappropriately, is the patient's age. A study using the medical records of nearly 1900 deceased adult cancer victims found that, among individuals with similar stages and sites of neoplasms, those over age 60 or so were much less likely than those under 60 to have received radiation or chemotherapy in their treatment (Mor et al. 1985).

Figure 14.5 Early cancer detection: examinations and warning signs

Examinations	**Warning signs of cancer: 'CAUTION'**
Doctor- or self-administered examinations are available for early detection of the following cancer sites:	If you have any of the following signs, see your doctor soon. Notice that the first letters spell 'caution'.
• breast • skin • colon or rectum • testes • prostate • uterus or cervix.	• **C**hange in bowel or bladder habits • **A** sore that does not heal • **U**nusual bleeding or discharge • **T**hickening or lump in the breast or elsewhere • **I**ndigestion or difficulty swallowing • **O**bvious change in a wart or mole • **N**agging cough or hoarseness.

Sources: ACS (1989, 1996).

From a medical standpoint, *surgery* is frequently the preferred treatment for eliminating a neoplasm, such as in breast or colorectal cancer (Laszlo 1987; Williams 1990). If the cancer is localised, surgery often can be completely effective by itself; if the cancer has spread, surgery may be useful in removing large clusters of cancerous cells, leaving the remainder for radiation or chemotherapy treatment. Sometimes the surgeon removes large portions of tissue near the neoplasm because of the possibility that the cancer has spread to those areas, too. In patients with colorectal cancer, for example, the surgeon may remove a long section of the colon even though the neoplasm seems to be restricted to a small area. But the practice of removing large amounts of nearby tissue is changing, particularly in the treatment of breast cancer: Research has shown that a *mastectomy* — the removal of the entire breast — is not necessary in many, if not most, cases (Jacobson et al. 1995; Laszlo 1987). Instead, a woman may choose to have a *lumpectomy*, in which just the tumour is removed, followed by radiation treatment.

Radiation in high doses alters body cells in such a way that they are either destroyed or cannot reproduce (Holum 1994). In treating cancer, radiation is used in two ways (Burish & Lyles 1983; Laszlo 1987; McNaull 1984). One approach, *external beam therapy*, involves directing a beam of intense radiation at the malignant tissue for a period of seconds or minutes. This is the most commonly used method and the one most people picture when the term 'radiation therapy' is used. External beam therapy is usually given several times in a week, and may be continued for up to several weeks. The second approach is called *internal radiation therapy* and involves placing a radioactive substance inside the body, near or into the tumour, by surgery or injection. Although radiation therapy is painless, it can have problematic side effects, depending on the area of the body radiated and the dose. Because radiation affects both healthy and malignant cells, the affected area may suffer irritation, burns or hair loss, for example. The person may experience nausea, vomiting, loss of appetite, sterility and reduced bone marrow function, particularly if the radiated area is large or is in the abdomen. In the day or two before undergoing radiation treatment, individuals often worry about these side effects and report heightened anxiety similar to that of people awaiting surgery (Andersen et al. 1984).

In *chemotherapy*, patients receive powerful drugs, usually orally or by injection, that circulate through the body to kill cells that divide very rapidly (Burish & Lyles 1983; Laszlo 1987; Williams 1990). The intended targets, of course, are cancerous cells, most of which reproduce rapidly. Some forms of cancer respond more readily than others to the drugs currently available; cancer of the testicles and some types of leukaemia are very responsive, but cancers of the brain and pancreas are not. One problem with chemotherapy is that the drugs also kill certain types of normal cells that divide rapidly — for example cells of the bone marrow, mouth and intestinal lining, and hair follicles, especially those of the scalp. Some programs of chemotherapy continue for a long time and can have several very adverse side effects, including reduced immunity to infection, sores in the mouth, hair loss, nausea and vomiting, and damage to internal organs (Williams 1990).

For many patients, the most unpleasant side effects of chemotherapy are the periods of nausea and vomiting they experience during and immediately after each treatment. These periods can be so aversive and prolonged for some patients that they have even discontinued treatment, knowing that doing so could shorten their lives (Carey & Burish 1988). Furthermore, after two or three treatments, some patients who are about to receive the drug begin vomiting before it is given — they develop *anticipatory nausea* — and may even become nauseated and throw up when they arrive at the hospital or while thinking about the upcoming treatment at home the night before.

Anticipatory nausea appears to develop in about 25 to 50 per cent of chemotherapy patients who have received the treatment repeatedly (Andrykowski 1990; Carey & Burish 1988). These patients seem to learn this reaction through classical conditioning, in which the drug itself is the unconditioned stimulus that reflexively produces the unconditioned response of nausea. Through association, other related events, such as seeing the hospital or thinking about the procedure, become conditioned stimuli and can elicit nausea in the absence of the drug (Bovbjerg et al. 1992; Jacobsen et al. 1995). Some evidence suggests that anticipatory nausea is more likely to develop in people who show a high degree of reactivity to conditioned stimuli in general than those who show less reactivity (Kvale, Psychol & Hugdahl 1994).

The psychologist David Horne and his colleagues in Melbourne also reported an interesting example of a conditioned phobia to injections in a cancer patient undergoing chemotherapy (Horne et al. 1986). The 50-year-old female patient undergoing chemotherapy following a radical mastectomy threatened to withdraw from treatment when she developed a phobia to injections following the unpleasant effects of chemotherapy. Horne and his colleagues successfully treated this phobia using a combination of relaxation and desensitisation techniques, and the patient was able to resume her course of chemotherapy.

Cancer treatment can not only be unpleasant, it can be complex and demanding. Most cancer patients must also take medications at home, and many must return to their clinics frequently for laboratory tests, keep diaries of their food intake, or adhere to dietary and other changes in living habits. Because of these conditions, we might expect cancer patients to show poor compliance with their treatment regimens. Studies of adherence to cancer regimens have produced mixed findings (Levy 1985; Nehemkis & Gerber 1986; Richardson et al. 1987; Tebbi et al. 1986). Although most adults seem to adhere closely to cancer treatments, adolescents and minority group individuals from the lower classes do not. Compliance to medical treatments depends on and influences a variety of psychosocial factors in patients' lives.

The psychosocial impact of cancer

Like all chronic illnesses, cancer involves a series of threats and difficulties that change, often getting worse over time. Cancer creates unique stresses for patients and their families. These patients have a disease they recognise as a 'real killer', and one that can lead to intense pain, disability and disfigurement. Even among patients who go into remission and adapt well during the first months or years, the threat of a recurrence looms — and if the disease flares up, some individuals are psychologically paralysed by their fear (Mages & Mendelsohn 1979). In addition, some patients experience medical procedures that, for them, can be more aversive than the disease itself. How well patients adapt to having cancer can have medical consequences and affect the progression of the disease. Individuals who experience high levels of stress and do not cope well show poor immune system activity, and some evidence suggests that patients' cancers worsen more quickly if their immune functions are impaired (Kiecolt-Glaser & Glaser 1986; Levy et al. 1985; Redd et al. 1991).

Given all of the stress associated with having cancer, most patients show a remarkable amount of resilience and adapt reasonably well. Even among hospitalised cancer patients, studies have generally found that fewer than half show significant emotional difficulties, and most of these involve relatively transient problems — chiefly anxiety and depressed mood — that are usually responsive to psychological therapy (Burish et al. 1987). This incidence of emotional problems may seem high, but there are a few points to keep in mind. First, these studies were done with hospitalised patients, and hospitalisation itself elevates anxiety and depression. Second, among patients hospitalised for all reasons, perhaps one-fourth have emotional disorders, and often these problems developed before the illness. Patients' emotional problems result from many factors other than their disease, such as experiencing other major stressful events and not having social support in their lives. Last, psychologists often consider it 'normal' for cancer patients to have some elevations in depression and anxiety. Given the life circumstances of these patients, our deciding when these reactions are appropriate and when they are dysfunctional is likely to be difficult and based on arbitrary criteria (Burish et al. 1987).

Although adaptation to cancer can be very difficult for patients during the first several months and when their conditions worsen, their ability to adjust to their illnesses appears to improve with time during remission or after a cure (Burish et al. 1987; Glanz & Lerman 1992). By two years or so, their psychosocial functioning stabilises at levels similar to those they had prior to the diagnosis. One study administered questionnaires regarding psychosocial adjustment to breast cancer patients and women from the general population (Craig, Comstock & Geiser 1974). All the subjects with breast cancer had been diagnosed and treated more than 9 months prior to the study. The patients and controls showed very similar levels of depression, happiness, optimism for the future and perceived health.

Adaptation among cancer patients depends on many aspects of their illness and psychosocial situation. For example, the emotional adjustment patients achieve depends on their age and physical condition — middle-aged or more physically impaired adults seem to fare worse than older or less impaired cancer patients (Vinocur et al. 1990). Patients who become most severely depressed tend to be those who are physically disabled by the disease or in pain (Burish et al. 1987; Spiegel, Sands & Koopman 1994). The site of the cancer is also important, and its impact often depends on the patient's age. Norman Mages and Gerald Mendelsohn have contrasted the situations of two men — one in young adulthood, the other middle-aged — with testicular cancer, each of whom had been made sterile by his treatment but had a good medical prognosis. The younger man had entered his career and developed a lasting and secure relationship with a woman two years before the diagnosis; the older man was married and had grown children.

> It is surely not surprising that the younger man was far more deeply distressed by his cancer than the older. His sterility was particularly painful for it meant that he could never have children of his own and, perhaps unrealistically, raised doubts about a future marriage and his sexual competence. . . . The older man, in contrast, was relatively little affected by his disease. Though he too had to face the issue of a potentially shortened life span, he had long since established a stable and satisfying adult existence and was securely embedded in a supportive social network. (1979, p. 277)

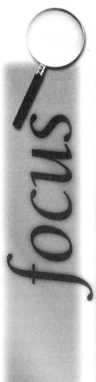

Focus on research
Chemotherapy and learned food aversions

When people with cancer begin chemotherapy, many experience a loss of appetite that can lead to excessive weight loss. This can create problems in their medical treatment and in their home lives. Families of patients who are not eating well become concerned about this situation — and eating may turn into a constant battle, with the patients feeling hounded to eat (Nevidjon 1984). Part of the reason for the loss of appetite such people experience may be that they develop a distaste for some foods they once liked. Cancer patients who receive chemotherapy or radiation therapy often report that this happens to them. Developing a strong dislike for foods they previously liked a lot, such as chocolate desserts, a morning cup of coffee, or a steak, can be demoralising to cancer victims, who may feel that their quality of life has suffered enough.

Why do these patients come to dislike foods they had liked? Since chemotherapy produces nausea and vomiting in many people, these symptoms may become associated with one or more foods they ingest before or after the symptoms occur (Horne 1997). A **learned food aversion** is a phenomenon in which a food becomes distasteful because the individual associates it with symptoms of illness or physical discomfort. Richard Mattes, Cathy Arnold and Marcia Boraas (1987a, 1987b) studied learned food aversions in 76 adult cancer patients who were beginning programs of chemotherapy. The subjects had no other physical conditions, such as diabetes, that might relate to their food preferences. During the hour preceding their first treatment, the patients were interviewed to determine their medical histories, the foods they had consumed during the prior 24 hours, their ratings of recently eaten foods, and any food aversions they already had.

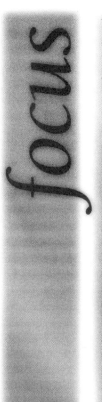

They were then given a form to fill out at home and return by mail. The form had the subjects list and rate all foods eaten during the 24 hours after the treatment.

At the next scheduled visit and at other visits during the next six months of treatment, the subjects provided information about their food preferences and any side effects they experienced from the treatment. The results revealed several interesting findings. First, 55 per cent of the patients developed aversions to foods consumed within the 24 hours preceding and following treatments. Second, many of these aversions formed after only one treatment, and subsequent treatments produced fewer and fewer new dislikes. Third, the amount of time (up to 24 hours) between eating the food and receiving the treatment did not affect whether an aversion would develop. Fourth, individuals whose side effects included vomiting developed more learned food aversions than those whose side effects did not, but receiving drugs to prevent vomiting did not help prevent aversions from forming. Fifth, the aversions generally lasted less than a month and included many of the foods the patients previously ate frequently and liked a great deal.

Can something be done to prevent cancer patients from learning to dislike foods they normally eat? One promising approach involves having a patient consume a strongly flavoured, unfamiliar food between his or her last meal and the chemotherapy treatment. Why? The purpose is to create a scapegoat — that is, to direct the learning process to this new food and allow *it* to become disliked, instead of foods in the patient's normal diet. Research has shown that this approach works for many adult and child cancer patients (Broberg & Bernstein 1987; Mattes, Arnold & Boraas 1987b). Individuals who form aversions to the scapegoat foods are much less likely to develop dislikes to foods in normal diets.

A similar pattern of concerns also affects women with cancer of the breast, cervix and uterus, but their difficulties may be compounded if surgery seriously disfigures their bodies or alters their physical ability to function sexually (Andersen & Hacker 1983; Glanz & Lerman 1992; Jacobsen & Holland 1991; Schain et al. 1994). As you might expect, sexual problems very frequently occur among men and women patients with cancers in sex-related organs, but many patients with cancers in other sites may also experience sexual problems as a result of their medical treatments, such as when chemotherapy causes fatigue (Burish et al. 1987; Redd et al. 1991).

Many cancer patients experience psychosocial problems that stem from changes in their relationships with family members and friends. In some cases, patients may begin to withdraw from social contact because they feel socially awkward or embarrassed by their conditions, especially if their bodies have become noticeably disfigured (Mages & Mendelsohn 1979). But two other reasons are probably more common (Bloom, Kang & Romano 1991). First, the patients' physical condition and treatment may interfere with their seeing their friends and families. Second, people may begin to avoid the patient. Although this sometimes occurs as a result of fear and ignorance, such as when people believe cancer is contagious, other reasons are often involved. For example, friends and family may experience conflicts between wanting to be cheerful and optimistic with the patient, while at the same time feeling very sad and personally vulnerable in his or her presence (Wortman & Dunkel-Schetter 1979). They may also worry that they will 'break down', or 'betray their feelings', or 'say the wrong thing' in front of the patient. When these people and the patient do get together, everyone may behave awkwardly.

Psychosocial interventions for cancer

Psychosocial approaches for helping individuals cope with their cancers can begin with the diagnostic interview (Roberts et al. 1994). Positive adaptation to the illness can be enhanced if the doctor discusses the diagnosis while the patient is alert with a spouse or other significant person present, expresses concern and gives the people some time to react emotionally and compose themselves, and then presents information about the prognosis and treatment options.

Several types of psychosocial interventions have been applied successfully to improve cancer patients' adjustment to their illness and quality of life (Meyer & Mark 1995). One focus of these approaches has been to help reduce patients' nausea from chemotherapy, and several techniques seem to be effective (Carey & Burish 1988). Two approaches with particularly strong support are relaxation training and systematic desensitisation. For example, one study found that training patients to use progressive muscle relaxation and imagery before and during chemotherapy sessions sharply reduced the development of nausea after the first session (Burish & Jenkins 1992). Another study showed that systematic desensitisation can help patients who have already developed anticipatory nausea (Morrow et al. 1992). Patients used relaxation techniques while they imagined increasingly difficult scenes relating to chemotherapy, such as having breakfast on the morning of treatment, driving to the clinic, and entering the waiting room. These individuals reported much less nausea and vomiting in subsequent chemotherapy sessions. Not all patients benefit from these techniques, partly because they don't believe psychosocial approaches will help (Carey & Burish 1988).

Other interventions have had broader focuses and shown that psychosocial methods not only enhance patients' adjustment to cancer, but may improve their survival, too. In one study, psychological and immunological assessments were made on cancer patients before serving in one of two research conditions, after serving in the condition, and six months later (Fawzy, Cousins et al. 1990; Fawzy, Kemeny et al. 1990). Subjects in the intervention condition met in groups for $1\frac{1}{2}$ hours in each of six weeks to discuss their concerns and problems and to learn health-promotion activities, positive coping strategies and stress management techniques. Subjects in the control condition received no psychosocial intervention. The results at the six-month assessment revealed that the intervention subjects had better immune function and reported more vigour, better coping behaviour, and less depression than the controls. A follow-up six years later revealed that 29 per cent of the controls and only 9 per cent of the intervention subjects had died (Fawzy et al. 1993). Another study assessed the survival of cancer patients after a year-long intervention in which they attended weekly group meetings that were led by therapists who had cancers that were in remission (Spiegel et al. 1989). The meetings enabled the patients to discuss their feelings and coping strategies and to learn self-hypnosis to manage pain. Compared with a control group, the patients who received the psychosocial intervention lived nearly 18 months longer during a 10-year follow-up period.

Because of the social problems cancer patients face, they and their families may benefit from family therapy and attending support groups that include education and group discussion (Helgeson & Cohen 1996; Tovian 1991). In one study, cancer patients in a support group received counselling sessions, training in relaxation and information about diet, exercise and their illnesses (Cain et al. 1986). Subsequent comparisons with control subjects revealed that those in the support group were less depressed and anxious, had fewer sexual problems and participated more in leisure activities. All Australian cancer societies and councils offer support and education programs for those suffering from cancer in each of the States and Territories. These vary from general information services and 'help lines' offering information on cancer to those needing it (sufferers or their families) to support groups for people in the varying stages of many types of cancer. A good example of this, and one that may be seen across the country, focuses on breast cancer. Groups for those with diagnosed breast cancer, whether under active treatment or not, provide a venue for sharing information and experiences, receiving emotional support for such ongoing problems as nausea (arising from chemotherapy or radiotherapy) and pain, and dealing with the disfiguring effects of breast surgery. These services can be easily accessed through the web sites of the various cancer societies and councils.

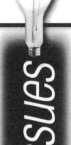

Highlight on issues

Can patients 'will away' their cancer?

The mind is a powerful instrument, and what people think can affect their health. How powerful is this instrument? Could cancer patients use it to recruit the soldiers of the immune system to seek and destroy malignant cells? The notion that the mind could do this forms the basis of a controversial approach for helping cancer patients control their disease.

O. Carl Simonton developed a therapy program in which patients receive group counselling and training in muscle relaxation while also receiving medical treatment (Simonton & Simonton 1975; see also Scarf 1980). The main feature of the program is an 'imaging' exercise in which the patients imagine that they can see their white blood cells attack and destroy cancer cells. One patient, for instance, imagined her white cells were sharks that would chase her cancer cells (small fish) 'and then pounce upon them, rending them to bits with their long, jagged teeth and destroying them' (Scarf 1980, p. 40).

Does this therapy program work? Little or no evidence exists to support the notion that the imaging exercise helps in curing cancer (P. H. Blaney 1985; Laszlo 1987). But other aspects of the program are quite promising. As adjuncts to medical treatment, counselling and relaxation can benefit patients' psychosocial adjustment, which is likely to enhance their immune function, improve their quality of life, increase their self-efficacy and resilience, help them become more involved in their treatment, and encourage them to maintain a 'fighting spirit'.

Childhood cancer

Australia had 971 new cases of cancer diagnosed in children in the years 1993 to 1997, with slightly more boys than girls. Of these, leukaemias accounted for 29 per cent while a further 22 per cent affected the central nervous system (AIHW 1999b). Improved treatment methods have reduced the death rate from cancer in childhood by over 60 per cent since 1960. Chemotherapy is the main form of treatment, but radiation may be used to prevent the disease from developing in the brain. These treatments produce much the same side effects in children as they do in adults, including chronic nausea and vomiting. Losing their hair is a very traumatic and embarrassing experience to most children and teenagers even though it does grow back eventually (Spinetta 1982). But if a child receives treatment and a relapse does not occur in the five years after diagnosis, the chances are very high that the leukaemia will never recur (Laszlo 1987).

The treatment program for leukaemia begins on an in-patient basis with an 'induction' phase, in which the patients receive combinations of drugs in high doses to produce a full remission (Eiser 1985; Williams 1990). Because of the high risk of relapse without continued treatment during the next three years, the program continues with a 'maintenance' phase on an out-patient basis. During this time, patients receive chemotherapy, weekly or bi-weekly blood tests, and frequent bone marrow examinations to check for the presence of cancer cells. One of these examinations — called a *bone marrow aspiration* — is extremely painful. It involves inserting a large needle into the child's hip bone, and then suctioning out a sample of marrow. The whole procedure is painful, but the most excruciating pain occurs as the marrow is withdrawn. Although pain-killing drugs help somewhat, the patients still feel intense pain. Researchers have found that children's pain and distress can be reduced with psychological methods, such as showing them a film of a child coping realistically with the procedure and teaching them to use techniques to distract their attention from the pain (Jay et al. 1985; Jay et al. 1987).

What are the psychosocial effects of having cancer on childhood patients and their families? In an overall sense, the effects are like those with adult patients. The initial trauma is extremely difficult, but the patient's and family's adjustment tends to improve over time (Eiser 1985; Koocher et al. 1980). Two factors that are important in children's psychosocial adaptation to cancer are the age at the onset of the disease and the time since the diagnosis. The earlier the diagnoses and treatment occurred in the children's lives and the longer the patients survive in remission, the better their long-term adjustment tends to be. Another psychosocial issue in childhood cancer is that these patients often lag behind other children in academic skills, particularly during the first few years of school (Allen & Zigler 1986; Eiser 1985). These deficits probably result from their missing many school days and the psychosocial and physical effects of their medical treatment.

AIDS

Acquired immune deficiency syndrome — AIDS — is a very different high-mortality chronic illness from the others we have discussed. For one thing, AIDS is a new disease and was virtually unknown before 1980. Also, it is an infectious disease that is caused by a virus (HIV) and is spread through the shared contact of blood and semen. The number of people who have died from AIDS in each of the last several years is only a small fraction of the number who have died of stroke. But AIDS is an epidemic, its annual mortality statistics are skyrocketing, many millions of people around the world are already infected with the virus, and the large majority of these people will probably die as a result of AIDS. Most of these people are heterosexuals who do not use drugs but live in countries with high rates of promiscuity and uncontrolled prostitution (Johnson & Laga 1990).

Risk factors, effects and treatment of AIDS

The risk factors for AIDS involve ways by which an infected person's blood or semen contacts the body fluid of an uninfected person. This contact almost always occurs in one of three main ways. These are:

- sexual activity that exposes each person's body fluids to the other's. Exposure is more likely if the genital area has wounds or inflammation from a sexually transmitted disease (Peterman 1990).
- sharing contaminated syringes during drug use
- birth by an infected mother.

We saw in chapter 6 that public health efforts have reduced these risks, especially among gay men and drug users in technologically advanced countries. But many people around the world still engage in risky behaviour.

Age, gender and sociocultural factors in AIDS

Despite the fact that AIDS has been with us now for almost two decades, in Australia it remains a disease largely, though not exclusively, of men aged between 20 and 40 years old. AIDS almost certainly originated in Africa, where the main burden of the disease is still evident. Its introduction to Australia, however, is most likely to have occurred through the United States and Europe. Australia has a high level of HIV (the virus causing AIDS) screening, most likely as a result of rigorous cautionary procedures associated with blood donorship. Routine HIV antibody testing commenced in Australia in 1985 and by 1992 quite comprehensive data on rates of HIV positive tests and of AIDS were available. The cumulative number of positive HIV tests (but not diagnosed cases of AIDS) to the middle of 1992 was 16 458 of whom the overwhelming proportion (96 per cent) were men. Statistical analyses to project these data both backwards and forwards in time suggests that new HIV infections peaked between 1983 and 1988 and then began to decline, levelling out at about 600 new cases each year from 1990. To mid-1992 Australia had seen a cumulative total of 3421 cases of AIDS itself, with 97 per cent of these being in males. This had resulted in 2259 AIDS-related deaths (Australian Department of Health 1993). By 1997 these figures had risen to around 17 600 cumulative HIV infections, with 8182 cases of AIDS and 5756 deaths from AIDS (National Centre in HIV Epidemiology and Clinical Research 1998).

Male homosexual activity accounted for about 86 per cent of all reported positive HIV tests to 1990, while HIV infection from needle sharing among intravenous drug users appeared to be increasing. HIV infection from heterosexual activity was still low in Australia, as was transmission from infected mothers to newborn babies via foetal blood (National Evaluation Steering Committee 1993). By 1998 HIV infection through male homosexual contact had declined to 78.9 per cent of all cases, but infection through heterosexual contact had increased to 9.2 per cent (National Centre in HIV Epidemiology and Clinical Research 1998). HIV infection of recipients of blood or blood products during medical procedures continues to occur but at lower rates than were evident a decade ago.

HIV infection and AIDS among indigenous Australians occurs at around the same rates as it does for white Australians, although there is a suggestion that transmission through heterosexual contact is more prominent among indigenous Australians than it is among whites (National Centre in HIV Epidemiology and Clinical Research 1998).

From HIV infection to AIDS

Once HIV infection occurs, several years may pass before the person's immune function is impaired — mainly from reduced numbers of helper T cells — and symptoms appear (Benjamini & Leskowitz 1991). During the period before symptoms emerge, the virus appears to hide in the person's lymph tissue, multiplying there and battling the immune system (Embretson et al. 1993; Ho et al. 1995; Pantaleo et al. 1993).

The diagnosis of AIDS is made only once the victim's condition meets a certain criterion. Before 1993 the criterion required that the person have contracted one of several opportunistic diseases associated with the loss of immune function. These illnesses include *Pneumocystis carinii pneumonia* and *Kaposi's sarcoma*, a form of cancer previously rare in developed countries. In 1993 the US Centers for Disease Control changed the criterion to involve a low level of helper T cells (also called CD4 cells) in the person's blood. Years before meeting either of these criteria, however, the victim might have learned from a blood test that he or she was infected with HIV. There is now an accurate method to test a person's 'viral load', an assessment of the number of viral particles in a blood sample, which reflects the amount of HIV in the body.

Between the time of infection and the AIDS diagnosis, the victim's immune system begins to falter, producing a variety of recurrent symptoms, such as spiking fever, night sweats, diarrhoea, fatigue and swollen lymph glands. At this stage, the victim is classified as having **AIDS-related complex** (ARC) and may develop AIDS within a few years. Before developing ARC, individuals infected with HIV have no symptoms of the disease. The only way they can tell they are infected is by having a blood test. By the time they are diagnosed with AIDS, their immune system is severely and chronically weakened. From that point on, the disease progresses with repeated bouts of opportunistic diseases.

Medical treatment for people with HIV/AIDS

Most of the opportunistic diseases in AIDS can be treated effectively with medications, such as antibiotics, but sometimes victims become hypersensitive, or allergic, to the medications and no therapy is available that their bodies will tolerate. For patients who survive repeated bouts of diseases, the prognosis is still poor (Osborn 1988; Tross & Hirsch 1988). Their bodies become severely weakened, and they gradually waste away. Many AIDS patients develop a brain disorder when the HIV invades the central nervous system. This invasion causes the brain to deteriorate — a condition called *encephalopathy*. These patients gradually lose their cognitive functions, become disoriented and confused, and may also become mute and have seizures. Eventually, they lapse into a coma.

The main medical treatment for AIDS from the mid-1980s to the mid-1990s was the drug AZT (*azidothymidine*, also called *zidovudine*), one of several *nucleosides* that can slow HIV reproduction in the early stages. AZT prolongs survival but does not cure the disease or reduce the occurrence of opportunistic diseases (Hamilton et al. 1992; Osborn 1988; Young 1987). By the mid-1990s, researchers developed a new class of drugs called *protease inhibitors* (brand names Crixivan and Invirase) that interfere with HIV reproduction at a later stage. In 1996 researchers reported preliminary evidence that a combined treatment with a protease inhibitor and two nucleosides dramatically reduces the viral load in many, but not all, HIV-infected individuals (Altman 1996; Leland 1996). Although these results have produced a great deal of optimism and hope that we may have a truly effective long-term treatment, it is too early to tell. Even if it is successful, the treatment is very expensive and can have difficult side effects.

AIDS has been fatal to virtually all of its victims, and most people with AIDS die within one or two years of its diagnosis. A minority of patients survive more than three years, and some are still living and active more than five years after the diagnosis (Gavzer 1988). Why do some individuals survive so much longer than most others? No-one really knows why for sure. A major part of the answer must involve biological differences between those who do and those who do not continue to survive, and some psychosocial relationships have been discovered. George Solomon and Lydia Temoshok (1987) conducted a long-term follow-up study of patients who filled out questionnaires to assess a variety of psychosocial factors soon after being diagnosed with AIDS or ARC. Longer survival was associated with higher scores on measures of personal control, problem-focused coping and social support. Because AIDS is such a new disease, most of the little knowledge that exists about patients' treatment and survival is very tentative. Research has begun to move quickly now after a slow start.

The psychosocial impact of AIDS

Every epidemic arouses fear — but when so little is known about the disease except that it is so deadly, people tend to react in extreme ways to protect themselves and the people they love. The Australian news media in the mid-1980s had frequent stories of AIDS patients being sacked from their jobs, children with AIDS not being allowed to attend school, families with an AIDS patient being driven from their homes, and health care workers refusing to treat AIDS patients.

Most of these stories have disappeared. Perhaps panic has mellowed to caution, as it should. But many continue to believe that AIDS patients are being punished by God for their misbehaviour (Herek & Capitanio 1993). Assaults and other hate crimes against gay males appeared to increase in the late 1980s and continue at high levels today (Freiberg 1995; Herek 1989). Some irrationality is likely to continue, even among people who are well informed. A beautifully written and sensitive example of this comes from Buffie Kaufman, a medical editor who attended an AIDS volunteer group meeting and met her first AIDS patient named Tom, who

> was literally skin and bones. He walked slowly, unsteadily, and sat down very gingerly on a cushioned chair that was brought in especially for him. He saw the large bowl of jelly beans that I had brought for the group and said, 'Great! I have no appetite anymore, but I can always eat candy.' 'Be my guest,' I replied, not looking directly at him. Would I eat any more jelly beans after he had his hand in the bowl? . . .
>
> Tom has had *Pneumocystis carinii* pneumonia twice, and almost died the second time. Currently he has a fungus infection, tuberculosis, and Kaposi's sarcoma. . . . I felt an overwhelming anxiety, which peaked and diminished often throughout the presentation. I had to control it. . . . Part of me wanted to hug this man; part of me wanted to leave. Can you be compassionate from a distance? (1988, pp. 31–32)

If people recognise the irrationality of their feelings, as Ms. Kaufman did, and are willing to discuss those feelings, they can overcome them. Of course, AIDS patients realise the fears other people have of them and must cope with people treating them 'like a leper'.

Because of the fears about AIDS, and because the disease is often associated with homosexuality and drug abuse in industrialised countries, AIDS patients and their families — which includes lovers — often feel stigmatised (Flaskerud 1988; Herek & Glunt 1988). One of the first questions they consider is, 'Should I tell anyone — and if so, who?' Many with HIV infections don't even tell their immediate family (Simoni et al. 1995). They worry that they will be rejected by family, friends, neighbours, and co-workers. This may lead to their being secretive and withdrawn, thereby cutting off the social support they will need as the disease progresses. For some families, learning of the AIDS diagnosis comes at the same time they first learn that the patient — their child or spouse — is gay, or bisexual, or a drug abuser. Moreover, spouses or lovers fear that the patient has already infected them, too. All of these factors add to the shock family and friends experience when they learn the diagnosis. Sometimes the stigma associated with the disease or the anger these people feel causes them to abandon the person.

The emotional distress of people with HIV and AIDS varies from one person to the next, but most seem to adapt well to their condition (Pugh et al. 1994; Rotheram-Borus et al. 1996). One victim, who had begun to experience some joy as his anxiety faded, said:

> 'This forces you to investigate what you really want your life to be. . . . What's there to be afraid of now?' he asked. 'I live with my greatest fear all the time.' (Hall 1990, p. 1)

Others don't fare as well, fearing they will be abandoned by those they love and suffer pain, debilitation and disfigurement (Flaskerud 1988). The cycles of AIDS-related diseases can arouse feelings of hopelessness and helplessness. Depression may become very severe, especially among those patients who try to cope mainly with avoidance strategies, believe their illness is punishment for past wrongdoings, and have been rejected by people they care about (Maj 1990; Nichols & Santelli 1990; Temoshok 1990a). Preventing and treating emotional distress is important because research has found that depressed HIV patients subsequently show faster disease progression and shorter survival than those who are not depressed (Ironson et al. 1994; Mayne et al. 1996; Patterson et al. 1996). Families and friends can help by trying to maintain a reasonably cheerful but realistic outlook, talking about their feelings and worries, and enlisting the aid of a social network.

Psychosocial interventions for AIDS

Psychosocial efforts for AIDS need to begin when patients are tested for HIV (Sheridan 1991). These individuals usually decide to get tested because they believe they could have the virus. They need carefully presented information to help reduce anxiety during the time before getting the results. Those who test HIV-positive will need counselling regarding the illness, treatment, and the many organisations and support groups available today to help AIDS patients and their families cope. Many HIV-positive individuals eventually provide services for these organisations when they cannot continue in their regular jobs.

People with HIV and AIDS need psychosocial interventions for a variety of problems, including pain management, sleep disorders and adherence to their medical treatments (Sikkema & Kelly 1996). So far, most interventions have focused on using stress management training, exercise and cognitive therapy to promote adaptation, reduce anxiety and depression, and enhance patients' immune function. Studies have shown that these interventions can help HIV-positive patients when begun in the early stages of HIV infection or long after. Research by Michael Antoni and his colleagues (1990, 1991) recruited gay men who did not know their HIV status and randomly assigned them to intervention and control groups. Intervention began weeks before HIV testing and consisted of aerobic exercise, relaxation training and group meetings that included cognitive restructuring methods to modify self-defeating beliefs. Psychological and immunological assessments were made at various points in the weeks before and after notification of the HIV test results. For individuals who tested positive, those who had received the intervention subsequently showed substantially less anxiety and depression and much stronger immune function, and these benefits increased with the amount of relaxation practice they did. Other studies have found that similar interventions also enhance immune function and reduce anxiety and depression for people with advanced levels of HIV or AIDS (Green & Hedge 1991; Lutgendorf et al. 1997; Maj 1990).

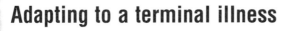

Adapting to a terminal illness

In this chapter we have examined what it is like to live with and adapt to four very different high-mortality health problems. Each of these diseases can disable its victims and progress to the point that the patients and their loved ones are aware that the disease is terminal and death is imminent.

When people talk about the hypothetical prospect of dying, you will often hear them say, 'I hope I go quickly and without pain.' Some people might argue that there are no good ways to die, but almost everyone would agree that a slow and painful death is the worst way. By definition, a terminal illness entails a slow death. The patient typically suffers a progressive deterioration in wellbeing and ability to function and may also experience chronic pain. Although dying from a terminal illness generally takes several weeks, it sometimes takes as little as a few days or as long as several months (Hinton 1984). One factor that affects how people adapt to a terminal illness is the age of the victim.

The patient's age

'Tragic' and 'untimely' are words people often use to describe a young person's terminal illness or death. Psychiatrist Avery Weisman (1976) has outlined several distinctions between *timely* and *untimely* deaths, one of which is whether death is 'appropriate' to the person's age. An 80-year-old's death is more appropriate than a 20-year-old's. Let's consider how people adapt to terminal illness at different times in the life span.

A terminally ill child

Do children know what dying means? Death is a very abstract concept and, as such, it is not well understood by young children (Lonetto 1980; Speece & Brent 1984). Prior to about five years of age, children think death is like living in another place and the person can come back. They may also believe people can avoid death. For instance, a child might conceive of death as a monster and argue that 'you won't die if you run faster than the monster or trick it'. By about eight years of age, most children understand that death happens to everyone, is final and involves the absence of bodily functions.

Most children at an early age have some experience with dying — for instance in the death of a close person, such as a grandparent or neighbour, or of a pet. Dying is not an easy topic for many adults to discuss, and they usually try to spare children the realities of death, saying that the dead person 'has gone away', or 'is in heaven, with Jesus', or 'is only sleeping' (Koch 1977; Sarafino 1986). When a child has a terminal illness, parents sometimes decide not to tell him or her so that the child will have less emotional suffering. But dying school-age children seem to realise the seriousness of their illnesses even when they are not told, and they exhibit far greater anxiety than seriously ill children who are not dying (Spinetta 1974).

Terminally ill children's awareness that they are dying develops gradually: at first, these children recognise that they are seriously ill but believe they will recover; later, they realise that they are continuously ill and will not get better; and then, when they learn of the death of a peer, especially one with a similar illness, they realise that they are dying, too (Bluebond-Langner 1977). Child specialists today generally believe children should know as much about their illnesses as they can comprehend. Because preschool-age children do not understand the meaning of death, there is little need to discuss death with them; the important thing is to allay their concerns about separation from their parents. With older children, an open, honest and sensitive approach seems to reduce their anxiety and maintain a trusting relationship with their parents (La Greca & Stone 1985).

A terminally ill adolescent or young adult

Although some adolescents and young adults, particularly those of the lower classes, think their odds of dying at a young age are fairly high, they envision their deaths as being sudden and violent (Kastenbaum & Costa 1977). If they develop terminal illnesses at this time of life, they realise how unlikely dying at their ages is and feel angry about the 'senselessness' and 'injustice' of it and about not having a chance to develop their lives. As one dying university student put it, 'Now a perfectly good person with an awful lot to give is going to die. A young person is going to die. His death is going to be senseless' (Shneidman 1977, p. 77).

This young man was having a very difficult time coping with his impending death, and his shouting and quarrelsome behaviour were creating problems on the hospital ward. Edwin Shneidman, a therapist whom the patient's doctor called in, has described their meetings.

> When I first saw him, he was sitting up in bed, behaving in a rather feisty and imperious way to the others in the room. . . . In my own heart I decided to see him because I felt that he was in for a rough time, and with his own defenses and alienating behavior, he might turn people away from him and have an unnecessarily psychologically painful death. I began to see him almost every day, alone, just he and I. It developed that he was an only child, his father was dead, and his relationship with his mother for the past several years could be characterized as a running verbal hostile fight. The content of our sessions grew more serious as he became increasingly ill. He sobered and matured enormously in a matter of weeks. (1977, p. 75)

During this time this young man's relationship with his mother became very close, and he noted, 'I have let her love me. I have let her be a mother. She has been so beautiful. I get more comfort from her than anybody else' (p. 76).

Having a terminal illness seems especially untimely when victims have young children. This condition is a threat to the family unit, and the patients feel guilty at not being able to care for their children and cheated out of the joys of seeing them develop. Because of the untimeliness of death at this point in the life span, young adults appear to experience more anger and emotional distress when they have life-threatening illnesses than older individuals do (Leventhal, Leventhal & Van Nguyen 1985).

Terminal illness in middle-aged and older adults

As people develop beyond the early adulthood years, the likelihood of contracting a high-mortality chronic illness — especially heart disease, cancer or stroke — increases sharply. Although dying may not be easy at any point in the life span, it seems to become less difficult as people progress from middle age to old age. Studies have found, for instance, that adults become less and less afraid of death as they get older (Bengston, Cuellar & Ragan 1977; Kalish & Reynolds 1976). Why is this?

Researcher Richard Kalish (1985) has outlined several reasons why the elderly have an easier time than younger individuals in facing impending death. As people get older, developing a terminal illness becomes less unexpected, less of a shock. The elderly know their remaining years are few, they realise that they will probably die of a chronic illness, and they think and talk more about poor health and death than most younger people do. Most of their peers and many relatives are suffering from declining health or have died. They often have made financial preparations, and some have even made plans or given instructions regarding the terminal care they would prefer and their funeral arrangements. In addition, older individuals have a longer past than younger people, which has allowed them the time to achieve more. Patients who have reviewed their past and believe they have accomplished important things and lived their lives well tend to have less difficulty adapting to terminal illnesses than those who do not (Mages & Mendelsohn 1979).

Psychosocial adjustments to terminal illness

As we have seen, most people with life-threatening chronic illnesses manage to adapt reasonably well to their condition over time after the initial crisis, and so do the closest people in their lives. But when their condition worsens and progresses to a terminal phase, new crises emerge that require intense coping efforts.

How people cope with terminal illness

How do terminally ill people and their families cope, and what stresses do they experience? The principal coping mechanism people use during the phase of terminal illness is denial (Hackett & Weisman 1985; Hinton 1984). As we saw in chapter 5, emotion-focused coping is especially useful when the individuals cannot do anything to change their situations. Unfortunately, when people mutually avoid facing the imminent death, they may not discuss with each other how they feel or have any way to 'say their goodbyes'.

Psychiatrist John Hinton (1984) has described three types of stress terminal patients experience. First, they must cope with the physical effects of their worsening conditions, such as pain, difficulty breathing, sleeplessness or loss of bowel control. Second, their condition severely alters their style of living, restricting their activity and making them highly dependent on others. Perhaps two-thirds of dying people are restricted in their activities during the last three months of their lives, and one-fifth of these patients are confined to bed. Third, they typically realise that the end of their lives is near, even when they are not told so. If they are in hospital, as most dying people are, they may think about never going home again or no longer being able to experience the intimacy they used to have with those they love.

Thinking about someone who is dying typically arouses feelings of sadness in people. According to Hinton (1984), healthy individuals who are unaccustomed to serious illness or the declining abilities of age may not realise how well many terminally ill people come to face and accept dying. He has noted by comparison that people with diminished lives — such as many elderly, disabled and bereaved individuals — still get pleasure from their lives

> despite any earlier view that such an existence would be intolerable. The same applies to people who have only a very limited life left. If their obvious stresses are relieved, they may still be capable of enjoyment. It helps if there is a sense of fulfillment; that sense depends on the individual's own values. People may derive their greatest satisfaction from their past family life, their career or the children they are leaving behind. . . . Some have the sense that they need struggle no longer and they can now find peace or believe that their life is now reasonably complete. There may be the conviction that they will rejoin a loved person in immortal existence. . . . With good care many people do achieve a positive acceptance of dying and have a peaceful death. (p. 245)

Patients who are likely to adapt to dying with the least amount of anger or depression are those individuals who are in little pain, receive sensitive and caring social support, feel satisfied with their lives, and have a history of coping well with life's problems and crises (Carey 1975; Hinton 1984; Kalish 1985). Often the person adapts better than his or her loved ones. For instance, spouses of dying people often experience increased health problems, depression and memory difficulties (Howell 1986). Support groups and family therapy can be of great help to dying individuals and their families.

Does adapting to dying happen in 'stages'?

'Time changes things,' people say. Since time passes in the process of dying from a terminal illness, we might expect that patients' reactions would change as they come to terms with their impending deaths. Do these changes occur in a predictable pattern, as a series of stages?

On the basis of interviews with more than 200 terminally ill people, Elisabeth Kübler-Ross (1969) proposed that people's adjustment to dying usually follows a predictable pattern, passing through a sequence of *five stages*. Figure 14.6 describes these stages. Not all the patients she interviewed showed this pattern — a few, for example, continued to deny that they were dying to the very last. But the pattern of adjustments seemed sufficiently regular for Kübler-Ross to propose that coping in most dying people begins with denial and advances through the stages in order.

Do Kübler-Ross's stages correctly reflect the emotional reactions most dying patients experience as they cope with terminal illnesses? Although many people believe most individuals adjust to dying with a predictable and orderly sequence of coping reactions, the evidence from subsequent research does not support this belief (Hinton 1984; Kalish 1985; Silver & Wortman 1980; Zisook et al. 1995). An overview of this evidence indicates that some terminal patients do follow an orderly and predictable sequence of adjustment, but most people's emotions and coping patterns fluctuate back and forth. Some people may go through a specific stage, such as anger, more than once during their adjustment; others experience more than one emotional reaction simultaneously; and some seem to skip stages. Some evidence indicates that people who achieve an 'acceptance' of their impending death die much sooner than those who do not reach this stage (Reed et al. 1994).

Figure 14.6 Kübler-Ross's stages of adjustment to dying

1. *Denial.* The first reaction to the prognosis of death involves refusing to believe it is true. Terminally ill patients say, 'No, it can't be true,' or 'There must be some mistake,' or 'The lab reports must have gotten mixed up.' Denial can be a valuable first reaction by giving patients time to mobilise other coping strategies and motivation to get second opinions. According to Kübler-Ross, denial soon fades in most patients and is replaced by anger.

2. *Anger.* The patients now realise, 'Oh, yes, it is me, it was not a mistake,' and are outraged and irate, asking, 'Why me?' or, 'Why couldn't it have been that miserable no-good guy down the street?' They resent others who are healthy and may show their anger in outbursts towards almost anyone — nurses, doctors and family.

3. *Bargaining.* At this point, patients try to change their circumstances by offering to 'make a deal'. Most of the bargains they try to negotiate are with God, for example thinking, 'Oh, God I promise to be a better person if you'll just make me well.'

4. *Depression.* When bargaining no longer helps and patients feel their time is running out, hopelessness and depression set in. They grieve for things they had in the past and for things they will miss in the future. According to Kübler-Ross, even though depression is painful and may last for a prolonged period, it is helpful because part of the grieving process involves becoming detached from the things in the patient's world. Being detached enables the last stage — acceptance — to occur.

5. *Acceptance.* Patients who live long enough may reach the last stage, in which they are no longer depressed but feel a quiet calm and readiness for death.

Source: Kübler-Ross (1969).

Despite these shortcomings, Kübler-Ross's work has had many positive effects. For one thing, it has been influential in stimulating people's awareness and discussion of the dying process and the needs of terminal patients. It has also led to important and very beneficial changes in the care and treatment of dying people, thereby improving the quality of the last weeks and days of their lives.

The quality of life in death

The medical community and patients' families face one dilemma after another in trying to do what's best for a dying person. Medical technology has made it possible to keep some patients alive only in a legal sense, and societies have begun to question whether these people are alive in a humane sense. The news media describe patients lying in comas for years, dependent on life-support systems to stay alive, but with virtually no likelihood of recovery. An artificial respirator can make a person breathe, and other devices can keep the heart going. The vast majority of American doctors favour withdrawing life-support systems from hopelessly ill or irreversibly comatose individuals if the patients or their families request it (Shogren 1988). In most of the United States, a person who anticipates these circumstances may issue a 'living will' that instructs practitioners not to use extraordinary life-support measures. In Australia, where the 'living will' concept has yet to be firmly established, the situation is somewhat less clear-cut. Forty-five per cent of a sample of South Australian doctors reported that they were in favour of legalised euthanasia under limited circumstances (Stevens & Hassan 1994) and 68 per cent of the same sample believed that formalised guidelines for withholding and withdrawal of treatment in the terminally ill should be available to guide medical practice. Most Australian doctors, however, believe that this should be limited to the withdrawal of ventilator-supported breathing to the unconscious patient suffering massive and irreversible brain damage (Pollard 1991); withdrawal of tube feeding is a much more contentious issue for Australian medicine. Both the ethical (Bates 1992) and legal (Gerber 1994) ramifications of withholding or withdrawal of treatment have been matters of vigorous debate in this country, perhaps signalling that neither doctor-initiated nor patient-initiated termination of treatment to hasten death where continued life is no longer feasible have yet reached the level of certainty which seems to apply in North America. The feature on the next page presents an example of a simple American living will, and offers Australians a possible strategy for the future.

A principal issue that enters into people's judgements about maintaining life support is the patient's quality of life. This is actually an issue that is relevant to all terminally ill people, not just the extreme cases. What kind of medical and psychological care do dying patients need? Who should be responsible for that care, and where should it be given? These are the main issues we consider in this section.

Medical and psychological care of dying patients

The terminal phase of care begins when medical judgement indicates that the patient's condition is worsening and no treatment is available to reverse or arrest the progress towards death (Benoliel 1977). At this point, medical treatment is mainly *palliative*, that is, it focuses on reducing pain and discomfort. This phase of treatment can be very distressing not only to the patients and their families, but to medical personnel, who entered the medical field to save lives. Terminally ill people in the United States can request that the specific instruction 'Do Not Resuscitate' be entered on their hospital charts. If they begin to die — for instance if the person's heart stops beating — the medical staff is not to interfere. The legal situation in Australia is far more ambiguous (Gerber 1994) and the patient's rights in such situations are not yet resolved in this country.

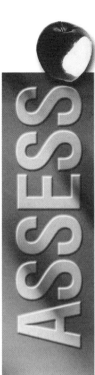

Assess yourself

YOUR LIVING WILL CHOICES

Fill out the *Health Care Living Will and Proxy* below, indicating what your wishes would be if you were unable to make decisions about your medical treatment, such as if you were in a coma. What specific treatments would you *want* or *not want* to receive? Whom would you choose as your agent or 'proxy' in making decisions if you were unable to make them? This person should be an adult who is familiar with your personal and health care views — someone you would trust to make the decisions you would make.

HEALTH CARE LIVING WILL AND PROXY

TO MY FAMILY, DOCTORS, AND OTHER CONCERNED PARTIES:

I, _____ (the *principal*), being of sound mind, make the following advance directives to be carried out if I become unable to make or communicate decisions about my medical treatment.

LIVING WILL

I request the withdrawal or withholding of life-sustaining procedures, consistent with my desire that I be permitted to die naturally if the situation occurs that I am either (1) near death with no reasonable likelihood of recovery or (2) in a coma or vegetative state and my doctors believe that there is no significant possibility of my ever regaining consciousness or higher functions of my brain. Under these circumstances, I specifically:

1. *DO NOT* want the following treatments I have *initialled*.
   - Cardiac resuscitation _____
   - Artificial respiration _____
   - Artificial feeding or fluids _____
   - Other (specify) _____

2. *DO* want the following conditions I have *initialled*.
   - Medication to relieve pain _____
   - To die at home, if possible _____
   - Other (specify) _____

PROXY

I designate here (1) a *first proxy*, _____ (name), to make decisions in accordance with the wishes and conditions specified above, or as he or she otherwise knows, and (2) a *second proxy*, _____ (name), as a substitute if the first proxy is unable, unwilling or unavailable to act as my health care proxy.

If this were a legal document, you and two witnesses would need to sign it.

Some living wills are much more complicated than this one, having the person make dozens of choices regarding many different medical procedures that might be considered in very different scenarios. One concern in being so specific is that knowledge about treatments can change: Suppose evidence on the effectiveness of a treatment changes between the time a patient rejects it in the will and the scenario actually occurs. What then?

Individuals who work with dying people on a daily basis must come to grips with the feelings of failure and loss they experience when patients die (Benoliel 1977; Maguire 1985). In an effort to protect themselves from this pain and to perform efficiently given their heavy work loads, medical staff often distance themselves psychologically from terminally ill people. By doing this, doctors and nurses avoid dealing with the psychological problems these patients have. How do staff members distance themselves? They may simply not ask about the person's feelings or adjustment, or they may provide false reassurance, saying, 'I'm sure you'll feel better soon,' when they believe otherwise. The staff may also use selective attention, as illustrated in the following interaction.

SURGEON: Well, how are you today?

PATIENT: (dying of breast cancer): I'm very worried about what is happening to me. I'm beginning to think I'm not going to get better this time. The pain in my hip is getting worse.

SURGEON: Tell me more about this pain in your hip. (Maguire 1985, p. 1711)

Although this patient mentioned both physical and psychological difficulties, the physician followed up only on the physical one. This may lead the patient to conclude that it is not appropriate to discuss psychological problems with medical staff.

Should terminally ill people be told they are dying? This is a controversial question, and medical personnel often face the dilemma of believing people have the right to know and being instructed by the patient's family not to tell (Maguire 1985). Some doctors and psychiatrists take the view that the issue of whether to tell the patient is moot, since terminally ill people generally realise they are dying and that the prognosis should be given to the patient and family together (Weisman 1977; White 1977). In his view, practitioners should be 'compassionately candid' for medical reasons, to give the person the right to choose or refuse treatments, and to encourage the patient and family to be prepared psychologically and legally. Other doctors note that some patients would prefer not to know, and these wishes should take precedence. To follow this approach, doctors need to probe sensitively to assess the person's wishes. Those who prefer not to know may be given the option of having their families handle all decisions (Blackhall et al. 1995).

Although many people are able to approach death with a feeling of acceptance and peace, others become very troubled. What can be done to help dying patients cope? In some cases, hospitals may provide individual psychotherapy for those individuals who are clearly having difficulty (Shneidman 1977). Health care workers may also be able to provide information about support groups that have been developed specifically to improve the quality of life for people with terminal illnesses. In addition, professionally led group therapy appears to be effective in helping terminal patients face their impending deaths with less anxiety and depression and a greater sense of control over their remaining life span (Levy 1983; Solomon & Temoshok 1987). In Australia each of the State and Territory cancer councils provide both group-based and help line (telephone) based support services for those with terminal cancer to assist both with living the remaining time to its fullest potential and with preparing for death. The comprehensive programs offered by the Anti-Cancer Council of Victoria (which can be seen on the Web at www.accv.org.au) and the New South Wales Cancer Council (www.nswcc.org.au) provide excellent examples of this.

A place to die — hospital, home or hospice?

Most people in Australia die in hospitals. Although hospitals can provide a great deal of expertise, technical equipment and efficient caretaking, they are usually not 'psychologically comfortable' places for people. The environment there is unfamiliar, and often it is mechanical and impersonal. Patients have little control over their daily routine and activities, and they lack access to such things as photo albums or musical recordings, for example, that they have relied on in the past for enjoyment and to enrich their experiences. Moreover, most of the people there are strangers, not family or friends. As a result, many terminally ill people would rather die at home, and many do. Is this a reasonable alternative?

Home care for the dying patient

Whether home care is a reasonable alternative for a dying person depends on his or her condition and the quality of care available at home. Although few terminal patients require prolonged, complex care, some do and may be better off at the hospital (Garfield 1978). Can patients receive good terminal care at home? Yes, they can. Studies have found that terminally ill people who have regular contact at home with a medical team and whose family members are trained receive very good care (Malkin 1976; Zimmer, Juncker & McCusker 1985). Unfortunately, many dying patients may not have the option of home care because they lack family members who are able to provide the care they need or financial resources that may be required.

Caring for a terminally ill person at home can be a physically and emotionally exhausting experience (Hinton 1984). There may be only one individual at home who can provide the care, and all of the burden falls on that person's shoulders. If the patient requires continuous attention, the life of that one caretaker may become limited to coping with the dying person's needs. This may go on for weeks or, sometimes, months. Even when there is more than one person available to help, their lives are to some extent restricted by the needs of the patient. Some terminally ill people are bedridden and need to be fed and bathed, for instance. Despite these hardships, many people who have cared for dying persons at home claim it is extremely rewarding to know they have done everything they could to make the last days or weeks as pleasant as possible for someone they love.

Hospice care for the dying patient

Is it possible to combine the strengths of a professional support system with the warm and loving care one can get at home, thereby helping terminal patients die comfortably and with dignity? This question led to the development of the concept of **hospice care**, which involves a medical and social support system to provide an enriched quality of life — through physical, psychosocial and spiritual care — for terminally ill people and their families (Cioppa 1984; Drake 1990). In the hospice approach, the staff consists of a medically supervised team of professionals and volunteers. Much of the physical care the staff provides is designed to reduce discomfort and pain, often with the use of drugs.

The hospice care approach to caring for dying people originated in Great Britain, largely through the efforts of physician Cicely Saunders, who was originally trained as a nurse and social worker (Saunders 1977; Torrens 1985). After working at a hospice in Ireland, she founded St. Christopher's Hospice near London in 1967. Originally, hospices were designed as separate institutions for the purpose of caring for dying patients on an in-patient basis. But as the philosophy of hospice care spread to

Australia, the organisational structure for delivering this care began to broaden. Hospice services in Australia are available today both *at home* and at many *in-patient facilities*, a lot of which are housed in hospitals or nursing homes. When home hospice care is used, services are provided on a part-time, regularly scheduled basis and staff are available on call 24 hours a day, seven days a week (Cioppa 1984).

In-patient facilities generally try to make the environment as much like home as possible, often including a kitchen and family room area. If the facility is in a hospital, existing policies need to be adjusted to satisfy the goals of the program. These adjustments often include:

- flexibility in visiting hours, including regulations that permit children and pets to visit
- freedom to wear one's own clothes
- provision of alcoholic beverages and meals prepared by family members
- expertise in palliative care and management of symptoms, especially the relief of pain
- psychologic and spiritual counselling for patients as well as family members
- arrangements with family members for assisting patients and their families in completing unfinished business (Cioppa 1984, p. 597).

In the hospice care approach, the patient and his or her family are considered to be the 'unit of care'. What this means is that all of these people together form a system, with each individual affecting the others and each needing hospice attention. Therefore, patients and their families actively participate in the development of a plan for the care of the whole unit (Cioppa 1984). Cicely Saunders (1986) has outlined several 'essential elements' in the hospice approach, some of which deal with psychosocial issues. First, people who are dying should be in a *place of choice* as they end their lives. They and their families should decide whether that place should be at home or in an in-patient setting. Second, the care given during the terminal phase should enable patients to *maximise their potential*, so that they perform to the limits of their physical, cognitive and social potential, particularly as active members of their families. Third, the care should *address all family members' needs*, which may involve help resolving interpersonal discord and feelings of anxiety, guilt and depression. Fourth, *follow-up care* is available, and family members can continue to receive help through and after the period of bereavement.

Does hospice care help patients and their families cope better with the dying process than conventional care does? The testimonials from patients and family members are massive and glowing, describing the programs as enormously supportive and enriching. A study has found that the quality of life is better with in-patient hospice care than standard hospital care (Viney et al. 1994). Evidence from the small number of carefully controlled studies of in-patient hospice and conventional care suggests that both provide similar pain control and daily activities, but hospice patients show less anxiety and greater satisfaction with their care (Torrens 1985).

The survivors: and life goes on

Whether a person dies suddenly and unexpectedly or with warning over a long period of time, the survivors must then come to terms with the death and eventually pick up the pieces of their lives. The state of having lost someone through death is called *bereavement*; this state is characterised by feelings of *grief* and the expression of these feelings in *mourning*.

People adapt to their bereavement in their own individual ways. This process takes time, usually at least a year, but it does not seem to follow any particular pattern or stages, and there is no good rule of thumb to predict how long it will take (Joyce 1984; Silver & Wortman 1980; Zisook et al. 1995). Each grieving person needs to adjust at his or her own pace, and urgings to 'start living again' may be both insensitive and unproductive when they occur early in the adjustment process. A longitudinal study of individuals whose spouses either survived or succumbed to serious illnesses revealed that the psychological distress of individuals whose spouses died was similar before and soon after the death, remained high for about a year, and was greater for middle-aged than elderly individuals (Hays, Kasl & Jacobs 1994). Several types of psycho-social interventions, such as individual therapy and support groups, can help people adjust to their losses (Zisook et al. 1995).

The AIDS epidemic has revealed two important issues about bereavement in gay individuals. First, many experience long series of bereavements within a few years, without time to complete their mourning between deaths. This has happened to many gay men in big cities who have experienced multiple losses — often losing their lovers and most of their friends — to AIDS. Coping with terminal illness repeatedly takes a severe emotional toll, and each death adds to the toll with increased demoralisation, sleep problems and stress reactions (Martin 1988; Martin & Dean 1993). Second, gay individuals who have lost their lovers receive less social support from others, such as bosses and co-workers, than heterosexuals do. For example, a man who was troubled by his lover's death and was performing below par at work reported that his getting little understanding from his boss 'makes me feel depressed, angry, and used. ... I really loved him and I do miss him' (Moskowitz et al. 1996, p. 49). People in the larger society probably do not realise that gay couples' relationships can be so strong and loving.

Some people think coming to terms with the loss of someone we love means we forget that person — he or she no longer means anything to us. This is not so. People who eventually adapt to the loss may feel recurrent moments or periods of sadness years later, especially on anniversaries or other significant dates (Joyce 1984). A mother who lost her infant child years ago wrote:

My mind does not mourn yesterday
It mourns today
The images that pass before my eyes
Do not recall the infant son
But see you running through my house
A teenage child in search of food and gym shoes and maybe me.
I do not mourn you for what you were,
But for what can't be . . .
(Anonymous, cited in Silver & Wortman 1980, p. 337)

The death of a child is one of the most tragic events that can happen to a family, and parents often experience grief for many years after the loss (Knapp 1987).

When a parent dies, the surviving children need special attention and under-standing. Often the surviving parent is so caught up in his or her own shock and grief that the children's emotional needs are not adequately addressed. Many surviving parents say little about the death and exclude their children from the mourning process. It is not unusual for children to show little sense of loss or outward grief when a close family member dies (Koch 1977; Sarafino 1986). Young children do not understand fully what death is, and this may account for their seeming lack of concern. Older children may be so confused and shocked by the tragedy that they are simply numbed emotionally. Their outward calmness should not be mistaken as a sign that they do not love the dead person. Sometimes their grief comes out later, and sometimes it happens privately.

During the first weeks after the death of a spouse, the surviving husband or wife usually receives a great deal of attention from friends and relatives. But soon this changes, and the bereaved person may feel isolated in efforts to organise his or her life and make decisions alone. A widow or widower must gradually become involved again in work and leisure activities, in maintaining old friendships and developing new ones, and, perhaps, in finding a new mate. One man described his experience as a widower in the following way.

> Having to 'date' in the early 40s, or older, and after long years of marriage is, for many, an unnerving experience. I suggest there is something even worse — not getting out and having companionship.
>
> How the widower chooses to begin his new social and sex life depends, of course, on his personality, his philosophy, and the sort of companionship he wants. Some widowers prefer to join Parents Without Partners, where they are sure to meet people with common interests. Like the majority of widowers, I had friends and relatives who put forward suggestions and invited me to dinner parties. I found most of these either tedious or painful. One night . . . however, I did meet a beautiful woman. She was a widow, with one child. . . . We are a complete household again and throughout the home there once again is the sound of laughter, of music and, best of all, the rich sound of meaningful conversation between children and their parents. (Lindeman 1976, pp. 285–6)

Of course, not all stories of people's coping with the loss of someone they love have happy endings. Some bereaved individuals never adjust to the loss. But with the help and support of others and a determined drive on their own part, most people can build a new and once again enriching life. The social support bereaved people need can come from family and friends, but support groups may be especially helpful.

Summary

People with high-mortality illnesses do not know for sure what the course of their diseases will be or if or when they will die. But their lives are threatened, and they and their families must adapt to living with uncertainty. Convalescing people tend to be optimistic about their future health, but watchful for symptoms and changes in their condition. Families can help patients adapt by encouraging them to develop reasonable plans and to carry them out, rather than encouraging helplessness and dependence. In adapting to illness over a long period of time, patients make cognitive adjustments by finding meaning in their illness experiences, gaining a sense of control over their illnesses, and restoring their self-esteem. A recurrence or relapse of the condition creates a new, and often very difficult, crisis.

Heart disease is the leading cause of death in Australia and cancer is second. Coronary heart disease may show up in an episode of angina pectoris or of myocardial infarction. The prevalence rate for heart disease is greater in men than in women and increases with age. Cardiac rehabilitation involves the use of medication, a program of exercise, stress management, and changes in diet and other aspects of lifestyle, especially if the person smokes, drinks too much or is overweight. Many heart patients fail to comply with the exercise programs and lifestyle changes. Most cardiac patients who were employed before the illness eventually return to work, often in less demanding jobs. Some people with heart disease need special interventions to enhance adaptation.

A stroke can cause damage to the brain through either an infarction or a haemorrhage. Depending on the amount and location of neurological damage, patients may suffer motor and cognitive deficits. Some impairments recover with time and rehabilitation, but others are permanent. Deficits may involve motor action, aphasia, visual disorders and emotional disorders. Stroke patients are very prone to depression.

Although there are many varieties of cancer, they can be classified into four types: carcinomas, lymphomas, sarcomas and leukaemias. Untreated neoplasms eventually metastasise and spread to other parts of the body. The most common sites of cancer are the skin, prostate gland, breast, lungs, colon or rectum, and uterus or cervix. Medical treatment consists of surgery, radiation and chemotherapy, each of which has important drawbacks. Chemotherapy, in particular, causes nausea and vomiting that is associated with learned food aversions. Despite the great stress cancer victims experience, most show a remarkable ability to adapt with time during remission or after a cure. Some, however, become very depressed and withdraw from social contact but usually benefit from psychosocial interventions. Leukaemia is the most common form of cancer in childhood.

AIDS and its precursor, ARC, are caused by HIV infection, which impairs the immune system, leaving the victims subject to opportunistic diseases. Most people with AIDS die within one or two years of reaching that stage of their disease. Because AIDS is an infectious disease, many people have reacted to its outbreak with alarm and discrimination, making adaptation all the more difficult. Psychosocial intervention can reduce anxiety and depression and enhance immune function.

If and when a chronic condition deteriorates and no cure is likely, the illness is considered terminal. One factor that affects how people adapt to terminal illness is the age of the patient. Adults see the death of a young person as particularly tragic and untimely. Young children have little understanding of the meaning of death; by about eight years of age, children's understanding is fairly complete. Adolescents and young adults react to their impending deaths with very strong feelings of anger and emotional distress. As adults get older, they become less fearful of death. Dying people may react to their condition with denial, anger, bargaining, depression and acceptance. The hospice care approach provides physical, psychosocial and spiritual care for dying patients and their families during the terminal phase and in bereavement.

Key terms

acquired immune deficiency syndrome	angina pectoris	hospice care	myocardial infarction
AIDS-related complex	cancer	learned food aversion	stroke

PART 7

Looking to the future

Chapter 15
What's ahead for health psychology?

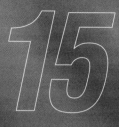

15 What's ahead for health psychology?

Prologue

'Oh, this looks very good,' the palm reader said as she studied Rick's hand. She explained: 'Your life line is very long, which usually means you will have a long and prosperous life. At first I thought this break here in the line meant you might have a serious health problem in your 50s, but these lines here at your wrist suggest otherwise. You'll have a long and healthy life!' Rick was relieved. He had come to have his fortune told rather than being tested for HIV. He knew that his past behaviour put him at risk for HIV infection, but he couldn't bring himself to reveal this to the palm reader. Unreasoned behaviour is not uncommon when people are very anxious.

Predicting the future is always a chancy enterprise. Still, because the field of health psychology is at an early stage in its development, many people wonder what the field and its goals will be like in the future. This chapter will try to predict what's ahead for health psychology, and our crystal ball will involve the views of noted researchers and trends that seem clear in recent research. As we consider what the crystal ball suggests, we will try to answer questions you may have about the field's prospects. What role will future health psychologists play in medical care? Are career opportunities and training programs for health psychologists likely to expand? How will the field's goals, issues and perspectives change? What factors will affect the success and direction of health psychology in the coming years?

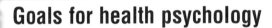

Goals for health psychology

Health and health care systems around the world have changed dramatically over the past several decades. People in most parts of the world today are living longer and are more likely to develop chronic illnesses than ever before. Many current health problems result from or are aggravated by people's long-standing habits, such as smoking cigarettes and coping poorly with stress, that medical professionals lack sufficient skills and time to change. The field of health psychology has made enormous advances in the past 15 to 20 years in Australia, generating new knowledge and applying information gained from many disciplines to supplement medical efforts in promoting health. Let's look at some major goals that lie ahead for health psychology.

Enhancing efforts to prevent illness

We have seen that efforts to prevent health problems should try to reduce unhealthy behaviours. These efforts can be directed towards three stages of health-protective activity: *health behaviours* before an illness occurs, *illness behaviours* after symptoms appear, or *sick-role behaviours* once the illness is identified and treatment starts.

Health-related behaviours that become features of people's lifestyles have received a great deal of attention in health psychology. Many of the health problems people develop result at least partly from lifestyle behaviours, and efforts have been directed towards preventing these behaviours from developing and changing unhealthy behaviours that have already developed. Unhealthy lifestyles seem to be harder to change than to prevent (Wright & Friedman 1991). We have seen that psychologists' efforts to change lifestyle behaviours such as smoking, exercising and eating habits have focused mainly on cognitive and behavioural approaches. Although these approaches are often very effective in producing initial changes, the behaviours frequently revert back to the unhealthy patterns after the interventions end. Relapse is a critical problem that researchers are working to reduce (Mattick & Baillie 1992), and it will certainly be an important focus for health psychology in the future.

Once people notice symptoms or are diagnosed with serious health conditions, they often — but by no means always — engage in illness and sick-role behaviours to protect their health. For instance, they may go to doctors, take medication or even follow medical advice that involves changing their lifestyles. Researchers have identified many psychosocial factors that influence whether people will seek health care and adhere to medical treatments. We know, for example, that individuals often decide to reject or delay seeking medical attention because they don't know the symptoms of serious diseases, such as cancer or diabetes. And people are less likely to adhere to medical advice if the treatments involve complex or long-term behavioural changes and if their doctors do not seem caring or explain the illnesses and treatment clearly. Although we know some methods to reduce these problems, these methods often require extra time or effort that medical professionals are just beginning to incorporate into their practices. Health psychologists in the future will continue their search for ways to improve patients' use of health care services and adherence to medical treatments.

Since the mid-1980s important theoretical advances regarding why people do or do not change unhealthy behaviours have built on the knowledge gained from earlier theories, especially the health belief model. The *stages of change model* outlines a series of stages in people's readiness to change health-related behaviours. Another recent theory is the *biobehavioural model* of cigarette smoking. It takes a biopsychosocial view, proposing that individuals continue to smoke cigarettes and have difficulty quitting because they depend on nicotine to regulate their cognitive and emotional states. These and other theories are beginning to generate important research that will undoubtedly contribute to our understanding of ways to promote healthier lifestyles. The findings from this research will enable psychologists to apply techniques with individuals and in community programs for health promotion more effectively.

One other issue relating to future efforts in health promotion should be mentioned: it is possible for people to become *overly concerned* with preventing illness (Becker 1990; Brownell 1991). This issue can take two forms. First, individuals may struggle to achieve impossible goals that require overriding strong biological forces, as often happens when obese adults set their sights on having slim, athletic bodies. Second, some healthy people become obsessive in trying to adhere to too many restrictions, worrying if they occasionally have a piece of cheesecake or fail to exercise. Future health promotion efforts need to identify and emphasise the most important risk factors that people can change.

Improving efforts for helping patients cope

Major advances have been made since the 1970s in using psychosocial methods to help people cope with various difficulties in their lives. Stress management programs are being applied widely with non-patient populations, such as in work-site wellness programs, to help prevent illness.

People with serious medical conditions often must cope with pain, anxiety and fear, and depression. Psychosocial interventions are being applied more and more widely with patients in pain centres, hospitals and other medical settings. Years ago the main function of psychologists in medical settings involved administering and interpreting tests of patients' emotional and cognitive functioning (Wright & Friedman 1991). But this situation has changed, and psychologists are focusing much more on a broader array of activities, such as training medical students and doctors and applying interventions to help patients cope with illnesses and medical treatment (Johnstone et al. 1995). The future is likely to see the role of health psychologists expand substantially in hospitals and out-patient rehabilitation programs for people with chronic health problems, such as heart disease and nervous system injuries (Frank, Gluck & Buckelew 1990).

Documenting the efficacy and cost–benefit ratio of care

Should health care organisations and employers provide psychosocial interventions to prevent illness and help patients cope? Perhaps most people would answer, 'Yes, because it's the humane thing to do.' But with today's spiralling medical costs, the answer is more commonly based on two factors: the intervention's *efficacy*, or the degree to which it accomplishes what is needed, and its *cost–benefit ratio*, or the extent to which providing the intervention saves more money in the long run than it costs (Jospe, Shueman & Troy 1991; Kaplan 1989). These 'bottom line' issues often are weighed heavily in deciding whether to offer wellness programs or psychosocial interventions at work at the community level and in medical settings.

Primary prevention is undoubtedly the most cost-effective approach in averting illness before it develops. In chapter 6 we saw that the PRECEDE/PROCEED model offers guidelines on how to evaluate the efficacy of a health program in terms of its impact and achievement of goals.

Health psychologists recognise the importance of documenting the efficacy of approaches they use, and they do careful research to compare different approaches against each other and control groups. But psychologists are not accustomed to calculating the financial costs and benefits of interventions and, with some exceptions (Milgrom, Walter & Green 1994), seldom do these analyses. Often the costs of providing an intervention are easily assessed, but the full benefits are not. At a work site, for instance, what benefits of a wellness program could you assess in dollars to compare with the costs of running it? You might assess worker absenteeism or medical insurance claims, but these variables would reflect only part of the benefits. They wouldn't reflect other important financial gains, such as in workers' improved job satisfaction and resulting increases in productivity. In medical settings, measuring the benefits of psychosocial interventions can be easier — for example, you could assign dollar values to the reduced time intervention patients spend recovering in the hospital and compare these data with the cost of the program.

Many psychosocial interventions for promoting health and helping patients cope have the potential for producing far more financial benefits than costs (Cummings 1991). More and more evidence is becoming available to document these effects (Friedman et al. 1995; Sobel 1995). We considered research in chapter 10 showing, for example, that hospital patients who receive help in coping with medical procedures recover more quickly and use less medication than those who don't receive such help. Other studies have shown that the financial savings are far greater than the costs of providing psychosocial and educational interventions to help pregnant women stop smoking and other patients manage their pain and control their asthma (Stieg & Turk 1988; Taitel et al. 1994; Windsor et al. 1993). Educating people about the benefits of cancer screening may lead to increased screening, and thus earlier detection of some cancers, although this needs to be weighed against any adverse effects (e.g. colonic perforation resulting from screening procedures for colon cancer).

Australian health psychologists have played an invaluable role in their work on psychological aspects of, and behavioural strategies for, the prevention of many cancers. The Centre for Behavioural Research in Cancer (CBRC) of the Anti-Cancer Council of Victoria has been prominent in research into the behavioural epidemiology of smoking. The centre is well-known for its studies on smoking prevalence and smoking cessation. The CBRC is also actively involved in consultative and advisory activities relating to health education, health promotion and program evaluation for the Anti-Cancer Council's health programs, one of which is the quit smoking campaign. Apart from its preventive health focus on smoking, the CBRC has conducted extensive population prevalence studies in the areas of skin-protection behaviour, Pap-smear testing, breast self-examination and screening mammography.

Significant contributions have also been made by Australian health psychologists in the area of clinical oncology practice. For instance, Foot and Sanson-Fisher (1995) have conducted needs assessment research among cancer patients that identified unmet needs for health information and psychological issues. Attention has been given to the factors influencing cancer screening (Cockburn et al. 1991), outcomes of breast self-examination (Hill et al. 1988), patients' beliefs about cancer management (Buchanan et al. 1996) and patient perceptions of cancer treatment (Rassaby & Hill 1983).

Australian health psychologists have been prominent in many other areas of research and intervention of benefit for patients and their families. Some of these areas include cardiac rehabilitation (Byrne 1987), psychological interventions for migraine sufferers (Martin 1993), and improving doctor–patient communication (Feletti, Firman & Sanson-Fisher 1986; Redman et al. 1989). Viney and associates have conducted extensive research using a phenomenological approach to understanding the patient's experience of chronic illness (Viney & Westbrook 1982; Westbrook & Viney 1981; 1982), reactions to heart disease (Viney & Westbrook 1980); reactions to diabetes (Viney & Westbrook 1982), and the role of biographical and illness-related factors in preferences for strategies for coping with chronic illness (Viney & Westbrook 1982).

Although most psychosocial methods with documented efficacy have not yet been subjected to cost–benefit analyses, health psychologists in the future will probably give much more attention to these analyses than they have in the past. They will also need to develop more effective methods to help people change unhealthy lifestyles — particularly with regard to using tobacco, eating healthy diets, exercising and solar protection — and demonstrate that the benefits of these methods outweigh the costs.

Enhancing psychologists' acceptance in medical settings

In an article in the late 1980s a woman described her experience when she developed breast cancer. Her doctors advised her to get treatment from a variety of medical professionals but did not recommend the involvement of a psychologist.

At no point did anyone in the medical fraternity recommend that I see a mental health professional to help me cope with the emotional impact of breast cancer. Perhaps they didn't realise that breast cancer had an emotional impact. But I did. So, I went to see a psychologist, ironically the one specialist not covered by my insurance. It was worth the cash out of pocket. (Kaufman, cited in Cummings 1991, p. 119)

Although gaining acceptance by the medical profession has progressed steadily since the early 1980s, it continues to be a major challenge for health psychology.

Part of the difficulty health psychologists have faced in gaining acceptance in medical settings stems from their past role and training. Before the mid-1980s in Australia psychological services were usually seen as tangential to the medical needs of most patients, and psychologists had little or no training in physiological systems, medical illnesses and treatments, and the organisation and protocols of hospitals. But these conditions have been changing quickly. Today health psychologists are receiving the training they need to work effectively in medical settings. More and more doctors are coming to recognise the importance of psychosocial factors in their patients' health, adherence to treatment regimens and rehabilitation. They also realise that they do not have the skills or time to address many of these factors.

But initial relations between medical staff and health psychologists still tend to be strained in some settings, particularly when one function of the psychologist may be to teach doctors and interns the 'people skills' that are important for interviewing patients and communicating with them effectively. This kind of training may get a mixed reception, especially from some medical staff who feel these skills are not part of medicine (Christensen & Levinson 1991). Even after medical and psychological staff have collaborated for a long time and seen that a biopsychosocial approach to health care can benefit patients, be intellectually stimulating and lead to developing new techniques, their different styles and points of view can lead to conflicts (McDaniel & Campbell 1986). For example, psychologists generally want to talk directly with the attending physician to describe subtle and complex issues relating to a patient's treatment plan, but medical specialists typically communicate with each other

through notes in the hospital chart, which follow a particular pattern, showing the person who referred the case, the reason for the referral, the consultant's observation of the patient, the tests performed, the results of the tests, the conclusions reached, and the recommendations for the patient's care. (Huszti & Walker 1991)

These kinds of differences can be resolved, and future relations between medical and psychological staff will become increasingly integrated. Physicians who have called upon the services of psychologists in hospitals appear to be satisfied with the outcome, but would like their patients to receive more follow-up services after being discharged (Huszti & Walker 1991).

What about patients — how do they feel about receiving psychological services? Their view is likely to depend on the way the doctor and psychologist introduce these services. If a patient thinks the services are offered because his or her doctor thinks he or she is 'crazy' or that the problem 'is all in your head', the patient is likely to have negative attitudes and fail to cooperate. People are more likely to view psychosocial interventions positively if the services are introduced as *part* of a *standard* 'team approach' with a biopsychosocial orientation.

Frank and Ross (1995) best sum up the process that is required for collaborative health care delivery in medical settings involving the health psychologist and other professionals as one of

> clearly defining and establishing psychology's role in health care [which] requires efforts at delineating psychology's unique contributions amid an increasing supply of other health-related professions. Caution must be used to avoid creating or perpetuating turf wars among professionals. Rather, efforts to establish clear professional boundaries and identities among the various health care groups should be based on dialogue, coordination, and cooperation to ensue that the health care needs of the population are met by qualified, ethical, and competent professionals. (p. 524)

Careers and training in health psychology

Most health psychologists follow one of two career categories: those who work mainly in a clinical capacity with patients and those who work mainly in community health promotion. Other health psychologists work in an academic or research capacity, training students in clinical and population health intervention skills, and conducting research that informs the conceptual basis of health services (Nathan, Milgrom & Martin 1996; Sweet, Rozensky & Tovian 1991). Health psychologists are guided in their work by the scientist-practitioner model, so it is common for many health psychologists to have careers that combine the above areas, being involved in both clinical and academic or research activities, and some do administrative work such as in government agencies or programs to promote health.

Career opportunities

The opportunities for careers in health psychology in Australia have generally been good, especially in health care settings — in hospitals and clinics and in community health promotion (Milgrom, Nathan & Martin 1996; Sanson-Fisher & Newell 1996; Touyz et al. 1992). For example, the number of psychologists in health care has increased greatly since Carlson and Sheppard's (1992) reporting of 60 per cent of the 3197 surveyed psychologists with membership in the Australian Psychological Society indicating research, teaching or clinical activities in health psychology. However, many barriers remain to the effective use of health psychology in the Australian health care system, particularly in the areas of (a) breaking the medical hierarchy and (b) public health care funding. While the use of health psychologists in the management of post–heart attack patients has been well established, many hospitals still do not use psychologists effectively but prefer to employ nurses or social workers in roles for which psychologists are better trained. A very recent report from the Cancer Strategy Working Group of the Commonwealth Department of Health and Aged Care (2001) has only now advocated the explicit employment of psychologists to deal with the management of anxiety and depression in patients newly diagnosed with cancer. What the job market will be in the future for health psychologists is hard to predict, but career opportunities in a variety of settings will probably continue to grow.

Besides hospitals, where else do health psychologists work? Some of the more prominent sites are:
• universities
• medical schools

- rehabilitation centres
- pain centres
- private practice and consultancy offices
- government departments and agencies.

Sometimes job descriptions for these settings are broad, opening them even to professionals from non-psychology fields, such as nursing, public health or social work. Although this can increase the competition for those jobs, broad job descriptions can increase the number of opportunities for psychologists, too. Being able to adapt psychological skills to diversified roles within the health system will be crucial for health psychologists seeking employment in the future (Frank & Ross 1995).

Training programs

What kind of training is available and necessary in health psychology? Training is offered at two educational levels: (1) At the undergraduate level, health psychology has been taught as a unit within the generic psychology degree program at most Australian universities. Currently, there is no undergraduate degree in health psychology. Undergraduate programs specifically targeted towards health psychology would be unacceptable to the accreditation process run by the Australian Psychological Society, since the Society believes that the first four years of study should contain basic science and not professional specialisation. (2) Health psychologists typically hold doctoral degrees, and many graduate programs now exist in Australia and other countries specifically for that training. Several master's programs in health and clinical psychology in Australia offer specialist training. Doctoral-level supervision in a health psychology area of research is also common in Australia along similar lines to the European apprenticeship model (Richards 1992). As the field develops, postdoctoral programs will be made available in health psychology or behavioural medicine, particularly for individuals with doctoral degrees that did not focus on the relationship between health and psychology.

Graduate and postdoctoral training programs in health psychology are diverse (Altman & Green 1988; Belar 1988, 1991). Some are highly interdisciplinary programs that are designed solely for this field. They often specialise in training students either for research careers or for direct clinical service to patients. Other programs provide graduate training in traditional psychology areas, such as clinical or social psychology, and contain special tracks or emphases relating to health. Common to all these programs is a solid grounding in psychology, along with training in research methods, biopsychosocial processes in health and disease, and health care terminology and organisation. Programs that educate students for direct clinical service to patients generally include medical courses, such as in physiology and pharmacology. The future may see greater standardisation of health psychology training programs in Australia and around the world, as some professionals have recommended (Maes & Kittel 1990; Methorst, Jansen & Kerkhof 1991; Richards 1992).

Information about graduate and postdoctoral training programs in health psychology can be obtained by contacting the following professional organisations:
- College of Health Psychologists, Australian Psychological Society Ltd, P.O. Box 126, Carlton South, Victoria 3053. Telephone: (03) 8662 3300 or 1800 333 497 (Freecall). E-mail: natloff@psychsociety.com.au. Web site: http://www.aps.psychsociety.com.au.
- Australasian Society of Behavioural Health and Medicine, Cancer Control Research Institute, 100 Drummond Street, Carlton VIC 3053. E-mail: Michael.Fotheringham@accv.org.au

Issues and controversies for the future

Findings from research and clinical experience will enable health psychologists to help societies resolve important issues and controversies in the future. We will look at several examples, beginning with the impact of environmental conditions on health and psychology.

Environment, health and psychology

Each of the varied environments in which people live around the world contains conditions that have the potential to harm the health and psychological status of its inhabitants. We read and hear in the news media that the environment is becoming increasingly polluted with toxic substances, which may be released accidently or deliberately into the air, ground or bodies of water. The environments in which people live are also becoming more crowded and noisy. What effects do these conditions have? How can we reduce harmful environmental conditions? Some answers use a public health approach: Because cigarette smoke pollutes the air and can lead to illnesses in those who breathe it, some psychologists have called for government control of tobacco products and regulation of smoking behaviour (Borland et al. 1994; Owen & Halford 1988). Workplace smoking bans in Australia have been effective in reducing smoking by up to 25 per cent (Borland, Owen & Hocking 1991; Borland & Owen 1995).

Many toxic environmental pollutants are produced as by-products either of manufacturing or of generating energy. For instance, some manufacturing industries produce highly toxic cyanide or mercury as by-products, which have made their ways into the environment. Power plants and automobiles generate energy along with potentially harmful by-products such as sulfur dioxide, carbon monoxide and nuclear radiation. What direct effects on health does long-term exposure to low levels of these pollutants have? How stressful is it to live or work in contaminated environments, and how much does this stress affect health? How much do the stresses of crowding and noise affect health? Health psychologists can help in efforts to answer these questions and find ways to change behaviours that produce these problems (Weinman 1990). Although we have some information on these questions, much more research will be needed in the future before we can provide accurate answers.

Quality of life

People's *quality of life* has become a significant issue in medical care because (1) it is reduced when they become sick and stay sick, and (2) it is an important consideration in prevention efforts before and after an illness occurs. Efforts to maintain people's good health also maintain their quality of life, and efforts to help patients recover quickly and fully lessen the negative impact of the illness on their lives. For people who are ill, their quality of life enters into decisions about the medical and psychological treatment they will receive. Are they in pain? If so, what type of pain-killing medication should they get, and how much? If they're distressed, what psychosocial methods are likely to improve their emotional status?

Life-or-death medical decisions are often heavily influenced by appraisals of patients' current and future quality of life. Current quality of life is especially important if there is virtually no hope of the patient's recovery. In such cases, the views of the patient, family and medical staff are likely to come down to a judgement of whether living in the current state is better than not living at all. Future quality of life is important in medical decisions that can enable the patient to survive, but will leave him or her with seriously impaired physical, psychological and social capacities. For example, the family of an elderly man with a disabling cardiovascular condition felt he would be better off not living

> if he was just going to be a vegetable. They said his whole life revolved around working in his yard and playing bridge; these were the things in life that gave him joy. Now the doctors were not giving any hope that he would ever get back to what he was before; the best that could be hoped for was that he would be able to sit in a wheelchair. They said they didn't want that for him, and … he wouldn't want that for himself either. (Degner & Beaton 1987, p. 64)

Decisions to withhold heroic medical efforts clearly involve humane concerns, but financial considerations are important, too (Spurgeon et al. 1990). Heroic medical efforts and aftercare are extremely expensive. With the enormous pressures to contain the cost of health care, are these expenses always justified even when the resulting quality of life will be poor?

Making medical and psychological decisions based on a patient's current or future quality of life is difficult, partly because researchers need to determine the best ways to measure it. The 'well-year' proposed by Kaplan and Bush (1982) is a useful indicator of wellbeing. It represents 'a year of completely well life, or a year of life free of dysfunction, symptoms and health-related problems' (p. 64). For each person, the number of well-years can be calculated beyond a certain age — say, 65 years — or after a medical event, for example the number of years a coronary heart patient lives free from chest pain or a second infarction. A related approach uses a scale called *quality-adjusted life years* (QALYs, pronounced 'QUAL-eez'). To calculate the QALYs for a medical treatment, we would assess how long a person is likely to live after receiving the treatment, multiply each year by its quality of life, and total these data (Bradley 1993; Kaplan 1994). Using QALYs, we could rank the value of different treatments for a particular person or in general, perhaps even taking the cost per QALY into account, and decide whether to provide the treatment. At the heart of this approach is the measurement of quality of life. Although there are dozens of questionnaires to assess quality of life, the qualities they measure vary widely (Gill & Feinstein 1995; Wilson & Cleary 1995). Which should we use? Health psychologists will play an important role in resolving measurement problems and how best to use quality of life assessments in making treatment decisions.

Ethical decisions in medical care

Suppose you were an obstetrician delivering a baby when you realised that complications you see developing will surely kill the baby and maybe the mother, too. Suppose also that the mother flatly refuses a Caesarean delivery for religious reasons. What do you do? The typical medical response is to seek an immediate court order to override her decision. The decisions made in this case and the ones we have just considered relating to quality of life all involve ethical issues. Many hospitals today have *bioethics committees* to discuss ethical issues in health care, make policy and recommend action regarding specific cases. The ethical issues these committees consider often involve the patient's right to choose treatments, to withhold or withdraw treatment (Bouton 1990). We will now examine two other important issues: the role of technology in medical decisions and the role of doctors in helping patients die.

Technology and medical decisions

The technological advances we have seen in our lives over the past few decades have been quite remarkable. Many of these advances have been in medical technology, and they have sometimes raised important ethical questions.

One of these technological advances is a computer program called APACHE III that calculates the odds that individual patients will die in intensive care or after they leave it (Seligmann & Sulavik 1992). Why might this be a problem? Decisions about continuing to provide intensive care treatment are made every day based on the likelihood that it will help the patient survive. The alternative decision is to transfer the person to a regular hospital ward. These decisions are based on doctors' broad estimates, such as, 'Her chances look bleak.' With the computer program, doctors can get precise estimates of the person's odds of dying if he or she continues in intensive care (say, 42 per cent) versus if he or she were transferred (say, 78 per cent). In this example, transferring the patient would greatly increase the odds that he or she would die. The comparison helps in making the decision. The ethical problems relate to how these numbers will be used. Should doctors tell families these numbers? Will doctors and families weigh these data too heavily in their decisions? Will hospitals release these data to insurance companies, which could then decide to limit coverage when scores drop below some level? Health psychologists can play a role in some of these decisions, especially those relating to families having and using these data (Weinman 1990).

Other ethical dilemmas arise in deciding whether to provide an organ transplant for patients. In 1998, 517 kidney transplant operations were performed in Australia (AIHW 2000). Health psychologists help medical practitioners to select candidates who are best able to benefit from the surgery and the scarce organs because these people are able to cope with the stress and behave appropriately to maintain their health with the new organ. To help make these decisions, psychologists screen potential candidates; some will be clearly up to the task, and some will not — for example candidates for liver transplant who have not been able to control their drinking. Others will be in between and may benefit from interventions of behavioural contracting and therapy to help them cope better (Olbrisch 1996).

Advances in genetics technology may also present ethical problems. For instance, geneticists are now able to identify individuals who are likely to develop serious diseases, such as cystic fibrosis and some forms of cancer, and may soon be able to identify individuals who are vulnerable to environmental causes of cancer and heart disease (Detjen 1991; Lerman, Audrain & Croyle 1994). Who should be tested for these risks, and who should have access to the results? Insurance companies would like this information, and some are already turning down applicants for insurance on the basis of known family histories of certain diseases.

Assisted suicide and euthanasia

Some people with serious illnesses come to the decision that they want to end their lives. Should doctors help them in their wishes? This is a very controversial issue for society in general and in the medical community. Among doctors, some feel they should not help because of certain beliefs they hold, such as that life is sacred or that medical workers should only save lives and not take them. Other doctors feel they should participate in this act if the patient 'is indeed beyond all help and not merely suffering from a treatable depression of the sort common to people with terminal illnesses. Such a depression requires therapeutic intervention' (Wanzer et al. 1989, p. 848). Depressed people who want to end their lives may change their minds if the depression is reduced (Zisook et al. 1995). This was found to be the case in Australian research, which indicated that while 44 per cent of elderly patients with depression wanted to end their lives, this figure declined to 11 per cent after treatment for depression (Hooper et al. 1997).

Some doctors have helped patients end their lives in two ways (Wanzer et al. 1989). In *assisted suicide* the patient takes the final act, but the doctor knowingly prescribes the needed drugs or describes the methods and doses required. Because of the legal consequences for doctors who help people take their lives, a book called *Final Exit* was published in 1991 describing the procedures doctors would recommend. In *euthanasia* the doctor (or someone else) takes the final act, usually by administering a drug that ends the life. Euthanasia is permitted under certain circumstances in the Netherlands. While euthanasia was legal for a brief time in the Northern Territory, in 1997 legislation to allow euthanasia was overturned.

In 1998 the Australian Psychological Society released a discussion paper, 'Psychological Perspectives on Euthanasia and the Terminally Ill', in which arguments for and against euthanasia were put forward for debate (Sanson et al. 1998). Some of the arguments for euthanasia centred on respect for sufferers' autonomy, to end suffering and to reduce reliance on life-support systems. Arguments against euthanasia included respect for human life, to eliminate the possibility of coercion or loss of autonomy in sufferers, impaired decision-making in the sufferer, conflicts of interest and misuse, as in genocide or ethnic cleansing. If societies decide in the future that it is acceptable for doctors to help a patient end his or her life, psychologists should be consulted to assess the person's emotional status and ability to make sound decisions, and to determine if psychosocial intervention might be helpful (Clay 1997).

Future focuses in health psychology

Although the research that contributes to our knowledge in health psychology comes from many different fields, early studies gave a relatively narrow view of the bio-psychosocial processes involved in health and illness because of the people researchers tended to recruit as subjects: They often were 18- to 60-year-old white American males. This focus existed for many reasons — for instance, these subjects often were more readily available, and some researchers incorrectly believed that the findings with these subjects would easily generalise to other populations. In the 1980s, studies began to broaden their focus to include subjects representing a wider range of people. This trend will surely continue in the future.

Also neglected in health research have been physiological measures in favour of psychological measures (Maes & Kittel 1990; Stone 1990). This most likely reflects the training of psychologists who have come to health psychology from the related fields of clinical and social psychology. In the future, health psychologists will have received the necessary training in endocrinology, immunology and other medical subspecialties to allow for a greater emphasis on physiological parameters. A greater focus in research is also needed on macro-level social factors and how these are related to behaviour, health and disease. While multivariate prospective research has increased over the past fifteen years, longitudinal research should continue to establish patterns of health behaviour and changes to illness resulting from psychological intervention.

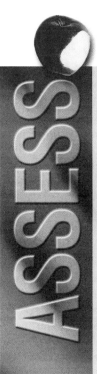

Assess yourself

SOME ETHICAL DILEMMAS: WHAT DO YOU THINK?

Each of the following cases describes a decision involving an ethical dilemma that is related to health. Circle the 'Yes' or 'No' preceding each case to indicate whether you agree with the decision.

Yes No A 47-year-old woman developed cirrhosis of the liver as a result of long-term alcoholism. She promised to stop drinking if she could receive a liver transplant. Her request was denied because of likely future drinking.

Yes No An overweight, chain-smoking, sedentary 51-year-old man with high blood pressure had his first heart attack seven years ago. His request for a heart transplant was denied because of continuing risk factors.

Yes No A 28-year-old married woman with a hereditary crippling disease that is eventually fatal decided to become pregnant, knowing that there was a 50 per cent chance that she would pass on the disease to her baby and that she would not consider having an abortion.

Yes No A 37-year-old executive was told by his boss that he would have to pay half of the costs of his employer provided health insurance if he did not quit smoking and lower his cholesterol.

Yes No An obese 20-year-old woman who refused to try to lose weight was expelled from nursing school, despite having good grades and clinical evaluations, because it was said she would 'set a poor example for patients'.

Yes No A 24-year-old man was denied employment as a bank clerk because he was overweight and smoked cigarettes.

Yes No A 30-year-old woman was denied a promotion to a job that involved working in an area with gases that could harm an embryo if she were to become pregnant.

Yes No A year after a boy developed leukaemia, the company that provided his family's health insurance quadrupled their premium.

These dilemmas are all based on examples that have appeared in the news media. Because they all involve controversies, there is no key to the 'right' answers. But you might want to ask friends or classmates what they think.

Life-span health and illness

We have seen that the health problems people have and the extent to which they use health services change with age. Individuals who are either very young or elderly use health services more than others do, and the elderly are much more likely to have chronic health problems than younger people are.

From conception to adolescence

Children's prenatal environments have a major effect on their health. Large numbers of babies are born each year in Australia with illnesses or defects that develop because of prenatal exposure to harmful conditions or chemicals, particularly when mothers use alcohol, drugs or tobacco during pregnancy. The health problems these babies develop can last for years or for life. Health psychologists are studying ways to improve babies' prenatal environments, such as by educating and counselling prospective parents (Weinman 1990). Although these approaches help, we need to find more effective ways to prevent these health problems from developing.

Childhood and adolescence are important periods in the life span because many health beliefs and habits form during these years. But very little research has examined how these beliefs and habits develop (Weinman 1990). We do know that efforts to promote health should be introduced early, before unhealthy beliefs and habits develop. Early childhood is clearly the time to intervene for some behaviours, such as for proper diets, exercise, dental care and seat-belt use. In later childhood, interventions should focus on preventing accidents, cigarette and drug use, and unsafe sex. We saw in chapter 7, for example, that programs to prevent children from starting to smoke cigarettes have had some success. We have also seen that behaviours that put people at high risk for AIDS can be changed substantially, thereby reducing their risk. Efforts to prevent the spread of HIV need to be intensified in the larger population. To design more effective health promotion programs, we will need to focus more research — especially longitudinal studies — on how health behaviours form and change in childhood and adolescence.

Adulthood and old age

By the time people reach adulthood, most health-related values and behaviours are ingrained and difficult to change. People's lifestyles during the early adulthood and middle-age years tend to continue and affect whether or when they will develop major chronic illnesses, particularly heart disease and cancer. The earlier they change unhealthy behaviours, the lower their risks become.

People in most areas of the world are living longer, and the proportion of elderly individuals in the population is increasing. As the population ages, the proportion of individuals with disabling or life-threatening illnesses will surely grow, thereby requiring more health services and psychosocial interventions. In Australia, for example, an unusually high birth rate after World War II created a very large generation of people called 'baby boomers', who now are swelling the ranks of the middle-aged. What happens down the road when their risk of serious health problems increases? How will the Australian health care system respond to the added load? This potential makes it even more crucial that we find ways to help people prevent or change risky lifestyles, particularly with regard to diet, exercise and substance use. Health psychologists may be called on to use their clinical expertise in the management of behaviours in the elderly residing in nursing homes, or for those in rehabilitation care (Johnstone et al. 1995; Kneebone 1996). They will also need to improve ways to help families cope with the difficulties of caring for elderly relatives. The number of studies dealing with health issues in old age published each year has increased since the early 1980s and will continue to be a major focus of health psychologists in the future to ensure that the elderly enjoy quality of life despite loss of sensory capacities, and that they are treated with dignity as they adjust to any chronic debilitating conditions.

Sociocultural factors in health

We have seen in many chapters that sociocultural differences in Australia and around the world are related to health and health behaviour. For instance, socioeconomically disadvantaged Australians and indigenous people tend to have poorer health and health habits than whites and the more economically advantaged. Lower socioeconomic groups are also less likely to take advantage of preventive services such as addiction treatment programs or screening (National Health Strategy 1992). These differences have been clear for a very long time. Although researchers have begun to investigate why these differences exist and what can be done to reduce them, our knowledge on these issues is not yet very specific. For example, we don't know how cultural customs and socio-economic factors shape the everyday lives of different ethnic groups (Anderson & Armstead 1995; Kaplan 1995), so we tend to draw broad conclusions, as when we say people in a minority group 'live in environments that do not encourage the practice of health-protective behaviour'. Health psychology must give greater emphasis to socio-cultural issues so that we can provide more specific and useful solutions in the future.

Cross-cultural research also needs more emphasis. We have scanty information about cultural differences in lifestyles, conceptions of health, perceiving symptoms of illness, and using health services, but most research on these differences is old and very incomplete. Notions of health determine how people perceive symptoms, whether they seek medical care and how they approach treatment recommendations. For instance, the concept of health for Australian indigenous people

> embraces spiritual, religious and social aspects which are very different to the non-indigenous biomedical model of health. The inclusion of issues relating to land rights, the number of Aboriginal people in gaol, restoration of dignity, pride and respect, as well as stronger cultural laws are indicative of the need to address social justice and cultural issues within the concept of health held by Aboriginal people in Australia. (Perkins et al. 1995; p. 274)

Indigenous people in some regions of Australia believe that they are powerless to affect health outcomes, attributing sudden illness or death to supernatural forces (Brady 1995). Health care delivery for indigenous people needs to be sensitive to these different views of disease causation and conceptions of health.

A related issue concerns the notion of health promotion for indigenous people. At the basis of health promotion is the assumption that individuals are responsible for their own health. Marks et al. (2000) argue that personal responsibility is based on a Westernised cultural value of individualism. For Aboriginal Australians, this focus on one's own health over that of the wider group with which they identify is discordant with the essence of Aboriginality. Health promotion may be impeded in indigenous communities if the emphasis is on individual health rather than community health.

The study of health psychology outside North America and Australia is advancing slowly, even in Europe (Schmidt & Dlugosch 1991; Stone 1991). In developing countries, where infectious diseases and malnutrition are often rampant, more than 16 million children under the age of five die each year (Elder et al. 1989). The number of people infected with the HIV virus in Africa and other developing areas of the world is astounding and growing rapidly (Cowley 1994). The countries with the most urgent need to change behavioural risk factors have not yet recognised that principles of health psychology can help promote public health. In addition, health psychologists need to conduct research to determine how to adapt the principles that work in Australia and other industrialised countries to the needs of other cultures (Elder et al. 1989).

Gender differences and women's health issues

Health issues relating to women and gender differences were also neglected in health psychology research until the early 1980s (Blechman 1983; Matthews 1989). Since that time, studies have begun to examine health issues that are specific to women, such as menstrual problems and reactions to breast cancer, and differences between males and females in a wide variety of characteristics, such as reactions to stress, Type A and B behaviour patterns, risk of AIDS and of heart disease, weight regulation, and tobacco and alcohol use. On the issue of breast cancer, for instance, researchers have shown that mammography screening markedly reduces breast cancer mortality and that certain types of programs are more effective than others in promoting women's screening use (Kerlikowske et al. 1995; Rimer 1994).

Gender-related research has become a main focus of health psychology today and for the future. This research is making clearer the uniqueness of women and men in their health and health-protective behaviours and the special interventions they are likely to need to promote their health.

Factors affecting health psychology's future

The picture of health psychology's future that we have considered is based on trends and needs that seem clear today. But trends and needs can change, and the prospects for our discipline will depend on forces and events in society, medical fields and psychology (Pattishall 1989; Weinman 1990). What factors are likely to affect the role and direction of health psychology in the future?

Some factors are likely to have a broad impact on health psychology, affecting the amount and type of research, clinical intervention and health promotion activities that we do. One of these factors is monetary: How much financial support will there be for these activities? During hard economic times, cutbacks in government and private funding may reduce this support. But there is another side to this issue — health care costs around the world are increasing, and many experts in health believe that two of the best ways to decrease these costs involve improving people's health behaviours and helping those individuals who become ill to recover quickly. Research findings have enabled health psychologists to help reduce costs in both of these ways. Funding will also depend on how health insurance and services are structured. Health care systems are changing rapidly in many countries. The changes that emerge will probably continue or strengthen support for psychosocial interventions with favourable research evidence regarding their cost–benefit ratios.

Another factor that can have a broad impact on health psychology's future is education and training in this discipline (Weinman 1990). Undergraduate courses in health psychology can reach students from various non-psychology fields, such as nursing, pre-med and sociology. Students who have a positive view of the role and success of health psychology are likely to promote its research, application and inter-disciplinary contacts in the future. If these students go into medical fields, they are likely to be receptive to learning about psychosocial methods by which they and health psychologists can promote the health of their patients. These circumstances can enhance acceptance of health psychologists in medical settings.

Developments in medicine will also influence the future of health psychology (Weinman 1990). New and growing health problems generally require psychosocial interventions to reduce people's risk factors for these illnesses and help patients and their families cope. This can be seen clearly in the role of health psychology in addressing these kinds of issues in AIDS and Alzheimer's disease, for instance. Health psychologists often have an important role to play when new medical treatments are found, particularly if these treatments are unpleasant or if they may impair the patient's quality of life.

As you can see, many factors will affect the future of health psychology. Although a significant number of psychologists, both clinicians and academic researchers, have been offering health services and conducting research in health-related areas for several years, the profession of health psychology in Australia is still in its infancy. The field has made dramatic advances in its short history, but we still have much to learn. As we enter the new millennium, Australian health psychologists are in the unique position of creating and shaping this field to reflect the health priorities of Australians and to work towards a healthier nation. We hope that this book will inspire students, clinicians and other health professionals to take up the challenge. The future of health psychology in Australia is now!

Summary

Major changes have occurred in health and health care systems around the world in the past several decades. People are living longer today and are more likely to develop chronic illnesses that result from or are aggravated by their longstanding health habits. Health psychology has made major advances in helping to prevent or change these behaviours. The field has also developed effective psychosocial methods to help patients and their families cope with these illnesses. For many of the interventions health psychologists use, favourable cost–benefit ratios have been demonstrated through research. These successes have helped to promote the acceptance of health psychologists in medical settings.

Career opportunities for health psychologists have expanded rapidly, and the employment outlook for the future continues to look good. The availability of training in health psychology has grown at undergraduate, graduate and postgraduate levels. This training is solidly based in psychology and includes a substantial amount of information on biopsychosocial processes in health and illness and on medical terminology and procedures.

Health psychology has begun to address important health issues and controversies that societies will need to resolve in the future. These issues and controversies include the impact of environmental pollutants on people's health and psychological status, patients' quality of life and ethical decisions in medical care. Some ethical questions relate to the use of technological advances in health care and whether physicians should participate, through assisted suicide or euthanasia, in helping hopelessly ill patients end their lives. Health psychology has also begun to focus its attention on life-span, socio-cultural and gender issues in health. The future role and direction of health psychology will be affected by forces and events in society, medicine and psychology.

Appendix

Requirements for the training of health psychologists and membership of the APS College of Health Psychologists (appendix to table 1.1, pp. 19–21)

Core and specialist competencies

Core competencies

All Health Psychologists demonstrate competencies to permit:

(a) the development and application of psychological theory (including cognitive and behavioural theory) to physical health promotion and/or illness prevention, diagnosis, rehabilitation and/or treatment.

(b) understanding and advancement of the health system, including knowledge of relevant Commonwealth and State health regulations and priorities, professional communication to optimise biopsychosocial health care and advance health system organisation.

Specialist competencies

The organisation of the College anticipates and encourages the increasing specialisation of Health Psychologists. Health Psychologists are currently employed across a continuum spanning two main areas — Health Psychologists working in the Health Promotion area concerned with illness prevention and health promotion, and Health Psychologists working in the Clinical Health area applying psychology in illness diagnosis, treatment and rehabilitation. Health Psychologists are expected to evidence competence in one or both of these specialisations described below.

(a) Health Psychologists in the Health Promotion area work at the family, community and organisational level and are engaged in risk factor research, health promotion, disease prevention and public health advocacy. Training and experience should evidence competence in the following: assessment of health risks; system level health intervention design, delivery and evaluation; public health advocacy.

(b) Health Psychologists in the Clinical Health area typically work with individuals or families and are engaged in the application of psychology in the diagnosis, treatment and rehabilitation of illnesses in in-patient or out-patient medical settings, or community or organisation health settings. Training and experience should evidence competence in the following: psychological assessment and diagnosis relevant to physical illness; psychological and behavioural management and treatment of illness; treatment of health risk behaviours; enhancement of medical investigation and treatment; encouragement of illness adaptation; provision of psychological support for health professionals and carers of patients.

Source: APS (2001).

Glossary

abstinence-violation effect   a cognitive process in which a relapse occurs when people feel guilt and reduced self-efficacy as they experience a lapse in efforts to change their behaviour

acquired immune deficiency syndrome (AIDS)   an infectious disease that disables the immune system. Individuals with AIDS are susceptible to a variety of life-threatening diseases.

acupuncture   a pain-control technique in which fine metal needles are inserted under the skin at certain locations and then activated

acute pain   the discomfort patients experience with temporary medical conditions, lasting less than about six months

adaptation   the changes people undergo in making adjustments to circumstances in their lives

addiction   the condition of physical and psychological dependence on using a substance

adherence   the degree to which patients follow the medical recommendations of practitioners; also called *compliance*

adoption studies   research with subjects adopted at very early ages, comparing their characteristics with corresponding traits of their adoptive and natural parents to assess the influence of heredity

adrenal glands   endocrine glands that secrete several hormones, such as cortisol, epinephrine and norepinephrine, that are involved in stress reactions

aerobic exercise   (air-OH-bik) sustained and energetic physical activity in which the body uses high volumes of oxygen over many minutes

AIDS-related complex (ARC)   a stage in the development of AIDS during which the immune system begins to falter and some disease symptoms appear

alarm reaction   the first stage in the general adaptation syndrome when the body's resources are mobilised

alcoholics   people who drink alcohol heavily and are addicted to it

algogenic substances   (al-go-JEN-ik) chemicals released at the site of tissue damage that cause inflammation and signal injury

Alzheimer's disease   a chronic and progressive brain disorder marked by a loss of cognitive functions, such as memory

angina pectoris   (AN-ji-nah PEK-to-ris) a condition marked by chest pain that generally results from a brief or incomplete blockage of the blood supply to heart tissue

anorexia nervosa   (an-or-EX-ee-ah ner-VOE-sah) an eating disorder marked by self-starvation and an extreme and unhealthy loss of weight

antibodies   protein molecules created to protect against specific antigens in body fluids

antibody-mediated immunity   the immune process that employs antibodies to attack antigens while they are still in body fluids and before they have invaded the cells

antigen   any substance that can trigger the immune system to respond

arteriosclerosis   (ar-TEER-ee-o-sklehROE-sis) a condition in which fatty patches have accumulated and hardened on artery walls, thereby reducing the elasticity of these walls

arthritis   a category of painful and potentially disabling chronic conditions that involve inflammation of the joints

asthma   a psychophysiological disorder of the respiratory system in which bronchial inflammation and spasms lead to episodes of breathing difficulty

atherosclerosis   (ATH-eh-roe-skleh-ROE-sis) the condition in which fatty patches (plaques) form on artery walls

attribution   the process by which people attempt to judge or explain events or their own or others' behaviour

autonomic nervous system   a division of the peripheral nervous system that carries messages between the central nervous system and the internal organs. It has two parts: the sympathetic and parasympathetic nervous systems.

aversion strategies   methods that use unpleasant stimuli to discourage undesirable behaviours

B cells   lymphocytes that lead to the formation of antibodies

behavioural control   a form of personal control involving the ability to reduce the impact of a stressor by taking concrete action

behavioural medicine   an interdisciplinary field introduced in the early 1970s to study the relationships between behaviour and health

biobehavioural model   the theory that people who smoke, e.g., come to depend on nicotine to regulate their cognitive and emotional states in coping processes

biofeedback   a process by which individuals can acquire voluntary control over a physiological function by monitoring its status

biomedical model   the view that illness results from physical causes, such as infection or injury; psychosocial processes are not viewed as causal factors

biopsychosocial model   the view that health and illness involve the interplay of biological, psychological and social factors in people's lives

blood pressure   the force of the blood against the inner walls of the arteries

brainstem   the lowest portion of the brain, located at the top of the spinal cord, consisting of the midbrain, reticular system, pons and medulla

buffering hypothesis   the view that the health benefits of social support come from its reducing the negative health effects of high stress levels

bulimia nervosa   (buh-LIM-ee-ah ner-VOE-sah) an eating disorder marked by repeated binge eating, usually followed by purging

burnout   an emotional and behavioural impairment resulting from exposure to high levels of occupational stress

cancer   a class of malignant diseases in which cells proliferate in an unrestricted manner, usually forming a tumour

carbon monoxide   a gas that is a constituent of cigarette smoke

carcinogens   chemical or physical agents that can cause cancer

cardiovascular system   a network of organs that circulates blood to supply oxygen and nutrients to the body's cells and removes wastes and other substances

casemix   a type of managed care in which diseases are classified into diagnostic related groups (DRGs), with hospital funding determined by the cost of treating certain diseases

case study   a non-experimental method in which a researcher uses interviews, past records and current observations to construct a biography of a single subject

catecholamines   (kat-eh-KOL-a-meenz) a class of hormones, including epinephrine and norepinephrine, secreted by the adrenal glands

cell-mediated immunity   the immune process that operates at the cellular level, using T cells to attack infected cells

central nervous system   that part of the nervous system consisting of the brain and spinal cord

cerebellum   (ser-uh-BEL-um) a large portion of the brain that coordinates motor activities and maintains body balance

cerebrum   (ser-EE-brum) the upper and largest portion of the human brain. It has primary control over motor and mental activity.

chromosomes   threadlike structures in the nucleus of each cell that contain genes that carry hereditary information

chronic diseases   illnesses that persist and generally get worse over a long period of time

chronic/intractable/benign pain   long-term continuous, but variable, discomfort stemming from benign causes

chronic/progressive pain   long-term continuous discomfort that worsens as the underlying malignant condition progresses

chronic/recurrent pain   long-term repeated and intense episodes of discomfort stemming from benign causes

clinical pain   any pain symptoms that receive or require professional treatment

cognitive appraisal   the mental process people use in assessing whether a demand is threatening and what resources are available to meet the demand

cognitive control   a form of personal control involving the ability to reduce the impact of a stressor by using thought processes

cognitive restructuring   a therapeutic process for replacing thoughts that provoke stress with ones that do not

cognitive therapy   a cognitive restructuring approach that has clients test hypotheses about maladaptive beliefs they hold about events in their lives

cohort effect   the influence of different subjects having been born and raised in different eras

commonsense models   cognitive representations people develop regarding specific illnesses

compliance   see *adherence*

conflict theory   an explanation of health-related behaviour that includes both rational and emotional factors

coping   the process by which people try to manage the stress they experience

coronary heart disease (CHD)   a class of illnesses that result when a narrowing or blockage of the coronary arteries restricts the blood supply to the heart muscle (myocardium)

correlation coefficient   a statistic that reflects the degree and direction of relationship between two variables; it can range from +1.00, through 0.00, to −1.00

correlational studies   non-experimental research conducted to determine the degree and direction of relationship between variables

corticosteroids   (cor-ti-koe-STEH-royds) a class of hormones, including cortisol, secreted by the adrenal glands

counter-irritation   a technique whereby one pain is reduced by creating another

crisis theory a model describing the factors that affect people's adjustment to having serious illnesses. The theory proposes that coping processes are influenced by three types of factors: illness-related, background and personal, and physical and social environmental.

critical incident stress debriefing (CISD) a type of crisis intervention, recommended to take place in the first 72 hours following a critical incident, in which the incident and associated thoughts and emotions are discussed, symptoms recorded and coping strategies considered

cross-sectional approach method of studying developmental trends by observing different groups of subjects of different ages within a relatively short period of time

daily hassles everyday annoyances or unpleasant events

decisional control a form of personal control involving the ability to reduce the impact of a stressor by choosing between alternative courses of action

depersonalisation a behavioural style of some practitioners that involves treating a patient as if he or she were not there or not a person

depressants drugs that induce relaxation and sleep

detoxification the process of getting an addicted individual safely through withdrawal after discontinuing the use of a substance

diagnostic related group a classification system used for grouping certain medical conditions for casemix funding

dietary diseases illnesses that result from poor nutrition

digestive system the network of organs that processes ingested food by breaking it down for the body's use and excreting the remains

direct effects hypothesis the view that the health benefits of social support accrue regardless of whether people experience high or low levels of stress

distraction a pain management technique in which people divert their focus to non-pain stimuli in the environment

doctor-centred the behavioural style of some doctors in which interactions with patients are highly controlled by the practitioner and focus on the symptoms or treatment rather than the person

double-blind an experimental procedure whereby neither the subject nor the researcher knows which research treatment the subject is receiving

dynamic approach an approach to understanding reactions to disaster that considers factors before, during and following the impact

emetic drug (eh-MEH-tik) a chemical that induces nausea when a person drinks alcohol

emotion-focused coping approaches people use for managing stress that are aimed at regulating their emotional responses

endocrine system an array of glands that secrete hormones into the bloodstream

endogenous opioids (en-DAH-je-nus OH-pee-oydz) opiatelike substances the body produces naturally that reduce the sensation of pain

enzymes (EN-zymz) substances that increase the speed of chemical reactions in cells

epidemic the situation in which the occurrence of a health problem has increased rapidly

epilepsy a chronic condition of the nervous system that produces recurrent seizures

essential hypertension persistent high blood pressure with no known organic cause

experiment a controlled study in which variables are manipulated and observed to assess cause–effect relationships

extinction in operant conditioning, a process by which a previously reinforced behaviour no longer receives reinforcement, making it less likely to occur in the future

gate-control theory an explanation of pain perception that proposes that a neural gate in the spinal cord can modulate incoming pain signals. The opening and closing of the gate is influenced by messages that descend from the brain and by the amount of activity in pain fibres and in other peripheral fibres.

general adaptation syndrome (GAS) the sequence of physiological reactions to prolonged and intense stress. The sequence consists of the alarm reaction, the stage of resistance and the stage of exhaustion.

genetic counselling a service in which prospective and expectant parents may receive information regarding their risks of giving birth to children with genetic defects

group norm the expected behaviour of members of a group, and the attitudes towards the behaviour demonstrated by that group

hallucinogens (ha-LOO-sin-a-jins) drugs that can produce perceptual and cognitive distortions

hardiness an array of personality characteristics that enable individuals to withstand stress and not succumb to its negative health effects

health a positive state of physical, mental and social wellbeing that changes in degree over time

health behaviour activity undertaken by people who believe they are healthy to prevent future health problems

health belief model an explanation of people's health-related behaviour based on their perception of the threat of illness or injury and the pros and cons of taking action

health-protective behaviour any behaviour people perform with the intention of promoting or maintaining wellbeing regardless of the state of their health

health psychology a field of psychology introduced in the late 1970s to examine the causes of illnesses and to study ways to promote and maintain health, prevent and treat illness, and improve the health care system

healthy migrant effect the better health status of some migrant groups, compared with Australian-born individuals, due to factors such as the staple diet of the group or Australian immigrant selection criteria based on health status

high-density lipoprotein (HDL) a cholesterol-carrying protein that is associated with decreased cholesterol deposits in blood vessels

hormones chemical substances secreted by endocrine glands that affect body functions and behaviour

hospice care a philosophy and procedure for enriching the quality of life of terminally ill patients and their families

hypertension the condition of persistent high blood pressure

hypochondriasis (hy-poe-kon-DRY-uhsis) the tendency of some individuals to be excessively concerned and vigilant regarding their health and body sensations

hypothalamus a part of the forebrain that contains control centres for many body functions, such as eating, drinking and sexual activity

iatrogenic conditions (eye-a-tro-JEN-ik) health problems that develop as a result of medical treatment

illness behaviour activity by people who feel ill with the purpose of determining the state of their health or finding a remedy

illness/wellness continuum a model that describes health and sickness as overlapping concepts that vary in degree, rather than being separate categories

immune system the organs and structures that protect the body against harmful substances or agents such as bacteria and viruses

impact evaluation assessment of the achievement of health program objectives; that is, whether behavioural and environmental factors were altered successfully as a result of implementing the program

incidence the number of *new* cases reported during a given period of time, such as the previous year

infectious diseases illnesses caused by the body being invaded by micro-organisms such as bacteria or viruses

inflammatory bowel disease a psychophysiological disorder involving wounds in the large or small intestine

informational control a form of personal control involving the ability to reduce the impact of a stressor by acquiring knowledge about impending events

insulin a hormone secreted by the pancreas that speeds the conversion of blood sugar to fat

insulin-dependent diabetes mellitus (IDDM) the health problem of having chronically elevated blood sugar levels because the pancreas produces little or no insulin. IDDM patients typically require daily insulin supplements

irritable bowel syndrome a digestive system disease with symptoms of pain, diarrhoea and constipation but no evidence of organic disorder

isokinetic exercise (eye-so-kin-EH-tic) a type of activity that involves exerting muscle force in more than one direction while moving an object

isometric exercise (eye-so-MET-rik) a type of activity that involves exerting muscle force against an object that does not move

isotonic exercise (eye-so-TAH-nik) a type of activity that involves exerting most of the muscle force in one direction

Lamaze training an educational and procedural program for natural childbirth that involves preparation, participation and minimal medication

lay referral system an informal network of individuals who provide advice or information regarding a person's symptoms and health

learned food aversion a phenomenon in which a food becomes disliked as a result of being associated with symptoms of illness

learned helplessness a condition of apathy or inactivity that results from repeated experiences with unavoidable stress

life events major occurrences in people's lives that require some degree of psychological adjustment

life-span perspective the viewpoint that considers the individual's prior development, current level of development and likely development in the future

limbic system a set of structures in the forebrain that seems to play a role in emotional expression

lipids (LIH-pidz) fatty materials, such as the cholesterol found in blood

lipoproteins (LIP-oh-pro-teenz or LY-po-pro-teenz) proteins that transport cholesterol in the blood

locus of control a generalised belief people have about the causes of events in their lives — whether the causes are within or outside their control

longitudinal approach a method of studying developmental changes in the same subjects by making repeated observations over a long period of time

low-density lipoprotein (LDL) a cholesterol-carrying protein that is associated with increased cholesterol deposits in blood vessels

lymphocytes (LIM-foe-sites) various types of white blood cells that have several important functions in the body's immune response

McGill Pain Questionnaire (MPQ) a self-report instrument for assessing people's pain

medulla (meh-DULL-ah) a part of the brainstem that contains control centres for such vital functions as breathing and heartbeat rate

meta-analysis a statistical technique that combines the results from earlier studies to generate an overview of those findings

metabolism the chemical reactions of the body's cells that synthesise new cell material, regulate body processes and create energy

methadone a chemical agent used in treating narcotic addiction that blocks the euphoric effects of opiates

midbrain a portion of the brainstem that plays an important role in vision, hearing and muscle movement

migraine headache recurrent head pain that results from the constriction and dilation of blood vessels in the head

Millon Behavioural Health Inventory (MBHI) a test that assesses several relevant characteristics of medical patients, such as their basic coping styles and hypochondriacal tendencies

mind/body problem the issue in psychology and philosophy regarding the relationship between processes and functions of the mind and those of the body

Minnesota Multiphasic Personality Inventory (MMPI) a lengthy test that assesses a variety of psychological problems, such as hypochondriasis, depression and hysteria

modelling learning by watching the behaviour of other people

morbidity the condition of illness, injury or disability

mortality death, usually with reference to large populations

motivated reasoning cognitive process whereby people's desires or preferences influence their decisions about the validity and utility of new information

motivational interviewing a form of interviewing that increases the person's motivation to change health risk behaviour and facilitates a readiness to enter the action stage of change

myocardial infarction (my-oh-KAR-dee-al in-FARK-shun) damage to the heart muscle (myocardium) that results from severe or prolonged blockage of blood supply to the tissue; commonly called a *heart attack*

narcotics drugs that relieve pain, act as sedatives and may produce euphoria. These substances are also called *opiates* and usually lead to addiction with continued use.

network resolution processing activating the fear network in memory (information on the cognitive, behavioural and physiological reactions to the event) as a traumatic event is relived. High-level intrusions (recurring thoughts, flashbacks) following a traumatic event, and avoidance coping, indicate that the person is reappraising the event and actively working through the trauma.

neurons specialised cells that provide for communication within the nervous system

neurotransmitter a chemical involved in the transmission of impulses across the synapse from one neuron to another

nicotine a chemical in cigarette smoke that appears to produce physical dependence

nicotine fading a treatment strategy that involves getting the smoker to switch to cigarette brands with progressively lower nicotine content while self-monitoring nicotine intake in order to achieve complete abstinence over a number of weeks

nicotine regulation model an explanation of continued cigarette smoking based on the body's dependence on nicotine

nociceptors (noe-see-SEP-torz) afferent nerve endings that respond to pain stimuli in the damaged region of the body

non-insulin-dependent diabetes mellitus (NIDDM) the health problem of having chronically elevated blood sugar levels even though the pancreas does produce at least some insulin. Most NIDDM patients can manage their conditions without insulin supplements.

non-pain imagery a pain management method that involves mentally picturing a scene that is unrelated to or incompatible with feeling discomfort

nosocomial infection (noe-soe-KOE-mee-al) an infection a patient acquires while in hospital

obese the weight classification of individuals whose weight exceeds their desirable range by more than 20 per cent as a result of excess fat

outcome evaluation assessing the achievement of a health program's goals; specifically, was the intervention successful in improving the health and life quality of participants?

overweight the weight classification of individuals whose weight exceeds their desirable range by 10 to 20 per cent

pain sensory and emotional discomfort, usually related to actual or threatened tissue damage

pain behaviours characteristic ways people behave when they are in pain

pain clinics centres specialising in the treatment of chronic pain

pain redefinition a pain management technique in which thoughts about pain that arouse a sense of threat are replaced with other thoughts that are more constructive or realistic

parasympathetic nervous system a division of the autonomic nervous system that helps the body conserve energy and restore the normal body state after arousal

passive smoking breathing the smoke in the environment from someone else's cigarette or other smoking product

patient-centred the behavioural style of some doctors in which their interactions encourage patients to share information and participate in medical decisions

periaqueductal grey area of the brainstem (per-ee-ak-weh-DUK-tal) a region of the midbrain that plays a major role in the perception of and reaction to pain stimuli

peripheral nervous system the network of nerve fibres that carry messages between the central nervous system and the skin, skeletal muscles and internal organs. This network has two parts: the somatic and autonomic nervous systems.

personal control the feeling people have that they can make decisions and take action to produce favourable events and avoid unfavourable ones

personality cognitive, affective or behavioural predispositions of people in different situations and over time

Peter Principle the stress experienced by a worker who has been promoted to perform at a higher level within an organisation, but who lacks the requisite skills to perform at that level

phagocytes (FAG-oh-sites) certain types of white blood cells that engulf and ingest any kind of invading particles

physical dependence a state in which the body has become accustomed to the presence of a substance in its physiological functioning

pituitary gland an endocrine gland that has connections to the brain and secretes hormones that stimulate other endocrine glands to secrete

placebo an inactive substance or procedure that may cause a change in an individual's behaviour or health

polygraph an electromechanical device that assesses the body's arousal by measuring and recording several physiological indexes, such as blood pressure and respiration rate, simultaneously

pons a portion of the brainstem involved in the control of eye movements and facial expressions

post-traumatic stress disorder a disorder resulting from exposure to a traumatic event, and characterised by flashbacks and distressing recurrent dreams about the event; avoidance symptoms such as psychological numbing or diminished responsiveness to external stimuli; inability to recall the event, or emotional detachment; and increased arousal, manifested by startle reactions, sleeping problems, difficulty concentrating, mood changes or violent behaviour — symptoms that must have been present for more than three months

PRECEDE/PROCEED model a model that provides guidelines for health promoters designing, implementing and evaluating programs involving a large number of people

prevalence the total number of cases existing at a given moment in time

primary appraisal the cognitive process people use in assessing the meaning of an event or situation for their wellbeing

primary prevention actions undertaken to avoid health problems before they occur

problem drinkers people who are psychologically dependent on alcohol and drink heavily

problem-focused coping approaches people use for managing stress aimed at reducing the discrepancy between their resources and the demands of the situation

process evaluation evaluation of the activities of a health-promotion program, in which an assessment is made of how well the program was delivered

progressive muscle relaxation a stress reduction technique in which people are trained to alternate between tightening and relaxing specific muscle groups

prospective approach a research strategy by which characteristics of subjects are measured and later examined for their relationships to future conditions, such as health problems

psychological dependence a state in which a person feels compelled to use a substance for the pleasant effect it produces

psychoneuroimmunology (psy-ko-nooroe-ih-myu-NOL-oh-jee) a field of study focusing on relationships between psychosocial processes and nervous, endocrine and immune system functioning

psychophysiological disorders physical symptoms or illnesses resulting from some combination of psychosocial and physiological processes

Psychosocial Adjustment to Illness Scale (PAIS) a test of several psychosocial aspects of a patient's life that are related to adjustment to medical illness

psychosomatic medicine a field introduced in the 1930s to study the relationships between people's symptoms of illness and their emotions

punishment a process by which a consequence of an operant behaviour suppresses that response

quality of life individuals' appraisals of the degree to which their lives contain features that they find satisfying or meaningful

quasi-experimental studies non-experimental research in which subjects are categorised or separated into two or more groups on the basis of existing characteristics and then compared regarding other variables

rational-emotive therapy (RET) a cognitive restructuring approach for replacing irrational thought patterns that provoke stress with thought patterns that are more realistic

rational non-adherence non-compliance with medical regimens for valid, but not necessarily medically beneficial, reasons

reactance people's angry responses to restrictions on their freedom of action or choice

reactivity the physiological component of the response to stress

referred pain the experience of discomfort as coming from an area of the body other than where the injury exists

reinforcement a process whereby a consequence of an operant response strengthens or maintains that behaviour

relapse regression to the full-blown pattern of an unwanted behaviour after beginning to change it

respiratory system a network of organs that supply oxygen for metabolism and expel carbon dioxide

restraint theory an explanation of eating regulation that proposes that people who constantly try to resist eating what they want tend to develop abnormal eating patterns in which they vacillate between inhibited and disinhibited consumption

reticular system a portion of the brainstem that contains control centres for sleep, arousal and attention

retrospective approach a research strategy through which the histories of subjects are examined for their relationships to recent conditions, such as health problems

risk factors characteristics or conditions that occur more often among individuals who develop particular diseases or injuries than among those who do not

secondary appraisal the cognitive process people use in assessing the resources they have to meet demands

secondary prevention actions undertaken to identify or treat a health problem early with the aim of arresting or reversing the condition

self-efficacy people's belief that they can succeed at something they want to do

self-management strategies methods used in helping people gain control over the conditions in their environment that encourage undesirable behaviours

separation distress emotional upset often shown by infants and young children when separated from their primary caretakers, typically their parents

set-point theory an explanation of weight regulation that proposes that each person has a 'set' physiologically based weight level that the body strives to maintain

sick-role behaviour activity by individuals who consider themselves to be ill for the purpose of becoming well

single-subject designs research approaches in which a variable is observed in one individual during two or more research conditions

social network a person's linkages with other people, as assessed by various qualitative and quantitative measures of social contacts

social support the perceived comfort, caring, esteem or help an individual receives from other people or groups

sociocultural relating to or involving social and cultural features or processes

somatic nervous system a division of the peripheral nervous system that transmits sensory and motor impulses

spinal cord the major neural pathway that carries impulses between the brain and the peripheral nervous system

spinal cord injury neurological damage in the spine that impairs motor and sensory function

stage of exhaustion the third stage in the general adaptation syndrome, when the body's energy reserves are severely depleted

stage of resistance the second stage in the general adaptation syndrome, when the body tries to adapt to the stressor

stages of change model a theory of intentional behaviour that describes people's readiness to change with five potential stages: precontemplation, contemplation, preparation, action and maintenance

stimulants drugs that activate the nervous system, producing physiological and psychological arousal

stimulation-produced analgesia (SPA) a phenomenon in which stimulation to the brainstem causes insensitivity to pain

strain the psychological and physiological response to a stressor

stress the condition that results when person–environment transactions lead the individual to perceive a discrepancy between the demands of a situation and his or her resources

stress-inoculation training a cognitive-behavioural approach for stress management that teaches people a variety of skills for alleviating stress and achieving personal goals

stressors events or circumstances a person perceives as threatening or harmful

stroke a condition involving brain damage that results from a disruption in the blood supply to that area of the brain

structural approach an approach used to describe the properties or dimensions of a disaster, such as the degree of impact, the duration, the preparedness of the community, the proportion of the community affected and the nature of suffering involved

subjective norm a construct in the theories of reasoned action and planned behaviour that refers to an individual's motivation to comply with perceived pressure from significant others to perform a behaviour, and is thought to influence behavioural intentions

substance abuse the prolonged overuse of a substance, involving a clear pattern of pathological use and heightened social and occupational problems

sudden death the abrupt death from cardiac dysfunction of a person who seemed healthy

sympathetic nervous system a division of the autonomic nervous system that enables the body to mobilise and expend energy during physical and emotional arousal

system a continuously changing entity that consists of constantly interrelated components

systematic desensitisation a classical conditioning technique for reducing fear or anxiety by replacing it with a calm response

tars tiny particles in cigarette smoke

technostress the strain experienced by workers who must adapt to changes associated with the introduction of new technology in the workplace and the development of new skills to keep up with these changes

T cells a class of lymphocytes; some attack antigens directly, and some work to regulate other immune functions

temperaments basic personality characteristics or dispositions that individuals show from birth, allowing many of them to be classified broadly as 'easy' or 'difficult'

tension-type headache recurrent head pain that results from persistent muscle tension in the head and neck; also called *muscle-contraction* headache

tertiary prevention actions undertaken to contain or slow the progress of damage from a serious or established health problem

thalamus a structure in the forebrain that serves as a relay station for sensory impulses to and commands from the cerebrum

theory a tentative explanation of phenomena

theory of planned behaviour an explanation of health-related behaviour that argues that behaviour depends on a person's behavioural intention, which is determined by attitudes and beliefs regarding the behaviour, the subjective norm and perceived control

theory of reasoned action an explanation of people's health-related behaviour. Their behaviour depends on their intention, which is based on their attitudes and beliefs regarding the behaviour and the subjective norm.

time management methods for managing stress that involve organising one's time

tolerance a gradual decrease in the body's response to a drug, thereby requiring larger and larger doses to achieve the same effect

transactions the continuous interplay and adjustments of the person and environment

transcutaneous electrical nerve stimulation (TENS) (tranz-kyu-TAIN-ee-us) a counter-irritation pain control technique that involves electrically stimulating an area near where the patient feels pain

treatment delay the elapsed time between noticing a symptom and getting medical care

twin studies research to assess the influence of heredity in determining a characteristic by focusing on differences between identical and fraternal twins

Type A behaviour pattern a behavioural or emotional style characterised by high levels of competitiveness, time urgency, and anger or hostility

Type B behaviour pattern a behavioural or emotional style characterised by low levels of competitiveness, time urgency, and anger or hostility

ulcers a psychophysiological disorder involving wounds to the stomach or upper section of the small intestine

variable a measurable characteristic of people, objects or events that may change in quantity or quality

very-low-density lipoproteins (VLDL) a cholesterol-carrying protein that is associated with increased deposits of cholesterol in blood vessels

withdrawal physical and psychological symptoms that occur when people stop taking a substance on which the body has become physically dependent

References*

* Authorship for references with more than 10 authors is cited with the format: first four authors et al.

Abbott, K. (1990). Therapeutic use of play in the psychological preparation of preschool children undergoing cardiac surgery. *Issues in Comprehensive Pediatric Nursing,* 13(4), 265–77.

Abdulwadud, O., Abramson, M., Forbes, A., James, A., Light, L., Thein, F., & Walters, E. H. (1997). Attendance at an asthma educational intervention: characteristics of participants and non-participants. *Respiratory Medicine,* 91, 524–9.

Abele, A., & Brehm, W. (1993). Mood effects of exercise versus sports games: findings and implications for well-being and health. In S. Maes, H. Leventhal & M. Johnston (Eds), *International review of health psychology* (Vol. 2). New York: John Wiley & Sons.

Abraham, S., & Llewellyn-Jones, D. (1992). *Eating disorders: the facts.* Oxford, NY: Oxford University Press.

Abrams, D. B., Niaura, R. S., Carey, K. B., Monti, P. M., & Binkoff, J. A. (1986). Understanding relapse and recovery in alcohol abuse. *Annals of Behavioral Medicine,* 8(2–3), 27–32.

Abramson, L. Y., Seligman, M. E. P., & Teasdale, J. D. (1978). Learned helplessness in humans: critique and reformulation. *Journal of Abnormal Psychology,* 87, 49–74.

ABS (Australian Bureau of Statistics) (1995). *National Health Survey: summary of results.* ABS Cat. No. 4360.0. Canberra: ABS.

ABS (1996a). *Children's immunisation, Australia, 1995.* ABS Cat. No. 4352.0. Canberra: ABS.

ABS (1996b). *National Health Survey 1995, First Results Australia.* Canberra: AGPS.

ABS (1997a). *1995 National Health Survey: summary of results, Australia.* ABS Cat. No. 4364.0. Canberra: ABS.

ABS (1997b). *1997 Year Book Australia.* ABS Cat. No. 1302.0. Canberra: AGPS.

ABS (1998). *Apparent consumption of foodstuffs, Australia, 1996–97.* ABS Cat. No. 4306.0. Canberra: ABS.

ABS (1999a). *Causes of death, Australia, 1998.* ABS Cat. No. 3303.0. Canberra: ABS.

ABS (1999b). *How Australians measure up — health: overweight and obesity.* Cat. No. 4359.0. Canberra: ABS.

ACCV (Anti-Cancer Council of Victoria) (1989). *SunSmart Evaluation Studies # 1. Skin Cancer Control Program 1988–89.* ACCV.

ACCV (1995). *SunSmart Evaluation Studies # 4.* ACCV.

Acevedo, H. F., Tong, J. Y., & Hartsock, R. J. (1995). Human chorionic gonadotropin-beta subunit gene expression in cultured human fetal cells of different types and origins. *Cancer,* 76, 1467–75.

Achterberg-Lawlis, J. (1988). Musculoskeletal disorders. In E. A. Blechman & K. D. Brownell (Eds), *Handbook of behavioral medicine for women.* New York: Pergamon.

ACIL (1994). *Smoking: costs and benefits for Australia.* Report commissioned by the Tobacco Institute of Australia.

ACS (American Cancer Society) (1989). *Cancer facts and figures — 1989.* Atlanta: Author.

ACS (1996). *Cancer facts and figures — 1996.* Atlanta: Author.

ADA (American Diabetes Association) (1991). *Set your sights: your future in dietetics.* Chicago: Author.

Adams, J. E., & Lindemann, E. (1974). Coping with long-term disability. In G. V. Coelho, D. A. Hamburg, & J. E. Adams (Eds), *Coping and adaptation.* New York: Basic Books.

Ader, R., & Cohen, N. (1975). Behaviorally conditioned immunosuppression. *Psychosomatic Medicine,* 37, 333–40.

Ader, R., & Cohen, N. (1982). Behaviorally conditioned immunosuppression and murine systemic lupus erythematosus. *Science,* 215, 1534–6.

Ader, R., & Cohen, N. (1985). CNS-immune system interactions: conditioning phenomena. *Behavioral and Brain Sciences,* 8, 379–95.

Adesso, V. J. (1985). Cognitive factors in alcohol and drug use. In M. Galizio & S. A. Maisto (Eds), *Determinants of substance abuse: biological, psychological, and environmental factors.* New York: Plenum.

Adler, N. E., Boyce, T., Chesney, M. A., Cohen, S., Folkman, S., Kahn, R. L., & Syme, S. L. (1994). Socioeconomic status and health: the challenge of the gradient. *American Psychologist,* 49, 15–24.

Adler, N. E., & Stone, G. C. (1979). Social science perspectives on the health system. In G. C. Stone, F. Cohen & N. E. Adler (Eds), *Health psychology — a handbook.* San Francisco: Jossey-Bass.

Affleck, G., Tennen, H., Keefe, F. J., Lefebvre, J. C., Kashikar-Zuck, S., Wright, K., Starr, K., & Caldwell, D. S. (1999). Everyday life with osteoarthritis or rheumatoid arthritis: independent effects of disease and gender on daily pain, mood and coping. *Pain,* 83(3), 601–9.

Affleck, G., Tennen, H., Pfeiffer, C., & Fifield, J. (1987). Appraisals of control and predictability in adapting to a chronic disease. *Journal of Personality and Social Psychology,* 53, 273–9.

Affleck, G., Tennen, H., Urrows, S., & Higgins, P. (1991). Individual differences in the day-to-day experience of chronic pain: a prospective daily study of rheumatoid arthritis patients. *Health Psychology,* 10, 419–26.

Agars, J., & McMurray, A. (1993). An evaluation of comparative strategies for teaching breast self-examination. *Journal of Advanced Nursing,* 18(10), 1595–1603.

Agosti, J. M., Sprenger, J. D., Lum, L. G., Witherspoon, R. P., Fisher, L. D., Storb, R., & Henderson, W. R. (1988). Transfer of allergen-specific IgE-mediated hypersensitivity with allogenic bone marrow transplantation. *New England Journal of Medicine,* 319, 1623–8.

Agras, W. S. (1984). The behavioral treatment of somatic disorders. In W. D. Gentry (Ed.), *Handbook of behavioral medicine.* New York: Guilford.

Agras, W. S. (1987). *Eating disorders: management of obesity, bulimia, and anorexia nervosa.* New York: Pergamon.

AHA (American Heart Association) (1994). *Heart and stroke facts.* Dallas, TX: Author.

AHMAC (Australian Health Ministers' Advisory Council) (1991). Cervical Cancer Screening Evaluation Steering Committee. *Cervical cancer screening in Australia: options for change.* Australian Institute of Health: Prevention Program Evaluation Series No. 2. Canberra: AGPS.

AIHW (Australian Institute of Health & Welfare) (1996). *Australia's health, 1996: 5th biennial health report of the Australian Institute of Health and Welfare.* Canberra: AGPS.

AIHW (1998). *Australia's health, 1998: 6th biennial health report of the Australian Institute of Health and Welfare.* Canberra: AGPS.

AIHW (1999a). *Australian hospital statistics, 1997–98.* Cat. No. HSE 6. Canberra: AGPS.

AIHW (1999b). *Cancer in Australia 1996 — incidence and mortality data for 1996 and selected data for 1997 and 1998.* Canberra: AIHW.

AIHW (1999c). *Heart, stroke and vascular diseases: Australian facts.* Canberra: AIHW.

AIHW (1999d). *Private Hospitals, Australia, 1997–98.* Cat. No. 4390.0. Canberra: AGPS.

AIHW (2000). *Australia's health, 2000: 7th biennial health report of the Australian Institute of Health and Welfare.* Canberra: AGPS.

AIHW: Harrison, J. E., & Cripps, R. A. (1994). *Injury in Australia: an epidemiological review.* Canberra: AGPS.

AIHW: Mathers, C., & Penm, R. (1999). *Health system costs of injury, poisoning and musculoskeletal disorders in Australia, 1993–94.* Cat. No. HWE 12. Canberra: AIHW.

Aiken, L. H. (1983). Nurses. In D. Mechanic (Ed.), *Handbook of health, health care, and the health professions.* New York: Free Press.

Ainsworth, M. D. S. (1973). The development of infant-mother attachment. In B. M. Caldwell & H. N. Ricciuti (Eds), *Review of child development research* (Vol. 3). Chicago: University of Chicago Press.

Ainsworth, M. D. S. (1979). Infant–mother attachment. *American Psychologist, 34,* 932–7.

Ajzen, I. (1991). The theory of planned behavior. *Organizational Behavior and Human Decision Processes, 50,* 179–211.

Ajzen, I., & Fishbein, M. (1980). *Understanding attitudes and predicting social behavior.* Englewood Cliffs, NJ: Prentice Hall.

Ajzen, I., & Madden, T. J. (1986). Prediction of goal-directed behavior: attitudes, intentions and perceived behavioural control. *Journal of Experimental Social Psychology, 22,* 453–74.

Akil, H., Mayer, D. J., & Liebeskind, J. C. (1976). Antagonism of stimulation-produced analgesia by naloxone, a narcotic antagonist. *Science, 191,* 961–2.

ALA (American Lung Association) (1994). *Facts about asthma.* New York: Author.

al'Absi, M., Lovallo, W. R., McKey, B. S., & Pincomb, G. A. (1994). Borderline hypertensives produce exaggerated adrenocortical responses to sustained mental stress. *Psychosomatic Medicine, 56,* 245–50.

Alagna, S. W., & Reddy, D. M. (1984). Predictors of proficient technique and successful lesion detection in breast self-examination. *Health Psychology, 3,* 113–27.

Alaranta, H., Rytökoski, U., Rissanen, A., Talo, S., Rönnemaa, T., Puukka, P., Karppi, S.-L., Videman, T., Kallio, V., & Slätis, P. (1994). Intensive physical and psychosocial training program for patients with chronic low back pain: a controlled clinical trial. *Spine, 19,* 1339–49.

Alberink, A. M., Casarolli Valery, P., Russell, A., & Green, A. (2000). Do forecasts of UV indexes influence people's outdoor behaviour? *Australian and New Zealand Journal of Public Health, 24*(5), 488–91.

Alderman, M. H. (1984). Worksite treatment of hypertension. In J. D. Matarazzo, S. M. Weiss, J. A. Herd, N. E. Miller & S. M. Weiss (Eds), *Behavioral health: a handbook of health enhancement and disease prevention.* New York: John Wiley & Sons.

Alexander, C. J. (1994, August). Effects of spinal cord injury on female sexual response. Paper presented at the meeting of the American Psychological Association in Los Angeles.

Alexander, F. (1950). *Psychosomatic medicine: its principles and applications.* New York: Norton.

Alexander, J. A. (1984). Blood pressure and obesity. In J. D. Matarazzo, S. M. Weiss, J. A. Herd, N. E. Miller & S. M. Weiss (Eds), *Behavioral health: a handbook of health enhancement and disease prevention.* New York: John Wiley & Sons.

Alexy, B. B. (1991). Factors associated with participation and non-participation in a workplace wellness center. *Research in Nursing & Health, 14,* 33–40.

Allan, R., & Scheidt, S. (1990). Life style: its effect and modification for the prevention of sudden cardiac death. In J. B. Kostis & M. Sanders (Eds), *The prevention of sudden cardiac death.* New York: John Wiley & Sons.

Allen, L., & Zigler, E. (1986). Psychosocial adjustment of seriously ill children. *Journal of the American Academy of Child Psychiatry, 25,* 708–712.

Allsop, S., & Saunders, B. (1989). Relapse and alcohol problems. In M. Gossop (Ed.), *Relapse and addictive behaviour* (pp. 11–40). London: Tavistock/Routledge.

Alpert, B., Field, T., Goldstein, S., & Perry, S. (1990). Aerobics enhances cardiovascular fitness and agility in preschoolers. *Health Psychology, 9,* 48–56.

Altman, D. G., & Green, L. W. (1988). Area review: education and training in behavioral medicine. *Annals of Behavioral Medicine, 10,* 4–7.

Altman, L. K. (1988, January 26). Cocaine's many dangers: the evidence mounts. *New York Times,* p. C1.

Altman, L. K. (1996, July 12). Scientists display substantial gains in AIDS treatment. *New York Times,* pp. A1, 16.

AMA (American Medical Association) (1989). *The American Medical Association encyclopedia of medicine.* New York: Random House.

Ames, B. N., & Gold, L. S. (1990). Too many rodent carcinogens: Mitogenisis increases mutogenesis. *Science, 249,* 970–71.

Amos, C. I., Hunter, S. M., Zinkgraf, S. A., Miner, M. H., & Berenson, G. S. (1987). Characterization of a comprehensive Type A measure for children in a biracial community: the Bogalusa Heart Study. *Journal of Behavioral Medicine, 10,* 425–39.

Anastasi, A. (1982). *Psychological testing* (5th ed.). New York: Macmillan.

Anda, R. F., Remington, P. L., Sienko, D. G., & Davis, R. M. (1987). Are physicians advising smokers to quit? The patient's perspective. *Journal of the American Medical Association, 257,* 1916–19.

Andersen, B. L., & Hacker, N. F. (1983). Treatment for gynecologic cancer: a review of the effects on female sexuality. *Health Psychology, 2,* 203–221.

Andersen, B. L., Karlsson, J. A., Anderson, B., & Tewfik, H. H. (1984). Anxiety and cancer treatment: response to stressful radiotherapy. *Health Psychology, 3,* 535–51.

Anderson, A. (1982, July). Neurotoxic follies. *Psychology Today,* pp. 30–42.

Anderson, B. J., Auslander, W. F., Jung, K. C., Miller, J. P., & Santiago, J. V. (1990). Assessing family sharing of diabetes responsibilities. *Journal of Pediatric Psychology, 15,* 477–92.

Anderson, K. O., Bradley, L. A., Young, L. D., McDaniel, L. K., & Wise, C. M. (1985). Rheumatoid arthritis: review of psychological factors related to etiology, effects, and treatment. *Psychological Bulletin, 98,* 358–87.

Anderson, K. O., & Masur, F. T. (1983). Psychological preparation for invasive medical and dental procedures. *Journal of Behavioral Medicine, 6,* 1–40.

Anderson, N. B., & Armstead, C. A. (1995). Toward understanding the association of socioeconomic status and health: a new challenge for the biopsychosocial approach. *Psychosomatic Medicine, 57,* 213–25.

Andrasik, F., Blake, D. D., & McCarran, M. S. (1986). A biobehavioral analysis of pediatric headache. In N. A. Krasnegor, J. D. Araster & M. F. Cataldo (Eds), *Child health behavior: a behavioral pediatrics perspective.* New York: John Wiley & Sons.

Andrasik, F., & Holroyd, K. A. (1980). A test of specific and non-specific effects in the biofeedback treatment of tension headache. *Journal of Consulting and Clinical Psychology, 48,* 575–86.

Andrew, J. M. (1970). Recovery from surgery with and without preparatory instruction for three coping styles. *Journal of Personality and Social Psychology, 15,* 223–6.

Andrews, H. B., & Jones, S. (1990). Eating behaviour in obese women: a test of two hypotheses. *Australian Psychologist*, 25(3), 351–7.

Andrykowski, M. A. (1990). The role of anxiety in the development of anticipatory nausea in cancer chemotherapy: a review and synthesis. *Psychosomatic Medicine*, 52, 458–75.

Ansari, Z., Brosi, J., Booth, J., & Collopy, B. (1994). *Measurement of care in Australian hospitals: 1994 hospital wide medical indicator results and comparisons to 1993 results*. Sydney: Australian Council on Healthcare Standards.

Anshel, M. H. (1991). A psycho-behavioral analysis of addicted versus non-addicted male and female exercisers. *Journal of Sport Behavior*, 14(2), 145–54.

Antoni, M. H. (1987). Neuroendocrine influences in psychoimmunology and neoplasia: a review. *Psychology and Health*, 1, 3–24.

Antoni, M. H., Baggett, L., Ironson, G., La-Perriere, A., August, S., Klimas, N., Schneiderman, N., & Fletcher, M. A. (1991). Cognitive-behavioral stress management intervention buffers distress responses and immunologic changes following notification of HIV-1 seropositivity. *Journal of Consulting and Clinical Psychology*, 59, 906–915.

Antoni, M. H., Schneiderman, N., Fletcher, M. A., Goldstein, D. A., Ironson, G., & Laperriere, A. (1990). Psychoneuroimmunology and HIV-1. *Journal of Consulting and Clinical Psychology*, 58, 38–49.

Antonovsky, A. (1979). *Health, stress, and coping*. San Francisco: Jossey-Bass.

Antonovsky, A. (1987). *Unraveling the mystery of health: how people manage stress and stay well*. San Francisco: Jossey-Bass.

Antonucci, T. C. (1985). Personal characteristics, social support, and social behavior. In R. H. Binstock & E. Shanas (Eds), *Handbook of aging and the social sciences* (2nd ed.). New York: Van Nostrand-Reinhold.

Antonuccio, D. O., & Lichtenstein, E. (1980). Peer modeling influences on smoking behavior of heavy and light smokers. *Addictive Behaviors*, 5, 299–306.

AOTA (American Occupational Therapy Association) (1994). *Occupational therapy careers*. Bethesda, MD: Author.

APA (American Psychiatric Association) (1994). *Diagnostic and statistical manual of mental disorders* (4th ed.). Washington, DC: APA.

APS (Australian Psychological Society) (2001). *The APS College of Health Psychologists table of competencies, October 2001*. Carlton South: APS.

APTA (American Physical Therapy Association) (1995). *A future in physical therapy*. Alexandria, VA: Author.

Arbuckle, T. Pushkar, D., Chaikelson, J., & Andres, D. (1999). Coping and control processes: do they contribute to individual differences in health in older adults? *Canadian Journal on Aging*, 18(3), 285–312.

Armor, D. J., Polich, J. M., & Stambul, H. B. (1978). *Alcoholism and treatment*. New York: John Wiley & Sons.

Armstrong, B. K., & English, D. R. (1996). Cutaneous malignant melanoma. In D. Schottenfeld & J. F. Fraumeni, Jr (Eds), *Cancer epidemiology and prevention*. New York: Oxford University Press.

Armstrong, C. A., Sallis, J. F., Hovell, M. F., & Hofstetter, C. R. (1992, March). Predicting exercise adoption: a stages of change analysis. Paper presented at the meeting of the Society of Behavioral Medicine, New York.

Arnow, B., Kenardy, J., & Agras, W. S. (1992). Binge eating among the obese. *Journal of Behavioral Medicine*, 15, 155–70.

Aronoff, G. M., Wagner, J. M., & Spangler, A. S. (1986). Chemical interventions for pain. *Journal of Consulting and Clinical Psychology*, 54, 769–75.

Arroll, B., & Beaglehole, R. (1992). Does physical activity lower blood pressure: a critical review of the clinical trials. *Journal of Clinical Epidemiology*, 45, 439–47.

Arthritis Foundation of Western Australia (2000) (http://www.arthritiswa.org.au, accessed August 2000).

Ary, D. V., & Biglan, A. (1988). Longitudinal changes in adolescent cigarette smoking behavior: Onset and cessation. *Journal of Behavioral Medicine*, 11, 361–82.

Ary, D. V., Biglan, A., Glasgow, R., Zoref, L., et al. (1990). The efficacy of social-influence prevention programs versus 'standard care': are new initiatives needed? *Journal of Behavioral Medicine*, 13, 281–96.

Ashburn, S. S. (1986). Biophysical development of the toddler and the preschooler. In C. S. Schuster & S. S. Ashburn (Eds), *The process of human development: a holistic life-span approach* (2nd ed.). Boston: Little, Brown.

Ashenberg, Z. S., Porzelius, J. E., Gorski-Simon, K., Kriegler, J. S. (1990, April). The efficacy of aerobic exercise training in the treatment of chronic back pain. Paper presented at the meeting of the Society of Behavioral Medicine, Chicago.

Ashley, M. J., & Rankin, J. G. (1988). A public health approach to the prevention of alcohol-related health problems. In L. Breslow, J. E. Fielding & L. B. Lave (Eds), *Annual review of public health* (Vol. 9). Palo Alto, CA: Annual Reviews.

Ashton, H., & Stepney, R. (1983). *Smoking: psychology and pharmacology*. New York: Routledge.

Askevold, F. (1975). Measuring body image. *Psychotherapy and Psychosomatics*, 26, 71–7.

Atkins, E., Solomon, L. J., Worden, J. K., & Foster, R. S. (1991). Relative effectiveness of methods of breast self-examination. *Journal of Behavioral Medicine*, 14, 357–67.

Atkinson, R. (1994, June 23). Germans wonder if health-care model can survive an aging population. *International Herald Tribune*, p. 2.

Atrens, D. M. (1994). The questionable wisdom of a low-fat diet and cholesterol reduction. *Social Science and Medicine*, 39(3), 433–47.

Attie, I., & Brooks-Gunn, J. (1987). Weight concerns as chronic stressors in women. In R. C. Barnett, L. Biener & G. K. Baruch (Eds), *Gender and stress*. New York: Free Press.

Auerbach, S. M., Martelli, M. F., & Mercuri, L. G. (1983). Anxiety, information, interpersonal impacts, and adjustment to a stressful health care situation. *Journal of Personality and Social Psychology*, 44, 1284–96.

Australian Encyclopaedia (1996) (6th ed.). Volume 5: 'Hospitals'. Terrey Hills: Australian Geographic Pty Ltd.

Australian Sports Commission, Participation Division. (1999). *Active Australia Physical Activity Survey, 1997*. Canberra: ASC.

Averill, J. R. (1973). Personal control over aversive stimuli and its relationship to stress. *Psychological Bulletin*, 80, 286–303.

Avlund, K. Damsgaard, M.-T., & Holstein, B. E. (1998). Social relations and mortality: an eleven year follow-up study of 70-yr-old men and women in Denmark. *Social Science and Medicine*, 47(5), 635–43.

Azar, B. (1994, November). Eating fat: Why does the brain say, 'Ahhh'? *American Psychological Association Monitor*, p. 20.

Bachen, E., Cohen, S., & Marsland, A. L. (1997). Psychoimmunology. In A. Baum, S. Newman, J. Weinman, R. West & C. McManus (Eds), *Cambridge handbook of psychology, health and medicine* (pp. 35–9). Cambridge: Cambridge University Press.

Baer, J. S., Kamarck, T., Lichtenstein, E., & Ransom, C. C. (1989). Prediction of smoking relapse: analyses of temptations and transgressions after initial cessation. *Journal of Consulting and Clinical Psychology*, 57, 623–7.

Baer, P. E., Garmezy, L. B., McLaughlin, R. J., Pokorny, A. D., & Wernick, M. J. (1987). Stress, coping, family conflict, and adolescent alcohol use. *Journal of Behavioral Medicine*, 10, 449–66.

Baghurst, K., Baghurst, P., & Record, S. (1994). Demographic and dietary profiles of high and low fat consumers in Australia. *Journal of Epidemiology and Community Health*, 48(1), 26–32.

Bagozzi, R. P. (1981). Attitudes, intentions, and behavior: a test of some key hypotheses. *Journal of Personality and Social Psychology*, 41, 606–627.

Baillie, A. J., Mattick, R. P., & Hall, W. (1995). Quitting smoking: estimation by meta-analysis of the rate of unaided smoking cessation. *Australian Journal of Public Health*, 19(2), 129–31.

Baillie, A. J., Mattick, R. P., Hall, W., & Webster, P. (1994). Meta-analytic review of the efficacy of smoking cessation interventions. *Drug and Alcohol Review*, 13, 157–70.

Bakal, D. A. (1979). *Psychology and medicine: psychological dimensions of health and illness*. New York: Springer.

Baker, R. (1989, January 29). The cholesterol thing. *New York Times*, p. A31.

Bakwin, H., & Bakwin, R. M. (1972). *Behavior disorders in children*. Philadelphia: Saunders.

Ball, J. F. (1976–77). Widow's grief: the impact of age and mode of health. *Omega*, 7, 307–333.

Bammer, G. (2000). What can a trial contribute to the debate about supervised injecting rooms? *Australian and New Zealand Journal of Public Health*, 24(2), 214–15.

Bandura, A. (1965a). Influence of model's reinforcement contingencies on the acquisition of imitative responses. *Journal of Personality and Social Psychology*, 1, 589–95.

Bandura, A. (1965b). Vicarious processes: a case of no-trial learning. In L. Berkowitz (Ed.), *Advances in experimental social psychology* (Vol. 2). New York: Academic Press.

Bandura, A. (1969). *Principles of behavior modification*. New York: Holt, Rinehart & Winston.

Bandura, A. (1977). Self-efficacy: toward a unifying theory of behavioral change. *Psychological Review*, 84, 191–215.

Bandura, A. (1986). *Social foundations of thought and action: a social cognitive theory*. Englewood Cliffs, NJ: Prentice Hall.

Bandura, A., O'Leary, A., Taylor, C. B., Gauthier, J., & Gossard, D. (1987). Perceived self-efficacy and pain control: Opioid and non-opioid mechanisms. *Journal of Personality and Social Psychology*, 53, 563–71.

Bandura, A., Reese, L., & Adams, N. E. (1982). Microanalysis of action and fear arousal as a function of differential levels of perceived self-efficacy. *Journal of Personality and Social Psychology*, 43, 5–21.

Bandura, A., Taylor, C. B., Williams, S. L., Mefford, I. N., & Barchas, J. D. (1985). Catecholamine secretion as a function of perceived coping self-efficacy. *Journal of Consulting and Clinical Psychology*, 53, 406–414.

Banks, S. M., Salovey, P., Greener, S., Rothman, A. J., Moyer, A., Beauvais, J., & Eppel, E. (1995). The effects of message framing on mammography utilization. *Health Psychology*, 14, 178–84.

Baranowski, T., & Nader, P. R. (1985). Family health behavior. In D. C. Turk & R. D. Kerns (Eds), *Health, illness, and families: a life-span perspective*. New York: John Wiley & Sons.

Barbee, A. P. (1990). Interactive coping: the cheering-up process in close relationships. In S. Duck with R. C. Silver (Eds), *Personal relationships and social support*. London: Sage.

Barbee, A. P., & Cunningham, M. R. (1988). The effects of mood on the cheering-up process in romantic couples. Paper presented at the annual convention of the American Psychological Association, Atlanta, GA, August.

Barber, J. (1986). Hypnotic analgesia. In A. D. Holzman & D. C. Turk (Eds), *Pain management: a handbook of psychological treatment approaches*. New York: Pergamon.

Barber, T. X. (1982). Hypnosuggestive procedures in the treatment of clinical pain: implications for theories of hypnosis and suggestive therapy. In T. Millon, C., Green & R. B. Meagher (Eds), *Handbook of clinical health psychology*. New York: Plenum.

Bardo, M. T., & Risner, M. E. (1985). Biochemical substrates of drug abuse. In M. Galizio & S. A. Maisto (Eds), *Determinants of substance abuse: biological, psychological, and environmental factors*. New York: Plenum.

Barefoot, J. C., Dahlstrom, W. G., & Williams, R. B. (1983). Hostility, CHD incidence and total mortality: a 25-year follow-up study of 255 physicians. *Psychosomatic Medicine*, 45, 559–63.

Barina, M. (1995). 'Obese' protein slims mice. *Science*, 269, 475–6.

Barlow, D. H., & Rapee, R. M. (1997). *Mastering stress: a lifestyle approach*. Killara: Lifestyle Press.

Baron, R. A. (1986). *Behavior in organizations: understanding and managing the human side of work* (2nd ed.). Boston: Allyn & Bacon.

Barrera, M., Jr. (1986). Distinctions between social support concepts, measures, and models. *American Journal of Community Psychology*, 14, 413–45.

Barrett, R. J. (1985). Behavioral approaches to individual differences in substance abuse. In M. Galizio & S. A. Maisto (Eds), *Determinants of substance abuse: biological, psychological, and environmental factors*. New York: Plenum.

Barsky, A. J., & Klerman, G. L. (1983). Overview: hypochondriasis, bodily complaints, and somatic styles. *American Journal of Psychiatry*, 140, 273–83.

Barton, A. H. (1969). *Communities in disaster: a sociological analysis of collective stress situations*. New York: Doubleday.

Barton, J., Chassin, L., Presson, C. C., & Sherman, S. J. (1982). Social image factors as motivators of smoking initiation in early and middle adolescence. *Child Development*, 53, 1499–1511.

Bartone, P. T. (1999). Hardiness protects against war-related stress in Army Reserve forces. *Consulting Psychology Journal: Practice and Research*, 51(2), 72–82.

Bashford, A. (1994). Respectability, morality, cleanliness: the feminisation of hospitals in colonial Australia. In K. Darian-Smith (Ed.), *Working papers in Australian studies*. Nos. 88–96 (pp. 85–96). London: Sir Robert Menzies Centre for Australian Studies, Institute of Commonwealth Studies, University of London.

Bastone, E. C., & Kerns, R. D. (1995). Effects of self-efficacy and perceived social support on recovery-related behaviors after coronary artery bypass graft surgery. *Annals of Behavioral Medicine*, 17, 324–30.

Batchelor, W. F. (1988). AIDS 1988: the science and the limits of science. *American Psychologist*, 43, 853–8.

Bates, P. (1992). Defining death, natural death legislation and withdrawal of treatment. *Australian Health Review*, 15, 392–421.

Battista, R. N., & Grover, S. A. (1988). Early detection of cancer: an overview. In L. Breslow, J. E. Fielding & L. B. Lave (Eds), *Annual review of public health* (Vol. 9). Palo Alto, CA: Annual Reviews.

Baum, A. (1988, April). Disasters, natural & otherwise. *Psychology Today*, pp. 56–60.

Baum, A. (1990). Stress, intrusive imagery, and chronic distress. *Health Psychology*, 9, 653–75.

Baum, A. (1994). Behavioral, biological, and environmental interactions in disease processes. In S. J. Blumenthal, K. Matthews & S. M. Weiss (Eds), *New research frontiers in behavioral medicine: proceedings of the national conference*. Washington: U.S. Government Printing Office.

Baum, A., Aiello, J. R., & Calesnick, L. E. (1978). Crowding and personal control: social density and the development of learned helplessness. *Journal of Personality and Social Psychology*, 36, 1000–1011.

Baum, A., & Gatchel, R. J. (1981). Cognitive determinants of reaction to uncontrollable events: development of reactance and learned helplessness. *Journal of Personality and Social Psychology*, 40, 1078–89.

Baum, A., Grunberg, N. E., & Singer, J. E. (1982). The use of physiological and neuroendocrinological measurements in the study of stress. *Health Psychology*, 1, 217–36.

Bauman, A. (1993). Effects of asthma patient education upon psychological and behavioural outcomes. In S. Maes, H. Leventhal & M. Johnston (Eds), *International review of health psychology* (Vol. 2). New York: John Wiley & Sons.

Bauman, A., Cooper, C., Bridges-Webb, C., Tse, M., Miles, D., Bhasale, A., & Pollock, M. (1995). Asthma management and morbidity in Australian general practice: the relationship between patient and doctor estimates. *Respiratory Medicine*, 89, 665–72.

Baumann, L. J., & Leventhal, H. (1985). 'I can tell when my blood pressure is up, can't I?' *Health Psychology*, 4, 203–218.

Beach, D. L., & Mayer, J. A. (1990). The effects of social demand on breast self-examination self-report. *Journal of Behavioral Medicine*, 13, 195–205.

Bean-Bayog, M. (1991). Alcoholics anonymous. In D. A. Ciraulo & R. I. Shader (Eds), *Clinical manual of chemical dependence*. Washington, DC: American Psychiatric Press.

Beck, A. T (1976). *Cognitive therapy and the emotional disorders*. New York: International Universities Press.

Beck, A. T., Freeman, A., & associates (1990). *Cognitive therapy of personality disorders*. New York: Guilford.

Beck, A. T., & Shaw, B. F. (1977). Cognitive approaches to depression. In A. Ellis & R. Grieger (Eds), *Handbook of rational-emotive therapy*. New York: Springer.

Beck, M., Springen, K., Beachy, L., Hager, M., & Buckley, L. (1990, April 30). The losing formula. *Newsweek*, pp. 52–8.

Becker, M. H. (1979). Understanding patient compliance: The contributions of attitudes and other psychosocial factors. In S. J. Cohen (Ed.), *New directions in patient compliance*. Lexington, MA: Heath.

Becker, M. H. (1990). In hot pursuit of health promotion: Some admonitions. In S. M. Weiss, J. E. Fielding & A. Baum (Eds), *Perspectives in behavioral medicine: health at work*. Hillsdale, NJ: Erlbaum.

Becker, M. H., Maiman, L. A., Kirscht, J. P., Haefner, D. P., & Drachman, R. H. (1977). The health belief model and prediction of dietary compliance: a field experiment. *Journal of Health and Social Behavior*, 18, 348–66.

Becker, M. H., & Rosenstock, I. M. (1984). Compliance with medical advice. In A. Steptoe & A. Mathews (Eds), *Health care and human behaviour*. London: Academic Press.

Beecher, H. K. (1956). Relationship of significance of wound to pain experienced. *Journal of the American Medical Association*, 161, 1609–1613.

Begley, S. (1994, February 7). One pill makes you larger, and one pill makes you small. *Newsweek*, pp. 36–40.

Begley, S. (1995, October 9). Promises, promises. *Newsweek*, pp. 60–62.

Beglin, S. J., & Fairburn, C. G. (1992). Women who choose not to participate in surveys on eating disorders. *International Journal of Eating Disorders*, 12, 113–16.

Bekkers, M. J. T. M., Van Knippenberg, F. C. E., Van Den Borne, H. W., Poen, H., Bergsma, J., & Vanbergehenegouwen, G. P. (1995). Psychosocial adaptation to stoma surgery: a review. *Journal of Behavioral Medicine*, 18, 1–31.

Belar, C. D. (1988). Education in behavioral medicine: Perspectives from psychology. *Annals of Behavioral Medicine*, 10, 11–14.

Belar, C. D. (1991). Issues in training clinical health psychologists. In M. A. Jansen & J. Weinman (Eds), *The international development of health psychology*. Chur, Switzerland: Harwood.

Belar, C. D., & Kibrick, S. A. (1986). Biofeedback in the treatment of chronic back pain. In A. D. Holzman & D. C. Turk (Eds), *Pain management: a handbook of psychological treatment approaches*. New York: Pergamon.

Bélisle, M., Roskies, E., & Lévesque, J. (1987). Improving adherence to physical activity. *Health Psychology*, 6, 159–72.

Belloc, N. B., & Breslow, L. (1972). Relationship of physical health status and health practices. *Preventive Medicine*, 1, 409–421.

Belluck, P. (1996, May 9). Mingling two worlds of medicine. *New York Times*, pp. B1, 4.

Bengston, V. L., Cuellar, J. B., & Ragan, P. K. (1977). Stratum contrasts and similarities in attitudes toward death. *Journal of Gerontology*, 32, 76–88.

Benjamini, S., & Leskowitz, S. (1991). *Immunology: a short course* (2nd ed.). New York: John Wiley & Sons.

Bennett, E. (1991). Weight-loss practices of overweight adults. *American Journal of Clinical Nutrition*, 53, S1519–21.

Bennett, H. L. (1989, Fall/Winter). Report of the First International Symposium on Memory and Awareness in Anaesthesia. *Health Psychologist*, pp. 3–4.

Bennett, P. (1995). Disorders of the gut. In A. Broome & S. Llewellyn (Eds), *Health psychology: process and applications* (2nd ed.) (pp. 225–44). London: Chapman & Hall.

Bennett, P., Wallace, L., Carroll, D., & Smith, N. (1991). Treating Type A behaviours and mild hypertension in middle-aged men. *Journal of Psychosomatic Research*, 35, 209–223.

Bennett, S. (1995). Cardiovascular risk factors in Australia: trends in socioeconomic inequalities. *Journal of Epidemiology and Community Health*, 49, 363–72.

Bennett, S. (1996). Socioeconomic inequalities in coronary heart disease and stroke mortality among Australian men, 1979–1993. *International Journal of Epidemiology*, 25, 266–75.

Bennett, S. A., & Magnus, P. (1994). Trends in cardiovascular risk factors in Australia: results from the National Heart Foundation's Risk Factor Prevalence Study, 1980–1989. *The Medical Journal of Australia*, 161, 519–27.

Bennett, T. L., Gottlieb, B. H., & Cadman, D. (1987). Social support for parents of children with chronic illness: Preliminary development of the CCISS. Unpublished manuscript.

Bennett, W. I. (1987, December 13). Monitoring drugs for the aged. *New York Times Magazine*, pp. 73–4.

Bennett, W., & Gurin, J. (1982). *The dieter's dilemma: eating less and weighing more*. New York: Basic Books.

Benoliel, J. Q. (1977). Nurses and the human experience of dying. In H. Feifel (Ed.), *New meanings of death*. New York: McGraw-Hill.

Benson, H. (1984). The relaxation response and stress. In J. D. Matarazzo, S. M. Weiss, J. A. Herd, N. E. Miller & S. M. Weiss (Eds), *Behavioral health: a handbook of health enhancement and disease prevention*. New York: John Wiley & Sons.

Benson, H. (1991). Mind/body interactions including Tibetan studies. In The Dalai Lama, H. Benson, R. A. F. Thurman, H. E. Gardner & D. Goleman (Eds), *Mind-science: an East–West dialogue*. Boston, MA: Wisdom.

Benson, H., Malhotra, M. S., Goldman, R. F., Jacobs, G. D., & Hopkins, P. J. (1990). Three case reports of the metabolic and electroencephalographic changes during advanced Buddhist meditation techniques. *Behavioral Medicine*, 16, 90–94.

Bentler, P. M., & Speckart, G. (1979). Models of attitude — behavior relations. *Psychological Review*, 86, 452–64.

Ben-Tovim, D. & Walker, M. (1991). Women's body attitudes: a review of measurement techniques. *International Journal of Eating Disorders*, 10(2), 155–67.

Ben-Zur, H., Rappaport, B., Ammar, R., & Uretzky, G. (2000). Coping strategies, life style changes and pessimism after open heart surgery. *Health and Social Work*, 25(3), 201–9.

Beran, R. G., Hall, L., & Michelazzi, J. (1985). An accurate assessment of the prevalence ratio of epilepsy adequately adjusted by influencing factors. *Neuroepidemiology*, 4, 71–81.

Bergman, L. R., & Magnusson, D. (1986). Type A behavior: a longitudinal study from childhood to adulthood. *Psychosomatic Medicine*, 48, 134–42.

Berkman, L. F. (1995). The role of social relations in health promotion. *Psychosomatic Medicine*, 57, 245–54.

Berkman, L. F., & Syme, S. L. (1979). Social networks, host resistance, and mortality: a nine-year follow-up study of Alameda County residents. *American Journal of Epidemiology*, 109, 186–204.

Berren, M. R., Beigel, A., & Ghertner, S. (1980). A topology for the classification of disasters. *Community Mental Health Journal*, 16, 103–111.

Bertalanffy, L. von (1968). *General systems theory*. New York: Braziller.

Best, J. A., Thomson, S. J., Santi, S. M., Smith, E. A., & Brown, K. S. (1988). Preventing cigarette smoking among school children. In L. Breslow, J. E. Fielding & L. B. Lave (Eds), *Annual review of psychology* (Vol. 9). Palo Alto, CA: Annual Reviews.

Bibace, R., & Walsh, M. E. (1979). Developmental stages in children's conceptions of illness. In G. C. Stone, F. Cohen & N. E. Adler (Eds), *Health psychology — a handbook*. San Francisco: Jossey-Bass.

Bien, T. H., Miller, W. R., & Boroughs, J. M. (1993). Motivational interviewing with alcohol outpatients. *Behavioural and Cognitive Psychotherapy*, 21, 347–56.

Biglan, A., McConnell, S., Severson, H. H., Bavry, J., & Ary, D. (1984). A situational analysis of adolescent smoking. *Journal of Behavioral Medicine*, 7, 109–114.

Biglan, A., Severson, H., Ary, D., Faller, C., Gallison, C., Thompson, R., Glasgow, R., & Lichtenstein, E. (1987). Do smoking prevention programs really work? Attrition and the internal and external validity of an evaluation of a refusal skills training program. *Journal of Behavioral Medicine*, 10, 159–71.

Billings, A. G., & Moos, R. H. (1981). The role of coping responses and social resources in attenuating the stress of life events. *Journal of Behavioral Medicine*, 4, 139–57.

Biondi, M., & Pancheri, P. (1995). Clinical research strategies in psychoimmunology: a review of 46 human research studies (1972–92). In B. Leonard & K. Miller (Eds), *Stress, the immune system and psychiatry*. New York: John Wiley & Sons.

Birch, L. L. (1989). Developmental aspects of eating. In R. Shepherd (Ed.), *Handbook of the psychophysiology of human eating*. Chichester: John Wiley & Sons.

Birren, J. E., & Zarit, J. M. (1985). Concepts of health, behavior, and aging. In J. E. Birren & J. Livingston (Eds), *Cognition, stress, and aging*. Englewood Cliffs, NJ: Prentice Hall.

Bishop, G. D., & Converse, S. A. (1986). Illness representations: a prototype approach. *Health Psychology*, 5, 95–114.

Black, F. L. (1992). Why did they die? *Science*, 258, 1739–40.

Blackburn, H., Luepker, R., Kline, F. G., Bracht, N., Carlaw, R., Jacobs, D., Mittelmark, M., Stauffer, L., & Taylor, H. L. (1984). The Minnesota Heart Health Program: a research and demonstration project in cardiovascular disease prevention. In J. D. Matarazzo, S. M. Weiss, J. A. Herd, N. E. Miller & S. M. Weiss (Eds), *Behavioral health: a handbook of health enhancement and disease prevention*. New York: John Wiley & Sons.

Blackhall, L. J., Murphy, S. T., Frank, G., Michel, V., & Azen, S. (1995). Ethnicity and attitudes toward patient autonomy. *Journal of the American Medical Association*, 274, 820–25.

Blair, S. N., Kohl, H. W., Gordon, N. F., & Paffenbarger, R. S. (1992). How much physical activity is good for health? In G. S. Omenn, J. E. Fielding & L. B. Lave (Eds), *Annual review of public health* (Vol. 13). Palo Alto, CA: Annual Reviews.

Blakeslee, S. (1994, April). Black smokers' higher risk of cancer may be genetic. *New York Times*, p. C14.

Blakey, R., & Baker, R. (1980). An exposure approach to alcohol abuse. *Behaviour Research and Therapy*, 18, 319–25.

Blanchard, E. B. (1987). Long-term effects of behavioral treatment of chronic headache. *Behavior Therapy*, 18, 375–85.

Blanchard, E. B., & Andrasik, F. (1985). *Management of chronic headaches: a psychological approach*. New York: Pergamon.

Blanchard, E. B., Andrasik, F., Appelbaum, K. A., Evans, D. D., Myers, P., & Barron, K. D. (1986). Three studies of the psychologic changes in chronic headache patients associated with biofeedback and relaxation therapies. *Psychosomatic Medicine*, 48, 73–83.

Blanchard, E. B., Andrasik, F., Guarnieri, P., Neff, D. F., & Rodichok, L. D. (1987). Two-, three-, and four-year follow-up on the self-regulatory treatment of chronic headache. *Journal of Consulting and Clinical Psychology*, 55, 257–9.

Blanchard, E. B., Appelbaum, K. A., Guarnieri, P., Morrill, B., & Dentinger, M. P. (1987). Five year prospective follow-up on the treatment of chronic headache with biofeedback and/or relaxation. *Headache*, 27, 580–83.

Blanchard, E. B., Buckley, T. C., Hickling, E. J., & Taylor, A. E. (1998). Posttraumatic stress disorder and comorbid major depression: Is the correlation an illusion? *Journal of Anxiety Disorders*, 12(1), 21–37.

Blanchard, E. B., McCoy, G. C., Wittrock, D., Musso, A., Gerardi, R. J., & Pangburn, L. (1988). A controlled comparison of thermal biofeedback and relaxation training in the treatment of essential hypertension: II. Effects on cardiovascular reactivity. *Health Psychology*, 7, 19–33.

Bland, S. H., O'Leary, E. S., Farinaro, E., Jossa, F., & Trevisan, M. (1996). Long-term psychological effects of natural disasters. *Psychosomatic Medicine*, 58, 18–24.

Blaney, N. T. (1985). Smoking: Psychophysiological causes and treatments. In N. Schneiderman & J. T. Tapp (Eds), *Behavioral medicine: the biopsychosocial approach*. Hillsdale, NJ: Erlbaum.

Blaney, P. H. (1985). Psychological considerations in cancer. In N. Schneiderman & J. T. Tapp (Eds), *Behavioral medicine: the biopsychosocial approach*. Hillsdale, NJ: Erlbaum.

Blechman, E. (1983). Behavioral medicine and women's health issues: responding to the challenges of biological events. *Behavioral Medicine Update*, 5, 7–10.

Bleiberg, J. (1986). Psychological and neuropsychological factors in stroke management. In P. E. Kaplan & L. J. Cerullo (Eds), *Stroke rehabilitation*. Boston: Butterworth.

Bleiberg, J., Ciulla, R., & Katz, B. I. (1991). Psychological components of rehabilitation programs for brain-injured and spinal-cord-injured patients. In J. J. Sweet, R. H. Rozensky & S. M. Tovian (Eds), *Handbook of clinical psychology in medical settings*. New York: Plenum.

Block, A. R., Kremer, E., & Gaylor, M. (1980a). Behavioral treatment of chronic pain: the spouse as a discriminative cue for pain behavior. *Pain*, 9, 243–52.

Block, A. R., Kremer, E., & Gaylor, M. (1980b). Behavioral treatment of chronic pain: variables affecting treatment efficacy. *Pain*, 8, 367–75.

Block, J. H. (1983). Differential premises arising from differential socialization of the sexes: some conjectures. *Child Development*, 54, 1335–54.

Block, M. A. (1976). Don't place alcohol on a pedestal. *Journal of the American Medical Association*, 235, 2103–4.

Bloom, F. E., Lazerson, A., & Hofstadter, L. (1985). *Brain, mind, and behavior*. New York: Freeman.

Bloom, J. R., Kang, S. H., & Romano, P. (1991). Cancer and stress: the effect of social support as a resource. In C. L. Cooper & M. Watson (Eds), *Cancer and stress: psychological, biological and coping studies*. Chichester: John Wiley & Sons.

Bloom, J. W., Kaltenborn, W. T., Paoletti, P., Camilli, A., & Lebowitz, M. D. (1987). Respiratory effects of non-tobacco cigarettes. *British Medical Journal*, 295, 1516–18.

Blount, R., Sturges, J., & Powers, S. (1990). Analysis of child and adult behavioral variations by phase of medical procedure. *Behavior Therapy*, 21, 33–48.

Bluebond-Langner, M. (1977). Meanings of death to children. In H. Feifel (Ed.), *New meanings of death*. New York: McGraw-Hill.

Blumenthal, J. A., & McCubbin, J. A. (1987). Physical exercise as stress management. In A. Baum & J. E. Singer (Eds), *Handbook of psychology and health* (Vol. 5). Hillsdale, NJ: Erlbaum.

Blumenthal, J. A., Williams, R. S., Wallace, A. G., Williams, R. B., & Needles, T. L. (1982). Physiological and psychological variables predict compliance to prescribed exercise therapy in patients recovering from myocardial infarction. *Psychosomatic Medicine*, 44, 519–27.

Blumer, D., & Heilbronn, M. (1982). Chronic pain as a variant of depressive disease: the pain-prone disorder. *Journal of Nervous and Mental Disease*, 170, 381–406.

Bodmer, W. F., Bailey, C. J., Bodmer, J., Bussey, H. J. R., et al. (1987). Localization of the gene for familial adenomatous polyposis on chromosome 5. *Nature*, 328, 614–16.

Bogaards, M. C., & ter Kuile, M. M. (1994). Treatment of recurrent tension headache: a meta-analytic review. *Clinical Journal of Pain*, 10, 174–90.

Bohm, L. C., & Rodin, J. (1985). Aging and the family. In D. C. Turk & R. D. Kerns (Eds), *Health, illness, and families: a life-span perspective*. New York: John Wiley & Sons.

Boldero, J. & Fallon, B. (1995). Adolescent help-seeking: what do they get help for and from whom? *Journal of Adolescence*, 18, 193–209.

Boldero, J., Moore, S., & Rosenthal, D. (1992). Intention, context and safe sex: Australian adolescents' responses to AIDS. *Journal of Applied Social Psychology*, 22(17), 1374–96.

Bond, G. G., Aiken, L. S., & Somerville, S. C. (1992). The health belief model and adolescents with insulin-dependent diabetes mellitus. *Health Psychology*, 11, 190–98.

Booth, M. L., Macaskill, P., Owen, N., Oldenburg, B., Marcus, B. H., & Bauman, A. (1993). Population prevalence and correlates of stages of change in physical activity. *Health Education Quarterly*, 20(3), 431–40.

Booth-Kewley, S., & Friedman, H. (1987). Psychological predictors of heart disease: a quantitative review. *Psychological Bulletin*, 101(3), 343–62.

Borland, R., Hill, D., & Noy, S. (1990). Being SunSmart: changes in community awareness and reported behaviour following a primary prevention program for skin cancer control. *Behaviour Change*, 7, 126–35.

Borland, R., & Owen, N. (1995). Need to smoke in the context of workplace smoking bans. *Preventive Medicine*, 24, 56–60.

Borland, R., Owen, N., Hill, D., & Chapman, S. (1994). Regulatory innovations, behavior and health: implications of research on workplace smoking bans. *International Review of Health Psychology*, 3, 167–85.

Borland, R., Owen, N., & Hocking, B. (1991). Changes in smoking behavior following the implementation of a total workplace smoking ban. *Australian Journal of Public Health*, 15, 130–34.

Borushek, A. (1986). *The 1986 Australian pocket calorie counter*. Singapore: Family Health Publications.

Borushek, A. (2001). *Allan Borushek's Calorie and fat counter*. Nedlands, WA: Family Health Publications.

Borysenko, J. (1984). Stress, coping, and the immune system. In J. D. Matarazzo, S. M. Weiss, J. A. Herd, N. E. Miller & S. M. Weiss (Eds), *Behavioral health: a handbook of health enhancement and disease prevention*. New York: John Wiley & Sons.

Bosley, C. M., Fosbury, J. A., & Cochrane, G. M. (1995). The psychological factors associated with poor compliance with treatment in asthma. *European Respiratory Journal*, 8, 899–904.

Bosma, H., Peter, R., Siegrist, J., & Marmot, M. (1998). Two alternative job stress models and the risk of coronary heart disease. *American Journal of Public Health*, 88(1), 68–74.

Botvin, G. J., Baker, E., Dusenbury, L., Tortu, S., & Botvin, E. M. (1990). Preventing adolescent drug abuse through a multimodal cognitive-behavioral approach: results of a 3-year study. *Journal of Consulting and Clinical Psychology*, 58, 437–46.

Botvin, G. J., Renick, N. L., & Baker, E. (1983). The effects of scheduling format and booster sessions on a broad-spectrum psychosocial approach to smoking prevention. *Journal of Behavioral Medicine*, 6, 359–79.

Botvin, G. J., & Wills, T. A. (1985). Personal and social skills training: cognitive-behavioral approaches to substance abuse prevention. In C. S. Bell & R. Battjes (Eds), *Prevention research: deterring drug abuse among children and adolescents* (NIDA Research Monograph 63). Washington, DC: US Government Printing Office.

Bou-Holaigah, I., Rowe, P. C., Kan, J., & Calkins, H. (1995). The relationship between neurally mediated hypotension and the chronic fatigue syndrome. *Journal of the American Medical Association*, 274, 961–7.

Boutcher, S. H. (1991). The influence of aerobic exercise on illness. In S. H. Boutcher, *Psychology of sports, exercise and fitness: social and personal issues* (pp. 103–118). New York: Hemisphere.

Bouton, K. (1990, August 5). Painful decisions: the role of the medical ethicist. *New York Times Magazine*, pp. 22–25, 53, 65.

Bovbjerg, D. H., Redd, W. H., Jacobsen, P. B., Manne, S. L., et al. (1992). An experimental analysis of classically conditioned nausea during cancer chemotherapy. *Psychosomatic Medicine*, 54, 623–37.

Bowen, A. M., & Trotter, R. (1995). HIV risk in intravenous drug users and crack cocaine smokers: predicting stage of change for condom use. *Journal of Consulting and Clinical Psychology*, 63, 238–48.

Bowes, W. A., Brackbill, Y., Conway, E., & Steinschneider, A. (1970). The effects of obstetrical medication on fetus and infant. *Monographs of the Society for Research in Child Development*, 35 (4, Whole No. 137).

Bowlby, J. (1969). *Attachment and loss. Vol. 1: Attachment*. New York: Basic Books.

Bowlby, J. (1973). *Attachment and loss. Vol. 2: Separation*. New York: Basic Books.

Bowman, J. A. (1991). *Screening for cancer of the cervix: barriers to utilisation and strategies for promotion*. Newcastle: University of Newcastle.

Boyce, L., & Graff, J. (1983). *Social work in the health field in Australia*. Brisbane: Department Social Work, University of Queensland.

Bracco, L., Gallato, R., Grigoletto, F., Lippi, A., et al. (1994). Factors affecting the course and survival in Alzheimer's disease. *Archives of Neurology*, 51, 1213–19.

Bradford, L. P. (1986). Can you survive retirement? In R. H. Moos (Ed.), *Coping with life crises: an integrated approach*. New York: Plenum.

Bradley, G. W. (1993). *Disease, diagnosis, & decisions*. New York: John Wiley & Sons.

Bradley, L. A. (1983). Coping with chronic pain. In T. G. Burish & L. A. Bradley (Eds), *Coping with chronic disease: research and applications*. New York: Academic Press.

Bradley, L. A. (1994). Pain measurement in arthritis. *Arthritis Care and Research*, 6, 178–86.

Bradley, L. A., & Van der Heide, L. H. (1984). Pain-related correlates of MMPI profile subgroups among back pain patients. *Health Psychology*, 3, 157–74.

Bradley, L. A., Young, L. D., Anderson, K. O., Turner, R. A., Agudelo, C. A., McDaniel, L. K., Pisko, E. J., Semble, E. L., & Morgan, T. M. (1987). Effects of psychological therapy on pain behavior of rheumatoid arthritis patients. *Arthritis and Rheumatism*, 30, 1105–1114.

Brady, M. (1995). Culture in treatment, culture as treatment: a critical appraisal of developments in addictions programs for indigenous North Americans and Australians. *Social Science and Medicine*, 11, 1487–98.

Braith, R. W., Pollock, M. L., Lowenthal, D. T., Graves, J. E., & Limacher, M. C. (1994). Moderate- and high-intensity exercise lowers blood pressure in normotensive subjects 60 to 79 years of age. *American Journal of Cardiology*, 73, 1124–8.

Braithwaite, V. A. (1990). *Bound to care*. Sydney: Allen & Unwin.

Braitman, L. E., Adlin, E. V., & Stanton, J. L. (1985). Obesity and caloric intake: The National Health and Nutrition Examination Survey of 1971–1975 (Hanes I). *Journal of Chronic Diseases*, 9, 727–32.

Brand, E. F., Lakey, B., & Berman, S. (1995). A preventive, psychoeducational approach to increase perceived support. *American Journal of Community Psychology*, 23, 117–36.

Brandon, T. H., Zelman, D. C., & Baker, T. B. (1987). Effects of maintenance sessions on smoking relapse: delaying the inevitable? *Journal of Consulting and Clinical Psychology*, 55, 780–82.

Brandsma, J. M., Maultsby, M. C., & Welsh, R. J. (1980). *Outpatient treatment of alcoholism: a review and comparative study*. Baltimore: University Park Press.

Brannon, L., & Feist, J. (1992). *Health psychology: an introduction to behaviour and health* (2nd ed.). Belmont, CA: Wadsworth.

Brantley, P. J., & Jones, G. N. (1993). Daily stressors and stress-related disorders. *Annals of Behavioral Medicine*, 15, 17–25.

Braveman, N. S. (1987). Immunity and aging: immunologic and behavioral perspectives. In M. W. Riley, J. D. Matarazzo & A. Baum (Eds), *Perspectives in behavioral medicine: the aging dimension*. Hillsdale, NJ: Erlbaum.

Bray, G. A. (1984). The role of weight control in health promotion and disease prevention. In J. D. Matarazzo, S. M. Weiss, J. A. Herd, N. E. Miller & S. M. Weiss (Eds), *Behavioral health: a handbook of health enhancement and disease prevention*. New York: John Wiley & Sons.

Brehm, J. W. (1966). *A theory of psychological reactance*. New York: Academic Press.

Brennan, A. F., Barrett, C. L., & Garretson, H. D. (1987). The utility of McGill Pain Questionnaire subscales for discriminating psychological disorder in chronic pain patients. *Psychology and Health*, 1, 257–72.

Breslow, L. (1983). The potential of health promotion. In D. Mechanic (Ed.), *Handbook of health, health care, and the health professions*. New York: Free Press.

Breslow, L. & Somers, A. R. (1977). The lifetime health-monitoring program. *New England Journal of Medicine*, 296, 601–8.

Brezinka, V. (1992). Conservative treatment of childhood and adolescent obesity. In S. Maes, H. Leventhal & M. Johnston (Eds), *International review of health psychology* (Vol. 1). New York: John Wiley & Sons.

Brindle, R. (1992). Local street speed management in Australia: is it 'traffic calming'? *Accident Analysis and Prevention*, 24, 29–38.

Bristol, J. B., Emmett, P. M., Heaton, K. W., & Williamson, R. C. N. (1985). Sugar, fat, and the risk of colorectal cancer. *British Medical Journal*, 291, 1467–70.

Broadhead, W. E., Kaplan, B. H., James, S. A., Wagner, E. H., Schoenbach, V. J., Grimson, R., Heyden, S., Tibblin, G., & Gehlbach, S. H. (1983). The epidemiologic evidence for a relationship between social support and health. *American Journal of Epidemiology*, 117, 521–37.

Broadstock, M., Borland, R., & Gason, R. (1992). Effects of suntan on judgements of healthiness and attractiveness by adolescents. *Journal of Applied Social Psychology*, 22, 157–72.

Broberg, D. J., & Bernstein, I. L. (1987). Candy as a scapegoat in the prevention of food aversions in children receiving chemotherapy. *Cancer*, 60, 2344–7.

Brod, C. (1988). *Technostress: human cost of the computer revolution*. Reading, MA: Addison-Wesley.

Brody, D. S., Miller, S. M., Lerman, C. E., Smith, D. G., & Caputo, G. C. (1989). Patient perception on involvement in medical care: relationship to illness attitudes and outcomes. *Journal of General Internal Medicine*, 4, 506–511.

Brody, J. E. (1987, March 11). Personal health. *New York Times*, p. C10.

Brody, J. E. (1993, March 24). Clarifying studies on cholesterol and fat. *New York Times*, p. C13.

Broman, C. L. (1993). Social relationships and health-related behavior. *Journal of Behavioral Medicine*, 16, 335–50.

Brook, J. S., Whiteman, M., & Gordon, A. S. (1983). Stages in drug use in adolescence: personality, peer, and family correlates. *Developmental Psychology*, 19, 269–77.

Brook, J. S., Whiteman, M., Gordon, A. S., & Cohen, P. (1986). Dynamics of childhood and adolescent personality traits and adolescent drug use. *Developmental Psychology*, 22, 403–414.

Brooks, P. (1999). Medicare is fundamental to the health care of Australia. *Australian and New Zealand Journal of Public Health*, 23(4), 339–41.

Brower, K. J., Eliopulos, G. A., Blow, F. C., Catlin, D. H., & Beresford, T. P. (1990). Evidence for physical and psychological dependence on anabolic steroids in eight weight lifters. *American Journal of Psychiatry*, 147, 510–12.

Brown, D. (1995, July 3–9). Weakening wonder drugs. *Washington Post National Weekly Edition*, pp. 6–9.

Brown, J. M., O'Keeffe, J., Sanders, S. H., & Baker, B. (1986). Developmental changes in children's cognition to stressful and painful situations. *Journal of Pediatric Psychology*, 11, 343–57.

Brown, P. L. (1991). The burden of caring for a husband with Alzheimer's disease. *Home Healthcare Nurse*, 9(3), 33–8.

Brown, W. J., & Bauman, A. E. (2000). Comparison of estimates of population levels of physical activity using two measures. *Australian and New Zealand Journal of Public Health*, 24(5), 520–25.

Brownell, K. D. (1982). Obesity: understanding and treating a serious, prevalent, and refractory disorder. *Journal of Consulting and Clinical Psychology*, 50, 820–40.

Brownell, K. D. (1986a). Public health approaches to obesity and its management. In L. Breslow, J. E. Fielding & L. B. Lave (Eds), *Annual review of public health* (Vol. 7). Palo Alto, CA: Annual Reviews.

Brownell, K. D. (1986b). Social and behavioral aspects of obesity in children. In N. A. Krasnegor, J. D. Arasteh & M. F. Cataldo (Eds), *Child health behavior: a behavioral pediatrics perspective*. New York: John Wiley & Sons.

Brownell, K. D. (1988, January). Yo-yo dieting. *Psychology Today*, pp. 20–23.

Brownell, K. D. (1989, June). When and how to diet. *Psychology Today*, pp. 40–46.

Brownell, K. D. (1991). Personal responsibility and control over our bodies: When expectation exceeds reality. *Health Psychology*, 10, 303–310.

Brownell, K. D., Cohen, R. Y., Stunkard, A. J., Felix, M. R. J., & Cooley, N. B. (1984). Weight loss competitions at the work site: impact on weight, morale and cost-effectiveness. *American Journal of Public Health*, 74, 1283–5.

Brownell, K. D., Marlatt, G. A., Lichtenstein, E., & Wilson, G. T. (1986). Understanding and preventing relapse. *American Psychologist*, 41, 765–82.

Brownell, K. D., & Rodin, J. (1994). The dieting maelstrom: Is it possible and advisable to lose weight? *American Psychologist*, 49, 781–91.

Brownell, K. D., & Wadden, T. A. (1991). The heterogeneity of obesity: fitting treatments to individuals. *Behavior Therapy*, 22, 153–77.

Brubaker, R. G., & Wickersham, D. (1990). Encouraging the practice of testicular self-examination: a field application of the theory of reasoned action. *Health Psychology*, 9, 154–63.

Brucker, B. S. (1983). Spinal cord injuries. In T. G. Burish & L. A. Bradley (Eds), *Coping with chronic disease: research and applications*. New York: Academic Press.

Bruehl, S., Carlson, C. R., Wilson, J. F., Norton, J. A., Colclough, G., Brady, M. J., Sherman, J. J., & McCubbin, J. A. (1996). Psychological coping with acute pain: an examination of the role of endogenous opioid mechanisms. *Journal of Behavioral Medicine*, 19, 129–41.

Brugha, T. S., Bebbington, P. E., Stretch, D. D., & MacCarthy, B., & Wykes, T. (1997). Predicting the short-term outcome of first episodes and recurrences of clinical depression: a prospective study of life events, difficulties and social support networks. *Journal of Clinical Psychiatry*, 58(7), 298–306.

Bruhn, J. G., & Phillips, B. U. (1987). A developmental basis for social support. *Journal of Behavioral Medicine*, 10, 213–29.

Brunswick, A. F., & Merzel, C. R. (1986). Biopsychosocial and epidemiologic perspectives on adolescent health. In N. A. Krasnegor, J. D. Arasteh & M. F. Cataldo (Eds), *Child health behavior: a behavioral pediatrics perspective*. New York: John Wiley & Sons.

Bruvold, W. H. (1993). A meta-analysis of adolescent smoking prevention programs. *American Journal of Public Health*, 83, 872–80.

Bryer, K. B. (1986). The Amish way of death: a study of family support systems. In R. H. Moos (Ed.), *Coping with life crises: an integrated approach*. New York: Plenum.

Buchanan, J., Borland, R., Cosolo, W., Millership, R., Haines, I., Zimet, A., & Zalcberg, J. (1996). Patients' beliefs about cancer management. *Support Care Cancer*, 4, 110–17.

Buchkremer, G., Bents, H., Horstmann, M., Opitz, K., & Tolle, R. (1989). Combination of behavioural smoking cessation with transdermal nicotine substitution. *Addictive Behaviours*, 14, 229–38.

Buchner, D. M., Beresford, S. A. A., Larson, E. B., Lacroix, A. Z., & Wagner, E. H. (1992). Effects of physical activity on health status in older adults II: intervention studies. In G. S. Omenn, J. E. Fielding & L. B. Lave (Eds), *Annual review of public health* (Vol. 13). Palo Alto, CA: Annual Reviews.

Buchwald, H., Varco, T. L., Matts, J. P., Long, J. M., et al. (1990). Effect of partial ileal bypass surgery on mortality and morbidity from coronary heart disease in patients with hypercholesterolemia. *New England Journal of Medicine*, 323, 946–55.

Buck, R. (1988). *Human motivation and emotion* (2nd ed.). New York: John Wiley & Sons.

Budzynski, T. H., Stoyva, J. M., Adler, C. S., & Mullaney, D. J. (1973). EMG biofeedback and tension headache: a controlled outcome study. *Psychosomatic Medicine*, 35, 484–96.

Buetow, S. A. (1995). What do general practitioners and their patients want from general practice and are they receiving it? a framework. *Social Science and Medicine*, 40(2), 213–21.

Bulcourf, B. B., Unrod, M. E., & Adams, S. G. (1996, March). Daily stress and upper respiratory illness. Paper presented at the meeting of the Society of Behavioral Medicine in Washington.

Bull, F., Schipper, E., Jamrozik, K., & Blanksby, B. (1995). Beliefs and behaviour of general practitioners regarding promotion of physical activity. *Australian Journal of Public Health*, 19(3), 300–304.

Bullock, K. D., Reed, R. J., & Grant, I. (1992). Reduced mortality risk in alcoholics who achieve long-term abstinence. *Journal of the American Medical Association*, 267, 668–72.

Bulman, R. J., & Wortman, C. B. (1977). Attributions of blame and coping in the 'real world': severe accident victims react to their lot. *Journal of Personality and Social Psychology*, 35, 351–63.

Bundy, C., Carroll, D., Wallace, L., & Nagle, R. (1994). Psychological treatment of chronic stable angina pectoris. *Psychology and Health*, 10, 69–77.

Burbach, D. J., & Peterson, L. (1986). Children's concepts of physical illness: a review and critique of the cognitive-developmental literature. *Health Psychology*, 5, 307–325.

Burg, I. N., & Ingall, C. G. (1985). The immune system. In L. L. Hayman & E. M. Sporing (Eds), *Handbook of pediatric nursing*. New York: John Wiley & Sons.

Burg, M. M., & Seeman, T. E. (1994). Families and health: the negative side of social ties. *Annals of Behavioral Medicine*, 16, 109–115.

Burish, T. G., & Jenkins, R. A. (1992). Effectiveness of biofeedback and relaxation training in reducing the side effects of cancer chemotherapy. *Health Psychology*, 11, 17–23.

Burish, T. G., & Lyles, J. N. (1983). Coping with the adverse effects of cancer treatments. In T. G. Burish & L. A. Bradley (Eds), *Coping with chronic disease: research and applications*. New York: Academic Press.

Burish, T. G., Meyerowitz, B. E., Carey, M. P., & Morrow, G. R. (1987). The stressful effects of cancer in adults. In A. Baum & J. E. Singer (Eds), *Handbook of psychology and health* (Vol. 5). New York: Erlbaum.

Burnett, K. F., Taylor, C. B., & Agras, W. S. (1985). Ambulatory computer-assisted therapy for obesity: a new frontier for behavior therapy. *Journal of Consulting and Clinical Psychology*, 53, 698–703.

Burns, E. M., & Arnold, L. E. (1990). Biological aspects of stress: effects on the developing brain. In L. E. Arnold (Ed.), *Childhood stress*. New York: John Wiley & Sons.

Burroughs, B. R., & Dieterle, P. (1985). The respiratory system. In L. L. Hayman & E. M. Sporing (Eds), *Handbook of pediatric nursing*. New York: John Wiley & Sons.

Bush, J. P. (1987). Pain in children: a review of the literature from a developmental perspective. *Psychology and Health*, 1, 215–36.

Bush, J. P., Holmbeck, G. N., & Cockrell, J. L. (1989). Patterns of PRN analgesic drug administration in children following elective surgery. *Journal of Pediatric Psychology*, 14, 433–48.

Bush, J. P., Melamed, B. G., Sheras, P. L., & Greenbaum, P. E. (1986). Mother–child patterns of coping with Anticipatory Medical Stress. *Health Psychology*, 5, 137–57.

Buss, A. H., & Plomin, R. (1975). *A temperamental theory of personality development*. New York: John Wiley & Sons.

Buss, A. H., & Plomin, R. (1986). The EAS approach to temperament. In R. Plomin & J. Dunn (Eds), *The study of temperament: changes, continuities and challenges*. Hillsdale, NJ: Erlbaum.

Buss, A. R. (1973). An extension of developmental models that separate ontogenetic changes and cohort differences. *Psychological Bulletin*, 80, 466–79.

Busse, W. W. (1990, May/June). What is asthma? *Advance Plus*, pp. 1–2.

Butler, C., & Steptoe, A. (1986). Placebo responses: an experimental study of psychophysiological processes in asthmatic volunteers. *British Journal of Clinical Psychology*, 25, 173–83.

Butler, N. (1997). Hyperthyroidism. In A. Baum, S. Newman, J. Weinman, R. West & C. McManus (Eds), *Cambridge handbook of psychology, health and medicine*, pp. 502–3. Cambridge: Cambridge University Press.

Butlin, N. G. (1983). Yo ho ho and how many bottles of rum? *Australian Economic History Review*, 23, 23 March.

Byers, T. E., Graham, S., Haughey, B. P., Marshall, J. R., & Swanson, M. K. (1987). Diet and lung cancer risk: findings from the Western New York Diet Study. *American Journal of Epidemiology*, 125, 351–63.

Byles, J. E., & Sanson-Fisher, R. W. (1996). Mass mailing campaigns to promote screening for cervical cancer: do they work, and do they continue to work? *Australian and New Zealand Journal of Public Health*, 20(3), 254–60.

Byrne, D. G. (1987). *The behavioural management of the cardiac patient*, pp. xi, 206. Norwood, NJ: Ablex.

Byrne, D. G. (1992). The Type A behavior pattern and coronary heart disease. In D. G. Bryne & G. R. Caddy (Eds), *Behavioural medicine: international perspectives* (Vol. 1). Norwood, NJ: Ablex.

Byrne, D. G. (1996). Type A behaviour, anxiety and neuroticism: reconceptualising the patho-physiological paths and boundaries of coronary-prone behaviour. *Stress Medicine*, 12, pp. 227–38.

Byrne, D. G. (1999). Stress, personality interactions and hypertension. In B. Raphael, P. Morris & A. Bordujenko (Eds), *Stress and challenge: health and disease* (pp. 133–55). Brisbane: AGPS.

Byrne, D. G. (2000). The frustration of success: Type A behaviour, occupational stress and cardiovascular disease. In D. Kenny, J. Carlson, F. J. McGuigan & J. L. Sheppard (Eds), *Stress and health: research and clinical applications*, pp. 411–36. Sydney: Harwood Academic Publishers.

Byrne, D.G., Byrne, A. E., & Reinhart, M. I. (1993). Psychosocial correlates of adolescent cigarette smoking: personality or environment. *Australian Journal of Psychology*, 45(2), 87–95.

Byrne, D.G., & Reinhart, M. I. (1990). Self-reported distress, job dissatisfaction and the Type A behaviour pattern in a sample of full-time employed Australians. *Work Stress*, 4, 155–66.

Byrne, D. G., & Rosenman, R. H. (1986). The Type A behaviour pattern as a precursor to stressful life-events: a confluence of coronary risks. *British Journal of Medical Psychology*, 59, 75–82.

Byrne, D. G., & Whyte, H. M. (1978). Dimensions of illness behaviour in survivors of myocardial infarction. *Journal of Psychosomatic Research*, 22, 485–91.

Byrne, D. G., & Whyte, H. M. (1979). A typology of responses to illness in survivors of myocardial infarction. *International Journal of Psychiatry in Medicine*, 9, 135–45.

Byrne, D. G., & Whyte, H. M. (1987). The efficacy of community based smoking cessation strategies: a long term follow-up study. *International Journal of Addictions*, 22, 791–801.

Byrne, D. G., Whyte, H. M., & Buttler, K. L. (1981). Illness behaviour and outcome following survived myocardial infarction: a prospective study. *Journal of Psychosomatic Research*, 25, 97–107.

Byrne, D. G., Whyte, H. M., & Lance, G. N. (1979). A typology of responses to illness in survivors of myocardial infarction. *International Journal of Psychiatry in Medicine*, 13, 1–9.

Byrne, P. S., & Long, B. E. L. (1976). Doctors talking to patients. London: Her Majesty's Stationery Office.

Cacioppo, J. T., Petty, R. E., & Marshall-Goodell, B. (1985). Physical, social, and inferential elements of psychophysiological measurement. In P. Karoly (Ed.), *Measurement strategies in health psychology*. New York: John Wiley & Sons.

Caddy, G. R., & Block, T. (1985). Individual differences in response to treatment. In M. Galizio & S. A. Maisto (Eds), *Determinants of substance abuse: biological, psychological, and environmental factors*. New York: Plenum.

Cadman, D., Rosenbaum, P., Boyle, M., & Offord, D. R. (1991). Children with chronic illness: family and parent demographic characteristics and psychosocial adjustment. *Pediatrics*, 87, 884–9.

Caggiula, A. R., Epstein, L. H., Siegel, S., Vezina, P., Bovbjerg, D. (1992, March). The role of conditioning in chronic drug effects: implications for theories of drug abuse and therapeutic drug efficacy. Symposium conducted at the meeting of the Society of Behavioral Medicine, New York.

Caggiula, A. W., Christakis, G., Farrand, M., Hulley, S. B., Johnson, R., Lasser, N. L., Stamler, J., & Widdowson, G. (1981). The Multiple Risk Intervention Trial (MRFIT): IV. Intervention on blood lipids. *Preventive Medicine*, 10, 443–75.

Cahill, L., Prins, B., Weber, M., & McGaugh, J. L. (1994). β-adrenergic activation and memory for emotional events. *Nature*, 371, 702–4.

Cain, E. N., Kohorn, E. I., Quinlan, D. M., Latimer, K., & Schwartz, P. E. (1986). Psychosocial benefits of a cancer support group. *Cancer*, 57, 183–9.

Cairl, R. E., & Kosberg, J. I. (1993). The interface of burden and level of task performance in caregivers of Alzheimer's disease patients: an examination of clinical profiles. *Journal of Gerontological Social Work*, 19, 133–51.

Calderone, K. (1990). The influence of gender on the frequency of pain and sedative medication administered to postoperative patients. *Sex Roles*, 23(11–12), 713–25.

Calhoun, D. A., Mutinga, M. L., Collins, A. S., Wyss, J. M., & Oparil, S. (1993). Normotensive blacks have heightened sympathetic response to cold pressor test. *Hypertension*, 22, 801–5.

Calhoun, K. S., & Burnette, M. M. (1983). Etiology and treatment of menstrual disorders. *Behavioral Medicine Update*, 5(4), 21–6.

Callahan, E. J. (1980). Alternative strategies in the treatment of narcotic addiction: a review. In W. R. Miller (Ed.), The addictive behaviors: treatment of alcoholism, drug abuse, smoking, and obesity. New York: Pergamon.

Caltabiano, M. L. (1995). Main and stress-moderating health benefits of leisure. *Society and Leisure*, 18(1), 27–42.

Caltabiano, M. L., & Caltabiano, N. J. (1992). The experience of daily hassles for university young people. *Transitions*, 2(3), 46–50.

Caltabiano, M. L., & Holzheimer, M. (1999). Dispositional factors: coping and adaptation during menopause, *Climacteric*, 2, 21–8.

Cameron, I. D., & Quine, S. (1994). External hip protectors: likely non-compliance among high risk elderly people living in the community. *Archives of Gerontology and Geriatrics*, 19(3), 273–81.

Cameron, L., Leventhal, E. A., & Leventhal, H. (1995). Seeking medical care in response to symptoms and life stress. *Psychosomatic Medicine*, 57, 1–11.

Cameron, M. H., Vulcan, A. P., Finch, C. F., & Newstead, S. V. (1994). Mandatory bicycle helmet use following a decade of helmet promotion in Victoria, Australia: an evaluation. *Accident Analysis and Prevention*, 26, 325–37.

Cameron, P., Dziukas, L., Hadj, A., Clark, P., & Hooper, S. (1995). Patterns of injury from major trauma in Victoria. *Australian New Zealand Journal of Surgery*, 65, 848–52.

Cameron, R., & Shepel, L. F. (1986). The process of psychological consultation in pain management. In A. D. Holzman & D. C. Turk (Eds), *Pain management: a handbook of psychological treatment approaches*. New York: Pergamon.

Cameron, S. (1986). *Kidney disease: the facts* (2nd ed.). Oxford, NY: Oxford University Press.

Campbell, T., & Chang, B. (1981). Health care of the Chinese in America. In G. Henderson & M. Primeaux (Eds), *Transcultural health care*. Menlo Park, CA: Addison-Wesley.

Cannon, J. T., Prieto, G. J., Lee, A., & Liebeskind, J. C. (1982). Evidence for opioid and non-opioid forms of stimulation-produced analgesia in the rat. *Brain Research*, 243, 315–21.

Cannon, W. B. (1929). *Bodily changes in pain, hunger, fear and rage* (2nd ed.). New York: Appleton.

Cannon, W. B. (1942). Voodoo death. *American Anthropologist*, 44, 169–81.

Cantor, M., & Little, V. (1985). Aging and social care. In R. H. Binstock & E. Shanas (Eds), *Handbook of aging and the social sciences*. New York: Van Nostrand-Reinhold.

Caplan, L. R. (1986). Care of the patient with acute stroke. In P. E. Kaplan & L. J. Cerullo (Eds), *Stroke rehabilitation*. Boston: Butterworth.

Caplan, R. D., Cobb, S., & French, J. R. P. (1975). Relationships of cessation of smoking with job stress, personality, and social support. *Journal of Applied Psychology*, 60, 211–19.

Cappell, H., & Greeley, J. (1987). Alcohol tension reduction: an update on research and theory. In H. Blane & K. E. Leonard (Eds), *Psychological theories of drinking and alcoholism* (pp. 15–54). New York: Guilford.

Carey, M. P., & Burish, T. G. (1988). Etiology and treatment of the psychological side effects associated with cancer chemotherapy: a critical review and discussion. *Psychological Bulletin*, 104, 307–325.

Carey, M. P., Kalra, D. L., Carey, K. B., Halperin, S., & Richards, C. S. (1993). Stress and unaided smoking cessation: a prospective investigation. *Journal of Consulting and Clinical Psychology*, 61, 831–8.

Carey, R. G. (1975). Living until death: a program of service and research for the terminally ill. In E. Kübler-Ross (Ed.), *Death: the final stage of growth*. Englewood Cliffs, NJ: Prentice Hall.

Carey, W. B., & McDevitt, S. C. (1978). Stability and change in individual temperament diagnoses from infancy to early childhood. *Journal of the American Academy of Child Psychiatry*, 17, 331–7.

Carlson, C. R., & Hoyle, R. H. (1993). Efficacy of abbreviated muscle relaxation training: a quantitative review of behavioral medicine research. *Journal of Consulting and Clinical Psychology*, 61, 1059–67.

Carlson, J.G., & Sheppard, J. L. (1992). Health psychology/behavioural medicine in Australia: a survey. *Australian Psychologist*, 27(2), 83–6.

Carlsson, C. P. O., & Sjölund, B. H. (1994). Acupuncture and subtypes of chronic pain: assessment of long-term results. *Clinical Journal of Pain*, 10, 290–95.

Carmargo, C. A., Vranizan, K. M., Thoresen, C. E., & Wood, P. D. (1986). Type A behavior pattern and alcohol intake in middle-aged men. *Psychosomatic Medicine*, 48, 575–81.

Carmelli, D., Dame, A., Swan, G., & Rosenman, R. (1991). Long-term changes in Type A behavior: a 27-year follow-up of the Western Collaborative Group Study. *Journal of Behavioral Medicine*, 14, 593–606.

Carmelli, D., Rosenman, R. H., & Chesney, M. A. (1987). Stability of the Type A structured interview and related questionnaires in a 10-year follow-up of an adult cohort of twins. *Journal of Behavioral Medicine*, 10, 513–25.

Carmody, T. P., Fey, S. G., Pierce, D. K., Connor, W. E., & Matarazzo, J. D. (1982). Behavioral treatment of hyperlipidemia: techniques, results, and future directions. *Journal of Behavioral Medicine*, 5, 91–116.

Carney, R. M., Freedland, K. E., Eisen, S. A., Rich, M. W., Skala, J. A., & Jaffe, A. S. (1998). Adherence to a prophylactic medication regimen in patients with symptomatic versus asymptomatic ischemic heart disease. *Behavioral Medicine: An Interdisciplinary Journal of Research and Practice*, 24(1), 35–9.

Carney, R. M., Freedland, K. E., Rich, M. W., & Jaffe, A. S. (1995). Depression as a risk factor for cardiac events in established coronary heart disease: a review of possible mechanisms. *Annals of Behavioral Medicine*, 17, 142–9.

Carney, R. M., Rich, M. W., Freedland, K. E., Saini, J., Tevelde, A., Simeone, C., & Clark, K. (1988). Major depressive disorder predicts cardiac events in patients with coronary artery disease. *Psychosomatic Medicine*, 50, 627–33.

Carpenter, D. J., Gatchel, R. J., & Hasegawa, T. (1994). Effectiveness of a videotaped behavioral intervention for dental anxiety: the role of gender and need for information. *Behavioral Medicine*, 20, 123–32.

Carr, D. B., Bullen, B. A., Skrinar, G. S., Arnold, M. A., Rosenblatt, M., Beitins, I. Z., Martin, J. B., & McArthur, J. W. (1981). Physical conditioning facilitates the exercise-induced secretion of beta-endorphin and beta-lipotropin in women. *New England Journal of Medicine*, 305, 560–63.

Carr, V. J., Lewin, T. J., Carter, G. L., & Webster, R. A. (1992). Patterns of service utilisation following the 1989 Newcastle earthquake: findings from phase 1 of the quake impact study. *Australian Journal of Public Health*, 16(4), 360–69.

Carruthers, M. (1983). Instrumental stress tests. In H. Selye (Ed.), *Selye's guide to stress research* (Vol. 2). New York: Van Nostrand-Reinhold.

Carson, D. K., Council, J. R., & Gravley, J. E. (1991). Temperament and family characteristics as predictors of children's reactions to hospitalisation. *Developmental and Behavioral Pediatrics*, 12, 141–7.

Carson, D. K., Gravley, J. E., & Council, J. R. (1992). Children's prehospitalisation conceptions of illness, cognitive development and personal adjustment. *Children's Health Care*, 21, 103–110.

Carver, C. S., Coleman, A. E., & Glass, D. C. (1976). The coronary-prone behavior pattern and the suppression of fatigue on a treadmill test. *Journal of Personality and Social Psychology*, 33, 460–66.

Carver, C. S., DeGregorio, E., & Gillis, R. (1981). Challenge and Type A behavior among intercollegiate football players. *Journal of Sport Psychology*, 3, 140–48.

Carver, C. S., Diamond, E. L., & Humphries, C. (1985). Coronary prone behavior. In N. Schneiderman & J. T. Tapp (Eds), *Behavioral medicine: the biopsychosocial approach*. Hillsdale, NJ: Erlbaum.

Castro, F. G., Newcomb, M. D., McCreary, C., & Baezconde-Garbanati, L. (1989). Cigarette smokers do more than just smoke cigarettes. *Health Psychology*, 8, 107–129.

Cataldo, M. F., Dershewitz, R. A., Wilson, M., Christophersen, E. R., Finney, J. W., Fawcett, S. B., & Seekins, T. (1986). Childhood injury control. In N. A. Krasnegor, J. D. Arasteh & M. F. Cataldo (Eds), *Child health behavior: a behavioral pediatrics perspective*. New York: John Wiley & Sons.

Catania, J. A., Coates, T. J., Stall, R., Bye, L., et al. (1991). Changes in condom use among homosexual men in San Francisco. *Health Psychology*, 10, 190–99.

CDC (Centers for Disease Control and Prevention, U.S. Public Health Service) (1995). HIV/AIDS surveillance report (Vol. 7, No. 1). Washington, DC: Author.

Cepeda-Benito, A. (1993). Meta-analytical review of the efficacy of nicotine chewing gum in smoking treatment programs. *Journal of Consulting and Clinical Psychology*, 61, 822–30.

Chambless, D. L., & Gillis, M. M. (1993). Cognitive therapy of anxiety disorders. *Journal of Consulting and Clinical Psychology*, 61, 248–60.

Champion, V. L. (1990). Breast self-examination in women 35 and older: a prospective study. *Journal of Behavioral Medicine*, 13, 523–38.

Chan, J. M., Rimm, E. B., Colditz, G. A., Stampfer, M. J., & Willett, W. C. (1994). Obesity, fat distribution, and weight gain as risk factors for clinical diabetes in men. *Diabetes Care*, 17, 961–9.

Chandra, R. K. (1991). Interactions between early nutrition and the immune system. In D. J. P. Barker (Chair, Ciba Foundation Symposium, No. 156), *The childhood environment and adult disease*. New York: John Wiley & Sons.

Chaney, E. F. (1989). Social skills training. In R. K. Hester & W. R. Miller (Eds), *Handbook of alcoholism treatment approaches: effective alternatives*. New York: Pergamon.

Chaney, E. F., O'Leary, M. R., & Marlatt, G. A. (1978). Skill training with alcoholics. *Journal of Consulting and Clinical Psychology*, 46, 1092–1104.

Chang, E. C. (1998). Dispositional optimism and primary and secondary appraisal of a stressor: Controlling for confounding influences and relations to coping and psychological and physical adjustment. *Journal of Personality and Social Psychology*, 74(4), 1109–1120.

Chapman, C. R. (1984). New directions in the understanding and management of pain. *Social Science and Medicine*, 19, 1261–77.

Chapman, C. R., Casey, K. L., Dubner, R., Foley, K. M., Gracely, R. H., & Reading, A. E. (1985). Pain measurement: an overview. *Pain*, 22, 1–31.

Chapman, S. L. (1991). Chronic pain: psychological assessment and treatment. In J. J. Sweet, R. H. Rozensky & S. M. Tovian (Eds), *Handbook of clinical psychology in medical settings*. New York: Plenum.

Chapman, S. L., & Brena, S. F. (1985). Pain and society. *Annals of Behavioral Medicine*, 7(3), 21–4.

Chapman, S., Leng Wong, W., & Smith, W. (1993). Self-exempting beliefs about smoking and health: differences between smokers and ex-smokers. *American Journal of Public Health*, 83(2), 215–19.

Chassin, L., Presson, C. C., Sherman, S. J., & Edwards, D. A. (1991). Four pathways to young-adult smoking status: adolescent social-psychological antecedents in a Midwestern community sample. *Health Psychology*, 10, 409–418.

Chelune, G. J. (1987). Epilepsy. In R. J. Corsini (Ed.), *Concise encyclopedia of psychology*. New York: John Wiley & Sons.

Chen, Y., Chen, C.-F., Riley, D. J., Allred, D. C., Chen, P.-H., Von Hoff, D., Osborne, C. K., & Lee, W.-H. (1995). Aberrant subcellular localization of BRCA1 in breast cancer. *Science*, 270, 789–91.

Cheng, T. L., Savageau, J. A., Sattler, A. L., & Dewitt, T. G. (1993). Confidentiality in health care: a survey of knowledge, perceptions, and attitudes among high school students. *Journal of the American Medical Association*, 269, 1404–7.

Cherkin, D. C., Deyo, R. A., Loeser, J. D., Bush, T., & Waddell, G. (1994). An international comparison of back surgery rates. *Spine*, 19, 1201–6.

Chesney, M. A. (1984). Behavior modification and health enhancement. In J. D. Matarazzo, S. M. Weiss, J. A. Herd, N. E. Miller & S. M. Weiss (Eds), *Behavioral health: a handbook of health enhancement and disease prevention*. New York: John Wiley & Sons.

Chesney, M. A., Frautschi, N. M., & Rosenman, R. H. (1985). Modifying Type A behavior. In J. C. Rosen & L. J. Solomon (Eds), *Prevention in health psychology*. Hanover, NH: University Press of New England.

Chilcoat, H. D., Dishion, T. J., & Anthony, J. C. (1995). Parent monitoring and the incidence of drug sampling in urban elementary school children. *American Journal of Epidemiology*, 141, 25–31.

Childress, A. R. (1996, March). Cue reactivity and drug craving. Paper presented at the meeting of the Society of Behavioral Medicine, Washington, DC.

Chrisman, N. J., & Kleinman, A. (1983). Popular health care, social networks, and cultural meanings: the orientation of medical anthropology. In D. Mechanic (Ed.), *Handbook of health, health care, and the health professions*. New York: Free Press.

Christensen, A. J., Edwards, D. L., Wiebe, J. S., Benotsch, E. G., McKelvey, L., Andrews, M., & Lubaroff, D. M. (1996). Effect of verbal self-disclosure on natural killer cell activity: moderating influence of cynical hostility. *Psychosomatic Medicine*, 58, 150–55.

Christensen, A. J., & Smith, T. W. (1995). Personality and patient adherence: correlates of the five-factor model in renal dialysis. *Journal of Behavioral Medicine*, 18, 305–313.

Christensen, J., & Levinson, W. (1991). Implementing a behavioral medicine program in an internal medicine residency: a description of curriculum content, resources and barriers encountered. In M. A. Jansen & J. Weinman (Eds), *The international development of health psychology*. Chur, Switzerland: Harwood.

Christie, M. D., & Shultz, K. S. (1998). Gender differences on coping with job stress and organizational outcomes. *Work and Stress*, 12(4), 351–61.

Ciaranello, R. D. (1983). Neurochemical aspects of stress. In N. Garmezy & M. Rutter (Eds), *Stress, coping, and development in children*. New York: McGraw-Hill.

Cinciripini, P. M., & Floreen, A. (1982). An evaluation of a behavioral program for chronic pain. *Journal of Behavioral Medicine*, 5, 375–89.

Cinciripini, P. M., Lapitsky, L., Seay, S., Wallfisch, A., Kitchens, K., & Van Vunakis, H. (1995). The effects of smoking schedules on cessation outcome: Can we improve on common methods of gradual and abrupt nicotine withdrawal? *Journal of Consulting and Clinical Psychology*, 63, 388–99.

Cioppa, A. L. (1984). Hospice care. In S. N. McIntire & A. L. Cioppa (Eds), *Nursing care: a developmental approach*. New York: John Wiley & Sons.

Ciraulo, D. A., & Renner, J. A. (1991). Alcoholism. In D. A. Ciraulo & R. I. Shader (Eds), *Clinical manual of chemical dependence*. Washington, DC: American Psychiatric Press.

Ciraulo, D. A., & Shader, R. I. (Eds) (1991). *Clinical manual of chemical dependence*. Washington, DC: American Psychiatric Press.

Citron, M. L., Johnston-Early, A., Boyer, M., Krasnow, S. H., Hood, M., & Cohen, M. H. (1986). Patient-controlled analgesia for severe cancer pain. *Archives of Internal Medicine*, 146, 734–6.

Clark, D. O., Patrick, D. L., Grembowski, D., & Durham, M. L. (1995). Socioeconomic status and exercise self-efficacy in late life. *Journal of Behavioral Medicine*, 18, 355–76.

Clarke, V., Hill, D., Rassaby, J., White, V., & Hirst, S. (1991). Determinants of continued breast self-examination practice in women 40 years and over after personalized instruction. *Health Education Research*, 6(3), 297–306.

Clarkson, T. B., Manuck, S. B., & Kaplan, J. R. (1986). Potential role of cardiovascular reactivity in atherogenesis. In K. A. Matthews, S. M. Weiss, T. Detre, T. M. Dembroski, B. Falkner, S. B. Manuck, & R. B. Williams (Eds), *Handbook of stress, reactivity, and cardiovascular disease*. New York: John Wiley & Sons.

Clay, R. A. (1997, April). Is assisted suicide even a rational choice? *American Psychological Association Monitor*, pp. 1, 43.

Clayer, J. (1984). Evaluation of the outcome of disaster. Unpublished report of the Health Commission of South Australia.

Cleeland, C. S., Gonin, R., Hatfield, A. K., Edmonson, J. H., Blum, R. H., Stewart, J. A., & Pandya, K. J. (1994). Pain and its treatment in outpatients with metastatic cancer. *New England Journal of Medicine*, 330, 592–6.

Clever, L. H., & Leguyader, Y. (1995). Infectious health risks for health care workers. In G. S. Omen, J. E. Fielding & L. B. Lave (Eds), *Annual review of public health* (Vol. 16). Palo Alto, CA: Annual Reviews.

Clever, L. H., & Omenn, G. S. (1988). Hazards for health care workers. In L. Breslow, J. E. Fielding & L. B. Lave (Eds), *Annual review of public health* (Vol. 9). Palo Alto, CA: Annual Reviews.

Cluss, P. A., & Epstein, L. H. (1985). The measurement of medical compliance in the treatment of disease. In P. Karoly (Ed.), *Measurement strategies in health psychology*. New York: John Wiley & Sons.

Cluss, P. A., & Fireman, P. (1985). Recent trends in asthma research. *Annals of Behavioral Medicine*, 7(4), 11–16.

Coates, T. J. (1990). Strategies for modifying sexual behavior for primary and secondary prevention of HIV disease. *Journal of Consulting and Clinical Psychology*, 58, 57–69.

Cobb, S. (1976). Social support as a moderator of stress. *Psychosomatic Medicine*, 38, 300–314.

Cobb, S., & Rose, R. M. (1973). Hypertension, peptic ulcer, and diabetes in air traffic controllers. *Journal of the American Medical Association*, 224, 489–92.

Coble, H. M., Gantt, D. L., & Mallinckrodt, B. (1996). Attachment, social competency, and the capacity to use social support. In G. R. Pierce, B. R. Sarason & I. G. Sarason (Eds), *Handbook of social support and the family* (pp. 141–72). New York: Plenum.

Cockburn, J., Murphy, B., Schofield, P., Hill, D., & Borland, R. (1991). Development of a strategy to encourage attendance for screening mammography. *Health Education Research*, 6(3), 279–90.

Coddington, R. D. (1972a). The significance of life events as etiological factors in the diseases of children — I: A survey of professional workers. *Journal of Psychosomatic Research*, 16, 7–18.

Coddington, R. D. (1972b). The significance of life events as etiological factors in the diseases of children — II: A study of a normal population. *Journal of Psychosomatic Research*, 16, 205–213.

Cody, R., & Lee, C. (1990). Behaviors, beliefs, and intentions in skin cancer prevention. *Journal of Behavioral Medicine*, 13(4), 373–89.

Cogan, R., Cogan, D., Waltz, W., & McCue, M. (1987). Effects of laughter and relaxation on discomfort thresholds. *Journal of Behavioral Medicine*, 10, 139–44.

Cohen, F., & Lazarus, R. S. (1979). Coping with the stresses of illness. In G. C. Stone, F. Cohen & N. E. Adler (Eds), *Health psychology — a handbook*. San Francisco: Jossey-Bass.

Cohen, F., & Lazarus, R. S. (1983). Coping and adaptation in health and illness. In D. Mechanic (Ed.), *Handbook of health, health care, and the health professions*. New York: Free Press.

Cohen, J. B., Syme, S. L., Jenkins, C. D., & Kagan, A. (1975). The cultural context of Type A behavior and the risk of CHD. *American Journal of Epidemiology*, 102, 434 (abstract).

Cohen, R. J., & Swerdlik, M. E. (1999) *Psychological testing and assessment: an introduction to tests and measurement*. Mountain View: Mayfield.

Cohen, R. Y., Brownell, K. D., & Felix, M. R. J. (1990). Age and sex differences in health habits and beliefs of schoolchildren. *Health Psychology*, 9, 208–224.

Cohen, S. (1980). After effects of stress on human performance and social behavior: a review of research and theory. *Psychological Bulletin*, 88, 82–108.

Cohen, S., Evans, G. W., Stokols, D., & Krantz, D. S. (1986). *Behavior, health, and environmental stress*. New York: Plenum.

Cohen, S., Glass, D. C., & Singer, J. E. (1973). Apartment noise, auditory discrimination, and reading ability in children. *Journal of Experimental Social Psychology*, 9, 407–422.

Cohen, S., Kamarck, T., & Mermelstein, R. (1983). A global measure of perceived stress. *Journal of Health and Social Behavior*, 24, 385–96.

Cohen, S., Kessler, R., & Underwood Gordon, L. (1995). Strategies for measuring stress in studies of psychiatric and physical disorders. In S. Cohen, R. Kessler & L. Underwood Gordon (Eds), *Measuring stress: a guide for health and social scientists* (pp. 3–26). New York: Oxford University Press.

Cohen, S., & Lichtenstein, E. (1990). Perceived stress, quitting smoking, and smoking relapse. *Health Psychology*, 9, 466–78.

Cohen, S., Lichtenstein, E., Prochaska, J. O., Rossi, J. S., et al. (1989). Debunking myths about self-quitting: evidence from 10 prospective studies of persons who attempt to quit smoking by themselves. *American Psychologist*, 44, 1355–65.

Cohen, S., & McKay, G. (1984). Social support, stress and the buffering hypothesis: a theoretical analysis. In A. Baum, J. E. Singer & S. E. Tayler (Eds), *Handbook of psychology and health* (pp. 253–67). Hillsdale, NJ: Erlbaum.

Cohen, S., & Rodriguez, M. S. (1995). Pathways linking affective disturbances and physical disorders. *Health Psychology*, 14, 374–80.

Cohen, S., & Spacapan, S. (1978). The aftereffects of stress: an attentional interpretation. *Environmental Psychology and Nonverbal Behavior*, 3, 43–57.

Cohen, S., Tyrrell, D. A. J., Russell, M. A. H., Jarvis, M. J., & Smith, A. P. (1993). Smoking, alcohol consumption, and susceptibility to the common cold. *American Journal of Public Health*, 83, 1277–83.

Cohen, S., Tyrrell, D. A. J., & Smith, A. P. (1991). Psychological stress and susceptibility to the common cold. *New England Journal of Medicine*, 325, 606–612.

Cohen, S., & Wills, T. A. (1985). Stress, social support and the buffering hypothesis. *Psychological Bulletin*, 98, 310–57.

Cohen, S. M., & Ellwein, L. B. (1990). Cell proliferation in carcinogenesis. *Science*, 249, 1007–1011.

Cohen, W. S. (1985). Health promotion in the workplace: a prescription for good health. *American Psychologist*, 40, 213–16.

Cohn, L. D., Macfarlane, S., Yanez, C., & Imai, W. K. (1995). Risk-perception: differences between adolescents and adults. *Health Psychology*, 14, 217–22.

Coker, L. (1998). Caregiving activities for cardiac surgery patients and emotional outcomes for spousal caregivers. *Dissertation Abstracts International: Section B — Sciences and Engineering*, 59(5-B), 2452.

Colerick, E. J. (1985). Stamina in later life. *Social Science and Medicine*, 21, 997–1006.

Colletti, G., & Brownell, K. D. (1983). The physical and emotional benefits of social support: application to obesity, smoking, and alcoholism. In M. Hersen, R. M. Eisler & P. M. Miller (Eds), *Progress in behavior modification*. New York: Academic Press.

Colligan, M. J., Urtes, M., Wisseman, C., Rosensteel, R. E., Anania, T. L., & Hornung, R. W. (1979). An investigation of apparent mass psychogenic illness in an electronics plant. *Journal of Behavioral Medicine*, 2, 297–309.

Collins, A., & Frankenhaeuser, M. (1978). Stress responses in male and female engineering students. *Journal of Human Stress*, 4, 43–8.

Collins, C., & Lipman, T. H. (1985). The endocrine system. In L. L. Hayman & E. M. Sporing (Eds), *Handbook of pediatric nursing*. New York: John Wiley & Sons.

Commonwealth Department of Community Services and Health (1990). *Statistics on Drug Abuse in Australia, 1989*. Canberra: AGPS.

Commonwealth Department of Health and Aged Care (2001). Priorities for action on cancer control (2001–2003). Cancer Strategy Working Group, Consultation Draft, January 2001 (chaired by Professor Bruce Armstrong). Commonwealth Department of Health and Aged Care.

Compas, B. E., Worsham, N. L., Ey, S., & Howell, D. C. (1996). When mom or dad has cancer: II. Coping, cognitive appraisals, and psychological distress in children of cancer patients. *Health Psychology*, 15, 167–75.

Conel, J. L. (1939–63). *The postnatal development of the human cerebral cortex* (Vols. 1–7). Cambridge, MA: Harvard University Press.

Conger, J. J., & Petersen, A. C. (1984). *Adolescence and youth: psychological development in a changing world* (3rd ed.). New York: Harper & Row.

Connell, C. M., & D'Augelli, A. R. (1990). The contribution of personality characteristics to the relationship between social support and perceived physical health. *Health Psychology*, 9, 192–207.

Connell, R., Crawford, J., Kippax, S., Dowsett, G., Baxter, D., Watson, L., & Berg, R. (1989). Facing the epidemic: changes in the sexual and social lives of gay and bisexual men in response to the Aids crisis, and their implications for Aids prevention strategies. *Social Problems*, 36, 384–402.

Conner, M., Fitter, M., & Fletcher, W. (1999). Stress and snacking: a diary study of daily hassles and between-meal snacking. *Psychology and Health*, 14(1), 51–63.

Conrad, B., Weidmann, E., Trucco, G., Rudert, W. A., Behboo, R., Ricordi, C., Rodriquez-Rilo, H., Finegold, D., & Trucco, M. (1994). Evidence for superantigen involvement in insulin-dependent diabetes mellitus aetiology. *Nature*, 371, 351–5.

Constable, J. F., & Russell, D. W. (1986). The effect of social support and the work environment upon burnout among nurses. *Journal of Human Stress*, 12, 20–26.

Contrada, R. J., & Krantz, D. S. (1988). Stress, reactivity, and Type A behavior: current status and future directions. *Annals of Behavioral Medicine*, 10, 64–70.

Contrada, R. J., Krantz, D. S., & Hill, D. R. (1988). Type A behavior, emotion, and psychophysiologic reactivity: psychological and biological interactions. In B. K. Houston & C. R. Snyder (Eds), *Type A behavior pattern: research, theory, and intervention*. New York: John Wiley & Sons.

Conway, T. L., Vickers, R. R., Ward, H. W., & Rahe, R. H. (1981). Occupational stress and variation in cigarette, coffee, and alcohol consumption. *Journal of Health and Social Behavior*, 22, 155–65.

Cook, P. S., Petersen, R. C., & Moore, D. T. (1990). *Alcohol, tobacco, and other drugs may harm the unborn*. Rockville, MD: U.S. Department of Health and Human Services.

Cook, W. W., & Medley, D. M. (1954). Proposed hostility and pharisaic-virtue scores for the MMPI. *Journal of Applied Psychology*, 38, 414–18.

Cooper, K. H. (1988). *Controlling cholesterol*. New York: Bantam.

Cooper, M. L., Peirce, R. S., & Huselid, R. F. (1994). Substance use and sexual risk taking among black adolescents and white adolescents. *Health Psychology*, 13, 251–62.

Cooper, P. J., Bawden, H. N., Camfield, P. R., & Camfield, C. S. (1987). Anxiety and life events in childhood migraine. *Pediatrics*, 79, 999–1004.

Cooper, S. (1987). The fetal alcohol syndrome. *Journal of Child Psychology and Psychiatry*, 28, 223–7.

Copeman, R. C., Swannell, R. J., Pincus, D. F., & Woodhead, K. A. (1989). Utilization of the 'Smokescreen' smoking-cessation program by general practitioners and their patients. *Medical Journal of Australia*, 151, 83–7.

Corah, N. L., O'Shea, R. M., Bissell, G. D., Thines, T. J., & Mendola, P. (1988). The dentist–patient relationship: perceived dentist behaviors that reduce patient anxiety and increase satisfaction. *Journal of the American Dental Association*, 116, 73–6.

Costa, P. T., & McCrae, R. R. (1980). Somatic complaints in males as a function of age and neuroticism: a longitudinal analysis. *Journal of Behavioral Medicine*, 3, 245–57.

Costa, P. T., & McCrae, R. R. (1985). Hypochondriasis, neuroticism, and aging. *American Psychologist*, 40, 19–28.

Costa, P. T., Somerfield, M. R., & McCrae, R. R. (1996). Personality and coping. In M. Zeidner & N. S. Endler (Eds), *Handbook of coping: theory, research, applications* (pp. 44–61). New York: John Wiley & Sons.

Costakis, C. E., Dunnagan, T., & Haynes, G. (1999). The relationship between the stages of exercise adoption and other health behaviors. *American Journal of Health Promotion*, 14(1), 22–30.

Costello, R. M., Baillargeon, J. G., Biever, P., & Bennett, R. (1980). Therapeutic community treatment for alcohol abusers: a one-year multivariate outcome evaluation. *International Journal of the Addictions*, 15, 215–32.

Cottington, E. M., & House, J. S. (1987). Occupational stress and health: a multivariate relationship. In A. Baum & J. E. Singer (Eds), *Handbook of psychology and health* (Vol. 5). Hillsdale, NJ: Erlbaum.

Cottington, E. M., Matthews, K. A., Talbott, E., & Kuller, L. H. (1986). Occupational stress, suppressed anger, and hypertension. *Psychosomatic Medicine*, 48, 249–60.

Cotton, M., & Anderson, R. V. (1991). The psychological impact of the Newcastle earthquake and counselling needs. *Australian Counselling Psychologist*, 7(2), 8–22.

Counter, C. M., Hirte, H. W., Bacchetti, S., & Harley. C. B. (1994). Telomerase activity in human ovarian carcinoma. *Proceedings of the National Academy of Sciences*, 91, 2900–2904.

Cousins, M. J. (2000). Relief of pain: a basic human right. *Medical Journal of Australia*, 172, 3–4.

Cousins, N. (1979). *Anatomy of an illness*. New York: Norton.

Cowley, G. (1994, August 22). The ever-expanding plague. *Newsweek*, p. 37.

Cox, D. J., Gonder-Frederick, L., Antoun, B., Cryer, P. E., & Clarke, W. L. (1993). Preceived symptoms in the recognition of hypoglycemia. *Diabetes Care*, 16, 519–27.

Cox, G. B., Chapman, C. R., & Black, R. G. (1978). The MMPI and chronic pain: the diagnosis of psychogenic pain. *Journal of Behavioral Medicine*, 1, 437–43.

Cox, T. (1978). *Stress*. Baltimore: University Park Press.

Cox, W. M. (1985). Personality correlates of substance abuse. In M. Galizio & S. A. Maisto (Eds), *Determinants of substance abuse: biological, psychological, and environmental factors*. New York: Plenum.

Coyne, J. C., & Holroyd, K. (1982). Stress, coping, and illness: a transactional perspective. In T. Millon, C. Green & R. Meagher (Eds), *Handbook of clinical health psychology*. New York: Plenum.

Craig, T. G., Comstock, G. W., & Geiser, P. B. (1974). The quality of survival in breast cancer: a case-control comparison. *Cancer*, 33, 1451–7.

Craun, A. M., & Deffenbacher, J. L. (1987). The effects of information, behavioral rehearsal, and prompting on breast self-exams. *Journal of Behavioral Medicine*, 10, 351–65.

Creamer, M., Burgess, P., & Pattison, P. (1992). Reaction to trauma: a cognitive processing model. *Journal of Abnormal Psychology*, 101, 452–9.

Criqui, M. H., & Ringel, B. L. (1994). Does diet or alcohol explain the French paradox? *The Lancet*, 344, 1719–23.

Crisp, A. H., & Kalucy, R. S. (1974). Aspects of the perceptual disorder in anorexia nervosa. *British Journal of Medical Psychology*, 47, 349–61.

Critelli, J. W., & Neumann, K. F. (1984). The placebo: conceptual analysis of a construct in transition. *American Psychologist*, 39, 32–9.

Crofford, O. B. (1995). Diabetes control and complications. In C. H. Coggins, E. W. Hancock & L. J. Levitt (Eds), *Annual review of medicine* (Vol. 46). Palo Alto, CA: Annual Reviews.

Croog, S. H. (1983). Recovery and rehabilitation of heart patients: psychosocial aspects. In D. S. Krantz, A. Baum & J. E. Singer (Eds), *Handbook of psychology and health* (Vol. 3). Hillsdale, NJ: Erlbaum.

Croog, S. H., & Fitzgerald, E. F. (1978). Subjective stress and serious illness of a spouse: wives of heart patients. *Journal of Health and Social Behavior*, 19, 166–78.

Croyle, R. T., & Barger, S. D. (1993). Illness cognition. In S. Maes, H. Leventhal & M. Johnston (Eds), *International review of health psychology* (Vol. 2). New York: John Wiley & Sons.

Croyle, R. T., & Ditto, P. H. (1990). Illness cognition and behavior: an experimental approach. *Journal of Behavioral Medicine*, 13, 31–52.

CSA (Council on Scientific Affairs) (1983). Medical evaluations of healthy persons. *Journal of the American Medical Association*, 249, 1626–33.

CSIRO (1993). *What are Australians eating? Results from the 1985 and 1990 Victorian Nutrition Surveys*. Adelaide: CSIRO Division of Human Nutrition.

CU (Consumers Union) (1990, October). Chronic fatigue: all in the mind? *Consumer Reports*, pp. 671–5.

CU (1994a, January). Acupuncture. *Consumer Reports*, pp. 54–9.

CU (1994b, January). Alternative medicine: the facts. *Consumer Reports*, pp. 51–3.

CU (1994c, September). Taking vitamins: can they prevent disease? *Consumer Reports*, pp. 561–4.

CU (1996a, August). How good is your health plan? *Consumer Reports*, pp. 28–42.

CU (1996b, August). Will a pill take your pounds off? *Consumer Reports*, pp. 15–17.

Cummings, N. A. (1991). Arguments for the financial efficacy of psychological services in health care settings. In J. J. Sweet, R. H. Rozensky & S. M. Tovian (Eds), *Handbook of clinical psychology in medical settings*. New York: Plenum.

Cummins, R. A., McCabe, M. P., Romeo, A., & Gullone, E. (1995). The Comprehensive Quality of Life (ComQol) Scale: instrument development and psychometric evaluation on college staff and students. *Educational and Psychological Measurement*, 54, 372–82.

Cumpston, J. H. L. (ed. M. J. Lewis) (1989). *Health and disease in Australia: a history*. Canberra: AGPS.

Cunningham, J., & Paradies, Y. (2000). *Occasional paper: mortality of indigenous Australians*. ABS Cat. No. 3315.0. Canberra: ABS.

Curry, S., Marlatt, G. A., & Gordon, J. R. (1987). Abstinence violation effect: validation of an attributional construct with smoking cessation. *Journal of Consulting and Clinical Psychology*, 55, 145–9.

Curry, S., Wagner, E. H., & Grothaus, L. C. (1990). Intrinsic and extrinsic motivation for smoking cessation. *Journal of Consulting and Clinical Psychology*, 58, 310–16.

Curry, S. J., & Emmons, K. M. (1994). Theoretical models for predicting and improving compliance with breast cancer screening. *Annals of Behavioral Medicine*, 16, 302–316.

Curry, S. J., & McBride, C. M. (1994). Relapse prevention for smoking cessation: review and evaluation of concepts and interventions. In G. S. Omenn, J. E. Fielding & L. B. Lave (Eds), *Annual review of public health* (Vol. 15). Palo Alto, CA: Annual Reviews.

Curry, S. J., Taplin, S. H., Anderman, C., Barlow, W. E., & McBride, C. (1993). A randomized trial of the impact of risk assessment and feedback on participation in mammography screening. *Preventive Medicine*, 22, 350–60.

Cutler, R. B., Fishbain, D. A., Rosomoff, H. L., Abdel-Moty, E., Khalil, T. M., & Rosomoff, R. S. (1994). Does nonsurgical pain center treatment of chronic pain return patients to work? A review and meta-analysis of the literature. *Spine*, 19, 643–52.

Cutrona, C. E., & Russell, D. W. (1990). Type of social support and specific stress: toward a theory of optimal matching. In B. R. Sarason, I. G. Sarason & G. R. Pierce (Eds), *Social support: an interactional view*. New York: John Wiley & Sons.

Cutrona, C. E. (1996). Social support as a determinant of marital quality: the interplay of negative and supportive behaviors. In G. R. Pierce, B. R. Sarason & I. G. Sarason, *Handbook of social support and the family* (pp. 17–94). New York: Plenum.

Cutrona, C. E. (1986). Behavioral manifestations of social support: a microanalytic investigation. *Journal of Personality and Social Psychology*, 51, 201–8.

Cutrona, C. E., & Russell, D. W. (1987). The provisions of social relationships and adaptation to stress. In W. H. Jones & D. Perlman (Eds), *Perspectives on interpersonal behavior and relationships* (pp. 37–67). Greenwich, CN: JAI Press.

Cutrona, C. E., & Troutman, B. R. (1986). Social support, infant temperament, and parenting self-efficacy: a mediational model of postpartum depression. *Child Development*, 57, 1507–1518.

Dahlberg, C. C. (1977, June). Stroke. *Psychology Today*, pp. 121–8.

Dahlquist, L. M., Gil, K. M., Armstrong, F. D., Delawyer, D. D., Greene, P., & Wuori, D. (1986). Preparing children for medical examinations: the importance of previous medical experience. *Health Psychology*, 5, 249–59.

Dalessio, D. J. (1994). Diagnosing the severe headache. *Neurology*, 44(Suppl. 3), S6–12.

Daltroy, L. H. (1993). Doctor–patient communication in rheumatological disorders. *Ballire's Clinical Rheumatology*, 7, 221–39.

Daltroy, L. H., Katz, J. N., Morlino, C. I., & Liang, M. H. (1991). Improving doctor–patient communication. *Arthritis Care and Research*, 4, 19.

Daniel, M., Rowley, K. G., McDermott, R., Mylvaganam, A., & O'Dea, K. (1999). Diabetes incidence in an Australian Aboriginal population: an 8-year follow-up study. *Diabetes Care*, 22, 1993–8.

Darrow, W. W., Echenberg, D. F., Jaffe, H. W., O'Malley, P. M., Byers, R. H., Getchell, J. P., & Curran, J. W. (1987). Risk factors for human immunodeficiency virus (HIV) infections in homosexual men. *American Journal of Public Health*, 77, 479–83.

Datillo, A. M., & Kris-Etherton, P. M. (1992). Effects of weight reduction on blood lipids and lipoproteins: a meta-analysis. *American Journal of Clinical Nutrition*, 56, 320–28.

Davidson, R. S. (1985). Behavioral medicine and alcoholism. In N. Schneiderman & J. T. Tapp (Eds), *Behavioral medicine: the bio-psychosocial approach*. Hillsdale, NJ: Erlbaum.

Davies, D. L. (1962). Normal drinking in recovered alcohol addicts. *Quarterly Journal of Studies on Alcohol*, 23, 94–104.

Davies, R. F., Linden, W., Habibi, H., Klinke, P., et al. (1993). Relative importance of psychologic traits and severity of ischemia in causing angina during treadmill exercise. *Journal of the American College of Cardiology*, 21, 331–6.

Davis, M. S. (1966). Variations in patients' compliance with doctors' orders: analysis of congruence between survey responses and results of empirical investigations. *Journal of Medical Education*, 41, 1037–48.

Davison, G. C., & Neale, J. M. (1994). *Abnormal psychology* (6th ed.). New York: John Wiley & Sons.

DeAngelis, T. (1990, October). Psychologists involved with epilepsy treatment. *American Psychological Association Monitor*, p. 24.

DeBenedittis, G., Lorenzetti, A., & Pieri, A. (1990). The role of stressful life events in the onset of chronic primary headache. *Pain*, 40, 65–75.

DeBenedittis, G., Panerai, A. A., & Villamira, M. A. (1989). Effects of hypnotic analgesia and hypnotizability on experimental ischemic pain. *International Journal of Clinical and Experimental Hypnosis*, 35, 55–69.

Degner, L. F., & Beaton, J. I. (1987). *Life–death decisions in health care*. New York: Hemisphere.

de-Groot, K., Boeke, S., van-den Berge, H. J., Duivenvoorden, H. J., Bonke, B., & Passchier, J. (1997). Assessing short and long term recovery from lumbar surgery with pre-operative biographical, medical and psychological variables. *British Journal of Health Psychology*, 2(3), 229–43.

DeJong, W. (1980). The stigma of obesity: the consequences of naive assumptions concerning the causes of physical deviance. *Journal of Health and Social Behavior*, 21, 75–87.

Delahanty, D. L., Dougall, A. L., Hawken, L., Trakowski, J. H., Schmitz, J. B., Jenkins, F. J., & Baum, A. (1996). Time course of natural killer cell activity and lymphocyte proliferation in response to two acute stressors in healthy men. *Health Psychology*, 15, 48–55.

DeLongis, A., Coyne, J. C., Dakof, G., Folkman, S., & Lazarus, R. S. (1982). Relationship to daily hassles, uplifts, and major life events to health status. *Health Psychology*, 1, 119–36.

Denissenko, M. F., Pao, A., Tang, M.-S., & Pfeifer, G. P. (1996). Preferential formation of benzo[a]pyrene adducts at lung cancer mutational hotspots in P53. *Science*, 274, 430–32.

Dennerstein, L., Lehert, P., Burger, H., & Dudley, E. (1999). Mood and the menopausal transition. *Journal of Nervous and Mental Disease*, 187(11), 685–91.

Dennis, C., Houston-Miller, N., Schwartz, R. G., Ahn, D. K., Kraemer, H. C., Gossard, D., Juneau, M., Taylor, C. B., & Debusk, R. F. (1988). Early return to work after uncomplicated myocardial infarction: results of a randomized trial. *Journal of the American Medical Association*, 260, 214–20.

Denton, D., Weisinger, R., Mundy, N. I., Wickings, E. J., et al. (1995). The effect of increased salt intake on blood pressure of chimpanzees. *Nature Medicine*, 1, 1009–1016.

DePalma, A. (1996, June 19). In Mexico, pain relief is a medical and political issue. *New York Times*, p. A6.

Department of Community Services and Health (DCSH) (1986). *National dietary survey of schoolchildren (aged 10–15 years): 1985. Report No 1, Foods consumed.* Canberra: AGPS.

Derogatis, L. R. (1977). *Psychological Adjustment to Illness Scale.* Baltimore: Clinical Psychometric Research.

Derogatis, L. R. (1986). The Psychological Adjustment to Illness Scale (PAIS). *Journal of Psychosomatic Research,* 30, 77–91.

Derogatis, L. R., Fleming, M. P., Sudler, N. C., & Dellapietra, L. (1995). Psychological assessment. In P. M. Nicassio & T. W. Smith (Eds), *Managing chronic illness: a biopsychosocial perspective.* Washington, DC: American Psychological Association.

Des Jarlais, D. C., & Friedman, S. R. (1988). The psychology of preventing AIDS among intravenous drug users: a social learning conceptualization. *American Psychologist,* 43, 865–70.

Des Jarlais, D. C., Friedman, S. R., & Casriel, C. (1990). Target groups for preventing AIDS among intravenous drug users: 2. The 'hard' data studies. *Journal of Consulting and Clinical Psychology,* 58, 50–56.

Descartes, R. (1664). *Traite de l'Homme.* Paris: Angot.

Desharnais, R., Jobin, J., Côté, C., Lévesque, L., & Godin, G. (1993). Aerobic exercise and the placebo effect: a controlled study. *Psychosomatic Medicine,* 55, 149–54.

Deshields, T., Carmin, C., Ross, L., & Mannen, K. (1995, March). Diagnosis of psychological disorders in primary care patients by medicine residents. Paper presented at the meeting of the Society of Behavioral Medicine, San Diego.

Detjen, J. (1991, November 10). Will genetics revolution mark some as victims? *Philadelphia Inquirer,* pp. A1, 18.

Devins, G. M., Binik, Y. M., Hollomby, D. J., Barré, P. E., & Guttmann, R. D. (1981). Helplessness and depression in end-stage renal disease. *Journal of Abnormal Psychology,* 90, 531–45.

Dew, M. A. (1994). Behavioral factors in heart transplantation: quality of life and medical compliance. *Journal of Applied Biobehavioral Research,* 2(1), 28–54.

Deyo, R. A., Cherkin, D., Conrad, D., & Volinn, E. (1991). Cost, controversy, crisis: low back pain and the health of the public. In G. S. Omenn, J. E. Fielding & L. B. Lave (Eds), *Annual review of public health* (Vol. 12). Palo Alto: Annual Reviews.

Diamond, E. L. (1982). The role of anger and hostility in essential hypertension and coronary heart disease. *Psychological Bulletin,* 92, 410–33.

Diamond, E. L., Massey, K. L., & Covey, D. (1989). Symptom awareness and blood glucose estimation in diabetic adults. *Health Psychology,* 8, 15–26.

Diamond, M. (1983). Social adaptation of the chronically ill. In D. Mechanic (Ed.), *Handbook of health, health care, and the health professions,* New York: Free Press.

Dickinson, J. A. (1989). Preventive activities in general practice consultations. Unpublished doctoral dissertation, University of Newcastle, Newcastle.

Dickinson, J. A., Leeder, S. R., & Sanson-Fisher, R. W. (1988). Frequency of cervical smear tests among patients of general practitioners. *Medical Journal of Australia,* 148, 128–31.

DiClemente, C. C., Prochaska, J. O., & Gilbertini, M. (1985). Self-efficacy and the stages of self-change of smoking. *Cognitive Therapy and Research,* 9, 181–200.

DiClemente, C. C., Prochaska, J. O., Velicer, W. F., Fairhurst, S., Rossi, J. S., & Velasquez, M. (1991). The process of smoking cessation: an analysis of precontemplation, contemplation and preparation stages of change. *Journal of Consulting and Clinical Psychology,* 59, 295–304.

DiClemente, R. J., Zorn, J., & Temoshok, L. (1987). The association of gender, ethnicity, and length of residence in the Bay Area to adolescents' knowledge and attitudes about acquired immune deficiency syndrome. *Journal of Applied Social Psychology,* 17, 216–30.

Dielman, T. E., Leech, S. L. Miller, M. V., & Moss, G. E. (1991). Sex and age interactions with the structured interview global Type A behavior pattern and hostility in the prediction of health behaviors. *Multivariate Experimental Clinical Research,* 10(1), 67–83.

DiFranza, J. R., & Lew, R. A. (1995). Effect of maternal cigarette smoking on pregnancy complications and sudden infant death syndrome. *Journal of Family Practice,* 40, 385–94.

DiMatteo, M. R. (1985). Physician–patient communication: promoting a positive health care setting. In J. C. Rosen & L. J. Solomon (Eds), *Prevention in health psychology.* Hanover, NH: University Press of New England.

DiMatteo, M. R., & DiNicola, D. D. (1982). *Achieving patient compliance: the psychology of the medical practitioner's role.* New York: Pergamon.

DiMatteo, M. R., Friedman, H. S., & Taranta, A. (1979). Sensitivity to bodily nonverbal communication as a factor in practitioner–patient rapport. *Journal of Nonverbal Behavior,* 4, 18–26.

DiMatteo, M. R., Hays, R. D., & Prince, L. M. (1986). Relationship of physicians' nonverbal communication skill to patient satisfaction, appointment noncompliance, and physician workload. *Health Psychology,* 5, 581–94.

DiMatteo, M. R., Linn, L. S., Chang, B. L., & Cope, D. W. (1985). Affect and neutrality in physician behavior: a study of patients' values and satisfaction. *Journal of Behavioral Medicine,* 8, 397–409.

Dimsdale, J. E., Alpert, B. S., & Schneiderman, N. (1986). Exercise as a modulator of cardiovascular reactivity. In K. A. Matthews, S. M. Weiss, T. Detre, T. M. Dembroski, B. Falkner, S. B. Manuck & R. B. Williams (Eds), *Handbook of stress, reactivity, and cardiovascular disease.* New York: John Wiley & Sons.

Dingle, A. E. (1978). Drink and drinking in nineteenth century Australia: a statistical commentary. *Monash Papers in Economic History,* 6, 1–41.

Dingle, A. E. (1980). The truly magnificent thirst: an historical survey of Australian drinking habits. *Historical Studies,* 19, 227–49.

Dinh, K. T., Sarason, I. G., Peterson, A. V., & Onstad, L. E. (1995). Children's perception of smokers and nonsmokers: a longitudinal study. *Health Psychology,* 14, 32–40.

DISC (Writing Group for the Disc Collaborative Research Group) (1995). Efficacy and safety of lowering dietary intake of fat and cholesterol in children with elevated low-density lipoprotein cholesterol: the Dietary Intervention Study in Children (DISC). *Journal of the American Medical Association,* 273, 1429–35.

Dishman, R. K. (1981). Biologic influences on exercise adherence. *Research Quarterly for Exercise and Sport,* 52, 143–59.

Dishman, R. K. (1982). Compliance/adherence in health-related exercise. *Health Psychology,* 1, 237–67.

Dishman, R. K. (1986). Mental health. In V. Seefeldt (Ed.), *Physical activity and well-being.* Reston, VA: American Alliance for Health, Physical Education, Recreation, and Dance.

Dishman, R. K. (1991). Increasing and maintaining exercise and physical activity. *Behavior Therapy,* 22, 345–78.

Dishman, R. K., Sallis, J. F., & Orenstein, D. R. (1985). The determinants of physical activity and exercise. *Public Health Reports,* 100, 158–71.

Ditto, B. (1993). Familial influences on heart rate, blood pressure, and self-report anxiety responses to stress: results from 100 twin pairs. *Psychophysiology,* 30, 635–45.

Doherty, K., Militello, F. S., Kinnunen, T., & Garvey, A. J. (1996). Nicotine gum dose and weight gain after smoking cessation. *Journal of Consulting and Clinical Psychology,* 64, 799–807.

Dohrenwend, B. P. (Ed.) (1998). *Adversity, stress and psychopathology.* New York: Oxford University Press.

Dohrenwend, B. S. (1973). Social status and stressful life events. *Journal of Personality and Social Psychology,* 28(2), 225–35.

Dohrenwend, B. S., & Dohrenwend, B. P. (1981). Life stress and illness: formulation of the issues. In B. S. Dohrenwend & B. P. Dohrenwend (Eds), *Stressful life events and their contexts*. New York: Prodist.

Dohrenwend, B. S., Krasnoff, L., Askenasy, A. R., & Dohrenwend, B. P. (1978). Exemplification of a method for scaling life events: the PERI Life Events Scale. *Journal of Health and Social Behavior*, 19, 205–229.

Dolbier, C. L., & Steinhardt, M. A. (2000). The development and validation of the sense of support scale. *Behavioral Medicine*, 25(4), 169–79.

Dolecek, T. A., Milas, N. C., Van Horn, L. V., Farrand, M. E., Gorder, D. D., Duchene, A. G., Dyer, J. R., Stone, P. A., & Randall, B. L. (1986). A long-term nutrition experience: lipid responses and dietary adherence patterns in the Multiple Risk Factor Intervention Trial. *Journal of the American Dietetic Association*, 86, 752–8.

Dolinski, D., Gromski, W., & Zawisza, E. (1987). Unrealistic pessimism. *Journal of Social Psychology*, 127, 511–16.

Dolman, J., Shackleton, G., Ziaian, T., Gay, J., & Yeboah, D. (1996). A survey of health agencies' responses to non-English speaking women's health needs in South Australia. *Australian and New Zealand Journal of Public Health*, 20(2), 155–60.

Donnerstein, E., & Wilson, D. W. (1976). Effects of noise and perceived control on ongoing and subsequent aggressive behavior. *Journal of Personality and Social Psychology*, 34, 774–81.

Dorman, S. M., & Rienzo, B. A. (1988). College students' knowledge of AIDS. *Health Values*, 12(4), 33–8.

Douglas, R. M., & Saltman, D. C. (1991). *Whither Australian general practice?* Canberra: National Centre for Epidemiology and Population Health.

Dowling, J. (1983). Autonomic measures and behavioral indices of pain sensitivity. *Pain*, 16, 193–200.

Downey, G., Silver, R. C., & Wortman, C. B. (1990). Reconsidering the attribution-adjustment relation following a major negative event: coping with the loss of a child. *Journal of Personality and Social Psychology*, 59, 925–40.

Doyle, L. W., Ford, G. W., Olinsky, A., Knoches, A. M., & Callanan, C. (1996). Passive smoking and respiratory function in very low birthweight children. *Medical Journal of Australia*, 164(4), 266–9.

Drake, D. C. (1990, August 19). Choosing a better way to die. *Philadelphia Inquirer Magazine*, pp. 12–21, 33–34.

Draper, B. M., Poulos, C. J., Cole, A. D., Poulos, R. G., & Ehrlich, F. (1992). A comparison of caregivers for elderly stroke and dementia victims. *Journal of the American Geriatrics Society*, 40, 896–901.

Drapkin, R. G., Wing, R. R., & Shiffman, S. (1995). Responses to hypothetical high risk situations: Do the predict weight loss in a behavioral treatment program or the context of dietary lapses? *Health Psychology*, 14, 427–34.

Drossman, D. A. (1994). Irritable bowel syndrome: the role of psychosocial factors. *Stress Medicine*, 10, 49–55.

Drummond, D. C., & Glautier, S. (1994). A controlled trial of cue exposure treatment in alcohol dependence. *Journal of Consulting and Clinical Psychology*, 62, 809–817.

Dua, J., & Hargreaves, L. (1992). Effect of aerobic exercise on negative affect, positive affect, stress and depression. *Perceptual and Motor Skills*, 75, 355–61.

Duck, S., & R. C. Silver (Eds) (1990). *Personal relationships and social support*. London: Sage.

Dula, A. (1994). African American suspicion of the healthcare system is justified: what do we do about it? *Cambridge Quarterly of Healthcare Ethics*, 3, 347–57.

Dunbar-Jacob, J. M., Schlenk, E. A., Burke, L.E., & Matthews, J. T. (1998). Predictors of patient adherence: patient characteristics. In S. A. Shumaker, E. B. Schron, J. K. Ockene & W. L. McBee (Eds), *The handbook of health behavior change* (2nd ed.). New York: Springer.

Dunkel-Schetter, C., & Bennett, T. L. (1990). Differentiating the cognitive and behavioral aspects of social support. In B. R. Sarason, I. G. Sarason & G. R. Pierce (Eds), *Social support: an interactional view*. New York: John Wiley & Sons.

Dunn, A. J. (1995). Psychoneuroimmunology: introduction and general perspectives. In B. Leonard & K. Miller (Eds), *Stress, the immune system and psychiatry*. New York: John Wiley & Sons.

Dunne, M. P., Yeo, M. A., Keane, J., & Elkins, D. B. (2000). Substance use by indigenous and non-indigenous primary school students. *Australian and New Zealand Journal of Public Health*, 24(5), 546–9.

DuRant, R. H., Rickert, V. I., Ashworth, C. S., Newman, C., & Slavens, G. (1993). Use of multiple drugs among adolescents who use anabolic steroids. *New England Journal of Medicine*, 328, 922–6.

Dusseldorp, E., van Elderen, T., Maes, S., Meulman, J., & Kraaij, V. (1999). A meta-analysis of psychoeducational programs for coronary heart disease patients. *Health Psychology*, 18(5), 506–519.

Dweck, C. S., Davidson, W., Nelson, S., & Enna, B. (1978). Sex differences in learned helplessness: II. The contingencies of evaluative feedback in the classroom, and III. An experimental analysis. *Developmental Psychology*, 14, 268–76.

Dweck, C. S., & Elliott, E. S. (1983). Achievement motivation. In P. H. Mussen (Ed.), *Handbook of child psychology* (4th ed., Vol. 4). New York: John Wiley & Sons.

Dweck, C. S., & Repucci, N. D. (1973). Learned helplessness and reinforcement responsibility in children. *Journal of Personality and Social Psychology*, 25, 109–116.

Dwyer, J. T. (1991). Nutritional consequences of vegetarianism. In R. E. Olson, D. M. Bier & D. B. McCormick (Eds), *Annual review of nutrition*. Palo Alto, CA: Annual Reviews.

Easterbrook, G. (1987, January 26). The revolution. *Newsweek*, pp. 40–74.

Edell, B. H., Edington, S., Herd, B., O'Brien, R. M., & Witkin, G. (1987). Self-efficacy and self-motivation as predictors of weight loss. *Addictive Behaviors*, 12, 63–6.

Edelstein, L. (1984). *Maternal bereavement: coping with the unexpected death of a child*. New York: Praeger.

Edgar, N. C., & Knight, R. G. (1994). Gender and alcohol-related expectancies for self and others. *Australian Journal of Psychology*, 46(3), 144–9.

Egger, G., Fitzgerald, W., Frape, G., Monaem, A., Rubinstein, P., Tyler, C., & McKay, B. (1983). Results of large scale media antismoking campaign, in Australia: North Coast 'Quit for Life' programme. *British Medical Journal*, 287, 1125–8.

Eichenwald, K. (1987, January 11). Braving epilepsy's storm. *New York Times Magazine*, pp. 30–36.

Eisenberg, J. M., Kitz, D. S., & Webber, R. A. (1983). Development of attitudes about sharing decision-making: a comparison of medical and surgical residents. *Journal of Health and Social Behavior*, 24, 85–90.

Eisenberg, M. G. (1984). Spinal cord injuries. In H. B. Roback (Ed.), *Helping patients and their families cope with medical problems*. San Francisco: Jossey-Bass.

Eiser, C. (1985). *The psychology of childhood illness*. New York: Springer-Verlag.

Eiser, E. (1997). Children's perceptions of illness and death. In A. Baum, S. Newman, J. Weinman, R. West & C. McManus (Eds), *Cambridge Handbook of psychology, health and medicine* (pp. 81–3). Cambridge: Cambridge University Press.

Elder, J. P., Schmid, T. L., Hovell, M. F., Molgaard, C. A., & Graeff, J. A. (1989). The global relevance of behavioral medicine: health and child survival in the developing world. *Annals of Behavioral Medicine*, 11, 12–17.

Eliopoulos, C., Klein, J., Phan, M. K., Knie, B., Greenwald, M., Chitayat, D., & Koren, G. (1994). Hair concentrations of nicotine and cotinine in women and their newborn infants. *Journal of the American Medical Association*, 271, 621–3.

Elizur, Y., & Hirsh, E. (1999). Psychosocial adjustment and mental health two months after coronary artery bypass surgery: a multisystemic analysis of patients' resources. *Journal of Behavioral Medicine*, 22(2), 157–77.

Ellington, L., & Wiebe, D. J. (1999). Neuroticism, symptom presentation and medical decision making. *Health Psychology*, 6(18), 634–43.

Elliott, D. J., Trief, P. M., & Stein, N. (1986). Mastery, stress, and coping in marriage among chronic pain patients. *Journal of Behavioral Medicine*, 9, 549–58.

Ellis, A. (1962). *Reason and emotion in psychotherapy*. New York: Lyle Stuart.

Ellis, A. (1977). The basic clinical theory of rational–emotive therapy. In A. Ellis & R. Grieger (Eds), *Handbook of rational–emotive therapy*. New York: Springer.

Ellis, A. (1987). The impossibility of achieving consistently good mental health. *American Psychologist*, 42, 364–75.

Elton, D., & Stanley, G. (1982). Cultural expectations and psychological factors in prolonged disability. In J. L. Sheppard (Ed.), *Advances in Behavioural Medicine* (Vol. 2, pp. 33–42). Sydney: Cumberland College of Health Sciences.

Embretson, J., Zupancic, M., Ribas, J. L., Burke, A., Racz, P., Tenner-Racz, K., & Haase, A. T. (1993). Massive covert infection of helper T lymphocytes and macrophages by HIV during the incubation period of AIDS. *Nature*, 359–62.

Emery, A. E. H., & Pullen, I. M. (1986). A contemporary approach to genetic counseling. In M. J. Christie & P. G. Mellett (Eds), *The psychosomatic approach: contemporary practice of whole-person care*. New York: John Wiley & Sons.

Emery, C. F., Hauck, E. R., & Blumenthal, J. A. (1992). Exercise adherence or maintenance among older adults: 1-year follow-up study. *Psychology and Aging*, 7, 466–70.

Emrick, C. (1975). A review of psychologically oriented treatment of alcoholism. II: The relative effectiveness of different treatment approaches and the effectiveness of treatment versus no treatment. *Journal of Studies on Alcohol*, 36, 88–108.

Emrick, C. D., & Hansen, J. (1983). Assertions regarding effectiveness of treatment for alcoholism. *American Psychologist*, 38, 1078–88.

Engel, G. L. (1977). The need for a new medical model: a challenge for biomedicine. *Science*, 196, 129–36.

Engel, G. L. (1980). The clinical application of the biopsychosocial model. *American Journal of Psychiatry*, 137, 535–44.

Engel, G. L., Reichsman, R., & Segal, H. L. (1956). A study of an infant with a gastric fistula: I. Behavior and the rate of total hydrochloric acid secretion. *Psychosomatic Medicine*, 18, 374–98.

Engels, G. I., Garnefski, N., & Diekstra, R. F. W. (1993). Efficacy of rational-emotive therapy: a quantitative analysis. *Journal of Consulting and Clinical Psychology*, 61, 1083–90.

Engstrom, D. (1984). A psychological perspective of prevention in alcoholism. In J. D. Matarazzo, S. M. Weiss, J. A. Herd, N. E. Miller & S. M. Weiss (Eds), *Behavioral health: a handbook of health enhancement and disease prevention*. New York: John Wiley & Sons.

Epilepsy Foundation of Victoria (2000) (http://www.epinet.org.au, accessed August 2000).

Epstein, L. H., & Cluss, P. A. (1982). A behavioral medicine perspective on adherence to long-term medical regimens. *Journal of Consulting and Clinical Psychology*, 50, 950–71.

Epstein, L. H., & Cluss, P. A. (1986). Behavioral genetics of childhood obesity. *Behavior Therapy*, 17, 324–34.

Epstein, L. H., & Jennings, J. R. (1986). Smoking, stress, cardiovascular reactivity, and coronary heart disease. In K. A. Matthews, S. M. Weiss, T. Detre, T. M. Dembroski, B. Faulkner, S. B. Manuck & R. B. Williams (Eds), *Handbook of stress, reactivity and cardiovascular disease*. New York: John Wiley & Sons.

Epstein, L. H., Saelens, B. E., & O'Brien, J. G. (1995). Effects of reinforcing increases in active behavior versus decreases in sedentary behavior for obese children. *International Journal of Behavioral Medicine*, 2, 41–50.

Epstein, L. H., Valoski, A., Vara, L. S., McCurley, J., Wisniewski, L., Kalarhian, M. A., Klein, K. R., & Shrager, L. R. (1995). Effects of decreasing sedentary behavior and increasing activity on weight change in obese children. *Health Psychology*, 14, 109–115.

Epstein, L. H., Valoski, A., Wing, R. R., & McCurley, J. (1995). Ten-year outcomes of behavioral family-based treatment for childhood obesity. *Health Psychology*, 13, 373–83.

Epstein, L. H., Wing, R. R., Penner, B. C., & Kress, M. J. (1985). Effect of diet and controlled exercise on weight loss in obese children. *Journal of Pediatrics*, 107, 358–61.

Epstein, L. H., Wing, R. R., Valoski, A., & Devos, D. (1988). Long-term relationship between weight and aerobic-fitness change in children. *Health Psychology*, 7, 47–53.

Erdman, R. A. M. (1990). Myocardial infarction and cardiac rehabilitation. In A. A. Kaptein, H. M. Van Der Ploeg, B. Garssen, P. J. G. Schreurs & R. Beunderman (Eds), *Behavioural medicine: psychological treatment of somatic disorders*. Chichester: John Wiley & Sons.

Eriksen, M. P., Lemaistre, C. A., & Newell, G. R. (1988). Health hazards of passive smoking. In L. Breslow, J. E. Fielding & L. B. Lave (Eds), *Annual review of public health* (Vol. 9). Palo Alto, CA: Annual Reviews.

Esterling, B. A., Antoni, M. H., Fletcher, M. A., Margulies, S., & Schneiderman, N. (1994). Emotional disclosure through writing or speaking modulates latent Epstein-Barr virus antibody titers. *Journal of Consulting and Clinical Psychology*, 62, 130–40.

Esterling, B. A., Kiecolt-Glaser, J. K., & Glaser, R. (1996). Psychosocial modulation of cytokine-induced natural killer cell activity in older adults. *Psychosomatic Medicine*, 58, 264–72.

Estey, A., Musseau, A., & Keehn, L. (1994). Patients' understanding of health information: a multihospital comparison. *Patient Education and Counseling*, 24, 73–8.

European Collaborative Study (1991). Children born to women with HIV-1 infection: natural history and risk of transmission. *The Lancet*, 337, 253–60.

Evans, B. J., Coman, G. J., Stanley, R. O., & Burrows, G. D. (1993). Police officers' coping strategies: an Australian police survey. *Stress Medicine*, 9(4), 237–46.

Evans, C., & Richardson, P. H. (1988). Improved recovery and reduced postoperative stay after therapeutic suggestions during general anaesthesia. *The Lancet*, 332, 491–3.

Evans, G. W., Hygge, S., & Bullinger, M. (1995). Chronic noise and psychological stress. *Psychological Science*, 6, 333–8.

Evans, G. W., & Lepore, S. J. (1993). Nonauditory effects of noise on children: a critical review. *Children's Environments*, 10, 31–51.

Evans, R. (1990, August/September). What you should know about childhood asthma. *Asthma and Allergy Advance* (reprint), pp. 1–4.

Evans, R. I. (1976). Smoking in children: developing a social psychological strategy of deterrence. *Preventive Medicine*, 5, 122–7.

Evans, R. I. (1984). A social inoculation strategy to deter smoking in adolescents. In J. D. Matarazzo, S. M. Weiss, J. A. Herd, N. E. Miller & S. M. Weiss (Eds), *Behavioral health: a handbook of health enhancement and disease prevention*. New York: John Wiley & Sons.

Evans, R. I., Rozelle, R. M., Mittelmark, M. B., Hansen, W. B., Bane, A. L., & Havis, J. (1978). Deterring the onset of smoking in children: knowledge of immediate physiological effects and coping with peer pressure, media pressure, and parent modeling. *Journal of Applied Social Psychology*, 8, 126–35.

Evans, R. L., Hendricks, R. D., Haselkorn, J. K., Bishop, D. S., & Baldwin, D. (1992). The family's role in stroke rehabilitation: a review of the literature. *American Journal of Physical Medicine & Rehabilitation*, 71, 135–9.

Everson, S. A., Goldberg, D. E., Kaplan, G. A., Cohen, R. D., Pukkala, E., Tuomilehto, J., & Salonen, J. T. (1996). Hopelessness and risk of mortality and incidence of myocardial infarction and cancer. *Psychosomatic Medicine*, 58, 113–21.

Everson, S. A., McKey, B. S., & Lovallo, W. R. (1995). Effect of trait hostility on cardiovascular responses to harrassment in young men. *International Journal of Behavioral Medicine*, 2, 172–91.

Ewart, C. K. (1991a). Familial transmission of essential hypertension: genes, environments, and chronic anger. *Annals of Behavioral Medicine*, 13, 40–47.

Ewart, C. K. (1991b). Social action theory for a public health psychology. *American Psychologist*, 46, 931–46.

Facchini, F., Chen, Y.-D. I., & Reaven, G. M. (1994). Light-to-moderate alcohol intake is associated with enhanced insulin sensitivity. *Diabetes Care*, 17, 115–19.

Fairburn, C. G., Jones, R., Peveler, R. C., Carr, S.J., Solomon, B. A., O'Connor, M. E., Burton, J., & Hope, R. A. (1991). Three psychological treatments for bulimia nervosa. *Archives of General Psychiatry*, 48, 463–9.

Falkner, B., & Light, K. C. (1986). The interactive effects of stress and dietary sodium on cardiovascular reactivity. In K. A. Matthews, S. M. Weiss, T. Detre, T. M. Dembroski, B. Falkner, S. B. Manuck & R. B. Williams (Eds), *Handbook of stress, reactivity, and cardiovascular disease*. New York: John Wiley & Sons.

Fallon, B. J. (1997). The balance between paid work and home responsibilities: personal problem or corporate concern? *Australian Psychologist*, 32(1), 1–9.

FAO (Food and Agricultural Organisation) (1993). *Production Yearbook* (Vol. 23). Geneva: FAO.

Farquhar, J. W., Fortmann, S. P., MacCoby, N., Wood, P. D., et al. (1984). The Stanford Five City Project: an overview. In J. D. Matarazzo, S. M. Weiss, J. A. Herd, N. E. Miller & S. M. Weiss (Eds), *Behavioral health: a handbook of health enhancement and disease prevention*. New York: John Wiley & Sons.

Farquhar, J. W., MacCoby, N., & Solomon, D. S. (1984). Community applications of behavioral medicine. In W. D. Gentry (Ed.), *Handbook of behavioral medicine*. New York: Guilford.

Farquhar, J. W., MacCoby, N., Wood, P. D. Alexander, J. K., et al. (1977, June 4). Community education for cardiovascular health. *The Lancet*, 1192–5.

Fathalla, M. F. (1990). Relationship between contraceptive technology and HIV transmission: an overview. In N. J. Alexander, H. L. Gabelnick & J. M. Spieler (Eds), *Heterosexual transmission of AIDS*. New York: John Wiley & Sons–Liss.

Fawzy, F. I., Cousins, N. Fawzy, N. W., Kemeny, M. E., Elashoff, R., & Morton, D. (1990). A structured psychiatric intervention for cancer patients: I. Changes over time in methods of coping and affective disturbance. *Archives of General Psychiatry*, 47, 720–25.

Fawzy, F. I., Fawzy, N. W., Hyun, C. S., Elashoff, R., Guthrie, D., Fahey, J. L., & Morton, D. L. (1993). Effects of an early structured psychiatric intervention, coping, and affective state on recurrence and survival 6 years later. *Archives of General Psychiatry*, 50, 681–9.

Fawzy, F. I., Kemeny, M. E., Fawzy, N. W., Elashoff, R., Morton, D., Cousins, N., & Fahey, J. L. (1990). A structured psychiatric intervention for cancer patients: II. Changes over time in immunological measures. *Archives of General Psychiatry*, 47, 729–35.

Feldman, M., & Richardson, C. T. (1986). Role of thought, sight, smell, and taste of food in the cephalic phase of gastric acid secretion in humans. *Gastroenterology*, 90, 428–33.

Feletti, G., Firman, D., & Sanson-Fisher, R. (1986). Patient satisfaction with primary-care consultations. *Journal of Behavioral Medicine*, 9, 389–400.

Felton, B. J., & Revenson, T. A. (1984). Coping with chronic illness: a study of illness controllability and the influence of coping strategies on psychological adjustment. *Journal of Consulting and Clinical Psychology*, 52, 343–53.

Fernandez, E. (1986). A classification system of cognitive coping strategies for pain. *Pain*, 26, 141–51.

Fernandez, E., & Milburn, T. W. (1994). Sensory and affective predictors of overall pain and emotions associated with affective pain. *Clinical Journal of Pain*, 10, 3–9.

Fernandez, E., & Turk, D. C. (1989). The utility of cognitive coping strategies for altering pain perception: a meta-analysis. *Pain*, 38, 123–35.

Ferrante, F. M., & Covino, B. G. (1990). Patient-controlled analgesia: a historical perspective. In F. M. Ferrante, G. W. Ostheimer & B. G. Covino (Eds), *Patient-controlled analgesia* (pp. 4–5). Boston: Blackwell Scientific Publications.

Feuerstein, M., Carter, R. L., & Papciak, A. S. (1987). A prospective analysis of stress and fatigue in recurrent low back pain. *Pain*, 31, 333–44.

Feuerstein, M., & Gainer, J. (1982). Chronic headache: etiology and management. In D. M. Doleys, R. L. Meredith & A. R. Ciminero (Eds), *Behavioral medicine: assessment and treatment strategies*. New York: Plenum.

Fiatarone, M. A., Morley, J. E., Bloom, E. T., Benton, D., Solomon, G. F. & Makinodan, T. (1989). The effect of exercise on natural killer cell activity in young and old subjects. *Journal of Gerontology: Medical Sciences*, 44, M37–45.

Fielding, J. E., & Piserchia, P. V. (1989). Frequency of worksite health promotion activities. *American Journal of Public Health*, 79, 16–20.

Fields, H. L., & Levine, J. D. (1984). Placebo analgesia — a role for endorphins? *Trends in Neurosciences*, 7, 271–3.

Filsinger, E. E. (1987). Social class. In R. J. Corsini (Ed.), *Concise encyclopedia of psychology*. New York: John Wiley & Sons.

Finch, J. F., Okun, M. A., Pool, G. J., & Ruehlman, L. S. (1999). A comparison of the influence of conflictual and supportive social interactions on psychological distress. *Journal of Personality*, 67(4), 581–622.

Finn, P. E., & Alcorn, J. D. (1986). Noncompliance to hemodialysis dietary regimens: literature review and treatment recommendations. *Rehabilitation Psychology*, 31, 67–78.

Fiore, M. C., Newcomb, P., & McBride, P. (1993). Natural history and epidemiology of tobacco use and addiction. In C. T. Orleans & J. Slade (Eds), *Nicotine addiction: principles and management*. New York: Oxford University Press.

Fiore, M. C., Smith, S. S., Jorenby, D. E., & Baker, T. B. (1994). The effectiveness of the nicotine patch for smoking cessation: a meta-analysis. *Journal of the American Medical Association*, 271, 1940–47.

Fishbein, M. (1980). A theory of reasoned action: some applications and implications. In M. M. Page (Ed.), *Nebraska symposium on motivation, 1979*. Lincoln, NB: University of Nebraska Press.

Fishbein, M. (1982). Social psychological analysis of smoking behavior. In J. R. Eiser (Ed.), *Social psychology and behavioral medicine*. New York: John Wiley & Sons.

Fisher, E. B., Lichtenstein, E., & Haire-Joshu, D. (1993). Multiple determinants of tobacco use and cessation. In C. T. Orleans & J. Slade (Eds), *Nicotine addiction: principles and management*. New York: Oxford University Press.

Fisher, J. D., Fisher, W. A., Misovich, S. H., Kimble, D. L., & Malloy, T. E. (1996). Changing AIDS risk behavior: effects of an intervention emphasizing AIDS risk reduction information, motivation, and behavioral skills in a college student population. *Health Psychology*, 15, 114–23.

Fiske, D. W., & Maddi, S. R. (1961). A conceptual framework. In D. W. Fiske & S. R. Maddi (Eds), *Functions of varied experience*. Homewood, IL: Dorsey.

Fitzpatrick, R., & Scambler, G. (1984). Social class, ethnicity, and illness. In R. Fitzpatrick, J. Hinton, S. Newman, G. Scambler, & J. Thompson (Eds), *The experience of illness*. London: Tavistock.

Flack, J. M., Amaro, H., Jenkins, W., Kunitz, S., Levy, J., Mixon, M., & Yu, E. (1995). Panel I: Epidemiology of minority health. *Health Psychology*, 14, 592–600.

Flaskerud, J. H. (1988). AIDS: psychosocial aspects. *Health Values*, 12(4), 44–52.

Flavell, H. A., Carrafa, G. P., Thomas, C. H., & Disler, P. B. (1996). Managing chronic pain: impact of an interdisciplinary team approach. *Medical Journal of Australia*, 165, 253–5.

Flay, B. R. (1985). Psychosocial approaches to smoking prevention: a review of findings. *Health Psychology*, 4, 449–88.

Flay, B. R. (1987). Mass media and smoking cessation: a critical review. *American Journal of Public Health*, 77, 153–60.

Flay, B. R., Koepke, D., Thomson, S. J., Santi, S., Best, A., & Brown, K. S. (1989). Six-year follow-up of the first Waterloo school smoking prevention trial. *American Journal of Public Health*, 79, 1371–6.

Fleming, I., Baum, A., Davidson, L. M., Rectanus, E., & McArdle, S. (1987). Chronic stress as a factor in physiologic reactivity to challenge. *Health Psychology*, 6, 221–37.

Fleming, R., Baum, A., Gisriel, M. M., & Gatchel, R. J. (1982). Mediating influences of social support on stress at Three Mile Island. *Journal of Human Stress*, 8, 14–22.

Flinn, W. R., Dalsing, M. C., & White, J. V. (1986). Carotid endarterectomy: indications, technique, and results. In P. E. Kaplan & L. J. Cerullo (Eds), *Stroke rehabilitation*. Boston: Butterworth.

Flodmark, C-E., Ohlsson, T., Rydén, O., & Sveger, T. (1993). Prevention of progression to severe obesity in a group of obese schoolchildren treated with family therapy. *Pediatrics*, 91, 880–84.

Flor, H., & Birbaumer, N. (1993). Comparison of the efficacy of electromyographic biofeedback, cognitive-behavioral therapy, and conservative medical interventions in the treatment of chronic musculoskeletal pain. *Journal of Consulting and Clinical Psychology*, 61, 653–8.

Flor, H., Fydrich, T., & Turk, D. C. (1992). Efficacy of multidisciplinary pain treatment centers: a meta-analytic review. *Pain*, 49, 221–30.

Flor, H., Kerns, R. D., & Turk, D. C. (1987). The role of spouse reinforcement, perceived pain, and activity levels of chronic pain patients. *Journal of Psychosomatic Research*, 31, 251–9.

Flor, H., & Turk, D. C. (1985). Chronic illness in an adult family member: pain as a prototype. In D. C. Turk & R. D. Kerns (Eds), *Health, illness, and families: a life-span perspective*. New York: John Wiley & Sons.

Florian, V., & Elad, D. (1998). The impact of mothers' sense of empowerment on the metabolic control of their children with juvenile diabetes. *Journal of Pediatric Psychology*, 23(4), 239–47.

Foa, E. B., Steketee, G., & Rothbaum, B. O. (1989). Behavioural/cognitive conceptualisations of post-traumatic stress disorder. *Behaviour Therapy*, 20, 155–76.

Foley, K. M. (1985). The medical treatment of cancer pain. *New England Journal of Medicine*, 313, 84–95.

Folkins, C. E., & Sime, W. E. (1981). Physical fitness training and mental health. *American Psychologist*, 36, 373–89.

Folkman, S. (1984). Personal control and stress and coping processes: a theoretical analysis. *Journal of Personality and Social Psychology*, 46, 839–52.

Folkman, S., & Lazarus, R. S. (1988). Coping as a mediator of emotion. *Journal of Personality and Social Psychology*, 54, 466–75.

Folkman, S., Lazarus, R. S., Dunkel-Schetter, C., Delongis, A., & Gruen, R. J. (1986). Dynamics of a stressful encounter: cognitive appraisal, coping, and encounter outcomes. *Journal of Personality and Social Psychology*, 50, 992–1003.

Folkman, S., Lazarus, R. S., Pimley, S., & Novacek, J. (1987). Age differences in stress and coping processes. *Psychology and Aging*, 2, 171–84.

Follick, M. J., Ahern, D. K., & Aberger, E. W. (1985). Development of an audiovisual taxonomy of pain behavior: reliability and discriminant validity. *Health Psychology*, 4, 555–68.

Follick, M. J., Ahern, D. K., Attanasio, V., & Riley, J. F. (1985). Chronic pain programs: current aims, strategies, and needs. *Annals of Behavioral Medicine*, 7(3), 17–20.

Follick, M. J., Gorkin, L., Smith, T. W., Capone, R. J., Visco, J., & Stablein, D. (1988). Quality of life post-myocardial infarction: effects of a transtelephonic coronary intervention system. *Health Psychology*, 7, 169–82.

Folsom, A. R., Kaye, S. A., Sellers, T. A., Hong, C.-P., Cerhan, J. R., Potter, J. D., & Prineas, R. J. (1993). Body fat distribution and 5-year risk of death in older women. *Journal of the American Medical Association*, 269, 483–7.

Folstein, M. F., Folstein, S. E., & McHugh, P. R. (1975). Mini-Mental State: a practical method for grading the cognitive state of patients for the clinician. *Journal of Psychiatric Research*, 12, 189–98.

Fontana, A. F., Kerns, R. D., Rosenberg, R. L., & Colonese, K. L. (1989). Support, stress, and recovery from coronary heart disease: a longitudinal causal model. *Health Psychology*, 8, 175–93.

Foot, G., & Sanson-Fisher, R. (1995). Measuring the unmet needs of people living with cancer. *Cancer Forum*, 19(2), 131–5.

Foote, S. (1999). Designing new drugs through DNA. *Australian Family Physician*, 28(10), 1011–16.

Fordyce, W. E. (1976). *Behavioral methods for chronic pain and illness*. St. Louis, MO: Mosby.

Fordyce, W. E., & Steger, J. C. (1979). Behavioral management of chronic pain. In O. F. Pomerleau & J. P. Brady (Eds), *Behavioral medicine: theory and practice*. Baltimore, MD: Williams & Wilkins.

Forero, R., Baumann, A., Chen, J., Flaherty, B. (1999). Substance use and socio-demographic factors among Aboriginal and Torres Strait Islander students in New South Wales. *Australian and New Zealand Journal of Public Health*, 23, 295–300.

Foreyt, J. P., & Leavesley, G. (1991). Behavioral treatment of obesity at the work site. In S. M. Weiss, J. E. Fielding & A. Baum (Eds), *Perspectives in behavioral medicine: health at work*. Hillsdale, NJ: Erlbaum.

Foreyt, J. P., Scott, L. W., Mitchell, R. E., & Gotto, A. M. (1979). Plasma lipid changes in the normal population following behavioral treatment. *Journal of Consulting and Clinical Psychology*, 47, 440–52.

Fosson, A., Martin, J. & Haley, J. (1990). Anxiety among hospitalised latency-age children. *Developmental and Behavioral Pediatrics*, 11, 324–7.

Fox, B. H. (1978). Premorbid psychological factors as related to cancer incidence. *Journal of Behavioral Medicine*, 1, 45–133.

Foxx, R. M., & Brown, R. A. (1979). Nicotine fading and self-monitoring for cigarette abstinence or controlled smoking. *Journal of Applied Behavior Analysis*, 12, 111–25.

Fradkin, B., & Firestone, P. (1986). Premenstrual tension, expectancy, and mother–child relations. *Journal of Behavioral Medicine*, 9, 245–59.

France, C., & Ditto, B. (1988). Caffeine effects on several indices of cardiovascular activity at rest and during stress. *Journal of Behavioral Medicine*, 11, 473–82.

Francis, D. P., & Chin, J. (1987). The prevention of acquired immunodeficiency syndrome in the United States: an objective strategy for medicine, public health, business, and the community. *Journal of the American Medical Association*, 257, 1357–66.

Francis, V., Korsch, B. M., & Morris, M. J. (1969). Gaps in doctor–patient communication. *New England Journal of Medicine*, 280, 535–40.

Frank, E., Winkleby, M. A., Altman, D. G., Rockhill, B., & Fortmann, S. P. (1991). Predictors of physicians' smoking cessation advice. *Journal of the American Medical Association*, 266, 3139–44.

Frank, R. G., & Ross, M. J. (1995). The changing workforce: the role of health psychology. *Health Psychology*, 14(6), 519–25.

Frank, R. G., Gluck, J. P., & Buckelew, S. P. (1990). Rehabilitation: psychology's greatest opportunity. *American Psychologist*, 45, 757–61.

Frank, R. G., Umlauf, R. L., Wonderlich, S. A., Askanazi, G. S., Buckelew, S. P., & Elliott, T. R. (1987). Differences in coping styles among persons with spinal cord injury: a cluster-analytic approach. *Journal of Consulting and Clinical Psychology*, 55, 727–31.

Frankenhaeuser, M. (1986). A psychobiological framework for research on human stress and coping. In M. H. Appley & R. Trumbull (Eds), *Dynamics of stress: physiological, psychological, and social perspectives*. New York: Plenum.

Frankenhaeuser, M. (1991). The psychophysiology of workload, stress, and health: comparison between the sexes. *Annals of Behavioral Medicine*, 13, 197–204.

Frankish, J., & Linden, W. (1991). Is response adaptation a threat to the high–low reactor distinction among female college students? *Health Psychology*, 10, 224–7.

Frasure-Smith, N., Lespérance, F., & Talajic, M. (1993). Depression following myocardial infarction: impact on 6-month survival. *Journal of the American Medical Association*, 270, 1819–25.

Frasure-Smith, N., Lespérance, F., & Talajic, M. (1995). Depression and 18-month prognosis after myocardial infarction. *Circulation*, 91, 999–1005.

Frazier, L. D., & Waid, L. D. (1999). Influences on anxiety in later life: the role of health status, health perceptions and health locus of control. *Aging and Mental Health*, 3(3), 213–20.

Fredrikson, M., & Matthews, K. A. (1990). Cardiovascular responses to behavioral stress and hypertension: a meta-analytic review. *Annals of Behavior Medicine*, 12, 30–39.

Freeman, A. (1990). Cognitive therapy. In A. S. Bellack & M. Hersen (Eds), *Handbook of comparative treatments for adult disorders*. New York: John Wiley & Sons.

Freeman, H. L., & Stansfeld, S. A. (1998). Psychosocial effects of urban environments, noise, and crowding. In A. Lundberg et al. (Eds), *The environment and mental health: a guide for clinicians* (pp. 147–73). Mahwah, NJ: Erlbaum.

Freeman, R., Touyz, S., Sara, G., Rennie, C., Gordon, E., & Beumont, P. (1991). In the eye of the beholder: processing body shape information in anorexic and bulimic patients. *International Journal of Eating Disorders*, 10(6), 709–714.

Freemon, B., Negrete, V. F., Davis, M., & Korsch, B. M. (1971). Gaps in doctor–patient communication: doctor–patient interaction analysis. *Pediatric Research*, 5, 298–311.

Freiberg, P. (1995, June). Psychologists examine attacks on homosexuals. *American Psychological Association Monitor*, pp. 30–31.

Freidson, E. (1961). *Patients' views of medical practice*. New York: Russell Sage Foundation.

French, D. J., & Carroll, A. (1997). Western Australian primary school teachers' knowledge about childhood asthma and its management. *Journal of Asthma*, 34, 469–75.

French, D. J., Christie, M. J., & West, A. (1994). Quality of life in childhood asthma: development of the Childhood Asthma Questionnaires. In M. J. Christie & D. J. French (Eds), *Assessment of Quality of Life in Childhood Asthma* (pp. 157–80). Chur, Switzerland: Harwood Academic Publishers.

French, S. A., & Jeffery, R. W. (1994). Consequences of dieting to lose weight: effects on physical and mental health. *Health Psychology*, 13, 195–212.

Frick, M. H., Elo, O., Haapa, K., Heinonen, O. P., et al. (1987). Helsinki Heart Study: primary-prevention trial with gemfibrozil in middle-aged men with dyslipidemia. *New England Journal of Medicine*, 317(20), 1237–45.

Friedman, H. S., & Booth-Kewley, S. (1987). The 'disease-prone' personality. *American Psychologist*, 42, 539–55.

Friedman, H. S., Tucker, J. S., & Reise, S. P. (1995). Personality dimensions and measures potentially relevant to health: a focus on hostility. *Annals of Behavioral Medicine*, 17, 245–53.

Friedman, H. S., Tucker, J. S., Schwartz, J. E., Tomlinson-Keasey, C., Martin, L. R., Wingard, D. L., & Criqui, M. H. (1995). Psychosocial and behavioral predictors of longevity. the aging and death of the 'Termites'. *American Psychologist*, 50, 69–78.

Friedman, L. A., & Kimball, A. W. (1986). Coronary heart disease mortality and alcohol consumption in Framingham. *American Journal of Epidemiology*, 124, 481–9.

Friedman, L. C., Webb, J. A., Bruce, S., Weinberg, A. D., & Cooper, H. P. (1995). Skin cancer prevention and early detection intentions and behavior. *American Journal of Preventive Medicine*, 11, 59–65.

Friedman, M., & Rosenman, R. H. (1974). *Type A behavior and your heart*. New York: Knopf.

Friedman, M., Thoresen, C. E., Gill, J. J., Ulmer, D., et al. (1986). Alteration of Type A behavior and its effect on cardiac recurrences in post myocardial infarction patients: summary results of the Recurrent Coronary Prevention Project. *American Heart Journal*, 112, 653–65.

Friis, R., & Taff, G. A. (1986). Social support and social networks, and coronary heart disease and rehabilitation. *Journal of Cardiopulmonary Rehabilitation*, 6, 132–47.

Friman, P. C., Finney, J. W., Glasscock, S. G., Weigel, J. W., & Christophersen, E. R. (1986). Testicular self-examination: validation of a training strategy for early cancer detection. *Journal of Applied Behavior Analysis*, 19, 87–92.

Frydenberg, E., & Lewis, R. (1993). *Manual: the Adolescent Coping Scale*. Melbourne: Australian Council for Educational Research.

Frydenberg, E., & Lewis, R. (1996). The Adolescent Coping Scale: multiple forms and applications of a self report inventory in a counselling and research context. *European Journal of Psychological Assessment*, 12(3), 216–27.

Frydenberg, E., & Lewis, R. (1999). Things don't get better just because you're older: a case for facilitating reflection. *British Journal of Educational Psychology*, 69(1), 81–94.

Fullerton, J. T., Kritz-Silverstein, D., Sadler, G. R., & Barrett-Connor, E. (1996). Mammography usage in a community-based sample of older women. *Annals of Behavioral Medicine*, 18, 67–72.

Fullilove, M. T., Fullilove, R. E., Haynes, K., & Gross, S. (1990). Black women and AIDS prevention: a view towards understanding the gender rules. *Journal of Sex Research*, 27, 47–64.

Funk, S. C. (1992). Hardiness: a review of theory and research. *Health Psychology*, 11, 335–45.

Futterman, A. D., Kemeny, M. E., Shapiro, D., & Fahey, J. L. (1994). Immunological and physiological changes associated with induced positive and negative mood. *Psychosomatic Medicine*, 56, 499–511.

Galavotti, C., Cabral, R. J., Lansky, A., Grimley, D. M., Riley, G. E., & Prochaska, J. O. (1995). Validation of measures of condom and other contraceptive use among women at high risk for HIV infection and unintended pregnancy. *Health Psychology*, 14, 570–78.

Galizio, M., & Maisto, S. A. (1985). Toward a biopsychosocial theory of substance abuse. In M. Galizio & S. A. Maisto (Eds), *Determinants of substance abuse: biological, psychological, and environmental factors*. New York: Plenum.

Gallagher, E. J., Viscoli, C. M., & Horwitz, R. I. (1993). The relationship of treatment adherence to the risk of death after myocardial infarction in women. *Journal of the American Medical Association*, 270, 742–4.

Gallois, C., Terry, D., Timmins, P., Kashima, Y., & McCamish, M. (1994). Safe sexual intentions and behavior among heterosexuals and homosexual men: testing the theory of reasoned action. *Psychology and Health*, 10(1), 1–16.

Gannon, L. R., Haynes, S. N., Cuevas, J., & Chavez, R. (1987). Psychophysiological correlates of induced headaches. *Journal of Behavioral Medicine*, 10, 411–23.

Ganora, A. (1986). Rehabilitation of work related back injury. *Australian Family Physician*, 15, 430–37.

Garcia-Vera, M. P., Labrador, F. J., & Sanz, J. (1997). Stress-management training for essential hypertension: A controlled study. *Applied Psychophysiology and Biofeedback*, 22(4), 261–83.

Gardner, E. J., Simmons, M. J., & Snustad, D. P. (1991). *Principles of genetics* (8th ed.). New York: John Wiley & Sons.

Garfield, C. (1978). *Psychosocial care of the dying patient*. New York: McGraw-Hill.

Garmezy, N. (1983). Stressors of childhood. In N. Garmezy & M. Rutter (Eds), *Stress, coping, and development in children*. New York: McGraw-Hill.

Garner, D. M., & Olmsted, M. P. (1984). *Manual of the eating disorders inventory*. Toronto: Psychological Assessment Resources.

Garrity, T. F., & Marx, M. B. (1979). Critical life events and coronary disease. In W. D. Gentry & R. B. Williams (Eds), *Psychological aspects of myocardial infarction and coronary care* (2nd ed.). St. Louis, MO: Mosby.

Gatchel, R. J. (1980). Effectiveness of two procedures for reducing dental fear: group-administered desensitization and group education and discussion. *Journal of the American Dental Association*, 101, 634–8.

Gatchel, R. J., Mayer, T. G., Capra, P., Diamond, P., & Barnett, J. (1986). Millon Behavioral Health Inventory: its utility in predicting physical function in low back pain patients. *Archives of Physical Medicine and Rehabilitation*, 67, 878–82.

Gaughwin, M. (2000). Just who is 'wrong' about the implications of heroin trials? *Australian and New Zealand Journal of Public Health*, 24(6), 640.

Gauthier, J. G., Bois, R., Allaire, D., & Drolet, M. (1981). Evaluation of skin temperature biofeedback training at two different sites for migraine. *Journal of Behavioral Medicine*, 4, 407–419.

Gauthier, J., Côté, G., & French, D. (1994). The role of home practice in the thermal biofeedback treatment of migraine headache. *Journal of Consulting and Clinical Psychology*, 62, 180–84.

Gavzer, B. (1988, September 18). Why do some people survive AIDS? *Parade Magazine*, pp. 4–7.

Gaziano, J. M., Buring, J. E., Breslow, J. L., Goldhaber, S. Z., Rosner, B., Vandenburgh, M., Willett, W., & Hennekens, C. H. (1993). Moderate alcohol intake, increased levels of high-density lipoprotein and its subfractions, and decreased risk of myocardial infarction. *New England Journal of Medicine*, 329, 1829–34.

Gentry, W. D. (1984). Behavioral medicine: a new research paradigm. In W. D. Gentry (Ed.), *Handbook of behavioral medicine*. New York: Guilford.

Gentry, W. D., & Kobasa, S. C. O. (1984). Social and psychological resources mediating stress — illness relationships in humans. In W. D. Gentry (Ed.), *Handbook of behavioral medicine*. New York: Guilford.

Gentry, W. D., & Owens, D. (1986). Pain groups. In A. D. Holzman & D. C. Turk (Eds), *Pain management: a handbook of psychological treatment approaches*. New York: Pergamon.

George, J., & Davis, A. (1998). *States of health: health and illness in Australia* (3rd ed.). Melbourne: Addison-Wesley Longman.

Gerace, R. A., & Vorp, R. (1985). Epidemiology and behavior. In N. Schneiderman & J. T. Tapp (Eds), *Behavioral medicine: the biopsychosocial approach*. Hillsdale, NJ: Erlbaum.

Gerber, P. (1994). Withdrawing treatment from patients in a persistent vegetative state. *Journal of Medical Ethics*, 161, 715–17.

Gerits, P., & Ce-Brabander, B. (1999). Psychosocial predictors of psychological, neurochemical and immunological symptoms of acute stress among breast cancer patients. *Psychiatry Research*, 85(1), 95–103.

Gervasio, A. H. (1986). Family relationships and compliance. In K. E. Gerber & A. M. Nehemkis (Eds), *Compliance: the dilemma of the chronically ill*. New York: Springer.

Geschwind, N. (1979, September). Specializations of the human brain. *Scientific American*, 241, 180–99.

Gibbons, F. X., McGovern, P. G., & Lando, H. A. (1991). Relapse and risk perception among members of a smoking cessation clinic. *Health Psychology*, 10, 42–5.

Gil, K. M., Ginsberg, B., Muir, M., Sykes, D., & Williams, D. A. (1990). Patient-controlled analgesia in postoperative pain: the relation of psychological factors to pain and analgesic use. *Clinical Journal of Pain*, 6, 137–42.

Gil, K. M., Keefe, F. J., Crisson, J. E., & Van Dalfsen, P. J. (1987). Social support and pain behavior. *Pain*, 29, 209–217.

Gil, K. M., Keefe, F. J., Sampson, H. A., McCaskill, C. C., Rodin, J., & Crisson, J. E. (1988). Direct observation of scratching behavior in children with atopic dermatitis. *Behavior Therapy*, 19, 213–27.

Gilbert, A., Luszcz, M., & Owen, N. (1993). Medication use and its correlates among the elderly. *Australian Journal of Public Health*, 17, 18–22.

Gilbert, D. G., & Spielberger, C. D. (1987). Effects of smoking on heart rate, anxiety, and feelings of success during social interaction. *Journal of Behavioral Medicine*, 10, 629–38.

Giles, G., Hill, D. J., & Silver, B. (1991). The lung cancer epidemic in Australia, 1910 to 1989. *Australian Journal of Public Health*, 15, 245–7.

Giles, G., Thursfield, V., & Staples, M. (1994, March). The bottom line: trends in cancer mortality, Australia 1950-1991. *Cancer Forum*, 18(1), 12–23.

Gill, T. M., & Feinstein, A. R. (1995). A critical appraisal of the quality of quality-of-life measurements. *Journal of the American Medical Association*, 272, 619–26.

Gillum, R. F. (1987a). The association of body fat distribution with hypertension, hypertensive heart disease, coronary heart disease, diabetes and cardiovascular risk factors in men and women aged 18–79 years. *Journal of Chronic Diseases*, 40, 421–8.

Gillum, R. F. (1987b). The association of the ratio of waist to hip girth with blood pressure, serum cholesterol and serum uric acid in children and youths aged 6–17 years. *Journal of Chronic Diseases*, 40, 413–420.

Ginzberg, E. (1983). Allied health resources. In D. Mechanic (Ed.), *Handbook of health, health care, and the health professions*. New York: Free Press.

Giovanucci, E., Rimm, E. B., Colditz, G. A., Stampfer, M. J., Ascherio, A., Chute, C. C., & Willett, W. C. (1993). A prospective study of dietary fat and risk of prostate cancer. *Journal of the National Cancer Institute*, 85, 1571–9.

Girodo, M., & Wood, D. (1979). Talking yourself out of pain: the importance of believing that you can. *Cognitive Therapy and Research*, 3, 23–33.

Gladis, M. M., Michela, J. L., Walter, H. J., & Vaughan, R. D. (1992). High school students' perceptions of AIDS risk: realistic appraisal or motivated denial? *Health Psychology*, 11, 307–316.

Glanz, K., & Lerman, C. (1992). Psychosocial impact of breast cancer: a critical review. *Annals of Behavioral Medicine*, 14, 204–212.

Glaser, R., Thorn, B. E., Tarr, K. L., Kiecolt-Glaser, J. K., & D'Ambrosio, S. M. (1985). Effects of stress on methyltransferase synthesis: an important DNA repair enzyme. *Health Psychology*, 4, 403–412.

Glaser, S. B. (1980). Anybody got a match? Treatment research and the matching hypothesis. In G. Edwards & M. Grant (Eds), *Alcoholism treatment in transition* (pp. 178–96). London: Croom Helm.

Glasgow, R. E., Klesges, R. C., Mizes, J. S., & Pechacek, T. F. (1985). Quitting smoking: strategies used and variables associated with success in a stop-smoking contest. *Journal of Consulting and Clinical Psychology*, 53, 905–912.

Glasgow, R. E., & Lichtenstein, E. (1987). Long-term effects of behavioral smoking cessation interventions. *Behavior Therapy*, 18, 297–324.

Glasgow, R. E., McCaul, K. D., & Schafer, L. C. (1986). Barriers to regimen adherence among persons with insulin-dependent diabetes. *Journal of Behavioral Medicine*, 9, 65–77.

Glasgow, R. E., McCaul, K. D., & Schafer, L. C. (1987). Self-care behaviors and glycemic control in Type I diabetes. *Journal of Chronic Diseases*, 40, 399–412.

Glass, D. C. (1977). *Behavior patterns, stress, and coronary heart disease*. Hillsdale, NJ: Erlbaum.

Glass, D. C., Krakoff, L. R., Contrada, R., Hilton, W. F., Kehoe, K., Mannucci, E. G., Collins, C., Snow, B., & Elting, E. (1980). Effect of harassment and competition upon cardiovascular and plasma catecholamine responses in Type A and Type B individuals. *Psychophysiology*, 17, 453–63.

Glass, T. A., Kasl, S. V., & Berkman, L. F. (1997). Stressful life events and depressive symptoms among the elderly. *Journal of Aging and Health*, 9(1), 70–89.

Glasser, W. (1976). *Positive addiction*. New York: Harper & Row.

Gleser, E. C., Green, B. L., & Winget, C. (1981). *Prolonged psychosocial effects of disaster: a study of Buffalo Creek*. New York: Academic Press.

Glick, R., & Cerullo, L. J. (1986). Subarachnoid and parenchymal hemorrhage. In P. E. Kaplan & L. J. Cerullo (Eds), *Stroke rehabilitation*. Boston, MA: Butterworth.

Glicksman, M., Dwyer, T., Wlodarczyk, J., & Pierce, J. (1989). Cigarette smoking in Australian schoolchildren. *Medical Journal of Australia*, 150, 81–4.

Glynn, S. M., Gruder, C. L., & Jegerski, J. A. (1986). Effects of biochemical validation of self-reported cigarette smoking on treatment success and on misreporting abstinence. *Health Psychology*, 5, 125–36.

Glynn, S. M., & Ruderman, A. J. (1986). The development and validation of an eating self-efficacy scale. *Cognitive Therapy and Research*, 10, 403–420.

Godin, G., Desharnais, R., Jobin, J., & Cook, J. (1987). The impact of physical fitness and health-age appraisal upon exercise intentions and behavior. *Journal of Behavioral Medicine*, 10, 241–50.

Godin, G., Desharnais, R., Valois, P., Lepage, L., Jobin, J., & Bradet, R. (1992, March). Perceived barriers to exercise among different populations. Paper presented at the meeting of the Society of Behavioral Medicine, New York.

Goetsch, V. L. (1989). Stress and blood glucose in diabetes mellitus: a review and methodological commentary. *Annals of Behavioral Medicine*, 11, 102–7.

Goffman, E. (1961). *Asylums*. Garden City, NY: Doubleday.

Gold, P. W., Gwirtsman, H., Avgerinos, P. C., Nieman, L. K., et al. (1986). Abnormal hypothalamic-pituitary-adrenal function in anorexia nervosa: pathophysiologic mechanisms in underweight and weight-corrected patients. *New England Journal of Medicine*, 314, 1335–42.

Gold, R. (1995). Why we need to rethink AIDS education for gay men. *Aids Care*, 7(1), 11–19.

Gold, R. S., Skinner, M. J., & Ross, M. W. (1994). Unprotected anal intercourse in HIV-infected and non-HIV-infected gay men. *Journal of Sex Research*, 31, 59–77.

Goldberg, E. L., & Comstock, G. W. (1980). Epidemiology of life events: frequency in general populations. *American Journal of Epidemiology*, 111, 736–52.

Golding, J. F., & Cornish, A. M. (1987). Personality and life-style in medical students: psychopharmacological aspects. *Psychology and Health*, 1, 287–301.

Goldman, M. S. (1983). Cognitive impairment in chronic alcoholics. *American Psychologist*, 38, 1045–54.

Goldsmith, D., & Parks, M. R. (1990). Communicative strategies for managing the risks of seeking social support. In S. Duck with R. C. Silver (Eds), *Personal relationships and social support* (pp. 104–121). London: Sage.

Goldstein, I. B., Jamner, L. D., & Shapiro, D. (1992). Ambulatory blood pressure and heart rate in healthy male paramedics during a workday and a non-workday. *Health Psychology*, 11, 48–54.

Goldstein, L. H. (1990). Behavioural and cognitive-behavioural treatments for epilepsy: a progress review. *British Journal of Clinical Psychology*, 29, 257–69.

Goldston, D. B., Kovacs, M., Obrosky, D. S., & Iyengar, S. (1995). A longitudinal study of life events and metabolic control among youths with insulin-dependent diabetes mellitus. *Health Psychology*, 14, 409–414

Goldwater, B. C., & Collis, M. L. (1985). Psychologic effects of cardiovascular conditioning: a controlled experiment. *Psychosomatic Medicine*, 47, 174–81.

Gomel, M., Oldenburg, B., Simpson, J. M., Owen, N. (1993). Work-site cardiovascular risk reduction: a randomized trial of health risk assessment, education, counselling and incentives. *American Journal of Public Health*, 83(9), 1231–8.

Gomez, R. (1998). Impatience-aggression, competitiveness and avoidant coping: direct and moderating effects on maladjustment among adolescents. *Personality and Individual Differences*, 25(4), 649–61.

Gonder-Frederick, L. A., Carter, W. R., Cox, D. J., & Clarke, W. L. (1990). Environmental stress and blood glucose change in insulin-dependent diabetes mellitus. *Health Psychology*, 9, 503–515.

Gonder-Frederick, L., Cox, D. J., Pohl, S. L., & Carter, W. (1984). Patient blood glucose monitoring: use, accuracy, adherence, and impact. *Behavioral Medicine Update*, 6(1), 12–16.

Goodall, T. A., & Halford, W. K. (1991). Self-management of diabetes mellitus: a critical review. *Health Psychology*, 10, 1–8.

Goodman, J. E., & McGrath, P. J. (1991). The epidemiology of pain in children and adolescence: a review. *Pain*, 46, 247–64.

Gorder, D. D., Dolecek, T. A., Coleman, G. G., Tillotson, J. L., Brown, H. B., Lenz-Litzow, K., Bartsch, G. E., & Grandits, G.(1986). Dietary intake in the Multiple Risk Factor Intervention Trial (MRFIT): nutrient and food group changes over 6 years. *Journal of the American Dietetic Association*, 86, 744–51.

Gordon, C. M., & Carey, M. P. (1996). Alcohol's effects on requisites for sexual risk reduction in men: an initial experimental investigation. *Health Psychology*, 15, 56–60.

Gordon, D. J., Probstfield, J. L., Garrison, R. J., Neaton, J. D., Castelli, W. P., Knoke, J. D., Jacobs, D. R., Bangdiwala, S., & Tyroler, H. A. (1989). High-density lipoprotein cholesterol and cardiovascular disease: four prospective American studies. *Circulation*, 79, 8–15.

Gordon, G. (1976). *Health, sickness and society*. Brisbane: University of Queensland Press.

Gordon, T., & Doyle, J. T. (1987). Drinking and mortality: the Albany Study. *American Journal of Epidemiology*, 125, 263–70.

Gordon, T., & Kannel, W. B. (1984). Drinking and mortality: the Framingham Study. *American Journal of Epidemiology*, 120, 97–107.

Gordon, W. A., & Diller, L. (1983). Stroke: coping with a cognitive deficit. In T. G. Burish & L. A. Bradley (Eds), *Coping with chronic disease: research and applications*. New York: Academic Press.

Gorman, C. (1996, Fall). Damage control. *Time*, pp. 31–5.

Gortmaker, S. L., Dietz, W. H., & Cheung, L. W. Y. (1990). Inactivity, diet, and the fattening of America. *Journal of the American Dietetic Association*, 90, 1247–52, 1255.

Gortmaker, S. L., Dietz, W. H., Sobol, A. M., & Wehler, C. A. (1987). Increasing pediatric obesity in the United States. *American Journal of Diseases of Children*, 141, 535–40.

Gortmaker, S. L., Eckenrode, J., & Gore, S. (1982). Stress and the utilization of health services: a time series and cross-sectional analysis. *Journal of Health and Social Behavior*, 23, 25–38.

Gottlieb, B. H. (1985). Social support and the study of personal relationships. *Journal of Social and Personal Relationships*, 2, 351–75.

Gottlieb, B. H., & Wagner, F. (1991). Stress and support processes in close relationships. In J. Eckenrode (Ed.), *The social context of coping*. New York: Plenum.

Gottlieb, N. H. (1983). The effect of health beliefs on the smoking behavior of college women. *Journal of American College Health*, 31, 214–21.

Gottlieb, N. H., & Baker, J. A. (1986). The relative influence of health beliefs, parental and peer behaviors and exercise program participation on smoking, alcohol use and physical activity. *Social Science and Medicine*, 22, 915–27.

Gottlieb, N. H., & Green, L. W. (1987). Ethnicity and lifestyle health risk: some possible mechanisms. *American Journal of Health Promotion*, 2, 37–45, 51.

Gould, K. L., Ornish, D., Scherwitz, L., Brown, S., et al. (1995). Changes in myocardial perfusion abnormalities by positive emission tomography after long-term, intense risk factor modification. *Journal of the American Medical Association*, 274, 894–901.

Gracey, M. (1995). New World Syndrome in Western Australian Aborigines. *Clinical and Experimental Pharmacology and Physiology*, 22, 220–25.

Grant, C. (1985). *Australian hospitals: operation and management*. Melbourne: Churchill Livingstone.

Grant, J. C. B. (1972). *An atlas of anatomy*. Baltimore, MD: Williams & Wilkins.

Graugaard, P. K., & Finset, A. (2000). Trait anxiety and reactions to patient-centered and doctor-centered styles of communication: an experimental study. *Psychosomatic Medicine*, 62(1), 33–9.

Graveley, E. A., & Oseasohn, C. S. (1991). Multiple drug regimens: medication compliance among veterans 65 years and older. *Research in Nursing and Health*, 14, 51–8.

Gray, D., Morfitt, B., Ryan, K., & Williams, S. (1997). The use of tobacco, alcohol and other drugs by young Aboriginal people in Albany, Western Australia. *Australian and New Zealand Journal of Public Health*, 21, 71–6.

Greeley, J., Swift, W., & Heather, N. (1992). Depressed affect as a predictor of increased desire for alcohol in current drinkers of alcohol. *British Journal of Addiction*, 87, 1005–1012.

Greeley, J., Swift, W., Prescott, J., & Heather, N. (1993). Reactivity of alcohol-related cues in heavy and light drinkers. *Journal of Studies on Alcohol*, 54(3), 359–68.

Green, C. J. (1985). The use of psychodiagnostic questionnaires in predicting risk factors and health outcomes. In P. Karoly (Ed.), *Measurement strategies in health psychology*. New York: John Wiley & Sons.

Green, J., & Hedge, B. (1991). Counselling and stress in HIV infection and AIDS. In C. L. Cooper & M. Watson (Eds), *Cancer and stress: psychological, biological and coping studies*. Chichester: John Wiley & Sons.

Green, L. W., & Kreuter, M. W. (1991). *Health promotion planning: an educational and environmental approach*. London: Mayfield.

Green, P. J., & Suls, J. (1996). The effects of caffeine on ambulatory blood pressure, heart rate, and mood in coffee drinkers. *Journal of Behavioral Medicine*, 19, 111–28.

Greenberg, E. R., Baron, J. A., Tosteson, T. D., Freeman, D. H., et al. (1994). A clinical trial of antioxidant vitamins to prevent colorectal adenoma. *New England Journal of Medicine*, 331, 141–7.

Greenfield, D. (1985). Nutritional basis of health and disease. In N. Schneiderman & J. T. Tapp (Eds), *Behavioral medicine: the biopsychosocial approach*. Hillsdale, NJ: Erlbaum.

Greenglass, E. R., & Noguchi, K. (1996, August). Longevity, gender and health: a psychocultural perspective. Paper presented at the meeting of the International Society of Health Psychology in Montreal.

Greenwald, H. P., Bonica, J. J., & Bergner, M. (1987). The prevalence of pain in four cancers. *Cancer*, 60, 2563–9.

Grilo, C. M., Shiffman, S., & WING, R. R. (1989). Relapse crises and coping among dieters. *Journal of Consulting and Clinical Psychology*, 57, 488–95.

Gritz, E. R., Carr, C. R., & Marcus, A. C. (1991). The tobacco withdrawal syndrome in unaided quitters. *British Journal of Addiction*, 86, 57–69.

Grob, G. N. (1983). Disease and environment in American history. In D. Mechanic (Ed.), *Handbook of health, health care, and the health professions*. New York: Free Press.

Grobbee, D. E., Rimm, E. B., Giovannucci, E., Colditz, G., Stampfer, M., & Willett, C. (1990). Coffee, caffeine, and cardiovascular disease in men. *New England Journal of Medicine*, 323, 1026–32.

Groseclose, S. L., Weinstein, B., Jones, T. S., Valleroy, L. A., Fehrs, L. J., & Kassler, W. J. (1995). Impact of increased legal access to needles and syringes on practices of injecting drug users and police officers — Connecticut, 1992–1993. *Journal of Acquired Immune Deficiency Syndromes and Human Retrovirology*, 10, 82–9.

Grossbart, T. A. (1982, February). Bringing peace to embattled skin. *Psychology Today*, pp. 55–60.

Grossi, G., Perski, A., Feleke, E., & Jakobson, U. (1998). State anxiety predicts poor psychosocial outcome after coronary bypass surgery. *International Journal of Behavioral Medicine*, 5(1), 1–16.

Grossi, G., Theorell, T., Jurisoo, M., & Setterlind, S. (1999). Psychophysiological correlates of organizational change and threat of unemployment among police inspectors. *Integrative Physiological and Behavioral Science*, 34(1), 30–42.

Groth-Marnat, G. (1988). A survey of the current and future directions of professional psychology in acute general hospitals in Australia. *Australian Psychologist*, 23(2), 127–35.

Grove, J. R., Wilkinson, A., & Dawson, B. T. (1993). Effects of exercise on selected correlates of smoking withdrawal. *International Journal of Sport Psychology*, 24, 217–36.

Grube, J. W., & Wallack, L. (1994). Television beer advertising and drinking knowledge, beliefs, and intentions among schoolchildren. *American Journal of Public Health*, 84, 254–9.

Gruen, W. (1975). Effects of brief psychotherapy during the hospitalization period on the recovery process in heart attacks. *Journal of Consulting and Clinical Psychology*, 43, 223–32.

Gruetzner, H. (1992). *Alzheimer's: a caregiver's guide and sourcebook*. New York: John Wiley & Sons.

Grunau, R. V. E., & Craig, K. D. (1987). Pain expression in neonates: facial action and cry. *Pain*, 28, 395–410.

Grunberg, N. E., & Bowen, D. J. (1985). Coping with the sequelae of smoking cessation. *Journal of Cardiopulmonary Rehabilitation*, 5, 285–9.

Grych, J. H., & Fincham, F. D. (1990). Marital conflict and children's adjustment: a cognitive contextual framework. *Psychological Bulletin*, 108, 267–90.

Guccione, A. A., Felson, D. T., Anderson, J. J., Anthony, J. M., Zhang, Y., Wilson, P. W. F., Kelly-Hayes, M., Wolf, P. A., Kreger, B. E., & Kannel, W. B. (1994). The effects of specific medical conditions on the functional limitations of elders in the Framingham Study. *American Journal of Public Health*, 84, 351–8.

Gullone, E., & Cummins, R. A. (1999). The Comprehensive Quality of Life Scale: a psychometric evaluation with an adolescent sample. *Behaviour Change*, 16, 127–39.

Guyton, A. C. (1985). *Anatomy and physiology*. Philadelphia, PA: Saunders.

Haaga, D. A. F., & Davison, G. C. (1993). An appraisal of rational-emotive therapy. *Journal of Consulting and Clinical Psychology*, 61, 215–20.

Haapanen, A., Koskenvuo, M., Kaprio, J., Kesäniemi, Y. A., & Heikkilä, K. (1989). Carotid arteriosclerosis in identical twins discordant for cigarette smoking. *Circulation*, 80, 10–16.

Haas, F., & Haas, S. S. (1990). *The chronic bronchitis and emphysema handbook*. New York: John Wiley & Sons.

Hackett, T. P., & Weisman, A. D. (1985). Reactions to the imminence of death. In A. Monat & R. S. Lazarus (Eds), *Stress and coping: an anthology* (2nd ed.). New York: Columbia University Press.

Haddock, C. K., Shadish, W. R., Klesges, R. C., & Stein, R. J. (1994). Treatments for childhood and adolescent obesity. *Annals of Behavioral Medicine*, 16, 235–44.

Hafen, B. Q. (1981). *Nutrition, food, and weight control*. Boston, MA: Allyn & Bacon.

Hall, S. M., Rugg, D., Tunstall, C., & Jones, R. T. (1984). Preventing relapse to cigarette smoking by behavioral skill training. *Journal of Consulting and Clinical Psychology*, 52, 372–82.

Hall, T. (1990, June 17). After AIDS diagnosis, some embrace life. *New York Times*, pp. 1, 20.

Halpern, D. F., & Coren, S. (1991). Handedness and life span. *New England Journal of Medicine*, 324, 998.

Hamilton, J. D., Hartigan, P. M., Simberkoff, M. S., Day, P. L., et al. (1992). A controlled trial of early versus late treatment with zidovudine in symptomatic human immunodeficiency virus infection: results of the Veterans Affairs Cooperative Study. *New England Journal of Medicine*, 326, 437–43.

Hammond, S. K., Sorenson, G., Youngstrom, R., & Ockene, J. K. (1995). Occupational exposure to environmental tobacco smoke. *Journal of the American Medical Association*, 274, 956–60.

Hansen, W. B., Graham, J. W., Sobel, J. L., Shelton, D. R., Flay, B. R., & Johnson C. A. (1987). The consistency of peer and parent influences on tobacco, alcohol, and marijuana use among young adolescents. *Journal of Behavioral Medicine*, 10, 559–79.

Hansen, W. B., Raynor, A. E., & Wolkenstein, B. H. (1991). Perceived personal immunity to the consequences of drinking alcohol: the relationship between behavior and perception. *Journal of Behavioral Medicine*, 14, 205–224.

Hanson, C. L., Henggeler, S. W., & Burghen, G. A. (1987). Social competence and parental support as mediators of the link between stress and metabolic control in adolescents with insulin-dependent diabetes mellitus. *Journal of Consulting and Clinical Psychology*, 55, 529–33.

Hardy, G. E., West, M. A., & Hill, F. (1996). Components and predictors of patient satisfaction. *British Journal of Health Psychology*, 1, 65–85.

Hare, B. D., & Milano, R. A. (1985). Chronic pain: perspectives on physical assessment and treatment. *Annals of Behavioral Medicine*, 7(3), 6–10.

Harkavy, J., Johnson, S. B., Silverstein, J., Spillar, R., McCallum, M., & Rosenbloom, A. (1983). Who learns what at diabetes summer camp. *Journal of Pediatric Psychology*, 8, 143–54.

Harley, H. G., Brook, J. D., Rundle, S. A., Crow, S., Reardon, W., Buckler, A. J., Harper, P. S., Housman, D. E., & Shaw, D. J. (1992). Expansion of an unstable DNA region and phenotypic variation in myotonic dystrophy. *Nature*, 355, 545–6.

Harper, P. S. (1981). *Practical genetic counselling*. Baltimore, MD: University Park Press.

Harris, D. M., & Guten, S. (1979). Health-protective behavior: an exploratory study. *Journal of Health and Social Behavior*, 20, 17–29.

Harris, J., & Liebert, R. (1991). *The child: A contemporary view of development* (3rd ed.). Upper Saddle River, NJ: Prentice Hall.

Harris, J. R., Pederson, N. L., McClearn, G. E., Plomin, R., & Nesselroade, J. R. (1992). Age differences in genetic and environmental influences for health from the Swedish Adoption/Twin Study of Aging. *Journal of Gerontology*, 47, 213–20.

Harris, T. (1991). Life stress and illness: the question of specificity. *Annals of Behavioral Medicine*, 13, 211–19.

Harris, T. (1997). Life events and health. In A. Baum, S. Newman, J. Weinman, R. West & C. McManus (Eds), *Cambridge handbook of psychology, health and medicine* (pp. 136–8). Cambridge: Cambridge University Press.

Harrison, S. L., Maclennan, R., Speare, R., & Wronski, I. (1994). Sun exposure and melanocytic naevi in young Australian children. *The Lancet*, 1994, 1529–32.

Hart, P. M. (1999). Predicting employee life satisfaction: a coherent model of personality, work and nonwork experiences and domain satisfactions. *Journal of Applied Psychology*, 84(4), 564–84.

Hart, W. (1987). *The art of living: Vipassana meditation*. New York: HarperCollins.

Harter, S. (1983). Developmental perspectives on the self-system. In P. H. Mussen (Ed.), *Handbook of child psychology* (4th ed., Vol. 4). New York: John Wiley & Sons.

Hartz, A. J., Rupley, D. C., & Rimm, A. A. (1984). The association of girth measurements with disease in 32,856 women. *American Journal of Epidemiology*, 119, 71–80.

Harvey, A. S., Nolan, T., & Carlin, J. B. (1993). Community based study of mortality in children with epilepsy. *Epilepsia*, 34, 597–603.

Harvey, P. G. (1984). Lead and children's health — recent research and future questions. *Journal of Child Psychology and Psychiatry*, 25, 517–22.

Harvey, P. W., Steele, J., Bruggemann, J. N., & Jeffery, R. W. (1998). The development and evaluation of Lighten Up, an Australian community-based weight management program. *American Journal of Health Promotion*, 13(1), 8–11.

Haskell, W. L. (1984). Overview: health benefits of exercise. In J. D. Matarazzo, S. M. Weiss, J. A. Herd, N. E. Miller & S. M. Weiss (Eds), *Behavioral health: a handbook of health enhancement and disease prevention*. New York: John Wiley & Sons.

Haskell, W. L. (1985). Exercise programs for health promotion. In J. C. Rosen & L. J. Solomon (Eds), *Prevention in health psychology*. Hanover, NH: University Press of New England.

Haskell, W. L., Alderman, E. L., Fair, J. M., Maron, D. J., et al. (1994). Effects of intensive multiple risk factor reduction on coronary atherosclerosis and clinical cardiac events in men and women with coronary artery disease: the Stanford Coronary Risk Intervention Project (SCRIP). *Circulation*, 89, 975–90.

Hatch, J. P., Gatchel, R. J., & Harrington, R. (1982). Biofeedback: clinical applications in medicine. In R. J. Gatchel, A. Baum & J. E. Singer (Eds), *Handbook of psychology and health* (Vol. 1). Hillsdale, NJ: Erlbaum.

Haug, M. R., & Lavin, B. (1981). Practitioner or patient — who's in charge? *Journal of Health and Social Behavior*, 22, 212–29.

Hauser, W. A., & Hesdorffer, D. C. (1990). *Facts about epilepsy*. Landover, MD: Epilepsy Foundation of America.

Hawks, D., & Lenton, S. (1995). Harm reduction in Australia: has it worked? A review. *Drug and Alcohol Review*, 14, 291–304.

Hay, D., & Oken, D. (1985). The psychological stresses of intensive care unit nursing. In A. Monat & R. S. Lazarus (Eds), *Stress and coping* (2nd ed.). New York: Columbia University Press.

Hayes, R. D., Kravitz, R. L., Mazel, R. M., Sherbourne, C. D., DiMatteo, M. R., Rogers, W. H., & Greenfield, S. (1994). The impact of patient adherence on health outcomes for patients with chronic disease in the Medical Outcomes Study. *Journal of Behavioral Medicine*, 17, 347–60.

Haynes, R. B. (1976). A critical review of the 'determinants' of patient compliance with therapeutic regimens. In D. L. Sackett & R. B. Haynes (Eds), *Compliance with therapeutic regimens*. Baltimore, MD: Johns Hopkins University Press.

Haynes, S. G., & Matthews, K. A. (1988). Review and methodological critique of recent studies on Type A behavior and cardiovascular disease. *Annals of Behavioral Medicine*, 10, 47–59.

Haynes, S. N., Griffin, P., Mooney, D., & Parise, M. (1975). Electromyographic biofeedback and relaxation instructions in the treatment of muscle contraction headaches. *Behaviour Therapy*, 6, 672–8.

Hays, J. C., Kasl, S. V., & Jacobs, J. C. (1994). The course of psychological distress following threatened and actual conjugal bereavement. *Psychological Medicine*, 24, 917–27.

Hays, K. F. (1999). *Working it out: using exercise in psychotherapy*. Washington, DC: American Psychological Association.

Heath, A.C., & Martin, N.G. (1994). Genetic influences on alcohol consumption patterns and problem drinking: results from the Australian NHMRC Twin Panel follow-up survey. *Annals New York Academy of Sciences*, 72–85.

Heather, N. (1987). DRAMS for problem drinkers: the potential of a brief intervention by general practitioners and some evidence of its effectiveness . In T. Stockwell & S. Clement (Eds), *Helping the problem drinker: new initiatives in community care* (pp. 83–104). London: Croom Helm.

Heather, N. (1989a). Brief intervention strategies. In R. K. Hester & W. R. Miller (Eds), *Handbook of alcoholism treatment approaches: effective alternatives*. Pergamon general psychology series, Vol. 157 (pp. 93–116). Elmsford: Pergamon Press.

Heather, N. (1989b). Treatment of alcohol problems: with special reference to the behavioral approach. In R. K. Hester & W. R. Miller (Eds), *Handbook of alcoholism treatment approaches: effective alternatives*. Pergamon general psychology series, Vol. 157 (pp. 283–312). Elmsford, NY: Pergamon.

Heather, N., & Tebbutt, J. (Eds) (1989). *The effectiveness of treatment for drug and alcohol problems: an overview*. NCADA Monograph Series No. 11. Canberra: AGPS.

Heaven, P. (1989). Adolescent smoking, toughmindedness and attitudes to authority. *Australian Psychologist*, 24, 27–35.

Heaven, P. (1996). *Adolescent health: the role of individual differences*. London: Routledge.

Hebb, D. O. (1955). Drives and the C.N.S. (conceptual nervous system). *Psychological Review*, 62, 243–54.

Hegsted, D. M. (1984). What is a healthful diet? In J. D. Matarazzo, S. M. Weiss, J. A. Herd, N. E. Miller & S. M. Weiss (Eds), *Behavioral health: a handbook of health enhancement and disease prevention*. New York: John Wiley & Sons.

Heiby, E. M., Onorato, V. A., & Sato, R. A. (1985, August). A cognitive-behavioral model of adherence to health-related exercise. Poster session presented at the American Psychological Association 93rd Annual Convention, Los Angeles, CA.

Heinrich, R. L., Cohen, M. J., Naliboff, B. D., Collins, G. A., & Bonnebakker, A. D. (1985). Comparing physical and behavior therapy for chronic low back pain on physical abilities, psychological distress, and patients' perceptions. *Journal of Behavioral Medicine*, 8, 61–78.

Heitzmann, C. A., & Kaplan, R. M. (1988). Assessment of methods for measuring social support. *Health Psychology*, 7, 75–109.

Helgeson, V. S., & Cohen, S. (1996). Social support and adjustment to cancer: reconciling descriptive, correlational, and intervention research. *Health Psychology*, 15, 135–48.

Helgeson, V. S., & Fritz, H. L. (1999). Cognitive adaptation as a predictor of new coronary events after percutaneous transluminal coronary angioplasty. *Psychosomatic Medicine*, 61(4), 488–95.

Heller, K. (1979). The effects of social support: prevention and treatment implications. In A. P. Goldstein & F. H. Kanfer (Eds), *Maximizing treatment gains: transfer enhancement in psychotherapy* (pp. 253–382). New York: Academic Press.

Heller, K., Price, R. H., & Hogg, J. R. (1990). The role of social support in community and clinical interventions. In B. R. Sarason, I. G. Sarason & G. R. Pierce (Eds), *Social support: an interactional view*. New York: John Wiley & Sons.

Henderson, D. K., Fahey, B. J., Willy, M., Schmitt, J. M., Carey, K., Koziol, D. E., Lane, H. C., Fedio, J., & Saah, A. J. (1990). Risk for occupational transmission of human immunodeficiency virus type 1 (HIV-1) associated with clinical exposures: a prospective evaluation. *Annals of Internal Medicine*, 113, 740–46.

Henderson, G., & Primeaux, M. (1981). Religious beliefs and healing. In G. Henderson & M. Primeaux (Eds), *Transcultural health care*. Menlo Park, CA: Addison-Wesley.

Hendler, N. H. (1984). Chronic pain. In H. B. Roback (Ed.), *Helping patients and their families cope with medical problems*. San Francisco: Jossey-Bass.

Hendrick, S. S. (1985). Spinal cord injury and neuromuscular reeducation. In N. Schneiderman & J. T. Tapp (Eds), *Behavioral medicine: the biopsychosocial approach*. Hillsdale, NJ: Erlbaum.

Henig, R. M. (1988, February 28). The high cost of thinness. *New York Times Magazine*, pp. 41–2.

Hennig, P., & Knowles, A. (1990). Factors influencing women over 40 years to take precautions against cervical cancer. *Journal of Applied Social Psychology*, 20 (19), 1612–21.

Henningfield, J. E., Cohen, C., & Pickworth, W. B. (1993). Psychopharmacology of nicotine. In C. T. Orleans & J. Slade (Eds), *Nicotine addiction: principles and management*. New York: Oxford University Press.

Henry, J. H., Liu, Y-Y., Nadra, W. E., Qian, C.-G., Mormede, P., Lemaire, V., Ely, D., & Hendley, E. D. (1993). Psychosocial stress can induce chronic hypertension in normotensive strains of rats. *Hypertension*, 21, 714–23.

Herbert, T. B., & Cohen, S. (1993). Stress and immunity in humans: a meta-analytic review. *Psychosomatic Medicine*, 55, 364–79.

Herd, J. A., & Weiss, S. M. (1984). Overview of hypertension: its treatment and prevention. In J. D. Matarazzo, S. M. Weiss, J. A. Herd, N. E. Miller & S. M. Weiss (Eds), *Behavioral health: a handbook of health enhancement and disease prevention*. New York: John Wiley & Sons.

Herek, G. M. (1989). Hate crimes against lesbians and gay men. *American Psychologist*, 44, 948–55.

Herek, G. M., & Capitanio, J. P. (1993). Public reactions to AIDS in the United States: a second decade of stigma. *American Journal of Public Health*, 83, 574–7.

Herek, G. M., & Glunt, E. K. (1988). An epidemic of stigma: public reactions to AIDS. *American Psychologist*, 43, 886–91.

Herman, C. P., & Mack, D. (1975). Restrained and unrestrained eating. *Journal of Personality*, 43, 647–60.

Herman, C. P., Olmstead, M. P., & Polivy, J. (1983). Obesity, externality, and susceptibility to social influence: an integrated analysis. *Journal of Personality and Social Psychology*, 45, 926–34.

Herman, C. P., & Polivy, J. (1980). Restrained eating. In A. J. Stunkard (Ed.), *Obesity*. Philadelphia: Saunders.

Hernandez, J. T., & Smith, F. J. (1990). Inconsistencies and misperceptions putting college students at risk of HIV infection. *Journal of Adolescent Health Care*, 11, 295–7.

Hester, R. K., & Miller, W. R. (1989). Self-control training. In R. K. Hester & W. R. Miller (Eds), *Handbook of alcoholism treatment approaches: effective alternatives*. New York: Pergamon.

Hewitt, P., & Flett, G. L. (1996). Personality traits and the coping process. In M. Zeidner & N. S. Endler (Eds), *Handbook of coping: theory, research, applications* (pp. 410–33). New York: John Wiley & Sons.

Hier, D. B. (1986). Recovery from behavioral deficits after stroke. In P. E. Kaplan & L. J. Cerullo (Eds), *Stroke rehabilitation*. Boston, MA: Butterworth.

Hilgard, E. R. (1967). Individual differences in hypnotizability. In J. E. Gordon (Ed.), *Handbook of clinical and experimental hypnosis*. New York: Macmillan.

Hilgard, E. R., & Hilgard, J. R. (1983). *Hypnosis in the relief of pain* (rev. ed.). Los Altos, CA: Kaufmann.

Hill, D., White, V., & Letcher, T. (1999). Tobacco use among Australian secondary students in 1996. (1999). *Australian and New Zealand Journal of Public Health*, 23(3), 252–9.

Hill, D., White, V., Jolley, D., & Mapperson, K. (1988). Self-examination of the breast: is it beneficial? Meta-analysis of studies investigating breast self-examination and extent of disease in patients with breast cancer. *British Medical Journal*, 297, 271–5.

Hill, D., White, V., Marks, R., & Borland, R. (1993). Changes in sun-related attitudes and behaviours and reduced sunburn prevalence in a population at high risk of melanoma. *European Journal of Cancer Prevention*, 2, 447–56.

Hill, D., Willcox, S., Gardner, G., & Houston, J. (1987). Tobacco and alcohol use among Australian secondary schoolchildren. *Medical Journal of Australia*, 146, 125–30.

Hill, D. J., & White, V. M. (1995). Australian adult smoking prevalence in 1992. *Australian Journal of Public Health*, 19(3), 305–8.

Hill, J. O., Sparling, P. B., Shields, T. W., & Heller, P. A. (1987). Effects of exercise and food restriction on body composition and metabolic rate in obese women. *American Journal of Clinical Nutrition*, 46, 622–30.

Himes, J., & Dietz, W. (1994). Guidelines for overweight in adolescent preventive services: recommendations from an expert committee. *American Journal of Clinical Nutrition*, 59, 307–316.

Hinton, J. (1984). Coping with terminal illness. In R. Fitzpatrick, J. Hinton, S. Newman, G. Scambler & J. Thompson (Eds), *The experience of illness*. London: Tavistock.

Hiroto, D. S., & Seligman, M. E. P. (1975). Generality of learned helplessness in man. *Journal of Personality and Social Psychology*, 31, 311–27.

Hitchcock, L. S., Ferrell, B. R., & McCaffery, M. (1994). The experience of chronic nonmalignant pain. *Journal of Pain and Symptom Management*, 9, 312–18.

Ho, D. D., Neumann, A. U., Perelson, A. S., Chen, W., Leonard, J. M., & Markowitz, M. (1995). Rapid turnover of plasma virons and CD4 lymphocytes in HIV-1 infection. *Nature*, 373, 123–6.

Ho, R. (1989). Why do people smoke? Motives for the maintenance of smoking behaviour and its possible cessation. *Australian Psychologist*, 24(3), 385–400.

Ho, R. (1994). Cigarette advertising and cigarette health warnings: what role do adolescents' motives for smoking play in their assessment? *Australian Psychologist*, 29(1), 49–56.

Hobfoll, S. E. (1989). Conservation of resources: a new attempt at conceptualizing stress. *American Psychologist*, 44, 513–24.

Hobson, C. J., Kamen, J., Szostek, J., Nethercut, C. M., Tiedmann, J. W., & Wojnarowicz, S. (1998). Stressful life events: a revision and update of the social readjustment rating scale. *International Journal of Stress Management*, 5(1), 1–23.

Hodgins, D. C., El-Guebaly, N., & Armstrong, S. (1995). Prospective and retrospective reports of mood states before relapse to substance abuse. *Journal of Consulting and Clinical Psychology*, 63, 400–407.

Hoek, H. W., Bartelds, A. I. M., Bosveld, J. J. F., Van Der Graaf, Y., Limpens, V. E. L., Maiwald, M., & Spaaij, C. J. K. (1995). Impact of urbanization on detection rates of eating disorders. *American Journal of Psychiatry*, 152, 1272–8.

Hoelscher, T. J., Lichstein, K. L., & Rosenthal, T. L. (1986). Home relaxation practice in hypertension treatment: objective assessment and compliance induction. *Journal of Consulting and Clinical Psychology*, 54, 217–21.

Hoffman, M. (1993, June 28). Killing the pain. *Philadelphia Inquirer*, pp. C1, 4.

Hofman, A., Walter, H. J., Connelly, P. A., & Vaughn, R. D. (1987). Blood pressure and physical fitness in children. *Hypertension*, 9, 188–91.

Hogg, R. S. (1992). Indigenous mortality rates and causes: an international comparison between Australia, Canada and New Zealand. *Aboriginal and Islander Health Worker Journal*, 16(3), 13–17.

Holahan, C. K., Holahan, C. J., & Belk, S. S. (1984). Adjustment in aging: the roles of life stress, hassles, and self-efficacy. *Health Psychology*, 3, 315–28.

Holahan, C. J., & Moos, R. H. (1985). Life stress and health: personality, coping, and family support in stress resistance. *Journal of Personality and Social Psychology*, 49, 739–47.

Holahan, C. J., Moos, R. H., Holahan, C. K., & Brennan, P. L. (1995). Social support, coping, and depressive symptoms in a late-middle-aged sample of patients reporting cardiac illness. *Health Psychology*, 14, 152–63.

Holbrook, T. (1985). The hematopoietic system. In L. L. Hayman & E. M. Sporing (Eds), *Handbook of pediatric nursing*. New York: John Wiley & Sons.

Holder, H., Longabaugh, R., Miller, W. R., & Rubonis, A. V. (1991). The cost effectiveness of treatment for alcoholism: a first approximation. *Journal of Studies on Alcohol*, 52, 517–40.

Holland, A. J., Sicotte, N., & Treasure, J. (1988). Anorexia nervosa: evidence for a genetic basis. *Journal of Psychosomatic Research*, 32, 561–71.

Hollis, J. F., Lichtenstein, E., Vogt, T. M., Stevens, V. J., & Biglan, A. (1993). Nurse-assisted counseling for smokers in primary care. *Annals of Internal Medicine*, 118, 521–5.

Hollon, S. D., Shelton, R. C., & Davis, D. D. (1993). Cognitive therapy for depression: conceptual issues and clinical efficacy. *Journal of Consulting and Clinical Psychology*, 61, 270–75.

Holmes, D. M. (1986). The person and diabetes in psychosocial context. *Diabetes Care*, 9, 194–206.

Holmes, D. S. (1984). Meditation and somatic arousal reduction. *American Psychologist*, 39, 1–10.

Holmes, D. S. (1993). Aerobic fitness and the response to psychological stress. In P. Seraganian (Ed.), *Exercise psychology: the influence of physical exercise on psychological processes*. New York: John Wiley & Sons.

Holmes, T. H., & Masuda, M. (1974). Life change and illness susceptibility. In B. S. Dohrenwend & B. P. Dohrenwend (Eds), *Stressful life events: their nature and effects*. New York: John Wiley & Sons.

Holmes, T. H., & Rahe, R. H. (1967). The Social Readjustment Rating Scale. *Journal of Psychosomatic Research*, 11, 213–18.

Holroyd, K. A., & Penzien, D. B. (1985). Client variables and the behavioral treatment of recurrent tension headache: a meta-analytic review. *Journal of Behavioral Medicine*, 9, 515–36.

Holroyd, K. A., & Penzien, D. B. (1990). Pharmacological versus non-pharmacological prophylaxis of recurrent migraine headache: a meta-analytic review of clinical trials. *Pain*, 42, 1–13.

Holroyd, K. A., France, J. L., Cordingley, G. E., Rokicki, L. A., Kvaal, S. A., Lipchik, G. L., & McCool, H. R. (1995). Enhancing the effectiveness of relaxation-thermal biofeedback training with propranolol hydrochloride. *Journal of Consulting and Clinical Psychology*, 63, 327–30.

Holroyd, K. A., France, J. L., Nash, J. M., & Hursey, K. G. (1993). Pain state as artifact in the psychological assessment of recurrent headache sufferers. *Pain*, 53, 229–35.

Holroyd, K. A., Nash, J. M., Pingel, J. D., Cordingley, G. E., & Jerome, A. (1991). A comparison of pharmacological (amitriptyline HCL) and nonpharmacological (cognitive-behavioral) therapies for chronic tension headaches. *Journal of Consulting and Clinical Psychology*, 59, 387–93.

Holroyd, K. A., Penzien, D. B., Hursey, K. G., Tobin, D. L., Rogers, L., Holm, J. E., Marcille, P. J., Hall, J. R., & Chila, A. G. (1984). Change mechanisms in EMG biofeedback training: cognitive changes underlying improvements in tension headache. *Journal of Consulting and Clinical Psychology*, 52, 1039–53.

Holt, J. (1995, December). Motivating Beth. *American Journal of Nursing*, 95, pp. 60, 62.

Holtzman, D., Lowry, R., Kann, L., Collins, J. L., & Kolbe, L. J. (1994). Changes in HIV-related information sources, instruction, knowledge, and behaviors among US high school students, 1989 and 1990. *American Journal of Public Health*, 84, 388–93.

Holubowycz, O., Kloeden, C. N., & McLean, A. J. (1994). Age, sex, and blood alcohol concentration of killed and injured drivers, riders, and passengers. *Accident Analysis and Prevention*, 26(4), 483–92.

Holum, J. R. (1994). *Fundamentals of general, organic, and biological chemistry* (5th ed.). New York: John Wiley & Sons.

Holusha, J. (1991, October 13). The nation's polluters — who emits what, and where. *New York Times*, p. 10.

Holzheimer, L., Mohay, H., & Masters, I. B. (1998). Educating young children about asthma: comparing the effectiveness of a developmentally appropriate asthma education video tape and picture book. *Child Care and Health Development*, 24, 85–99.

Honig, A. S. (1987). Stress and coping in children. In H. E. Fitzgerald & M. G. Walraven (Eds), *Annual editions: human development 87/88*. Guilford, CT: Dushkin.

Hooper, S., Vaughan, K., Tennant, C., & Perz, J. (1997). Preferences for voluntary euthanasia during major depression and following improvement in an elderly population. *Australian Journal on Ageing*, 16(1), 3–7.

Hopkins, P. N. (1992). Effects of dietary cholesterol on serum cholesterol: a meta-analysis and review. *American Journal of Clinical Nutrition*, 55, 1060–70.

Horn, J. C., & Meer, J. (1987, May). The vintage years. *Psychology Today*, pp. 76–84, 89–90.

Horne, D. J. DeL (1997) Vomiting and nausea as side-effects of drugs. In A. Baum, S. Newman, J. Weinman, R. West & C. McManus (Eds), *Cambridge handbook of psychology, health and medicine* (pp. 618—20). Cambridge: Cambridge University Press.

Horne, D. J. DeL, McCormack, H. M., Collins, J. P., Forbes, J. F., & Russell, I. S. (1986). Psychological treatment of phobic anxiety associated with adjuvant chemotherapy. *Medical Journal of Australia*, 145, 346–8.

Horne, R. (1998). Adherence to medication: a review of existing research. In L. B. Myers & K. Midence, *Adherence to treatment in medical conditions* (pp. 285–310). Amsterdam: Harwood Academic Publishers.

Horne, R., & Weinman, J. (1999). Patients' beliefs about prescribed medicines and their role in adherence to treatment in chronic physical illness. *Journal of Psychosomatic Research*, 47(6), 555–67.

Horner, K. L. (1998). Individuality in vulnerability: influences on physical health. *Journal of Health Psychology*, 3(1), 71–85.

Horowitz, M. J. (1975). Intrusive and repetitive thoughts after stress. *Archives of General Psychiatry*, 32, 1457–63.

Hosoi, J., Murphy, G. F., Egan, C. L., Lerner, E. A., Grabbe, S., Asahina, A., & Granstein, R. D. (1993). Regulation of Langerhans cell function by nerves containing calcitonin gene-related peptide. *Nature*, 363, 159–63.

Hossack, K. F., & Leff, N. B. (1987). Influence of education and work history on patient perception of cardiovascular risk factors. *Journal of Cardiopulmonary Rehabilitation*, 7, 540–46.

Hough, R. L., Fairbank, D. T., & Garcia, A. M. (1976). Problems in the ratio measurement of life stress. *Journal of Health and Social Behavior*, 17, 70–82.

House, J. S., & Kahn, R. L. (1985). Measures and concepts of social support. In S. Cohen & S. L. Syme (Eds), *Social support and health* (pp. 83–108). New York: Academic Press.

House, J. S., Robbins, C., & Metzner, H. L. (1982). The association of social relationships and activities with mortality: prospective evidence from the Tecumseh Community Health Study. *American Journal of Epidemiology*, 116, 123–40.

Houston, B. K. (1986). Psychological variables and cardiovascular and neuroendocrine reactivity. In K. A. Matthews, S. M. Weiss, T. Detre, T. M. Dembroski, B. Falkner, S. B. Manuck & R. B. Williams (Eds), *Handbook of stress, reactivity, and cardiovascular disease*. New York: John Wiley & Sons.

Houston, B. K., & Vavak, C. R. (1991). Cynical hostility: developmental factors, psychosocial correlates, and health behaviors. *Health Psychology*, 10, 9–17.

Howard, J. H., Rechnitzer, P. A., Cunningham, D. A., & Donner, A. P. (1986). Change in Type A behavior a year after retirement. *The Gerontologist*, 26, 643–9.

Howell, D. (1986). The impact of terminal illness on the spouse. *Journal of Palliative Care*, 2, 22–30.

Hudgel, H. D., Cooperson, D. M., & Kinsman, R. A. (1982). Recognition of added resistive loads in asthma: the importance of behavioral styles. *American Review of Respiratory Disease*, 126, 121–5.

Huffman, L. C., & Del Carmen, R. (1990). Prenatal stress. In L. E. Arnold (Ed.), *Childhood stress*. New York: John Wiley & Sons.

Hughes, J. R. (1986). Genetics of smoking: a brief review. *Behavior Therapy*, 17, 335–45.

Hull, J. G., & Bond, C. F. (1986). Social and behavioral consequences of alcohol consumption and expectancy: a meta-analysis. *Psychological Bulletin*, 99, 347–60.

Hull, J. G., Van Treuren, R. R., & Virnelli, S. (1987). Hardiness and health: a critique and alternative approach. *Journal of Personality and Social Psychology*, 53, 518–30.

Hull, J. G., Young, R. D., & Jouriles, E. (1986). Applications of the self-awareness model of alcohol consumption: predicting patterns of use and abuse. *Journal of Personality and Social Psychology*, 51, 790–96.

Humble, C., Croft, J., Gerber, A., Casper, M., Hames, C. G., & Tyroler, H. A. (1990). Passive smoking and 20-year cardiovascular disease mortality among nonsmoking wives, Evans County, Georgia. *American Journal of Public Health*, 80, 599–601.

Hunt, W. A., & Matarazzo, J. D. (1982). Changing smoking behavior: a critique. In R. J. Gatchel, A. Baum & J. E. Singer (Eds), *Handbook of psychology and health* (Vol. 1). Hillsdale, NJ: Erlbaum.

Hunt, W. A., Matarazzo, J. D., Weiss, S. M., & Gentry, W. D. (1979). Associative learning, habit, and health behavior. *Journal of Behavioral Medicine*, 2, 111–24.

Hunter, E., Hall, W., & Spargo, R. (1991). Patterns and correlates of alcohol use among Aborigines of the Kimberley. Monograph of the National Drug and Alcohol Research Centre, Sydney.

Hurley, D. (1987, August). A sound mind in an unsound body. *Psychology Today*, pp. 34–43.

Hussussian, C. J., Struewing, J. P., Goldstein, A. M., Higgins, P. A. T., Ally, D. S., Sheahan, M. D., Clark, W. H., Tucker, M. A., & Dracopoli, N. C. (1994). Germline p16 mutations in familial melanoma. *Nature Genetics*, 8, 15–21.

Huston, A. C. (1983). Sex-typing. In P. H. Mussen (Ed.), *Handbook of child psychology* (4th ed., Vol. 4). New York: John Wiley & Sons.

Huszti, H. C., & Walker, C. E. (1991). Critical issues on consultation and liaison. In J. J. Sweet, R. H. Rozensky & S. M. Tovian (Eds), *Handbook of clinical psychology in medical settings*. New York: Plenum.

Hygge, S. (1996). The effects of combined noise sources on long-term memory in children aged 12–14 years. In A. Schick & M. Klatte (Eds), *Contributions to psychological acoustics. Result of the seventh Oldenburg symposium on psychological acoustics.* Oldenburg, Germany: Bibliotheks-und Informationssystem der Universität Oldenburg.

Hygge, S., Evans, G. W., & Bullinger, M. (1996). The Munich airport noise study: cognitive effects on children from before to after the change over of airports. Invited paper to Inter Noise 96, Liverpool, 30 July – 2 August 1996.

Hyson, M. C. (1983). Going to the doctor: a developmental study of stress and coping. *Journal of Child Psychology and Psychiatry*, 24, 247–59.

ICNIRP (International Commission on Non-Ionizing Radiation Protection) (1995). *Global Solar UVI.* Oberschleinsheim: Budesamt für Strahlenschutz Institut für Stahlenhygiene, ICNIRP, January.

Ilfeld, F. W. (1980). Coping styles of Chicago adults: description. *Journal of Human Stress*, 6, 2–10.

Inui, T. S., Yourtee, E. L., & Williamson, J. W. (1976). Improved outcomes in hypertension after physician tutorials. *Annals of Internal Medicine*, 84, 646–51.

Ironson, G., Friedman, A., Klimas, N., Antoni, M., Fletcher, M. A., Laperriere, A., Simoneau, J., & Schneiderman, N. (1994). Distress, denial, and low adherence to behavioral interventions predict faster disease progression in gay men infected with human immunodeficiency virus. *International Journal of Behavioral Medicine*, 1, 90–105.

Ironson, G., Taylor, C. B., Boltwood, M., Bartzokis, T., Dennis, C., Chesney, M., Spitzer, S., & Segall, G. M. (1992). Effects of anger on left ventricular ejection fraction in coronary artery disease. *American Journal of Cardiology*, 70, 281–5.

Irwin, M., Mascovich, A., Gillin, J. C., Willoughby, R., Pike, J., & Smith, T. L. (1994). Partial sleep deprivation reduces natural killer cell activity in humans. *Psychosomatic Medicine*, 56, 493–8.

Izard, C. E. (1979). Emotions as motivations: an evolutionary developmental perspective. In H. E. Howe & R. A. Dienstbier (Eds), Nebraska Symposium on Motivation 1978 (Vol. 27). Lincoln, NE: University of Nebraska Press.

Izard, C. E., Hembree, E. A., Dougherty, L. M., & Spizzirri, C. C. (1983). Changes in facial expressions of 2- to 19-month-old infants following acute pain. *Developmental Psychology*, 19, 418–26.

Jaccard, J., & Turrisi, R. (1987). Cognitive processes and individual differences in judgments relevant to drunk driving. *Journal of Personality and Social Psychology*, 53, 135–45.

Jacob, R. G., & Chesney, M. A. (1986). Psychological and behavioral methods to reduce cardiovascular reactivity. In K. A. Matthews, S. M. Weiss, T. Detre, T. M. Dembroski, B. Falkner, S. B. Manuck & R. B. Williams (Eds), *Handbook of stress, reactivity, and cardiovascular disease.* New York: John Wiley & Sons.

Jacobsen, P. B., & Holland, J. C. (1991). The stress of cancer: Psychological responses to diagnosis and treatment. In C. L. Cooper & M. Watson (Eds), *Cancer and stress: psychological, biological and coping studies.* Chichester: John Wiley & Sons.

Jacobson, A. M., Hauser, S. T., Lavori, P., Willett, J. B., Cole, C. F., Wolfsdorf, J. I., Dumont, R. H., & Wertlieb, D. (1994). Family environment and glycemic control: a four-year prospective study of children and adolescents with insulin-dependent diabetes mellitus. *Psychosomatic Medicine*, 56, 401–9.

Jacobson, A. M., Hauser, S. T., Wolfsdorf, J. I., Houlihan, J., Milley, J. E., Herskowitz, R. D., Wertlieb, D., & Watt, E. (1987). Psychologic predictors of compliance in children with recent onset of diabetes mellitus. *Journal of Pediatrics*, 110, 805–811.

Jacobson, E. J. (1938). *Progressive relaxation.* Chicago: University of Chicago Press.

Jacobson, J. A., Danforth, D. N., Cowan, K. H., D'angelo, T., Steinberg, S. M., Pierce, L., Lippman, M. E., Lichter, A. S., Glatstein, E., & Okunieff, P. (1995). Ten-year results of a comparison of conservation with mastectomy in the treatment of stage I and II breast cancer. *New England Journal of Medicine*, 332, 907–911.

Jadad, A. R., Carroll, D., Glynn, C. J., Moore, R. A., & McQuay, H. J. (1992). Morphine responsiveness of chronic pain: double-blind randomised crossover study with patient-controlled anesthesia. *The Lancet*, 339, 1367–71.

Jamal, M. (1999). Job stress, Type A behavior and well-being: a cross-cultural examination. *International Journal of Stress Management*, 6(1), 57–67.

James, G. D., Yee, L. S., Harshfield, G. A., Blank, S. G., & Pickering, T. G. (1986). The influence of happiness, anger, and anxiety on the blood pressure of borderline hypertensives. *Psychosomatic Medicine*, 48, 502–8.

James, J. (1990–91). The influence of user status and anxious disposition on the hypertensive effects of caffeine. *International Journal of Psychophysiology*, 10 (20), 171–9.

James, J. (1991). Pressor effects of caffeine and cigarette smoking. *British Journal of Clinical Psychology*, 30 (3), 276–8.

James, J. E. (1994). Health care, psychology, and the scientist-practitioner model. *Australian Psychologist*, 29, 5–11.

Jamner, L. D., & Tursky, B. (1987). Syndrome-specific descriptor profiling: a psychophysiological and psychophysical approach. *Health Psychology*, 6, 417–30.

Janal, M. N., Glusman, M., Kuhl, J. P., & Clark, W. C. (1994). On the absence of correlation between responses to noxious heat, cold, electrical, and ischemic stimulation. *Pain*, 58, 403–411.

Janis, I. L. (1958). *Psychological stress.* New York: John Wiley & Sons.

Janis, I. L. (1967). Effects of fear arousal on attitude change: recent developments in theory and experimental research. In L. Berkowitz (Ed.), *Advances in experimental social psychology* (Vol. 3). New York: Academic Press.

Janis, I. L. (1984). The patient as decision maker. In W. D. Gentry (Ed.), *Handbook of behavioral medicine.* New York: Guilford.

Janis, I. L., & Mann, L. (1977). *Decision making: a psychological analysis of conflict, choice, and commitment.* New York: Free Press.

Janson-Bjerklie, S., Carrieri, V. K., & Hudes, M. (1986). The sensations of pulmonary dyspnea. *Nursing Research*, 35, 154–9.

Jaret, P. (1986, June). Our immune system: the wars within. *National Geographic*, 169, 702–735.

Jaret, P. (1994, July). Viruses. *National Geographic*, 186, 58–91.

Jarvik, M. E., & Henningfield, J. E. (1993). Pharmacological adjuncts for the treatment of tobacco dependence. In C. T. Orleans & J. Slade (Eds), Nicotine addiction: principles and management. New York: Oxford University Press.

Javitt, J. C., Aiello, L. P., Chiang, Y., Ferris, F. L., Canner, J. K., & Greenfield, S. (1994). Preventive eye care in people with diabetes is cost-saving to the federal government. *Diabetes Care*, 17, 909–917.

Jay, S. M., Elliott, C. H., Katz, E., & Siegel, S. E. (1987). Cognitive-behavioral and pharmacologic interventions for children's distress during painful medical procedures. *Journal of Consulting and Clinical Psychology*, 55, 860–65.

Jay, S. M., Elliott, C. H., Ozolins, M., Olson, R. A., & Pruitt, S. D. (1985). Behavioral management of children's distress during painful medical procedures. *Behavior Research and Therapy*, 23, 513–20.

Jeans, M. E. (1983). Pain in children — a neglected area. In P. Firestone, P. J. McGrath & W. Feldman (Eds), *Advances in behavioral medicine for children and adolescents.* Hillsdale, NJ: Erlbaum.

Jeffery, R. W. (1991). Weight management and hypertension. *Annals of Behavioral Medicine*, 13, 18–22.

Jeffery, R. W. (1992). Is obesity a risk factor for cardiovascular disease? *Annals of Behavioral Medicine*, 14, 109–112.

Jeffery, R. W., French, S. A., & Schmid, T. L. (1990). Attributions for dietary failures: problems reported by participants in the Hypertension Prevention Trial. *Health Psychology*, 9, 315–29.

Jemmott, J. B., Croyle, R. T., & Ditto, P. H. (1988). Commonsense epidemiology: self-based judgments from laypersons and physicians. *Health Psychology*, 7, 55–73.

Jemmott, J. B., Ditto, P. H., & Croyle, R. T. (1986). Judging health status: effects of perceived prevalence and personal relevance. *Journal of Personality and Social Psychology*, 50, 899–905.

Jemmott, J. B., & Locke, S. E. (1984). Psychosocial factors, immunologic mediation, and human susceptibility to infectious diseases: how much do we know? *Psychological Bulletin*, 95, 78–108.

Jenkins, C. D. (1979). An approach to the diagnosis and treatment of problems of health related behaviour. *International Journal of Health Education*, 22 (Suppl. 2), 1–24.

Jenkins, C. D., Zyzanski, S. J., & Rosenman, R. H. (1979). *The Jenkins Activity Survey for Health Prediction.* New York: The Psychological Corporation.

Jenner, D. A.,& Miller, M. R. (1991). Intakes of selected nutrients in year 7 Western Australian children: comparison between weekend days and relationships with socio-economic status. *Australian Journal of Nutrition and Dietetics*, 48, 50–56.

Jennings, G., Nelson, L., Nestel, P., Esler, M., Korner, P., Burton, D., & Bazelmans, J. (1986). The effects of changes in physical activity on major cardiovascular risk factors, hemodynamics, sympathetic function, and glucose utilization in man: a controlled study of four levels of activity. *Circulation*, 73, 30–40.

Jensen, G. M., & Lorish, C. D. (1994). Promoting patient cooperation with exercise programs. *Arthritis Care and Research*, 7, 181–9.

Jensen, M. P., Karoly, P., O'Riordan, E. F., Bland, F., & Burns, R. S. (1989). The subjective experience of acute pain: an assessment of the utility of 10 indices. *Clinical Journal of Pain*, 5, 153–9.

Jensen, M. P., & McFarland, C. A. (1993). Increasing the reliability and validity of pain intensity measurement in chronic pain patients. *Pain*, 55, 195–203.

Jessor, R. (1984). Adolescent development and behavioral health. In J. D. Matarazzo, S. M. Weiss, J. A. Herd, N. E. Miller & S. M. Weiss (Eds), *Behavioral health: a handbook of health enhancement and disease prevention.* New York: John Wiley & Sons.

Jessor, R., & Jessor, S. L. (1977). *Problem behavior and psychosocial development: a longitudinal study of youth.* New York: Academic Press.

Jette, A. M. (1984). Understanding and enhancing patient cooperation with arthritis treatments. In G. K. Riggs & E. P. Gall (Eds), *Rheumatic diseases: rehabilitation and management.* Boston, MA: Butterworth.

Jobling, I., & Cotterell, J. (1990). Adolescent leisure: sport and physical recreation. In Heaven, P., & Callan, V., *Adolescence: Australian perspectives* (pp. 184–97). Marrickville: Harcourt Brace Jovanovich.

Johns, K. R., & Littlejohn, G. O. (1999). The role of sex hormones in pain response. *Pain*, 83(1), 112–13.

Johnson, A. M., & Laga, M. (1990). Heterosexual transmission of HIV. In N. J. Alexander, H. L. Gabelnick & J. M. Spieler (Eds), *Heterosexual transmission of AIDS.* New York: John Wiley & Sons–Liss.

Johnson, B. G. (1984). Biofeedback, transcutaneous electrical nerve stimulation, acupuncture, and hypnosis. In G. K. Riggs & E. P. Gall (Eds), *Rheumatic diseases: rehabilitation and management.* Boston, MA: Butterworth.

Johnson, C. A., Hansen, W. B., Collins, L. M., & Graham, J. W. (1986). High-school smoking prevention: results of a three-year longitudinal study. *Journal of Behavioral Medicine*, 9, 439–52.

Johnson, J. E. (1983). Psychological interventions and coping with surgery. In A. Baum, S. E. Taylor & J. E. Singer (Eds), *Handbook of psychology and health* (Vol. 4). Hillsdale, NJ: Erlbaum.

Johnson, J. E., & Leventhal, H. (1974). Effects of accurate expectations and behavioral instructions on reactions during a noxious medical examination. *Journal of Personality and Social Psychology*, 29, 710–18.

Johnson, J. E., Rice, V. H., Fuller, S. S., & Endress, M. P. (1978). Sensory information, instruction in a coping strategy, and recovery from surgery. *Research in Nursing and Health*, 1, 4–17.

Johnson, J. H. (1986). *Life events as stressors in childhood and adolescence.* Newbury Park, CA: Sage.

Johnson, K., Anderson, N. B., Bastida, E., Kramer, B. J., Williams, D., & Wong, M. (1995). Panel II. Macrosocial and environmental influences on minority health. *Health Psychology*, 14, 601–612.

Johnson, S. B. (1985). The family and the child with chronic illness. In D. C. Turk & R. D. Kerns (Eds), *Health, illness, and families: A life-span perspective.* New York: John Wiley & Sons.

Johnson, S. B., Freund, A., Silverstein, J., Hansen, C., & Malone, J. (1990). Adherence: health status relationships in childhood diabetes. *Health Psychology*, 9, 606–631.

Johnson, S. B., Kelly, M., Henretta, J. C., Cunningham, W. R., Tomer, A., & Silverstein, J. H. (1992). A longitudinal analysis of adherence and health status in childhood diabetes. *Journal of Pediatric Psychology*, 17, 537–53.

Johnston, D. W. (1992). The management of stress in the prevention of coronary heart disease. In S. Maes, H. Leventhal & M. Johnston (Eds), *International review of health psychology* (Vol. 1). New York: John Wiley & Sons.

Johnston, L. D., O'Malley, P. M., & Bachman, J. G. (1995). *National survey results on drug use from the Monitoring the Future Study, 1975–1994* (NIH Publication No. 95-4026). Rockville, MD: National Institute on Drug Abuse.

Johnston, M. (1997). Hospitalization in adults. In A. Baum, S. Newman, J. Weinman, R. West & C. McManus (Eds), *Cambridge handbook of psychology, health and medicine* (pp. 121–3). Cambridge: Cambridge University Press.

Johnston, M., & Vögele, C. (1993). Benefits of psychological preparation for surgery: a meta-analysis. *Annals of Behavioral Medicine*, 15, 245–56.

Johnston, M., Wright, S., & Weinman, J. (Eds) (1995). *Measures in health psychology: a user's portfolio.* Windsor, UK: NFER-Nelson.

Johnstone, B., Frank, R., Belar, C., Berk, S., Bieliauskas, L., Bigler, E., et al. (1995). Psychology in health care: future directions. *Professional Psychology: Research and Practice*, 26(4), 341–65.

Jonas, H. A., Dobson, A. J., & Brown, W. J. (2000). Patterns of alcohol consumption in young Australian women: socio-demographic factors, health-related behaviours and physical health. *Australian and New Zealand Journal of Public Health*, 24(2), 185–91.

Jones, D. M., & Macken, W. J. (1993). Irrelevant tones produce an irrelevant speech effect: implications for coding in phonological memory. *Journal of Experimental Psychology: Learning, Memory and Cognition*, 19, 369–81.

Jones, D. M., & Morris, N. (1992). Irrelevant speech and cognition. In A. P. Smith & D. M. Jones (Eds), *Handbook of human performance: Vol 1. The physical environment* (pp. 29–54). London: Academic Press.

Jones, L. M., Halford, W. K., & Dooley, R. T. (1993). Long term outcome of anorexia nervosa. *Behaviour Change*, 10(2), 93–102.

Jones, L. R., Mabe, P. A., & Riley, W. T. (1989). Physician interpretation of illness behavior. *International Journal of Psychiatry in Medicine*, 19, 237–48.

Jones, R. T. (1991). Tobacco. In D. A. Ciraulo & R. I. Shader (Eds), *Clinical manual of chemical dependence.* Washington, DC: American Psychiatric Press.

Jones, T. F., Craig, A. S., Hoy, D., Gunter, E. W., Ashley, D. L., Barr, D. B., Brock, J. W., & Schaffner, W. (2000). Mass psychogenic illness attributed to toxic exposure at a high school. *New England Journal of Medicine,* 342(2), 96–100.

Jorm, A. F., & Henderson, A. S. (1993). *The Problem of Dementia in Australia* (3rd ed.). Canberra: AGPS.

Joseph, J. G., Montgomery, S. B., Emmons, C., Kessler, R. C., Ostrow, D. G., Wortman, C. B., O'Brien, K., Eller, M., & Eshleman, S. (1987). Magnitude and determinants of behavioral risk reduction: longitudinal analysis of a cohort at risk for AIDS. *Psychology and Health,* 1, 73–96.

Joseph, S., Williams, R., & Yule, W. (1997). *Understanding posttraumatic stress: a psychosocial perspective on PTSD and treatment.* Chichester: John Wiley & Sons.

Jospe, M., Shueman, S. A., & Troy, W. G. (1991). Quality assurance and the clinical health psychologist: a programmatic approach. In J. J. Sweet, R. H. Rozensky & S. M. Tovian (Eds), *Handbook of clinical psychology in medical settings.* New York: Plenum.

Jousilahti, P., Vartiainen, E., Tuomilehto, J., Pekkanen, J., & Puska, P. (1995). Effect of risk factors and changes in risk factors on coronary mortality in three cohorts of middle-aged people in Eastern Finland. *American Journal of Epidemiology,* 141, 50–60.

Joyce, C. (1984, November). A time for grieving. *Psychology Today,* pp. 42–6.

Köhler, T., & Haimerl, C. (1990). Daily stress as a trigger of migraine attacks: results of thirteen single-subject studies. *Journal of Consulting and Clinical Psychology,* 58, 870–72.

Kabat-Zinn, J. (1982). An outpatient program in behavioral medicine for chronic pain patients based on the practice of mindfulness meditation: theoretical considerations and preliminary results. *General Hospital Psychiatry,* 4, 33–47.

Kabat-Zinn, J., Lipworth, L., & Burney, R. (1985). The clinical use of mindfulness meditation for the self-regulation of chronic pain. *Journal of Behavioral Medicine,* 8, 163–90.

Kahn, K. L., Keeler, E. B., Sherwood, M. J., Rogers, W. H., Draper, D., Bentow, S. S., Reinisch, E. J., Rubenstein, L. V., Kosecoff, J., & Brook, R. H. (1990). Comparing outcomes of care before and after implementation of the DRG-based prospective payment system. *Journal of the American Medical Association,* 264, 1984–8.

Kahn, K. L., Rogers, W. H., Rubenstein, L. V., Sherwood, M. J., Reinisch, E. J., Keeler, E. B., Draper, D., Kosecoff, J., & Brook, R. H. (1990). Measuring quality of care with explicit process criteria before and after implementation of the DRG-based prospective payment system. *Journal of the American Medical Association,* 264, 1969–73.

Kalichman, S. C., Carey, M. P., & Johnson, B. T. (1996). Prevention of sexually transmitted HIV infection: a meta-analytic review of the behavioral outcome literature. *Annals of Behavioral Medicine,* 18, 6–15.

Kalichman, S. C., & Coley, B. (1995). Context framing to enhance HIV-antibody-testing messages targeted at African American women. *Health Psychology,* 14, 247–54.

Kalichman, S. C., Kelly, J. A., Hunter, T. L., Murphy, D. A., & Tyler, R. (1993). Culturally tailored HIV-AIDS risk-reduction messages targeted to African-American urban women: impact on risk sensitization and risk reduction. *Journal of Consulting and Clinical Psychology,* 61, 291–5.

Kalichman, S. C., Rompa, D., & Coley, B. (1996). Experimental component analysis of a behavioral HIV-AIDS prevention intervention for inner-city women. *Journal of Consulting and Clinical Psychology,* 64, 687–93.

Kalish, R. A. (1985). The social context of death and dying. In R. H. Binstock & E. Shanas (Eds), *Handbook of aging and the social sciences.* New York: Van Nostrand-Reinhold.

Kalish, R. A., & Reynolds, D. K. (1976). *Death and ethnicity: a psychocultural study.* Los Angeles: University of Southern California Press.

Kaloupek, D. G., White, H., & Wong, M. (1984). Multiple assessment of coping strategies used by volunteer blood donors: implications for preparatory training. *Journal of Behavioral Medicine,* 7, 35–60.

Kamarck, T. W., & Lichtenstein, E. (1985). Current trends in clinic-based smoking control. *Annals of Behavioral Medicine,* 7(2), 19–23.

Kamarck, T. W., Manuck, S. B., & Jennings, J. R. (1990). Social support reduces cardiovascular reactivity to psychological challenge: a laboratory model. *Psychosomatic Medicine,* 52, 42–58.

Kamen, L. P., & Seligman, M. E. P. (1989). Explanatory style and health. In M. Johnston & T. Marteau (Eds), *Applications in health psychology.* New Brunswick, NJ: Transaction.

Kandel, D. (1974). Inter- and intragenerational influences of adolescent marijuana use. *Journal of Social Issues,* 30, 107–135.

Kandel, D., & Faust, R. (1975). Sequence and stages in patterns of adolescent drug use. *Archives of General Psychiatry,* 32, 923–32.

Kandel, D. B., Wu, P., & Davies, M. (1994). Maternal smoking during pregnancy and smoking by adolescent daughters. *American Journal of Public Health,* 84, 1407–1413.

Kang, D. H., Coe, C. L., Karaszewski, J., & McCarthy, D. O. (1998). Relationship of social support to stress responses and immune function in healthy and asthmatic adolescents. *Research in Nursing and Health,* 21(2), 117-28.

Kanner, A. D., Coyne, J. C., Schaefer, C., & Lazarus, R. S. (1981). Comparison of two modes of stress measurement: daily hassles and uplifts versus major life events. *Journal of Behavioral Medicine,* 4, 1–39.

Kanner, R. (1986). Pain management. *Journal of the American Medical Association,* 256, 2110–14.

Kaplan, B. J., & Wyler, A. R. (1983). Coping with epilepsy. In T. G. Burish & L. A. Bradley (Eds), *Coping with chronic disease: research and applications.* New York: Academic Press.

Kaplan, G. A. (1995). Where do shared pathways lead? Some reflections on a research agenda. *Psychosomatic Medicine,* 57, 208–212.

Kaplan, N. M. (1986). Dietary aspects of the treatment of hypertension. In L. Breslow, J. E. Fielding & L. B. Lave (Eds), *Annual review of public health* (Vol. 7). Palo Alto, CA: Annual Reviews.

Kaplan, R. M. (1989). Health outcome models for policy analysis. *Health Psychology,* 8, 723–35.

Kaplan, R. M. (1994). The Ziggy theorem: toward an outcomes-focused health psychology. *Health Psychology,* 13, 451–60.

Kaplan, R. M., Atkins, C. J., & Reinsch, S. (1984). Specific efficacy expectations mediate exercise compliance in patients with COPD. *Health Psychology,* 3, 223–42.

Kaplan, R. M., & Bush, J. W. (1982). Health-related quality of life measurement for evaluation research and policy analysis. *Health Psychology,* 1, 621–80.

Kaplan, R. M., & Simon, H. J. (1990). Compliance in medical care: reconsideration of self-predictions. *Annals of Behavioral Medicine,* 12, 66–71.

Kaplan, R. M., & Toshima, M. (1990). The functional effects of social relationships on chronic illnesses and disability. In B. R. Sarason, I. G. Sarason & G. R. Pierce, *Social support: an interactional view* (pp. 427–53). New York: John Wiley & Sons.

Kapust, L. R., & Weintraub, S. (1984). Living with a family member suffering from Alzheimer's disease. In H. B. Roback (Ed.), *Helping patients and their families cope with medical problems.* San Francisco: Jossey-Bass.

Karasek, R., & Theorell, T. (1990). *Healthy work: stress, productivity and the reconstruction of working life.* New York: Basic Books.

Karoly, P. (1985). The assessment of pain: concepts and procedures. In P. Karoly (Ed.), *Measurement strategies in health psychology.* New York: John Wiley & Sons.

Karvonen, M., Tuomilehto, J., Libman, I., & Laports, R. (1993). A review of recent epidemiological data on the world-wide incidence of Type 1 (insulin-dependent) diabetes mellitus. World Health Organisation DIAMOND Project Group. *Diabetologia*, 36, 883–92.

Kasch, F. W., Wallace, J. P., & Van Camp, S. P. (1985). Effects of 18 years of endurance exercise on the physical work capacity of older men. *Journal of Cardiopulmonary Rehabilitation*, 5, 308–312.

Kashima, Y., Gallois, C., & McCamish, M.(1992). Predicting the use of condoms: past behavior, norms and the sexual partner. In T. Edgar, M. A. Fitzpatrick & V. S. Freimuth (Eds), *Aids: a communication perspective. Communication.* (pp. 21–46). Hillsdale, NJ: Erlbaum.

Kasl, S. (1997). Unemployment and health. In A. Baum, S. Newman, J. Weinman, R. West & C. McManus (Eds), *Cambridge handbook of psychology, health and medicine* (pp. 186–8). Cambridge: Cambridge University Press.

Kasl, S. V., & Cobb, S. (1966a). Health behavior, illness behavior, and sick role behavior: I. Health and illness behavior. *Archives of Environmental Health*, 12, 246–66.

Kasl, S. V., & Cobb, S. (1966b). Health behavior, illness behavior, and sick role behavior: II Sick role behavior. *Archives of Environmental Health*, 12, 531–41.

Kastenbaum, R., & Costa, P. T. (1977). Psychological perspectives on death. In M. R. Rosenzweig & L. W. Porter (Eds), *Annual review of psychology* (Vol. 28). Palo Alto, CA: Annual Reviews.

Katz, J., & Melzack, R. (1990). Pain 'memories' in phantom limbs: review and clinical observations. *Pain*, 43, 319–36.

Kaufman, B. (1988). A distant compassion. *Health Values*, 12(4), 31–2.

Kavanagh, D. J., Pierce, J., Kai Lo, S., & Shelley, J. (1993). Self-efficacy and social support as predictors of smoking after a quit attempt. *Psychology and Health*, 8, 231–42.

Kavanaugh, D. J., Gooley, S., & Wilson, P. H. (1993). Prediction of adherence and control in diabetes. *Journal of Behavioral Medicine*, 16(5), 509–522.

Kawachi, I., Colditz, G. A., Stampfer, M. J., Willett, W. C., Manson, J. E., Rosner, B., Speizer, F. E., & Hennekens, C. H. (1993). Smoking cessation and decreased risk of stroke in women. *Journal of the American Medical Association*, 269, 232–6.

Kawachi, I., Colditz, G. A., & Stone, C. B. (1994). Does coffee drinking increase the risk of coronary heart disease? Results from a meta-analysis. *British Heart Journal*, 72, 269–75.

Keefe, F. J. (1982). Behavioral assessment and treatment of chronic pain: current status and future directions. *Journal of Consulting and Clinical Psychology*, 50, 896–911.

Keefe, F. J., & Block, A. R. (1982). Development of an observation method for assessing pain behavior in chronic low back pain patients. *Behavior Therapy*, 13, 363–75.

Keefe, F. J., & Dolan, E. (1986). Pain behavior and pain coping strategies in low back pain and myofascial pain dysfunction syndrome patients. *Pain*, 24, 49–56.

Keefe, F. J., & Gil, K. M. (1985). Recent advances in the behavioral assessment and treatment of chronic pain. *Annals of Behavioral Medicine*, 7(3), 11–16.

Keefe, F. J., Hauck, E. R., Egert, J., Rimer, B., & Kornguth, P. (1994). Mammography pain and discomfort: a cognitive-behavioral perspective. *Pain*, 56, 247–60.

Keesey, R. E. (1986). A set point theory of obesity. In K. D. Brownell & J. P. Foreyt (Eds), *The physiology, psychology, and treatment of the eating disorders*. New York: Basic Books.

Keesey, R. E., & Powley, T. L. (1975). Hypothalamic regulation of body weight. *American Scientist*, 63, 558–65.

Kegeles, S. M., Adler, N. E., & Irwin, C. E. (1989). Adolescents and condoms: associations of beliefs with intentions to use. *American Journal of Diseases in Children*, 143, 911–15.

Kegeles, S. S. (1983). Behavioral methods for effective cancer screening and prevention. *Behavioral Medicine Update*, 5(2 & 3), 36–44.

Kellner, R. (1985). Functional somatic symptoms and hypochondriasis: a survey of empirical studies. *Archives of General Psychiatry*, 42, 821–33.

Kellner, R. (1987). Hypochondriasis and somatization. *Journal of the American Medical Association*, 258, 2718–22.

Kelly, J. A., Kalichman, S. C., Kauth, M. R., Kilgore, H. G., Hood, H. V., Campos, P. E., Rao, S. M., Brasfield, T. L., & St. Lawrence, J. S. (1991). Situational factors associated with AIDS risk behavior lapses and coping strategies used by gay men who successfully avoid lapses. *American Journal of Public Health*, 81, 1335–8.

Kelly, J. A., Sikkema, K. J., Winett, R. A., Solomon, L. J., Roffman, R. A., Heckman, T. G., Stevenson, L. Y., Perry, M. J., Norman, A. D., & Desiderato, L. J. (1995). Factors predicting continued high-risk behavior among gay men in small cities: psychological, behavioral, and demographic characteristics related to unsafe sex. *Journal of Consulting and Clinical Psychology*, 63, 101–7.

Kelly, J. A., St. Lawrence, J. S., Stevenson, Y., Hauth, A. C., Kalichman, S. C., Diaz, Y. E., Brasfield, T. L., Koob, J. J., & Morgan, M. G. (1992). Community AIDS/HIV risk reduction: the effects of endorsements by popular people in three cities. *American Journal of Public Health*, 82, 1483–9.

Kelsey, J. L., & Hochberg, M. C. (1988). Epidemiology of chronic musculoskeletal disorders. In L. Breslow, J. E. Fielding & L. B. Lave (Eds), *Annual review of public health* (Vol. 9). Palo Alto, CA: Annual Reviews.

Kempe, C. H. (1976). Child abuse and neglect. In N. B. Talbot (Ed.), *Raising children in modern America: problems and prospective solutions*. Boston, MA: Little, Brown.

Kendall, P. C., Williams, L., Pechacek, T. F., Graham, L. E., Shisslak, C., & Herzoff, N. (1979). Cognitive-behavioral and patient education interventions in cardiac catheterization procedures: The Palo Alto Medical Psychology Project. *Journal of Consulting and Clinical Psychology*, 47, 49–58.

Kendler, K. S., Maclean, C., Neale, M., Kessler, R., Heath, A., & Eaves, L. (1991). The genetic epidemiology of bulimia nervosa. *American Journal of Psychiatry*, 148, 1627–37.

Kennedy, S., Kiecolt-Glaser, J. K., & Glaser, R. (1990). Social support, stress, and the immune system. In B. R. Sarason, I. G. Sarason & G. R. Pierce (Eds), *Social support: an interactional view*. New York: John Wiley & Sons.

Kennell, J., Klaus, M., McGrath, S., Robertson, S., & Hinkley, C. (1991). Continuous emotional support during labor in a U.S. hospital. *Journal of the American Medical Association*, 265, 2197–2201.

Kenny, D., & Adams, R. (1994). The relationship between eating attitudes, body mass index, age, and gender in Australian university students. *Australian Psychologist*, 29(2), 128–34.

Kent, G. (1985). Memory of dental pain. *Pain*, 21, 187–94.

Kerlikowske, K., Grady, D., Rubin, S. M., Sandrock, C., & Ernster, V. L. (1995). Efficacy of screening mammography: a meta-analysis. *Journal of the American Medical Association*, 273, 149–54.

Kern, P. A., Ong, J. M., Saffari, B., & Carty, J. (1990). The effects of weight loss on the activity and expression on adipose-tissue lipoprotein lipase in very obese humans. *New England Journal of Medicine*, 322, 1053–9.

Kerns, R. D. (1995). Family assessment and intervention. In P. M. Nicassio & T. W. Smith (Eds), *Managing chronic illness: a biopsychosocial perspective*. Washington, DC: American Psychological Association.

Kerns, R. D., & Curley, A. D. (1985). A biopsychosocial approach to illness and the family: neurological diseases across the life span. In D. C. Turk & R. D. Kerns (Eds), *Health, illness, and families: a life-span perspective*. New York: John Wiley & Sons.

Kerns, R. D., Turk, D. C., & Rudy, T. E. (1985). The West Haven–Yale Multidimensional Pain Inventory. *Pain*, 23, 345–56.

Kerns, R. D., & Weiss, L. H. (1994). Family influences on the course of chronic illness: a cognitive-behavioral transactional model. *Annals of Behavioral Medicine*, 16, 116–21.

Kessler, R. (1999). The consequences of individual differences in preparation for surgery and invasive medical procedures. *Australian Journal of Clinical and Experimental Hypnosis*, 27(1), 40–53.

Kett, J. F. (1977). *Rites of passage: adolescence in America 1790 to present*. New York: Basic Books.

Ketterer, M. W., Brymer, J., Rhoads, K., Kraft, P., Kenyon, L., Foley, B., Lovallo, W. R., & Voight, C. J. (1996). Emotional distress among males with 'syndrome X'. *Journal of Behavioral Medicine*, 19, 455–66.

Keys, A. (1970). Coronary heart disease in seven countries. *Circulation*, 225 (Suppl. 1), 1–211.

Keys, A. (1980). *Seven countries — a multivariate analysis of death and coronary heart disease*. Cambridge, MA: Harvard University Press.

Keys, A., Brozek, J., Henschel, A., Mickelsen, O., & Taylor, H. L. (1950). *The biology of human starvation*. Minneapolis, MN: University of Minnesota Press.

Khalid, R., & Sial, S. (1998). Personality factors and the recovery rate of heart patients after coronary artery bypass surgery. *Journal of Behavioural Sciences*, 9(1–2), 37–54.

Khaw, K., & Barrett-Connor, E. (1986). Family history of heart attack: a modifiable risk factor? *Circulation*, 74, 239–44.

Kiecolt-Glaser, J. K., Dura, J. R., Speicher, C. E., Trask, O. J., & Glaser, R. (1991) Spousal caregivers of dementia victims: longitudinal changes in immunity and health. *Psychosomatic Medicine*, 53, 345–62.

Kiecolt-Glaser, J. K., Dyer, C. S., & Shuttleworth, E. (1988). Upsetting social interactions and distress among Alzheimer's disease family caregivers: a replication and extension. *American Journal of Community Psychology*, 116, 825–37.

Kiecolt-Glaser, J. K., Fisher, L. D., Ogrocki, P., Stout, J. C., Speicher, C. E., & Glaser, R. (1987). Marital quality, marital disruption, and immune function. *Psychosomatic Medicine*, 49, 13–34.

Kiecolt-Glaser, J. K., Garner, W., Speicher, C., Penn, G. M., Holliday, J., & Glaser, R. (1984). Psychosocial modifiers of immunocompetence in medical students. *Psychosomatic Medicine*, 46, 7–14.

Kiecolt-Glaser, J. K., & Glaser, R. (1986). Psychological influences on immunity. *Psychosomatics*, 27, 621–4.

Kiecolt-Glaser, J. K., & Glaser, R. (1995). Psychoneuroimmunology and health consequences: data and shared mechanisms. *Psychosomatic Medicine*, 57, 269–74.

Kiecolt-Glaser, J. K., & Williams, D. A. (1987). Self-blame, compliance, and distress among burn patients. *Journal of Personality and Social Psychology*, 53, 187–93.

Killen, J. D., & Fortmann, S. P. (1994). Role of nicotine dependence in smoking relapse: results from a prospective study using population-based recruitment methodology. *International Journal of Behavioral Medicine*, 1, 320–34.

Killen, J. D., Taylor, C. B., Hayward, C., Wilson, D. M., et al. (1994). Pursuit of thinness and onset of eating disorder symptoms in a community sample of adolescent girls: a three-year prospective analysis. *International Journal of Eating Disorders*, 16, 227–38.

Killen, J. D., Taylor, C. B., Telch, M. J., Saylor, K. E., Maron, D. J., & Robinson, T. N. (1986). Self-induced vomiting and laxative and diuretic use among teenagers. *Journal of the American Medical Society*, 255, 1447–9.

Kilo, C., & Williamson, J. R. (1987). *Diabetes: the facts that let you regain control of your life*. New York: John Wiley & Sons.

Kippax, S., & Crawford, J. (1993). Flaws in the theory of reasoned action. In D. Terry, C. Gallois & M. McCamish (Eds), *The theory of reasoned action: its application to AIDS-preventive behaviour*. Oxford, NY: Pergamon.

Kirkby, R. J. (1995). Sport psychology in Australia: past myths and future directions. Special issue: Sport and exercise psychology. *Australian Psychologist*, 30(2), 75–7.

Kirkby, R. J. & Whelan, T. A. (1996). The effects of hospitalisation and medical procedures on children and their families. *Journal of Family Studies*, 2(1), 65–77.

Kirschbaum, D., Wüst, S., & Hellhammer, D. (1992). Consistent sex differences in cortisol responses to psychological stress. *Psychosomatic Medicine*, 54, 648–57.

Kirscht, J. P. (1983). Preventive health behavior: a review of research and issues. *Health Psychology*, 2, 277–301.

Kirscht, J. P., & Rosenstock, I. M. (1979). Patients' problems in following recommendations of health experts. In G. C. Stone, F. Cohen & N. E. Adler (Eds), *Health psychology — a handbook*. San Francisco: Jossey-Bass.

Kiser, L. J., Ostoja, E., & Pruitt, D. B. (1998). Dealing with stress and trauma in families. *Child and Adolescent Psychiatric Clinics of North America*, 7(1), 87–103.

Kivlahan, D. R., Marlatt, G. A., Fromme, K., Coppel, D. B., & Williams, E. (1990). Secondary prevention with college drinkers: evaluation of an alcohol skills training program. *Journal of Consulting and Clinical Psychology*, 58, 805–810.

Klag, M. J., Whelton, P. K., Coresh, J., Grim, C. E., & Kuller, L. H. (1991). The association of skin color with blood pressure in US blacks with low socioeconomic status. *Journal of the American Medical Association*, 265, 599–602.

Klapow, J. C., Slater, M. A., Patterson, T. L., Doctor, J. N., Atkinson, J. H., & Garfin, S. R. (1993). An empirical evaluation of multidimensional clinical outcome in chronic low back pain patients. *Pain*, 55, 107–118.

Kleinke, C. L., & Spangler, A. S. (1988). Psychometric analysis of the audiovisual taxonomy for assessing pain behavior in chronic back-pain patients. *Journal of Behavioral Medicine*, 11, 83–94.

Klepp, K.-I., Kelder, S. H., & Perry, C. L. (1995). Alcohol and marijuana use among adolescents: long-term outcomes of the Class of 1989 Study. *Annals of Behavioral Medicine*, 17, 19–24.

Klesges, R. C., Benowitz, N. L., & Meyers, A. W. (1991). Behavioral and biobehavioral aspects of smoking and smoking cessation: the problem of postcessation weight gain. *Behavior Therapy*, 22, 179–99.

Klesges, R. C., Eck, L. H., & Ray, J. W. (1995). Who underreports dietary intake in a dietary recall? Evidence from the Second National Health and Nutrition Examination Survey. *Journal of Consulting and Clinical Psychology*, 63, 438–44.

Klesges, R. C., Shuster, M. L., Klesges, L. M., & Werner, K. (1992, March). The effects of television viewing on metabolic rate in normal weight and obese children. Paper presented at the meeting of the Society of Behavioral Medicine, New York.

Klockenbrink, M. (1987, September 27). How to read a label. *New York Times Magazine*, pp. 67–72.

Klohn, L. S., & Rogers, R. W. (1991). Dimensions of the severity of a health threat: the persuasive effects of visibility, time of onset, and rate of onset on young women's intentions to prevent osteoporosis. *Health Psychology*, 10, 323–9.

Klose, K. J., Needham, B. M., Schmidt, D., Broton, J. G., & Green, B. A. (1993). An assessment of the contribution of electromyographic biofeedback as an adjunct therapy in the physical training of spinal cord injured persons. *Archives of Physical Medicine and Rehabilitation*, 74, 453–6.

Knapp, R. J. (1987, July). When a child dies. *Psychology Today*, pp. 60–67.

Kneebone, I. I. (1996). Teaching about ageing: the new challenge for Australian clinical psychology. *Australian Psychologist*, 31(2), 124–6.

Kneut, C. M. (1982). Legal, ethical, and moral considerations in pediatric nursing. In M. J. Smith, J. A. Goodman, N. L. Ramsey & S. B. Pasternack (Eds), *Child and family: concepts of nursing practice*. New York: McGraw-Hill.

Knittle, J., Merritt, R. J., Dixon-Shanies, D., Ginsberg-Fellner, F., Timmers, K. I., & Katz, D. P. (1981). Childhood obesity. In R. M. Suskind (Ed.), *Textbook of pediatric nutrition*. New York: Raven Press.

Knox, S. S. (1992). Psychophysiological mechanisms in the etiology and treatment of essential hypertension. In D. G. Byrne & G. R. Caddy, *Behavioural medicine: international perspectives* (Vol. 1). Norwood, MN: Ablex.

Kobasa, S. C. (1979). Stressful life events, personality, and health: an inquiry into hardiness. *Journal of Personality and Social Psychology*, 37, 1–11.

Kobasa, S. C., & Maddi, S. R. (1977). Existential personality theory. In R. Corsini (Ed.), *Current personality theories*. Itasca, IL: Peacock.

Kobasa, S. C., Maddi, S. R., & Puccetti, M. C. (1982). Personality and exercise as buffers in the stress–illness relationship. *Journal of Behavioral Medicine*, 5, 391–404.

Kobasa, S. C. O. (1986). How much stress can you survive? In M. G. Walraven & H. E. Fitzgerald (Eds), *Annual editions: human development 86/87*. Guilford, CT: Dushkin.

Kobasa, S. C. O., Maddi, S. R., Puccetti, M. C., & Zola, M. A. (1985). Effectiveness of hardiness, exercise and social support as resources against illness. *Journal of Psychosomatic Research*, 29, 525–33.

Koch, J. (1977, August). When children meet death. *Psychology Today*, pp. 64–66, 79–80.

Kofoed, L., Friedman, M. J., & Peck, R. (1993). Alcoholism and drug abuse in patients with PTSD. *Psychiatric Quarterly*, 64(2), 151–71.

Kohn, P. M., & Macdonald, J. E. (1992). The survey of recent life experiences: a decontaminated hassles scale for adults. *Journal of Behavioural Medicine*, 15, 221–36.

Kohn, P. M., & Milrose, J. A. (1993). The inventory of high-school students' recent life experiences: a decontaminated measure of adolescent hassles. *Journal of Youth and Adolescence*, 22, 43–55.

Kohn, P. M., Lafreniere, K., & Gurevich, M. (1990). The inventory of college students' recent life experiences: a decontaminated hassles scale for a special population. *Journal of Behavioural Medicine*, 13, 619–30.

Kohrt, W. M., Kirwan, J. P., Staten, M. A., Bourey, R. E., King, D. S., & Holloszy, J. O. (1993). Insulin resistance in aging is related to abdominal obesity. *Diabetes*, 42, 273–81.

Kokkinos, P. F., Narayan, P., Colleran, J. A., Pittaras, A., Notargiacomo, A., Reda, D., & Papademetriou, V. (1995). Effects of regular exercise on blood pressure and left ventricular hypertrophy in African-American men with severe hypertension. *New England Journal of Medicine*, 333, 1462–7.

Kolata, G. (1990, February 20). Wariness is replacing trust between health and patient. *New York Times*, pp. A1, D15.

Kolata, G. (1992a, September 3). A cancer legacy from Chernobyl. *New York Times*, p. A9.

Kolata, G. (1992b, May 10). Confronting new ideas, doctors often hold on to the old. *New York Times*, p. E6.

Kolata, G. (1996, February 27). New era of robust elderly belies the fears of scientists. *New York Times*, pp. A1, C3.

Kolbe, L. J., Green, L. Foreyt, J., Darnell, L., et al. (1986). Appropriate functions of health education in schools: improving health and cognitive performance. In N. A. Krasnegor, J. D. Arasteh & M. F. Cataldo (Eds), *Child health behavior: a behavioral pediatrics perspective*. New York: John Wiley & Sons.

Koocher, G. P., O'Malley, J. E., Gogan, J. L., & Foster, D. J. (1980). Psychological adjustment among pediatric cancer survivors. *Journal of Child Psychology and Psychiatry*, 21, 163–73.

Kopp, C. B. (1983). Risk factors in development. In P. H. Mussen (Ed.), *Handbook of child psychology* (4th ed., Vol. 2). New York: John Wiley & Sons.

Korotkov, D. L. (1998). The sense of coherence: making sense out of chaos. In P. T. P. Wong & P. S. Fry (Eds), *The human quest for meaning: a handbook of psychological research and clinical applications* (pp. 51–70). Mahwah, NJ: Erlbaum.

Kors, D., & Linden, W. (1995, March). The impact of 'non-evaluative' and 'evaluative' friends on cardiovascular stress reactivity. Paper presented at the meeting of the Society of Behavioral Medicine, San Diego.

Korsch, B. M., Fine, R. N., & Negrete, V. F. (1978). Noncompliance in children with renal transplants. *Pediatrics*, 61, 872–6.

Korsch, B. M., Gozzi, E. K., & Francis, V. (1968). Gaps in doctor–patient communication: I. Doctor–patient interaction and patient satisfaction. *Pediatrics*, 42, 855–71.

Kosten, T. R., Jacobs, S. C., & Kasl, S. V. (1985). Terminal illness, bereavement, and the family. In D. C. Turk & R. D. Kerns (Eds), *Health, illness, and families: a life-span perspective*. New York: John Wiley & Sons.

Koutsosimou, M., McDonald, A.S., & Davey, G. C. (1996). Coping and psychopathology in surgery patients: a comparison of accident patients with other surgery patients. *British Journal of Health Psychology*, 1, 357–64.

Kozlowski, L. T. (1984). Pharmacological approaches to smoking modification. In J. D. Matarazzo, S. M. Weiss, J. A. Herd, N. E. Miller & S. M. Weiss (Eds), *Behavioral health: a handbook of health enhancement and disease prevention*. New York: John Wiley & Sons.

Krajick, K. (1988, May). Private passions and public health. *Psychology Today*, pp. 50–58.

Krantz, D. C., Lundberg, U., & Frankenhaeuser, M. (1987). Stress and Type A behavior: interactions between environmental and biological factors. In A. Baum & J. E. Singer (Eds), *Handbook of psychology and health* (Vol. 5). Hillsdale, NJ: Erlbaum.

Krantz, D. S., Baum, A., & Wideman, M. V. (1980). Assessment for preferences for self-treatment and information in health care. *Journal of Personality and Social Psychology*, 39, 977–90.

Krantz, D. S., & Deckel, A. W. (1983). Coping with coronary heart disease and stroke. In T. G. Burish & L. A. Bradley (Eds), *Coping with chronic disease: research and applications*. New York: Academic Press.

Krantz, D. S., & Durel, L. A. (1983). Psychobiological substrates of the Type A behavior pattern. *Health Psychology*, 2, 393–411.

Krantz, D. S., Durel, L. A., Davia, J. E., Shaffer, R. T., Arabian, J. M., Dembroski, T. M., & Macdougall, J. M. (1982). Propranolol medication among coronary patients: relationship to Type A behavior and cardiovascular response. *Journal of Human Stress*, 8, 4–12.

Kranzler, H. R., & Anton, R. F. (1994). Implications of recent neuropsychopharmacologic research for understanding the etiology and development of alcoholism. *Journal of Consulting and Clinical Psychology*, 62, 1116–26.

Krause, J. S., & Crewe, N. M. (1991). Chronologic age, time since injury, and time of measurement: effect on adjustment after spinal cord injury. *Archives of Physical Medicine and Rehabilitation*, 72, 91–100.

Kreuter, M. W., & Strecher, V. J. (1995). Changing inaccurate perceptions of health risk: results from a randomized trial. *Health Psychology*, 14, 56–63.

Krieg, A. M., Yi, A.-K., Matson, S., Waldschmidt, T. J., Bishop, G. A., Teasdale, R., Koretzky, G. A., & Klinman, D. M. (1995). CpG motifs in bacterial DNA trigger direct B-cell activation. *Nature*, 374, 546–9.

Kristensen, T. S. (1996). Job stress and cardiovascular disease: a theoretic critical review. *Journal of Occupational Health Psychology*, 1(3), 246–60.

Krohne, H. W., de Bruin, J. T., El-Giamal, M., & Schmukle, S. C. (2000). The assessment of surgery-related coping: the Coping with Surgical Stress Scale. *Psychology and Health*, 15(1), 135–49.

Krumholz, H. M., Seeman, T. E., Merrill, S. S., Mendes de Leon, C. F., Vaccarino, V., Silverman, D. I., Tsukahara, R., Ostfeld, A. M., & Berkman, L. F. (1994). Lack of association between cholesterol and coronary heart disease mortality and morbidity and all-cause mortality in persons older than 70 years. *Journal of the American Medical Association*, 272, 1335–40.

Krupat, E., Rosenkranz, S. L., Yeager, C. M., Barnard, K., Putnam, S. M., & Inui, T. S. (2000). The practice orientations of physicians and patients: the effect of doctor–patient congruence on satisfaction. *Patient Education and Counseling*, 39(1), 49–59.

Ku, L., Sonenstein, F. L., & Pleck, J. H. (1993). Young men's risk behaviors for HIV infection and sexually transmitted diseases, 1988 through 1991. *American Journal of Public Health*, 83, 1609–1615.

Kübler-Ross, E. (1969). *On death and dying*. New York: Macmillan.

Kulik, J. A., & Carlino, P. (1987). The effect of verbal commitment and treatment choice on medication compliance in a pediatric setting. *Journal of Behavioral Medicine*, 10, 367–76.

Kulik, J. A., & Mahler, H. I. M. (1987a). Effects of preoperative roommate assignment on preoperative anxiety and recovery from coronary-bypass surgery. *Health Psychology*, 6, 525–43.

Kulik, J. A., & Mahler, H. I. M. (1987b). Health status, perceptions of risk, and prevention interest for health and nonhealth problems. *Health Psychology*, 6, 15–27.

Kulik, J. A., & Mahler, H. I. M. (1989). Social support and recovery from surgery. *Health Psychology*, 8, 221–38.

Kulik, J. A., Moore, P. J., & Mahler, H. I. M. (1993). Stress and affiliation: hospital roommate effects on preoperative anxiety and social interaction. *Health Psychology*, 12, 118–24.

Kunda, Z. (1990). The case for motivated reasoning. *Psychological Bulletin*, 108, 480–98.

Kusaka, Y., Kondou, H., & Morimoto, K. (1992). Healthy lifestyles are associated with higher natural killer cell activity. *Preventive Medicine*, 21, 602–615.

Kvale, G., Psychol, C., & Hugdahl, K. (1994). Cardiovascular conditioning and anticipatory nausea and vomiting in cancer patients. *Behavioral Medicine*, 20, 78–83.

Labarba, R. C. (1984). Prenatal and neonatal influences on behavioral health development. In J. D. Matarazzo, S. M. Weiss, J. A. Herd, N. E. Miller & S. M. Weiss (Eds), *Behavioral health: a handbook of health enhancement and disease prevention*. New York: John Wiley & Sons.

Lacey, J. H., & Birtchnell, S. A. (1986). Abnormal eating behavior. In M. J. Christie & P. G. Mellett (Eds), *The psychosomatic approach: contemporary practice of wholeperson care*. New York: John Wiley & Sons.

Lachman, M. E. (1986). Personal control in later life: stability, change, and cognitive correlates. In M. M. Baltes & P. B. Baltes (Eds), *The psychology of control and aging*. Hillsdale, NJ: Erlbaum.

Lacroix, A. Z., Lang, J., Scherr, P., Wallace, R. B., Cornoni-Huntley, J., Berkman, L., Curb, D., Evans, D., & Hennekens, C. H. (1991). Smoking and mortality among older men and women in three communities. *New England Journal of Medicine*, 324, 1619–25.

Laffrey, S. C. (1986). Normal and overweight adults: perceived weight and health behavior characteristics. *Nursing Research*, 35, 173–7.

Laforge, R. G., Willey, C., Prochaska, J. O., & Levesque, D. A. (1995, March). Naturalistic evidence for a synergistic effect of nicotine patch with a stage matched smoking cessation intervention. Paper presented at the meeting of the Society of Behavioral Medicine, San Diego.

La Gaipa, J. J. (1990). The negative effects of informal support systems. In S. Duck with R. C. Silver (Eds), *Personal relationships and social support* (pp. 122–39). London: Sage.

LA Greca, A. M., & Stone, W. L. (1985). Behavioral pediatrics. In N. Schneiderman & J. T. Tapp (Eds), *Behavioral medicine: the biopsychosocial approach*. Hillsdale, NJ: Erlbaum.

Lairson, D. R., Hindson, P., & Hauquitz, A. (1995). Equity of health care in Australia. *Social Science and Medicine*, 41(4), 475–82.

Lakein, A. (1973). *How to get control of your time and life*. New York: New American Library.

Lakey, B., & Heller, K. (1988). Social support from a friend, perceived support and social problem-solving. *American Journal of Community Psychology*, 16, 811–24.

Lakey, B., & Lutz, C. J. (1996). Social support and preventive and therapeutic interventions. In G. R. Pierce, B. R. Sarason & I. G. Sarason (Eds), *Handbook of social support and the family* (pp. 435–65). New York: Plenum.

Landers, A. (1992, August 9). Was it airline food that cut short a passenger's trip of a lifetime? *Philadelphia Inquirer*, p. L3.

Lando, H. A. (1993). Formal quit smoking treatments. In C. T. Orleans & J. Slade (Eds), *Nicotine addiction: principles and management*. New York: Oxford University Press.

Lando, H. A., & McGovern, P. G. (1985). Nicotine fading as a non-aversive alternative in a broad spectrum treatment for eliminating smoking. *Addictive Behavior*, 10, 153–61.

Landrine, H., & Klonoff, E. A. (1992). Culture and health-related schemas: a review and proposal for interdisciplinary integration. *Health Psychology*, 11, 267–76.

Lane, M. A., Baer, D. J., Rumpler, W. V., Weindruch, R., Ingram, D. K., Tilmont, E. M., Cutler, R. G., & Roth, G. S. (1996). Calorie restriction lowers body temperature in rhesus monkeys, consistent with a postulated anti-aging mechanism in rodents. *Proceedings of the National Academy of Sciences*, 93, 4159–64.

Lang, A. R., & Marlatt, G. A. (1982). Problem drinking: a social learning perspective. In R. J. Gatchel, A. Baum & J. E. Singer (Eds), *Handbook of psychology and health* (Vol. 1). Hillsdale, NJ: Erlbaum.

Langer, E. J. (1975). The illusion of control. *Journal of Personality and Social Psychology*, 32, 311–28.

Langer, E. J., Janis, I. L., & Wolfer, J. A. (1975). Reduction of psychological stress in surgical patients. *Journal of Experimental Social Psychology*, 11, 155–65.

Langer, E. J., & Rodin, J. (1976). The effects of choice and enhanced personal responsibility for the aged: a field experiment in an institutional setting. *Journal of Personality and Social Psychology*, 34, 191–8.

Langlie, J. K. (1977). Social networks, health beliefs, and preventive health behavior. *Journal of Health and Social Behavior*, 18, 244–60.

Langosch, W. (1984). Behavioural interventions in cardiac rehabilitation. In A. Steptoe & A. Mathews (Eds), *Health care and human behaviour*. London: Academic Press.

La Place, J. (1984). *Health* (4th ed.). Englewood Cliffs, NJ: Prentice Hall.

Larkin, K. T., Knowlton, G. E., & D'alessandri, R. (1990). Predicting treatment outcome to progressive relaxation training in essential hypertensive patients. *Journal of Behavioral Medicine*, 13, 605–618.

Larocco, J. M., House, J. S., & French, J. R. P. (1980). Social support, occupational stress, and health. *Journal of Health and Social Behavior*, 21, 202–218.

Larson, E. B., Kukull, W. A., & Katzman, R. L. (1992). Cognitive impairment: dementia and Alzheimer's disease. In G. S. Ommen, J. E. Fielding & L. B. Lave (Eds), *Annual review of public health* (Vol. 13). Palo Alto, CA: Annual Reviews.

Lasater, T., Abrams, D., Artz, L., Beaudin, P., et al. (1984). Lay volunteer delivery of a community-based cardiovascular risk factor change program: the Pawtucket experiment. In J. D. Matarazzo, S. M. Weiss, J. A. Herd, N. E. Miller & S. M. Weiss (Eds), *Behavioral health: a handbook of health enhancement and disease prevention*. New York: John Wiley & Sons.

Laszlo, J. (1987). *Understanding cancer*. New York: Harper & Row.

Lau, R. R., & Hartman, K. A. (1983). Common sense representations of common illnesses. *Health Psychology*, 2, 167–85.

Lau, R. R., Hartman, K. A., & Ware, J. E. (1986). Health as a value: methodological and theoretical considerations. *Health Psychology*, 5, 25–43.

Lau, R., Kane, R., Berry, S., Ware, J., & Roy, D. (1980). Channeling health: a review of the evaluation of televised health campaigns. *Health Education Quarterly*, 7, 56–89.

Lave, J. R. (1989). The effect of the Medicare prospective payment system. In L. Breslow, J. E. Fielding & L. B. Lave (Eds), *Annual review of public health* (Vol. 10). Palo Alto, CA: Annual Reviews.

Lavey, E. B., & Winkle, R. A. (1979). Continuing disability of patients with chest pain and normal coronary arteriograms. *Journal of Chronic Diseases*, 32, 191–6.

Lavigne, J. V., Schulein, M. J., & Hahn, Y. S. (1986a). Psychological aspects of painful medical conditions in children. I. Developmental aspects and assessment. *Pain*, 27, 133–46.

Lavigne, J. V., Schulein, M. J., & Hahn, Y. S. (1986b). Psychological aspects of painful medical conditions in children. II. Personality factors, family characteristics and treatment. *Pain*, 27, 147–69.

Law, M. R., Frost, C. D., & Wald, N. J. (1991). Analysis of data from trials of salt reduction. *British Medical Journal*, 302, 819–24.

Lawler, K. A., Allen, M. T., Critcher, E. C., & Standard, B. A. (1981). The relationship of physiological responses to the coronary-prone behavior pattern in children. *Journal of Behavioral Medicine*, 4, 203–216.

Lazarus, A. A. (1971). *Behavior therapy and beyond*. New York: McGraw-Hill.

Lazarus, R. S. (1983). The costs and benefits of denial. In S. Bresnitz (Ed.), *Denial of stress*. New York: International Universities Press.

Lazarus, R. S. (1987). Coping. In R. J. Corsini (Ed.), *Concise encyclopedia of psychology*. New York: John Wiley & Sons.

Lazarus, R. S., & DeLongis, A. (1983). Psychological stress and coping in aging. *American Psychologist*, 38, 245–54.

Lazarus, R. S., & Folkman, S. (1984a). Coping and adaptation. In W. D. Gentry (Ed.), *Handbook of behavioral medicine*. New York: Guilford.

Lazarus, R. S., & Folkman, S. (1984b). *Stress, appraisal, and coping*. New York: Springer.

Lazarus, R. S., & Launier, R. (1978). Stress-related transactions between person and environment. In L. A. Pervin & M. Lewis (Eds), *Perspectives in interactional psychology*. New York: Plenum.

Leach, J. (1994). *Survival psychology*. London: Macmillan.

Leahey, T. H. (1987). *A history of psychology: main currents in psychological thought* (2nd ed.). Englewood Cliffs, NJ: Prentice Hall.

Leary, W. E. (1992, March 6). U.S. urges doctors to fight surgical pain (and myths). *New York Times*, pp. A1, 17.

Leary, W. E. (1995, September 20). Report endorses needle exchanges as AIDS strategy. *New York Times*, pp. A1, B10.

Leboyer, F. (1977). *Birth without violence*. London: Fontana/Collins.

Lee, C. (1989). Perceptions of immunity to disease in adult smokers. *Journal of Behavioral Medicine*, 12(3), 267–77.

Lee, C. (1991). Women and aerobic exercise: directions for research development. *Annals of Behavioral Medicine*, 13(3), 133–40.

Lee, C. (1994). Health care, psychology and a healthy society: a comment on James (1994). *Australian Psychologist*, 29(1), 15–17.

Lee, G.-H., Proenca, R., Montez, J. M., Carroll, K. M., Darvishzadeh, J. G., Lee, J. I., & Friedman, J. M. (1996). Abnormal splicing of the leptin receptor in diabetic mice. *Nature*, 379, 632–5.

Lee, I.-M., Hsieh, C., & Paffenbarger, R. S. (1995). Exercise intensity and longevity in men: the Harvard Alumni Health Study. *Journal of the American Medical Association*, 273, 1179–84.

Lee, W.-H., Morton, R. A., Epstein, J. I., Brooks, J. D., Campbell, P. A., Bova, G. S., Hsieh, W.-S., Isaacs, W. B., & Nelson, W. G. (1994). Cytidine methylation of regulatory sequences near the ≤-class glutathione S-transferase gene accompanies human prostatic carcinogenesis. *Proceedings of the National Academy of Sciences USA*, 91, 11733–7.

Legrady, D., Dyer, A. R., Shekelle, R. B., Stamler, J., Liu, K., Paul, O., Lepper, M., & Shryock, A. M. (1987). Coffee consumption and mortality in the Chicago Western Electric Company Study. *American Journal of Epidemiology*, 126, 803–812.

Leibel, R. L., Rosenblum, M., & Hirsch, J. (1995). Changes in energy expenditure resulting from altered body weight. *New England Journal of Medicine*, 332, 621–8.

Leigh, B. C. (1990). The relationship of substance use during sex to high-risk sexual behavior. *Journal of Sex Research*, 27, 199–213.

Leigh, B. C., Morrison, D. M., Trocki, K., & Temple, M. T. (1994). Sexual behavior of American adolescents: results from a U.S. national survey. *Journal of Adolescent Health*, 15, 117–25.

Leino, P., Aro, S., & Hasan, J. (1987). Trunk muscle function and low back disorders: a ten-year follow-up study. *Journal of Chronic Diseases*, 40, 289–96.

Lekander, M., Fürst, C. J., Rotstein, S., Blomgren, H., & Fredrikson, M. (1995). Anticipatory immune changes in women treated with chemotherapy for ovarian cancer. *International Journal of Behavioral Medicine*, 2, 1–12.

Leland, J. (1996, December 2). The end of AIDS? *Newsweek*, pp. 64–73.

Lenneberg, E. H. (1967). *Biological foundations of language*. New York: John Wiley & Sons.

Lennon, M. C. (1999). Work and unemployment as stressors. In A. V. Horwitz & T. L. Scheid (Eds), *A handbook for the study of mental health: social contexts, theories and systems* (pp. 284–94). New York: Cambridge University Press.

Leonard, B. E. (1995). Stress and the immune system: immunological aspects of depressive illness. In B. E. Miller & K. Miller (Eds), *Stress, the immune system and psychiatry*. New York: John Wiley & Sons.

Leonard, E. A. (1990, April 9). How the brain recovers. *Newsweek*, pp. 48–50.

Leonard, R., & Alison, L. (1999). Critical incident stress debriefing and its effects on coping strategies and anger in a sample of Australian police officers involved in shooting incidents. *Work and Stress*, 13(2), 144–61.

Leonova, A. B. (1996). Occupational stress, personnel adaptation and health. In C. D. Spielberger & I. G. Sarason (Eds), *Stress and emotion: anxiety, anger and curiosity* (Vol. 16, pp. 109–125). Washington, DC: Taylor & Francis.

Lepore, S. J. (1995). Cynicism, social support, and cardiovascular reactivity. *Health Psychology*, 14, 210–216.

Lepore, S. J., Allen, K. A. M., & Evans, G. W. (1993). Social support lowers cardiovascular reactivity to an acute stressor. *Psychosomatic Medicine*, 55, 518–24.

Lerman, C., Audrain, J., & Croyle, R. T. (1994). DNA-testing for heritable breast cancer risks: lessons from traditional genetic counseling. *Annals of Behavioral Medicine*, 16, 327–33.

Lerman, C., Schwartz, M. D., Miller, S. M., Daly, M., Sands, C., & Rimer, B. (1996). A randomized trial of breast cancer risk counseling: interacting effects of counseling, educational level, and coping style. *Health Psychology*, 15, 75–83.

Lerman, C., Trock, B., Rimer, B. K., Boyce, A., Jepson, C., & Engstrom, P. F. (1991). Psychological and behavioral implications of abnormal mammograms. *Annals of Internal Medicine*, 114, 657–61.

Lester, N., Lefebvre, J. C., & Keefe, F. J. (1994). Pain in young adults: I. Relationship to gender and family history. *Clinical Journal of Pain*, 10, 282–9.

Levenson, R. W. (1986). Alcohol, reactivity, and the heart: implications for coronary health and disease. In K. A. Matthews, S. M. Weiss, T. Detre, T. M. Dembroski, B. Falkner, S. B. Manuck & R. B. Williams (Eds), *Handbook of stress, reactivity, and cardiovascular disease*. New York: John Wiley & Sons.

Leventhal, H., & Cleary, P. D. (1980). The smoking problem: a review of research and theory in behavioral risk modification. *Psychological Bulletin*, 88, 370–405.

Leventhal, E. A., Hansell, S., Diefenbach, M., Leventhal, H., & Glass, D. C. (1996). Negative affect and self-report of physical symptoms: two longitudinal studies of older adults. *Health Psychology*, 15, 193–9.

Leventhal, H., Leventhal, E. A., & Contrada, R. J. (1997). Self regulation, health, and behavior: a perceptual-cognitive approach. *Psychology & Health*, 13, 717–33.

Leventhal, H., Leventhal, E. A., & Van Nguyen, T. (1985). Reactions of families to illness: theoretical models and perspectives. In D. C. Turk & R. D. Kerns (Eds), *Health, illness, and families: a life-span perspective*. New York: John Wiley & Sons.

Leventhal, E. A., & Prohaska, T. R. (1986). Age, symptom interpretation, and health behavior. *Journal of the American Geriatrics Society*, 34, 185–91.

Leventhal, H., Prohaska, T. R., & Hirschman, R. S. (1985). Preventive health behavior across the life span. In J. C. Rosen & L. J. Solomon (Eds), *Prevention in health psychology*. Hanover, NH: University Press of New England.

Levey, J., McDermott, S., & Lee, C. (1989). Current issues in bulimia nervosa, *Australian Psychologist*, 24(2), 171–85.

Levin, D. N., Cleeland, C. S., & Dar, R. (1985). Public attitudes toward cancer pain. *Cancer*, 56, 2337–9.

Levine, J. D., Gordon, N. C., & Fields, H. L. (1978, September 23). The mechanism of placebo analgesia. *The Lancet*, 654–7.

Levine, M. A., Grossman, R. S., Darden, P. M., Jackson, S. M., et al. (1992). Dietary counseling of hypercholesterolemic patients by internal medicine residents. *Journal of General Internal Medicine*, 7, 511–16.

Levinson, W., Stiles, W. B., Inui, T. S., & Engle, R. (1993). Physician frustration in communicating with patients. *Medical Care*, 31, 285–95.

Levy, S. M. (1983). The process of death and dying: behavioral and social factors. In T. G. Burish & L. A. Bradley (Eds), *Coping with chronic disease: research and applications*. New York: Academic Press.

Levy, S. M. (1985). *Behavior and cancer*. San Francisco: Jossey-Bass.

Levy, S. M., & Heiden, L. (1991). Depression, distress, and immunity: risk factors for infectious disease. *Stress Medicine*, 7, 45–51.

Levy, S. M., Herberman, R. B., Maluish, A. M., Schlien, B., & Lippman, M. (1985). Prognostic risk assessment in primary breast cancer by behavioral and immunological parameters. *Health Psychology*, 4, 99–113.

Levy, S. M., Herberman, R. B., Whiteside, T., Sanzo, K., Lee, J., & Kirkwood, J. (1990). Perceived social support and tumor estrogen/progesterone receptor status as predictors of natural killer cell activity in breast cancer patients. *Psychosomatic Medicine*, 52, 73–85.

Levy-Lahad, E., Wasco, W., Poorkaj, P., Romano, D. M., et al. (1995). Candidate gene for the chromosome 1 familial Alzheimer's disease locus. *Science*, 269, 973–7.

Lewin, K. (1935). *A dynamic theory of personality*. New York: McGraw-Hill.

Ley, P. (1982). Satisfaction, compliance, and communication. *British Journal of Clinical Psychology*, 21, 241–54.

Ley, P. (1988). *Communicating with patients: improving communication, satisfaction and compliance*. London: Croom Helm.

Ley, P. (1989). Improving patients' understanding, recall, satisfaction and compliance. In A. K. Broome (Ed.), *Health psychology: processes and applications*, London: Chapman & Hall.

Lichstein, K. L. (1988). *Clinical relaxation strategies*. New York: John Wiley & Sons.

Lichtenstein, E., & Mermelstein, R. J. (1984). Review of approaches to smoking treatment: behavior modification strategies. In J. D. Matarazzo, S. M. Weiss, J. A. Herd, N. E. Miller & S. M. Weiss (Eds), *Behavioral health: a handbook of health enhancement and disease prevention*. New York: John Wiley & Sons.

Lichtenstein, E., Weiss, S. M., Hitchcock, J. L., Leveton, L. B., O'Connell, K. A., & Prochaska, J. O. (1986). Task Force 3: patterns of smoking relapse. *Health Psychology*, 5 (Suppl.), 29–40.

Lichtman, S. W., Pisarska, K., Berman, E. R., Pestone, M., Dowling, H., Offenbacher, E., Weisel, H., Heshka, S., Matthews, D. E., & Heymsfield, S. B. (1992). Discrepancy between self-reported and actual caloric intake and exercise in obese subjects. *New England Journal of Medicine*, 327, 1893–8.

Liebman, R., Minuchin, S., & Baker, L. (1974). The use of structural family therapy in the treatment of intractable asthma. *American Journal of Psychiatry*, 121, 535–40.

Lin, E. H., & Peterson, C. (1990). Pessimistic explanatory style and response to illness. *Behavior Research and Therapy*, 28, 243–8.

Lindeman, B. (1976). Widower, heal thyself. In R. H. Moos (Ed.), *Human adaptation: coping with life crises*. Lexington, MA: Heath.

Linden, W., & Chambers, L. (1994). Clinical effectiveness of non-drug treatment for hypertension: a meta-analysis. *Annals of Behavioral Medicine*, 16, 35–45.

Lindenberg, C. S., Alexander, E. M., Gendrop, S. C., Nencioli, M., & Williams, D. G. (1991). A review of the literature on cocaine abuse in pregnancy. *Nursing Research*, 40, 69–75.

Linton, S. J., Althoff, B., Melin, L., Lundin, A., Bodin, L., Mägi, A., Lindström, K., & Lihagen, T. (1994). Psychological factors related to health, back pain, and dysfunction. *Journal of Occupational Rehabilitation*, 4, 1–10.

Linton, S. J., & Buer, N. (1995). Working despite pain: factors associated with work attendance versus dysfunction. *International Journal of Behavioral Medicine*, 2, 252–62.

Lipkus, I. M., Barefoot, J. C., Williams, R. B., & Siegler, I. C. (1994). Personality measures as predictors of smoking initiation and cessation in the UNC Alumni Heart Study. *Health Psychology*, 13, 149–55.

Lipowski, Z. J. (1986). What does the word 'psychosomatic' really mean? a historical and semantic inquiry. In M. J. Christie & P. G. Mellett (Eds), *The psychosomatic approach: contemporary practice and wholeperson care*. New York: John Wiley & Sons.

Lipton, R. B., Silberstein, S. D., & Stewart, W. F. (1994). An update on the epidemiology of migraine. *Headache*, 34, 319–28.

Litt, M. D., Nye, C., & Shafer, D. (1995). Preparation for oral surgery: evaluating elements of coping. *Journal of Behavioral Medicine*, 18, 435–59.

Livermore, B. (1991, December). What reflexology can do for you. *Self*, p. 50.

Logue, A. W. (1991). *The psychology of eating and drinking: an introduction* (2nd ed.). New York: Freeman.

Lollis, C. M., Johnson, E. H., Antoni, M. H., & Hinkle, Y. (1996). Characteristics of African-Americans with multiple risk factors associated with HIV/AIDS. *Journal of Behavioral Medicine*, 19, 55–71.

Lombardo, T., & Carreno, L. (1987). Relationship of Type A behavior pattern in smokers to carbon monoxide exposure and smoking topography. *Health Psychology*, 6, 445–52.

Lonetto, R. (1980). *Children's conceptions of death*. New York: Springer.

Long, R. T., Lamont, J. H., Whipple, B., Bandler, L., Blom, G. E., Burgin, L., & Jessner, L. (1958). A psychosomatic study of allergic and emotional factors in children with asthma. *American Journal of Psychiatry*, 114, 890–99.

Lorber, J. (1975). Good patients and problem patients: conformity and deviance in a general hospital. *Journal of Health and Social Behavior*, 16, 213–25.

Lorenz, R., Christensen, N., & Pichert, J. (1985). Diet related knowledge, skill and adherence among children with IDDM. *Pediatrics*, 75, 872–6.

Lorish, C. D., Richards, B., & Brown, S. (1989). Missed medication doses in rheumatic arthritis patients: intentional and unintentional reasons. *Arthritis Care and Research*, 2, 3–9.

Lovallo, W. R. (1997). *Stress and health: biological and psychological interactions*. Thousand Oaks, CA: Sage.

Lovallo, W. R., Al'absi, M., Pincomb, G. A., Everson, S. A., Sung, B. H., Passey, R. B., & Wilson, M. F. (1996). Caffeine and behavioral stress effects on blood pressure in borderline hypertensive Caucasian men. *Health Psychology*, 15, 11–17.

Lovallo, W. R., Pincomb, G. A., Sung, B. H., Everson, S. A., Passey, R. B., & Wilson, M. F. (1991). Hypertension risk and caffeine's effect on cardiovascular activity during mental stress in young men. *Health Psychology*, 10, 236–43.

Lowry, R., Holtzman, D., Truman, B. I., Kann, L., Collins, J. L., & Kolbe, L. J. (1994). Substance use and HIV-related sexual behaviors among US high school students: are they related? *American Journal of Public Health*, 84, 1116–20.

Ludwick-Rosenthal, R., & Neufeld, R. W. J. (1993). Preparation for undergoing an invasive medical procedure: interacting effects of information and coping style. *Journal of Consulting and Clinical Psychology*, 61, 156–64.

Lumley, J., & Astbury, J. (1980). *Birth rites, birth rights: childbirth alternatives for Australian parents*. Melbourne: Thomas Nelson.

Lumley, M. A., Abeles, L. A., Melamed, B. G., Pistone, L.M., & Johnson, J. H. (1990). Coping outcomes in children undergoing stressful medical procedures: the role of child-environment variables. *Behavioral Assessment*, 12, 223–38.

Lund, A. K., & Kegeles, S. S. (1984). Rewards and adolescent health behavior. *Health Psychology*, 3, 351–69.

Lundberg, U. (1986). Stress and Type A behavior in children. *Journal of the American Academy of Child Psychiatry*, 25, 771–8.

Lundin, R. W. (1987). Locus of control. In R. J. Corsisi (Ed.), *Concise encyclopedia of psychology*. New York: John Wiley & Sons.

Luparello, T. J., Lyons, H. A., Bleecker, E. R., & McFadden, E. R. (1968). Influences of suggestion on airway reactivity in asthmatic subjects. *Psychosomatic Medicine*, 30, 819–25.

Lutgendorf, S. K., Antoni, M. H., Ironson, G., Klimas, N., Kumar, M., Starr, K., McCabe, P., Cleven, K., Fletcher, M. A., & Schneiderman, N. (1997). Cognitive behavioral stress management decreases dysphoric mood and herpes simplex virus-type 2 antibody titers in symptomatic HIV-seropositive gay men. *Journal of Consulting and Clinical Psychology*, 65, 31–43.

Lykken, D. T. (1987). Psychophysiology. In R. J. Corsini (Ed.), *Concise encyclopedia of psychology*. New York: John Wiley & Sons.

Mabe, A., Treiber, F. A., & Riley, W. T. (1991). Examining emotional distress during pediatric hospitalisation for school-aged children. *Children's Health Care*, 20, 162–9.

Mackay, C., & Cox, T. (1978). Stress at work. In T. Cox (Ed.), *Stress*. Baltimore, MD: University Park Press.

MacLennan, A. H., Wilson, D. H., & Taylor, A. W. (1996). Prevalence and cost of alternative medicine in Australia. *The Lancet*, 347, 569–73.

Maddi, S. R. (1999). The personality construct of hardiness: 1. Effects on experiencing, coping, and strain. *Consulting Psychology Journal: Practice and Research*, 51(2), 83–94.

Maddux, B. A., Sbraccia, P., Kumakura, S., Sasson, S., et al. (1995). Membrane glycoprotein PC-1 and insulin resistance in non-insulin-dependent diabetes mellitus. *Nature*, 373, 448–51.

Maddux, J. E., Roberts, M. C., Sledden, E. A., & Wright, L. (1986). Developmental issues in child health psychology. *American Psychologist*, 41, 25–34.

Maes, S., & Kittel, F. (1990). Training research health psychologists. *Psychology and Health*, 4, 39–50.

Magery, A., & Boulton, J. (1995). The Adelaide Nutrition Study. 3. Food sources of nutrients at ages 11, 13 and 15 years. *Australian Journal of Nutrition and Dietetics*, 52, 124–30.

Mages, N. L., & Mendelsohn, G. A. (1979). Effects of cancer on patients' lives: a personological approach. In G. C. Stone, F. Cohen & N. E. Adler (Eds), *Health psychology — a handbook*. San Francisco: Jossey-Bass.

Magni, G., Moreschi, C., Rigatti-Luchini, S., & Merskey, H. (1994). Prospective study on the relationship between depressive symptoms and chronic musculoskeletal pain. *Pain*, 56, 289–97.

Maguire, P. (1985). Barriers to psychological care of the dying. *British Medical Journal*, 291, 1711–13.

Mahler, H. I. M., & Kulik, J. A. (1991). Health care involvement preferences and social-emotional recovery of male coronary-artery-bypass patients. *Health Psychology*, 10, 399–408.

Maier, S. F., Watkins, L. R., & Fleshner, M. (1994). Psychoneuroimmunology: the interface between behavior, brain, and immunity. *American Psychologist*, 49, 1004–1017.

Maj, M. (1990). Psychiatric aspects of HIV-1 infection and AIDS. *Psychological Medicine*, 20, 547–63.

Makkai, T., & McAllister, I. (1998). *Patterns of drug use in Australia, 1985–95*. Canberra: AGPS.

Malik, A. K., & Sabharwal, M. (1999). Locus of control as determinant ororganizational role stress. *Journal of the Indian Academy of Applied Psychology*, 25(1–2), 61–4.

Malkin, S. (1976). Care of the terminally ill. *Canadian Medical Association Journal*, 115, 129–30.

Malkoff, S. B., Muldoon, M. F., Zeigler, Z. R., & Manuck, S. B. (1993). Blood platelet responsivity to acute mental stress. *Psychosomatic Medicine*, 55, 477–82.

Manne, S. L., Bakeman, R., Jacobsen, P. B., Gorfinkle, K., Bernstein, D., & Redd, W. H. (1992). Adult-child interaction during invasive medical procedures. *Health Psychology*, 11, 241–9.

Manne, S. L., Bakeman, R., Jacobsen, P. B., Gorfinkle, K., & Redd, W. H. (1994). An analysis of a behavioral intervention for children undergoing venipuncture. *Health Psychology*, 13, 556–66.

Manne, S. L., Jacobsen, P. B., Gorfinkle, K., Gerstein, F., & Redd, W. H. (1993). Treatment adherence difficulties among children with cancer: the role of parenting style. *Journal of Pediatric Psychology*, 18, 47–62.

Manne, S. L., & Zautra, A. J. (1990). Couples coping with chronic illness: women with rheumatoid arthritis and their healthy husbands. *Journal of Behavioral Medicine*, 13, 327–42.

Manniche, C., Hesselsoe, G., Bentzen, L., Christensen, I., & Lundberg, E. (1988). Clinical trial of intensive muscle training for chronic low back pain. *The Lancet*, 332, 1473–6.

Manning, M. R., & Fusilier, M. R. (1999). The relationship between stress and health care use: an investigation of the buffering roles of personality, social support and exercise. *Journal of Psychosomatic Research*, 47(2), 159–73.

Manson, J. E., Colditz, G. A., Stampfer, M. J., Willett, W. C., Rosner, B., Monson, R. R., Speizer, F. E., & Hennekens, C. H. (1990). A prospective study of obesity and risk of coronary heart disease in women. *New England Journal of Medicine*, 322, 882–9.

Manson, J. E., Willett, W. C., Stampfer, M. J., Colditz, G. A., Hunter, D. J., & Hankinson, S. E. (1995). Body weight and mortality among women. *New England Journal of Medicine*, 333, 677–85.

Manuck, S. B. (1994). Cardiovascular reactivity in cardiovascular disease: 'Once more unto the breach'. *International Journal of Behavioral Medicine*, 1, 4–31.

Manuck, S. B., Kaplan, J. R., Adams, M. R., & Clarkson, T. B. (1988). Effects of stress and the sympathetic nervous system on coronary artery atherosclerosis in the cynomolgus macaque. *American Heart Journal*, 116, 328–33.

Manuck, S. B., Marsland, A. L., Kaplan, J. R., & Williams, J. K. (1995). The pathogenicity of behavior and its neuroendocrine mediation: an example from coronary artery disease. *Psychosomatic Medicine*, 57, 275–83.

Marcus, B. H., & Simkin, L. R. (1994). The transtheoretical model: applications to exercise behavior. *Medicine and Science in Sports and Exercise*, 26(11), 1400–1404.

Margolis, L. H., McLeroy, K. R., Runyan, C. W., & Kaplan, B. H. (1983). Type A behavior: an ecological approach. *Journal of Behavioral Medicine*, 6, 245–58.

Mariano, A. J. (1992). Chronic pain and spinal cord injury. *Journal of Clinical Pain*, 8, 87–92.

Markovitz, J. H., & Matthews, K. A. (1991). Platelets and coronary heart disease: potential psychophysiologic mechanisms. *Psychosomatic Medicine*, 53, 643–68.

Markovitz, J. H., Matthews, K. A., Kiss, J., & Smitherman, T. C. (1996). Effects of hostility on platelet reactivity to psychological stress in coronary heart disease patients and healthy controls. *Psychosomatic Medicine*, 58, 143–9.

Marks, D. F., Murray, M., Evans, B., & Willig, C. (2000). *Health psychology: theory, research and practice*. London: Sage.

Marks, G., Richardson, J. L., Graham, J. W., & Levine, A. (1986). Role of health locus of control beliefs and expectations of treatment efficacy in adjustment to cancer. *Journal of Personality and Social Psychology*, 51, 443–50.

Marks, G., Richardson, J. L., & Maldonado, N. (1991). Self-disclosure of HIV infection to sexual partners. *American Journal of Public Health*, 81, 1321–3.

Marks, R. (1995). An overview of skin cancers: incidence and causation. *Cancer*, 75, 607–612.

Marlatt, G. A. (1983). The controlled-drinking controversy: a commentary. *American Psychologist*, 38, 1097–1110.

Marlatt, G. A., & Gordon, J. R. (1980). Determinants of relapse: implications for the maintenance of behavior change. In P. O. Davidson & S. M. Davidson (Eds), *Behavioral medicine: changing health lifestyles*. New York: Brunner/Mazel.

Marmot, M. G., Kogevinas, M., & Elston, M. A. (1987). Social/economic status and disease. In L. Breslow, J. E. Fielding & L. B. Lave (Eds), *Annual review of public health* (Vol. 8). Palo Alto, CA: Annual Reviews.

Maron, D. J., & Fortmann, S. P. (1987). Nicotine yield and measures of cigarette smoke exposure in a large population: are lower-yield cigarettes safer? *American Journal of Public Health*, 77, 546–9.

Marsh, N. V., Kersel, D. A., Havill, J. H., & Sleigh, J. W. (1998). Caregiver burden at 7 months following severe traumatic brain injury. *Brain Injury*, 12(3), 225–38.

Marshall, N. L., Barnett, R. C., & Sayer, A. (1997). The changing workforce, job stress, and psychological distress. *Journal of Occupational Health Psychology*, 2(2), 99–107.

Marsland, A. L., Manuck, S. B., Fazzari, T. V., Stewart, C. J., & Rabin, B. S. (1995). Stability of individual differences in cellular immune responses to acute psychological stress. *Psychosomatic Medicine*, 57, 295–8.

Marteau, T. M. (1990). Attitudes towards doctors and medicine: the preliminary development of a new scale. *Psychology and Health*, 4, 351–6.

Marteau, T. M., & Johnston, M. (1986). Determinants of beliefs about illness: a study of parents of children with diabetes, asthma, epilepsy, and no chronic illness. *Journal of Psychosomatic Research*, 30, 673–83.

Marteau, T. M., Johnston, M., Baum, J. D., & Bloch, S. (1987). Goals of treatment in diabetes: a comparison of doctors and parents of children with diabetes. *Journal of Behavioral Medicine*, 10, 33–48.

Martelli, M. F., Auerbach, S. M., Alexander, J., & Mercuri, L. G. (1987). Stress management in the health care setting: matching interventions with patient coping styles. *Journal of Consulting and Clinical Psychology*, 55, 201–7.

Martin, J. E., & Dubbert, P. M. (1985). Exercise in hypertension. *Annals of Behavioral Medicine*, 7(1), 13–18.

Martin, J. L. (1988). Psychological consequences of AIDS-related bereavement among gay men. *Journal of Consulting and Clinical Psychology*, 56, 856–62.

Martin, J. L. (1990). Drug use and unprotected anal intercourse among gay men. *Health Psychology*, 9, 450–65.

Martin, J. L., & Dean, L. (1993). Effects of AIDS-related bereavement and HIV-related illness on psychological distress among gay men: a 7-year longitudinal study, 1985–1991. *Journal of Consulting and Clinical Psychology*, 61, 94–103.

Martin, P. R. (1988). The teaching of health psychology in Australia. *Health Psychology Update*, 2, 3–6.

Martin, P. R. (1993). *Psychological management of chronic headaches*. New York: Guilford.

Martin, P. R. (1998). Headache. In A. S. Bellack & M. Hersen (Eds), *Comprehensive clinical psychology*, Vol. 8, pp. 529–56. Oxford, NY: Pergamon.

Martin, P. R., & Mathews, A. M. (1978). Tension headaches: psychophysiological investigation and treatment. *Journal of Psychosomatic Research*, 22, 389–99.

Martin, P. R., Milech, D., & Nathan, P. R. (1993). Towards a functional model of chronic headaches: investigation of antecedents and consequences. *Headache*, 33, 461–70.

Martin, P. R., & Seneviratne, H. M. (1997). Effects of food deprivation and a stressor on head pain. *Health Psychology*, 16, 1–9.

Martin, P. R., & Teoh, H.-J. (1999). Effects of visual stimuli and a stressor on head pain. *Headache*, 39, 705–715.

Martin, P. R., & Todd, J. (2001). Effects of noise and a stressor on head pain. Manuscript in preparation.

Martin, R., Davis, G. M., Baron, R. S., Suls, J., & Blanchard, E. B. (1994). Specificity in social support: perceptions of helpful and unhelpful provider behaviors among irritable bowel, headache, and cancer patients. *Health Psychology*, 13, 432–9.

Martinez, F. D., Wright, A. L., Taussig, L. M., & The Group Health Medical Associates (1994). The effect of paternal smoking on the birthweight of newborns whose mothers did not smoke. *American Journal of Public Health*, 84, 1489–91.

Marx, M. H., & Hillix, W. A. (1963). Systems and theories in psychology. New York: McGraw-Hill.

Maslach, C. (1979). Negative emotional biasing in unexplained arousal. *Journal of Personality and Social Psychology*, 37, 953–69.

Maslach, C., & Jackson, S. E. (1982). Burnout in health professions: a social psychological analysis. In G. S. Sanders & J. Suls (Eds), *Social psychology of health and illness*. Hillsdale, NJ: Erlbaum.

Mason, J. W. (1975). A historical view of the stress field. *Journal of Human Stress*, 1, 22–36.

Masters, J. C., Burish, T. G., Hollon, S. D., & Rimm, D. C. (1987). *Behavior therapy: techniques and empirical findings* (3rd ed.). San Diego, CA: Harcourt Brace Jovanovich.

Matarazzo, J. D. (1982). Behavioral health's challenge to academic, scientific, and professional psychology. *American Psychologist*, 37, 1–14.

Mathews, A., & Ridgeway, V. (1984). Psychological preparation for surgery. In A. Steptoe & A. Mathews (Eds), *Health care and human behaviour*. London: Academic Press.

Mathis, M., & Lecci, L. (1999). Hardiness and college adjustment: identifying students in need of services. *Journal of College Student Development*, 40(3), 305–9.

Maticka-Tyndale, E. (1991). Sexual scripts and AIDS prevention: variations in adherence to safer-sex guidelines by heterosexual adolescents. *Journal of Sex Research*, 28, 45–66.

Mattes, R. D., Arnold, C., & Boraas, M. (1987a). Learned food aversions among cancer chemotherapy patients. *Cancer*, 60, 2576–80.

Mattes, R. D., Arnold, C., & Boraas, M. (1987b). Management of learned food aversions in cancer patients receiving chemotherapy. *Cancer Treatment Reports*, 71, 1071–8.

Matthews, K. A. (1982). Psychological perspectives on the Type A behavior pattern. *Psychological Bulletin*, 91, 293–323.

Matthews, K. A. (1986). Summary, conclusions, and implications. In K. A. Matthews, S. M. Weiss, T. Detre, T. M. Dembroski, B. Falkner, S. B. Manuck & R. B. Williams (Eds), *Handbook of stress, reactivity, and cardiovascular disease*. New York: John Wiley & Sons.

Matthews, K. A. (1988). Coronary heart disease and Type A behaviors: update on and alternative to the Booth-Kewley and Friedman (1987) quantitative review. *Psychological Bulletin*, 104, 373–80.

Matthews, K. A. (1989). Are sociodemographic variables markers for psychological determinants of health? *Health Psychology*, 8, 641–8.

Matthews, K. A., & Angulo, J. (1980). Measurement of the Type A behavior pattern in children: assessment of children's competitiveness, impatience-anger, and aggression. *Child Development*, 51, 466–75.

Matthews, K. A., & Jennings, J. R. (1984). Cardiovascular responses of boys exhibiting the Type A behavior pattern. *Psychosomatic Medicine*, 46, 484–97.

Matthews, K. A., Rosenman, R. H., Dembroski, T. M., Harris, E. L., & MacDougall, J. M. (1984). Familial resemblance in components of the Type A behavior pattern: a reanalysis of the California Type A Twin Study. *Psychosomatic Medicine*, 46, 512–22.

Matthews, K. A., & Woodall, K. L. (1988). Childhood origins of overt Type A behaviors and cardiovascular reactivity to behavioral stressors. *Annals of Behavioral Medicine*, 10, 71–7.

Mattick, R. P., & Baillie, A. (1992). *An outline for approaches to smoking cessation*. Canberra: AGPS.

Mattick, R. P., & Jarvis, T. (1994). A summary of recommendations for the management of alcohol problems: the quality assurance in the treatment of drug dependence project. *Drug and Alcohol Review*, 13, 145–55.

Mattson, M. E., Pollack, E. S., & Cullen, J. W. (1987). What are the odds that smoking will kill you? *American Journal of Public Health*, 77, 425–31.

Maude, D., Wertheim, E. H., Paxton, S. J., Gibbons, K., & Szmukler, G.I. (1993). Body dissatisfaction, weight loss behaviours and bulimic tendencies in Australian adolescents with an estimate of female data representativeness. *Australian Psychologist*, 28, 128–32.

May, B. (1991). Diabetes. In M. Pitts & K. Phillips (Eds), *The Psychology of Health* (pp. 214–30). London: Routledge.

Maybery, D. J. (1998). Validity, reliability and generalizability of the Positive and Negative Event Scale (PANE). In *Proceedings of the 2nd World Congress on Stress*. Secretariate, International Convention Management Services, Melbourne.

Maybery, D. J., & Graham, D. (2001). Hassles and uplifts: including interpersonal events. *Stress and Health*, 17, 91–104.

Mayer, J. (1975). *A diet for living*. New York: David McKay.

Mayer, J. (1980). The best diet is exercise. In P. J. Collipp (Ed.), *Childhood obesity* (2nd ed.). Littleton, MA: PSG Publishing.

Mayer, W. (1983). Alcohol abuse and alcoholism: the psychologist's role in prevention, research, and treatment. *American Psychologist*, 38, 1116–21.

Mayne, T. J., Vittinghoff, E., Barrett, D. C., Chesney, M. A., & Coates, T. J. (1996, March). Depressive affect and HIV survival. Paper presented at the meeting of the Society of Behavioral Medicine in Washington, DC.

Mays, V. M., & Cochran, S. D. (1988). Issues in the perception of AIDS risk and risk reduction activities by black and Hispanic/Latina women. *American Psychologist*, 43, 949–57.

Mazze, R. S., Shamoon, H., Pasmantier, R., Lucido, D., Murphy, J., Hartmann, K., Kuykendall, V., & Lopatin, W. (1984). Reliability of blood glucose monitoring by patients with diabetes mellitus. *American Journal of Medicine*, 77, 211–17.

McAdoo, W. G., Weinberger, M. H., Miller, J. Z., Feinberg, N. S., & Grim, C. E. (1990). Race and gender influence hemodynamic responses to psychological and physical stimuli. *Journal of Hypertension*, 8, 961–7.

McBride, S., & Browne, J. (1993). The school canteen: advocate or adversary in school health promotion? *Health Promotion Journal of Australia*, 3(3), 15–19.

McCaffrey, R. J., & Blanchard, E. B. (1985). Stress management approaches to the treatment of essential hypertension. *Annals of Behavioral Medicine*, 7(1), 5–12.

McCahon, C. P. (1991). Why did Martha want her husband to deteriorate? *Nursing*, 21(4), 44–6.

McCamish, M., Timmins, P., Gallois, C., & Terry, D. (1993). *APES: a norm-based workshop for HIV prevention and safer sex*. Brisbane: The University of Queensland.

McCann, B. S., Bovbjerg, V. E., Brief, D. J., Turner, C., Follette, W. C., Fitzpatrick, V., Dowdy, A., Retzlaff, B., Walden, C. E., & Knopp, R. H. (1995). Relationship of self-efficacy to cholesterol lowering and dietary change in hyperlipidemia. *Annals of Behavioral Medicine*, 17, 221–6.

McCann, B. S., Bovbjerg, V. E., Curry, S. J., Retzlaff, B. M., Walden, C. E., & Knopp, R. H. (1996). Predicting participation in a dietary intervention to lower cholesterol among individuals with hyperlipidemia. *Health Psychology*, 15, 61–3.

McCarty, D. (1985). Environmental factors in substance abuse: the microsetting. In M. Galizio & S. A. Maisto (Eds), *Determinants of substance abuse: biological, psychological, and environmental factors*. New York: Plenum.

McCaul, K. D., & Malott, J. M. (1984). Distraction and coping with pain. *Psychological Bulletin*, 95, 516–33.

McCaul, K. D., Monson, N., & Maki, R. H. (1992). Does distraction reduce pain-produced distress among college students? *Health Psychology*, 11, 210–17.

McClearn, G. E. (1968). Behavioral genetics: an overview. *Merrill-Palmer Quarterly*, 14, 9–14.

McClelland, D. C., Floor, E., Davidson, R. J., & Saron, C. (1980). Stressed power motivation, sympathetic activation, immune function, and illness. *Journal of Human Stress*, 6, 11–19.

McClennan, A. T., Arndt, I. O., Metzger, D. S., Woody, G. E., & O'Brien, C. P. (1993). The effects of psychosocial services in substance abuse treatment. *Journal of the American Medical Association*, 269, 1953–9.

McClintic, J. R. (1985). *Physiology of the human body* (3rd ed.). New York: John Wiley & Sons.

McClowry, S. G., & McLeod, S. M. (1990). The psycho-social responses of school-age children to hospitalisation. *Children's Health Care*, 19, 155–61.

McColl, M., Hart, G., & Chung, D. (1996). Client follow-up at the Adelaide sexually transmitted disease clinic. *Australian and New Zealand Journal of Public Health*, 20(2), 161–4.

McConnell, S., Biglan, A., & Severson, H. H. (1984). Adolescents' compliance with self-monitoring and physiological assessment of smoking in natural environments. *Journal of Behavioral Medicine*, 7, 115–22.

McCoy, S. B., Gibbons, F. X., Reis, T. J., Gerrard, M., Luus, C. A. E., & Von Wald Sufka, A. (1992). Perceptions of smoking risk as a function of smoking status. *Journal of Behavioral Medicine*, 15, 469–88.

McCrady, B. S. (1988). Alcoholism. In E. A. Blechman & K. D. Brownell (Eds), *Handbook of behavioral medicine for women*. New York: Pergamon.

McCrady, B. S., & Irvine, S. (1989). Self-help groups. In R. K. Hester & W. R. Miller (Eds), *Handbook of alcoholism treatment approaches: effective alternatives*. New York: Pergamon.

McCubbin, H. I., & Patterson, J. M. (1983). The family stress process: the double ABCX model of adjustment and adaptation. *Marriage and Family Review*, 6, 7–37.

McDaniel, S., & Campbell, T. L. (1986). Physicians and family therapists: the risk of collaboration. *Family Systems Medicine*, 4, 4–8.

McElnay, J. C., & McCallion, C. R. (1998). Adherence and the elderly. In L. B. Myers & K. Midence (Eds), *Adherence to treatment in medical conditions*. Amsterdam: Harwood Academic Publishers.

McFarlane, A. C. (1992). Avoidance and intrusion in post-traumatic stress disorder. *Journal of Nervous and Mental Disease*, 180, 439–45.

McGee, D.S., & Cegala, D. J. (1998). Patient communication skills training for improved communication competence in the primary care medical consultation. *Journal of Applied Communication Research*, 26(4), 412–30.

McGehee, D. S., Heath, M. J. S., Gelber, S., Devay, P., & Role, L. W. (1995). Nicotine enhancement of fast excitatory transmission in CNS by presynaptic receptors. *Science*, 269, 1692–6.

McGinnis, J. M. (1994). The role of behavioral research in national health policy. In J. A. Blumenthal, K. Matthews & S. M. Weiss (Eds), *New frontiers in behavioral medicine*: Proceedings of the national conference. Washington, DC: National Institutes of Health.

McGinnis, J. M., Shopland, D., & Brown, C. (1987). *Tobacco and health: trends in smoking and smokeless tobacco consumption in the United States*. In L. Breslow, J. E. Fielding & L. B. Lave (Eds), *Annual review of public health* (Vol. 8). Palo Alto, CA: Annual Reviews.

McGrady, A., & Higgins, J. T. (1990). Effect of repeated measurements of blood pressure in essential hypertension: role of anxiety. *Journal of Behavioral Medicine*, 13, 93–101.

McGrady, A., Conran, P., Dickey, D., Garman, D., Farris, E., & Schumann-Brzezinski, C. (1992). The effects of biofeedback-assisted relaxation on cell-mediated immunity, cortisol, and white blood cell count in healthy adult subjects. *Journal of Behavioral Medicine*, 15, 343–54.

McGrath, J., & McGrath, G. (2000). *A love for life*. Sydney: Random House.

McGrath, P. A. (1987). An assessment of children's pain: a review of behavioral, physiological and direct scaling techniques. *Pain*, 31, 147–76.

McGuire, F. L. (1982). Treatment of the drinking driver. *Health Psychology*, 1, 137–52.

McIlwain, H. H., Silverfield, J. C., Burnette, M. C., & Bruce, D. F. (1991). *Winning with arthritis*. New York: John Wiley & Sons.

McInman, A. D., & Grove, J. R. (1991). Multidimensional self-concept, cigarette smoking and intentions to smoke in adolescents. *Australian Psychologist*, 26(3), 192–6.

McKeown, T. (1979). *The role of medicine: dream, mirage or nemesis?* Oxford, UK: Basil Blackwell.

McKinlay, J. B. (1975). Who is really ignorant — physician or patient? *Journal of Health and Social Behavior*, 16, 3–11.

McKinney, M. E., Hofschire, P. J., Buell, J. C., & Eliot, R. S. (1984). Hemodynamic and biochemical responses to stress: the necessary link between Type A behavior and cardiovascular disease. *Behavioral Medicine Update*, 6(4), 16–21.

McKnight, J. D., & Glass, D. C. (1995). Perceptions of control, burnout, and depressive symptomatology: a replication and extension. *Journal of Consulting and Clinical Psychology*, 63, 490–94.

McMurray, A. (1999). *Community health and wellness: a sociological approach*. Artarmon, NSW: Mosby.

McNamara, J. J., Molot, M. A., Stremple, J. F., & Cutting, R. T. (1971). Coronary artery disease in combat casualties in Vietnam. *Journal of the American Medical Association*, 216, 1185–7.

McNaull, F. W. (1984). Radiation therapy. In S. N. McIntire & A. L. Cioppa (Eds), *Cancer nursing: a developmental approach*. New York: John Wiley & Sons.

McSherry, W. C., & Holm, J. E. (1994). Sense of coherence: its effect on psychological and physiological processes prior to, during, and after a stressful situation. *Journal of Clinical Psychology*, 50(4), 476–87.

McSherry, W. C., Holm, J. E., & Popinga, M. (1991). Sense of coherence and hardiness: Comparing their abilities to predict physical symptoms and psychological distress. Paper presented at the meeting of the Association for Advancement of Behavior Therapy, New York.

MDBDF (March of Dimes Birth Defects Foundation) (1993). *March of Dimes statbook: statistics for healthier mothers and babies*. White Plains, NY: Author.

Mead, M., & Newton, N. (1967). Cultural patterning of perinatal behavior. In S. A. Richardson & A. F. Guttmacher (Eds), *Childbearing: its social and psychological aspects*. Baltimore, MD: Williams & Wilkins.

Mechanic, D. (1972). Social psychologic factors affecting the presentation of bodily complaints. *New England Journal of Medicine*, 286, 1132–9.

Mechanic, D. (1976). Stress, illness, and illness behavior. *Journal of Human Stress*, 2, 2–6.

Mechanic, D. (1979). The stability of health and illness behavior: results from a 16-year follow-up. *American Journal of Public Health*, 69, 1142–5.

Mechanic, D. (1980). The experience and reporting of common physical complaints. *Journal of Health and Social Behavior*, 21, 146–55.

Medley, G. (1995). Failures in screening for cervical cancer: who is to blame? *Medical Journal of Australia*, 7(3), 342.

Meichenbaum, D., & Cameron, R. (1983). Stress inoculation training: toward a general paradigm for training coping skills. In D. Meichenbaum & M. E. Jaremko (Eds), *Stress reduction and prevention*. New York: Plenum.

Meichenbaum, D., & Deffenbacher, J. L. (1988). Stress inoculation training. *Counseling Psychologist*, 16, 69–90.

Meichenbaum, D., & Turk, D. (1982). Stress, coping, and disease: a cognitive-behavioral perspective. In R. W. J. Neufield (Ed.), *Psychological stress and psychopathology*. New York: McGraw-Hill.

Melamed, B. G. (1993). Putting the family back in the child. *Behavioral Research and Therapy*, 31, 239–47.

Melamed, B. G., & Bush, J. P. (1985). Family factors in children with acute illness. In D. C. Turk & R. D. Kerns (Eds), *Health, illness, and families: a life-span approach*. New York: John Wiley & Sons.

Melamed, B. G., Dearborn, M., & Hermecz, D. A. (1983). Necessary conditions for surgery preparation: age and previous experience. *Psychosomatic Medicine*, 45, 517–25.

Melamed, B. G., & Siegel, L. J. (1975). Reduction of anxiety in children facing hospitalization and surgery by use of filmed modeling. *Journal of Consulting and Clinical Psychology*, 43, 511–21.

Melin, B., & Lundberg, U. (1997). A biopsychosocial approach to work-stress and musculosceletal disorders. *Journal of Psychophysiology*, 11(3), 238–47.

Mellors, V., Boyle, G. J., & Roberts, L. (1994). Effects of personality, stress and lifestyle on hypertension: An Australian twin study. *Personality and Individual Differences*, 16(6), 967–74.

Melzack, R. (1975). The McGill Pain Questionnaire: major properties and scoring methods. *Pain*, 1, 277–99.

Melzack, R., & Torgerson, W. S. (1971). On the language of pain. *Anesthesiology*, 34, 50–59.

Melzack, R., & Wall, P. D. (1965). Pain mechanisms: a new theory. *Science*, 150, 971–9.

Melzack, R., & Wall, P. D. (1982). *The challenge of pain*. New York: Basic Books.

Melzack, R., Weisz, A. Z., & Sprague, L. T. (1963). Strategems for controlling pain: contributions of auditory stimulation and suggestion. *Experimental Neurology*, 8, 239–47.

Menaghan, E. (1982). Measuring coping effectiveness: a panel analysis of marital problems and coping efforts. *Journal of Health and Social Behavior*, 23, 220–34.

Mendelson, B. K., & White, D. R. (1985). Development of self-body-esteem in overweight youngsters. *Developmental Psychology*, 21, 90–96.

Menefee, L. A., Haythornthwaite, J. A., Clark, M. R., & Koenig, T. (1996, March). The effect of social responses on pain coping strategies. Paper presented at the meeting of the Society of Behavioral Medicine, Washington, DC.

Menkes, M. S., Matthews, K. A., Krantz, D. S., Lundberg, U., Mead, L. A., Qaqish, B., & Liang, K.-Y. (1989). Cardiovascular reactivity to the cold pressor test as a predictor of hypertension. *Hypertension*, 14, 524–30.

Mentzer, S. J., & Snyder, M. L. (1982). The doctor and the patient: a psychological perspective. In G. S. Sanders & J. Suls (Eds), *Social psychology of health and illness*. Hillsdale, NJ: Erlbaum.

Meredith, C. N., & Dwyer, J. T. (1991). Nutrition and exercise: effects on adolescent health. In G. S. Omenn, J. E. Fielding & L. B. Lave (Eds), *Annual review of public health* (Vol. 12). Palo Alto, CA: Annual Reviews.

Meredith, H. V. (1978). *Human body growth in the first ten years of life*. Columbia, SC: The State Printing Company.

Mermelstein, R. J., Karnatz, T., & Reichmann, S. (1992). Smoking. In P. H. Wilson (Ed.), *Principles and practice of relapse prevention* (pp. 43–67). New York: Guilford.

Methorst, G. J., Jansen, M. A., & Kerkhof, A. J. F. M. (1991). Training in health psychology: an international look. In M. A. Jansen & J. Weinman (Eds), *The international development of health psychology*. Chur, Switzerland: Harwood.

Meyer, D., Leventhal, H., & Gutmann, M. (1985). Common-sense models of illness: the example of hypertension. *Health Psychology*, 4, 115–35.

Meyer, T. J., & Mark, M. M. (1995). Effects of psychosocial interventions with adult cancer patients: a meta-analysis of randomized experiments. *Health Psychology*, 14, 101–8.

Meyerowitz, B. E. (1983). Postmastectomy coping strategies and quality of life. *Health Psychology*, 2, 117–32.

Michela, J. L. (1987). Interpersonal and individual impacts of a husband's heart attack. In A. Baum & J. E. Singer (Eds), *Handbook of psychology and health* (Vol. 5). Hillsdale, NJ: Erlbaum.

Migliorelli, R., Tesón, A., Sabe, L., Petracchi, M., Leiguarda, R., & Starkstein, S. E. (1995). Prevalence and correlates of dysthymia and major depression among patients with Alzheimer's disease. *American Journal of Psychiatry*, 152, 37–44.

Miles, F., & Meehan, J. W. (1995). Visual discrimination of pigmented skin lesions. *Health Psychology*, 14, 171–7.

Milgrom, J., Nathan, P. R., & Martin, P. R. (1996). Overview and practice in a general hospital setting. In P. R. Martin & J. S. Birnbrauer (Eds), *Clinical psychology: profession and practice in Australia*. Hong Kong: Macmillan.

Milgrom, J. Walter, P., & Green, S. (1994). Cost savings following psychological intervention in a hospital setting: the need for Australian-based research. *Australian Psychologist*, 29(3), 194–200.

Millar, W. J., & Stephens, T. (1987). The prevalence of overweight and obesity in Britain, Canada, and the United States. *American Journal of Public Health*, 77, 38–41.

Miller, B., & Cafasso, L. (1992). Gender differences in caregiving: fact or artifact? *The Gerontologist*, 32, 498–507.

Miller, B. D., & Wood, B. L. (1994). Psychophysiologic reactivity in asthmatic children: a cholinergically mediated confluence of pathways. *Journal of the American Academy of Child and Adolescent Psychiatry*, 33, 1236–45.

Miller, M., Hamilton, M., & Flaherty, B. (1992). The evaluation of Australia's national campaign against drug abuse. *Journal of Drug Issues*, 22(3), 487–506.

Miller, N. E. (1959). Liberalization of basic S-R concepts: extensions to conflict behavior, motivation, and social learning. In S. Koch (Ed.), *Psychology: a study of a science* (Vol. 2). New York: McGraw-Hill.

Miller, N. E. (1978). Biofeedback and visceral learning. In M. R. Rosenzweig & L. W. Porter (Eds), *Annual review of psychology* (Vol. 29). Palo Alto, CA: Annual Reviews.

Miller, R. H., & Luft, H. S. (1994). Managed care plans: characteristics, growth, and premium performance. In G. S. Omenn, J. E. Fielding & L. B. Lave (Eds), *Annual review of public health* (Vol. 15). Palo Alto, CA: Annual Reviews.

Miller, S. B., Turner, J. R., Sherwood, A., Brownley, K. A., Hinderliter, A. L., & Light, K. C. (1995). Parental history of hypertension and cardiovascular response to stress in black and white men. *International Journal of Behavioral Medicine*, 2, 339–57.

Miller, S. M. (1979). Controllability and human stress: method, evidence and theory. *Behaviour Research and Therapy*, 17, 287–304.

Miller, S. M., & Green, M. L. (1984). Coping with stress and frustration: origins, nature, and development. In M. Lewis & C. Saarni (Eds), *Origins of behavior* (Vol. 5). New York: Plenum.

Miller, S. M., & Mangan, C. E. (1983). Interacting effects of information and coping style in adapting to gynecologic stress: should the doctor tell all? *Journal of Personality and Social Psychology*, 45, 223–36.

Miller, S. M., Brody, D. S., & Summerton, J. (1987). Styles of coping with threat: Implications for health. *Journal of Personality and Social Psychology*, 54, 142–8.

Miller, W. (1983). Motivational interviewing with problem drinkers. *Behavioural Psychotherapy*, 11, 147–72.

Miller, W. R. (1989a). Increasing motivation for change. In R. K. Hester & W. R. Miller (Eds), *Handbook of alcoholism treatment approaches: effective alternatives*. New York: Pergamon.

Miller, W. R. (1989b). Matching individuals with interventions. In R. K. Hester & W. R. Miller (Eds), *Handbook of alcoholism treatment approaches: effective alternatives*. New York: Pergamon.

Miller, W. R., & Hester, R. K. (1980). Treating the problem drinker: modern approaches. In W. R. Miller (Ed.), *The addictive behaviors: treatment of alcoholism, drug abuse, smoking, and obesity*. New York: Pergamon.

Miller, W. R., & Hester, R. K. (1985). Inpatient alcoholism treatment: who benefits? *American Psychologist*, 41, 794–805.

Miller-Johnson, S., Emery, R. E., Marvin, R. S., Clarke, W., Lovinger, R., & Martin, M. (1994). Parent–child relationships and the management of insulin-dependent diabetes mellitus. *Journal of Consulting and Clinical Psychology*, 62, 603–610.

Millon, T., Green, C., & Meagher, R. (1982). Millon Behavioral Health Inventory Manual. Minneapolis, MN: National Computer Systems.

Mills, N. M. (1989). Pain behaviors in infants and toddlers. *Journal of Pain and Symptom Management*, 4, 184–90.

Milne, E., English, D. R., Cross, D., Corti, B., Costa, C., Johnston, R. (1999). Evaluation of an intervention to reduce sun exposure in children: design and baseline results. *American Journal of Epidemiology*, 150, 164–73.

Milne, E., English, D. R., Johnston, R., Cross, D., Borland, R., Costa, C., & Giles-Corti, B. (2000). Improved sun protection behaviour in children after two years of the Kidskin intervention. *Australian and New Zealand Journal of Public Health*, 24(5), 481–7.

Milne, G. (1977a). Cyclone Tracy: I Some consequences of the evacuation for adult victims. *Australian Psychologist*, 12(1), 39–54.

Milne, G. (1977b). Cyclone Tracy: II The effects on Darwin children. *Australian Psychologist*, 12(1), 55–62.

Minor, M. A., & Sanford, M. K. (1993). Physical interventions in the management of pain in arthritis. *Arthritis Care and Research*, 6, 197–206.

Miro, J., & Raich, R. M. (1999). Preoperative preparation for surgery: an analysis of the effects of relaxation and information provision. *Clinical Psychology and Psychotherapy*, 6(3), 202–9.

Mitchell, H., Hirst, S., Cockburn, J., Reading, D. J., Staples, M. P., & Medley, G. (1991). Cervical cancer screening: a comparison of recruitment strategies among older women. *Medical Journal of Australia*, 155, 79–82.

Mitchell, J. C. (Ed.) (1969). *Social networks in urban situations*. Manchester, UK: Manchester University Press.

Mitchell, J. T. (1983). When disaster strikes: the critical incident stress debriefing process. *Journal of Emergency Medical Services*, January, 36–9.

Mittleman, M. A., Maclure, M., Sherwood, J. B., Mulry, R. P., Tofler, G. H., Jacobs, S. C., & Friedman, R. (1995). Triggering of acute episodes of myocardial infarction onset by episodes of anger. *Circulation*, 92, 1720–25.

Mizener, D., Thomas, M., & Billings, R. (1988). Cognitive changes of migraineurs receiving biofeedback training. *Headache*, 28, 339–43.

Mizoguchi, H., O'Shea, J. J., Longo, D. L., Loeffler, C. M., McVicar, D. W., & Ochoa, A. C. (1992). Alterations in signal transduction molecules in T lymphocytes from tumor-bearing mice. *Science*, 258, 1795–8.

Moberg, E., Kollind, M., Lins, P.-E., & Adamson, U. (1994). Acute stress impairs insulin sensitivity in IDDM patients. *Diabetologia*, 37, 247–51.

Monti, P. M., Rohsenow. D. J., Rubonis, A. V., Naiura, R. S., Sirota, A. D., Colby, S. M., Goddard, P., & Abrams, D. B. (1993). Cue exposure with coping skills treatment for male alcoholics: a preliminary investigation. *Journal of Consulting and Clinical Psychology*, 61, 1011–19.

Moore, D. C., (1993). Body image and eating behaviour in adolescents. *Journal of American College of Nutrition*, 12, 505–510.

Moore, M. L. (1983). *Realities of childbearing* (2nd ed.). Philadelphia, PA: Saunders.

Moore, S., & Rosenthal, D. (1991). Adolescent invulnerability and perceptions of AIDS risk. *Journal of Adolescent Research*, 6(2), 164–80.

Moos, R. H. (1982). Coping with acute health crises. In T. Millon, C. Green & R. Meagher (Eds), *Handbook of clinical health psychology*. New York: Plenum.

Moos, R. H., & Finney, J. W. (1983). The expanding scope of alcoholism treatment evaluation. *American Psychologist*, 38, 1036–44.

Moos, R. H., & Schaefer, J. A. (1986). Life transitions and crises: a conceptual overview. In R. H. Moos (Ed.), *Coping with life crises: an integrated approach*. New York: Plenum.

MOR, V., Masterson-Allen, S., Goldberg, R. J., Cummings, F. J., Glicksman, A. S., & Fretwell, M. D. (1985). Relationships between age at diagnosis and treatments received by cancer patients. *Journal of the American Geriatrics Society*, 33, 585–9.

Moreland, J., & Thompson, M. A. (1994). Efficacy of electromyographic biofeedback compared with conventional physical therapy for upper-extremity function in patients following stroke: a research overview and meta-analysis. *Physical Therapy*, 74, 534–47.

Morgan, D. L. (1990). Combining the strengths of social networks, social support and personal relationships. In. S. Duck with R.C. Silver (Eds), *Personal relationships and social support* (pp. 190–215). London: Sage.

Morris, P. L., Robinson, R. G., Raphael, B., & Bishop, D. (1991). The relationship between the perception of social support and post-stroke depression in hospitalised patients. *Psychiatry*, 54, 306–316.

Morris, R. J., & Kratochwill, T. R. (1983). *Treating children's fears and phobias: a behavioral approach*. New York: Pergamon.

Morris, S. (1999). Recovering from coronary artery bypass graft surgery: do depression, optimism and coping predict quality of recovery? *Dissertation Abstracts International: Section B: Sciences and Engineering*, 59(7-B): 3675.

Morrow, G. R., Asbury, R., Hammon, S., Dobkin, P., Caruso, L., Pandya, K., & Rosenthal, S. (1992). Comparing the effectiveness of behavioral treatment for chemotherapy-induced nausea and vomiting when administered by oncologists, oncology nurses, and clinical psychologists. *Health Psychology*, 11, 250–56.

Moser, D. K., & Dracup, K. (1996). Is anxiety early after myocardial infarction associated with subsequent ischemic and arrhythmic events? *Psychosomatic Medicine*, 58, 395–401.

Moskowitz, J. T., Folkman, S., Collette, L., & Vittinghoff, E. (1996). Coping and mood during AIDS-related caregiving and bereavement. *Annals of Behavioral Medicine*, 18, 49–57.

Mosley, T. H., Penzien, D. B., Johnson, C. A., Wittrock, D., Rubman, S., Payne, T. J., & Holroyd, K. A. (1990, April). Coping with stress in headache sufferers and no-headache controls. Paper presented at the meeting of the Society of Behavioral Medicine, Chicago.

Moss, G. E., Dielman, T. E., Campanelli, P. C., Leech, S. L., Harlan, W. R., van Harrison, R., & Horvath, W. J. (1986). Demographic correlates of SI assessments of Type A behavior. *Psychosomatic Medicine*, 48, 564–74.

Moyle, P., & Parkes, K. (1999). The effects of transition stress: a relocation study. *Journal of Organizational Behavior*, 20(5), 625–46.

Muldoon, M. F., & Manuck, S. B. (1992). Health through cholesterol reduction: are there unforeseen risks? *Annals of Behavioral Medicine*, 14, 101–8.

Muldoon, M. F., Manuck, S. B., & Matthews, K. A. (1990). Lowering cholesterol concentrations and mortality: a quantitative review of primary prevention trials. *British Medical Journal*, 301, 309–314.

Muller, J. E., Ludmer, P. L., Willich, S. N., Tofler, G. H., Aylmer, G., Klangos, I., & Stone, P. H. (1987). Circadian variation in the frequency of sudden cardiac death. *Circulation*, 75, 131–8.

Muller, J. E., Mittleman, M. A., Maclure, M., Sherwood, J. B., et al. (1996). Triggering myocardial infarction by sexual activity: low absolute risk and prevention by regular physical exertion. *Journal of the American Medical Association*, 275, 1405–9.

Mullins, R., & Borland, R. (1993). Evaluation of the 1993 media campaign: results from the pre- and post-campaign telephone surveys. *Quit Evaluation Studies No. 7*. Melbourne: VSHP.

Mumford, E., Schlesinger, H. J., & Glass, G. V. (1982). The effects of psychological intervention on recovery from surgery and heart attacks: an analysis of the literature. *American Journal of Public Health*, 72, 141–51.

Murdaugh, C. L. (1998). Problems with adherence in the elderly. In S. A. Shumaker, E. B. Schron, J. K. Ockene & W. L. McBee (Eds), *The handbook of health behavior change* (2nd ed.). New York: Springer.

Murray, D. M., Davis-Hearn, M., Goldman, A. I., Pirie, P., & Luepker, R. V. (1988). Four- and five-year follow-up results from four seventh-grade smoking prevention strategies. *Journal of Behavioral Medicine*, 11, 395–405.

Murray, D. M., Pirie, P., Leupker, R. V., & Pallonen, U. (1989). Five- and six-year follow-up results from four seventh-grade smoking prevention strategies. *Journal of Behavioral Medicine*, 12, 207–218.

Murray, D. M., Richards, P. S., Luepker, R. V., & Johnson, C. A. (1987). The prevention of cigarette smoking in children: two- and three-year follow-up comparisons of four prevention strategies. *Journal of Behavioral Medicine*, 10, 595–611.

Murray, M., Swan, A. V., Johnson, M. R. D., & Bewley, B. R. (1983). Some factors associated with increased risk of smoking by children. *Journal of Child Psychology and Psychiatry*, 24, 223–32.

Murray, P., Liddell, A., & Donohue, J. (1989). A longitudinal study of the contribution of dental experience to dental anxiety in children between 9 and 12 years of age. *Journal of Behavioral Medicine*, 12, 309–320.

Murrell, J., Farlow, M., Ghetti, B., & Benson, M. D. (1991). A mutation in the amyloid precursor protein associated with hereditary Alzheimer's disease. *Science*, 254, 97–9.

Muscat, J. E., Harris, R. E., Haley, N. J., & Wynder, E. L. (1991). Cigarette smoking and plasma cholesterol. *American Heart Journal*, 121, 121–41.

Myers, L. B., & Midence, K.(1998). *Adherence to treatment in medical conditions*. Amsterdam: Harwood Academic Publishers.

Nash, S. S., & Smith, M. J. (1982). Perception and coordination. In M. J. Smith, J. A. Goodman, N. L. Ramsey & S. B. Pasternack (Eds), *Child and family: concepts in nursing practice*. New York: McGraw-Hill.

Nathan, P. E. (1985). Prevention of alcoholism: a history of failure. In J. C. Rosen & L. J. Solomon (Eds), *Prevention in health psychology*. Hanover, NH: University Press of New England.

Nathan, P. E. (1986). Outcomes of treatment for alcoholism: current data. *Annals of Behavioral Medicine*, 8(2–3), 40–46.

Nathan, P. R., Milgrom, J., & Martin, P. R. (1996). Theoretical context and clinical applications. In P. R. Martin & J. S. Birnbrauer (Eds), *Clinical psychology: profession and practice in Australia*. Hong Kong: Macmillan.

National Center for HIV and TB Prevention, Divisions of HIV/AIDS Prevention (2001). *Basic statistics — international statistics* (http://www.hivmail@cdc.gov).

National Centre in HIV Epidemiology and Clinical Research (1998). *HIV/AIDS and related diseases in Australia. Annual Surveillance Report 1998* (http://www.med.unsw.edu.au/nchecr/downloads/98ansurvrpt.pdf, accessed August 2000).

National Coordinating Committee for Health Promotion in the Workplace (1992). *Health at Work Newsletter*, Issue No. 13, Winter.

National Evaluation Steering Committee (1993). *Report on the Evaluation of the National HIV/AIDS Strategy*. Canberra: Australian Department of Health.

National Health Strategy (1992). 'Enough to make you sick', *National Health Strategy*, Research Paper No. 1. Canberra: Australian Department of Health.

National Tobacco Campaign (2001). *Campaign fact file* (http://www.quitnow.info.au).

Negri, E., La Vecchia, C., D'Avanzo, B., Nobili, A., et al. (1994). Acute myocardial infarction: association with time since stopping smoking in Italy. *Journal of Epidemiology and Community Health*, 48, 129–33.

Nehemkis, A. M., & Gerber, K. E. (1986). Compliance and the quality of survival. In K. E. Gerber & A. M. Nehemkis (Eds), *Compliance: the dilemma of the chronically ill*. New York: Springer.

Nelson, E. C., Stason, W. B., Neutra, R. R., Solomon, H. S., & McArdle, P. J. (1978). Impact of patient perceptions on compliance with treatment for hypertension. *Medical Care*, 16, 893–906.

Nelson, G. E. (1989). *Biological principles with human applications* (3rd ed.). New York: John Wiley & Sons.

Neugarten, B. L., & Neugarten, D. A. (1987, May). The changing meanings of age. *Psychology Today*, pp. 29–33.

Neundorfer, M. M. (1991). Coping and health outcomes in spouse caregivers of persons with dementia. *Nursing Research*, 40, 260–65.

Nevidjon, B. M. (1984). Chemotherapy. In S. N. McIntire & A. L. Cioppa (Eds), *Cancer nursing: a developmental approach*. New York: John Wiley & Sons.

Newcomb, M. D., & Bentler, P. M. (1986). Cocaine use among adolescents: longitudinal associations with social context, psychopathology, and use of other substances. *Addictive Behaviors*, 11, 263–73.

Newcomb, M. D., Maddahian, E., & Bentler, P. M. (1986). Risk factors for drug use among adolescents: concurrent and longitudinal analyses. *American Journal of Public Health*, 76, 525–31.

Newcomb, P. A., Weiss, N. S., Storer, B. E., Scholes, D., Young, B. E., & Voigt, L. F. (1991). Breast self-examination in relation to the occurrence of advanced breast cancer. *Journal of the National Cancer Institute*, 83, 260–65.

Newlin, D. B., & Thomson, J. B. (1991). Chronic tolerance and sensitization to alcohol in sons of alcoholics. *Alcoholism: Clinical and Experimental Research*, 15, 399–405.

Newman, M. G., & Stone, A. A. (1996). Does humor moderate the effects of experimentally-induced stress? *Annals of Behavioral Medicine*, 18, 101–9.

Newman, S. (1984a). Anxiety, hospitalization, and surgery. In R. Fitzpatrick, J. Hinton, S. Newman, G. Scambler & J. Thompson (Eds), *The experience of illness*. London: Tavistock.

Newman, S. (1984b). The psychological consequences of cerebrovascular accident and head injury. In R. Fitzpatrick, J. Hinton, S. Newman, G. Scambler & J. Thompson (Eds), *The experience of illness*. London: Tavistock.

Ng, B., Dimsdale, J. E., Shragg, P., & Deutsch, R. (1996). Ethnic differences in analgesic consumption for postoperative pain. *Psychosomatic Medicine*, 58, 125–9.

Nguyen, M., Watanabe, H., Budson, A. E., Richie, J. P., Hayes, D. F., & Folkman, J. (1994). Elevated levels of an angiogenic peptide, basic fibroblast factor, in the urine of patients with a wide spectrum of cancers. *Journal of the National Cancer Institute*, 86, 356–61.

NHF (National Heart Foundation) (1987). *Update on diet and disease 1987: 1-news on cholesterol*. National Heart Foundation of Australia.

NHMRC (National Health & Medical Research Council) (1991). *Health implications of long term climate change*. Canberra: AGPS.

NHMRC (1993). *National Immunisation Strategy*. Canberra: AGPS.

NHMRC (1999). *Acute pain management: scientific evidence*. Canberra: NHMRC.

NIA (National Institute on Aging) (1995). *Progress report on Alzheimer's disease 1995*. Silver Spring, MD: Author.

NIAAA (National Institute on Alcohol Abuse and Alcoholism) (1993). Alcohol and health (8th Special Report to the U.S. Congress, Publication No. 94-3699). Washington, DC: U.S. Government Printing Office.

Nicassio, P. M., Radojevic, V., Weisman, M. H., Culbertson, A. L., Lewis, C., & Clemmey, P. (1993). The role of helplessness in the response to disease-modifying drugs in rheumatoid arthritis. *Journal of Rheumatology*, 20, 1114–20.

Nicassio, P. M., Wallston, K. A., Callahan, L. F., Herbert, M., & Pincus, T. (1985). The measurement of helplessness in rheumatoid arthritis: the development of the Arthritis Helplessness Index. *Journal of Rheumatology*, 12, 462–7.

Nicholas, M., Molloy, A., Tonkin, L., & Beeston, L. (2000). *Practical and positive ways of adapting to chronic pain: manage your pain.* Sydney: ABC Books.

Nichols, R. S., & Santelli, J. (1990, March). The AIDS patient: extreme elevation of MMPI scales. Paper presented at the meeting of the Eastern Psychological Association, Philadelphia, PA.

Nides, M. A., Rakos, R. F., Gonzales, D., Murray, R. P., et al. (1995). Predictors of initial smoking cessation and relapse through the first 2 years of the Lung Health Study. *Journal of Consulting and Clinical Psychology*, 63, 60–69.

NKF (National Kidney Foundation) (1990). *Dining out with confidence: a guide for renal patients.* New York: Author.

Noble, L. M. (1998). Doctor–patient communication and adherence to treatment. In L. B. Myers & K. Midence, *Adherence to treatment in medical conditions* (pp. 51–82). Amsterdam: Harwood Academic Publishers.

Norris, C. M. (1990). The work of getting well. *American Journal of Nursing*, 90, 47–50.

North, T. C., McCullagh, P., & Tran, Z. (1990). Effect of exercise on depression. *Exercise and Sport Science Reviews*, 18, 379–415.

Northcote, R. J., Flannigan, C., & Ballantyne, D. (1986). Sudden death and vigorous exercise — a study of 60 deaths associated with squash. *British Heart Journal*, 55, 198–203.

Novaco, R. W. (1975). *Anger control: the development and evaluation of an experimental treatment.* Lexington, MA: Heath.

Novaco, R. W. (1978). Anger and coping with stress: cognitive behavioral interventions. In J. P. Foreyt & D. P. Rathjen (Eds), *Cognitive behavior therapy: research and application.* New York: Plenum.

Nowack, K. M. (1989). Coping style, cognitive hardiness, and health status. *Journal of Behavioral Medicine*, 12, 145–58.

Nowak, M. (1998). The weight-conscious adolescent: body image, food intake and weight-related behavior. *Journal of Adolescent Health*, 23(6), 389–98.

Nowak, M., & Crawford, D. (1998). Getting the message across: adolescents' health concerns and views about the importance of food. *Australian Journal of Nutrition and Dietetics*, 55, 3–8.

Nowak, M., & Speare, R. (1996). Gender differences in food-related concerns, beliefs and behaviours of North Queensland adolescents. *Journal of Paediatric Child Health*, 32, 424–7.

Nowak, M., Speare, R., & Crawford, D. (1996). Gender differences in adolescent weight and shape-related beliefs and behaviours. *Journal of Paediatric Child Health*, 32, 148–52.

Nutbeam, D., Blakey, V., & Pates, R. (1991). The prevention of HIV infection from injecting drug use: a review of health promotion approaches. *Social Science and Medicine*, 33(9), 977–83.

Nutbeam, D., Wise, M., & Leeder, S. (1993). Achieving better health in Australia in the next five years. *Medical Journal of Australia*, 159, 503–4.

Nutbeam, D., Wise, M., Bauman, A., Harris, E., & Leeder, S. (1993). *Goals and targets for Australia's health in the year 2000 and beyond.* Canberra: AGPS.

Nyamathi, A., Bennett, C., Leake, B., Lewis, C., & Flaskerud, J. (1993). AIDS-related knowledge, perceptions, and behaviors among impoverished minority women. *American Journal of Public Health*, 83, 65–71.

Nystul, M. S. (1987). Transcendental meditation. In R. J. Corsini (Ed.), *Concise encyclopedia of psychology.* New York: John Wiley & Sons.

O'Brien, C. P. (1996). Recent developments in the pharmacotherapy of substance abuse. *Journal of Consulting and Clinical Psychology*, 64, 677–86.

O'Brien, S., & Lee, C. (1990). Effects of a videotape intervention on pap smear knowledge, attitudes and behaviour. *Behaviour Change*, 7(3), 143–50.

O'Connor, M. L., & Parker, E. (1995). *Health promotion: principles and practice in the Australian context.* St Leonards: Allen & Unwin.

Ockene, J. K., Hosmer, D., Rippe, J., Williams, J., Goldberg, R. J., Decosimo, D., Maher, P. M., & Dalen, J. E. (1985). Factors affecting cigarette smoking status in patients with ischemic heart disease. *Journal of Chronic Diseases*, 38, 985–94.

Ockene, J. K., Kristeller, J., Goldberg, R., Amick, T. L., Pekow, P. S., Hosmer, D., Quirk, M., & Kalan, K. (1991). Increasing the efficacy of physician-delivered smoking interventions. *Journal of General Internal Medicine*, 6, 1–8.

Ockene, J. K., Kristeller, J. L., Goldberg, R., Ockene, I., Merriam, P., Barrett, S., Pekow, P., Hosmer, D., & Gianelly, R. (1992). Smoking cessation and severity of disease: the Coronary Artery Smoking Intervention Study. *Health Psychology*, 11, 119–26.

Ockene, J. K., Kristeller, J. L., Pbert, L., Hebert, J. R., Luippold, R., Goldberg, R. J., Landon, J., & Kalan, K. (1994). The Physician-Delivered Smoking Intervention Project: Can short-term interventions produce long-term effects for a general outpatient population? *Health Psychology*, 13, 278–81.

Ockene, J. K., Kuller, L. H., Svendsen, K. H., & Meilahn, E. (1990). The relationship of smoking cessation to coronary heart disease and lung cancer in the Multiple Risk Factor Intervention Trial (MRFIT). *American Journal of Public Health*, 80, 954–8.

O'Connor, G. T., Buring, J. E., Yusuf, S., Goldhaber, S. Z., Olmstead, E. M., Paffenbarger, R. S., & Hennekens, C. H. (1989). An overview of randomized trials of rehabilitation with exercise after myocardial infarction. *Circulation*, 80, 234–44.

O'Donnell, L., O'Donnell, C. R., Pleck, J. H., Snarey, J., & Rose, R. M. (1987). Psychosocial responses of hospital workers to acquired immune deficiency syndrome (AIDS). *Journal of Applied Social Psychology*, 17, 269–85.

O'Dougherty, M., & Brown, R. T. (1990). The stress of childhood illness. In L. E. Arnold (Ed.), *Childhood stress.* New York: John Wiley & Sons.

Oei, T. P. S., & Burton, A. (1990). Attitudes toward smoking in 7 to 9 year old children. *International Journal of the Addictions*, 25(1), 43–52.

Oei, T. P. S., Lim B., & Young, R. M. (1991). Cognitive processes and cognitive behavior therapy in the treatment of problem drinking. *Journal of Addictive Diseases*, 10(3), 63–80.

Oginska-Bulik, N. (1998). Psychological correlates of the Type A behaviour pattern in children. *Polish Psychological Bulletin*, 29(4), 321–9.

Öhlund, C., Lindström, I., Areskoug, B., Eek, C., Peterson, L.-E., & Nachemson, A. (1994). Pain behavior in industrial subacute low back pain: Part I. Reliability: concurrent and predictive validity of pain behavior assessments. *Pain*, 58, 201–9.

Olafsson, O., & Svensson, P. (1986). Unemployment-related lifestyle changes and health disturbances in adolescents and children in the Western countries. *Social Science and Medicine*, 22, 1105–1113.

Olbrisch, M. E. (1996). Picking winners and grooming the dark horse: psychologists evaluate and treat organ transplant patients. *Health Psychologist*, 18(1), 10–11.

Oldenburg, B. (1994). Promotion of health: integrating the clinical and public health approaches. *International Review of Health Psychology*, 3, 121–43.

Oldenburg, B., & Owen, N. (1990). Health psychology in Australia. *Psychology and Health*, 4, 73–81.

Oldenburg, B., Andrews, G., & Perkins, R. J. (1985). Controlled trial of psychological intervention in myocardial infarction. *Journal of Consulting and Clinical Psychology*, 53, 852–9.

Oldenburg, B., & Perkins, R. (1984). Psychological intervention in myocardial infarction. Unpublished manuscript. Department of Psychiatry, Prince Henry Hospital, Sydney.

Oldenburg, B., Perkins, R. J., & Andrews, G. (1985). Controlled trial of psychological intervention in myocardial infarction. *Journal of Consulting and Clinical Psychology*, 53, 852–9.

Oldridge, N. B. (1984). Adherence to adult exercise fitness programs. In J. D. Matarazzo, S. M. Weiss, J. A. Herd, N. E. Miller & S. M. Weiss (Eds), *Behavioral health: a handbook of health enhancement and disease prevention*. New York: John Wiley & Sons.

Oldridge, N. B., & Spencer, J. (1985). Exercise habits and perceptions before and after graduation of dropout from supervised cardiac exercise rehabilitation. *Journal of Cardiopulmonary Rehabilitation*, 5, 313–19.

O'Leary, A., Shoor, S., Lorig, K., & Holman, H. R. (1988). Cognitive-behavioral treatment for rheumatoid arthritis. *Health Psychology*, 7, 527–44.

Olff, M., Brosschot, J. F., Godaert, G., Benschop, R. J., Ballieux, R. E., Heijnen, C. J., De Smet, M. B. M., & Ursin, H. (1995). Modulatory effects of defense and coping on stress-induced changes in endocrine and immune parameters. *International Journal of Behavioral Medicine*, 2, 85–103.

Olivet, L. W. (1982). Basic needs of the hospitalized child. In M. J. Smith, J. A. Goodman, N. L. Ramsey & S. B. Pasternack (Eds), *Child and family: concepts of nursing practice*. New York: McGraw-Hill.

Olshansky, S. J., Carnes, B. A., & Cassel, C. (1990). In search of Methuselah: estimating the upper limits to human longevity. *Science*, 250, 634–40.

Olson, D. H. (1997). Family stress and coping: a multisystem perspective. In S. Dreman (Ed.), *The family on the threshold of the 21st century: trends and implications* (pp. 259–80). Mahwah, NJ: Erlbaum.

Ong, L. M., Visser, M. R., Van Zuuren, F. J., Rietbroek, R. C., Lammes, F. B., de Haes, J. C. (1999). Cancer patients' coping styles and doctor–patient communication. *Psycho-oncology*, 8(2), 155–66.

Orford, J., & Edwards, G. (1977). *Alcoholism*. Maudsley Monographs No. 26. Oxford: Oxford University Press.

Orfutt, C., & Lacroix, J. M. (1988). Type A behavior pattern and symptom reports: a prospective investigation. *Journal of Behavioral Medicine*, 11, 227–37.

Orne, M. T. (1989). On the construct of hypnosis: how its definition affects research and its clinical application. In G. D. Burrows & L. Dennerstein (Eds), *Handbook of hypnosis and psychosomatic medicine*. Amsterdam: Elsevier.

Ornish, D., Brown, S. E., Scherwitz, L. W., Billings, J. H., Armstrong, W. T., Ports, T. A., McLanahan, S. M., Kirkeeide, R. L., Brand, R. J., & Gould, K. L. (1990). Can lifestyle changes reverse coronary heart disease: the Lifestyle Heart Trial. *The Lancet*, 336, 129–33.

O'Rourke, D. F., Houston, B. K., Harris, J. K., & Snyder, C. R. (1988). The Type A behavior pattern: summary, conclusions, and implications. In B. K. Houston & C. R. Snyder (Eds), *Type A behavior pattern: research, theory, and intervention*. New York: John Wiley & Sons.

Orpen, C. (1991). The effect of work stress on employee physical and psychological well-being: a study of Australian nurses. *Psychology — A Journal of Human Behavior*, 27(4)–28(1), 48–51.

Osborn, J. E. (1988). The AIDS epidemic: six years. In L. Breslow, J. E. Fielding & L. B. Lave (Eds), *Annual review of public health* (Vol. 9). Palo Alto, CA: Annual Reviews.

Owen, N., & Halford, K. (1988). Psychology, public health and cigarette smoking. *Australian Psychologist*, 23(2), 137–51.

Owen, N., & Oldenburg, B. (1992). Australian health psychology. In S. Maes, H. Leventhal & M. Johnston, *International Review of Health Psychology* (Vol. 1, pp. 211–25). Chichester: John Wiley & Sons.

Owen, N., James, R., Henrikson, D., & Van Beurden, E. (1990). Community cholesterol screenings: the impact of follow-up letters and incentives on retest rates and biometric changes in follow-up screenings. *American Journal of Health Promotion*, 5(1), 58–61.

Pallonen, U. E., Murray, D. M., Schmid, L., Pirie, P., Luepker, R. V. (1990). Patterns of self-initiated smoking cessation among young adults. *Health Psychology*, 9, 418–26.

Palmer, K. J., Langeluddecke, P. M., Jones, M., & Tennant, C. (1992). The relation of the Type A behaviour pattern, factors of the structured interview and anger to survival after myocardial infarction. *Australian Journal of Psychology*, 44(1), 13–19.

Pandey, S. (1999). Role of perceived control in coping with crowding. *Psychological Studies*, 44(3), 86–91.

Panico, S., Celentano, E., Krogh, V., Jossa, F., Farinaro, E., Trevisan, M., & Mancini, M. (1987). Physical activity and its relationship to blood pressure in school children. *Journal of Chronic Diseases*, 40, 925–30.

Pantaleo, G., Graziosi, C., Demarest, J. F., Butini, L., Montroni, M., Fox, C. H., Orenstein, J. M., Kotler, D. P., & Fauci, A. S. (1993). HIV infection is active and progressive in lymphoid tissue during the clinically latent stage of the disease. *Nature*, 362, 355–8.

Paoletti, P., Camilli, A. E., Holberg, C. J., & Lebowitz, M. D. (1985). Respiratory effects in relation to estimated tar exposure from current and cumulative cigarette consumption. *Chest*, 88, 849–55.

Parcel, G. S., Bruhn, J. G., & Cerreto, M. C. (1986). Longitudinal analysis of health and safety behaviors among school children. *Psychological Reports*, 59, 265–6.

Parfitt, R. R. (1977). *The birth primer*. Philadelphia, PA: Running Press.

Park, C. L. (1998). Stress-related growth and thriving through coping: the roles of personality and cognitive processes. *Journal of Social Issues*, 54(2), 267–77.

Parker, J. C. (1995). Stress management. In P. M. Nicassio & T. W. Smith (Eds), *Managing chronic illness: a biopsychosocial perspective*. Washington, DC: American Psychological Association.

Parker, J. C., Frank, R. G., Beck, N. C., Smarr, K. L., Buescher, K. L., Phillips, L. R., Smith, E. I., Anderson, S. K., & Walker, S. E. (1988). Pain management in rheumatoid arthritis patients: a cognitive-behavioral approach. *Arthritis and Rheumatism*, 31, 593–601.

Parker, J. C., Smarr, K. L., Walker, S. E., Hagglund, K. J., Anderson, S. K., Hewett, J. E., Bridges, A. J., & Caldwell, C. W. (1991). Biopsychosocial parameters of disease activity in rheumatoid arthritis. *Arthritis Care and Research*, 4, 73–80.

Parker, P. A., & Kulik, J. A. (1995). Burnout, self- and supervisor-rated job performance, and absenteeism among nurses. *Journal of Behavioral Medicine*, 18, 581–99.

Parker, S. K., & Sprigg, C. A. (1999). Minimizing strain and maximizing learning: the role of job demands, job control and proactive personality. *Journal of Applied Psychology*, 84(6), 925–39.

Parrish, J. M. (1986). Parent compliance with medical and behavioral recommendations. In N. A. Krasnegor, J. D. Arasteh & M. F. Cataldo (Eds), *Child health behavior: a behavioral pediatrics perspective*. New York: John Wiley & Sons.

Parsons, O. A. (1986). Alcoholics' neuropsychological impairment: current findings and conclusions. *Annals of Behavioral Medicine*, 8(2–3), 13–19.

Parsons, T. (1951). *The social system*. New York: Free Press.

Parsons, T. (1964). *Social structure and personality*. London: Collier-Macmillan & Co.

Partridge, C., & Johnston, M. (1989). Perceived control of recovery from physical disability: measurement and prediction. *British Journal of Clinical Psychology*, 28, 53–9.

Passer, M. W. (1982). Psychological stress in youth sports. In R. A. Magill, M. J. Ash & F. L. Smoll (Eds), *Children in sport* (2nd ed.). Champaign, IL: Human Kinetics.

Paterson, R. J., & Neufeld, R. W. J. (1987). Clear danger: situational determinants of the appraisal of threat. *Psychological Bulletin*, 101, 404–416.

Patrick, A. W., Gill, G. V., MacFarlane, I. A., Cullen, A., Power, E., & Wallymahmed, M. (1994). Home glucose monitoring in type 2 diabetes: is it a waste of time? *Diabetic Medicine*, 11, 62–5.

Patrick, K., Sallis, J. F., Long, B., Calfas, K. J., Wooten, W., Heath, G., & Pratt, M. (1994). A new tool for encouraging activity: Project PACE. *Physician and Sportsmedicine*, 22(11), 45–55.

Patterson, J. M., & Garwick, A. W. (1994). The impact of chronic illness on families: a family systems perspective. *Annals of Behavioral Medicine*, 16, 131–42.

Patterson, S. M., Matthews, K. A., Allen, M. T., & Owens, J. F. (1995). Stress-induced hemoconcentration of blood cells and lipids in healthy women during acute psychological stress. *Health Psychology*, 14, 319–24.

Patterson, S. M., Zakowski, S. G., Hall, M. H., Cohen, L., Wollman, K., & Baum, A. (1994). Psychological stress and platelet activation: differences in platelet reactivity in healthy men during active and passive stressors. *Health Psychology*, 13, 34–8.

Patterson, T. L., Shaw, W. S., Semple, S. J., Cherner, M., et al. (1996). Relationship of psychosocial factors to HIV disease progression. *Annals of Behavioral Medicine*, 18, 30–39.

Pattishall, E. G. (1989). The development of behavioral medicine: historical models. *Annals of Behavioral Medicine*, 11, 43–8.

Patton, G. C. (1992). Eating disorders: antecedents, evolution and course. *Annals of Medicine*, 24, 281–5.

Paulson, M. C. (1988, October). Fighting for your life. *Changing Times*, pp. 100–106.

Pavlov, I. P. (1927). *Conditioned reflexes*. New York: Oxford University Press.

Paxton, S. J., Wertheim, E. H., Gibbons, K., Szmukler, G. I., Hillier, L., & Petrovich, J. L. (1991). Body image satisfaction, dieting beliefs and weight loss behaviours in adolescent boys and girls. *Journal of Youth and Adolescence*, 20, 361–79.

Paykel, E. S., Prusoff, B. A., & Uhlenhuth, E. H. (1971). Scaling of life events. *Archives of General Psychiatry*, 25, 340–47.

Payne, R. L., & Jones, J. G. (1987). Measurement and methodological issues in social support. In S. V. Kasl & C. L. Cooper (Eds), *Stress and health: issues in research methodology*. New York: John Wiley & Sons.

Pearlin, L. I. (1991). The study of coping: an overview of problems and directions. In J. Eckenrode (Ed.), *The social context of coping* (pp. 261–76). New York: Plenum.

Pearlin, L. I. (1999). Stress and mental health: a conceptual overview. In A. V. Horwitz, T. L. Scheid (Eds), *A handbook for the study of mental health: social contexts, theories and systems*. New York: Cambridge University Press.

Pearlin, L. I., & McCall, M.E. (1990). Occupational stress and marital support: a description of microprocesses. In J. Eckenrode & S. Gore (Eds), *Stress between work and family* (pp. 39–60). New York: Plenum.

Pearlin, L. I., & Schooler, C. (1978). The structure of coping. *Journal of Health and Social Behavior*, 19, 2–21.

Pechacek, T. F., Fox, B. H., Murray, D. M., & Luepker, R. V. (1984). Review of techniques for measurement of smoking behavior. In J. D. Matarazzo, S. M. Weiss, J. A. Herd, N. E. Miller & S. M. Weiss (Eds), *Behavioral health: a handbook of health enhancement and disease prevention*. New York: John Wiley & Sons.

Pechacek, T. F., Murray, D. M., Luepker, R. V., Mittelmark, M. B., Johnson, C. A., & Shutz, J. M. (1984). Measurement of adolescent smoking behavior: rationale and methods. *Journal of Behavioral Medicine*, 7, 123–40.

Peck, A. (1972). Emotional reactions to having cancer. *American Journal of Roentgenology, Radium Therapy, and Nuclear Medicine*, 114, 591–9.

Peck, C. L., & King, N. J. (1985). Compliance and the doctor–patient relationship. *Drugs*, 30, 78–84.

Pedersen, N. L., Lichtenstein, P., Plomin, R., Defaire, U., McClearn, G. E., & Matthews, K. A. (1989). Genetic and environmental influences for Type A-like measures and related traits: a study of twins reared apart and twins reared together. *Psychosomatic Medicine*, 51, 428–40.

Pederson, L. L. (1982). Compliance with physician advice to quit smoking: a review of the literature. *Preventive Medicine*, 11, 71–84.

Peele, S. (1984). The cultural context of psychological approaches to alcoholism: can we control the effects of alcohol? *American Psychologist*, 39, 1337–51.

Peerbhoy, D., Hall, G., Parker, C., Shenkin, A., & Salmon, P. (1998). Patients' reactions to attempts to increase passive or active coping with surgery. *Social Science and Medicine*, 47(5), 595–601.

Peirce, R. S., Frone, M. R., Russell, M., & Cooper, M. L. (1996). Financial stress, social support, and alcohol involvement: a longitudinal test of the buffering hypothesis in a general population survey. *Health Psychology*, 15, 38–47.

Pendery, M. L., Maltzman, I. M., & West, L. J. (1982). Controlled drinking by alcoholics? New findings and a reevaluation of a major affirmative study. *Science*, 217, 169–75.

Penn, A., & Snyder, C. A. (1993). Inhalation of sidestream cigarette smoke accelerates development of arteriosclerotic placques. *Circulation*, 88 (Part 1), 1820–25.

Pennebaker, J. W. (1983). Accuracy of symptom perception. In A. Baum, S. E. Taylor & J. Singer (Eds), *Handbook of psychology and health* (Vol. 4). Hillsdale, NJ: Erlbaum.

Pennebaker, J. W. (1990). *Opening up: the healing power of confiding in others*. New York: William Morrow.

Pennebaker, J. W., & Watson, D. (1988). Blood pressure estimation and beliefs among normotensives and hypertensives. *Health Psychology*, 7, 309–328.

Perini, C., Nil, R., Bolli, P., Bättig, K., & Bühler, F. R. (1993). Ischemic ECG changes are found more often in asymptomatic men with coronary prone behaviour pattern. *Journal of Psychosomatic Research*, 37, 355–60.

Perkins, J. J., Sanson-Fisher, R. W., Blunden, S., Lunnay, D., Redman, S., & Hensley, M. J. (1994). The prevalence of drug use in urban Aboriginal communities. *Addiction*, 89, 1319–31.

Perkins, J. J., Sanson-Fisher, R. W., Girgis, A., Blunden, S., & Lunnay, D. (1995). The development of a new methodology to assess perceived needs among indigenous Australians. *Social Science and Medicine*, 41(2), 267–75.

Perkins, K. A. (1985). The synergistic effect of smoking and serum cholesterol on coronary heart disease. *Health Psychology*, 4, 337–60.

Perkins, K. A. (1994). Issues in the prevention of weight gain after smoking cessation. *Annals of Behavioral Medicine*, 16, 46–52.

Perkins, K. A., Rohay, J., Meilahn, E. N., Wing, R. R., Matthews, K. A., & Kuller, L. H. (1993). Diet, alcohol, and physical activity as a function of smoking status in middle-aged women. *Health Psychology*, 12, 410–15.

Perri, M. G., McAllister, D. A., Gange, J. J., Jordan, R. C., McAdoo, W. G., & Nezu, A. M. (1988). Effects of four maintenance programs on the long-term management of obesity. *Journal of Consulting and Clinical Psychology*, 56, 529–34.

Perri, M. G., Nezu, A. M., & Viegener, B. J. (1992). *Improving the long-term management of obesity*. New York: John Wiley & Sons.

Perz, C. A., DiClemente, C. C. & Carbonari, J. P. (1996). Doing the right thing at the right time? The interaction of stages and processes of change in successful smoking cessation. *Health Psychology*, 15, 462–8.

Pescatello, L. S., Fargo, A. E., Leach, C. N., & Scherzer, H. H. (1991). Short-term effect of dynamic exercise on arterial blood pressure. *Circulation*, 83, 1557–61.

Peter, L. J. (1969). *The Peter Principle*. New York: Morrow.

Peterman, T. A. (1990). Facilitators of HIV transmission during sexual contact. In N. J. Alexander, H. L. Gabelnick & J. M. Spieler (Eds), Heterosexual transmission of AIDS. New York: John Wiley & Sons.

Peterson, C., Beck, K., & Rowell, G. (1992). *Psychology: an introduction for nurses and allied health professionals*. New York: Prentice Hall.

Peterson, J. L., & Marán, G. (1988). Issues in the prevention of AIDS among black and Hispanic men. *American Psychologist*, 43, 871–7.

Peterson, L., & Mori, L. (1988). Preparation for hospitalisation. In D. K. Routh (Ed.), *Handbook of paediatric psychology* (pp. 460–91). New York: Guilford.

Petruzello, S. J., Landers, D. M., Hatfield, B. D., Kubitz, K. A., & Salazar, W. (1991). A meta-analysis on the anxiety-reducing effects of acute and chronic exercise. *Sports Medicine*, 11(3), 143–82.

Peveler, R. C., & Johnston, D. W. (1986). Subjective and cognitive effects of relaxation. *Behaviour Research and Therapy*, 24, 413–19.

Phares, E. J. (1984). *Introduction to personality*. Columbus, OH: Merrill.

Phares, E. J. (1987). Locus of control. In R. J. Corsini (Ed.), *Concise encyclopedia of psychology*. New York: John Wiley & Sons.

Philips, C. A. (1989). Rehabilitation of the patient with rheumatoid hand involvement. *Physical Therapy*, 69, 1091–8.

Pickard, B. (1986). Dairy products and red meat — villains or victims. In D. Anderson (Ed.), *A diet of reason* (pp. 21–39). London: Social Affairs Unit.

Pierce, G. R., Sarason, B. R., & Sarason, I. G. (1990). Integrating social support perspectives: working models, personal relationships and situational factors. In S. Duck with R. C. Silver (Eds), *Personal relationships and social support*. London: Sage.

Pierce, J. P., & Gilpin, E. A. (1995). A historical analysis of tobacco marketing and the uptake of smoking by youth in the United States: 1890–1977. *Health Psychology*, 14, 500–508.

Pilisuk, M. (1982). Delivery of social support: the social inoculation. *American Journal of Orthopsychiatry*, 52, 20–31.

Pillitteri, A. (1981). *Child health nursing: care of the growing family* (2nd ed.). Boston, MA: Little, Brown.

Pinkowish, M. D. (1999). Recognizing posttraumatic stress. *Patient Care*, 33(16), 171–83.

Pinto, R. P., & Hollandsworth, J. G. (1989). Using videotape modeling to prepare children psychologically for surgery: influence of parents and costs versus benefits of providing preparation services. *Health Psychology*, 8, 79–95.

Piotrowski, C., & Lubin, B. (1990). Assessment practices of health psychologists: survey of APA Division 38 clinicians. *Professional Psychology: Research and Practice*, 21, 99–106.

Place, M. (1984). Hypnosis and the child. *Journal of Child Psychology and Psychiatry*, 25, 339–47.

Plotnikoff, R. C., & Higginbotham, N. (1995). Predicting low-fat diet intentions and behaviours for the prevention of coronary heart disease: an application of protection motivation theory among an Australian population. *Psychology and Health*, 10, 397–408.

Pohl, S. L., Gonder-Frederick, L., & Cox, D. J. (1984). Diabetes mellitus: an overview. *Behavioral Medicine Update*, 6(1), 3–7.

Polich, J. M., Armor, D. J., & Braiker, H. B. (1981). *The course of alcoholism: four years after treatment*. New York: John Wiley & Sons.

Polivy, J., & Herman, C. P. (1985). Dieting and bingeing: a causal analysis. *American Psychologist*, 40, 193–201.

Polivy, J., & Thomsen, L. (1988). Dieting and other eating disorders. In E. A. Blechman & K. D. Brownell (Eds), *Handbook of behavioral medicine for women*. New York: Pergamon.

Pollack, A. C., & Steklis, H. D. (1986). Urinary catecholamines and stress in male and female police cadets. *Human Biology*, 58, 209–220.

Pollard, B. J. (1991). Withdrawing life sustaining treatment from severely brain damaged persons. *Medical Journal of Australia*, 154, 559–61.

Pollock, A. (1995). Where should health services go: local authorities versus the NHS. *British Medical Journal*, 310, 1580–84.

Pollock, S. E. (1989). The hardiness characteristic: a motivating factor in adaptation. *Advances in Nursing Science*, 11(2), 53–62.

Pollock, S. E., Christian, B. J., & Sands, D. (1990). Responses to chronic illness: analysis of psychological and physiological adaptation. *Nursing Research*, 39(5), 300–304.

Pollock, S. E., Christian, B. J., & Sands, D. (1991). Responses to chronic illness: analysis of psychological and physiological adaptation. *Nursing Research*, 39, 300–304.

Pollock, S. E., & Duffy, M. E. (1990). The health-related hardiness scale: development and psychometric analysis. *Nursing Research*, 39(4); 218–22.

Polonsky, W. H., Anderson, B. J., Lohrer, P. A., Aponte, J. E., Jacobson, A. M., & Cole, C. F. (1994). Insulin omission in women with IDDM. *Diabetes Care*, 17, 1178–85.

Pomerleau, O. F., Collins, A. C., Shiffman, S., & Pomerleau, C. S. (1993). Why some people smoke and others do not: new perspectives. *Journal of Consulting and Clinical Psychology*, 61, 723–31.

Pomerleau, O. F., & Pomerleau, C. S. (1989). A biobehavioral perspective on smoking. In T. Ney & A. Gale (Eds), *Smoking and human behavior*. New York: John Wiley & Sons.

Pope, M. K., & Smith, T. W. (1991). Cortisol excretion in high and low cynically hostile men. *Psychosomatic Medicine*, 53, 386–392.

Population Health Division (2000). *Australia HIV/AIDS Figures*. Commonwealth Department of Health and Aged Care. http:www.health.gov.au:80/pubhlth/strateg/hiv_hepc/hiv/figure.htm.

Porges, S. W. (1992). Vagal tone: a physiological marker of stress vulnerability. *Pediatrics*, 90, 498–504.

Porges, S. W. (1995). Cardiac vagal tone: a physiological index of stress. *Neuroscience and Behavioral Reviews*, 19, 225–33.

Porter, F. L., Miller, R. H., & Marshall, R. E. (1986). Neonatal pain cries: effects of circumcision on acoustic features and perceived urgency. *Child Development*, 57, 790–802.

Pothmann, R., Frankenberg, S. V., Müller, B., Sartory, G., & Hellmeier, W. (1994). Epidemiology of headache in children and adolescents: evidence of high prevalence of migraine among girls under 10. *International Journal of Behavioral Medicine*, 1, 76–89.

Powch, I. G., & Houston, B. K. (1996). Hostility, anger-in, and cardiovascular reactivity in white women. *Health Psychology*, 15, 200–208.

Powell, K. C. (1988). *Drinking and alcohol in colonial Australia 1788-1901 for the Eastern Colonies*. National Campaign Against Drug Abuse, Monograph Series No. 3. Canberra: AGPS.

Powell, K. E., Thompson, P. D., Caspersen, C. J., & Kendrick, J. S. (1987). Physical activity and the incidence of coronary heart disease. In L. Breslow, J. E. Fielding & L. B. Lave (Eds), *Annual review of public health* (Vol. 8). Palo Alto, CA: Annual Reviews.

Powell, L. H. (1984). The Type A behavior pattern: an update on conceptual, assessment, and intervention research. *Behavioral Medicine Update*, 6(4), 7–10.

Powell, L. H. (1987). Issues in the measurement of the Type A behaviour pattern. In S. V. Kasl & C. L. Cooper (Eds), *Stress and health: issues in research methodology*. Chichester: John Wiley & Sons.

Powell, L. H., & Friedman, M. (1986). Alteration of Type A behaviour in coronary patients. In M. J. Christie & P. G. Mellett (Eds), *The psychosomatic approach: contemporary practice of whole-person care*. New York: John Wiley & Sons.

Powell, L. H., Friedman, M., Thoresen, C. E., Gill, J. J., & Ulmer, D. K. (1984). Can the Type A behavior pattern be altered after myocardial infarction? A second year report from the Recurrent Coronary Prevention Project. *Psychosomatic Medicine*, 46, 293–313.

Praeger, S. G., & Liebenberg, A. (1994). Strategies for helping adolescents access health care in Western Australia. *Family and Community Health*, 17(2), 60–64.

Pratt, K., & Borland, R. (1994). Predictors of sun protection among adolescents at the beach. *Australian Psychologist*, 29(2), 135–9.

Presley, R. W., & Cousins, M. J. (1992). Current concepts in chronic pain management. *Current Therapeutics*, 18, 51–60.

Price, R. A., Cadoret, R. J., Stunkard, A. J., & Troughton, E. (1987). Genetic contributions to human fatness: an adoption study. *American Journal of Psychiatry*, 144, 1003–8.

Priest, R. G. (1986). Benzodiazepines: the search for tranquillity. In M. J. Christie & P. G. Mellett (Eds), The psychosomatic approach: contemporary practice of whole-person care. New York: John Wiley & Sons.

Pritchard, D. A., Straton, J. A., & Hyndman, J. (1995). Cervical screening in general practice. *Australian Journal of Public Health*, 19(2), 167–72.

Prochaska, J. O., & DiClemente, C. C. (1984). *The transtheoretical approach: crossing traditional boundaries of therapy*. Homewood, IL: Dow Jones/Irwin.

Prochaska, J. O., DiClemente, C. C., & Norcross, J. C. (1992). In search of how people change: applications to addictive behaviors. *American Psychologist*, 47, 1102–1114.

Prochaska, J. O., Johnson, S., & Lee, P. (1998). The transtheoretical model of behavior change. In S. A. Shumaker, E. B. Schron, J. K. Ockene & W. L. McBee (Eds), *The handbook of health behavior change* (2nd ed.) (pp. 59–83). New York: Springer.

Prohaska, T. R., Keller, M. L., Leventhal, E. A., & Leventhal, H. (1987). Impact of symptoms and aging attribution on emotions and coping. *Health Psychology*, 6, 495–514.

Ptacek, J., Smith R. E., & Dodge, K. L. (1994). Gender differences in coping with stress: when stressor and appraisals do not differ. *Personality and Social Psychology Bulletin*, 20, 421–30.

Ptacek, J., Smith, R., & Zanas, J. (1992). Gender, appraisal and coping: a longitudinal analysis. *Journal of Personality*, 60, 747–70.

Pugh, K., Riccio, M., Jadresic, D., Burgess, A. P., Baldeweg, T., Catalan, J., Lovett, E., Hawkins, D. A., Gruzelier, J., & Thompson, C. (1994). A longitudinal study of the neuropsychiatric consequences of HIV-1 infection in gay men. II. Psychological and health status at baseline and at 12–month follow-up. *Psychological Medicine*, 24, 897–904.

Puleo, P. R., Meyer, D., Wathen, C., & Tawa, C. B., et al. (1994). Use of rapid assay of subforms of creatine kinase MB to diagnose or rule out acute myocardial infarction. *New England Journal of Medicine*, 331, 561–6.

Purcell, K., Weiss, J., & Hahn, W. (1972). Certain psychosomatic disorders. In B. B. Wolman (Ed.), *Manual of child psychopathology*. New York: McGraw-Hill.

Quay, H. C., & La Greca, A. M. (1986). Disorders of anxiety, withdrawal, and dysphoria. In H. C. Quay & J. S. Werry (Eds), *Psychopathological disorders of childhood* (3rd ed.). New York: John Wiley & Sons.

Quick, J. C., & Quick, J. D. (1984). *Organizational stress and preventive management*. New York: McGraw-Hill.

Quine, S., & Stephenson, J. A. (1990). Predicting smoking and drinking intentions and behavior of pre-adolescents: the influence of parents, siblings, and peers. *Family Systems Medicine*, 8(2), 191–200.

Radecki, S. E., & Brunton, S. A. (1992). Health promotion/disease prevention in family practice residency training: results of a national survey. *Family Medicine*, 24, 534–7.

Ragland, D. R., & Brand, R. J. (1988). Type A behavior and mortality from coronary heart disease. *New England Journal of Medicine*, 318, 65–9.

Rahe, R. H. (1974). The pathway between subjects' recent life changes and their near-future illness reports: representative results and methodological issues. In B. S. Dohrenwend & B. P. Dohrenwend (Eds), *Stressful life events: their nature and effects*. New York: John Wiley & Sons.

Rahe, R. H., & Arthur, R. J. (1978). Life change and illness studies: past history and future directions. *Journal of Human Stress*, 4, 3–15.

Rainville, P., Feine, J. S., Bushnell, M. C., & Duncan, G. H. (1992). A psychophysical comparison of sensory and affective responses to four modalities of experimental pain. *Somatosensory and Motor Research*, 9, 265, 277.

Rakowski, W., Dube, C. E., Marcus, B. H., Prochaska, J. O., Velicer, W. F., & Abrams, D. B. (1992). Assessing elements of women's decisions about mammography. *Health Psychology*, 11, 111–18.

Ramsey, N. L. (1982). Effects of hospitalization on the child and family. In M. J. Smith, J. A. Goodman, N. L. Ramsey & S. B. Pasternack (Eds), *Child and family: concepts of nursing practice*. New York: McGraw-Hill.

Raphael, K. G., Cloitre, M., & Dohrenwend, B. P. (1991). Problems of recall and misclassification with checklist methods of measuring stressful life events. *Health Psychology*, 10, 62–74.

Rappaport, N. B., McAnulty, D. P., Waggoner, C. D., & Brantley, P. J. (1987). Cluster analysis of Minnesota Multiphasic Personality Inventory (MMPI) profiles in a chronic headache population. *Journal of Behavioral Medicine*, 10, 49–60.

Raps, C. S., Peterson, C., Jonas, M., & Seligman, M. E. P. (1982). Patient behavior in hospitals: helplessness, reactance, or both? *Journal of Personality and Social Psychology*, 42, 1036–41.

Rassaby, J., & Hill, D. (1983). Patient's perceptions of breast reconstruction following mastectomy. *Medical Journal of Australia*, 2, 173–6.

Ratliff-Crain, J., & Baum, A. (1990). Individual differences and health: gender, coping, and stress. In H. S. Friedman (Ed.), *Personality and disease*. New York: John Wiley & Sons.

Raven, B. H., & Haley, R. W. (1982). Social influence and compliance of hospital nurses with infection control policies. In J. R. Eiser (Ed.), *Social psychology and behavioral medicine*. New York: John Wiley & Sons.

Raymond, N. R., & D'Eramo-Melkus, G. (1993). Non-insulin-dependent diabetes and obesity in the black and Hispanic population: culturally sensitive management. *Diabetes Educator*, 19, 313–17.

Rector, N. A., & Roger, D. (1997). The stress buffering effects of self-esteem. *Personality and Individual Differences*, 23(5), 799–808.

Redd, W. H., Silberfarb, P. M., Andersen, B. L., Andrykowski, M. A., et al. (1991). Physiologic and psychobehavioral research in oncology. *Cancer*, 67, 813–22.

Reddy, D, M., Fleming, R., & Adesso, V. J. (1992). Gender and health. In S. Maes, H. Leventhal & M. Johnston (Eds), *International review of health psychology* (Vol. 1). New York: John Wiley & Sons.

Redman, S., Dickinson, J. A., Hennrikus, D. J., & Sanson-Fisher, R. W. (1989). The assessment of reactivity in direct observation studies of doctor–patient interactions. *Psychology and Health*, 3, 17–28.

Reed, G. M., Kemeny, M. E., Taylor, S. E., Wang, H.-Y., & Visscher, B. R. (1994). Realistic acceptance as a predictor of decreased survival time in gay men with AIDS. *Health Psychology*, 13, 299–307.

Rejeski, W.J., Thompson, A., Brubaker, P. H., & Miller, H. S. (1992). Acute exercise: buffering psychosocial stress responses in women. *Health Psychology*, 11, 355–62.

Reichman, W. E. (1990, Fall). Dementia of the Alzheimer type: identification and management of neuropsychiatric features. *The Older Patient*, pp. 4–8.

Reid, A., Lynskey, M., & Copeland, J. (2000). Cannabis use among Australian adolescents: findings of the 1998 National Drug Strategy Household Survey. *Australian and New Zealand Journal of Public Health*, 24(6), 596–602.

Reifman, A. (1995). Social relationships, recovery from illness, and survival: a literature review. *Annals of Behavioral Medicine*, 17, 124–31.

Reiman, E. M., Casellu, R. J., Yun, L. S., Chen, K., Bandy, D., Minoshima, S. L., Thibodeau, S. N., & Osborne, D. (1996). Preclinical evidence of Alzheimer's disease in persons homozygous for the ε4 allele for apolipoprotein E. *New England Journal of Medicine*, 334, 752–8.

Reinis, S., & Goldman, J. M. (1980). *The development of the brain: biological and functional perspectives*. Springfield, IL: Charles C. Thomas.

Reisch, L. M., Wiehl, L. G., & Tinsley, B. J. (1994, August). Health locus of control and health-related behaviours — a meta-analytic review. Paper presented at the meeting of the American Psychological Association in Los Angeles.

Reker, G. T., & Wong, P. T. P. (1985). Personal optimism, physical and mental health. In J. E. Birren & J. Livingston (Eds), Cognition, stress, and aging. Englewood Cliffs, NJ: Prentice Hall.

Retchin, S. M., Wells, J. A., Valleron, A.-J., & Albrecht, G. L. (1992). Health behavior changes in the United States, the United Kingdom, and France. *Journal of General Internal Medicine*, 7, 615–22.

Revenson, T. A. (1994). Social support and marital coping with chronic illness. *Annals of Behavioral Medicine*, 16, 122–30.

Revenson, T. A., & Majerovitz, S. D. (1991). The effects of chronic illness on the spouse: social resources as stress buffers. *Arthritis Care and Research*, 4, 63–72.

Reynolds, J. Dommers, E., & Spillman, D. (1994). Toward a framework for school-based food and nutrition education. *Journal of the HEIA*, 1(4), 19–32.

Reynolds, W. J., & Scott, B. (2000). Do nurses and other professional helpers normally display much empathy? *Journal of Advanced Nursing*, 31, 226–34.

Rhoades, R., & Pflanzer, R. (1996). *Human physiology* (3rd ed.). Fort Worth, TX: Saunders.

Ribisl, P. M. (1984). Developing an exercise prescription for health. In J. D. Matarazzo, S. M. Weiss, J. A. Herd, N. E. Miller & S. M. Weiss (Eds), *Behavioral health: a handbook of health enhancement and disease prevention*. New York: John Wiley & Sons.

Rice, P. L. (1992). *Stress and health* (2nd ed.). Pacific Grove: Brooks/Cole.

Richards, J. C. (1992). Training health psychologists: a model for the future. *Australian Psychologist*, 27, 87–90.

Richards, J. C. (1994). Giving psychology away? A comment on health care, psychology, and the scientist-practitioner model by James (1994). *Australian Psychologist*, 29(1), 12–14.

Richards, J. S., Nepomuceno, C., Riles, M., & Suer, Z. (1982). Assessing pain behavior: the UAB Pain Behavior Scale. *Pain*, 14, 393–8.

Richardson, J. L., Marks, G., Johnson, C. A., Graham, J. W., Chan, K. K., Selser, J. N., Kishbaugh, C., Barranday, Y., & Levine, A. M. (1987). Path model of multidimensional compliance with cancer therapy. *Health Psychology*, 6, 183–207.

Richardson, S. A., Goodman, N., Hastorf, A. H., & Dornbusch, S. M. (1961). Cultural uniformity in reaction to physical disabilities. *American Sociological Review*, 26, 241–7.

Richmond, R. L., & Webster, I. W. (1985). A smoking cessation programme for use in general practice. *Medical Journal of Australia*, 142, 190–94.

Rietveld, S., & Prins, P. J. (1998). Children's perception of physical symptoms: the example of asthma. *Advances in Clinical Child Psychology*, 20, 153–82.

Rietveld, S., Prins, P. J., & Kolk, A. M. (1996). The capacity of children with and without asthma to detect external restive loads on breathing. *Journal of Asthma*, 33, 221–30.

Rigby, K., Brown, M. Anagnostou, P., Ross, M. W., & Rosser, B. R. S. (1989). Shock tactics to counter AIDS: the Australian experience. *Psychology and Health*, 3, 145–59.

Rigotti, N. A., Singer, D. E., Mulley, A. G., & Thibault, G. E. (1991). Smoking cessation following admission to a coronary care unit. *Journal of General Internal Medicine*, 6, 305–311.

Rimer, B. K. (1994). Mammography use in the U.S.: trends and the impact of interventions. *Annals of Behavioral Medicine*, 16, 317–26.

Rimm, E. B., Giovannucci, E. L., Willett, W. C., Colditz, G. A., Ascherio, A., Rosner, B., & Stampfer, M. J. (1991). Prospective study of alcohol consumption and risk of coronary disease. *The Lancet*, 338, 464–8.

Risser, N. L., & Belcher, D. W. (1990). Adding spirometry, carbon monoxide, and pulmonary symptom results to smoking cessation counseling: a randomized trial. *Journal of General Internal Medicine*, 5, 16–22.

Roads and Traffic Authority. (1998). *Road traffic accidents in New South Wales, 1996*. Sydney: RTA.

Rob, M., Reynolds, I., & Finlayson, P. F. (1990). Adolescent marijuana use: risk factors and implications. *Australian and New Zealand Journal of Psychiatry*, 24, 47–56.

Roback, H. B. (1984). Introduction: The emergence of disease-management groups. In H. B. Roback (Ed.), *Helping patients and their families cope with medical problems*. San Francisco: Jossey-Bass.

Robbins, L. (1994). Precipitating factors in migraine: a retrospective review of 494 patients. *Headache*, 34, 214–16.

Roberts, A. H. (1986). The operant approach to the management of pain and excess disability. In A. D. Holzman & D. C. Turk (Eds), *Pain management: a handbook of psychological treatment approaches*. New York: Pergamon.

Roberts, A. H. (1995). The powerful placebo revisited: magnitude of nonspecific effects. *Mind/Body Medicine*, 1, 35–43.

Roberts, C. S., Cox, C. E., Reintgen, D. S., Baile, W. F., & Gilbertini, M. (1994). Influence of physician communication on newly diagnosed breast patients' psychologic adjustment and decision-making. *Cancer*, 74, 336–41.

Robins, C. J., & Hayes, A. M. (1993). An appraisal of cognitive therapy. *Journal of Consulting and Clinical Psychology*, 61, 205–214.

Robinson, C. H., & Lawler, M. R. (1977). *Normal and therapeutic nutrition* (15th ed.). New York: Macmillan.

Robinson, M. E., Wise, E. A., Riley, J. L., & Atchison, J. W. (1998). Sex differences in clinical pain: a multisample study. *Journal of Clinical Psychology in Medical Settings*, 5(4), 413–24.

Rodenhuis, S., Van De Wetering, M. L., Moor, W. J., Evers, S. G., Van Zandwijk, N., & Bos, J. L. (1987). Mutational activation of the K-ras oncogene. *New England Journal of Medicine*, 317, 929–35.

Rodin, J. (1981). Current status of the internal–external hypothesis for obesity: what went wrong? *American Psychologist*, 36, 361–372.

Rodin, J. (1985). Insulin levels, hunger, and food intake: an example of feedback loops in body weight regulation. *Health Psychology*, 4, 1–24.

Rodin, J. (1986). Health, control, and aging. In M. M. Baltes & P. B. Baltes (Eds), *The psychology of control and aging*. Hillsdale, NJ: Erlbaum.

Rodin, J. (1987). Personal control throughout the life course. In R. P. Abeles (Ed.), Life-span perspectives and social psychology. Hillsdale, NJ: Erlbaum.

Rodin, J., & Baum, A. (1978). Crowding and helplessness: potential consequences of density and loss of control. In A. Baum & Y. M. Epstein (Eds), Human response to crowding. Hillsdale, NJ: Erlbaum.

Rodin, J., & Janis, I. L. (1979). The social power of health-care practitioners as agents of change. Journal of Social Issues, 35, 60–81.

Rodin, J., & Langer, E. J. (1977). Long-term effects of a control-relevant intervention with the institutionalized aged. Journal of Personality and Social Psychology, 35, 897–902.

Rodriguez, B. L., Curb, J. D., Burchifiel, C. M., Abbott, R. D., Petrovitch, H., Masaki, K., & CHIU, D. (1994). Physical activity and 23-year incidence of coronary heart disease morbidity and mortality among middle-aged men: the Honolulu Heart Program. Circulation, 89, 2540–44.

Rogentine, G. N., Van Kammen, D. P., Fox, B. H., Docherty, J. P., Rosenblatt, J. E., Boyd, S. C., & Bunney, W. E. (1979). Psychological factors in the prognosis of malignant melanoma: a prospective study. Psychosomatic Medicine, 41, 647–55.

Rogers, M. P., Dubey, D., & Reich, P. (1979). The influence of the psyche and the brain on immunity and disease susceptibility: a critical review. Psychosomatic Medicine, 41, 147–64.

Rogers, P. (1994, September 19). Surviving the second wave. Newsweek, pp. 50–51.

Rogers, W. H., Draper, D., Kahn, K. L., Keeler, E. B., Rubenstein, L. V., Kosecoff, J., & Brook, R. H. (1990). Quality of care before and after implementation of the DRG-based prospective payment system. Journal of the American Medical Association, 264, 1989–94.

Rohling, M. L., Binder, L. M., & Langhinrichsen-Rohling, J. (1995). A meta-analytic review of the association between financial compensation and the experience and treatment of chronic pain. Health Psychology, 14, 537–47.

Rolls, B. J. (1995). Carbohydrates, fats, and satiety. American Journal of Clinical Nutrition, 61 (Suppl.), 960S–967S.

Rona, R. J., Angelico, F., Antonini, R., Arca, M., et al. (1985). Plasma cholesterol response to a change in dietary fat intake: a collaborative twin study. Journal of Chronic Diseases, 38, 927–34.

Rook, K. S., & Schuster, T. L. (1996). Compensatory processes in the social networks of older adults. In G. R. Pierce, B. R. Sarason & I. G. Sarason (Eds), Handbook of social support and the family (pp. 219–48). New York: Plenum.

Rose, J. S., Chassin, L., Presson, C. C., & Sherman, S. J. (1996). Prospective predictors of quit attempts and smoking cessation in young adults. Health Psychology, 15, 261–8.

Rose, K. J., Derry, P. A., & McLachlan, R. S. (1995). Patient expectations and postoperative depression, anxiety, and psychosocial adjustment after temporal lobectomy: a prospective study. International Journal of Behavioral Medicine, 2, 27–40.

Rose, R. J. (1986). Familial influences on cardiovascular reactivity to stress. In K. A. Matthews, S. M. Weiss, T. Detre, T. M. Dembroski, B. Falkner, S. B. Manuck & R. B. Williams (Eds), Handbook of stress, reactivity, and cardiovascular disease. New York: John Wiley & Sons.

Rosen, J. C., Grubman, J. A., Bevins, T., & Frymoyer, J. W. (1987). Musculoskeletal status and disability of MMPI profile subgroups among patients with low back pain. Health Psychology, 6, 581–98.

Rosenhan, D. L., & Seligman, M. E. P. (1984). Abnormal psychology. New York: Norton.

Rosenman, R. H. (1978). The interview method of assessment of the coronary-prone behavior pattern. In T. M. Dembroski, S. M. Weiss, J. L. Shields, S. G. Haynes & M. Feinleib (Eds), Coronary-prone behavior. New York: Springer-Verlag.

Rosenman, R. H., Brand, R. J., Jenkins, C. D., Friedman, M., Straus, R., & Wurm, M. (1975). Coronary heart disease in the Western Collaborative Group Study: final follow-up experience of $8\frac{1}{2}$ years. Journal of the American Medical Association, 233, 872–7.

Rosenman, R. H., Brand, R. J., Sholtz, R. I., & Friedman, M. (1976). Multivariate prediction of coronary heart disease during 8.5 year follow-up in the Western Collaborative Group Study. American Journal of Cardiology, 37, 903–910.

Rosenman, R. H., Swan, G. E., & Carmelli, D. (1988). Definition, assessment, and evolution of the Type A behavior pattern. In B. K. Houston & C. R. Snyder (Eds), Type A behavior pattern: research, theory, and intervention. New York: John Wiley & Sons.

Rosenstiel, A. K., & Keefe, F. J. (1983). The use of coping strategies in chronic low back pain patients: relationship to patient characteristics and current adjustment. Pain, 17, 33–44.

Rosenstock, I. M. (1966). Why people use health services. Millbank Memorial Fund Quarterly, 44, 94–127.

Rosenstock, I. M. (1985). Understanding and enhancing patient compliance with diabetic regimens. Diabetes Care, 8, 610–16.

Rosenstock, I. M., & Kirscht, J. P. (1979). Why people seek health care. In G. C. Stone, F. Cohen & N. E. Adler (Eds), Health psychology — a handbook. San Francisco: Jossey-Bass.

Rosenthal, D. A., Hall, C., & Moore, S. M. (1992). AIDS, Adolescents, and sexual risk taking: a test of the health belief model. Australian Psychologist, 27(3), 166–71.

Rosenthal, E. (1992, November 24). Commercial diets lack proof of their long-term success. New York Times, pp. A1, C11.

Roskies, E. (1983). Stress management for Type A individuals. In D. Meichenbaum & M. E. Jaremko (Eds), Stress reduction and prevention. New York: Plenum.

Roskies, E., Kearney, H., Spevack, M., Surkis, A., Cohen, C., & Gilman, S. (1979). Generalizability and durability of treatment effects in an intervention program for coronary-prone (Type A) managers. Journal of Behavioral Medicine, 2, 195–207.

Roskies, E., Seraganian, P., Oseasohn, R., Hanley, J. A., Collu, R., Martin, N., & Smilga, C. (1986). The Montreal Type A Intervention Project: major findings. Health Psychology, 5, 45–69.

Roskies, E., Spevack, M., Surkis, A., Cohen, C., & Gilman, S. (1978). Changing the coronary-prone (Type A) behavior pattern in a nonclinical population. Journal of Behavioral Medicine, 1, 201–216.

Ross, R., & Glomset, J. A. (1976a). The pathogenesis of atherosclerosis (part 1). New England Journal of Medicine, 295, 369–77.

Ross, R., & Glomset, J. A. (1976b). The pathogenesis of atherosclerosis (part 2). New England Journal of Medicine, 295, 420–25.

Ross, C. E., & Mirowsky, J. (1979). A comparison of life-event weighting schemes: change, undesirability and effect-proportional indices. Journal of Health and Social Behavior, 20(2), 166–77.

Ross, M. W., & McLaws, M. L. (1992). Subjective norms about condoms are better predictors of use and intention to use than attitudes. Health Education Research, 7(3), 335–9.

Ross, M. W., Rigby, K., Rosser, B. R. S., Anagnostou, P., & Brown, M. (1990), The effect of a national campaign on attitudes toward AIDS. Aids Care, 2(4), 339–46.

Ross, M. W., & Rosser, B. R. S. (1989). Education and AIDS risks: a review. Health Education Research, 4(3), 273–84.

Rosser, B. R. S. (1991). The effects of using fear in public AIDS education on the behaviour of homosexually active men. Journal of Psychology & Human Sexuality, 4(3), 123–34.

Rotem, T. R., Lawson, J. S., Wilson, S., Engel, A. Rutkowski, S. B., & Aisbett, C. W. (1998). Severe cervical spinal cord injuries related to rugby union and league football in New South Wales, 1984–1996. Medical Journal of Australia, 168, 379–81.

Roter, D. (1989). Which facets of communication have strong effects on outcome: a meta-analysis. In M. Stewart & D. Roter (Eds), Communicating with medical patients (pp. 183–96). Newbury Park, CA: Sage.

Roter, D. L., & Ewart, C. K. (1992). Emotional inhibition in essential hypertension: obstacle to communication during medical visits? *Health Psychology*, 11, 163–9.

Roter, D. L., & Hall, J. A. (1989). Studies of doctor–patient interaction. In L. Breslow, J. E. Fielding & L. B. Lave (Eds), *Annual review of public health* (Vol. 10). Palo Alto, CA: Annual Reviews.

Roth, D. L., & Holmes, D. S. (1985). Influence of physical fitness in determining the impact of stressful life events on physical and psychologic health. *Psychosomatic Medicine*, 47, 164–73.

Rotheram-Borus, M. J., Murphy, D. A., Reid, H. M., & Coleman, C. L. (1996). Correlates of emotional distress among HIV+ youths: health status, stress, and personal resources. *Annals of Behavioral Medicine*, 18, 16–23.

Rotter, J. B. (1966). Generalized expectancies for the internal versus external control of reinforcement. *Psychological Monographs*, 90(1), 1–28.

Rouse, K. A., Ingersoll, G. M., & Orr, D. P. (1998). Longitudinal health endangering behavior risk among resilient and nonresilient early adolescents. *Journal of Adolescent Health*, 23(5), 297–302.

Roviaro, S., Holmes, D. S., & Holmsten, R. D. (1984). Influence of a cardiac rehabilitation program on the cardiovascular, psychological, and social functioning of cardiac patients. *Journal of Behavioral Medicine*, 7, 61–81.

Rowbotham, M. C., & Lowenstein, D. H. (1990). Neurologic consequences of cocaine use. In W. P. Creger, C. H. Coggins & E. W. Hancock (Eds), *Annual review of medicine* (Vol. 41). Palo Alto, CA: Annual Reviews.

Roy, R. (1985). Chronic pain and marital difficulties. *Health and Social Work*, 10, 199–207.

Rozin, P. (1989). The role of learning in the acquisition of food preferences by humans. In R. Shepherd (Ed.), *Handbook of the psychophysiology of human eating*. Chichester: John Wiley & Sons.

Rozin, P., & Fallon, A. E. (1981). Th acquisition of likes and dislikes for foods (pp. 35–48). In J. Solms & R. L. Hall (Eds), *Criteria of food acceptance*. Zurich: Forster.

Rubin, J. Z., Provenzano, F. J., & Luria, Z. (1974). The eye of the beholder: parents' views on sex of newborns. *American Journal of Orthopsychiatry*, 44, 512–19.

Rubinfeld, A. R., & Pain, M. C. (1977). Conscious perception of bronchospasm as a protective phenomenon in asthma, *Chest*, 72, 154.

Ruderman, A. J. (1986). Dietary restraint: a theoretical and empirical review. *Psychological Bulletin*, 99, 247–62.

Ruffin, R. E., Wilson, D., Southcott, A. M., Smith, B., & Adams, R. J. (1999). A South Australian population survey of the ownership of asthma action plans. *Medical Journal of Australia*, 171, 348–51.

Ruge, A., & Lee, C. (1995). Inpatient cervical screening: a survey of patient acceptability. *Australian Journal of Public Health*, 19(1), 96–7.

Runyan, C. W. (1985). Health assessment and public policy within a public health framework. In P. Karoly (Ed.), *Measurement strategies in health psychology*. New York: John Wiley & Sons.

Rutter, M. (1983). Stress, coping, and development: some issues and some questions. In N. Garmezy & M. Rutter (Eds), *Stress, coping, and development in children*. New York: McGraw-Hill.

Ryan, R. S., & Travis, J. W. (1981). *The wellness workbook*. Berkeley, CA: Ten Speed Press.

Rybstein-Blinchik, E. (1979). Effects of different cognitive strategies on chronic pain experience. *Journal of Behavioral Medicine*, 2, 93–101.

Rzewnicki, R., & Forgays, D. G. (1987). Recidivism and self-cure of smoking and obesity: an attempt to replicate. *American Psychologist*, 42, 97–100.

Sabbioni, M. E. E. (1991). Cancer and stress: a possible role for psychoneuroimmunology in cancer research? In C. L. Watson & M. Watson (Eds), *Cancer and stress: psychological, biological, and coping studies*. New York: John Wiley & Sons.

Sacks, D. A., & Koppes, R. H. (1986). Blood transfusion and Jehovah's Witnesses: medical and legal issues in obstetrics and gynecology. *American Journal of Obstetrics and Gynecology*, 154, 483–6.

Safer, M. A., Tharps, Q. J., Jackson, T. C., & Leventhal, H. (1979). Determinants of three stages of delay in seeking care at a medical clinic. *Medical Care*, 17, 11–29.

Sallis, J. F., Patterson, T. L., Buono, M. J., Atkins, C. J., & Nader, P. R. (1988). Aggregation of physical activity habits in Mexican-American and Anglo families. *Journal of Behavioral Medicine*, 11, 31–41.

Sallis, J. F., Trevorrow, T. R., Johnson, C. C., Hovell, M. F., & Kaplan, R. M. (1987). Worksite stress management: a comparison of programs. *Psychology and Health*, 1, 237–55.

Salonen, J. T. (1987). Did the North Karelia project reduce coronary mortality? *The Lancet*, August, 1, 269.

Salvaggio, A., Periti, M., Miano, L., & Zambelli, C. (1990). Association between habitual coffee consumption and blood pressure levels. *Journal of Hypertension*, 8, 585–90.

Sanchez-Menegay, C., Hudes, E. S., & Cummings, S. R. (1992). Patient expectations and satisfaction with medical care for upper respiratory infections. *Journal of General Internal Medicine*, 7, 432–4.

Sandberg, G. G., & Marlatt, G. A. (1991). Relapse prevention. In D. A. Ciraulo & R. I. Shader (Eds), *Clinical manual of chemical dependence*. Washington, DC: American Psychiatric Press.

Sanders, G. S. (1982). Social comparison and perceptions of health and illness. In G. S. Sanders & J. Suls (Eds), *Social psychology of health and illness*. Hillsdale, NJ: Erlbaum.

Sanders, J. D., Smith, T. W., & Alexander, J. F. (1991). Type A behavior and marital interaction: hostile-dominant responses during conflict. *Journal of Behavioral Medicine*, 14, 567–80.

Sanders, S. H. (1985). Chronic pain: conceptualization and epidemiology. *Annals of Behavioral Medicine*, 7(3), 3–5.

Sanders, S. H., Brena, S. F., Spier, C. J., Beltrutti, D., McConnell, H., & Quintero, O. (1992). Chronic low back pain patients around the world: cross-cultural similarities and differences. *Journal of Clinical Pain*, 8, 317–23.

Sandler, I. N., & Guenther, R. T. (1985). Assessment of life stress events. In P. Karoly (Ed.), *Measurement strategies in health psychology*. New York: John Wiley & Sons.

Sanson, A., Dickens, E., Melita, B., Nixon, M., Rowe, J., Tudor, A., & Tyrrell, M. (1998). Psychological perspectives on euthanasia and the terminally ill: an Australian Psychological Society discussion paper. *Australian Psychologist*, 33(1), 1–11.

Sanson-Fisher, R. (1993). Primary and secondary prevention of cancer: opportunities for behavioural scientists. In S. Maes, H. Leventhal & M. Johnston (Eds), *Interdisciplinary review of health psychology* (Vol. 2). New York: John Wiley & Sons.

Sanson-Fisher, R. W., & Newell, S. (1996). Population health psychology: the new challenge. In In P. R. Martin & J. S. Birnbrauer (Eds), *Clinical psychology: profession and practice in Australia*. Hong Kong: Macmillan.

Sanson-Fisher, R. W., Schofield, M. J., & Perkins, J. (1993). Behaviour therapy's role in preventing physical illness. *Behaviour Change*, 10(1), 25–31.

Sanson-Fisher, R., Byrne, D., Cameron-Traub, E., Dunn, S., Goodall, T., Halford, K., Harris, R., Heather, N., Hill, D., Martin, P., Owen, N., Peck, C., & Sanders, M. (1990). Report to the Australian Psychological Society on the Status and future directions of Health Psychology in Australia. Unpublished report: Australian Psychological Society, Parkville, Victoria.

Sanson-Fisher, R., Redman, S., Homel, R., & Key, W. (1990). Drink driver rehabilitation programs: an Australian perspective. *Alcohol, Drugs and Driving*, 6(3–4), 133–45.

Santiago, J. V. (1984). Effect of treatment on the long term complications of IDDM. *Behavioral Medicine Update*, 6(1), 26–31.

Sapolsky, R. M. (1999). The physiology and pathophysiology of unhappiness. In D. Kahneman, E. Diener, N. Schwarz & E. Diener (Eds), *Well-being: the foundations of hedonic psychology* (pp. 453–69). New York: Russell Sage.

Sapon-Shevin, M. (1980). Teaching cooperation in early childhood settings. In G. Cartledge & J. F. Milburn (Eds), *Teaching social skills to children: innovative approaches*. New York: Pergamon.

Sarafino, E. P. (1986). *The fears of childhood: a guide to recognizing and reducing fearful states in children*. New York: Human Sciences Press.

Sarafino, E. P. (1987a). Personal space. In R. J. Corsini (Ed.), *Concise encyclopedia of psychology*. New York: John Wiley & Sons.

Sarafino, E. P. (1987b). Rewards and intrinsic interest. In R. J. Corsini (Ed.), *Concise encyclopedia of psychology*. New York: John Wiley & Sons.

Sarafino, E. P. (1996). *Principles of behavior change: understanding behavior modification techniques*. New York: John Wiley & Sons.

Sarafino, E. P. (1997a). *Behavioral approaches in the treatment of asthma*. Lewiston, NY: Edwin Mellon Press.

Sarafino, E. P. (1997b). Hassles Assessment Scale for Students in College (HASS/Col): preliminary version. Unpublished manuscript.

Sarafino, E. P., & Armstrong, J. W. (1986). *Child and adolescent development* (2nd ed.). St. Paul, MN: West.

Sarafino, E. P., & Dillon, J. M. (1996). Relationships among respiratory infections, triggers of attacks, and asthma severity in children. Paper submitted for publication.

Sarafino, E. P., & DiMattia, P. A. (1978). Does grading undermine intrinsic interest in a college course? *Journal of Educational Psychology*, 70, 916–21.

Sarafino, E. P., Eastlack, S. C., & McCarthy, C. P. (1994). Connections among parent and child atopic illnesses. Paper presented at the meeting of the Society of Behavioral Medicine in Boston.

Sarafino, E. P., & Goldfedder, J. (1995). Genetic factors in the presence, severity, and triggers of asthma. *Archives of Disease in Childhood*, 73, 112–16.

Sarason, B. R., Pierce, G. R., & Sarason, I. G. (1990). Social support: the sense of acceptance and the role of relationships. In B. R. Sarason, I. G. Sarason & G. R. Pierce (Eds), *Social support: an interactional view*. New York: John Wiley & Sons.

Sarason, B. R., Shearin, E. N., Pierce, G. R., & Sarason, I. G. (1987). Interrelations of social support measures: theoretical and practical implications. *Journal of Personality and Social Psychology*, 52, 813–32.

Sarason, I. G., & Sarason, B. R. (1981). The importance of cognition and moderator variables in stress,. In D. Magnusson (Ed.), *Toward a psychology of situations: an interactional perspective* (pp. 195–211). Hillsdale. NJ: Erlbaum.

Sarason, I. G., & Sarason, B. R. (1984). *Abnormal psychology* (4th ed.). Englewood Cliffs, NJ: Prentice Hall.

Sarason, I. G., Johnson, J. H., & Siegel, J. M. (1978). Assessing the impact of life changes: development of the Life Experiences Survey. *Journal of Consulting and Clinical Psychology*, 46, 932–46.

Sarason, I. G., Levine, H. M., Basham, R. B., & Sarason, B. R. (1983). Assessing social support: the Social Support Questionnaire. *Journal of Personality and Social Psychology*, 44, 127–39.

Sarason, I. G., Sarason, B. R., & Johnson, J. H. (1985). Stressful life events: measurement, moderators and adaptation. In S. R. Burchfield (Ed.), *Stress: psychological and physiological interactions* (pp. 241–61). Washington, DC: Hemisphere.

Sarason, I. G., Sarason, B. R., Potter, E. H., & Antoni, M. H. (1985). Life events, social support, and illness. *Psychosomatic Medicine*, 47, 156–63.

Sartory, G., Mueller, B., Metsch, J., & Pothmann, R. (1998). A comparison of psychological and pharmacological treatment of pediatric migraine. *Behaviour Research and Therapy*, 36(12), 1155–70.

Saunders, C. (1977). Dying they live: St. Christopher's Hospice. In H. Feifel (Ed.), *New meanings of death*. New York: McGraw-Hill.

Saunders, C. (1986). A philosophy of terminal care. In M. J. Christie & P. G. Mellett (Eds), *The psychosomatic approach: contemporary practice of whole-person care*. New York: John Wiley & Sons.

Saunders, K. J., Pilgrim, C. A., & Pennypacker, H. S. (1986). Increased proficiency of search in breast selfexamination. *Cancer*, 58, 2531–7.

Scambler, G. (1984). Perceiving and coping with stigmatizing illness. In R. Fitzpatrick, J. Hinton, S. Newman, G. Scambler & J. Thompson (Eds), *The experience of illness*. London: Tavistock.

Scambler, G. (1997). Epilepsy. In A. Baum, S. Newman, J. Weinman, R. West & C. McManus (Eds), *Cambridge handbook of psychology, health and medicine* (pp. 457–9). Cambridge: Cambridge University Press.

Scarf, M. (1980, September). Images that heal: a doubtful idea whose time has come. *Psychology Today*, pp. 33–46.

Scarr, S., & Kidd, K. K. (1983). Developmental behavior genetics. In P. H. Mussen (Ed.), *Handbook of child psychology* (4th ed., Vol. 2). New York: John Wiley & Sons.

Schachter, S. (1971). Some extraordinary facts about obese humans and rats. *American Psychologist*, 26, 129–44.

Schachter, S. (1980). Urinary pH and the psychology of nicotine addiction. In P. O. Davidson & S. M. Davidson (Eds), *Behavioral medicine: changing health lifestyles*. New York: Brunner/Mazel.

Schachter, S. (1982). Recidivism and self cure of smoking and obesity. *American Psychologist*, 37, 436–44.

Schachter, S., Silverstein, B., Kozlowski, L. T., Perlick, D., Herman, C. P., & Liebling, B. (1977). Studies of the interaction of psychological and pharmacological determinants of smoking. *Journal of Experimental Psychology: General*, 106, 3–40.

Schachter, S., & Singer, J. E. (1962). Cognitive, social, and physiological determinants of emotional state. *Psychological Review*, 69, 379–99.

Schachter, S., & Singer, J. E. (1979). Comments on the Maslach and Marshall-Zimbardo experiments. *Journal of Personality and Social Psychology*, 37, 989–95.

Schaefer, C., Coyne, J.C., & Lazarus, R. S. (1981). The health-related functions of social support. *Journal of Behavioral Medicine*, 4, 381-406.

Schafer, L. C., Glasgow, R. E., & McCaul, K. D. (1982). Increasing the adherence of diabetic adolescents. *Journal of Behavioral Medicine*, 5, 353–62.

Schaie, K. W. (1965). A general model for the study of developmental problems. *Psychological Bulletin*, 64, 92–107.

Schain, W. S., D'Angelo, T. M., Dunn, M. E., Lichter, A. S., & Pierce, L. J. (1994). Mastectomy versus conservative surgery and radiation therapy. *Cancer*, 73, 1221–8.

Schaubroeck, J., & Merritt, D. E. (1997). Divergent effects of job control on coping with work stressors: the key role of self-efficacy. *Academy of Management Journal*, 40(3), 738–54.

Schechter, N. L., Allen, D. A., & Hanson, K. (1986). Status of pediatric pain control: a comparison of hospital analgesic usage in children and adults. *Pediatrics*, 77, 11–15.

Scheier, L. M., Botvin, G. J., & Miller, N. L. (1999). Life events, neighborhood stress, psychosocial functioning and alcohol use among urban minority youth. *Journal of child and Adolescent Substance Abuse*, 9(1), 19–50.

Scheier, M. F., & Bridges, M. W. (1995). Person variables and health: personality predispositions and acute psychological states as shared determinants for disease. *Psychosomatic Medicine*, 57, 255–68.

Scherer, K. R. (1986). Voice, stress, and emotion. In M. H. Appley & R. Trumbull (Eds), *Dynamics of stress: physiological, psychological, and social perspectives*. New York: Plenum.

Schiffman, H. R. (1976). *Sensation and perception: an integrated approach*. New York: John Wiley & Sons.

Schifter, D. E., & Ajzen, I. (1985). Intention, perceived control, and weight loss: an application of the theory of planned behavior. *Journal of Personality and Social Psychology*, 45, 843–51.

Schleifer, S. J., Scott, B., Stein, M., & Keller, S. E. (1986). Behavioral and developmental aspects of immunity. *Journal of the American Academy of Child Psychiatry*, 26, 751–63.

Schmeider, R., Friedrich, G., Neus, H., Rüdel, H., & Von Eiff, A. W. (1983). The influence of beta-blockers on cardiovascular reactivity and Type A behavior pattern in hypertensives. *Psychosomatic Medicine*, 45, 417–23.

Schmidt, L. R., & Dlugosch, G. E. (1991). Health psychology within the European health care systems. In M. A. Jansen & J. Weinman (Eds), *The international development of health psychology*. Chur, Switzerland: Harwood.

Schmitt, F. E., & Wooldridge, P. (1973). Psychological preparation of surgical patients. *Nursing Research*, 22(2), 108–116.

Schnall, P. L., Pieper, C., Schwartz, J. E., Karasek, R. A., Schlussel, Y., Devereux, R. B., Ganau, A., Alderman, M., Warren, K., & Pickering, T. G. (1990). The relationship between 'job strain', workplace diastolic blood pressure, and left ventricular mass index: results of a case-control study. *Journal of the American Medical Association*, 263, 1929–35.

Schneider, A. M., & Tarshis, B. (1975). *An introduction to physiological psychology*. New York: Random House.

Schneiderman, N., & Hammer, D. (1985). Behavioral medicine approaches to cardiovascular disorders. In N. Schneiderman & J. T. Tapp (Eds), *Behavioral medicine: the biopsychosocial approach*. Hillsdale, NJ: Erlbaum.

Schoenberg, N. E., Amey, C.H., & Coward, R. T. (1998). Stories of meaning: lay perspectives on the origin and management of non-insulin dependent diabetes mellitus among older women in the United States. *Social Science and Medicine*, 47(12), 2113–25.

Schoenborn, C. A. (1993). The Alameda Study — 25 years later. In S. Maes, H. Leventhal & M. Johnston (Eds), *International review of health psychology* (Vol. 2). New York: John Wiley & Sons.

Schofield, H. L., Bloch, S., Nankervis, J., Murphy, B., Singh, B. S., & Herrman, H. E. (1999). Health and well-being of women family carers: a comparative study with a generic focus. *Australian New Zealand Journal of Public Health*, 23, 585–9.

Schofield, M. J., Sanson-Fisher, R., Halpin, S., & Redman, S. (1994). Notification and follow-up of pap test results: current practices and women's preferences. *Preventive Medicine: An International Journal Devoted to Practice and Theory*, 23(3), 276–83.

Schrader, H., Oelieniene, D., Bovim, G., Surkiene, D., Mickeviciene, D., Miseviciene, I., & Sand, T. (1996). Natural evolution of late whiplash syndrome outside the medicolegal context. *The Lancet*, 347, 1207–1211.

Schuckit, M. A. (1985). Genetics and the risk for alcoholism. *Journal of the American Medical Association*, 254, 2614–17.

Schuckit, M. A. (1996). Recent developments in the pharmacotherapy of alcohol dependence. *Journal of Consulting and Clinical Psychology*, 64, 669–76.

Schulz, R. (1976). Effects of control and predictability on the physical and psychological well-being of the institutionalized aged. *Journal of Personality and Social Psychology*, 33, 563–73.

Schulz, R., & Hanusa, B. H. (1978). Long-term effects of control and predictability-enhancing interventions: findings and ethical issues. *Journal of Personality and Social Psychology*, 36, 1194–1201.

Schultz, R., O'Brien, A. T., Bookwala, J., & Fleissner, K. (1995). Psychiatric and physical morbidity effects of dementia caregiving: prevalence, correlates and causes. *The Gerontologist*, 35(6), 771–91.

Schunk, D. H., & Carbonari, J. P. (1984). Self-efficacy models. In J. D. Matarazzo, S. M. Weiss, J. A. Herd, N. E. Miller & S. M. Weiss (Eds), *Behavioral health: a handbook of health enhancement and disease prevention*. New York: John Wiley & Sons.

Schuster, C. R., & Kilbey, M. M. (1992). Prevention of drug abuse. In J. M. Last & R. B. Wallace (Eds), *Maxcy-Rosenau-Last public health and preventive medicine* (13th ed.). Norwalk, CT: Appleton & Lange.

Schuster, C. S. (1986). Biophysical development of the adolescent. In C. L. Schuster & S. S. Ashburn (Eds), *The process of human development: a holistic life-span approach*. Boston: Little, Brown.

Schutz, H. G., & Diaz-Knauf, K. V. (1989). The role of the mass media in influencing eating. In R. Shepherd (Ed.), *Handbook of the psychophysiology of human eating*. Chichester: John Wiley & Sons.

Schwartz, G. E. (1982). Testing the biopsychosocial model: the ultimate challenge facing behavioral medicine? *Journal of Consulting and Clinical Psychology*, 50, 1040–53.

Schwartz, S. P., & Blanchard, E. B. (1990). Inflammatory bowel disease: a review of the psychological assessment and treatment literature. *Annals of Behavioral Medicine*, 12, 95–105.

Schwartzberg, N. S., & Dytell, R. S. (1996). Dual earner families: the importance of work stress and family stress for psychological well-being. *Journal of Occupational Health Psychology*, 1(2), 211–23.

Schwarzer, R., & Schroeder, K. (1997). Effects of self-efficacy and social support on postsurgical recovery of heart patients. *Irish Journal of Psychology*, 18(1), 88–103.

Scinto, L. F. M., Daffner, K. R., Dressler, D., Ransil, B. I., Rentz, D., Weintraub, S., Mesaulam, M., & Potter, H. (1994). A potential noninvasive neurobiological test for Alzheimer's disease. *Science*, 266, 1051–3.

Sears, S. J., & Milburn, J. (1990). School-age stress. In L. E. Arnold (Ed.), *Childhood stress*. New York: John Wiley & Sons.

Seddon, L., & Berry, N. (1996). Media-induced disinhibition of dietary restraint. *British Journal of Health Psychology*, 1, 27–33.

Seeman, M., & Seeman, T. E. (1983). Health behavior and personal autonomy: a longitudinal study of the sense of control in illness. *Journal of Health and Social Behavior*, 24, 144–60.

Seeman, T. E., & McEwen, B. S. (1996). Impact of social environment characteristics on neuroendocrine regulation. *Psychosomatic Medicine*, 58, 459–71.

Seidenberg, M., & Berent, S. (1992). Childhood epilepsy and the role of psychology. *American Psychologist*, 47, 1130–33.

Self, C. A., & Rogers, R. W. (1990). Coping with threats to health: effects of persuasive appeals on depressed, normal, and antisocial personalities. *Journal of Behavioral Medicine*, 13, 343–57.

Seliger, S. (1986). Stress can be good for you. In M. G. Walraven & H. E. Fitzgerald (Eds), *Annual editions: Psychology 86/87*. Guilford, CT: Dushkin.

Seligman, M. E. P. (1975). *Helplessness: on depression, development, and death*. San Francisco: Freeman.

Seligmann, J., & Sulavik, C. (1992, April 27). Software for hard issues. *Newsweek*, p. 55.

Selye, H. (1956). *The stress of life*. New York: McGraw-Hill.

Selye, H. (1974). *Stress without distress*. Philadelphia: Lippincott.

Selye, H. (1976). *Stress in health and disease*. Reading, MA: Butterworth.

Selye, H. (1985). History and present status of the stress concept. In A. Monat & R. S. Lazarus (Eds), *Stress and coping* (2nd ed.). New York: Columbia University Press.

Seraganian, P., Roskies, E., Hanley, J. A., Oseasohn, R., & Collu, R. (1987). Failure to alter psychophysiological reactivity in Type A men with physical exercise and stress management programs. *Psychology and Health*, 1, 195–213.

Serdula, M. K., Ivery, D., Coates, R. J., Freedman, D. S., Williamson, D. F., & Byers, T. (1993). Do obese children become obese adults? A review of the literature. *Preventive Medicine*, 22, 167–77.

Serdula, M. K., Williamson, D. F., Anda, R. F., Levy, A., Heaton, A., & Byers, T. (1994). Weight control practices in adults: results of a multistate telephone survey. *American Journal of Public Health*, 84, 1821–4.

Serfass, R. C., & Gerberich, S. G. (1984). Exercise for optimal health: strategies and motivational considerations. *Preventive Medicine*, 13, 79–99.

Severson, H. H. (1993). Smokeless tobacco: risks, epidemiology, and cessation. In C. T. Orleans & J. Slade (Eds), *Nicotine addiction: principles and management.* New York: Oxford University Press.

Severson, H. H., & Lichtenstein, E. (1986). Smoking prevention programs for adolescents: rationale and review. In N. A. Krasnegor, J. D. Arasteh & M. F. Cataldo (Eds), *Child health behavior: a behavioral pediatrics perspective.* New York: John Wiley & Sons.

Sgandurra, A., Cipolat, L., Petrini, F., & Martinelli, G. (1998). Anesthesia and psychology in the elderly patient. *Archives of Gerontology and Geriatrics*, 6, 487–90.

Shadel, W. G., & Mermelstein, R. (1993). Cigarette smoking under stress: the role of coping expectancies among smokers in a clinic-based smoking cessation program. *Health Psychology*, 12, 443–50.

Shah, M., & Jeffery, R. W. (1991). Is obesity due to overeating and inactivity, or to a defective metabolic rate? A review. *Annals of Behavioral Medicine*, 13, 73–81.

Shanas, E., & Maddox, G. L. (1985). Health, health resources, and the utilization of care. In R. H. Binstock & E. Shanas (Eds), *Handbook of aging and the social sciences.* New York: Van Nostrand-Reinhold.

Shapiro, A. P., Krantz, D. S., & Grim, C. E. (1986). Pharmacologic agents as modulators of stress. In K. A. Matthews, S. M. Weiss, T. Detre, T. M. Dembroski, B. Falkner, S. B. Manuck & R. B. Williams (Eds), *Handbook of stress, reactivity, and cardiovascular disease.* New York: John Wiley & Sons.

Shapiro, D., & Goldstein, I. B. (1982). Biobehavioral perspectives on hypertension. *Journal of Consulting and Clinical Psychology*, 50, 841–58.

Sharpley, C. F., Dua, J. K., Reynolds, R., & Acosta, A. (1995). The direct and relative efficacy of cognitive hardiness, Type A behaviour pattern, coping behaviour and social support as predictors of stress and ill-health. *Scandinavian Journal of Behaviour Therapy*, 24, 15–29.

Shaw, R. E., Cohen, F., Doyle, B., & Palesky, J. (1985). The impact of denial and repressive style on information gain and rehabilitation outcomes in myocardial infarction patients. *Psychosomatic Medicine*, 47, 262–73.

Shekelle, R. B., Hulley, S. B., Neaton, J. D., Billings, J. H., Borhani, N. O., Gerace, T. A., Jacobs, D. R., Lasser, N. L., Mittelmark, M. B., & Stamler, J. (1985). The MRFIT Behavior Pattern Study: II. Type A behavior and incidence of coronary heart disease. *American Journal of Epidemiology*, 122, 559–70.

Sheppard, J. L. (Ed.) (1982). *Advances in behavioural medicine* (Vol. 1). Sydney: Cumberland College of Health Sciences.

Sheppard, J. L. (Ed.). (1989). *Advances in behavioural medicine.* (Vol. 6). Sydney: Cumberland College of Health Sciences.

Shepperd, S. L., Solomon, L. J., Atkins, E., Foster, R. S., & Frankowski, B. (1990). Determinants of breast self-examination among women of lower income and lower education. *Journal of Behavioral Medicine*, 13, 359–71.

Sheridan, K. (1991). Psychosocial services for persons with human immunodeficiency virus disease. In J. J. Sweet, R. H. Rozensky & S. M. Tovian (Eds), *Handbook of clinical psychology in medical settings.* New York: Plenum.

Sherif, M., & Sherif, C. W. (1953). *Groups in harmony and tension.* New York: Harper.

Sherliker, L., & Steptoe, A. (2000).Coping with new treatment of cancer: a feasibility study of daily diary measures. *Patient Education and Counseling*, 40(1), 11–19.

Sherwood, A., & Turner, J. R. (1995). Hemodynamic responses during psychological stress: Implications for studying disease processes. *International Journal of Behavioral Medicine*, 2, 193–218.

Shewchuk, R. M., Elliott, T. R., MacNair-Semands, R. R., & Harkins, S. (1999). Triat influences on stress appraisal and coping: an evaluation of alternative frameworks. *Journal of Applied Social Psychology*, 29(4), 685–704.

Shiffman, S. (1986). A cluster-analytic classification of smoking relapse episodes. *Addictive Behaviors*, 11, 295–307.

Shiffman, S. (1993). Smoking cessation treatment: any progress? *Journal of Consulting and Clinical Psychology*, 61, 718–22.

Shiffman, S., Fischer, L. B., Zettler-Segal, M., & Benowitz, N. L. (1990). Nicotine exposure among nondependent smokers. *Archives of General Psychiatry*, 47, 333–6.

Shiffman, S., Hickcox, M., Paty, J. A., Gnys, M., Kassel, J. D., & Richards, T. J. (1996). Progression from a smoking lapse to relapse: prediction from abstinence violation effects, nicotine dependence, and lapse characteristics. *Journal of Consulting and Clinical Psychology*, 64, 993–1002.

Shiffman, S., Paty, J. A., Gnys, M., Kassel, J. D., & Elash, C. (1995). Nicotine withdrawal in chippers and regular smokers: subjective and cognitive effects. *Health Psychology*, 14, 301–9.

Shillitoe, R. (1995). Diabetes mellitus. In A. Broome & S. Llewellyn (Eds), *Health Psychology: process and applications* (2nd ed.) (pp. 187–204). London: Chapman & Hall.

Shilton, T. (1993). School heart health promotion: the National Heart Foundation (Western Australian) approach. *Journal of School Health*, 63(3), 136–40.

Shipley, R. H., Butt, J. H., Horwitz, B., & Farbry, J. E. (1978). Preparation for a stressful medical procedure: effect of amount of stimulus preexposure and coping style. *Journal of Consulting and Clinical Psychology*, 46, 499–507.

Shneidman, E. S. (1977). The college student and death. In H. Feifel (Ed.), *New meanings of death.* New York: McGraw-Hill.

Shogren, E. (1988, June 3). Physicians favor death with 'dignity'. *Philadelphia Inquirer*, p. D14.

Shontz, F. C. (1975). *The psychological aspects of physical illness and disability.* New York: Macmillan.

Shopland, D. R., & Burns, D. M. (1993). Medical and public health implications of tobacco addiction. In C. T. Orleans & J. Slade (Eds), *Nicotine addiction: principles and management.* New York: Oxford University Press.

Shuchman, M., & Wilkes, M. (1986, September 28). Challenging the annual physical. *New York Times Magazine*, pp. 36–40.

Shuchman, M., & Wilkes, M. S. (1989, February 12). Asking — and telling. *New York Times Magazine*, pp. 45–6.

Shupe, D. R. (1985). Perceived control, helplessness, and choice: their relationship to health and aging. In J. E. Birren & J. Livingston (Eds), *Cognition, stress, and aging.* Englewood Cliffs, NJ: Prentice Hall.

Siegel, L. J., & Peterson, L. (1980). Stress reduction in young dental patients through coping skills and sensory information. *Journal of Consulting and Clinical Psychology*, 48, 785–7.

Siegel, W. C., & Blumenthal, J. A. (1991). The role of exercise in the prevention and treatment of hypertension. *Annals of Behavioral Medicine*, 13, 23–30.

Siegler, I. C., Feaganes, J. R., & Rimer, B. K. (1995). Predictors of adoption of mammography in women under age 50. *Annals of Behavioral Medicine*, 14, 274–8.

Siegman, A. W. (1993). Cardiovascular consequences of expressing, experiencing, and repressing anger. *Journal of Behavioral Medicine*, 16, 539–69.

Sigelman, C., Maddock, A., Epstein, J., & Carpenter, W. (1993). Age differences in understandings of disease causality: AIDS, colds, and cancer. *Child Development*, 64, 272–84.

Sikkema, K. J., & Kelly, J. A. (1996). Behavioral medicine interventions can improve the quality-of-life and health of persons with HIV disease. *Annals of Behavioral Medicine*, 18, 40–48.

Silver, R. L., & Wortman, C. B. (1980). Coping with undesirable life events. In J. Garber & M. E. P. Seligman (Eds), *Human helplessness: theory and applications*. New York: Academic Press.

Simoni, J. M., Mason, H. R. C., Marks, G., Ruiz, M. S., Reed, D., & Richardson, J. L. (1995). Women's self-disclosure of HIV infection: rates, reasons, and reactions. *Journal of Consulting and Clinical Psychology*, 63, 474–8.

Simons-Morton, B. G., Parcel, G. S., O'Hara, N. M., Blair, S. N., & Pate, R. R. (1988). Health-related physical fitness in childhood: status and recommendations. In L. Breslow, J. E. Fielding & L. B. Lave (Eds), *Annual review of public health* (Vol. 9). Palo Alto, CA: Annual Reviews.

Simonton, O. C., & Simonton, S. S. (1975). Belief systems and the management of emotional aspects of malignancy. *Journal of Transpersonal Psychology*, 7, 29–47.

Sims, E. A. H. (1974). Studies in human hyperphagia. In G. A. Bray & J. E. Bethune (Eds), *Treatment and management of obesity*. New York: Harper & Row.

Sims, E. A. H. (1976). Experimental obesity, dietary-induced thermogenesis, and their clinical implications. *Clinics in Endocrinology and Metabolism*, 5, 377–95.

Sinclair, C., Borland, R., Davidson, M., & Noy, S. (1994). *From Slip! Slop! Slap! to SunSmart: a profile of a health education campaign*. Anti-Cancer Council of Victoria.

Singer, J. E., & Davidson, L. M. (1986). Specificity and stress research. In M. H. Appley & R. Trumbull (Eds), *Dynamics of stress: physiological, psychological, and social perspectives*. New York: Plenum.

Sisson, R. W., & Azrin, N. H. (1986). Family-member involvement to initiate and promote treatment of problem drinkers. *Journal of Behavior Therapy and Experimental Psychiatry*, 17, 15–21.

Skelly, A. H., Marshall, J. R., Haughey, B. P., Davis, P. J., & Dunford, R. G. (1995). Self-efficacy and confidence in outcomes as determinants of self-care practices in inner-city, African-American women with non-insulin-dependent diabetes. *Diabetes Educator*, 21, 38–46.

Skelton, J. A., & Pennebaker, J. W. (1982). The psychology of physical symptoms and sensations. In G. S. Sanders & J. Suls (Eds), *Social psychology of health and illness*. Hillsdale, NJ: Erlbaum.

Skevington, S. M. (1990). A standardised scale to measure beliefs about controlling pain (BPCQ): a preliminary study. *Psychology and Health*, 4, 221–32.

Sklar, L. S., & Anisman, H. (1981). Stress and cancer. *Psychological Bulletin*, 89, 369–406.

Skolnick, A. S. (1986). *The psychology of human development*. San Diego, CA: Harcourt Brace Jovanovich.

Smart, C. R. (1994). Highlights of the evidence of benefit for women aged 40–49 years from the 14-year follow-up of the Breast Cancer Detection Demonstration Project. *Cancer*, 74, 296–300.

Smart, J. L. (1991). Critical periods in brain development. In D. J. P. Barker (Chair, Ciba Foundation Symposium, No. 156), *The childhood environment and adult disease*. New York: John Wiley & Sons.

Smith, B., & Zautra, A. J. (2000). Purpose in life and coping with knee-replacement surgery. *Occupational Therapy Journal of Research*, 20(1), 96–9.

Smith, C. A., & Wallston, K. A. (1992). Adaptation in patients with chronic rheumatoid arthritis: application of a general model. *Health Psychology*, 11, 151–62.

Smith, C. E., Fernengel, K., Holcorft, C., Gerald, K., & Marien, L. (1994). Meta-analysis of the associations between social support and health outcomes. *Annals of Behavioral Medicine*, 16, 352–62.

Smith, E. L. (1984). Special considerations in developing exercise programs for the older adult. In J. D. Matarazzo, S. M. Weiss, J. A. Herd, N. E. Miller & S. M. Weiss (Eds), *Behavioral health: a handbook of health enhancement and disease prevention*. New York: John Wiley & Sons.

Smith, G. S., & Kraus, J. F. (1988). Alcohol and residential, recreational, and occupational injuries: a review of the epidemiologic evidence. In L. Breslow, J. E. Fielding & L. B. Lave (Eds), *Annual review of public health* (Vol. 9). Palo Alto, CA: Annual Reviews.

Smith, J. B., & Autman, S. H. (1985). The experience of hospitalization. In L. L. Hayman & E. M. Sporing (Eds), *Handbook of pediatric nursing*. New York: John Wiley & Sons.

Smith, N. A., Seale, J. P., & Shaw, J. (1984). Medication compliance in children with asthma. *Australian Paediatric Journal*, 20, 47–51.

Smith, R. C., & Zimny, G. H. (1988). Physicians' emotional reactions to patients. *Psychosomatics*, 29, 392–7.

Smith, T. W. (1992). Hostility and health: current status of a psychosomatic hypothesis. *Health Psychology*, 11, 139–50.

Smith, T. W., & Anderson, N. B. (1986). Models of personality and disease: an interactional approach to Type A behavior and cardiovascular risk. *Journal of Personality and Social Psychology*, 50, 1166–73.

Smith, T. W., Peck, J. R., & Ward, J. R. (1990). Helplessness and depression in rheumatoid arthritis. *Health Psychology*, 9, 377–89.

Smith, T. W., Turner, C. W., Ford, M. H., Hunt, S. C., Barlow, G. K., Stults, B. M., & Williams, R. R. (1987). Blood pressure reactivity in adult male twins. *Health Psychology*, 6, 209–220.

Snowdon, D. A. Greiner, L. H., Mortimer, J. A., Riley, K. P., Greiner, P. A., & Markesbery, W. R. (1997). Brain infarction and the clinical expression of Alzheimer's disease. *Journal of the American Medical Associations*, 277, 813–17.

Snyder, S. H. (1977). Opiate receptors and internal opiates. *Scientific American*, 236, 44–56.

Sobel, D. S. (1990). The placebo effect: using the body's own healing mechanisms. In R. Ornstein & C. Swencionis (Eds), *The healing brain: a scientific reader*. New York: Guilford.

Sobel, D. S. (1995). Rethinking medicine: improving health outcomes with cost-effective psychosocial interventions. *Psychosomatic Medicine*, 57, 234–44.

Sobel, L. C., Sobel, M. B., Toneatto, T., & Leo, G. I. (1993). What triggers the resolution of alcohol problems without treatment? *Alcoholism: Clinical and Experimental Research*, 17, 217–24.

Sobel, M. B., & Sobel, L. C. (1976). Second-year treatment outcome of alcoholics treated by individualized behavior therapy: results. *Behavior Research and Therapy*, 14, 195–215.

Sobel, M. B., & Sobel, L. C. (1978). *Behavioral treatment of alcohol problems*. New York: Plenum.

Solé-Leris, A. (1986). *Tranquility and insight*. Boston, MA: Shambhala.

Solomon, G. F., & Temoshok, L. (1987). A psychoneuroimmunologic perspective on AIDS research: questions, preliminary findings, and suggestions. *Journal of Applied Social Psychology*, 17, 286–308.

Somers, V. K., Dyken, M. E., Mark, A. L., & Abboud, F. M. (1993). Sympathetic-nerve activity during sleep in normal subjects. *New England Journal of Medicine*, 328, 303–7.

Sorbi, M., Tellegen, B., & Du Long, A. (1989). Long term effects of training in relaxation and stress-coping in patients with migraine: a 3-year follow-up. *Headache*, 29, 111–21.

Sorensen, G., Jacobs, D. R., Pirie, P., Folsom, A., Luepker, R., & Gillum, R. (1987). Relationships among Type A behavior, employment experiences, and gender: the Minnesota Heart Survey. *Journal of Behavioral Medicine*, 10, 323–36.

Sorensen, G., Pechacek, T., & Pallonen, U. (1986). Occupational and worksite norms and attitudes about smoking cessation. *American Journal of Public Health*, 76, 544–9.

Southard, D. R., Coates, T. J., Kolodner, K., Parker, F. C., Padgett, N. E., & Kennedy, H. L. (1986). Relationship between mood and blood pressure in the natural environment: an adolescent population. *Health Psychology*, 5, 469–80.

Spanos, N. P., Perlini, A. H., & Robertson, L. A. (1989). Hypnosis, suggestion, and placebo in the reduction of experimental pain. *Journal of Abnormal Psychology*, 98, 285–93.

Spark, R., Donovan, R. J., & Howat, P. (1991). Promoting health and preventing injury in remote Aboriginal communities: a case study. *Health Promotion Journal of Australia*, 1(2), 10–16.

Specter, M. (1996, March 31). 10 years later, through fear, Chernobyl still kills in Belarus. *New York Times*, pp. 1, 6.

Speece, M. W., & Brent, S. B. (1984). Children's understanding of death: a review of three components of a death concept. *Child Development*, 55, 1671–86.

Spiegel, D., Bloom, J. R., Kraemer, H. C., & Gottheil, E. (1989). Effect of psychosocial treatment on survival of patients with metastic breast cancer. *The Lancet*, 334, 888–91.

Spiegel, D., Sands, S., & Koopman, C. (1994). Pain and depression in patients with cancer. *Cancer*, 74, 2570–78.

Spiegel, D., Sephton, S. E., & Stites, D. P. (1998). Effects of psychosocial treatment in prolonging cancer survival may be mediated by neuroimmune pathways. In S. M. McCann, J. M. Lipton et al., *Annals of the New York Academy of Sciences, Vol. 840: Neuroimmunomodulation: molecular aspects, integrative systems, and clinical advances* (pp. 674–83). New York: New York Academy of Sciences.

Spiga, R. (1986). Social interaction and cardiovascular response of boys exhibiting the coronary-prone behavior pattern. *Journal of Pediatric Psychology*, 11, 59–69.

Spinetta, J. J. (1974). The dying child's awareness of death: a review. *Psychological Bulletin*, 81, 256–60.

Spinetta, J. J. (1982). Behavioral and psychological research in childhood cancer. *Cancer*, 50, 1939–43.

Spirduso, W., & Gilliam-MacRae, P. (1991). Physical activity and quality of life in the frail elderly. In J. E. Birren & J. E. Lubben (Eds), *The concept and measurement of quality of life in the frail elderly* (pp. 226–55). San Diego, CA: Academic Press.

Spiro III, A., Aldwin, C. M., Ward, K. D., & Mroczek, D. K., (1995). Personality and the incidence of hypertension among older men: longitudinal findings from the normative aging study. *Health Psychology*, 14(6), 563–9.

Spooner, C., Mattick, R. P., & Noffs, W. (2000). A study of the patterns and correlates of substance use among adolescents applying for drug treatment. *Australian and New Zealand Journal of Public Health*, 24(5), 492–502.

Spurgeon, P., Broome, A., Earll, L., & Harris, B. (1990). Health psychology in a broader context. In P. Bennett, J. Weinman & P. Spurgeon (Eds), *Current developments in health psychology*. Chur, Switzerland: Harwood.

St. Jeor, S. T., Sutnick, M. R., & Scott, B. J. (1988). Nutrition. In E. A. Blechman & K. D. Brownell (Eds), *Handbook of behavioral medicine for women*. New York: Pergamon.

St. Lawrence, J. S., Brasfield, T. L., Jefferson, K. W., Alleyne, E., O'Bannon, R. E., & Shirley, A. (1995). Cognitive-behavioral intervention to reduce African American adolescents' risk for HIV infection. *Journal of Consulting and Clinical Psychology*, 63, 221–37.

St. Lawrence, J. S., Jefferson, K. W., Alleyne, E., & Brasfield, T. L. (1995). Comparison of education versus behavioral skills training interventions in lowering sexual HIV-risk behavior of substance-dependent adolescents. *Journal of Consulting and Clinical Psychology*, 63, 154–7.

Staats, P., Hekmat, H., & Staats, A. (1998). Suggestion/placebo effects on pain: negative as well as positive. *Journal of Pain and Symptom Management*, 15(4), 235–43.

Stacy, A. W., Bentler, P. M., & Flay, B. R. (1994). Attitudes and health behavior in diverse populations: drunk driving, alcohol use, binge eating, marihuana use, and cigarette use. *Health Psychology*, 13, 73–85.

Stall, R. D., Coates, T. J., & Hoff, C. (1988). Behavioral risk reduction for HIV infection among gay and bisexual men: a review of results from the United States. *American Psychologist*, 43, 878–85.

Stallone, D. D., & Stunkard, A. J. (1991). The regulation of body weight: evidence and clinical implications. *Annals of Behavioral Medicine*, 13, 220–30.

Stamler, R., Stamler, J., Gosch, F. C., Civinelli, J., Fishman, J., McKeever, P., McDonald, A., & Dyer, A. R. (1989). Primary prevention of hypertension by nutritional-hygienic means: final report of a randomized, controlled trial. *Journal of the American Medical Association*, 262, 1801–7.

Stanton, A. L. (1987). Determinants of adherence to medical regimens by hypertensive patients. *Journal of Behavioral Medicine*, 10, 377–94.

Stanton, W. R., & Silva, P. A. (1992). A longitudinal study of the influence of parents and friends on children's initiation of smoking. *Journal of Applied Developmental Psychology*, 13(4), 423–34.

Stanton, W. R., Mahalski, P. A., McGee, R., & Silva, P. A. (1993). Reasons for smoking or not smoking in early adolescence. *Addictive Behaviors*, 18, 321–9.

Staudinger, U. M., Freund, A. M., Linden, M., & Maas, I. (1999). Self, personality, and life regulation: facets of psychological resilience in old age. In P. B. Baltes & K. U. Mayer (Eds), *The Berlin aging study: aging from 70 to 100* (pp. 302–328). New York: Cambridge University Press.

Steele, D. J., Jackson, T. C., & Gutmann, M. C. (1990). Have you been taking your pills? The adherence monitoring sequence in the medical interview. *Journal of Family Practice*, 30, 294–9.

Stein, J. A., Newcomb, M. D., & Bentler, P. M. (1987). An 8-year study of multiple influences on drug use and drug use consequences. *Journal of Personality and Social Psychology*, 53, 1094–1105.

Steinberg, L. (1985). Early temperamental antecedents of adult Type A behaviors. *Developmental Psychology*, 21, 1171–80.

Steiner, H., & Clark, W. R. (1977). Psychiatric complications of burned adults: a classification. *Journal of Trauma*, 17, 134–43.

Stephens, R. S., Roffman, R. A., & Simpson, E. E. (1994). Treating adult marijuana dependence: a test of the relapse prevention model. *Journal of Consulting and Clinical Psychology*, 62, 92–9.

Stephens, T., & Caspersen, C. J. (1994). The demography of physical activity. In C. Bouchard, R. J. Shephard & T. Stephens (Eds), *Physical activity, fitness and health: international proceedings and consensus statement* (pp. 204–213). Champaign, IL: Human Kinetics Publishers.

Steptoe, A., Fieldman, G., Evans, O., & Perry, L. (1993). Control over work pace, job strain and cardiovascular responses in middle-aged men. *Journal of Hypertension*, 11, 751–9.

Steptoe, A., Lipsey, Z., & Wardle, J. (1998). Stress, hassles and variations in alcohol consumption, food choice and physical exercise: a diary study. *British Journal of Health Psychology*, 3(1), 51–63.

Steptoe, A., Wardle, J., Vinck, J., Tuomisto, M., Holte, A., & Wichström, L. (1994). Personality and attitudinal correlates of healthy and unhealthy lifestyles in young adults. *Psychology and Health*, 9, 331–43.

Sterman, M. B. (1986). Epilepsy and its treatment with EEG feedback therapy. *Annals of Behavioral Medicine*, 8(1), 21–5.

Stevens, C. A., & Hassan, R. (1994). Management of death, dying and euthanasia: attitudes and practices of medical practitioners in South Australia. *Journal of Medical Ethics*, 161, 715–17.

Stevens-Long, J. (1984). *Adult life: developmental processes* (2nd ed.). Palo Alto, CA: Mayfield.

Stewart, A. L., & Ware, J. E. (1992). *Measuring functioning and well-being: the Medical Outcomes Study approach*. Chapel Hill, NC: Duke University Press.

Stewart, W. F., Shechter, A., & Lipton, R. B. (1994). Migraine heterogeneity: disability, pain intensity, and attack frequency and duration. *Neurology*, 44 (Suppl. 4), S24–39.

Stewart, W. F., Shechter, A., & Rasmussen, B. K. (1994). Migraine prevalence: a review of population-based studies. *Neurology*, 44 (Suppl. 4), S17–23.

Stieg, R. L., & Turk, D. C. (1988). Chronic pain syndrome: demonstrating the cost–benefit of treatment. *Clinical Journal of Pain*, 4, 58–63.

Stockton, W. (1988, March 7). Fresh research tells asthmatics to stay active. *New York Times*, p. C9.

Stockwell, T., & Town, C. (1989). Anxiety and stress management. In R. K. Hester & W. R. Miller (Eds), *Handbook of alcoholism treatment approaches: effective alternatives*. New York: Pergamon.

Stone, A. A., Kennedy-Moore, E., & Neale, J. M. (1995). Association between daily coping and end-of-day mood. *Health Psychology*, 14, 341–9.

Stone, A. A., Neale, J. M., Cox, D. S., Napoli, A., Valdimarsdottir, H., & Kennedy-Moore, E. (1994). Daily events are associated with a secretory immune response to an oral antigen in men. *Health Psychology*, 13, 440–46.

Stone, G. C. (1979). Health and the health system: a historical overview and conceptual framework. In G. C. Stone, F. Cohen & N. E. Adler (Eds), *Health psychology — a handbook*. San Francisco: Jossey-Bass.

Stone, G. C. (1990). An international review of the emergence and development of health psychology. *Psychology and Health*, 4, 3–17.

Stone, G. C. (1991). An international review of the emergence and development of health psychology. In M. A. Jansen & J. Weinman (Eds), *The international development of health psychology*. Chur, Switzerland: Harwood.

Story, M., & Faulkner, P. (1990). The prime time diet: a content analysis of eating behavior and food messages in television program content and commercials. *American Journal of Public Health*, 80, 738–40.

Strathern, A., & Stewart, P. J. (1999). *Curing and healing: medical anthropology in global perspective*. Durham, NC: Carolina Academic Press.

Straton, J. (1992). *A hospital-based Pap smear service: report of a pilot project*. University of Western Australia: Department of Public Health.

Strauss, L. M., Solomon, L. J., Costanza, M. C., Worden, J. K., & Foster, R. S. (1987). Breast self-examination practices and attitudes of women with and without a history of breast cancer. *Journal of Behavioral Medicine*, 10, 337–50.

Strauss, R. H., & Yesalis, C. E. (1991). Anabolic steroids in the athlete. In W. P. Creger, C. H. Coggins & E. W. Hancock (Eds), *Annual review of medicine* (Vol. 42). Palo Alto, CA: Annual Reviews.

Straw, M. K. (1983). Coping with obesity. In T. G. Burish & L. A. Bradley (Eds), *Coping with chronic disease: research and applications*. New York: Academic Press.

Strecher, V. J., Kreuter, M. W., & Kobrin, S. C. (1995). Do cigarette smokers have unrealistic perceptions of their heart attack, cancer, and stroke risks? *Journal of Behavioral Medicine*, 18(1), 45–54.

Strickland, B. R. (1978). Internal–external expectancies and health-related behaviors. *Journal of Consulting and Clinical Psychology*, 6, 1192–1211.

Striegel-Moore, R., & Rodin, J. (1985). Prevention of obesity. In J. C. Rosen & L. J. Solomon (Eds), *Prevention in health psychology*. Hanover, NH: University Press of New England.

Striegel-Moore, R. H., Silberstein, L. R., & Rodin, J. (1986). Toward an understanding of risk factors for bulimia. *American Psychologist*, 41, 246–63.

Stuart, K., Borland, R., & McMurray, N. (1994). Self-efficacy, health locus of control, and smoking cessation. *Addictive Behaviors*, 19(1), 1–12.

Stuart, R. B. (1967). Behavioral control of overeating. *Behavior Research and Therapy*, 5, 357–65.

Stunkard, A. J. (1987). Conservative treatments for obesity. *American Journal of Clinical Nutrition*, 45, 1142–54.

Stunkard, A. J., & Berthold, H. C. (1985). What is behavior therapy? a very short description of behavioral weight control. *American Journal of Clinical Nutrition*, 41, 821–3.

Stunkard, A. J., Felix, M. R. J., & Cohen, R. Y. (1985). Mobilizing a community to promote health: the Pennsylvania County Health Improvement Program (CHIP). In J. C. Rosen & L. J. Solomon (Eds), *Prevention in health psychology*. Hanover, NH: University Press of New England.

Stunkard, A. J., Foch, T. T., & Hrubec, Z. (1986). A twin study of human obesity. *Journal of the American Medical Association*, 256, 51–4.

Stunkard, A. J., Sorensen, T. I. A., Hanis, C., Teasdale, T. W., Chakraborty, R., Schull, W. J., & Schulsinger, F. (1986). An adoption study of human obesity. *New England Journal of Medicine*, 314, 193–8.

Stunkard, A. J., Stinnett, J. L., & Smoller, J. W. (1986). Psychological and social aspects of the surgical treatment of obesity. *American Journal of Psychiatry*, 143, 417–29.

Suarez, E. C., Williams, R. B., Kuhn, C. M., Zimmerman, E. H., & Schanberg, S. M. (1991). Biobehavioral basis of coronary-prone behavior in middle-aged men. Part II: Serum cholesterol, the Type A behavior pattern, and hostility as interactive modulators of physiological reactivity. *Psychosomatic Medicine*, 53, 528–37.

Suedfeld, P. (1990). Restricted environmental stimulation and smoking cessation: a 15-year progress report. *International Journal of the Addictions*, 25, 861–88.

Suedfeld, P., & Ikard, F. F. (1974). Use of sensory deprivation in facilitating the reduction of cigarette smoking. *Journal of Consulting and Clinical Psychology*, 42, 888–95.

Suinn, R. M. (1982). Intervention with Type A behavior. *Journal of Consulting and Clinical Psychology*, 50, 933–49.

Suitor, C. W., & Hunter, M. F. (1980). *Nutrition: principles and application in health promotion*. Philadelphia, PA: Lippincott.

Sullivan, J. M. (1991). Salt sensitivity: definition, conception, methodology, and long-term issues. *Hypertension*, 17 (Suppl. I), I61–8.

Suls, J. (1982). Social support, interpersonal relations, and health: benefits and liabilities. In G. S. Sanders & J. Suls (Eds), *Social psychology of health and illness*. Hillsdale, NJ: Erlbaum.

Suls, J. (1984). Levels of analysis and efforts to modify adolescent health behavior: a commentary on Lund and Kegeles. *Health Psychology*, 3, 371–5.

Suls, J., & Fletcher, B. (1985). The relative efficacy of avoidant and nonavoidant coping strategies: a meta-analysis. *Health Psychology*, 4, 249–88.

Suls, J., & Mullen, B. (1981). Life change and psychological distress: the role of perceived control and desirability. *Journal of Applied Social Psychology*, 11, 379–89.

Suls, J., & Sanders, G. S. (1988). Type A behavior as a general risk factor for physical disorder. *Journal of Behavioral Medicine*, 11, 210–26.

Suls, J., Sanders, G. S., & Labrecque, M. S. (1986). Attempting to control blood pressure without systematic instruction: when advice is counterproductive. *Journal of Behavioral Medicine*, 9, 567–76.

Suls, J., & Swain, A. (1993). Use of meta-analysis in health psychology. In S. Maes, H. Leventhal & M. Johnston (Eds), *International review of health psychology* (Vol. 2). New York: John Wiley & Sons.

Suls, J., Wan, C. K., & Blanchard, E. B. (1994). A multilevel data-analytic approach for evaluation of relationships between daily life stressors and symptomatology: Patients with irritable bowel syndrome. *Health Psychology*, 13, 103–113.

Suls, J., Wan, C. K., & Costa, P. T. (1995). Relationship of trait anger to resting blood pressure: a meta-analysis. *Health Psychology*, 14, 444–56.

Super, C. N. (1981). Cross-cultural research on infancy. In H. C. Trandis & A. Heron (Eds), *Handbook of cross-cultural psychology: developmental psychology* (Vol. 4). Boston, MA: Allyn & Bacon.

Superko, H. R., & Krauss, R. M. (1994). Coronary artery disease regression: convincing evidence for the benefit of aggressive lipoprotein management. *Circulation*, 90, 1056–69.

Surwit, R. S. (1993). Of mice and men: behavioral medicine in the study of type II diabetes. *Annals of Behavioral Medicine*, 15, 227–35.

Surwit, R. S., Feinglos, M. N., & Scovern, A. W. (1983). Diabetes and behavior: a paradigm for health psychology. *American Psychologist*, 38, 255–62.

Susser, M., Hopper, K., & Richman, R. (1983). Society, culture, and health. In D. Mechanic (Ed.), *Handbook of health, health care, and the health professions*. New York: Free Press.

Suter, P. O., Schutz, Y., & Jequier, E. (1992). The effect of ethanol on fat storage in healthy subjects. *New England Journal of Medicine*, 326, 983–7.

Sutton, S. R. (1982). Fear-arousing communications: a critical examination of theory and research. In J. R. Eiser (Ed.), *Social psychology and behavioral medicine*. New York: John Wiley & Sons.

Sutton, S., & Hallett, R. (1988). Understanding the effects of fear-arousing communications: the role of cognitive factors and the amount of fear aroused. *Journal of Behavioral Medicine*, 11, 353–60.

Svarstad, B. (1976). Physician–patient communication and patient conformity with medical advice. In D. Mechanic (Ed.), *The growth of bureaucratic medicine*. New York: John Wiley & Sons.

Swan, G. E., Carmelli, D., & Rosenman, R. H. (1986). Spouse-pair similarity on the California Psychological Inventory with reference to husband's coronary heart disease. *Psychosomatic Medicine*, 48, 172–86.

Swardson, A., (1995, October 16–22). In Canada's ailing system, the doctor is out. *Washington Post National Weekly Edition*, p. 29.

Sweet, J. J. (1991). Psychological evaluation and testing services in medical settings. In J. J. Sweet, R. H. Rozensky & S. M. Tovian (Eds), *Handbook of clinical psychology in medical settings*. New York: Plenum.

Sweet, J. J., Rozensky, R. H., & Tovian, S. M. (1991). *Handbook of clinical psychology in medical settings*. New York: Plenum.

Swigonski, M. E. (1987). Bio-psycho-social factors affecting coping and compliance with the hemodialysis treatment regimen. University Microfilms International (Order No. 8803518).

Syme, S. L. (1984). Sociocultural factors and disease etiology. In W. D. Gentry (Ed.), *Handbook of behavioral medicine*. New York: Guilford.

Taft, C. T., Stern, A. S., King, L. A., & King, D. W. (1999). Modeling physical health and functional health status: the role of combat exposure, posttraumatic stress disorder and personal resource attributes. *Journal of Traumatic Stress*, 12(1), 3–23.

Tagliacozzo, D. L., & Mauksch, H. O. (1972). The patient's view of the patient's role. In E. G. Jaco (Ed.), *Patients, physicians, and illness* (2nd ed.). New York: Free Press.

Taitel, M. S., Kotses, H., Bernstein, L., Bernstein, D., & Creer, T. L. (1994). A cost–benefit analysis of a self-management program for adult asthma. Paper presented at the meeting of the Society of Behavioral Medicine in Boston.

Takeda, W., & Wessel, J. (1994). Acupuncture for the treatment of pain in osteoarthritic knees. *Arthritis Care and Research*, 7, 118–22.

Tallmer, J., Scherwitz, L., Chesney, M., Hecker, M., Hunkeler, E., Serwitz, J., & Hughes, G. (1990). Selection, training, and quality control of Type A interviewers in a prospective study of young adults. *Journal of Behavioral Medicine*, 13, 449–66.

Tanner, J. M. (1970). Physical growth. In P. H. Mussen (Ed.), *Carmichael's manual of child psychology* (3rd ed.). New York: John Wiley & Sons.

Tanner, J. M. (1978). *Foetus into man*. Cambridge, MA: Harvard University Press.

Tapp, J. T. (1985). Multisystems interventions in disease. In N. Schneiderman & J. T. Tapp (Eds), *Behavioral medicine: the biopsychosocial approach*. Hillsdale, NJ: Erlbaum.

Tate, D. G., Maynard, F., & Forchheimer, M. (1993). Predictors of psychologic distress one year after spinal cord injury. *American Journal of Physical Medicine and Rehabilitation*, 72, 272–5.

Tausig, M. (1982). Measuring life events. *Journal of Health and Social Behavior*, 23, 52–64.

Taylor, R., & Quine, S. (1992). Differences in life expectancy: social factors in mortality rates. *Australian Journal on Ageing*, 11(1), 21–35.

Taylor, R., & Salkeld, G. (1996). Health care expenditure and life expectancy in Australia: how well do we perform? *Australian and New Zealand Journal of Public Health*, 20(3), 233–40.

Taylor, S. E. (1979). Hospital patient behavior: reactance, helplessness, or control? *Journal of Social Issues*, 35, 156–84.

Taylor, S. E. (1983). Adjustment to threatening events: a theory of cognitive adaptation. *American Psychologist*, 38, 1161–73.

Taylor, S. E., Lichtman, R. R., & Wood, J. V. (1984). Attributions, beliefs about control, and adjustment to breast cancer. *Journal of Personality and Social Psychology*, 46, 489–502.

Taylor, S. E., & Seeman, T. E. (1999). Psychosocial resources and the SES-health relationship. In N. Adler & M. Marmot (Eds), *Socioeconomic status and health in industrial nations: social, psychological and biological pathways. Annals of the New York Academy of Sciences* (Vol. 896, pp. 210–25). New York: New York Academy of Sciences.

Tebbi, C. K., Cummings, K. M., Zevon, M. A., Smith, L., Richards, M., & Mallon, J. (1986). Compliance of pediatric and adolescent cancer patients. *Cancer*, 58, 1179–84.

Tell, G. S., Polak, J. F., Ward, B. J., Kittner, S. J., et al. (1994). Relation of smoking with carotid artery wall thickness and stenosis in older adults: the Cardiovascular Health Study. *Circulation*, 90, 2905–8.

Temoshok, L. (1990a). Applying the biopsychosocial model to research on HIV/AIDS. In P. Bennett, J. Weinman & P. Spurgeon (Eds), *Current developments in health psychology*. Chur, Switzerland: Harwood.

Temoshok, L. (1990b). On attempting to articulate the biopsychosocial model: psychological-psychophysiological homeostasis. In H. S. Friedman (Ed.), *Personality and disease*. New York: John Wiley & Sons.

Temoshok, L., & Dreher, H. (1992). *The Type C connection: the behavioral links to cancer and your health.* New York: Random House.

Tennant, C., & Andrews, G. (1976). A scale to measure the stress of life events. *Australian and New Zealand Journal of Psychiatry,* 10(1), 27–32.

Tennes, K., & Kreye, M. (1985). Children's adrenocortical responses to classroom activities and tests in elementary school. *Psychosomatic Medicine,* 47, 451–60.

Teri, L., Hughes, J. P., & Larson, E. B. (1990). Cognitive deterioration in Alzheimer's disease: behavioral and health factors. *Journal of Gerontology: Psychological Sciences,* 45, P58–63.

Terry, D. Gallois, C., & McCamish, M. (1993). *The theory of reasoned action: its application to Aids-preventive behaviour.* Oxford, NY: Pergamon.

Terry, D. J. (1992). Stress, coping and coping resources as correlates of adaptation in myocardial infarction patients. *British Journal of Clinical Psychology,* 31(2), 215–25.

Terry, D. J. (1994). Determinants of coping: the role of stable and situational factors. *Journal of Personality and Social Psychology,* 66(5), 895–910.

Terry, D. J., Galligan, R. F., & Conway, V. J. (1993). The prediction of safe sex behaviour: the role of intentions, attitudes, norms and control beliefs. *Psychology and Health,* 8, 355–68.

Terry, D. Gallois, C., & McCamish, M. (1993). *The theory of reasoned action: its application to Aids-preventive behaviour.* Oxford, UK: Pergamon.

Terry, D., & O'Leary, J. E. (1995). The theory of planned behaviour: the effects of perceived behavioural control and self-efficacy. *British Journal of Social Psychology,* 34, 199–220.

Terry, R. D., Oakland, M. J., & Ankeny, K. (1991). Factors associated with adoption of dietary behavior to reduce heart disease risk among males. *Journal of Nutrition Education,* 23, 154–60.

Thackwray, D. E., Smith, M. C., Bodfish, J. W., & Meyers, A. W. (1993). A comparison of behavioral and cognitivebehavioral intervention for bulimia nervosa. *Journal of Consulting and Clinical Psychology,* 61, 639–45.

Thelen, M. H., Fry, R. A., Fehrenbach, P. A., & Frautschi, N. M. (1979). Therapeutic videotape and film modeling: a review. *Psychological Bulletin,* 86, 701–720.

Theorell, T., & Rahe, R. H. (1975). Life change events, ballistocardiography, and coronary death. *Journal of Human Stress,* 1, 18–24.

Thoits, P. (1983). Dimensions of life events that influence psychological distress: an evaluation and synthesis of the literature. In H. B. Kaplan (Ed.), *Psychological stress: trends in theory and research* (pp. 33–103). New York: Academic Press.

Thoits, P. A. (1982). Conceptual, methodological, and theoretical problems in studying social support as a buffer against life stress. *Journal of Health and Social Behavior,* 23, 145–59.

Thoits, P. A. (1994). Stressors and problem-solving: the individual as psychological activist. *Journal of Health and Social Behavior,* 35, 143–59.

Thompson, J. (1984). Communicating with patients. In R. Fitzpatrick, J. Hinton, S. Newman, G. Scambler & J. Thompson (Eds), *The experience of illness.* London: Tavistock.

Thompson, R. H., & Vernon, D. T. A. (1993). Research on children's behavior after hospitalistion: a review and synthesis. *Developmental and Behavioral Pediatrics,* 14, 28–35.

Thompson, S. C. (1981). Will it hurt less if I can control it? A complex answer to a simple question. *Psychological Bulletin,* 90, 89–101.

Thompson, S. C., Nanni, C., & Schwankovsky, L. (1990). Patient-oriented interventions to improve communication in a medical office visit. *Health Psychology,* 9, 390–404.

Thompson, W. R., & Thompson, D. L. (1987). Effects of exercise compliance on blood lipids in post-myocardial infarction patients. *Journal of Cardiopulmonary Rehabilitation,* 7, 332–41.

Thoresen, C. E. (1984). Overview. In J. D. Matarazzo, S. M. Weiss, J. A. Herd, N. E. Miller & S. M. Weiss (Eds), *Behavioral health: a handbook of health enhancement and disease prevention.* New York: John Wiley & Sons.

Thoresen, C. E., Friedman, M., Powell, L. H., Gill, J. J., & Ulmer, D. K. (1985). Altering the Type A behavior pattern in postinfarction patients. *Journal of Cardiopulmonary Rehabilitation,* 5, 258–66.

Thoresen, C. E., & Pattillo, J. R. (1988). Exploring the Type A behavior pattern in children and adolescents. In B. K. Houston & C. R. Snyder (Eds), *Type A behavior pattern: research, theory, and intervention.* New York: John Wiley & Sons.

Thun, M. J., Day-Lally, C. A., Calle, E. E., Flanders, W. D., & Heath, C. W. (1995). Excess mortality among cigarette smokers: changes in a 20-year interval. *American Journal of Public Health,* 85, 1223–30.

Tiggemann, M. (1996). 'Thinking' versus 'feeling' fat: correlates of two indices of body image dissatisfaction. *Australian Journal of Psychology,* 48(1), 21–5.

Timko, C. (1987). Seeking medical care for a breast cancer symptom: determinants of intentions to engage in prompt or delay behavior. *Health Psychology,* 6, 305–328.

Tims, F. M., Fletcher, B. W., & Hubbard, R. L. (1991). Treatment outcomes for drug abuse clients. In R. W. Pickens, C. G. Leukefeld & C. R. Schuster (Eds), *Improving drug abuse treatment.* Rockville, MD: National Institute on Drug Abuse.

Tinetti, M. E., Baker, D. I., McAvay, G., Claus, E. B., Garrett, P., Gottschalk, M., Koch, M. L., Trainor, K., & Horwitz, R. I. (1994). A multifactorial intervention to reduce the risk of falling among elderly people living in the community. *New England Journal of Medicine,* 331, 821–7.

Tomkins, S. (1966). Psychological model for smoking behavior. *American Journal of Public Health,* 56 (12, Suppl.), 17–20.

Tomkins, S. (1968). A modified model of smoking behavior. In E. F. Borgatta & R. R. Evans (Eds), *Smoking, health and behavior.* Chicago: Aldine.

Tooth, L., McKenna, K., & Colquhoun, D. (1993). Prediction of compliance with a post-myocardial infarction home-based walking programme. *Australian Occupational Therapy Journal,* 40(1), 17–22.

Torrens, P. R. (1985). Hospice care: what have we learned? In L. Breslow, J. E. Fielding & L. B. Lave (Eds), *Annual review of public health* (Vol. 6). Palo Alto, CA: Annual Reviews.

Tortora, G. J., & Grabowski, S. R. (1993). *Principles of anatomy and physiology* (7th ed.). New York: HarperCollins.

Toseland, R. W., Rossiter, C. M., & Labrecque, M. S. (1989). The effectiveness of peer-led and professionally led groups to support family caregivers. *The Gerontologist,* 29, 465–80.

Totman, R. (1982). Psychosomatic theories. In J. R. Eiser (Ed.), *Social psychology and behavioral medicine.* New York: John Wiley & Sons.

Touyz, S., & Beaumont, P. J. (1985). *Eating disorders: prevalence and treatment.* Sydney: Williams and Wilkins.

Touyz, S., Blaszczynski, A., Digiusto, E., & Byrne, D. (1992). The emergence of clinical psychology departments in Australian teaching hospitals. *Australian and New Zealand Journal of Psychiatry,* 26(4), 554–9.

Tovian, S. M. (1991). Integration of clinical psychology into adult and pediatric oncology programs. In J. J. Sweet, R. H. Rozensky & S. M. Tovian (Eds), *Handbook of clinical psychology in medical settings.* New York: Plenum.

Trabin, T., Rader, C., & Cummings, C. (1987). A comparison of pain management outcomes for disability compensation and non-compensation patients. *Psychology and Health,* 1, 341–51.

Tremblay, A., Wouters, E., Wenker, M., St-Pierre, S., Bouchard, C., & Després, J.-P. (1995). Alcohol and a high-fat diet: a combination favoring overfeeding. *American Journal of Clinical Nutrition,* 62, 639–44.

Trent, R. (1999). Diagnosing disease through DNA: an exciting new frontier. *Australian Family Physician*, 28(10), 1005–9.

Tross, S., & Hirsch, D. A. (1988). Psychological distress and neuropsychological complications of HIV infection and AIDS. *American Psychologist*, 43, 929–34.

Trotter, L., & Mullins, R. (1998). Environmental tobacco smoke: public opinions and behaviour. In L. Trotter & R. Mullins (Eds), *Quit Evaluation Studies 9*. Victoria: ACCV, 27–41.

Trumbull, R., & Appley, M. H. (1986). A conceptual model for examination of stress dynamics. In M. H. Appley & R. Trumbull (Eds), *Dynamics of stress: physiological, psychological, and social perspectives*. New York: Plenum.

TSC (Trenton State College) (1992). *Alcohol & drug education program*. Trenton, NJ: Author.

Tucker, J. S., Friedman, H. S., Wingard, D. L., & Schwartz, J. E. (1996). Marital history at midlife as a predictor of longevity: alternative explanations to the protective effect of marriage. *Health Psychology*, 15, 94–101.

Tucker, J. S., Schwartz, J. E., Clark, K. M., & Friedman, H. S. (1999). Age-related changes in the associations of social network ties with mortality risk. *Psychology and Aging*, 14(4), 564–71.

Tunks, E., & Bellissimo, A. (1991). *Behavioral medicine: concepts and procedures*. New York: Pergamon.

Turk, D. C., & Holzman, A. D. (1986). Commonalities among psychological approaches in the treatment of chronic pain: specifying the meta-constructs. In A. D. Holzman & D. C. Turk (Eds), *Pain management: a handbook of psychological treatment approaches*. New York: Pergamon.

Turk, D. C., Litt, M. D., Salovey, P., & Walker, J. (1985). Seeking urgent pediatric treatment: factors contributing to frequency, delay, and appropriateness. *Health Psychology*, 4, 43–59.

Turk, D. C., & Meichenbaum, D. (1991). Adherence to self-care regimens: the patient's perspective. In J. J. Sweet, R. H. Rosensky & S. M. Tovain (Eds), *Handbook of clinical psychology in medical settings*. New York: Plenum.

Turk, D. C., Meichenbaum, D. H., & Berman, W. H. (1979). Application of biofeedback for the regulation of pain: a critical review. *Psychological Bulletin*, 86, 1322–38.

Turk, D. C., Meichenbaum, D., & Genest, M. (1983). *Pain and behavioral medicine: a cognitive-behavioral perspective*. New York: Guilford.

Turk, D. C., & Rudy, T. E. (1986). Assessment of cognitive factors in chronic pain: a worthwhile enterprise? *Journal of Consulting and Clinical Psychology*, 54, 760–68.

Turk, D. C., Rudy, T. E., & Sorkin, B. A. (1992).Chronic pain: behavioural conceptualisations and interventions. In S. M. Turner, K. S. Calhoun & H. E. Adams (Eds), *Handbook of clinical behavior therapy* (2nd ed.). New York: John Wiley & Sons.

Turk, D. C., & Salovey, P. (1995). Cognitive-behavioral treatment of illness behavior. In P. M. Nicassio & T. W. Smith (Eds), *Managing chronic illness: a biopsychosocial perspective*. Washington, DC: American Psychological Association.

Turk, D. C., & Stacey, B. R. (1997). Multidisciplinary pain centers in the treatment of chronic back pain. In J. W. Frymoyer, T. B. Ducker, N. M. Hadler, J. P., Kostuik, J. N. Weinstein & T. S. Whitcloud (Eds), *The adult spine: principles and practice* (2nd ed.). New York: Raven Press.

Turk, D. C., Wack, J. T., & Kerns, R. D. (1985). An empirical examination of the 'pain-behavior' construct. *Journal of Behavioral Medicine*, 8, 119–30.

Turkkan, J. S., McCaul, M. E., & Stitzer, M. L. (1989). Psychophysiological effects of alcohol-related stimuli: II. Enhancement with alcohol availability. *Alcoholism: Clinical and Experimental Research*, 13, 392–8.

Turner, J. A. (1982). Comparison of group progressive-relaxation training and cognitive-behavioral group therapy for chronic low back pain. *Journal of Consulting and Clinical Psychology*, 50, 757–65.

Turner, J. A., Clancy, S., McQuade, K. J., & Cardenas, D. D. (1990). Effectiveness of behavioral therapy for chronic low back pain: a component analysis. *Journal of Consulting and Clinical Psychology*, 58, 573–9.

Turner, J. A., Clancy, S., & Vitaliano, P. P. (1987). Relationships of stress, appraisal and coping, to chronic low back pain. *Behavior Research and Therapy*, 25, 281–8.

Turner, J. R., & Hewitt, J. K. (1992). Twin studies of cardiovascular response to psychological challenge: a review and suggested future directions. *Annals of Behavioral Medicine*, 14, 12–20.

Turner, J. R., Ward, M. M., Gellman, M. D., Johnston, D. W., Light, K. C., & Van Doornen, L. J. P. (1994). The relationship between laboratory and ambulatory cardiovascular activity: current evidence and future directions. *Annals of Behavioral Medicine*, 16, 12–23.

Turner, R. J., & Avison, W. R. (1992). Innovations in the measurement of life stress: crisis theory and the significance of event resolution. *Journal of Health and Social Behavior*, 33, 36–50.

Turner, R. J., & Wheaton, B. (1995). Checklist measurement of stressful life events. In S. Cohen, R. Kessler & L. Underwood, Gordon (Eds), *Measuring stress: a guide for health and social scientists* (pp. 29–58). New York: Oxford University Press.

Turrell, G., & Najman, J. M. (1995). Collecting food-related data from low socioeconomic groups: how adequate are our current research designs? *Australian Journal of Public Health*, 19(4), 410–16.

Twisk, J. W. R., Snel, J., Kemper, H. C. G., & van Mechelen, W. (1999). Changes in daily hassles and life events and the relationship with coronary heart disease risk factors: a 2 year longitudinal study in 27–29 yr old males and females. *Journal of Psychosomatic Research*, 46(3), 229–40.

Tyhurst, J. S. (1951). Individual reactions to community disaster: the natural history of psychiatric phenomena. *American Journal of Psychiatry*, 107, 764–9.

Tyler, D. C. (1990). Patient-controlled analgesia in adolescents. *Journal of Adolescent Health Care*, 11, 154–8.

Uchino, B. N., Cacioppo, J. T., Malarkey, W., Glaser, R., & Kiecolt-Glaser, J. K. (1995). Appraisal support predicts age-related differences in cardiovascular function in women. *Health Psychology*, 14(6), 556–62.

Uchino, B. N., Uno, D., & Holt-Lunstad, J. (1999). Social support, physiological processes and health. *Current Directions in Psychological Science*, 8(5), 145–8.

Ugolini, K. (1999). The effects of social support type on psychosocial adjustment to low back pain: testing the optimal matching model. *Dissertation Abstracts International — Sciences and Engineering*, 60(2-B): 0845.

Ukestad, L. K., & Wittrock, D. A. (1996). Pain perception and coping in female tension headache sufferers and headache-free controls. *Health Psychology*, 15, 65–8.

Urban, B. J., France, R. D., Steinberger, E. K., Scott, D. L., & Maltbie, A. A. (1986). Long-term use of narcotic/antidepressant medication in the management of phantom limb pain. *Pain*, 24, 191–6.

USBC (United States Bureau of the Census) (1995). *Statistical Abstracts of the United States: 1994* (114th ed.). Washington, DC: U.S. Government Printing Office.

USDHHS (United States Department of Health and Human Services) (1981). *Medicines and you* (Publication No. NIH 81–2140). Washington, DC: U.S. Government Printing Office.

USDHHS (1986a). *Clinical opportunities for smoking intervention: a guide for the busy physician* (Publication No. NIH 86–2178). Washington, DC: U.S. Government Printing Office.

USDHHS (1986b). *The health consequences of involuntary smoking: a report of the Surgeon General* (Publication No. CDC 87–8398). Washington, DC: U.S. Government Printing Office.

USDHHS (1989). *Reducing the health consequences of smoking: 25 years of progress.* A report of the Surgeon General (DHHS Publication No. CDC 89–8411). Rockville, MD: Office on Smoking and Health.

USDHHS (1990). *Alcohol and health* (Publication No. ADM 90–1656). Rockville, MD: National Institute on Alcohol Abuse and Alcoholism.

USDHHS (1994). *Acute low back pain problems in adults: assessment and treatment* (quick reference guide for clinicians: No. 14). Washington, DC: U.S. Government Printing Office.

USDHHS (1995). *Health United States: 1994* (Publication No. PHS 95–1232). Washington, DC: U.S. Government Printing Office.

Valois, R. F., Adams, K. G., & Kammermann, S. K. (1996). One-year evaluation results from CableQuit: a community cable television smoking cessation pilot program. *Journal of Behavioral Medicine,* 19, 479–99.

van der Kolk, B. A. (1987). *Psychological trauma.* Washington, DC: American Psychiatric Press.

van der Voort, D. (1999). Quality of social support in mental and physical health. *Current Psychology: Developmental, Learning, Personality, Social,* 18(2), 205-222.

van Eck, M. M., & Nicolson, N. A. (1994). Perceived stress and salivary cortisol in daily life. *Annals of Behavioral Medicine,* 16, 221–7.

Van Egeren, L. F., Sniderman, L. D., & Roggelin, M. S. (1982). Competitive two-person interactions of Type-A and Type-B individuals. *Journal of Behavioral Medicine,* 5, 55–66.

Van Griensven, G. J. P., De Vroome, E. M. M., Goudsmit, J., & Coutinho, R. E. (1989). Changes in sexual behaviour and the fall in incidence of HIV infection among homosexual men. *British Medical Journal,* 298, 218–21.

van Zuuren, F. J., & Dooper, R. (1999). Coping style and self-reported health promotion and disease detection behaviour. *British Journal of Health Psychology,* 4, 81–9.

Varni, J. W., & Babani, L. (1986). Long-term adherence to health care regimens in pediatric chronic disorders. In N. A. Krasnegor, J. D. Arasteh & M. F. Cataldo (Eds), *Child health behavior: a behavioral pediatrics perspective.* New York: John Wiley & Sons.

Varni, J. W., Jay, S. M., Masek, B. J., & Thompson, K. L. (1986). Cognitive-behavioral assessment and management of pediatric pain. In A. D. Holzman & D. C. Turk (Eds), *Pain management: a handbook of psychological treatment approaches.* New York: Pergamon.

Varni, J. W., & Thompson, K. L. (1986). Biobehavioral assessment and management of pediatric pain. In N. A. Krasnegor, J. D. Arasteh & M. F. Cataldo (Eds), *Child health behavior: a behavioral pediatrics perspective.* New York: John Wiley & Sons.

Vecchio, P. C. (1994). Attitudes to alternative medicine by rheumatology outpatient attenders. *Journal of Rheumatology,* 21, 145–7.

Venn, J. R., & Short, J. G. (1973). Vicarious classical conditioning of emotional responses in nursery school children. *Journal of Personality and Social Psychology,* 28, 249–55.

Verbrugge, L. M. (1980). Sex differences in complaints and diagnoses. *Journal of Behavioral Medicine,* 3, 327–55.

Verbrugge, L. M. (1985). Gender and health: an update on hypotheses and evidence. *Journal of Health and Social Behavior,* 26, 156–182.

Veroni, M., Gracey, M., & Rouse, I. (1994). Patterns of mortality in Western Australian Aboriginals, 1983–1989. *International Journal of Epidemiology,* 23, 73–81.

Verrier, R. L., Desilva, R. A., & Lown, B. (1983). Psychological factors in cardiac arrhythmias and sudden death. In D. S. Krantz, A. Baum & J. E. Singer (Eds), *Handbook of psychology and health* (Vol. 3). Hillsdale, NJ: Erlbaum.

Vertinsky, P., & Auman, J. T. (1988). Elderly women's barriers to exercise, Part I: Perceived risks. *Health Values,* 12(4), 13–19.

VicHealth (1993). *Partnerships: partnerships with healthy industry.* Annual Review 1993, Health Partners Program. Melbourne: Victorian Health Promotion Foundation.

Viney, L. L., Walker, B. M., Robertson, T., Lilley, B., & Ewan, C. (1994). Dying in palliative care units and in hospital: a comparison of the quality of life of terminal cancer patients. *Journal of Consulting and Clinical Psychology,* 62, 157–64.

Viney, L. L., & Westbrook, M. T. (1980). Psychosocial reactions to heart disease: an application of content analysis methodology. *Proceedings of the Geigy Symposium on Behavioural Medicine,* Melbourne.

Viney, L. L., & Westbrook, M. T. (1982). Coping with chronic illness: the mediating role of biographic and illness-related factors. *Journal of Psychosomatic Medicine,* 26, 595–605.

Vinocur, A. D., Threatt, B. A., Vinokur-Kaplan, D., & Satariano, W. A. (1990). The process of recovery from breast cancer for younger and older patients: changes during the first year. *Cancer,* 65, 1242–54.

Virgili, M., Owen, N., & Severson, H. H. (1991). Adolescents' smoking behavior and risk perceptions. *Journal of Substance Abuse,* 3, 315–24.

Visintainer, P. F., & Matthews, K. A. (1987). Stability of overt Type A behaviors in children: results from a two- and five-year longitudinal study. *Child Development,* 58, 1586–91.

Visser, A., & Antoni, M. (1994). Current perspectives on AIDS/HIV education and counseling. *Patient Education and Counseling,* 24, 191–8.

Vita, P., & Owen, N. (1995). A perspective on the behavioural epidemiology, the determinants and the stages of exercise involvement. *Australian Psychologist,* 30(2), 135–40.

Vitaliano, P. P., Russo, J., Bailey, S. L., Young, H. M., & McCann, B. S. (1993). Psychosocial factors associated with cardiovascular reactivity in older adults. *Psychosomatic Medicine,* 55, 164–77.

Vitaliano, P. P., Russo, J., Breen, A. R., Vitiello, M. V., & Prinz, P. N. (1986). Functional decline in the early stages of Alzheimer's disease. *Journal of Psychology and Aging,* 1, 41–6.

Vitaliano, P. P., Russo, J., & Niaura, R. (1995). Plasma lipids and their relationships with psychosocial factors in older adults. *Journal of Gerontology,* 50B, P18–24.

Volinn, E., Turczyn, K. M., & Loeser, J. D. (1994). Patterns of low back pain hospitalizations: implications for the treatment of low back pain in an era of health care reform. *Clinical Journal of Pain,* 10, 64–70.

Wadden, T. A., & Anderton, C. H. (1982). The clinical use of hypnosis. *Psychological Bulletin,* 91, 215–43.

Wadden, T. A., & Brownell, K. D. (1984). The development and modification of dietary practices in individuals, groups, and large populations. In J. D. Matarazzo, S. M. Weiss, J. A. Herd, N. E. Miller & S. M. Weiss (Eds), *Behavioral health: a handbook of health enhancement and disease prevention.* New York: John Wiley & Sons.

Wadden, T. A., Stunkard, A. J., & Liebschutz, J. (1988). Three-year follow-up of the treatment of obesity by very low calorie diet, behavior therapy, and their combination. *Journal of Consulting and Clinical Psychology,* 56, 925–8.

Wagner, F. (1986). An exploratory study of parental coping in the context of chronic childhood illness. Unpublished master's thesis. Department of Psychology, University of Guelph, Ontario.

Wahlqvist, M. L. (Ed.) (1988). *Food and nutrition in Australia* (3rd ed.). Melbourne: Thomas Nelson.

Wakefield, M., Roberts, L., & Miller, C. (1999). Perceptions of the effect of an impending restaurant smoking ban on dining-out experience. *Preventive Medicine,* 29, 53–6.

Waldenstrom, U., & Lawson, J. (1998). Birth centre practices in Australia. *Australian New Zealand Journal of Obstetrics and Gynaecology*, 38, 50–52.

Walker, R. (1984). *Under fire: a history of tobacco smoking in Australia*. Melbourne: Melbourne University Press.

Wallace, L. M. (1986). Communication variables in the design of pre-surgical preparatory information. *British Journal of Clinical Psychology*, 25, 111–18.

Wallerstein, J. S. (1983). Children of divorce: stress and developmental tasks. In N. Garmezy & M. Rutter (Eds), *Stress, coping, and development in children*. New York: McGraw-Hill.

Wallerstein, J. S. (1986). Children and divorce: the psychological tasks of the child. In R. H. Moos (Ed.), *Coping with life crises: an integrated approach*. New York: Plenum.

Wallston, B. S., Alagna, S. W., Devellis, B. M., & Devellis, R. F. (1983). Social support and physical illness. *Health Psychology*, 2, 367–91.

Wallston, K. A. (1993). Health psychology in the USA. In S. Maes, H. Leventhal & M. Johnston (Eds), *International review of health psychology* (Vol. 2). Chichester: John Wiley & Sons.

Wallston, K. A., & Wallston, B. S. (1982). Who is responsible for your health? The construct of health locus of control. In G. S. Sanders & J. Suls (Eds), *Social psychology of health and illness*. Hillsdale, NJ: Erlbaum.

Walsh, J. (1988). Costs of spinal cord injury in Australia. *Paraplegia*, 26, 380–88.

Walsh, R. A., Paul, C. L., & Tzelepis, F. (2000). Overwhelming support for smoking bans. *Australian and New Zealand Journal of Public Health*, 24(6), 640.

Walters, E. E., & Kendler, K. S. (1995). Anorexia nervosa and anorexic-like syndromes in a population-based female twin sample. *American Journal of Psychiatry*, 152, 64–71.

Wang, P. H., Lau, J. & Chalmers, T. C. (1993). Meta-analysis of effects of intensive blood-glucose control on late complications of type I diabetes. *The Lancet*, 341, 1306–9.

Wang, Y., Corr, J. G., Thaler, H. T., Tao, Y., Fair, W. R., & Heston, W. D. W. (1995). Decreased growth of established human prostate LNCaP tumors in nude mice fed a low-fat diet. *Journal of the National Cancer Institute*, 87, 1456–62.

Wang, Z., Hoy, W., & McDonald, S. (2000). Body mass index in Aboriginal Australians in remote communities. *Australian and New Zealand Journal of Public Health*, 24(6), 570–75.

Wanzer, S. H., Federman, D. D., Adelstein, S. J., Cassel, C. K., et al. (1989). The physician's responsibility toward hopelessly ill patients: a second look. *New England Journal of Medicine*, 320, 844–9.

Ward, A., & Pratt, C. (1996). Psychosocial influences on the use of health care by children, *Australian and New Zealand Journal of Public Health*, 20(3), 309–316.

Ward, J. (1994). Concluding commentary: challenges and choices for health promotion in general practice. *Behaviour Change*, 11(3), 186–8.

Ward, J. E., Boyle, K., Redman, S., & Sanson-Fisher, R. W. (1991). Increasing women's compliance with opportunistic cervical cancer screening: a randomized trial. *American Journal of Preventive Medicine*, 7(5), 285–91.

Ward, S. E., Goldberg, N., Miller-McCaulry, V., Mueller, C., Nolan, A., Pawlik-Plank, D., Robbins, A., Stormoen, D., & Weissman, D. E. (1993). Patient-related barriers to management of cancer pain. *Pain*, 52, 319–24.

Wardle, F. J., Collins, W., Pernet, A. L., Whitehead, M. I., Bourne, T. H., & Campbell, S. (1993). Psychological impact of screening for familial ovarian cancer. *Journal of the National Cancer Institute*, 85, 653–7.

Wardle, J. (1990). Overeating: a regulatory behaviour in restrained eaters. *Appetite*, 14, 133–6.

Warga, C. (1987, August). Pain's gatekeeper. *Psychology Today*, pp. 50–56.

Warr, P. (1996). Job features and excessive stress. In J. Billsberry (Ed.), *The effective manager: perspectives and illustrations* (pp. 61–8). Milton Keynes, UK: Open University Press.

Warr, P. B., & Jackson, P. R. (1984). Men without jobs: some correlates of age and length of unemployment. *Journal of Occupational Psychology*, 57, 77–85.

Warr, P. B., & Jackson, P. R. (1985). Factors influencing the psychological impact of prolonged unemployment and of re-employment. *Psychological Medicine*, 15, 795–807.

Warshaw, R. (1992, March 8). Fat chance. *Philadelphia Inquirer Magazine*, pp. 26–31.

Watson, D., & Pennebaker, J. W. (1989). Health complaints, stress, and distress: exploring the central role of negative affectivity. *Psychological Review*, 96, 234–54.

Watson, M., & Ramirez, A. (1991). Psychological factors in cancer prognosis. In C. L. Cooper & M. Watson (Eds), *Cancer and stress: psychological, biological, and coping studies*. New York: John Wiley & Sons.

Watts, R. W., McLennan, G., Bassham, I., & El-Saadi, O. (1997). Do patients with asthma fill their prescriptions? A primary compliance study. *Australian Family Physician*, 26 (Suppl. 1), S4–6.

Watts, T. D., Elliott, D., & Mayadas, N. S. (Eds) (1995). *International handbook on social work education*. Westport, CT: Greenwood.

Weber, J. M., Klesges, R. C., & Klesges, L. M. (1988). Dietary restraint and obesity: their effects on dietary intake. *Journal of Behavioral Medicine*, 11, 185–99.

Weeda-Mannak, W. L. (1990). Bulimia nervosa. In A. A. Kaptein, H. M. Van Der Ploeg, B. Garssen, P. J. G. Schreurs & R. Beunderman (Eds), *Behavioural medicine: psychological treatment of somatic disorders*. Chichester: John Wiley & Sons.

Weekes, B. S., & Waterhouse, I. K. (1991). Hostile attitudes and the coronary prone personality. *Australian Psychologist*, 26(1), 33–6.

Weidner, G., Connor, S. L., Hollis, J. F., & Connor, W. E. (1992). Improvements in hostility and depression in relation to dietary change and cholesterol lowering: the Family Heart Study. *Annals of Internal Medicine*, 117, 820–23.

Weidner, G., & Matthews, K. A. (1978). Reported physical symptoms elicited by unpredictable events and the Type A coronary-prone behavior pattern. *Journal of Personality and Social Psychology*, 36, 1213–20.

Weinberger, M., Hiner, S. L., & Tierney, W. M. (1987). In support of hassles as a measure of stress in predicting health outcomes. *Journal of Behavioral Medicine*, 10, 19–31.

Weiner, H. (1977). *Psychobiology and human disease*. New York: Elsevier.

Weinman, J. (1990). Health psychology: progress, perspectives and prospects. In P. Bennett, J. Weinman & P. Spurgeon (Eds), *Current developments in health psychology*. Chur, Switzerland: Harwood.

Weinstein, N. D. (1982). Unrealistic optimism about susceptibility to health problems. *Journal of Behavioral Medicine*, 5, 441–60.

Weinstein, N. D. (1987). Unrealistic optimism about susceptibility to health problems: conclusions from a community-wide sample. *Journal of Behavioral Medicine*, 10, 481–500.

Weinstein, N. D. (1988). The precaution adoption process. *Health Psychology*, 7, 355–86.

Weinstein, N. D., & Klein, W. M. (1995). Resistance of personal risk perceptions to debiasing interventions. *Health Psychology*, 14, 132–40.

Weir, R., Browne, G., Roberts, J., Tunks, E., & Gafni, A. (1994). The Meaning of Illness Questionnaire: further evidence for its reliability and validity. *Pain*, 58, 377–86.

Weisenberg, M. (1977). Pain and pain control. *Psychological Bulletin*, 84, 1008–1044.

Weisman, A. D. (1976). Coping with untimely death. In R. H. Moos (Ed.), *Human adaptation: coping with life crises*. Lexington, MA: Heath.

Weisman, A. D. (1977). The psychiatrist and the inexorable. In H. Feifel (Ed.), *New meanings of death*. New York: McGraw-Hill.

Weisman, A. D. (1979). *Coping with cancer*. New York: McGraw-Hill.

Weiss, G. L., Larsen, D. L., & Baker, W. K. (1996). The development of health protective behaviors among college students. *Journal of Behavioral Medicine*, 19, 143–61.

Weiss, S. M. (1984). Health hazard/health risk appraisals. In J. D. Matarazzo, S. M. Weiss, J. A. Herd, N. E. Miller & S. M. Weiss (Ed.), *Behavioral health: a handbook of health enhancement and disease prevention*. New York: John Wiley & Sons.

Welborn, T. A., Glatthaar, C., Whittall, D., & Bennett, S. (1989). An estimate of diabetes prevalence from a national population sample: a male excess. *Medical Journal of Australia*, 150, 78–81.

Welin, L., Svärdsudd, K., Wilhelmsen, L., Larsson, B., & Tibblin, G. (1987). Analysis of risk factors for stroke in a cohort of men born in 1913. *New England Journal of Medicine*, 317, 521–6.

Wenneker, M. B., Weissman, J. S., & Epstein, A. M. (1990). The association of payer with utilization of cardiac procedures in Massachusetts. *Journal of the American Medical Association*, 264, 1255–60.

Wensing, M., Grol, R., & Smits, A. (1994). Quality judgements by patients on general practice care: a literature analysis. *Social Science and Medicine*, 38, 45.

Werner, E. E., & Smith, R. S. (1982). *Vulnerable but invincible: a study of resilient children*. New York: McGraw-Hill.

Werry, J. S. (1986). Physical illness, symptoms, and allied disorders. In H. C. Quay & J. S. Werry (Eds), *Psychopathological disorders of childhood* (3rd ed.). New York: John Wiley & Sons.

Westbrook, M. T., & Viney, L. L. (1981). Biographic and illness-related predictors of patients' reactions to the onset of chronic illness. *Advances in Behavioural Medicine*, 1, 57–74.

Westbrook, M. T., & Viney, L. L. (1982). Psychological reaction to the onset of chronic illness. *Social Science and Medicine*, 16, 899–906.

Westerdahl, J., Olsson, H., Måsbäck, A., Ingvar, C., Jonsson, N., Brandt, L., Jönsson, P.-E., & Möller, T. (1994). Use of sunbeds or sunlamps and malignant melanoma in Southern Sweden. *American Journal of Epidemiology*, 140, 691–9.

Westerink, J., & Giarratano, L. (1999). The impact of posttraumatic stress disorder on partners and children of Australian Vietnam veterans. *Australian and New Zealand Journal of Psychiatry*, 33(6), 841–7.

Wethington, E., Brown, G. W., & Kessler, R. C. (1995). Interview measurement of stressful life events. In S. Cohen, R. Kessler & L. Underwood Gordon (Eds), *Measuring stress: a guide for health and social scientists* (pp. 59–79). New York: Oxford University Press.

Wethington, E., & Kessler, R. C. (1986). Perceived support, received support, and adjustment to stressful life events. *Journal of Health and Social Behavior*, 27, 78–89.

Wetter, D. W., Fiore, M. C., Baker, T. B., & Young, T. B. (1995). Tobacco withdrawal and nicotine replacement influence objective measures of sleep. *Journal of Consulting and Clinical Psychology*, 63, 658–67.

Whalen, C. K., Henker, B., O'Neil, R., Hollingshead, J., Holman, A., & Moore, B. (1994). Optimism in children's judgements of health and environmental risks. *Health Psychology*, 13, 319–25.

Wheaton, B. (1978). The sociogenesis of psychological disorder: reexamining the causal issues with longitudinal data. *American Sociological Review*, 43, 383–403.

Whelan, T. A., & Kirkby, R. J. (1995). Children and their families: psychological preparation for hospital interventions. *Journal of Family Studies*, 1(2), 130–41.

Whisman, M. A., & Kwon, P. (1993). Life stress and dysphoria: the role of self-esteem and hopelessness. *Journal of Personality and Social Psychology*, 65, 1054–60.

Whitbread, J., & McGown, A. (1994). The treatment of bulimia nervosa: what is effective? A meta-analysis. *Indian Journal of Clinical Psychology*, 21, 32–44.

White, A. D. (1990). The use of sunscreens in Australia. *Journal of Clinical Medicine*, 33(1), 27–39.

White, K., Terry, D. J., & Hogg, M. A. (1994). Safer sex behavior: the role of attitudes, norms and control factors. *Journal of Applied Social Psychology*, 24(24), 2164–92.

White, L. P. (1977). Death and the physician: mortus vivos docent. In H. Feifel (Ed.), *New meanings of death*. New York: McGraw-Hill.

Whitehead, A. S., Gallagher, P., Mills, J. L., Kirke, P. N., Burke, H., Molloy, A. M., Weir, D. G., Shields, D. C., & Scott, J. M. (1995). A genetic defect in 5,10 methylenetetrahydrofolate reductase in neural tube defects. *Quarterly Journal of Medicine*, 88, 763–6.

Whitehead, W. E. (1986). Pediatric gastrointestinal disorders. In N. A. Krasnegor, J. D. Arasteh & M. F. Cataldo (Eds), *Child health behavior: a behavioral pediatrics perspective*. New York: John Wiley & Sons.

Whitehead, W. E., Busch, C. M., Heller, B. R., & Costa, P. T. (1986). Social learning influences on menstrual symptoms and illness behavior. *Health Psychology*, 5, 13–23.

Whitney, C. R. (1996, April 25). In France, socialized medicine meets a Gallic version of HMO. *New York Times*, p. A5.

WHO (1946). *Constitution of the World Health Organization*. Reprinted in basic documents, 37th ed. Geneva: WHO.

Wickersham, B. A. (1984). The exercise program. In G. K. Riggs & E. P. Gall (Eds), *Rheumatic diseases: rehabilitation and management*. Boston, MA: Butterworth.

Wideman, M. V., & Singer, J. E. (1984). The role of psychological mechanisms in preparation for childbirth. *American Psychologist*, 39, 1357–71.

Wiebe, D. J., & McCallum, D. M. (1986). Health practices and hardiness as mediators in the stress-illness relationship. *Health Psychology*, 5, 425–38.

Wielgosz, A. T., Fletcher, R. H., McCants, C. B., McKinnis, R. A., Haney, T. L., & Williams, R. B. (1984). Unimproved chest pain in patients with minimal or no coronary disease: a behavioral phenomenon. *American Heart Journal*, 108, 67–72.

Wiens, A. N., & Menustik, C. E. (1983). Treatment outcome and patient characteristics in an aversion therapy program for alcoholism. *American Psychologist*, 38, 1089–96.

Wiggers, J. H., Sanson-Fisher, R. W., & Halpin, S. J. (1995). Prevalence and frequency of health service use: associations with occupational prestige and educational attainment. *Australian Journal of Public Health*, 19(5), 512–19.

Wilcox, S., & Storandt, M. (1996). Relations among age, exercise, and psychological variables in a community sample of women. *Health Psychology*, 15, 110–13.

Wilcox, V. L., Kasl, S. V., & Berkman, L. F. (1994). Social support and physical disability in older people after hospitalization: a prospective study. *Health Psychology*, 13, 170–79.

Wilkinson, G. (1987). The influence of psychiatric, psychological and social factors on the control of insulin-dependent diabetes mellitus. *Journal of Psychosomatic Research*, 31, 277–86.

Wilkinson, S. (1991). Factors which influence how nurses communicate with cancer patients. *Journal of Advanced Nursing*, 16, 677–88.

Wilks, J. (1992). Adolescent views on risky and illegal alcohol use. *Drug and Alcohol Review*, 11(2), 137–43.

Wilks, J., & Callan, V. (1990). Adolescents and alcohol. In P. Heaven & V. Callan (Eds), *Adolescence: an Australian perspective*. Sydney: Harcourt Brace Jovanovich.

Wilks, J., Callan, V. J., & Forsyth, S. J. (1985). Cross-cultural perspectives on teenage attitudes to alcohol. *International Journal of the Addictions*, 20, 547–61.

Williams, C. J. (1990). *Cancer biology and management: an introduction.* New York: John Wiley & Sons.

Williams, D. A., & Keefe, F. J. (1991). Pain beliefs and the use of cognitive-behavioral coping strategies. *Pain*, 46, 185–90.

Williams, P. G., & Wiebe, D. J. (2000). Individual differences in self-assessed health: gender, neuroticism and physical symptom reports. *Personality and Individual Differences*, 28(5), 823–35.

Williams, P. G., Wiebe, D. J., & Smith, T. W. (1992). Coping processes as mediators of the relationship between hardiness and health. *Journal of Behavioral Medicine*, 15, 237–55.

Williams, R. (1989, January/February). The trusting heart. *Psychology Today*, pp. 36–42.

Williams, R. B., & Barefoot, J. C. (1988). Coronary-prone behavior: the emerging role of the hostility complex. In B. K. Houston & C. R. Snyder (Eds), *Type A behavior pattern: research, theory, and intervention.* New York: John Wiley & Sons.

Williams, R. B., Haney T. L., Lee, K. L., Kong, Y.-H., Blumenthal, J. A., & Whalen, R. E. (1980). Type A behavior, hostility, and coronary atherosclerosis. *Psychosomatic Medicine*, 42, 539–49.

Williams, R. B., Suarez, E. C., Kuhn, C. M., Zimmerman, E. A., & Schanberg, S. M. (1991). Biobehavioral basis of coronary-prone behavior in middle-aged men. Part I: Evidence for chronic SNS activation in Type As. *Psychosomatic Medicine*, 53, 517–27.

Williams, S., Weinman, J., & Dale, J. (1998). Doctor–patient communication and patient satisfaction: a review. *Family Practice*, 15(5), 480–92.

Williamson, D. A., Cubic, B. A., & Fuller, R. D. (1992). Eating disorders. In S. E. Turner, K. S., Calhoun & H. E. Adams (Eds), *Handbook of clinical behavior therapy* (2nd ed.). New York: John Wiley & Sons.

Williamson, D. F., Madans, J., Anda, R. F., Kleinman, J. C., Giovino, G. A., & Byers, T. (1991). Smoking cessation and severity of weight gain in a national cohort. *New England Journal of Medicine*, 324, 739–45.

Willich, S. N., Löwel, H., Lewis, M., Hörmann, A., Arntz, H.-R., & Keil, U. (1994). Weekly variation of acute myocardial infarction: increased Monday risk in the working population. *Circulation*, 90, 87–93.

Willis, L., Thomas, P., Garry, P. J., & Goodwin, J. S. (1987). A prospective study of response to stressful life events in initially healthy elders. *Journal of Gerontology*, 42, 627–30.

Wills, T. A. (1986). Stress and coping in early adolescence: relationships to substance use in urban school samples. *Health Psychology*, 5, 503–529.

Wilner, N. (1976). Field studies on the impact of life events. In M. J. Horowitz, *Stress response syndromes* (pp. 34–61). New York: Jason Aronson Inc.

Wilson, A., & Siskind, V. (1995). Coronary heart disease mortality in Australia: Is mortality starting to increase among young men? *International Journal of Epidemiology*, 24(4), 678–84.

Wilson, D. K., Holmes, S. D., Arheart, K., & Alpert, B. S. (1995). Cardiovascular reactivity in black and white siblings versus matched controls. *Annals of Behavioral Medicine*, 17, 207–212.

Wilson, D. P., & Endres, R. K. (1986). Compliance with blood glucose monitoring in children with type 1 diabetes mellitus. *Behavioral Pediatrics*, 108, 1022–4.

Wilson, G. T. (1984). Weight control treatments. In J. D. Matarazzo, S. M. Weiss, J. A. Herd, N. E. Miller & S. M. Weiss (Eds), *Behavioral health: a handbook of health enhancement and disease prevention.* New York: John Wiley & Sons.

Wilson, G. T., & Smith, D. (1987). Cognitive-behavioral treatment of bulimia nervosa. *Annals of Behavioral Medicine*, 9(4), 12–17.

Wilson, I. B., & Cleary, P. D. (1995). Linking clinical variables with health-related quality of life. *Journal of the American Medical Association*, 273, 59–65.

Wilson, W., Ary, D. V., Biglan, A., Glasgow, R. E., Toobert, D. J., & Campbell, D. R. (1986). Psychosocial predictors of self-care behaviors (compliance) and glycemic control in non-insulindependent diabetes mellitus. *Diabetes Care*, 9, 614–22.

Wincze, J. P. (1977). Sexual deviance and dysfunction. In D. C. Rimm & J. W. Somervill (Eds), *Abnormal psychology.* New York: Academic Press.

Windauer, U., Lennerts, W., Talbot, P., Touyz, S. W., & Beumont, P. J. V. (1993). How well are 'cured' anorexia nervosa patients? an investigation of 16 weight-recovered anorexic patients. *British Journal of Psychiatry*, 163, 195–200.

Windsor, R. A., Lowe, J. B., Perkins, L. L., Smith-Yoder, D., Artz, L., Crawford, M., Amburgy, K., & Boyd, N. R. (1993). Health education for pregnant smokers: its behavioral impact and cost benefit. *American Journal of Public Health*, 83, 201–6.

Winefield, H. R. (1991). Health psychology for medical students. In M. A. Jansen & J. Weinman (Eds), *The international development of health psychology.* Chur, Switzerland: Harwood Academic Publishers.

Winefield, H. R., & Murrell, T. G. (1991). Speech patterns and satisfaction in diagnostic and prescriptive stages of general practice consultations. *British Journal of Medical Psychology*, 64, 103–115.

Winefield, H. R., & Murrell, T. G. (1992). Verbal interactions in general practice: information, support and doctor satisfaction. *Medical Journal of Australia*, 157, 677–82.

Winefield, H. R., Murrell, T. G., & Clifford, J. (1995). Process and outcomes in general practice consultations: problems in defining high quality care. *Social Science and Medicine*, 41(7), 969–75.

Winefield, H. R., Winefield, A. H., Tiggemann, M., & Goldney, R. (1989). Psychological concomitants of tobacco and alcohol use in young Australian adults. *British Journal of Addiction*, 84, 1067–73.

Winett, R. A. (1995). A framework for health promotion and disease prevention programs. *American Psychologist*, 50, 341–50.

Winett, R. A., King, A. C., & Altman, D. G. (1989). *Health psychology and public health: an integrative approach.* New York: Pergamon.

Wing, R. R. (1992). Weight cycling in humans: a review of the literature. *Annals of Behavioral Medicine*, 14, 113–19.

Wing, R. R., Epstein, L. H., & Nowalk, M. P. (1984). Dietary adherence in patients with diabetes. *Behavioral Medicine Update*, 6(1), 17–21.

Wing, R. R., Epstein, L. H., Nowalk, M. P., & Lamparski, D. M. (1986). Behavioral self-regulation in the treatment of patients with diabetes mellitus. *Psychological Bulletin*, 99, 78–89.

Wing, R. R., Nowalk, M. P., & Guare, J. C. (1988). Diabetes mellitus. In E. A. Blechman & K. D. Brownell (Eds), *Handbook of behavioral medicine for women.* New York: Pergamon.

Winger, G., Hofmann, F. G., & Woods, J. H. (1992). *A handbook on drug and alcohol abuse: the biomedical aspects* (3rd ed.). New York: Oxford University Press.

Winn, M. (1991). The Grim Reaper: Australia's first mass media AIDS education campaign. *AIDS prevention through health promotion: facing sensitive issues*, 33–8.

Winstanley, M. H., & Woodward, S. D. (1992). Tobacco in Australia — an overview. *Journal of Drug Issues*, 22(3), 733–42.

Winters, R. (1985). Behavioral approaches to pain. In N. Schneiderman & J. T. Tapp (Eds), *Behavioral medicine: the biopsychosocial approach.* Hillsdale, NJ: Erlbaum.

Witryol, S. L. (1971). Incentives and learning in children. In H. W. Reese (Ed.), *Advances in child development and behavior* (Vol. 6). New York: Academic Press.

Wodak, A. (1992). HIV Infection and injecting drug use in Australia: responding to a crisis. *Journal of Drug Issues*, 22(3), 549–62.

Wodak, A. (1993). Policy issues relating to drug abuse and the human immunodeficiency virus (HIV). *Bulletin on Narcotics*, XLV(1), 48–60.

Wodak, A., & Des Jarlais, D. (1993). Strategies for the prevention of HIV infection among and from injecting drug uses. *Bulletin on Narcotics*, 45(1), 47–60.

Wolchik, S. A., West, S. G., Westover, S., Sandler, I. N., Martin, A., Lustig, J., Tein, J. Y., & Fisher, J. (1993). The children of divorce parenting intervention: outcome evaluation of an empirically based program. *American Journal of Community Psychology*, 21, 293–331.

Wolf, M. H., Putnam, S. M., James, S. A., & Stiles, W. B. (1978). The medical interview satisfaction scale: development of a scale to measure patient perceptions of physician behavior. *Journal of Behavioral Medicine*, 1, 391.

Wolf, S., & Wolff, H. G. (1947). *Human gastric function* (2nd ed.). New York: Oxford University Press.

Wolpe, J. (1958). Psychotherapy by reciprocal inhibition. Stanford, CA: Stanford University Press.

Wolpe, J. (1973). *The practice of behavior therapy* (2nd ed.). New York: Pergamon.

Woodall, K., & Epstein, L. H. (1983). The prevention of obesity. *Behavioral Medicine Update*, 5(1), 15–21.

Woods, A. M., & Birren, J. E. (1984). Late adulthood and aging. In J. D. Matarazzo, S. M. Weiss, J. A. Herd, N. E. Miller & S. M. Weiss (Eds), *Behavioral health: a handbook of health enhancement and disease prevention*. New York: John Wiley & Sons.

Woods, P. J., & Burns, J. (1984). Type A behavior and illness in general. *Journal of Behavioral Medicine*, 7, 411–15.

Woods, P. J., Morgan, B. T., Day, B. W., Jefferson, T., & Harris, C. (1984). Findings on a relationship between Type A behavior and headaches. *Journal of Behavioral Medicine*, 7, 277–86.

Woodward, N. J., & Wallston, B. S. (1987). Age and health care beliefs: self-efficacy as a mediator of low desire for control. *Psychology and Aging*, 2, 3–8.

Wooster, R., Bignell, G., Lancaster, J., Swift, S., et al. (1995). Identification of the breast cancer susceptibility gene BRCA2. *Nature*, 378, 789–92.

Wortman, C. B. (1975). Some determinants of perceived control. *Journal of Personality and Social Psychology*, 31, 282–94.

Wortman, C. B., & Dunkel-Schetter, C. (1979). Interpersonal relationships and cancer. *Journal of Social Issues*, 35, 120–55.

Wortman, C. B., & Dunkel-Schetter, C. (1987). Conceptual and methodological issues in the study of social support. In A. Baum & J. E. Singer (Eds), *Handbook of psychology and health* (Vol. 5). Hillsdale, NJ: Erlbaum.

Wright, L. (1988). The Type A behavior pattern and coronary artery disease. *American Psychologist*, 43, 2–14.

Wright, L., & Friedman, A. G. (1991). Challenge of the future: psychologists in medical settings. In J. J. Sweet, R. H. Rozensky & S. M. Tovian (Eds), *Handbook of clinical psychology in medical settings*. New York: Plenum.

Wulfert, E., Wan, C. K., & Backus, C. A. (1996). Gay men's safer sex behavior: an integration of three models. Journal of Behavioral Medicine, 19, 345–66.

Wurtele, S. K., & Maddux, J. E. (1987). Relative contributions of protection motivation theory components in predicting exercise intentions and behavior. *Health Psychology*, 6, 453–66.

Yarnold, P. R., Bryant, F. B., & Grimm, L. G. (1987). Comparing the long and short forms of the student version of the Jenkins Activity Survey. *Journal of Behavioral Medicine*, 10, 75–90.

Yeaton, W. H., Smith, D., & Rogers, K. (1990). Evaluating understanding of popular press reports of health research. *Health Education Quarterly*, 72, 223–34.

Young, A. E., & Murphy, G. C. (1998). Spinal cord injury rehabilitation outcomes: a comparison of agricultural and non-agricultural workers. *Australian Journal of Rural Health*, 6, 175–80.

Young, F. E. (1987, September). Special AIDS issue. *FDA Drug Bulletin*, 17 (2).

Young, K., & Zane, N. (1995). Ethnocultural influences in evaluation and management. In P. M. Nicassio & T. W. Smith (Eds), *Managing chronic illness: a biopsychosocial perspective*. Washington, DC: American Psychological Association.

Young, R., Oei, T., & Knight. R. (1990). Tension reduction hypothesis revisited: an expectancies perspective. *British Journal of Addiction*, 85, 31–40.

Zaldivar, R. A. (1993, March 12). Poll finds Americans fatter, more stressed out. Philadelphia Inquirer, pp. A1, A11.

Zamula, E. (1987). *A primer on high blood pressure* (HHS Publication No. FDA 87–3162). Washington, DC: U.S. Government Printing Office.

Zarski, J. J. (1984). Hassles and health: a replication. *Health Psychology*, 3, 243–51.

Zautra, A. J., Burleson, M. H., Smith, C. A., Blalock, S. J., Wallston, K. A., Devellis, R. F., DeVellis, B. M., & Smith, T. W. (1995). Arthritis and perceptions of quality of life: an examination of positive and negative affect in rheumatoid arthritis patients. *Health Psychology*, 14, 399–408.

Zautra, A. J., Okun, M. A., Robinson, S. E., Lee, D., Roth, S. H., & Emmanual, J. (1989). Life stress and lymphocyte alterations among patients with rheumatoid arthritis. *Health Psychology*, 8, 1–14.

Zhang, Y., Proenca, R., Maffei, M., Barone, M., Leopold, L., & Friedman, J. M. (1994). Positional cloning of the mouse obese gene and its human homologue. *Nature*, 372, 425–32.

Zhu, S.-H., Strech, V., Balabanis, M., Rosbrook, B., Sadler, G., & Pierce, J. P. (1996). Telephone counseling for smoking cessation: effects of single-session and multiple-session interventions. *Journal of Consulting and Clinical Psychology*, 64, 202–211.

Zigmond, A. S., & Snaith, R. P. (1983). The Hospital Anxiety and Depression Scale. *Acta Psychiatrica Scandinavica*, 67, 361–70.

Zimmer, J. G., Juncker, A. G., & McCusker, J. (1985). A randomized controlled study of a home health care team. *American Journal of Public Health*, 75, 134–41.

Zinman, B. (1984). Diabetes mellitus and exercise. *Behavioral Medicine Update*, 6(1), 22–5.

Zisook, S., Peterkin, J. J., Shuchter, S. R., & Bardone, A. (1995). Death, dying, and bereavement. In P. M. Nicassio & T. M. Smith (Eds), *Managing chronic illness: a biopsychosocial perspective*. Washington, DC: American Psychological Association.

Zola, I. K. (1973). Pathways to the doctor — from person to patient. *Social Science and Medicine*, 7, 677–89.

Zucker, R. A., & Gomberg, E. S. L. (1986). Etiology of alcoholism reconsidered: the case for a biopsychosocial process. *American Psychologist*, 41, 783–93.

Index

A

Aboriginal people *see* indigenous Australians
absorption   59
abstinence-violation effect   282
accidental injury   343–4
acetylcholine   270
acquired immune deficiency syndrome *see* AIDS
acupuncture   32, 490–1
acute pain   432, 452, 466
   chemical treatment   468–9
   in burn patients   434–5
adaptation
   to chronic health problems   507–8
   to dying   574–5
   to high-mortality illness   539–42
   to terminal illness   570–5
addiction   261
additives (food)   307–8
adherence to medical advice   377
   age, gender and sociocultural factors   380–1
   and doctor–patient communication   384
   and patient–practitioner relationship   384–5
   extent of non-adherence problem   377–8
      in diabetics   521
   increasing patient adherence   385–8
   medical treatments and illness characteristics   379–80
   methods for enhancing compliance   386–8
   non-adherence and health outcomes   385–6
   psychosocial aspects of the patient   381–3
   why patients do and do not adhere to medical
      advice   379–83
adolescents   598
   and alcohol abuse   287–8
   and drug use   300–1
   and health-related behaviour   237
   and HIV/AIDS   256–7
   and smoking   266–7
   diabetes in   525
   terminal illness in   571–2
adoption studies   40
adrenal glands   55
adrenocorticotropin hormone (ACTH)   54
adulthood   598
   and health-related behaviour   238
aerobic exercise   338
afferent neurons   50
age
   and adherence to medical advice   381
   and AIDS   567
   and alcohol use   283–5
   and cancer   557–8
   and drug use   300
   and heart disease   543
   and smoking habits   263–4
   and stroke   551
   of health service users   363
AIDS   74
   age, gender and sociocultural factors   567
   prevention programs   253–8
   psychological impact   569–70

   psychosocial interventions   570
   risk factors   556–7
   see also HIV/AIDS
AIDS-related complex   568
alarm reaction (GAS)   92
alcohol abuse treatment   293–8
   Alcoholics Anonymous   295
   behavioural and cognitive methods   296–7
   chemical therapies   297
   goals and criteria for success   294–5
   insight therapy   295–6
   setting for treatment   294
   treatment success and the relapse problem   297–8
alcohol use and abuse   283
   drinking and health   290–1
   prevention   291–3
   who drinks and how much   283–6
   why people use abuse alcohol   286–9
alcoholics   286
algogenic substances   433
allergies   71
alternative medicine   365, 366
alternative practitioners, usage of   363
alveoli   61
Alzheimer's disease   528–9
   causes and treatment   529–30
   education and support services   532
   psychosocial effects   530–1
ambiguity (stress appraisals)   90–1
amino acids   59
analgesics   469, 470
Ancient Greece and Rome, approach to illness   9
anger   95, 96, 149
angina pectoris   542
anorexia nervosa   331–3
   reasons for   333–4
   treatments   333–4
antecedent cues   211–12, 288
anthropology   28
antibodies   75
antibody-mediated 'humoral' immunity   72, 73, 75
anticipatory nausea   560
antidepressants   471
antigens   70–2, 75
anti-inflammatories   510
anxiety   95–6
aorta   66
apathy   137
appetite suppressants   329
appraising events as stressful   88–90
   determining factors   90–1
approach/approach conflict   98
approach/avoidance conflict   99
arteries   65
arteriosclerosis   69, 148
arthritis   525–6
   cognitive/behavioural management approaches   536
   effects and treatment   526–7
   psychosocial factors   527–8
   types and causes   526
assisted suicide   596